Clinical Endocrine Oncology

Clinical Endocrine Oncology

EDITED BY

IAN D. HAY, BSc, MB, PhD, FACE, FACP, FRCP, FRCPI (Hon)

Professor of Medicine and Dr R.F. Emslander Professor of Endocrinology Research
Mayo Clinic College of Medicine; and
Consultant in Endocrinology and Internal Medicine
Mayo Clinic
Rochester, Minnesota, USA

JOHN A.H. WASS, MA, MD, FRCP

Professor of Endocrinology
University of Oxford; and
Consultant Physician
Churchill Hospital
Oxford, UK

FOREWORD BY

ANTHONY P. WEETMAN, MD, DSc, FRCP, FMedSci

Dean of the School of Medicine and Biomedical Sciences
University of Sheffield
Sheffield, UK

SECOND EDITION

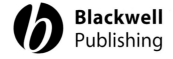

© 2008 by Blackwell Publishing

Blackwell Publishing, Inc., 350 Main Street, Malden, Massachusetts 02148-5020, USA
Blackwell Publishing Ltd, 9600 Garsington Road, Oxford OX4 2DQ, UK
Blackwell Publishing Asia Pty Ltd, 550 Swanston Street, Carlton, Victoria 3053, Australia

The right of the Author to be identified as the Author of this Work has been asserted in accordance with the Copyright, Designs and Patents Act 1988.

First published 2008
1   2008

Library of Congress Cataloging-in-Publication Data

Clinical endocrine oncology/edited by Ian D. Hay, John A. H. Wass.—2nd ed.
    p. ; cm.
    Includes bibliographical references and index.
    ISBN 978-1-4051-4584-8
    1. Endocrine glands—Tumors.   I. Hay, Ian D.   II. Wass, J. A. H.
    [DNLM: 1. Endocrine Gland Neoplasms.   2. Endocrine System Diseases. WK 140 C641 2008]
    RC280.E55C567 2008
    616.99′44—dc22

                                                                                    2007029820

ISBN: 978-1-4051-4584-8

A catalogue record for this title is available from the British Library

Set in 9.25/12 Minion by Graphicraft Limited, Hong Kong
Printed and bound in Singapore by COS Printers Pte Ltd

Commissioning Editor: Alison Brown
Editorial Assistant: Jennifer Seward
Development Editor: Elisabeth Dodds
Production Controller: Debbie Wyer

For further information on Blackwell Publishing, visit our website:
http://www.blackwellpublishing.com

The publisher's policy is to use permanent paper from mills that operate a sustainable forestry policy, and which has been manufactured from pulp processed using acid-free and elementary chlorine-free practices. Furthermore, the publisher ensures that the text paper and cover board used have met acceptable environmental accreditation standards.

Contents

List of Contributors, viii

Foreword, xiv

Preface, xv

Endocrinology, the Hertz Brothers, and the History of Cancer, xvi

Part 1: Endocrine Oncology and Therapeutic Options

1 Structure and Development of the Endocrine System, 3
John F. Morris

2 Epidemiology of Endocrine Tumors, 18
Amanda Nicholson

3 Inherited Cancers, Genes, and Chromosomes, 24
Emma R. Woodward and Eamonn R. Maher

4 Hormones, Growth Factors, and Tumor Growth, 32
Andrew G. Renehan

5 Genetic Counseling and Clinical Cancer Genetics, 41
Lucy Side

6 Prospects for Gene Therapy for Endocrine Malignancies, 49
Christine Spitzweg, Ian D. Hay, and John C. Morris

7 Tumor Targeting, 58
Mona Waterhouse and Ashley B. Grossman

8 Techniques in Radiation Medicine, 64
P. Nicholas Plowman

9 Interventional Radiology, 70
Jane Phillips-Hughes and Philip Boardman

10 Surgical Management of Endocrine Tumors, 78
Gustavo G. Fernandez Ranvier and Orlo H. Clark

11 Endocrine Tumor Markers, 86
Stefan K.G. Grebe

12 General Management of Cancer Patients, 102
Marcia Hall

Part 2: Thyroid and Parathyroid Tumors

13 Assessment of Thyroid Neoplasia, 111
Kristien Boelaert, Jayne A. Franklyn, and Michael Sheppard

14 Thyroid and Parathyroid Imaging, 116
Conor J. Heaney and Gregory A. Wiseman

15 Pathogenesis of Thyroid Cancer, 124
Jan Zedenius and Theodoros Foukakis

16 Papillary Thyroid Carcinoma, 130
Ian D. Hay

17 Follicular Thyroid Carcinoma, 143
Manisha H. Shah and Matthew D. Ringel

18 Anaplastic Thyroid Carcinoma, 155
Richard T. Kloos

19 Thyroid Lymphoma, 162
Christopher M. Nutting and Kevin J. Harrington

20 Radiation-induced Thyroid Tumors, 166
David H. Sarne and Arthur Schneider

21 Parathyroid Adenomas and Hyperplasia, 172
Bart L. Clarke

22 Parathyroid Carcinoma, 180
Göran Åkerström, Per Hellman, and Peyman Björklund

Part 3: Pituitary and Hypothalamic Lesions

23 Molecular Pathogenesis of Pituitary Adenomas, 187
Ines Donangelo and Shlomo Melmed

24 Functional Assessment of the Pituitary, 194
John S. Bevan

25 Imaging of the Pituitary and Hypothalamus, 200
James V. Byrne

Contents

26 Pathology of Tumors of the Pituitary, 215
Eva Horvath and Kalman Kovacs

27 Surgery for Pituitary Tumors, 222
Simon A. Cudlip

28 Pituitary Radiotherapy, 231
P. Nicholas Plowman

29 Prolactinomas, 237
Mary P. Gillam and Mark E. Molitch

30 Acromegaly, 246
John A.H. Wass

31 Cushing's Disease, 253
John Newell-Price

32 Non-functioning Pituitary Adenomas and
Gonadotropinomas, 262
Maarten O. van Aken, Aart Jan van der Lelij,
and Steven W.J. Lamberts

33 Thyrotropinomas, 268
Paolo Beck-Peccoz and Luca Persani

34 Pituitary Carcinoma, 274
Olaf Ansorge

35 Pituitary Incidentalomas, 278
Karin Bradley

36 Craniopharyngioma, 282
Niki Karavitaki

37 Benign Cysts: Rathke's Cleft Cysts, Mucoceles, Arachnoid
Cysts, and Dermoid and Epidermoid Cysts, 288
Niki Karavitaki

38 Hypothalamic Hamartomas and Gangliocytomas, 293
Lawrence A. Frohman

39 Cranial Ependymoma, 298
Silvia Hofer and Michael Brada

40 Perisellar Tumors including Chordoma, Optic Nerve
Glioma, Meningioma, Hemangiopericytoma, and
Glomus Tumors, 302
David Choi and Alan Crockard

41 Pineal Tumors: Germinomas and Non-germinomatous
Germ Cell Tumors, 310
Frank Saran and Sharon Peoples

42 Cavernous Sinus Hemangiomas, 318
Mark E. Linskey

43 Langerhans' Cell Histiocytosis, 325
Matthew F. Gorman, Michelle Hermiston, and
Katherine K. Matthay

44 Pituitary and Hypothalamic Sarcoidosis, 331
Damian G. Morris and Shern L. Chew

Part 4: Adrenal and Gonadal Tumors

45 Imaging of the Adrenal Glands, 339
Anju Sahdev and Rodney H. Reznek

46 Pheochromocytoma, 354
Andrew Solomon and Pierre Bouloux

47 Peripheral Neuroblastic Tumors, 360
Bruno De Bernardi, Vito Pistoia, Claudio Gambini,
and Claudio Granata

48 Primary Hyperaldosteronism, 370
Mark Sherlock and Paul M. Stewart

49 Adrenal Causes of Cushing's Syndrome, 378
John R. Lindsay and A. Brew Atkinson

50 Adrenal Incidentalomas, 384
Maria Verena Cicala, Pierantonio Conton, Anna Patalano,
and Franco Mantero

51 Androgen-secreting Tumors, 390
Quirinius Barnor, Tom R. Kurzawinski, and Gerard S. Conway

52 Functional Ovarian Tumors, 396
Nia Jane Taylor and Niall Richard Moore

53 Endocrine Aspects of Ovarian Tumors, 404
John H. Shepherd and Lisa Wong

54 Testicular Germ Cell Cancers, 412
R. Timothy D. Oliver

55 Neoplasia and Intersex States, 421
Sabine E. Hannema and Ieuan A. Hughes

56 Gestational Trophoblastic Neoplasia, 430
Tim Crook and Michael J. Seckl

**Part 5: Neuroendocrine Tumors and
the Clinical Syndromes**

57 Classification of Neuroendocrine Tumors, 437
Adeel Ansari, Karim Meeran, and Stephen R. Bloom

58 Imaging of Gastrointestinal Neuroendocrine Tumors, 443
Andrew F. Scarsbrook and Rachel R. Phillips

59 Insulinomas and Hypoglycemia, 455
Adrian Vella and F. John Service

60 Gastrinomas (Zollinger–Ellison Syndrome), 462
Matthew L. White and Gerard M. Doherty

61 VIPomas, 469
Vian Amber and Stephen R. Bloom

62 Glucagonomas, 474
Niamh M. Martin, Karim Meeran, and Stephen R. Bloom

63 Somatostatinomas, 479
John A.H. Wass

64 Lung and Thymic Neuroendocrine Tumors, 482
Dan Granberg and Kjell Öberg

65 Carcinoid Syndrome, 488
Thorvardur R. Halfdanarson and Timothy J. Hobday

66 Appendiceal and Hindgut Carcinoids, 498
Humphrey J.F. Hodgson

67 Chemotherapy for Neuroendocrine Tumors, 502
Rebecca L. Bowen and Maurice L. Slevin

Part 6: Medical Syndromes and Endocrine Neoplasia

68 Multiple Endocrine Neoplasia Type 1 (MEN 1), 507
Cornelis J.M. Lips, Koen M.A. Dreijerink, Gerlof D. Valk, and Jo W.M. Höppener

69 Medullary Thyroid Carcinoma and Associated Multiple Endocrine Neoplasia Type 2, 515
Clive S. Grant

70 von Hippel–Lindau Disease, 523
Shern L. Chew and Eamonn R. Maher

71 Neurofibromatosis Type 1, 528
Vincent M. Riccardi

72 Carney Complex, 532
Constantine A. Stratakis

73 McCune–Albright Syndrome, 537
William F. Schwindinger and Michael A. Levine

74 Cowden Syndrome, 545
Ingrid Witters and Jean-Pierre Fryns

75 Paraneoplastic Syndromes, 549
David William Ray

76 Syndrome of Inappropriate Antidiuretic Hormone Secretion, 556
Rachel K. Crowley and Chris Thompson

77 Hypercalcemia of Malignancy, 561
Gregory R. Mundy, Babatunde Oyajobi, Susan Padalecki, and Julie A. Sterling

78 Syndrome of Ectopic ACTH Secretion, 567
Marie-Laure Raffin-Sanson, Hélène Fierrard, and Xavier Bertagna

79 Insulin-like Growth Factors and Tumor Hypoglycemia, 576
Robert C. Baxter

80 Metastatic and Other Extraneous Neoplasms in Endocrine Organs, 582
Ian D. Buley

81 Endocrine Late Effects of Cancer Therapy, 588
Robert D. Murray

Part 7: Endocrine-responsive Tumors and Female Reproductive Hormone Therapy

82 Endocrine-responsive Tumors: Prostate Cancer, 601
Sarah Ngan, Ana Arance, and Jonathan Waxman

83 Endocrine Therapy in Breast Cancer Management, 609
Andrew M. Wardley

84 Female Reproductive Hormone Therapy: Risks and Benefits, 618
Toral Gathani, Jane Green, and Valerie Beral

Appendix of conversion units, 623
Index, 627

Color plate section is found facing p. 364

List of Contributors

Göran Åkerström, MD
Professor, Endocrine Surgery
Department of Surgery
University Hospital, Uppsala, Sweden

Vian Amber, MBChB, MSc, PhD,
MRCPath
Department of Metabolic Medicine
Hammersmith Hospital Campus
Imperial College London
London, UK

Adeel Ansari, MD
Department of Metabolic Medicine
Hammersmith Hospital Campus
Imperial College
London, UK

Olaf Ansorge, MD, MRCPath
Department of Neuropathology
John Radcliffe Hospital
Oxford, UK

Ana Arance, MD, PhD
Department of Oncology
The Gary Weston Cancer Centre
Hammersmith Hospital
London, UK

A. Brew Atkinson, DSc, MD, FRCP
Senior Endocrinologist and Professor
of Endocrinology
Regional Centre for Endocrinology
and Diabetes
Royal Victoria Hospital
Belfast, UK

Quirinius Barnor, MRCP
Department of Endocrinology
University College London Hospitals
London, UK

Robert C. Baxter, PhD, DSc
Director, Kolling Institute of Medical Research
University of Sydney
Royal North Shore Hospital
St Leonards, NSW, Australia

Paolo Beck-Peccoz, MD
Department of Medical Sciences
Fondazione Policlinico IRCCS
Milan, Italy

Valerie Beral, FRSI
Professor of Epidemiology
Director, Cancer Epidemiology Unit
University of Oxford
Oxford, UK

Xavier Bertagna, MD, PhD
Institut Cochin, Université Paris Descartes,
CNRS(UMR 8104);
INSEMR U567; and
AP-HP, Hôpital Cochin
Paris, France

John S. Bevan, MD, FRCPEd
Consultant Endocrinologist
Department of Endocrinology
Aberdeen Royal Infirmary
Foresterhill, Aberdeen, Scotland

Peyman Björklund, MSci
University of Uppsala
Uppsala, Sweden

Stephen R. Bloom, MB ChB, MA, FRCP,
FRCPath, DSc, MD
Professor of Medicine
Department of Metabolic Medicine
Imperial College London
London, UK

Philip Boardman, MRCP, FRCR
Consultant Radiologist
Churchill Hospital
Oxford, UK

Kristien Boelaert, MD, MRCP, PhD
Lecturer and MRC Clinician Scientist
Division of Medical Sciences
University of Birmingham
Queen Elizabeth Hospital
Birmingham, UK

Pierre-Marc G. Bouloux, BSc,
MBBS(Hons), MRCS, LRCP, MD, FRCP
Professor of Endocrinology
Royal Free and University College Medical School
London, UK

Rebecca L. Bowen, BMedSci,
BMBS, MRCP
Specialist Registrar, Medical Oncology
St Bartholomew's Hospital
London, UK

Michael Brada
Professor of Clinical Oncology
Academic Unit of Radiotherapy and Oncology
The Institute of Cancer Research; and
Neuro-Oncology Unit
The Royal Marsden NHS Trust
London and Sutton, UK

Karin Bradley, BSc, MBBS, MRCP, DPhil
Consultant Physician and Endocrinologist
Bristol Royal Infirmary
Bristol, UK

Ian D. Buley, FRCPath
Consultant Histopathologist
Honorary University Fellow Peninsula Medical
School
Torbay Hospital
Torquay, UK

James V. Byrne, MD, FRCS, FRCR
Professor of Neuroradiology
Department of Neuroradiology
University of Oxford
John Radcliffe Hospital
Oxford, UK

Shern L. Chew, BSc, MBBChir, MD, FRCP
Professor of Endocrine Medicine/Consultant
Physician
St Bartholomew's Hospital
London, UK

David Choi, MA, MBChB, FRCS(SN), PhD
Consultant Neurosurgeon
Victor Horsley Department of Neurosurgery
The National Hospital for Neurology and
Neurosurgery
London, UK

Maria Verena Cicala, MD
Division of Endocrinology
Department of Medical and Surgical Sciences
University of Padua
Padua, Italy

Orlo H. Clark, MD
Professor of Surgery
Department of Surgery
University of California, San Francisco
San Francisco, California, USA

Bart L. Clarke, MD
Division of Endocrinology, Diabetes/
Metabolism, and Nutrition
Mayo Clinic College of Medicine
Rochester, Minnesota, USA

Pierantonio Conton, MD
Division of Endocrinology
Department of Medical and Surgical Sciences
University of Padua
Padua, Italy

Gerard S. Conway, MD, FRCP
Department of Endocrinology
University College London Hospitals
London, UK

Alan Crockard, DSc, FRCS, FDS,
RCS (Eng), FRCP
Victor Horsley Department of Neurosurgery
The National Hospital for Neurology and
Neurosurgery
London, UK

Tim Crook, PhD, MRCP
Department of Medical Oncology
Charing Cross Hospital; and
Cancer Genetics and Epigenetics Laboratory
The Breakthrough Toby Robins Breast Cancer
Research Centre
at The Institute of Cancer Research
London, UK

Rachel K. Crowley, MB, MRCPI
Honorary Lecturer in Endocrinology
Academic Department of Diabetes &
Endocrinology
Beaumont Hospital/RCSI Medical School
Dublin, Ireland

Simon A. Cudlip, MB,BS, BSc, MD,
FRCS (SN)
Consultant Neurosurgeon
John Radcliffe Hospital
Oxford, UK

Bruno De Bernardi, MD
Department of Hematology/Oncology
Giannina Gaslini Children's Hospital
Genova, Italy

Gerard M. Doherty, MD
NW Thompson Professor of Surgery
Head, Section of General Surgery
Residency Program Director, Surgery
University of Michigan
Ann Arbor, Michigan, USA

Ines Donangelo, MD, PhD
Cedars-Sinai Research Institute
UCLA David Geffen School of Medicine at
University of California Los Angeles
Los Angeles, California, USA

Koen M.A. Dreijerink, MD
Department of Clinical Endocrinology
University Medical Center
Utrecht, The Netherlands

Hélène Fierrard
Unité d'Endocrinologie
Assistance Publique-Hôpitaux de Paris
Hôpital Ambroise Paré
Boulogne, France; and
INSERM
Institut Cochin
Département Endocrinologie Métabolisme &
Cancer
Paris, France

Theodoros Foukakis, MD, PhD
Department of Oncology
Karolinska University Hospital
Stockholm, Sweden

Jayne A. Franklyn, MD, PhD, FRCP,
FMedSci
Professor of Medicine
Department of Medicine
University of Birmingham
Birmingham, UK

Lawrence A. Frohman, MD
Professor Emeritus of Medicine
Section of Endocrinology, Diabetes and
Metabolism
University of Illinois at Chicago
Chicago, Illinois, USA

Jean-Pierre Fryns
Chairman, Genetics Department
Center for Human Genetics
University Hospital of Leuven
Leuven, Belgium

Claudio Gambini, MD
Service of Pathology
Giannina Gaslini Children's Hospital
Genova, Italy

Toral Gathani, MRCS(Eng), MBBS(Hons),
BSc(Hons)
Clinical Research Fellow
Cancer Epidemiology Unit
University of Oxford
Oxford, UK

Mary P. Gillam, MD
Division of Endocrinology, Metabolism and
Molecular Medicine
Northwestern University Feinberg School
of Medicine
Chicago, Illinois, USA

Matthew F. Gorman, MD
Clinical Fellow
Department of Pediatrics
Division of Hematology/Oncology
University of California, San Francisco
UCSF Children's Hospital
San Francisco, California, USA

Claudio Granata, MD
Service of Radiology
Giannina Gaslini Children's Hospital
Genova, Italy

Dan Granberg, MD, PhD
Department of Medical Sciences and Department
of Endocrine Oncology
University Hospital
Uppsala, Sweden

Clive S. Grant, MD
Professor of Surgery
Mayo Clinic
Rochester, Minnesota, USA

List of Contributors

Stefan K.G. Grebe, MD, FRACP, DABCC
Co-director, Endocrine and Automated
Immunoassay Laboratories
Chair, Division of Clinical Biochemistry and
Immunology
Departmental Vice-Chair for Information
Management and Supply Chain
Department of Laboratory Medicine & Pathology
Mayo Clinic
Rochester, Minnesota, USA

Jane Green, BM BCh, Dphil
Cancer Epidemiology Unit
University of Oxford
Oxford, UK

Ashley B. Grossman, BA, BSc, MD,
FRCP, FMedSci
Professor of Neuroendocrinology
Department of Endocrinology
St Bartholomew's Hospital
London, UK

Thorvardur R. Halfdanarson
Mayo Clinic College of Medicine
Department of Oncology
Division of Medical Oncology
Rochester, Minnesota, USA

Marcia Hall, MBBS, PhD, FRCP
Consultant in Medical Oncology
Department of Medical Oncology
Mount Vernon Cancer Centre
Northwood, Middlesex, UK

Sabine E. Hannema, MD, PhD
Department of Paediatrics
Juliana Children's Hospital
The Hague, The Netherlands

Kevin J. Harrington, FRCP, FRCR
The Institute of Cancer Research
Targeted Therapy Laboratory
Cancer Research UK Centre for Cell and Molecular
Biology
London, UK

Ian D. Hay, BSc, MB, PhD, FACE, FACP,
FRCP, FRCPI (Hon)
Professor of Medicine and Dr R.F. Emslander
Professor of Endocrinology Research
Mayo Clinic College of Medicine; and
Consultant in Endocrinology and
Internal Medicine
Mayo Clinic
Rochester, Minnesota, USA

Conor J. Heaney, MD
Clinical Fellow
Department of Radiology
Mayo School of Graduate Medical Education
Rochester, Minnesota, USA

Per Hellman, MD
University of Uppsala
Uppsala, Sweden

Michelle Hermiston, MD, PhD
Assistant Professor
Pediatric Hematology-Oncology
UCSF School of Medicine
San Francisco, California, USA

Timothy J. Hobday, MD
Assistant Professor of Oncology
Department of Oncology
Mayo Clinic
Rochester, Minnesota, USA

Humphrey J. F. Hodgson, FRCP,
DM, FMedSci
Sheila Sherlock Chair of Medicine
Royal Free and University College School
of Medicine
London, UK

Silvia Hofer, MD
Medical Oncology Department
University Hospital Zürich
Zürich, Switzerland

Jo W.M. Höppener, PhD
Associate Professor
Department of Metabolic and Endocrine Diseases
University Medical Center Utrecht
Utrecht, The Netherlands

Eva Horvath, PhD
Department of Laboratory Medicine
St. Michael's Hospital
Toronto, Ontario, Canada

Ieuan A. Hughes, MA, MD, FRCP, FRCP(C),
FRCPCH, FMedSci
Department of Paediatrics
University of Cambridge
Addenbrooke's Hospital
Cambridge, UK

Niki Karavitaki, MBBS, MSc, PhD
Department of Endocrinology
Oxford Centre for Diabetes, Endocrinology
and Metabolism
Churchill Hospital
Oxford, UK

Richard T. Kloos, MD
Divisions of Endocrinology & Nuclear Medicine
The Ohio State University Medical Center and
Comprehensive Cancer Center
The Arthur G James Cancer Hospital and Solove
Research Center
Columbus, Ohio, USA

Kalman Kovacs, MD, PhD
Professor of Pathology
St. Michael's Hospital
Toronto, Ontario, Canada

Tom R. Kurzawinski, FRCS
Department of Endocrinology
University College London Hospitals
London, UK

Steven W.J. Lamberts, MD, PhD
Professor of Medicine
Erasmus Medical Center
Department of Internal Medicine
Division of Endocrinology
Rotterdam, The Netherlands

Michael A. Levine, MD
Section of Pediatric Endocrinology
Division of Pediatrics
Cleveland Clinic Children's Hospital; and
Lerner College of Medicine of Case Western
Reserve University
Cleveland, Ohio, USA

John R. Lindsay, MD
Consultant Physician
Endocrinology & Diabetes
Altnagelvin Area Hospital
Londonderry
United Kingdom

Mark E. Linskey, MD, PhD
Associate Professor and Chairman
Department of Neurological Surgery
University of California, Irvine
UCI Medical Center
Orange, California, USA

Cornelis J.M. Lips, MD, PhD
Professor of Endocrinology and Internal Medicine
University Medical Center Utrecht
Utrecht, The Netherlands

D. Lynn Loriaux, MD, PhD
Chair
Department of Medicine
Oregon Health & Science University
Portland, Oregon, USA

Eamonn R. Maher, MD, FRCP, FMedSci
Professor of Medical Genetics
Department of Medical and Molecular Genetics
University of Birmingham School of Medicine; and
West Midlands Regional Genetics Service
Birmingham Women's Hospital
Birmingham, UK

Eamonn R. Maher, MD, FRCP, FMedSci
Professor of Medical Genetics
Department of Medical and Molecular Genetics
University of Birmingham School of Medicine; and
West Midlands Regional Genetics Service
Birmingham Women's Hospital
Birmingham, UK

Franco Mantero, MD
Professor of Endocrinology
Division of Endocrinology
Department of Medical and Surgical Sciences
University of Padua
Padua, Italy

Niamh M. Martin, MBChB PhD MRCP
Clinical Senior Lecturer
Department of Metabolic Medicine
Imperial College
London, UK

Katherine K. Matthay, MD
Professor of Pediatrics
Chief, Pediatric Hematology-Oncology
UCSF School of Medicine
San Francisco, CA, USA

Karim Meeran, MBBS, MD, FRCP
Professor of Endocrinology
Department of Metabolic Medicine
Imperial College
London, UK

Shlomo Melmed, MD
Cedars-Sinai Research Institute
UCLA David Geffen School of Medicine at
University of California Los Angeles
Los Angeles, California, USA

Mark E. Molitch, MD
Professor of Medicine
Division of Endocrinology, Metabolism and
Molecular Medicine
Northwestern University Feinberg School of
Medicine
Chicago, Illinois, USA

Niall R. Moore, FRCP, FRCR
Departments of Radiology and Nuffield
Department of Medicine
Oxford Radcliffe Hospital
University of Oxford
Oxford, UK

Damian G. Morris, MBBS, PhD, MRCP
Consultant Physician
Department of Diabetes & Endocrinology
The Ipswich Hospital NHS Trust
Ipswich, UK

John C. Morris, MD
Professor of Medicine
Division of Endocrinology
Mayo Clinic College of Medicine
Rochester, Minnesota, USA

John F. Morris, BSc, MB ChB, MD, MA, FMedSci
University Lecturer and Professor of Human
Anatomy
Director of Preclinical Studies
Department of Physiology, Anatomy & Genetics
University of Oxford
Oxford, UK

Gregory R. Mundy, MD
John A. Oates Chair in Translational Medicine
Director, Vanderbilt Center for Bone Biology
Professor of Medicine, Pharmacology,
Orthopaedics, Cancer Biology
Nashville, Tennessee, USA

Robert D. Murray, MD, MRCP
Department of Endocrinology
Leeds Teaching Hospitals NHS Trust
Leeds, UK

John Newell-Price, MA, PhD, FRCP
Senior Lecturer and Consultant Endocrinologist
Academic Unit of Diabetes and Endocrinology
University of Sheffield
Sheffield, UK

Sarah Ngan, MBBS, MRCP (UK)
Clinical Research Fellow
Department of Oncology
Imperial College
London, UK

Amanda Nicholson, MBBS, PhD
Clinical Research Fellow
Department of Epidemiology and Public Health
University College London
London, UK

Christopher M. Nutting, BSc, MRCP, FRCR, MD
Consultant and Hon. Senior Lecturer in Clinical
Oncology; and
Head of Head and Neck Unit
Royal Marsden Hospital
London, UK

Kjell Öberg, MD, PhD
Professor of Endocrine Oncology
Department of Medical Sciences and Department
of Endocrine Oncology
University Hospital
Uppsala, Sweden

R. Timothy D. Oliver, MD, FRCP
Professor of Medical Oncology
St Bartholomew's Hospital
Department of Medical Oncology
London, UK

Babatunde Oyajobi, MD, PhD
Assistant Professor
Department of Cellular and Structural Biology
Graduate School of Biomedical Sciences
University of Texas Health Science Center at
San Antonio
San Antonio, Texas, USA

Susan Padalecki, PhD
Department of Cellular and Structural Biology
University of Texas Health Science Center
San Antonio, Texas, USA

Anna Patalano, MD
Division of Endocrinology
Department of Medical and Surgical Sciences
University of Padua
Padua, Italy

Sharon Peoples, MBChB, MRCP, FRCR
Specialist Registrar
Edinburgh Cancer Centre
Western General Hospital
Edinburgh, UK

Luca Persani, MD, PhD
Associate Professor of Endocrinology
Department of Medical Sciences
University of Milan
Istituto Auxologico Italiano IRCCS
Milan, Italy

Rachel R. Phillips, FRCP, DCH, FRCR
Consultant Radiologist
Honorary Senior Clinical Lecturer in Radiology
University of Oxford
Oxford, UK

Jane Phillips-Hughes, MRCP, FRCR
Radiology Department
John Radcliffe Hospital
Oxford, UK

Vito Pistoia
Laboratory of Oncology
Giannina Gaslini Children's Hospital
Genova, Italy

**P. Nicholas Plowman, MA, MD,
FRCP, FRCR**
Department of Clinical Oncology
St Bartholomew's Hospital
London, UK

Marie-Laure Raffin-Sanson, MD, PhD
Unité d'Endocrinologie
Assistance Publique-Hôpitaux de Paris
Hôpital Ambroise Paré
Boulogne, France; and
INSERM
Institut Cochin
Département Endocrinologie Métabolisme
& Cancer
Paris, France

Gustavo G. Fernandez Ranvier, MD
Endocrine Oncology Surgical Fellow
Department of Surgery
University of California, San Francisco
San Francisco, California, USA

David William Ray, FRCP, PhD
Professor of Medicine, and Endocrinology
University of Manchester
Manchester, UK

Andrew G. Renehan, PhD, FRCS, FDS
Senior Lecturer in Cancer Studies and Surgery
University of Manchester
Department of Surgery
Christie Hospital NHS Trust
Manchester, UK

**Rodney H. Reznek, FRANZCR(Hon),
FRCP, FRCR**
Professor of Diagnostic Imaging
Institute of Cancer
Barts and The London School of Medicine
and Dentistry
London, UK

Vincent M. Riccardi, MD
The Neurofibromatosis Institute
La Crescenta, California, USA

Matthew D. Ringel, MD
Professor of Medicine
Divisions of Endocrinology, Metabolism,
and Diabetes and Oncology
Department of Internal Medicine
The Ohio State University
Columbus, Ohio, USA

Anju Sahdev, MBBS(Lon), MRCP, FRCR
Cancer Imaging
Department of Radiology
St Bartholomew's Hospital
London, UK

Frank Saran, MD, FRCR
Consultant Clinical Oncologist and
Honorary Senior Lecturer
Department of Radiotherapy
Royal Marsden NHS Foundation Trust
Sutton, Surrey, UK

David H. Sarne, MD
Associate Professor of Medicine
University of Illinois at Chicago
Chicago, Illinois, USA

**Andrew F. Scarsbrook, BMedSci,
BM.BS, FRCR**
Consultant Radiologist & Nuclear Medicine
Physician
Department of Radiology
St James's University Hospital
Leeds Teaching Hospitals
United Kingdom

Arthur B. Schneider, MD, PhD
Professor Emeritus of Medicine
University of Illinois at Chicago
Chicago, Illinois, USA

William F. Schwindinger, MD, PhD
Weis Center for Research, Geisinger Clinic
Danville, Pennsylvania, USA

Michael J. Seckl, PhD, FRCP
Professor of Medical Oncology
Head of Section of Molecular Oncology
Director of the Charing Cross Gestational
Trophoblastic Disease Centre
Head of Lung Cancer Biology Group
Hammersmith Hospitals Campus of Imperial
College London
London, UK

F. John Service, MD, PhD
Professor of Medicine
Division of Endocrinology & Metabolism
Department of Internal Medicine
Mayo Clinic College of Medicine
Rochester, Minnesota, USA

Manisha H. Shah, MD
Assistant Professor of Internal Medicine
Division of Hematology-Oncology
Department of Internal Medicine
The Ohio State University
Columbus, Ohio, USA

**John H. Shepherd, FRCS, FRCOG,
FACOG**
Professor of Surgical Gynaecology
St Bartholomew's and the Royal London School
of Medicine and Dentistry
Consultant Gynaecological Surgeon and
Oncologist
Royal Marsden Hospital
London, UK

Michael Sheppard, FMedSci
Dean of the School of Medicine
Department of Medicine
University of Birmingham
Birmingham, UK

Mark Sherlock, MB, MRCPI
MRC Clinical Research Fellow
University of Birmingham
Birmingham, UK

Lucy Side, MRCP(UK), MD
Consultant in Clinical Genetics
Department of Clinical Genetics
Churchill Hospital
Oxford, UK

Maurice L. Slevin, MD
St Bartholomew's Hospital
London, UK

**Andrew Solomon, MA (Cantab),
BM BCh (Oxon), MRCP**
Department of Endocrinology
Royal Free Hospital
London, UK

Christine Spitzweg, MD
Department of Internal Medicine II – Campus
Grosshadern
Ludwig-Maximilians-University Munich
Munich, Germany

Julie A. Sterling, PhD
Department of Medicine/Clinical Pharmacology
Center for Bone Biology
Vanderbilt University
Nashville, Tennessee, USA

Paul M. Stewart, FRCP, FMedSci
Professor of Medicine
University of Birmingham
Birmingham, UK

Constantine A. Stratakis, MD, D(med)Sci
Director, Pediatric Endocrinology Program
Chief, Heritable Disorders Branch
National Institute of Child Health and Human
Development (NICHD)
National Institutes of Health
Bethesda, Maryland, USA

Nia J. Taylor, MRCP, FRCR
Specialist Registrar
Department of Radiology
The John Radcliffe Hospital
Oxford, UK

Chris Thompson, MD, FRCPI
Professor of Endocrinology
Academic Department of Diabetes &
Endocrinology
Beaumont Hospital/RCSI Medical School
Dublin, Ireland

Gerlof D. Valk, MD, PhD
Department of Clinical Endocrinology
University Medical Center
Utrecht, The Netherlands

Maarten O. van Aken, MD, PhD
Internist-endocrinologist
Department of Internal Medicine
Erasmus Medical Center
Rotterdam, The Netherlands

Aart Jan van der Lelij, MD, PhD
Head of Section of Endocrinology
Erasmus Medical Center
Rotterdam, The Netherlands

Adrian Vella, MD, FRCP
Associate Professor of Medicine
Division of Endocrinology & Metabolism
Department of Internal Medicine
Mayo Clinic College of Medicine
Rochester, Minnesota, USA

Andrew M. Wardley, MD, FRCP
Consultant Medical Oncologist & Clinical
Research Lead Manchester Breast Centre
Cancer Research UK Department of Medical
Oncology
Christie Hospital
Manchester, UK

John A.H. Wass, MA, MD, FRCP
Professor of Endocrinology
University of Oxford
Consultant Physician
Churchill Hospital
Oxford, UK

Mona Waterhouse, MA, MRCP
Department of Endocrinology
St Bartholomew's Hospital
London, UK

Jonathan Waxman, BSc, MD, FRCP
Professor of Oncology
Imperial College
London, UK

Matthew L. White, MD
Research Fellow
Department of Surgery
University of Michigan; and
Resident
Department of Surgery
St. Joseph Mercy Hospital
Ann Arbor, Michigan, USA

Gregory A. Wiseman, MD
Assistant Professor of Medicine
Mayo Clinic College of Medicine
Rochester, Minnesota, USA

Ingrid Witters
Center for Human Genetics
University Hospital of Leuven
Leuven, Belgium

Lisa Wong MRCOG (London)
Gynaecological Oncology Fellow
Royal Marsden Hospital
London, UK

Emma R. Woodward, MD
Cancer Research UK Renal Molecular
Oncology Group
Section of Medical and Molecular Genetics
University of Birmingham, Institute of
Biomedical Research; and
West Midlands Regional Genetics Service
Birmingham Women's Hospital
Birmingham, UK

Jan Zedenius MD, PhD
Associate Professor of Surgery
Karolinska University Hospital
Stockholm, Sweden

Foreword

The aim of the first edition of this textbook, published 11 years ago, was to gather together a vast amount of information and present a scientifically sound approach to the management of endocrine tumors. Although its scope was broad, the book succeeded admirably and provided an invaluable resource covering topics that previously would have demanded consultation of several textbooks on endocrinology, oncology, radiology and pathology. Another important feature of the book was the wide range of illustrations from a number of different sources, which not only made the book a pleasure to read, but also served to enhance the integration of the various disciplines.

It is therefore a pleasure to be asked to write the foreword for this second edition which has built on the success of the original to provide a truly comprehensive, lucid and up-to-date account of this field. As before, the material is arranged in seven parts: Endocrine Oncology and Therapeutic Options, Thyroid and Para-thyroid Tumors, Pituitary and Hypothalamic Lesions, Adrenal and Gonadal Tumors, Neuroendocrine Tumors and the Clinical Syndromes, Medical Syndromes and Endocrine Neoplasia and, finally, Endocrine-responsive Tumors and Female Reproductive Hormone Therapy. Many of the authors of these chapters are new and their fresh approach has ensured that the present edition will serve the broad community of readers well for the next decade.

The editorship has also altered; John Wass continues as one of the editors and is now joined by Ian Hay. Both are widely acknowledged experts in this field and they are to be thanked for bringing together such a strong group of contributors and for ensuring that the tremendous recent advances in our under-standing of tumorigenesis are matched by coverage of the latest developments in patient management and treatment. This edition will be an invaluable resource to all who work in the field, be they scientists, endocrinologists, oncologists or surgeons. In addition, the book will appeal as a single resource to general physicians of all specialties, given the frequency with which some of these endocrine problems occur and the diverse ways in which they can present.

Anthony P. Weetman
Dean of the School of Medicine and Biomedical Sciences
University of Sheffield

Preface

Endocrinology is a wonderful medical subspecialty. One of the fascinations for a clinical endocrinologist is to observe the diverse ways in which patients with various endocrine problems can present. Another hugely enjoyable aspect relates to the expertise that is required, not only from endocrinologists, but also from a large number of other specialists who cooperate to deliver multi-disciplinary care to a patient with a tumor in an endocrine organ. It is now more generally recognized that the level of expertise and experience delivered has an important bearing on the outcome of such patients.

The first edition of this book was, happily, well reviewed. We now publish this second (and much extended) edition and are very pleased to welcome a number of new authors who have been selected from all over the world for their special expertise. We are very grateful to all of them for their excellent contributions.

The first edition aimed to provide, across the multiple disciplines, sound guidelines on the basic science, clinical presentation, investigation, and treatment of endocrine tumors. We believe this to be the most comprehensive book of its kind, bringing together the expertise necessary to permit delivery of multidisciplinary care to patients with endocrine tumors.

It has been a stimulating and enjoyable experience planning and preparing this treatise. We are particularly grateful to Elisabeth Dodds who, with great assiduity, has kept us on track with good nature and humor. We are also obliged to her many colleagues at Wiley-Blackwell for their support in the project.

Ian D. Hay
John A.H. Wass

Endocrinology, the Hertz Brothers, and the History of Cancer

D. Lynn Loriaux

The history of cancer is long. It is referred to in the oldest extant medical documents; for example the Ebers Papyrus, in which paragraphs 863 to 867 are devoted to tumors and other swellings. Similarly, in paragraph 811, we find the encantation for the breasts to protect them from discharge, blood, and "self consumption," suggesting carcinoma of the breast [1].

The concepts evolved slowly. Tumor, a local encapsulated swelling, often could be treated with surgery. Cancer, a locally invasive tumor, sometimes could be treated with surgery. Malignancy/distant spread, however, could never be treated adequately with surgery, or anything else for that matter. A couple of general concepts emerged along the way: Ehrlich's "magic bullet," a concept as true for cancer as it was for syphilis; and Knudson's two-hit hypothesis emerging from a careful study of retinoblastoma, still the most cogent argument for "mutations" underlying malignant transformation. This desultory state of affairs continued until the middle of the twentieth century when two American brothers, both endocrinologists, took the problem of cancer "head on" and changed the treatment of the disease forever.

The brothers were Saul and Roy Hertz (Fig. 1). Perhaps you have heard of one or the other; probably not. The Hertz family lived in Cleveland, Ohio, and were first-generation immigrants from Eastern Europe [2]. There were seven boys: Saul was the oldest, and Roy came fourth in line. The father owned a pawnshop and supplemented that income with construction jobs and property management. The boys were raised in the tradition of Orthodox Judaism. Their father held the highest position in the family synagogue and carried the Shopar for many years. One of the strongest family values was learning. All of the children were destined for a university education. Saul went to the University of Michigan where he graduated with a Phi Beta Kappa key and went on to Harvard Medical School. He returned to Cleveland for an internship and residency at the Mt. Sinai Hospital, and then returned to Boston to the Massachusetts General Hospital [3]. He returned to study metabolic disease. There was no stipend or salary. After three months, Francis Howard Means, Jackson Professor of Clinical Medicine at Harvard University and Chief of the Medical Service at the Massachusetts General Hospital, acquired a Dalton

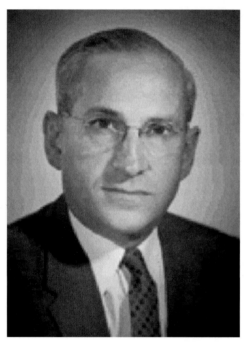

Figure 1 Roy Hertz, circa 1960. (Courtesy of Roy Hertz, July 2002.)

Scholarship for Hertz. Then, in 1934, he named Hertz the Director of Thyroid Clinic at the MGH but still there were no funds to support the position. Means would reappoint Hertz periodically. In modern parlance, he was on an annual contract.

On 12 November 1936, at a Harvard Medical School luncheon on the Longwood Campus, Karl Compton, the President of Massachusetts Institute of Technology, gave a presentation entitled "What Physics Can do for Biology and Medicine." In preparing for the talk, Compton asked one of his "young Turks," Robley Evans, for some ideas. Evans noted that "tracer" molecules for the study of metabolism might be a good idea. He supplemented the concept with the idea of using "artificially radioactive isotopes" for the tracer. This idea probably emanated from a *Nature* paper by Enrico Fermi, in which he described 22 new radioactive elements

[4]. One of the elements was iodine. It had a stable atomic weight of 127 but, after a neutron capture, it became I^{128} and very radioactive.

For his talk, Compton described how these radioactive tracer molecules were made, and how they could be used to follow metabolic sequences in living cells. In the "question-and-answer" period, Saul Hertz asked Compton if he could make enough radioactive iodine to do metabolic studies on the thyroid gland. Compton said he would find out, and assigned the problem to Robley Evans [5].

A month later, Compton wrote to Hertz explaining that iodine could be made radioactive and the isotope had a half-life of radioactive decay of about 25 minutes. Hertz wrote back that his idea was to use the radioactive iodine to develop a useful treatment for overactivity of the thyroid gland.

Compton assigned the task of making and purifying radioactive iodine to Robley Evans. Robley Evans, in turn, hired Arthur Roberts, newly graduated with a PhD in physics, to set up and oversee all of the "physics" needed for the experiment. At the same time, Howard Means designated Saul Hertz as director of the "radioiodine" project from the medical perspective. Hertz and Roberts became a team.

Roberts' challenge was to make adequate amounts of radioactive iodine. He used the radium–beryllium neutron source described by Fermi. The iodine to be radiated was in the form of ethyl iodide, a liquid at room temperature. He placed the neutron source next to the flask of ethyl iodide and let the neutrons do their work. When I^{128} is formed this way, the ethyl group is cleaved and I^{128} iodide is released. Iodide is soluble in water — ethyl iodide is not. Thus, radioactive iodine could be concentrated and isolated by a simple H_2O/ethyl iodide partition. Hertz did the first animal experiment that showed the I^{128} to be concentrated in rabbit thyroid glands and the rest excreted in the urine. The experiments were very rushed because of the short half-life of I^{128}. In collaboration with the Lawrence-Livermore Laboratory, I^{126} (13-day half-life), I^{130} (12.5-hour half-life), and I^{131} (8-day half-life) were prepared and isolated using a cyclotron as the heavy particle source. It became clear that if there was ever to be enough radioactive iodine to treat humans, a dedicated cyclotron was a must. The John and Mary Markle Foundation donated $30 000 to build a cyclotron at MIT for this purpose. It was completed in 1940, and the human work began in earnest.

In 1940 and 1941, Hertz and Roberts studied radioactive iodine uptake and tissue distribution in normal human beings and hyperthyroid patients. In March 1941, they made their first attempt to treat hyperthyroidism. By the end of the year, they had treated 18 hyperthyroid patients. Of these, Hertz concluded that five were cured, two improved, one had failed therapy, and the others were unchanged. The paper was presented at the Atlantic City meetings on 1 May 1942.

Hertz continued to treat hyperthyroid patients with radioactive iodine at the MGH for the remainder of 1942. When his appointment there ended in 1942, Means found a "partial" salary for him and he continued at the MGH part time, devoting the rest of his effort to building a private practice in Boston proper. Means replaced Hertz as head of the Thyroid Clinic with Rulon Rawson. By late 1943, Hertz and Roberts had treated 19 patients, 10 of whom were judged to be cured. One interesting aspect of the treatment plan for these 19 patients was that a large dose of non-radioactive iodine was given on the third post-treatment day. The idea was to "washout" the radioactive iodine. This would become an important issue down the line.

For reasons unknown, Hertz, now encumbered with a family and private practice, precipitously joined the Navy as a medical officer. Hertz asked Earle Chapman, who had been with him at the seminal lecture by Compton, to continue his work with the research patients, and to assume the care of his private practice while he was gone.

The ensuing period was one of misunderstanding, suspicion, duplicity, and, perhaps, betrayal — all of the things that can go wrong in a scientific collaboration around an issue that can lead to fame, if not fortune. Hertz was reluctant to reveal all of his data to Means. Chapman wanted to change the experimental protocol and drop the post-treatment non-radioactive iodine. He was reluctant to completely disclose the change to Means or Hertz. Means, feeling unappreciated and, perhaps, maligned, lost his sense of obligation to Hertz. When Hertz returned from the war in 1946, he found that Chapman and Robley Evans had written a paper on the treatment of hyperthyroidism that did not include Hertz or his patients. To add insult to injury, Means had no place for Hertz in his plans for the Thyroid Unit at MGH. In the end, after much travail, two papers describing the treatment of hyperthyroidism with radioactive iodine were sent to the same journal, *JAMA*, at the same time from the same laboratory [6, 7]. Both were published in the same journal issue and both were somewhat lost in the new enthusiasm for the thiouracils, a less "dangerous" therapy.

Hertz diverted his time to his practice and to some time spent at the Beth Israel on work with radioactive iodine. However, he never recovered his enthusiasm or his self-confidence. He became despondent and bitter. He died by his own hand on 2 August 1950, at 45 years of age.

Hertz's brilliant insight was that radioactive iodine could do more than act as a tracer, it could be Ehrlich's "magic bullet" when it came to treating hyperthyroidism. Even more, he was sure that radioactive iodine could be an effective treatment for metastatic thyroid cancer. He never had the chance to test this hypothesis.

Means, in his book on the history of clinical investigation at the MGH – "*Ward 4 – the Mallinckrodt Research Ward of the Massachusetts General Hospital*" gave the following pronunciumento:

Radioactive iodine was first used in the treatment of patients with Graves disease in 1941. This was in the thyroid clinic of the Massachusetts General Hospital. The original studies were conducted by Saul Hertz, and since 1943, they have been continued by Earle M. Chapman. The total number of patients treated at the MGH had reached about 1000 in 1957, and throughout the world the number would be about 50 000. Almost no untoward results have been reported.

The other condition in which radioactive iodine is used for treatment is cancer of the thyroid. Here it is of very secondary importance. Thus far, the rule in the treatment of cancer in general holds also for cancer of the thyroid, namely, that when sur-gical removal is possible, it takes precedence over all other forms of treatment [8].

As we all now know, radioactive iodine is the only effective treatment for metastatic thyroid cancer. This work was left to be done by others. It remains the first truly rational targeted therapy for any cancer – Ehrlich's vision realized.

Now, Roy Hertz, the little brother, enters the fray. Roy was born on 19 June 1909, the fourth of seven boys. He was much like his older brother, religious and studious with an innate interest in the natural sciences. Surprisingly, Roy majored in comparative literature at the University of Wisconsin. "He said that his move into physiology from comparative literature was serendipitous and was precipitated by receiving a 'C' grade in a Latin poetry course." "I'd never gotten a 'C' before in my life. I took that card and I sat under a tree for about one hour, and I decided if I got a 'C', I'm not a fit man for the study of comparative literature, I'd better turn to something else" [2].

That something else was graduate study in the laboratory of Fredrick Lee Hisaw. He was a professor of physiology at Wisconsin, and the discoverer of relaxin and of the requirement for proges-terone to maintain pregnancy. Hertz's assignment was to decipher the effects of pituitary LH and FSH on the reproductive cycle of the rabbit. He spent hours "harvesting" cow pituitary glands at the nearby Oscar-Mayer slaughter house. He was, in the end, able to demonstrate the need for sequential stimulation of the ovary by FSH and LH to complete the ovulatory cycle. He received his PhD in 1933.

Hertz's first job was teaching physiology at Howard University. That job lasted a year. His second job was teaching physiology at Brown University. That job lasted a year. Hertz decided that a life of science would require a separate source of income that he did not have. He returned to the University of Wisconsin as a medical student and earned his MD degree in three years.

Following a rotating internship, Hertz joined the U.S. Public Health Service. The first two years allowed him to earn an MPH at Johns Hopkins University. Then, his supervisor found him a position in the division of physiology at the nascent National Institutes of Health. Hertz began the appointment on 8 December 1941 – the day after the attack on Pearl Harbor.

Hertz began his NIH career in the nutrition research laboratory of Dr. Henry Sebrell. The focus of the work was the biologic inter-actions between avidin, biotin, progesterone, stilbestrol, and folic acid. In particular, he worked on the effects of folate and purine antagonists on the developing female urogenital tract. About this time, Hertz was appointed chief of the Endocrinology Section of the National Cancer Institute. In this role, Hertz developed a clinical research unit at George Washington University Hospital, which was moved to the new NIH Clinical Center in 1953. Hertz was now Chief of the Endocrinology Branch of the National Cancer Institute and admitted the first patient to the new NIH Clinical Center in that year, Mr. Charles Meredith, who had advanced prostate cancer (Fig. 2).

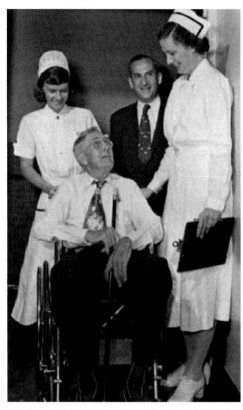

Figure 2 Charles Meredith, the first patient admitted to the NIH Clinical Center. Center, shown here with Roy Hertz, second from right. (Courtesy of Roy Hertz, 2002.)

Hertz needed a young doctor to help him manage the patients under his care. One of the applicants for this job was Dr. Min Chia Li. Unable to find a place at the NIH in 1952, Dr. Li went to the Memorial Sloan-Kettering Cancer Institute to work with Dr. Olaf Pearson. During his stay at Memorial, Dr. Li was involved in an interesting experiment designed by Dr. Von Gilse, a visiting oncologist from the Rotterdam Radiotherapy Institute. Dr. Von Gilse had read Hertz's papers showing that folate antagonists could interrupt the embryonic development of the female reproductive tract. She reasoned that the most likely reason for this was that the folate antagonist was also an estrogen antagonist. Von Gilse's primary interest was in breast cancer, and she was looking for an estrogen antagonist that might leave therapeutic value in the treat-ment of breast cancer. She designed a study to test the hypothesis. She planned to quantitate the effect of a folate antagonist on the cornification index of the vaginal epithelium of a patient being treated with methotrexate. The patient was a 35-year-old woman with a malignant melanoma. Von Gilse measured the vaginal cornification index over a period of 40 days. The first 20 days of methotrexate alone, and the second 20 days of methotrexate plus estinyl. Surprisingly, methotrexate did not antagonize the effects of vaginal cornification. As a chance observation, however, human chorionic gonadotropin fell dramatically over the course of the experiment. Li noted this effect, and concluded that methotrexate might be an effective treatment for patients with hCG-secreting

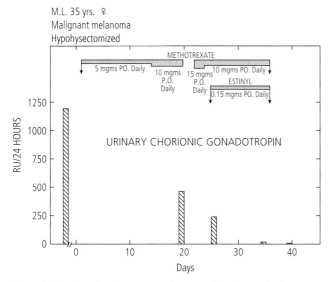

Figure 3 The effect of methotrexate on urinary gonadotropin excretion in a patient with malignant melanoma. (From Hertz R. et al. [9], with permission.)

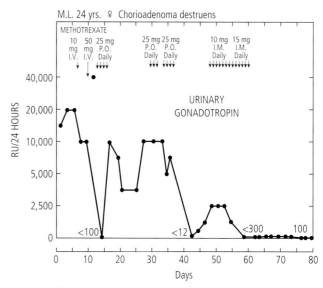

Figure 4 Effect of methotrexate on urinary gonadotropin excretion on a patient with metastatic choriocarcinoma. (From Hertz R. et al. [10], with permission.)

cancers, in particular, choriocarcinoma (Fig. 3) Hertz remembered Li and contacted him. Li took the job.

After being at the NIH for less than a month, a woman with choriocarcinoma was admitted to Dr. Li. Hertz was fascinated by the rare occurrence of spontaneous remission in choriocarcinoma and planned to study the phenomenon with daily urine hCG measurements. The young woman promptly died of a cerebral hemorrhage.

Li was very upset by this and believed that all of these patients should be treated with something and not just observed for the natural history of the disease. He went to Hertz with his "methotrexate" hypothesis that he developed at Sloan-Kettering. He proposed to Hertz that they treat the next patient with choriocarcinoma with methotrexate. Hertz agreed. They did not have to wait long. Two months later, Bill Lucas from the National Naval Medical Center admitted a 24-year-old woman with choriocarcinoma and a large hemopneumothorax. She appeared to be at death's door. Li gave her 10 mg of methotrexate intravenously. She survived the first day, and Li gave her 50 mg methotrexate intravenously the next day. She seemed better. Li then gave her 25 mg of methotrexate orally for four days, followed by "short courses" of 10 or 15 mg of methotrexate over the next 60 days. All of the urinary gonadotropins disappeared from the urine. Pulmonary metastases seen on standard chest radiograph dis-appeared. She was discharged from the hospital at 80 days. She was seen four months later and was in excellent health. She lived a long and healthy life. This is the first known cure of a metastatic solid tumor. Two more cases were treated in the ensuing months with similar results — apparent cure.

Hertz told Li that he thought this must be "beginner's luck". He thought the findings probably represented some unlikely "cluster" of spontaneous remission. Even so, the results were published in the Proceedings of the Society for Experimental Biology and Medicine in 1956 (Fig. 4).

With the ongoing success in treating gestational choriocarcinoma, the two men turned their attention to the problem of testicular choriocarcinoma. This tumor, however, was far more resistant to treatment. No remissions were achieved. Hertz and Li concluded that the different results between men and women could be explained by the "genetic" nature of the tumor. Gestational choriocarcinoma is a cancer of fetal origin. Half of the chromosomes are paternal. The cancer is subject to immunologic rejection by the host. This is not the case with non-gestational choriocarcinoma. Very insightful for the time.

Roy Hertz went on to become the scientific director of NICHD, Associate Director of the Population Council, Rockefeller University, Professor of Pharmacology at George Washington University, and, finally, Adjunct Scientist at the National Institutes of Health, ending his scientific career where it had begun many years before.

Hertz and Min Li won the Lasker Award in 1972, and Hertz was elected to the National Academy of Sciences in the same year. Hertz finally found his way to a quiet retirement in Hollywood Maryland on the shores of the Patuxent River. When asked what achievement in his life he was most proud of, he answered, "The reciprocation of my children's and my wife's love for me, the reciprocation of my love for them. That's the whole story. Everything else is minor" [2].

Roy Hertz died of a stroke on 28 October 2002, eleven days after the death of his wife Dorothy.

So, there you have it. Two brothers, sons of a pawnbroker finding their way to science through the suffering of mankind, devoting their lives to the "hard problems." The older brother paved the way for Ehrlich's "magic bullet" in the treatment of cancer. The younger brother was the first to cure metastatic cancer by any means. This achievement was the motive force behind Richard Nixon's "*War on Cancer.*" Both brothers were physicians first, endocrinologists second, and scientists third. Their work in cancer treatment was revelatory and an inflection point in the history of the disease. Nothing quite like it has happened since.

References

1. Nunn, JF. *Ancient Egyptian Medicine.* Norman, OK: University of Oklahoma Press, Red River Books, 2002, pp. 33 and 197.

2. Yarris JD, Hunter AJ. Roy Hertz, MD (1909–2002): the cure of choriocarcinoma. *Gynecol. Oncol.* 2003;89:193–198.

3. Sawin CT, Becker DV. Radioiodine and the treatment of hyperthyroidism: the early history. *Thyroid* 1997;7:63–176.

4. Fermi E. Radioactivity induced by neutron bombardment. *Nature* 1934;133:757.

5. Adelstein SJ. Robley Evans and what physics can do for medicine. *Cancer Biother. Radiopharm.* 2001;16:179–185.

6. Hertz S, Roberts A. The use of radioactive iodine therapy in hyperthyroidism. *Trans. Am. Assoc. Study. Goiter* 1946, p. 62.

7. Chapman EW. Treatment of Grave's Disease with radioactive iodine. *Trans. Am. Assoc. Study. Goiter* 1946, p. 74.

8. Means, JH. Ward 4 – the Mallinckrodt Research Ward of the Massachusetts General Hospital. Cambridge, MA: Harvard University Press, 1958, p. 66.

9. Hertz R, Bergenstal DM, Lipsett MB, Price EB, Hilbish TF. Chemotherapy of choriocarcinoma and related trophoblastic tumors in women. *Ann. N.Y. Acad. Sci.* 1959;80:262–264.

10. Hertz R, Li MC, Spencer DB. Effect of methotrexate therapy upon choriocarcinoma and chorioadenoma. *Proc. Soc. Exp. Biol. Med.* 1956;93:361–366.

1 Endocrine Oncology and Therapeutic Options

1 Structure and Development of the Endocrine System

John F. Morris

Key points

- Endocrine gland normal gross and microscopic structure is well known.
- Peptides and amines are released by exocytosis; steroids are now known to be transported out of cells.
- Mechanisms involved in "constitutive" secretion of hormones remain poorly understood; in tumors, both "regulated" and "constitutive" secretion can occur.
- Understanding of molecular aspects of the development of endocrine tissues has increased dramatically recently. Mutations in the molecular signals identified in developing animal models have, in many cases (e.g., pituitary development), been shown to be associated with the expected human endocrine developmental anomalies, showing that these signalling mechanisms are well conserved in mammals.
- Increased understanding of these molecular aspects could help elucidate the role of dysdifferentiation and stem cells in endocrine tumors. It is possible, for example, that the molecular signal(s) which normally down-regulate(s) gastrin production in the pancreas are themselves switched off when gastrinomas develop.

Introduction

Concepts of what comprises the endocrine system are rapidly expanding. Classically thought of as the discrete endocrine glands and their products, the concept has broadened to include the diffuse endocrine systems of the gut, respiratory tract, heart and endothelium. The term "cytokines" originally covered the products of the immune system but it is now clear that they are produced more widely; similarly, growth factors are chemical signals which are produced by many tissues and generally have local actions, although liver insulin-like growth factor may have much wider effects. Therefore, it is now clear that most if not all tissues produce signal molecules that act over longer or shorter distances. To the original concept of an endocrine action via the bloodstream have thus been added paracrine, juxtacrine, autocrine, and even intracrine modes of action. Indeed any one hormonal signal may act in many of these ways.

Endocrine cells produce, in addition to their principal hormone(s), many different compounds in differing amounts. Some, such as the neurophysins, are produced as part of the hormone precursor; others, such as the chromogranin group of proteins, are produced rather widely in peptide- and amine-secreting cells; both can serve as useful markers of hormone-producing tumors.

Some have signalling activity, some do not. Co-secreted molecules which are not part of the main prohormone are usually produced in very much smaller (0.1–1.0%) amounts than the main product; the amounts vary physiologically and their actions are largely autocrine or paracrine. Many molecules produced by endocrine cells are not restricted to one tissue; for example, many "gut" peptides are also found in the brain. Apparent "ectopic" production is even more marked in endocrine tumors.

Endocrine tissues can conveniently be divided into those secreting peptide/protein, amine, steroid and iodothyronine signals. To these can be added the eicosanoids (prostaglandins, thromboxanes, leukotrienes, hydroxyeicosatetraenoic acid), nitric oxide and carbon monoxide; such compounds are produced by many different cell types and will not be considered further here. It is now clear that most steroid- and amine-secreting endocrine cells also produce protein peptide/protein secretory products. It is also clear that some tissues, especially the brain, can produce and/or modify steroid to new active compounds – the neurosteroids.

Whereas the general structure and development of the endocrine system have been well understood for many years, our understanding of molecular and developmental endocrinology has mushroomed [1]. The genes for most hormones and hormone-producing enzymes have been identified and their chromosomal location determined. For this reason, most of the references quoted are to reviews of genetic and molecular aspects of development. Although original concepts of the formation of various glands from ectodermal, endodermal or mesodermal tissues still largely hold true, we now have a much better understanding of the

Clinical Endocrine Oncology, 2nd edition. Edited by Ian D. Hay and John A.H. Wass. © 2008 Blackwell Publishing. ISBN 978-1-4051-4584-8.

diverse contributions made by the neural crest, and are beginning to understand the induction processes and molecular switches that lead to the differentiation of endocrine tissues and thereby determine the tissue-specific production of hormones. Indeed, the concept of dysdifferentiation [2] involving tumor formation by clonal expansion offers perhaps the best explanation of the variety of hormones produced by tumors. Equally, understanding of the receptors and postreceptor mechanisms that lead to hormone release allows insight into how autonomous secretion of hormone can result from defects in these mechanisms.

This basic science, combined with clinical experience of endocrine system dysfunction, now permits a better understanding of the development of endocrine tumors and the products they secrete.

Chemically different hormones: "regulated" and "constitutive" release

The chemically different types of hormone necessarily have different cellular mechanisms for their production and release (Fig. 1.1).

The *peptide/protein/glycoprotein* group of hormones are products of genes that usually code for much larger precursors. The mRNAs are translated by ribosomes and simultaneously sequestered in the rough endoplasmic reticulum where the signal sequence is removed, primary glycosylation occurs and disulfide bridges are formed. The immature products (prohormones) are then translocated to the Golgi apparatus where any terminal

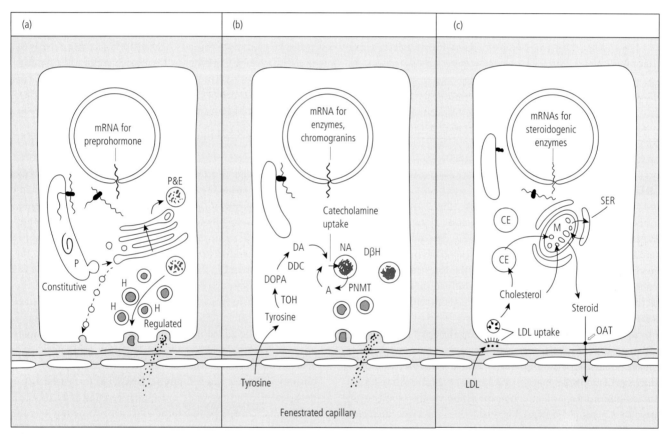

Figure 1.1 Different cellular mechanisms of hormone secretion. (a) Production of peptide, protein and glycoprotein hormones (H). mRNA for the preprohormone and processing enzymes attach first to free ribosomes, then are translated into the rough endoplasmic reticulum. The signal is removed co-translationally to yield the prohormone (P) which may be core-glycosylated in the RER; this is passed to the Golgi where, in the "regulated" pathway, the prohormone is packaged into vesicles in a concentrated form with processing enzymes (E) then transported to the plasma membrane or stored until a secretagogue stimulus is received by the cell which causes exocytosis of the dense-cored vesicles. In the "constitutive" pathway the hormone is packaged apparently unconcentrated into small vesicles which are then immediately transported to the membrane and exocytosed. Constitutive release may predominate in tumors. (b) In catecholamine-secreting cells secretory vesicles are produced in the same way but the DOPA and dopamine (DA) precursors are produced in the cytoplasm by the enzymes tyrosine hydroxylase (TOH) and DOPA decarboxylase (DDC), and pumped into the vesicles where DA is converted to noradrenaline (NA) by dopamine β-hydroxylase (DβH); amine leaks slowly out of the vesicles and, in adrenaline-producing cells, NA is converted by phenylethanolamine-*N*-methyl transferase (PNMT) to adrenaline (A) which is pumped back into vesicles which are stored prior to release. (c) Steroid-producing cells are characterized by distinctive mitochondria (M) surrounded by smooth endoplasmic reticulum (SER). These organelles contain the enzymes which convert cholesterol derived from low-density lipoprotein (LDL) uptake or from stored cholesterol ester (CE) into steroids, which are transported out of the cells by organic anion transporters (OATs).

glycosylation occurs and proteolytic cleavage of the prohormone commences. The Golgi apparatus packages the prohormones and converting enzymes (prohormone convertase; PC1–3) into vesicles which are then transported to the plasma membrane for release by exocytosis. For the "regulated" secretory pathway the prohormones and convertases are concentrated within the vesicles so that the vesicles have an electron-dense core in which cleavage of the prohormone continues. Variable numbers of the dense-cored vesicles are stored in the cytoplasm awaiting the signal for release (or if not released, for lysosomal degradation). The membranes of dense-cored vesicles have a proton pump which maintains an acidic intravesicular pH which stabilizes the peptides near their isoelectric point and is optimal for intravesicular proteolysis.

Some peptide hormones, in particular the growth factors and cytokines, are not stored but released immediately via the "constitutive" pathway. The vesicles that transport the peptide to the membrane in the constitutive pathway are not well understood. They are difficult to identify because the peptide is not concentrated and the vesicles are short-lived. In the "regulated" pathway the extracellular concentration of the hormone is controlled by signals that stimulate release from the stored pool of vesicles, usually within seconds of the stimulus; at the same time synthesis is stimulated more slowly to replenish the stores. By contrast, the extracellular concentration of peptides released by the "constitutive" pathway is determined by control of their synthesis and usually takes several hours to reach peak levels.

In cells that normally release hormone by the regulated pathway, the number of hormone-containing vesicles that are stored in the cytoplasm varies depending, in part, on the demand for the acute release of large amounts of hormone. Thus, for hormones controlling parameters that vary only slowly (e.g., parathyroid hormone (PTH) controlling plasma calcium) the store is small and hormone-containing vesicles are sparse; by contrast, where the demand can be large (e.g., insulin) the cytoplasmic dense-cored vesicles are plentiful.

All endocrine cells have the cellular machinery for both the regulated and constitutive secretory pathways and in some normal endocrine cells both pathways may operate. For example, there is evidence that, while luteinizing hormone (LH) is released predominantly by the regulated pathway, most follicle-stimulating hormone (FSH) is released constitutively [3]. It is therefore not surprising that in some endocrine tumors a peptide normally released by the regulated pathway is released constitutively, with virtually no dense-cored vesicles in the tissue. In tumorous endocrine cells that do contain dense-cored vesicles these may be of a different size to the vesicles that characterize the normal tissue (indeed, little is known about how vesicle size is determined). It is also not surprising that the peptide produced may be abnormal in some way so that, even it if is detectable by radioimmunoassay of the plasma, it may not be bioactive. Finally, tumor cells may have defects in their secretory mechanisms such that hormone can be identified within the cells but is not secreted in detectable amounts.

Cells secreting *catecholamine* hormones also contain numerous dense-cored vesicles, which is not surprising considering their role as acute stress hormones. However, the synthetic pathway is very different. Tyrosine is converted in the cytoplasm first to dihydroxyphenylalanine (DOPA) and then to dopamine (DA). The amine is then pumped into Golgi-derived vesicles which already contain proteins such as chromogranin, co-packaged peptides such as corticotropin-releasing hormone (CRH) and enkephalin, the enzyme dopamine β-hydroxylase, together with ATP and calcium accumulated from the cytoplasm. Dopamine is converted to noradrenaline within the vesicles, but the amines leak slowly through the vesicle membrane and, in adrenaline-producing cells, the noradrenaline is converted to adrenaline by the cytoplasmic enzyme phenylethanolamine-N-methyl transferase. The amine pump on the membrane of the vesicles ensures that only about 1% of the amine is free in the cytoplasm. The membrane of catecholamine vesicles also has a proton pump which, by protonating the intravesicular amines, slows their diffusion out of the vesicles. Production of mature amine-containing vesicles takes about 20 h; they are released by exocytosis as in the regulated pathway for peptide hormones, immature vesicles tend not to be released. The stores of catecholamine-containing vesicles, although large, can become exhausted if severe stress is prolonged, depriving the body of its ability to respond to shock.

Cells secreting *steroid* hormones are characterized by mitochondria with tubulo-vesicular cristae, surrounded by large amounts of smooth endoplasmic reticulum. These two organelles contain the enzymes of the steroid-synthesizing pathways. Cholesterol, derived from low-density lipoprotein (LDL) uptake or from cholesterol esters stored as lipid droplets in the cytoplasm, is transported into the mitochondria by a steroid acute regulatory (STAR) protein. In the mitochondria the rate-limiting side-chain cleavage enzyme ($P450_{SCC}$) converts the cholesterol to pregnenolone. Which other steroids are produced from the pregnenolone depends on which other enzymes the cells express. Steroids are not stored to any significant extent (though a small amount may be retained in sulfated form) and were thought to diffuse from the cell through the plasma membrane. However, recent evidence indicates that organic anion transporters (OATs) are responsible for releasing the majority of the steroid. Some steroid-producing cells also secrete proteins (some corpus luteum cells secrete both oxytocin and a progesterone-binding protein) which are packaged in dense-cored vesicles. It is therefore likely that in cells secreting both steroid and protein some steroid is associated with hydrophobic regions of the secreted proteins.

The mechanisms involved in the secretion of *iodothyronines* are described in the section on the thyroid gland.

Many hormones of all chemical types are secreted in pulses; the amplitude and frequency of these pulses are often critical for the action of the hormone.

The normal histological characteristics of endocrine cells are given in Table 1.1.

Table 1.1 Cellular characteristics of hormone-secreting cells

Organ	Principal hormones: cell types	Cellular characteristics	Secretory vesicles: diameter, form
Hypothalamus			
Magnocellular (neurohypophysis)	Oxytocin Vasopressin	Large neurons (50 μm), prominent RER, Golgi; both beaded axons and dendrites contain peptide; axonal dilatations (Herring bodies) and nerve terminals in neural lobe	Spherical, 160–200 nm
Parvocellular (median eminence)	CHR (+ AVP) TRH GHRH GnRH Somatostatin Dopamine	Small neurons (15 μm), modest RER, Golgi, both fine beaded axons and dendrites contain peptide; axons terminate on portal capillaries in median eminence	Spherical, 100–110 nm
Pituitary adenohypophysis	Growth hormone: somatotroph (50%)*	Rounded cells (acidophil), often perivascular; perinuclear RER, Golgi	Profuse, spherical, 350–600 nm
	Prolactin: lactotroph (10–25%; proliferate in pregnancy)	Rounded or irregular (acidophil) cells, modest RER, prominent Golgi. Sparsely and profusely granulated types; types I, II, III	Type I, ovoid, 275–600 nm Type II, spherical , 200–300 nm Type III, spherical, 100–200 nm
	TSH, thyrotropin: thyrotroph (<10%)	Small, irregular (basophilic) cells; sparse peripheral secretory vesicles	Spherical, 100–150 nm
	LH, FSH; gonadotropins: gonadotroph (10–15%)	Type 1: large, oval basophilic cells; plentiful RER, Golgi, many large secretory vesicles Type 2: smaller (basophilic) cells; scant RER, Golgi; fewer, smaller secretory vesicles	Type 1: most 300–400 nm, some smaller Type 2: 200 nm
	ACTH; corticotropin (with other POMC products): corticotroph (15–20%)	Medium-sized stellate (basophilic) cells; perinuclear bundles of cytokeratin filaments; peripheral secretory vesicles	Spherical, 250–350 nm
Thyroid	T$_4$, T$_3$ (thyroxine, triiodothyronine): thyroid follicular cells	Cuboidal (normal), columnar (active) or flattened (inactive) cells around follicular lumen containing, respectively, modest, little or much colloid. Cells have basal RER, supranuclear Golgi, active apical membrane with microvilli, pino- and phagocytosis of colloid, fusion with lysosomes	Vesicles of thyroglobulin exocytosed at apical membrane into the colloid
	Calcitonin: parafollicular "C" cells; a few also in parathyroids, thymus	Large, ovoid cells between or in base of follicular epithelium; rich in mitochondria and secretory vesicles, which also contain 5-HT	Spherical, 150 nm
Parathyroid	PTH: chief cells	Chief cells: round or polygonal (8–12 μm), glycogen-rich; rather small numbers of peripherally placed secretory vesicles Oxyphil cells (10–18 μm): cytoplasm rich in mitochondria, scanty RER, glycogen	Irregular, 200–400 nm
Pancreatic islets	Insulin (and IAPP): B or β cells (70%)	Large cells with well developed RER and Golgi; numerous vesicles with pale, (immature) or crystalloid (mature) content	300 nm; electron-dense crystalloid core or pale core
	Glucagon: A or α cells (20%)	Similar to B cells; more peripherally placed in islets; eccentric dense-cored secretory vesicles	Spherical, 200 nm, eccentric electron-dense core
	Somatostatin: D or δ cells (15–20%)	Scattered cells, well developed RER, Golgi	Spherical, 350 nm; rather pale core
	Pancreatic polypeptide: F or PP cells (1–2%)	The predominant cell in the uncinate lobe of pancreas; sparse in dorsal pancreas	Spherical, 150–170 nm; dense-cored vesicles with wide halo
	VIP: EC cells	Occasional scattered cells in islets and exocrine tissue	Spherical, 250 nm, variable electron density
	Gastrin: G cells	In fetus and gastrinomas only	
Gastrointestinal tract†	Different peptide and/or amine hormones produced in different parts of the GI tract	Cells stain less than most enterocytes. All contact basal lamina; most ("open") also contact GI tract lumen with receptive microvillous border. Prominent RER and Golgi; granules located basally	
	Gastrin: G cells	Pyramidal cells in neck and middle third of pyloric antral glands; "open". Also numerous in duodenal crypts, villi and Brunner's glands. Also in fetal pancreas	Spherical, 200–400 nm, variable electron density

Table 1.1 (*Continued*)

Organ	Principal hormones: cell types	Cellular characteristics	Secretory vesicles: diameter, form
	Secretin: S cells	Scattered in duodenal and jejunal mucosa	Spherical, 200 nm
	Cholecystokinin I cells	Cells in duodenum and jejunum; also in enteric neurons in distal intestine	Spherical or slightly irregular, 250 nm
	GIP: K cells	In duodenum and jejunum, a few in ileum	Irregular, 350 nm
	Enteroglucagon: L cells	In ileum and colon	Spherical, 260 nm
	VIP	In subepithelial neurons of the GI and respiratory tracts	Dense-cored vesicles in nerves; 150 nm
	Somatostatin: D cells	In stomach and small bowel. Fundic D cells are "closed"; antral D cells are "open". Cells often have basal processes which contact other endocrine cells. Also in enteric neurons	Spherical, 260–370 nm, weakly electron-dense
	Serotonin, substance P, motilin: Enterochromaffin cells	EC_1 and EC_2 forms throughout the bowel	EC_1: large, very pleomorphic EC_2: irregular, large
	Histamine, 5-HT: Enterochromaffin cells	Widely distributed through bowel. In stomach, source of histamine	
Adrenal medulla	Epinephrine and norepinephrine (also chromogranins, enkephalins)	Large, polarized columnar cells, moderate RER and Golgi. Cholinergic synapses contact apical pole; secretory vesicles concentrated toward capillary pole. Noradrenaline vesicles more electron-dense than those containing adrenaline	250–300 nm; noradrenaline often ellipsoidal
Adrenal cortex	Adrenal corticosteroids	Variable cells. Characteristic mitochondria with distinctive cristae; abundant SER often encircling mitochondria. "Lipid" droplets of cholesterol ester more prominent in inactive than in active cells	Dense-cored vesicles in some steroid-secreting cells reflect co-secretion of peptides
Zona glomerulosa	Aldosterone	Small polyhedral cells arranged in spherical clusters; dense nuclei, little cytoplasm, few lipid droplets, elongated mitochondria	
Zona fasciculata	Cortisol	Large polyhedral cells arranged in sheets, two cells thick, between vascular sinusoids; spherical mitochondria with tubular cristae; abundant lipid droplets	
Zona reticularis	Androgens (DHEA)	Rounded cells arranged in a network; abundant SER, lysosomes and pigment granules, possibility indicating senescence	
Fetal zone	DHEA-sulfate	The major part of the gland in the fetus	
Testis	Androgens (testosterone) Leydig cells	Angular shaped cells in interstices of seminiferous tubules. Scanty cytoplasm filled with SER, lipid droplets, 20-μm-long crystals of Reinke	
	Inhibin, steroid interconversion Sertoli cells	Variable shape and nuclear configuration, long cytoplasmic processes among developing germ cells. Abundant cytoplasmic organelles including RER, SER, but very few secretory vesicles	
Ovary	Androgens (mainly androstenedione): Theca interna cells	Vascularized layer of spindle-shaped steroid-secreting cells clustered around the follicle basal lamina	Type II cells: 250–450 nm
	Activin, inhibin, follistatin, IGF-1, steroid conversion to estrogen: Granulosa cells	Non-vascularized cells lining basal lamina of follicle and surrounding the oocyte. Regionally variable cells with abundant organelles including RER, SER but few secretory vesicles	
	Progesterone, estrogen, relaxin, oxytocin, progesterone-binding protein: Corpus luteum	Vascularized steroid-secreting cells produced by luteinization of the follicle. Type I: small cells (<25 μm), irregular nuclei, abundant SER, mitochondria, lipid droplets, no dense-cored secretory vesicles. Type II: very large (up to 40 μm) polyhedral cells with abundant SER, variously shaped mitochondria, sparse lipid droplets; extensive RER, Golgi, dense-cored secretory vesicles	

* Proportion of total endocrine cells in the gland. NB this varies in different physiological conditions.

† Only the major gastrointestinal hormones are included, in particular those which give rise to tumors.

ACTH, adrenocorticotropic hormone; AVP, arginine vasopressin; CRH, corticotropin-releasing hormone; DHEA, dehydroepiandrosterone; EC, enterochromaffin; GHRH, growth hormone-releasing hormone; GI, gastrointestinal; GnRH, gonadotropin-releasing hormone; 5-HT, 5-hydroxytryptamine; IAPP, islet-associated polypeptide (amylin); POMC, pro-opiomelanocortin; PTH, parathyroid hormone; RER, rough endoplasmic reticulum; SER, smooth endoplasmic reticulum; TRH, thyrotropin-releasing hormone; TSH, thyroid-stimulating hormone; VIP, vasoactive intestinal polypeptide.

Hypothalamus and pituitary gland

The hypothalamus is that part of the forebrain on either side of the ventral part of the third cerebral ventricle. Its floor comprises the optic chiasm and tract, the pituitary stalk, mamillary bodies and posterior perforated substance; anteriorly it is limited by the lamina terminalis and anterior commissure; posteriorly it blends with the midbrain; superiorly it is continuous with the thalamus and epithalamus; and laterally it blends with the zona incerta and internal capsule. Its neuroendocrine neurons are situated in its medial zone (Fig. 1.2): magnocellular neurons secreting vasopressin or oxytocin as their primary product are located mostly in the supraoptic and paraventricular nuclei; parvocellular neurons secreting the releasing factors that control the anterior pituitary are more widely distributed but many are located in the ventromedial part of the paraventricular nucleus (CRH, thyrotropin-releasing hormone (TRH)), in the arcuate nucleus (dopamine, growth hormone-releasing hormone (GHRH)), in the adjacent medial basal hypothalamus (gonadotropin-releasing hormone (GnRH)) and in the periventricular zone (somatostatin). Parts of the hypothalamus,

notably the arcuate nucleus and lateral hypothalamus, contain the cells producing neuropeptide Y (NPY) and agouti-related protein (AgRP), α-melanocyte-stimulating hormone (α-MSH), ghrelin and orexin peptides, all of which are involved in the control of appetite. Vasopressin and oxytocin are released into the systemic circulation from the axons of the magnocellular neurons which form the bulk of the posterior pituitary; the releasing factors are secreted from axons of parvocellular neurons into the portal capillary plexus in the median eminence. Central branches of the internal carotid artery enter the ventral surface of the hypothalamus to supply it; superior hypophysial branches form a capillary plexus in the neurohemal contact zone of the median eminence from which the hypophysial portal veins pass down the pituitary stalk to perfuse the anterior pituitary. It is now clear, however, that many neurosecretory peptides can be released, not only from the axon terminals of the neurosecretory neurons, but also from their dendrites into the extracellular fluid of the brain [4] and the same may be true for peptidergic neurons in general. They are therefore capable of diffusing over considerable distances (perhaps via the cerebrospinal fluid) in the CNS and producing organized behaviors such as nest-building (oxytocin), and appetitive behavior (NPY), in a way quite

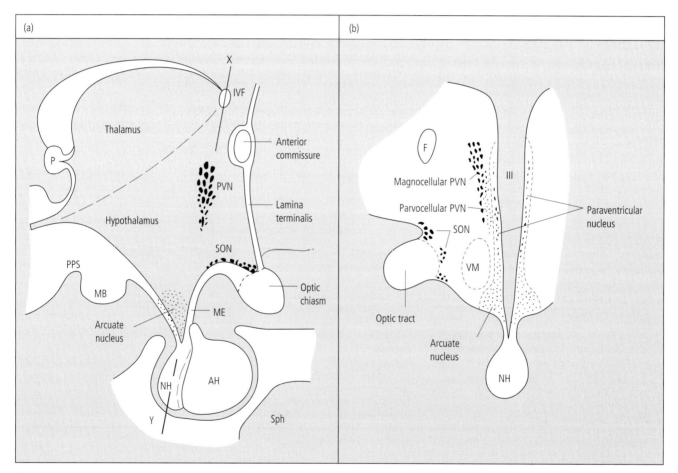

Figure 1.2 Location of cells producing hypothalamic hormones. (a) Midline and (b) near coronal (along plane X–Y in (a)) sections through the human diencephalon. PVN, paraventricular nucleus; SON, supraoptic nucleus; AH, adenohypophysis; F, fornix; IVF, interventricular foramen; MB, mamillary body; ME, median eminence (infundibulum); NH, neurohypophysis; P, pineal; PPS, posterior perforated substance; Sph, sphenoid air sinus; III, third ventricle; VM, ventromedial nucleus.

different from the cellular responses resulting from activation of postsynaptic target cell membranes [5] but analogous to paracrine or even endocrine actions in the peripheral endocrine systems.

The pituitary gland is situated in the pituitary fossa of the sphenoid. Below is the sphenoid air sinus, on either side the internal carotid artery, abducent nerve and cavernous sinus, and above the posterior pituitary is continuous with the pituitary stalk of the basal hypothalamus which, with the pituitary portal veins, passes down through the dura mater which roofs the pituitary fossa. The pituitary gland is composed of two very different types of endocrine tissue: the individual endocrine cells of the adenohypophysis; and the axonal terminals of magnocellular hypothalamic neurons which, with the glial pituicytes, form the neurohypophysis. The posterior pituitary is supplied by inferior hypophysial branches of the internal carotid artery; the anterior pituitary by the hypothalamo-hypophysial portal veins. Both parts drain into the internal jugular venous system.

The hypothalamus is formed from the floor of the diencephalic forebrain vesicle (Fig. 1.3) in the region of prosomeres P4–P6. Expression of fibroblast growth factor 8 (FGF-8) by the anterior neural ridge induces expression of brain factor-1 (BF-1) which regulates the development of the forebrain. Sonic hedgehog induces and organizes the ventral forebrain. Steroidogenic factor

1 (SF-1) is important in the development of the hypothalamic ventromedial nucleus. GnRH neurons, however, do not originate in the neural tube, but in the nasal placode; they migrate centrally into the hypothalamus controlled by glycoprotein neural adhesion molecule anosmin-1 coded for by the *KAL1* gene on the X chromosome (failure of this migration is the origin of the hypogonadism of Kallmann syndrome). The neurohypophysis develops from the neuroectodermal floor of the forebrain vesicle which, at 3.5 weeks' development, lies adjacent to the roof of the ectodermal stomodeum, just anterior to the oropharyngeal membrane. By about 3 weeks' gestation, the forebrain induces this ectoderm (which originally lay just anterior to the neural plate but was carried beneath it by embryonic folding) to form an adenohypophysial (Rathke's) pouch which then forms a vesicle that separates from the roof of the developing mouth. The anterior wall of the vesicle forms trabeculae of proto-endocrine cells which interact with the surrounding mesoderm to form the pars distalis, an extension of which grows up around the developing neurohypophysial stalk as the pars tuberalis; the posterior wall of the pouch apposed to the developing neurohypophysis remains small and free of blood vessels to form the pars intermedia; and the original cavity of the vesicle becomes the pituitary cleft. Axonal terminals of the hypothalamic magnocellular neurons

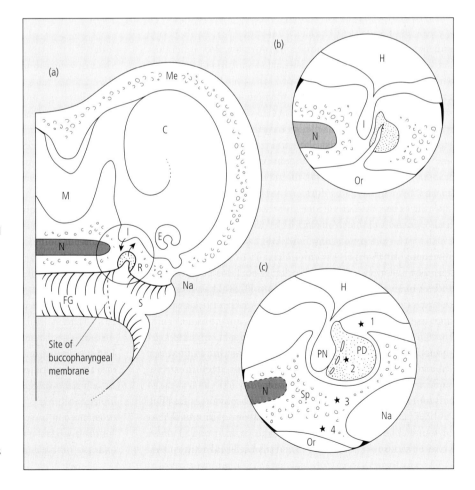

Figure 1.3 Development of the pituitary gland and sites of associated tumors. Diagrams showing the progressive development of the infundibular process (I) downward from the floor of the forebrain vesicle and of Rathke's pouch (R) upward from the roof of the ectodermal stomodeum (S) to form, respectively, the pars nervosa (LPN) and pars distalis (PD) or the pituitary gland. (a) A low power view of early stage; (b, c) area circled in (a) at progressively later stages. Developing structures: C, cerebral cortex; E, eye; F, foregut; H, hypothalamus; M, midbrain; Me, mesenchyme destined to form skull; N, notochord; Na, nasal cavity; Or, oral cavity; Sp, sphenoid bone. Asterisks mark the position of (1) suprasellar, (2) intrasellar, (3) intrasphenoid and (4) palatal cysts or tumors attributed to Rathke's pouch remnants.

grow to contact systemic capillaries in the posterior pituitary part of the neurohypophysis. This is continuous with a similar neuro-hemal contact zone in the base of the hypothalamus, where parvo-cellular neurosecretory axon terminals, which secrete the various releasing factors and thereby control the adenohypophysial cells, end on portal capillaries that descend the stalk to perfuse the ade-nohypophysis. The anterior pituitary and neurosecretory systems become active around the middle of prenatal life.

Our understanding of the molecular signals which transform the anterior ectoderm into the different cell types of the anterior pituitary has increased markedly in recent years. Formation of Rathke's pouch involves the homeodomain genes Rpx (Hesx1) and Pitx (three different transcription factors); mutations in Rpx are associated with septo-optic dysplasia, isolated pituitary hypoplasia and with holoprosencephaly; mutations in the equivalent of Pitx2 (RIEG) are associated with Rieger syndrome, which includes pitu-itary anomalies. Animal studies suggest that expression of a fibro-blast growth factor (FGF-8) and a bone morphogenetic protein (BMP-4) control the initial derivation of Pit-1-independent thyrotrophs from ectodermal stem cells. Where FGF influence declines definitive Pit-1-independent thyrotrophs are formed but disappear by birth. The continuing presence of FGF maintains the progenitor state. Corticotroph differentiation requires expression of NeuroD1 and the T box factor Tpit which, with Pitx1, activate POMC transcription. Pitx1 (with LIM homeobox genes *Lhx3* and *Lhx4*) directly activates the promoter of the α-subunit gene of the glycoprotein hormones. Humans with mutations in *Lhx3* com-pletely lack GH, PRL, TSH, and gonadotropins. Proper develop-ment of gonadotrophs, thyrotrophs, lactotrophs and somatotrophs also requires the transcription factor Prop-1, which is restricted to the anterior pituitary. Formation of gonadotrophs also involves steroidogenic factor 1 (SF-1) and GATA2. Tissue-specific expres-sion of growth hormone (GH) prolactin (PRL) and thyroid-stimulating hormone (TSH) in definitive anterior pituitary cells and proliferation of these cells is controlled by the POU-domain transcription factor Pit-1 (POUF1) [6]. Humans with mutations in the Pit-1 gene have a syndrome of postnatal growth retardation, PRL deficiency, and congenital hypothyroidism. Somatotrophs and prolactotrophs develop from a common stem cell and differ-entiate to form the two "acidophil" cell types and somatomam-motrophs which express both GH and PRL. It is therefore not surprising that many acidophil tumors produce both GH and PRL. Other pituitary tumors produce TSH, gonadotropins, pro-opiomelanocortin (POMC) products and peptides with no apparent endocrine effects, and not infrequently produce more than one of these. It is thought that most pituitary tumors are monoclonal [7] though it is possible that a few arise as a result of hyperstimulation from the hypothalamus but, once tumorous, secretion of hormone becomes autonomous.

Asymptomatic cystic remnants of Rathke's pouch are found in 13–23% of autopsies, and traces of the oral end of the pouch may be found at the junction of the nasal septum and palate. Tumors (craniopharyngiomas) containing epithelial cells and a brown fluid rich in cholesterol have been thought to derive from such remnants. However, the fact that >75% occur in a suprasellar position rather than within the pituitary fossa (sella) casts doubt on this origin. Like many adenohypophysial tumors, Rathke's pouch tumors signal their presence by pressure on the optic chiasm or hypotha-lamus. The tip of the notochord lies near the developing pituitary; chordomas can therefore occur in the region of the pituitary.

The cells secreting the releasing factors and the neurohy-pophysial hormones oxytocin and vasopressin are non-dividing hypothalamic neurons, so tumors in the hypothalamus and poste-rior pituitary are derived from glia (gliomas), ependymal cells (ependymomas), or pituicytes (pituicytomas). However, tumors in other sites can secrete releasing factors (e.g. GHRH in pancre-atic tumor) and lung tumors not infrequently secrete vasopressin and neurophysin, causing the Schwartz–Bartter syndrome.

Pineal gland

The pineal is a small midline gland projecting backward from the epithalamus above the posterior commissure and midbrain. It is derived from cells in the roof of the forebrain (3rd) ventricle. It comprises two types of cell: pinealocytes (derived from primordial photoreceptive cells) and interstitial glial-like cells. The pineal synthesizes melatonin from tryptophan and secretes it in the dark phase. It responds to light by an indirect route which involves a special class of photoreceptive retinal ganglion cells which innervate the suprachiasmatic nucleus (the intrinsic body clock) which in turn innervates cells in the paraventricular nucleus of the hypothalamus that project to the sympathetic preganglionic neurons in the upper thoracic cord. The preganglionic neurons synapse on neurons of the superior cervical ganglion which innervate the pineal (the only part of the CNS to receive auto-nomic innervation). The melatonin is released into both the CSF and bloodstream. It acts on melatonin receptors in the sup-rachiasmatic nucleus, providing a feedback loop which explains its ability to reset the internal body clock in jet-lag, in "free-running" blind subjects and in circadian-based sleep disorders. It also acts on the tuberal part of the pituitary and exerts powerful regulatory actions on the reproductive axis of many animals, in particular seasonal breeders, but any role on human reproduction is uncertain. With increasing age calcified deposits appear in the pineal but these have little effect on its function.

Despite the uncertain relation between melatonin and human reproduction, pineal tumors (which are rare) can cause precoci-ous puberty as well as local neurological abnormalities such as Parinaud syndrome. However, the precocious puberty is probably also the result of local effects of the tumor on the hypothalamus, or of secretion of human chorionic gonadotropin from pineal choriocarcinomas. Tumors of pinealocytes are primitive neuroec-todermal tumors of variable differentiation, but immunopositive for the neuronal marker synaptophysin. Pineoblastomas are basi-cally neuroblastomas. Germinomas also occur in the pineal.

Thyroid gland and parafollicular C-cells

The thyroid gland is normally situated in the neck and comprises a midline isthmus which lies anterior to the second and third tracheal rings, and two lateral lobes that extend upward over the lower half of each thyroid cartilage lamina. The gland lies deep to the strap muscles of the neck, enclosed in pretracheal fascia which anchors it to the trachea, so that the thyroid moves upward on swallowing. Its lateral lobes receive the superior thyroid branches of the external carotid artery and inferior thyroid branches from the thyrocervical trunk of the subclavian artery; a small thyroidea ima artery from the arch of the aorta may pass up to the isthmus. Superior and middle thyroid veins follow, respectively, the superior and inferior thyroid arteries; inferior thyroid veins drain downward within the pretracheal fascia to the left brachiocephalic vein. Histologically the thyroid is a unique endocrine gland because its epithelial cells form follicles. The cells secrete a protein (thyroglobulin) into the follicular lumen where certain of its tyrosine residues are complexed with iodine produced by the apical membrane peroxidase from iodide that is pumped into the cells by the basal sodium-iodide transporter. The peroxidase also catalyses the linkage of iodotyrosyl residues in the thyroglobulin to form "colloid." The iodothyronines (principally T_4 if sufficient iodide is available) are produced by proteolytic (lysosomal) cleavage of endocytosed iodinated colloid. The system contains huge reserves of iodinated colloid and secretion of iodothyronines is slow, starting only about 30 minutes after stimulation by TSH. Release of T_4, once thought to be by diffusion, is probably due to a specific transporter. After release the T_4 is converted by peripheral tissues (mainly the liver) to the metabolically active T_3 or to inactive (reverse) T_3.

The human thyroid gland starts to develop at 3 weeks' gestation from thickened endoderm in the midline of the floor of the pharynx between pharyngeal arches 1 and 2 (Fig. 1.4). Its cells form a bilobed mass connected to the pharynx by a stalk (thyroglossal duct) which, at 6 weeks, migrates caudally through the mesoderm anterior to (sometimes through) the developing hyoid bone, thyrohyoid membrane, thyroid and cricoid cartilages to reach its adult position by the 7th week. During development its posterior aspect becomes associated with the developing parathyroid glands (and sometimes thymic tissue), and parafollicular (C) cells derived from neural crest cells in the ultimobranchial body become incorporated into its substance. In the 7th week the epithelial cells begin to organize themselves into follicles; colloid formation starts one week later and iodothyronines are formed at 10–12 weeks.

The thyroid gland or remnants may be found at any position along this route, i.e. in the tongue (lingual thyroid), in relation to the hyoid, as a pyramidal lobe (thyroglossal duct remnant), or it can descend too far and reach the superior mediastinum. The thyroid may fail to form (congenital cretinism), a thyroglossal cyst may form along the duct, and the duct may persist to form a thyroglossal fistula that develops an opening in the midline of the neck. Accessory thyroid tissue may be found elsewhere in the neck, presumably as a result of anomalous attachment to adjacent developing organs, though it must also be borne in mind that apparently ectopic thyroid tissue is usually a secondary deposit of a well-differentiated thyroid tumor. For unknown reasons, thyroid tissue may rarely also develop in the ovary.

The thyroid transcription factors TTF-1 and -2 and the paired domain factor PAX8 are expressed in thyroid follicular cells from the start of their differentiation. Mice in which TTF-1 is deleted lack both follicular and C-cells; heterozygous TTF-1 mutations in humans produce only mild thyroid dysfunction. Homozygous mutations in TTF-2 prevent thyroid formation, but heterozygous parents are euthyroid; heterozygous PAX-8 mutations cause thyroid hypoplasia. Upstream genes controlling these three transcription factors and commitment to a thyroid cell lineage are presently unknown [8, 9]. Mutations in the TSH receptor gene also cause thyroid hypoplasia with associated TSH resistance and congenital hypothyroidism.

Hyperplasia and benign or malignant tumors can develop in thyroid tissue at any location. In the neck there is usually plenty of room for enlargement (goiter). However, if thyroid tissue expands behind the hyoid or manubrium, it will compress the larynx or trachea. Hyperplastic adenomatous nodules are organized like normal thyroid follicles. They may secrete autonomously and cause thyrotoxicosis but never become malignant. Their distinction from true adenomas is difficult, as is the distinction between true adenomas (which are of a number of different morphological subtypes) and well-differentiated follicular carcinomas. Invasion of the capsule or blood vessels distinguishes the carcinomas. Follicular and papillary carcinomas obviously originate from malignant change in thyroid epithelial cells (possibly stem cells) [10] and the epithelial markers low molecular weight (cyto)keratin and lactoferrin are usually expressed. The very aggressive, undifferentiated anaplastic thyroid carcinomas probably share the same origin as they may express the same markers and anaplastic areas can be found in otherwise well-differentiated carcinomas; also, about 50% produce iodothyronines and thyroglobulin. The so-called "small cell carcinomas" are not of thyroid origin but probably represent either thyroid lymphomas or occasionally thyroid metastases of small cell lung carcinomas [11].

The parafollicular C-cells form isolated or small groups of cells at the periphery of thyroid follicles. They secrete calcitonin. They are derived from neural crest cells which become incorporated into the ultimobranchial body of the caudal pharyngeal complex (Fig. 1.4) and thus into the thyroid gland in which they disperse, principally in the upper two-thirds of the lateral lobes. Tumors of parafollicular cells (medullary thyroid carcinoma) can occur sporadically or as part of multiple endocrine neoplasia (MEN) 2a or 2b associated with a mutation in chromosome 10. The unregulated secretion of calcitonin does not disturb calcium homeostasis partly because osteoclasts down-regulate their calcitonin receptor mechanisms ("calcitonin escape") and partly because of the overriding control by parathyroid hormone.

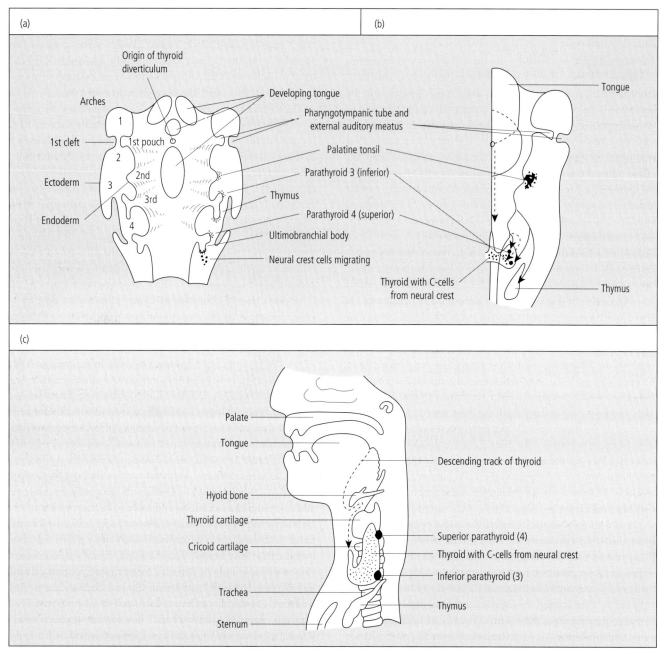

Figure 1.4 Development of the thyroid, parathyroid and thymus. (a) Floor of the mouth showing the first four branchial arches (1–4) and the corresponding endodermal pouches. Note that the 4th and more caudal pouches open as a single complex. (b) Right side of the floor of the mouth at a later stage of development. The thymus has migrated caudally carrying parathyroid 3 caudal to parathyroid 4. Neural crest cells have entered the thyroid gland, which has also migrated caudally, where they will produce C-cells. (c) Lateral view to show the course of descent of the thyroid gland. Ectopic thyroid and tumors can appear anywhere along the tract; the thymus and parathyroid 3 are most likely to be ectopic and can be either more cranially or more caudally situated.

Parathyroid glands and thymus

There are usually four parathyroid glands (two superior and two inferior) embedded in the posterior aspect of the lateral lobes of the thyroid close to the anastomotic vessel linking the superior and inferior thyroid arteries, all of which can supply the glands.

Each gland is a ball of cells: principally cells which secrete parathyroid hormone (PTH), and oxyphil cells of unknown function.

The adult thymus gland comprises two more or less joined lobes of lymphoid tissue situated in the upper part of the anterior mediastinum above the pericardium and usually extending into the neck. In addition to its key role in the development and maintenance of cell-mediated immune responses, the thymus also produces a number of associated hormones (e.g. thymosin, thymopoietin). The thymus grows in size until puberty but thereafter atrophies progressively. This age-associated involution is accelerated by glucocorticoids.

The parathyroid glands develop in the region of the 3rd and 4th pharyngeal pouches (Fig. 1.4). They are usually said to arise from the pouch endoderm but more recently it has been suggested that they arise from the adjacent cleft ectoderm. Parathyroid 3 arises as a cellular mass from the dorsal and the thymus from the ventral part of the 3rd pharyngeal pouch. As the thymus descends into the anterior mediastinum parathyroid 3 is carried part-way with it so that it forms the inferior parathyroid gland. It is much more variable in position than parathyroid 4 which becomes the superior parathyroid. The number of parathyroids can vary from 2 to 6; they frequently contain cysts. In the DiGeorge syndrome, the thymus and parathyroids are absent, apparently as a result of agenesis of the 3rd and 4th pharyngeal pouches. The absence of the parathyroids causes hypocalcemia; absence of the thymus immunological incompetence. The frequently associated aortic arch and facial defects are of neural crest origin (see below).

The master gene regulating parathyroid development appears to be (glial cell missing) *GCMB* and *GCMB* expression is increased in parathyroid adenomas [12] but mouse knockouts suggest that both *Six* and (eyes absent) *Eya1* genes are required for the development of not only parathyroid but other pharyngeal pouch tissue such as thymus [13].

Tumors of the parathyroids may be restricted to the parathyroids or be associated with tumors of the pancreatic islets and pituitary (MEN 1; autosomal dominant, chromosome 11) or with medullary carcinoma of the thyroid and phaeochromocytoma (MEN 2a; chromosome 10). In MEN 1 two mutations are involved: the first leads to hyperplasia, the second to tumor formation. Of the tumor-prone tissues in MEN 2, the C-cells and adrenal medulla derive from the neural crest, whereas the parathyroids are apparently of endodermal origin. However, occipital neural crest cells migrate through the 3rd and 4th arches and all three tissues express the *ret* (receptor-type tyrosine kinase) proto-oncogene.

Parathyroid hormone-related protein

This molecule, which acts like PTH on the PTH receptor, is produced by a wide variety of tumors (particularly lung and breast) and is the cause of the hypercalcemia of malignancy. It is also secreted constitutively by a similarly wide variety of fetal and adult tissues. Its physiological autocrine and paracrine function in these tissues has yet to be determined. In the placenta it is suggested to help activate the placental calcium pump.

Adrenal glands

The adrenal glands are situated on the medial aspect of the upper pole of each kidney. Each comprises a steroid-secreting cortex and a catecholamine-secreting medulla. They receive a profuse blood supply from the adjacent aorta, phrenic and renal arteries and drain by a large central vein into the inferior vena cava (right) or left renal vein (left). Each also receives a profuse innervation largely composed of preganglionic cholinergic sympathetic fibers from the thoracic splanchnic nerves and celiac plexus; some postganglionic fibers also enter the gland. Many of the preganglionic fibers synapse on the chromaffin cells of the medulla to control the secretion of catecholamines. It is now clear that splanchnic nerves also modulate the secretion from and sensitivity of the adrenal cortex, at least in part by controlling blood flow through the gland. In sympathetic arousal, when most of the splanchnic vascular bed is constricted, blood flow through the adrenals is increased.

The adult adrenal cortex comprises an outer zone (about 5%) of balls of cells, the zona glomerulosa; a large mid-zone (about 65%) of radially arranged sheets of cells interspersed with blood vessels, the zona fasciculata; and an inner network of cells (about 5%), the zona reticulata. Cells of the zona glomerulosa express the enzyme 18-hydroxylase and secrete aldosterone; cells of the zona fasciculata secrete largely cortisol in humans; and cells of the zona reticulata secrete weak androgens, principally dehydroepiandrosterone (DHEA). The medulla is composed of the adrenaline- and noradrenaline-secreting (epinephrine, norepinephrine) chromaffin cells and their associated cholinergic innervation; adrenaline-secreting cells predominate. Chromaffin cells also secrete numerous peptides including met-enkephalin, CRH and chromogranins.

The cortex and medulla develop from quite different primordia (Fig. 1.5). The cortical cells develop from the intermediate mesoderm which forms the celomic epithelium between the mesonephros and dorsal mesogastrium. Cords of endocrine cells form between the developing vascular sinuses. The first cells to develop form that large *fetal zone* of the cortex; this then becomes surrounded by cells that will form the definitive cortex. The fetal cortex cells do not express 3-β-hydroxysteroid oxidoreductase and therefore produce largely DHEA (which is sulfated). At birth the adrenal glands are relatively large (about 30% of the size of the kidneys); this is because the fetal zone is very large but the definitive zone and medulla are both small. The fetal cortex decreases in size during the first 2–3 postnatal months by a non-inflammatory involution process; the definitive cortex increases rapidly at first, then more slowly up to 20 years of age. The chromaffin cells of the medulla are derived from migrating neural crest cells (and are the equivalent of sympathetic ganglion cells without neuritic processes). At 5–6 weeks' development, neural crest cells migrate into the developing adrenal cortex and eventually become surrounded by cortical tissue. The cortical cells probably induce the neural crest cells to form chromaffin cells; also cortisol stimulates the expression of phenylethanolamine-*N*-methyl transferase (PNMT) which converts noradrenaline to adrenaline. Other neural crest cells migrate further to form the midline sympathetic ganglia, the ganglion cells of the enteric nervous system, and the chromaffin cells of the organ of Zuckerkandl, which is thought to be the major source of catecholamines in the first postnatal year.

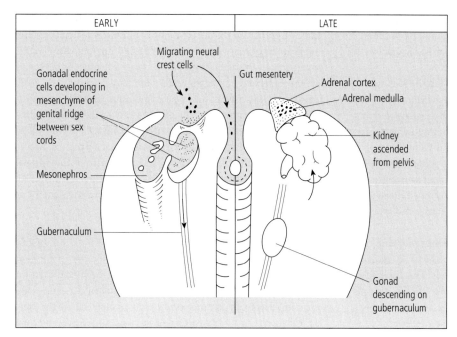

Figure 1.5 Development of the suprarenals and gonads. Diagrammatic views of early (left) and later (right) stages in the development of the adrenal glands and gonads. Celomic epithelium between the mesonephros and the gut mesentery develops to form adrenal cortical tissue which comes to surround neural crest cells which have migrated into the region and which will form the adrenal medulla. Other neural crest cells migrate into the gut mesentery where they form sympathetic ganglion and enteric nervous system cells. Endocrine cells of the gonads develop in the mesenchyme of the genital ridge between the sex cords or primordial follicles.

The development of the intermediate mesoderm which forms the adrenals and gonads depends on a number of genes including (Wilms tumor) WT1, (steroidogenic factor) SF1, LIM1 and EMX2. Formation of the primordial adrenal requires the continued presence of SF1 which regulates a number of genes involved in steroidogenesis. Growth and zonation of the adrenal cortex and regression of the fetal adrenal require (dosage-sensitive sex-reversal, adrenal hypoplasia) DAX1 which interacts with SF1 (see also development of gonads) and insulin-like growth factor-2 (IGF-2) and its receptor. Mutations in SF1 are associated with adrenal insufficiency or failure; high expression of IGF-2 occurs in human fetal adrenal and 85% of adrenocortical tumors and alterations in genomic imprinting appear to be partly responsible for the overexpression of IGF-2 [14, 15].

Considering the extent to which neural crest cells migrate it is not surprising that ectopic clusters of chromaffin cells can be found outside the adrenal glands, along the abdominal aorta and almost anywhere that sympathetic ganglion cells are located. Accessory cortical tissue is also common near the kidneys and along the track of the descending gonads (all of which form from intermediate mesoderm). Abdominal accessory chromaffin and cortical tissue often coexists. Very occasionally suprarenal (cortex and medulla) tissue is found intracranially – the cause for this is unknown.

Developmental defects occur in the expression of most of the steroid-processing enzymes of the adrenal cortex. The most common – an autosomal recessive defect in 21-hydroxylase – leads to the failure of cortisol and aldosterone production. The lack of corticosteroid feedback causes increased ACTH secretion and thus congenital adrenal hyperplasia; the shunting of precursors into androgen production causes the associated virilization of female fetuses.

Tumors of cortical tissue can secrete aldosterone (Conn syndrome), cortisol (Cushing syndrome) or sex steroids, and steroid intermediates. Well-differentiated tumors usually secrete only one major steroid; carcinomas frequently secrete multiple steroids. Tumors of adrenal medullary or ectopic chromaffin tissue (pheochromocytomas) secrete catecholamines (mostly epinephrine) and a wide variety of normally co-secreted peptides (e.g. met-enkephalin, ACTH, vasoactive intestinal polypeptide [VIP]), neural crest-associated peptides (e.g. calcitonin, substance P), and unexpected peptides (e.g. gastrin). Chromaffin tumors may be isolated or part of the MEN 2a (medullary thyroid carcinoma, parathyroid tumors, pheochromocytomas) or MEN 2b (medullary thyroid carcinoma, pheochromocytoma, mucosal neuromas) syndromes. Ganglioneuromas (usually well differentiated) and neuroblastomas (malignant) are tumors of neural crest-derived sympathetic ganglion or more primitive adrenal neuroblast cells; dopamine is the major catecholamine secreted.

Endocrine tissue of the gonads

In the adult male, each testis is an ovoid organ normally located in a pouch of peritoneum within the scrotum. Each consists of a mass of seminiferous tubules comprising the germ cell series and the sustentacular (Sertoli) cells and connected to the rete testis, epididymis and vas deferens. Around the tubules are myoid cells which produce local controlling signals. Between the seminiferous tubules are the interstitial (Leydig) cells and blood and lymph vessels derived from the spermatic cord. Leydig cells secrete androgens, particularly testosterone; Sertoli cells secrete inhibin and Müllerian-inhibiting factor (MIF), and convert testosterone to both dihydrotestosterone and estrogen.

The testes develop at about 6 weeks from indifferent gonadal primordia formed after primordial germ cells (which are first specified in the epiblast) migrate from the yolk sac wall, via the gut mesentery into the thickened celomic epithelium on the medial aspect of the intermediate mesoderm forming the urogenital ridge (Fig. 1.5). Formation of the urogenital ridge involves the autosomal Wilms' tumor suppressor gene WT1, the gene for the "orphan receptor" steroidogenic factor 1 (SF1), LIM1, LX9 and probably GATA4 [16]. Lack of any of these results in failure of formation of gonads of either sex. If the DNA-binding protein coded for by the Y-specific (SRY) gene for the testis-determining factor is expressed, the celomic epithelium proliferates markedly and becomes organized around the germ cells to form primary testicular cords which separate from the surface epithelium, the mesodermal cells becoming differentiated to form pre-Sertoli cells and, later, Leydig cells. It is clear from the insertion of SRY into mouse XX oocytes that SRY can switch the bipotential tissue into forming a testis, but mutations in SRY only account for a minority of human XY sex reversal. Other factors must therefore be involved, but progress in understanding the mechanism of SRY action has been disappointingly slow. As the sex cords form, vascular endothelial cells migrate from the mesonephros to surround the cords and form a testis-specific vasculature. Shortly after this SRY expression declines and the homeobox gene SOX9 assumes control. SOX9 is initially expressed in both XX and XY gonads, but is upregulated in XY gonads and downregulated in XX gonads [17]. An appropriate expression of the orphan nuclear receptor DAX1, which was originally proposed to act as an "anti-testis" factor, is now known to be necessary for proper testis development, and in mice DAX1 deficiency disrupts developmental events between expression of SRY and SOX9. In humans DAX1 mutations cause (in addition to adrenal hypoplasia) hypogonadism which may result from gonadal dysgenesis [18, 19]. SOX9 induces the production of MIF from the Sertoli cells. This directs the involution of the paramesonephric ducts and assists testicular descent in the male; later the Sertoli cells also produce inhibin and androgen-converting enzymes. Mesonephric tubules in the hilus of the developing testis form the rete testis tissue but do not fuse with the developing seminiferous tubules till mid-gestation. Various growth factors and their receptors, including fibroblast growth factor (FGF), platelet-derived growth factor (PDGF), insulin and IGF, WNT, and transforming growth factor-β (TGF-β), are also crucial to correct gonadal development [17]. The interstitial Leydig cells develop in two waves. The first forms at 8 weeks' gestation when testosterone secretion starts and promotes the development of the mesonephric duct system into the epididymis and vas deferens; later most of these early Leydig cells degenerate, but a second wave of Leydig cell formation gives rise to the definitive interstitial cells of the postnatal male. Desert hedgehog (DHH) is required for the differentiation and multiplication of Leydig cells; mutations in human DHH in 46,XY individuals are associated with partial or complete pure gonadal dysgenesis.

Male differentiation of the external genitalia (at 9−11 weeks' gestation) is dependent on 5α-dihydrotestosterone (DHT) produced by 5α-reductase in those tissues. Testicular descent down the gubernaculum on the posterior abdominal wall and into the scrotum is partly the product of differential growth; descent from the pelvic brim and into the scrotum requires androgens and MIF. The current increase in undescended testes is thought to be due to estrogenic chemicals in the environment. Genetic defects causing the absence of any of these genes, hormones, receptors or enzymes result in defects of the masculinization process.

The ovaries in the adult are small ovoid organs lying on the posterior aspect of the broad ligament in the recto-uterine pouch, close to the fimbriated opening of the Fallopian tube. The ovarian artery, pampiniform plexus of veins, and some nerves reach the ovary in the "suspensory ligament" which descends over the pelvic brim. The ovary is attached to the uterotubal junction by the ovarian ligament component of the gubernaculum; the rest of the gubernaculum forms the round ligament which passes out of the abdomen through the inguinal canal to end in the labia majora.

The initial development of the ovary also involves the migration of primordial germ cells from the yolk sac wall into the thickened celomic epithelium of the intermediate mesoderm (the indifferent gonadal primordium). If SRY is not expressed, the celomic epithelial cells do not separate from the surface to form primary sex cords but, somewhat later, differentiate to form pregranulosa cells which surround the germ cells to form primordial ovarian follicles in which the germ cells enter and arrest in prophase 1 [17]. Thereafter obvious morphological differentiation of the ovary occurs at later stages. The intermediate mesoderm forms the interstitial thecal tissue which remains undifferentiated until puberty. Formation of an ovary rather than a testis requires the expression of the X-associated DAX1 and WNT4 genes. WNT4 appears to control expression of (bone morphogenetic protein) BMP2 and (follistatin) FST, both of which are expressed specifically in XX gonads. The pregranulosa cells appear to be of two types which either induce or inhibit meiosis of the germ cells. Female internal and external genitalia develop independently of any ovarian hormone production, provided that MIF and testosterone are not present. Estrogen secretion starts at about 8 weeks' gestation but in very small amounts and its cellular origin is unclear. The arrest of meiosis in the primordial germ cells in early fetal life involves local signals; thereafter unknown mechanisms regularly cause a few primordial follicles to start their developmental trajectory, but until puberty all are destined to become atretic. Mutations in the forkhead gene *FOXL2* are associated with premature ovarian failure in women, and in mice *FOXL2* is expressed early in and is necessary for the function of pregranulosa cells [20].

At puberty, when pulsatile GnRH and gonadotroph secretion has become established, androgen-secreting theca interna cells become organized around developing follicles and the growing definitive granulosa cells of the follicles produce activins, inhibins, follistatin, growth factors such as IGF-1, and aromatase to convert androgens from the theca to estradiol. After ovulation, cells of both thecal and granulosa origin contribute to the formation of the corpus luteum.

In males, tumors can form from both Leydig and Sertoli cells. Leydig cell tumors can produce androgens, estrogens and progestins; the very rare Sertoli cell tumors usually cause feminization, presumably because of increased aromatase activity. In females, tumors can likewise form from granulosa or thecal cells and also from hilar cells; these can produce androgens (especially hilar cell tumors), estrogens or progestins.

Endocrine tissues of the gut and pancreas

Endocrine cells are found scattered throughout the epithelium of the gut from the stomach to the colon, and are collected as islets of Langerhans in the pancreas.

The islets of Langerhans comprise about 2×10^6 roughly spherical balls of endocrine cells surrounded by a capsule of glia-like cells; they are distributed widely throughout the pancreas. Those in the body and tail of the pancreas contain ~60% insulin-producing B cells located mainly centrally, 15% glucagon-secreting A cells located peripherally, and 10% somatostatin-secreting D cells scattered between. Islets in the uncinate process, which develops from the ventral pancreatic rudiment, also contain pancreatic polypeptide-secreting F cells. Each islet has a rich blood supply which enters it centrally and a rich innervation from both sympathetic and parasympathetic nerves.

The endocrine cells of the gut epithelium are mostly located within the crypts. In the body of the stomach enterochromaffin (ECL) cells produce the histamine that controls gastric acid production and both ghrelin (appetite-stimulating) and adipostatin (appetite-suppressing) are produced from the same gene expressed by the acid-secreting parietal cells; gastrin-secreting (G) cells are located in the pyloric antrum and duodenum. In the small bowel, secretin (S) cells occur from duodenum to distal ileum, cholecystokinin (I) cells and GIP (glucose-dependent insulinotropic peptide/gastric inhibitory peptide) (K) cells are located in duodenum and jejunum, glucagon-like peptide (GLP) in the duodenum, and neurotensin (N) cells in distal ileum. In the colon enteroglucagon is produced by L cells (also by gastric A cells). Somatostatin (D) cells, motilin cells and VIP (H) cells are distributed throughout the tract. Enterochromaffin cells secreting serotonin are also distributed throughout the tract and are the largest single endocrine cell group; they also produce a variety of peptides (e.g. substance P, motilin).

It was at one time thought that gut and pancreatic endocrine cells originated from the neural crest, but transplantation studies in animal fetuses have shown that they originate from endodermal cells of the developing gut. The pancreas develops from two different primordia: a smaller ventral pancreas which forms the lower part of the head and uncinate process from a bud which also forms the hepatic diverticulum; and a larger dorsal pancreas which forms from dorsal gut endoderm under the influence of activin and FGF-2 signals from the adjacent notochord and which represses sonic hedgehog expression in the underlying endoderm to permit the expression of transcription factors Pdx-1 (pancreatic-duodenal-homeobox) and Hlxb-9 which are necessary for pancreatic differentiation. Endocrine cells of the islets of Langerhans differentiate early as cells budding off the branching endodermal tubules that will form the exocrine ducts and secretory acini of the pancreas, and it would appear that the ducts can continue to provide a source of islet cells throughout life. In the endocrine progenitor cells Notch signaling is inactivated and transcription factors neurogenin 3 and Isl-1 are expressed. These then give rise to two groups of endocrine cells: glucagon- and pancreatic polypeptide-producing cells differentiate early under the influence of Pax6; insulin- and somatostatin-producing cells a little later under the influence of Pax4 [21, 22]. It is therefore not surprising that exo-endocrine cells with characteristics of both acinar and endocrine cells can be found. Co-expression of different hormones is also common in early stages. During fetal life activin A- and gastrin-producing cells are prominent in the islets, but these disappear after birth. Abnormal multifocal proliferation of islet cells during development (nesidioblastosis) causes profound uncontrolled hypoglycemia in infants.

The gut endocrine cells develop from multipotential progenitors – common stem cells in the crypt compartment of the intestine. The enteroendocrine cells differentiate as the cells migrate up the crypt–villus axis, turning over every 3–4 days. Unlike endocrine cells in many other glands that differentiate early on and turn over only very slowly, gut endocrine cells are formed throughout life from a stem cell reservoir [23]. As in the pancreas, Notch signaling blocks endocrine differentiation in gut stem cells. Deletion in mice of a gene controlled by Notch increased the number of endocrine cells in the stomach and small bowel and increased expression of pro-endocrine beta helix-loop-helix (bHLH) proteins Math1, NGN3 and Beta2. Deletion of Math1 prevents the development of all gut endocrine cells; deletion of NGN3 prevents their formation in the small intestine but not the stomach. Further downstream, Beta2(NeuroD1) is necessary for the development of secretin- and cholecystokinin-secreting cells; Pax6 for glucagon (GLP-1 and GLP-6), gastrin and somatostatin in the antrum and GIP in the duodenum; Pax4-null mice lack serotonin and somatostatin cells in the antrum and most endocrine cells in the proximal small intestine. Clearly, much remains to be discovered about how the individual endocrine cell types become differentiated [24].

Most, if not all these endocrine cells can form tumors. Interestingly, most gastrinomas arise in the pancreas, not the stomach. Also, the original discovery of GHRH in a pancreatic tumor emphasizes the apparent ectopic expression that can occur in tumors. Tumors secreting somatostatin, enteroglucagon, VIP and serotonin all produce characteristic syndromes. Pancreatic tumors occur in MEN 1; insulinomas produce characteristic hypoglycemic episodes.

References

1. Larsen PR, Kronenberg HM, Melmed S, Polonsky K (eds). *Williams Textbook of Endocrinology*, 10th edn. New York: Saunders, 2002.

2. Baylis SB, Mendelsohn G. Ectopic (inappropriate) hormone production by tumours: Mechanisms involved and the biological and clinical implications. *Endocr. Rev.* 1980;1:45–77.

3. McNeilly AS, Crawford JL, Taragnat C, Nicol L, McNeilly JR. The differential secretion of FSH and LH: regulation through genes, feedback and packaging. *Reproduction* 2003; 61(Suppl.):463–476.

4. Morris JF. Morphological studies of dendrites and dendritic secretion. In Ludwig M (ed.) *Dendritic Neurotransmitter Release.* New York: Springer Science+Business Media, Inc., 2005: 15–33.

5. Leng, G, Ludwig, M. Information processing in the hypothalamus: Peptides and analogue computation. *J. Neuroendocrinol.* 2006;18: 379–392.

6. Cohen LE, Radovick S. Molecular basis of combined pituitary hormone deficiencies. *Endocr. Rev.* 2002; 23:431–442.

7. Korbonits M, Morris DG, Nanzer A, Kola B, Grossman AB. Role of regulatory factors in pituitary tumour formation. *Front. Horm. Res.* 2004;32:63–95.

8. Polak M, Sura-Trueba S, Chauty A, Szinnai, Carré A, Castanet M. Molecular mechanisms of thyroid dysgenesis. *Hormone Res.* 2004;62(Suppl 3):14–21.

9. Xu P-X, Zheng W, Laclef C, et al. *Eya1* is required for the morphogenesis of mammalian thymus, parathyroid and thyroid. *Development* 2002;129:3033–3044.

10. Takano T, Amino N. Fetal cell carcinogenesis: A new hypothesis for better understanding of thyroid carcinoma. *Thyroid* 2005;15:432–438.

11. Mazzferri EL Classification of thyroid tumours. In Mazzaferri EL, Samaan MA (eds). *Endocrine Tumours.* Oxford: Blackwell Science, 1993:223–227.

12. Kebebew E, Peng M, Wong MG. *GCMB* gene, a master regulator of parathyroid gland development, expression, and regulation in hyperparathyroidism. *Surgery* 2004;136:1261–1266.

13. Zhou D, Silvius D, Davenport J, Grifone R, Maire P, Xu P-X. Patterning of the third pharyngeal pouch into thymus/parathyroid by Six and Eya1. *Dev. Biol.* 2006;293:499–512.

14. Ozisik G, Achermann JC, Meeks JJ, Jameson JL. SF1 in the development of the adrenal glands and gonads. *Hormone Res.* 2003;59(Suppl 1): 94–98.

15. Coulter CL. Fetal adrenal development: insight gained from adrenal tumors. *Trends Endocrinol. Metab.* 2005;16:235–242.

16. Lovell-Badge R, Canning C, Sekido R. Sex-determining genes in mice: building pathways. In *The Genetics and Biology of Sex Determination.* Chichester, Wiley, Novartis Foundation Symposium 2002;244:4–22.

17. Ross AJ, Capel B. Signaling at the crossroads of gonad development. *Trends Endocrinol. Metab.* 2005;16:19–25.

18. Meeks JJ, Crawford SE, Russell TA, Morohashi K-I, Weiss J, Jameson JL. Dax 1 regulates testis cord organization during gonadal development. *Development* 2003;130:1029–1036.

19. Meeks JJ, Weiss J, Jameson JL. Dax 1 is required for testis determination. *Nat. Genet.* 2003;34:32–33.

20. Uhlenhaut NH, Trier M. Foxl2 function in ovarian development. *Molec. Genet. Metab.* 2006;88:225–234.

21. Habener JF, Kemp DM, Thomas MK. Minireview: Transcriptional regulation in pancreatic development. *Endocrinology* 2005;146:1025–1034.

22. Murtaugh LC, Melton DA. Genes, signals and lineages in pancreas development. *Annu. Rev. Cell Dev. Biol.* 2003;19:71–90.

23. Oldham KT, Thompson JC. Ontogeny of gut peptides. In Thompson JC, Greeley GH Jr, et al. (eds). *Gastrointestinal Endocrinology.* New York: McGraw Hill, 1987:158–77.

24. Schonhoff SE, Giel-Moloney M, Leiter AB. Minireview: Development and differentiation of gut endocrine cells. *Endocrinology* 2004;145: 2639–2644.

2 Epidemiology of Endocrine Tumors

Amanda Nicholson

Key points

- Endocrine tumors are rare compared to other cancers. Parathyroid adenomas, ovarian carcinomas and testicular tumors are the most common.
- Many lesions of the parathyroid, thyroid, adrenal and pituitary glands are undiagnosed in the population.
- Reported incidence rates depend on medical services available and hence increasing incidence rates may be due to increased ascertainment of asymptomatic tumors, so-called incidentalomas, rather than a true increase in incidence.
- Testicular cancer incidence is rising in the developed world.
- There is marked geographical variation in incidence of cancers of testis and thyroid, but the environmental risk factors involved are poorly understood.

Introduction

Epidemiology is the quantitative study of distribution, determinants and control of disease in human populations. It seeks to describe the burden of disease; its distribution by time, person and place; its causes and how it might be prevented. This chapter aims to place endocrine tumors in a population perspective, giving an estimate of their frequency in comparison to other tumors and summarizing what is known of their etiological risk factors.

Two measures are commonly used to describe the burden of disease in a population. *Incidence* is the number of new cases occurring in a given population in a given period of time, often described as *x cases/100 000/year*. For diseases with a high case fatality rate, mortality may be used as a measure of incidence. *Prevalence* is the number of cases (both old and new) in a given population at a given point in time. Incidence is used most commonly to describe the frequency of neoplasms and is a useful measure for planning hospital services.

Epidemiological study of endocrine tumors is limited by certain characteristics of the diseases [1].

1 A major problem is that for many endocrine systems, such as pituitary and adrenal, many small tumors do not lead to clinical presentation but may be discovered in the course of other investigations – so-called incidentalomas – so that hospital-based studies will only assess the tip of the iceberg. Issues of case definition and completeness of ascertainment arise in nearly all published work and may account for some of the large variations in estimates of incidence and prevalence seen both geographically and over time.

2 Related to these asymptomatic cases, questions remain unanswered about what should be considered as a disease state for some conditions and what action should be taken when they are diagnosed.

3 Endocrine disease is rare, necessitating large studies, but investigations are costly, thus precluding true community-based work.

4 Since many of these tumors are, fortunately, amenable to treatment, mortality statistics cannot be used as a measure of incidence as they can for more lethal cancers. Cancer registries must be used which are not universal and vary in completeness.

Register and other incidence data will not differentiate between cases presenting clinically and those discovered incidentally. International comparisons become difficult under these circumstances as apparent differences in incidence may reflect differences in ascertainment or register deficiencies. Data are most reliable for the life-threatening tumors affecting ovary and testes. Discussion of other tumors (such as those of the adrenal, parathyroids, neuroendocrine) is severely hampered by the sparse and sometimes poor-quality data available.

Scale of the problem

Endocrine tumors are rare. Only ovarian cancer features in estimates of worldwide incidence of 12 major cancers, where it is the sixth most frequent cancer in women [2, 3]. Some endocrine malignancies show marked geographical variation but even in countries with high incidence, endocrine tumors represent a small fraction of the burden of malignant disease. Cancers of the lung, gastrointestinal tract and breast pose a far greater challenge to health services.

Clinical Endocrine Oncology, 2nd edition. Edited by Ian D. Hay and John A.H. Wass. © 2008 Blackwell Publishing. ISBN 978-1-4051-4584-8.

Ovarian cancer

There are three types of ovarian neoplasm: epithelial (66%), germ cell (25–30%) and sex-cord stromal tumors (6%). Hormone secretion and feminizing effects are seen with stromal tumors. It has been estimated that 80–90% of malignant tumors are epithelial in origin and most of the epidemiological evidence applies to epithelial tumors [4].

There is considerable geographical variation in the incidence of ovarian cancer. It is generally more common in developed countries with incidence rates in northern Europe and North America of between 8–12/100 000/year. The incidence rate rises with age to reach a peak at 75 years, with an earlier peak due to germ cell tumors in teenage years. Rates are lower in southern Europe, with lowest rates seen in Japan and Africa. Within countries, there are differences between ethnic groups with rates highest in white populations compared to African populations. The life-threatening nature of the disease means that these geographical differences are likely to reflect real differences in incidence rather than ascertainment effects. Ovarian cancer is more common in urban populations and in earlier studies was found to be more common in women of higher social status [4]. Incidence rates appear to be fairly stable in developed countries with falling mortality due to better treatment. The overall incidence rate may mask a rising incidence of teratoma in younger women in developed countries.

The causes of ovarian cancer remain unclear. Similar geographic patterns are seen in breast, ovarian and endometrial cancer – suggesting common risk factors. Overall, 5 to 10% of ovarian cancers are familial, but this proportion is higher in younger age groups. Family history is the most significant risk factor for ovarian cancer, with a relative risk of 9. *BRCA1* and *BRCA2* mutations account for the majority of hereditary disease. Hormonal factors are also most important, with lifetime number of ovulations related to risk – the incessant ovulation hypothesis. Nulliparity, low parity, infertility and late menopause increase risk, whereas use of the oral contraceptive pill is protective [5].

International differences in rates led to suggestions that a low fat diet may be protective but recent epidemiological evidence, including individual level studies, has not confirmed a role for diet in the etiology of ovarian cancer. Similarly, exposure to talc or asbestos has not been proven to be a risk factor.

Testicular cancer

Testicular cancer is uncommon, with incidence rates of between 3.1 and 10/100 000 per year in white men and much lower rates in Africans and Asians. Rates are highest in northern Europe, notably Switzerland and Denmark, with rates of 10/100 000/year. African Americans have much lower rates than white Americans (1.1 versus 4.1/100 000/year) and there is no evidence of migration increasing risk, suggesting a genetic component. There are several different histological groupings of testicular cancer, but epidemiologically the most useful is seminoma and non-seminoma (the majority of which are germ cell tumors). Testicular cancer has a distinct pattern with age, with few cases before puberty, followed by a peak for non-seminoma in the late 20s and for seminoma in the 30s. These peaks are followed by a marked fall and then a modest increase after the age of 65. In older men non-germ cell tumors predominate. Testicular cancers have been increasing in white populations in Europe and North America, with some suggestion that the increase may now be leveling off [6]. Both seminoma and non-seminoma are increasing although advances in treatment mean that mortality is falling despite this rise. A similar rise in incidence has not been seen in non-white populations (see Fig. 2.1 [7]) and there are important differences between countries as close as Finland and Denmark. Although there may be some element of ascertainment effects in the data, as in ovarian cancer these trends are thought to reflect true variation in the incidence of the disease.

The major established risk factor is maldescended testis (MDT), with a 2–4-fold increase in risk. It appears that risk is raised only in the maldescended testis and not in the opposite. There is

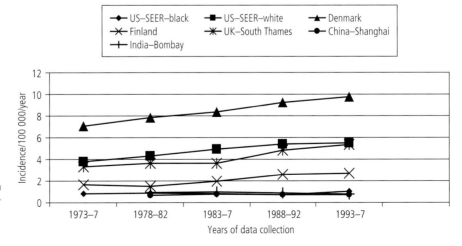

Figure 2.1 Secular trends in testicular cancer. (Data from Parkin DM, Whelan SL, Ferlay J, Storm H. Cancer Incidence in Five Continents, Vol. I to VIII, IARC CancerBase No. 7, Lyon, 2005 [7].)

evidence that testicular cancer is also associated with reduced fertility (although the temporal sequence may be difficult to establish). A spectrum of disorders including testicular cancer, low sperm count and MDT termed testicular dysgenesis syndrome (TDS) has been suggested, with a possible common origin in fetal life. There is some evidence that the prevalence of MDT and low sperm count is increasing in some countries in parallel with the rising incidence of testicular cancer (but questions remain about the methodology and comparability of measures). No satisfactory explanation is available for the rise in incidence rates in recent decades or for the disparity seen between countries. *In utero* exposure to estrogens has been associated with testicular cancer but evidence is less robust for MDT. The source of estrogens is unclear.

Increased exposure to environmental estrogens is now largely discounted as an explanation due to weak estrogenicity of the compounds implicated. Alternative explanations are environmental agents decreasing endogenous androgens [6], increasing maternal age, lower parity and premature birth. Secular trends suggest an environmental cause but the large differences between ethnic groups within countries and lack of migration effect suggest a genetic component, perhaps with gene–environment interactions [8, 9].

Thyroid cancer

Thyroid cancer is by far the most common cancer of endocrine glands, accounting for 92% in data from the United States [10]. There are four different histological types of thyroid cancer which have distinct epidemiological features. The vast majority are derived from follicular cells and are differentiated or undifferentiated anaplastic. The differentiated cancers are subdivided into papillary (40–70% of reported series) and follicular (10–40% of reported series). The ratio of papillary to follicular carcinoma

varies geographically but in Europe and the USA papillary carcinomas are most common and show a peak incidence in women in middle age. The sex differential in incidence is widest for papillary carcinoma. The incidence of follicular carcinomas rises steadily with age in men and women. Anaplastic carcinomas are less common (approximately 10%) and typically occur in men and women over 50 years old. Medullary carcinoma, derived from the parafollicular cells, is rare (less than 5%) and may be sporadic or in approximately 25% of cases familial, associated with multiple endocrine neoplasia (MEN) 2. Although many data treat thyroid cancer as one group, this is likely to be masking important biological differences in etiology and prognosis. There have been considerable changes in diagnosis, so-called "papillarization," with both the inclusion of previously designated adenomas into the malignant group and also the shift of malignant tumors with papillary features into the papillary cancer group. In addition clinical practice has altered with increasing investigation of cold nodules in the thyroid, including fine-needle biopsy, radio-isotope scanning and ultrasound.

There is a marked sex difference, with annual incidence rates higher in women, and a marked geographical variation with a ten-fold variation in incidence rates (see Fig. 2.2), largely due to differences in papillary carcinomas. Rates are high in Iceland, Switzerland and the Nordic countries. Exceptionally high rates are seen in Filipino women in Hawaii (19.4/100 000/year) but incidence is also high in Filipinos in the USA (12.1/100 000/year) and is lower in the Philippines (7.5 /100 000/year), but still raised compared to other countries in Asia [2]. Not all evidence from migration is consistent, with high rates in Jews in Israel regardless of their origin. Differences in ascertainment and access to medical services undoubtedly contribute to these differences, as well as true variations in incidence.

There is good evidence that thyroid cancer incidence has been increasing in countries with sophisticated medical services [7]. An earlier suggestion that the rise was leveling off since the late

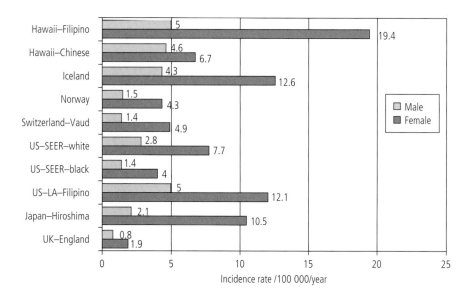

Figure 2.2 Geographical variation in incidence of thyroid cancer. (Data for 1993–1997 from Cancer in Five Continents, Volume VIII [2].)

1970s [11] or earlier [12] has not been confirmed, with recent reports from the USA and Scotland of a continuing rise into the 2000s [13–15]. The rise seems to be accounted for by an increase in small papillary carcinoma [13]. One possible explanation is that increased investigation of solitary thyroid nodules is leading to increased diagnosis of occult papillary tumors. Secular changes in follicular carcinoma have been less marked, with contradictory reports of rise or fall over time. This rise in incidence in developed countries has not been accompanied by rising mortality, due to effective treatment.

Risk factors for the development of thyroid tumors are not well understood. Radiation, perhaps in very low doses, is clearly related to thyroid cancers, particularly papillary. This is demonstrated by the large rise in thyroid cancer seen in Belarus since the Chernobyl disaster [7]. Benign thyroid disease is probably associated with a higher risk of developing a malignancy. Genetic factors are important in the development of medullary cancer, related to MEN 2, but most cases of medullary cancer are sporadic. Iodine deficiency in the diet has been linked to the development of thyroid cancer, particularly follicular cancer, with a suggestion that excess associated iodine may lead to papillary cancer. Reproductive factors have been considered in light of the large sex differences, but evidence for any effect is weak. The striking geographic differences remain unexplained.

Parathyroid tumors

Issues concerning case ascertainment and the extent of undiagnosed disease are of paramount importance in parathyroid tumors. The introduction of automated serum calcium measurement in the early 1970s, led to a huge rise in the number of cases of primary hyperparathyroidism (PHP) being detected. PHP is caused by an adenoma in 85% of cases and therefore PHP can be used as a marker for parathyroid adenomas. Data from Rochester, MN in the US, have provided an accurate indicator of trends in the developed world. Incidence rates increased from 16/100 000/year before automated screening was introduced in 1974, reaching a peak of 83 and falling to 21 in the most recent time-period, 1993–2001 [16]. Automated calcium screening was withdrawn in 1996 but measurement of calcium levels remains more common than pre-1974 due to awareness of osteoporosis. Hence, incidence rates of adenomas are higher. Incidence is higher in women and rises with age in both sexes. The dramatic secular trends are largely explained by calcium screening policy, but the sustained fall since 1983 may suggest that some other etiological factor has declined. Both head and neck irradiation (widespread in the 1930s for childhood conditions) and radioactive fallout have been suggested [16, 17].

These figures suggest that parathyroid tumors are the most common endocrine tumor but there are many geographical variations which may reflect real differences in incidence or, more likely, patterns of care. Issues of effectiveness and cost-benefit of treating asymptomatic PHP remain unresolved. Parathyroid carcinoma is extremely rare, causing less than 5% of PHP.

Independent incidence data for parathyroid carcinoma are not available.

Neuroendocrine tumors

Neuroendocrine tumors include carcinoid tumors and other tumors of the gastrointestinal endocrine system. Incidence data for these rare tumors are exquisitely sensitive to random variation and differences in case ascertainment, which makes international comparisons very difficult. Some series only focus on gastrointestinal tumors. Recent estimates of the incidence of all carcinoid tumors vary from 0.5 to 2.0 /100 000/year. There is good evidence that incidence rates have been rising, largely due to increased detection, but rates may now be leveling off [18, 19]. The proportion of carcinoids found in the lung varies from 9% in Sweden, 30% in Italy to 50% in the US, probably related to the underlying incidence rate of lung cancer. Incidence of the carcinoid syndrome (dependent on the presence of hepatic metastases) is much lower, certainly less than 0.5/100 000/year, estimated from published data. Sex and age trends are difficult to assess due to the diagnostic bias from varying rates of surgery and autopsy. Incidence rates appear to increase with age, with tumors uncommon before 40 years, although an increase in appendiceal carcinoids has been reported in younger women in Sweden [19]. The etiology of these tumors is uncertain. MEN 1 contributed only 1% of cases in the Swedish study. Higher social class and urban living were associated with higher incidence, perhaps related to detection bias.

Data on other gastrointestinal endocrine tumors come from the Northern Ireland register [20] and are based on clinically apparent cases. Insulinomas occur in 1.2/million/year with all other tumors occurring less than 1/million /year.

Adrenal cortical adenomas and carcinomas

Prior to the widespread use of computerized tomography (CT) or magnetic resonance imaging scanning, the discovery of adrenal cortical tumors depended on either secretion of hormones secreted by the tumor (corticosteroids [resulting in adrenocorticotropic hormone (ACTH)-independent Cushing syndrome], aldosterone [resulting in Conn syndrome] or androgens [resulting in virilization]), or on mass effects. Carcinomas eventually present with mass effects and symptoms of malignancy but non-functioning adenomas are often undiagnosed in life. The detection of adrenal masses as incidentalomas is increasing. Prevalence estimates for adrenal masses of at least 0.5 cm diameter from CT studies are 0.35–4.6%, with much higher rates from autopsy studies [21]. In one report, 12% of such incidentalomas were malignant and 10% proved to be pheochromocytomas [22]. Any such estimates will depend on the size of adrenal masses investigated and on the age of the patient. Other than an estimate of 0.8/million/year for the incidence of Conn syndrome [23], there are no incidence data for functioning adenomas.

Adrenocortical carcinoma remains a very rare disease, and despite the possibility of increased detection via incidentalomas, national incidence rates are steady [7]. Histological diagnosis of malignancy can be difficult. One population-based study in Norway in 1970–1980s indicated that adrenal cortical carcinoma has an incidence of 1.5/million/year [24]. There is a bimodal age distribution, with peaks in the first 5 years of life (incidence of 6.67/million/year[25]) and then in the sixth and seventh decades. Incidence is similar in both sexes. Geographical differences are not apparent for overall incidence but have been reported for childhood adrenocortical carcinoma, with high incidence in Brazil potentially linked to a P53 germline mutation [26].

Pheochromocytomas

Population-based estimates of the incidence of pheochromocytoma indicate an incidence of approximately 1.5–2/million/year Higher estimates have been given where the autopsy rate is high, as up to half of cases may be initially diagnosed at post-mortem [23, 27]. Recent reports that 50% of clinical series had been detected by the imaging of adrenal masses suggest that the incidence may rise [28]: 10% are malignant and 10% bilateral. Although up to 40% of MEN 2 patients develop pheochromocytomas, approximately 10% of all pheochromocytomas, are associated with MEN syndromes.

Pituitary adenomas

A recent meta-analysis found that the population prevalence of pituitary adenomas was 17% (14% in CT, 23% in autopsy studies) [29], hence clinical incidence rates will vary depending on ascertainment and there have been some reports that they are increasing. Estimates based on registers of intracranial neoplasms are in the order of 1–2/100 000/year with rises in recent decades. The majority of tumors are non-functioning, with prolactinomas the most common hormone-secreting tumors, followed by growth hormone (GH)-secreting and with ACTH-secreting tumors less common. Tumors are more common in women than men and clinical incidence appears to peak in middle age but other risk factors for their development are poorly understood. Life expectancy is impaired in patients with an adenoma, related to excess hormone secretion and to the impact of hypopituitarism, but the distinction between normal and disease state is blurred [30, 31].

The incidence of acromegaly is described in population studies as between 3 and 4 cases per million per year [32, 33], although recent registry data from Spain gave a lower figure of 2.1/million/year [34]. Cushing disease is less common with an incidence of 2/million/year [35]. The available data indicate that the incidence of both acromegaly and Cushing disease is rising, with estimates for most recent time periods (1985 onwards) of 5.6 and 3.9/million/year, respectively.

Conclusion

Within the constraints of available data, Table 2.1 gives the estimated incidences of clinically apparent endocrine tumors. These figures must be treated as approximate at best. By comparison with other neoplasms all these tumors are rare and some are very rare indeed. With the exception of ovarian and testicular cancer, the tumors discussed here present somewhat of a dilemma to public health practice. There is good evidence that increased investigation will lead to increased detection and raised incidence rates since it is obvious that many tumors are not detected during life. The effectiveness and cost-benefit of subsequent treatment have often not been evaluated. It is unclear whether the hidden iceberg really represents a "disease" state. However, the rise in testicular cancer appears to be real and requires further explanation. Despite an increasing interest in the genetic component to endocrine disease, the available data suggest that environmental risk factors are important in the etiology of these tumors.

Table 2.1 Approximate incidences of endocrine tumors in the UK (cases/100 000/year)

	Males	Females
Lung*	51.1	21.9
Breast*		74.4
Ovary*		12.4
Testis*	5.1	
Thyroid*	0.8	1.9
	Both sexes	
Parathyroid adenoma	20	
Pituitary adenoma	1.5	
Carcinoid tumors	1.5	
Insulinoma	0.1	
Other GI endocrine tumors	<0.1	
Adrenocortical carcinoma	0.15	
Pheochromocytoma	0.15	

Rates may be taken from small studies where published rates were not age-standardized.

* Data for 1993–1997 for UK – England [2].

References

1. Monson JP. The epidemiology of endocrine tumours. *Endocr. Relat. Cancer* 2000;7:29–36.
2. Parkin DM, Whelan SL, Ferlay J, Teppo L, Thomas DB. *Cancer Incidence in Five Continents*, Vol VIII. Lyon: IARC, 2002.
3. Parkin DM. Global cancer statistics in the year 2000. *Lancet Oncology* 2001;2:533–543.
4. Parazzini F, Franceschi S, La Vecchia C, Fasoli M. The epidemiology of ovarian cancer. *Gynecol. Oncol.* 1991;43:9–23.
5. Holschneider CH, Berek JS. Ovarian cancer: epidemiology, biology, and prognostic factors. *Semin. Surg. Oncol.* 2000;19:3–10.

6. Sharpe RM. The "oestrogen hypothesis" – where do we stand now? *Int. J. Androl.* 2003;26:2–15.

7. Parkin DM, Whelan SL, Ferlay J, Storm H. *Cancer Incidence in Five Continents*, Volumes I to VIII, 2006. Available from: http://www-dep.iarc.fr/

8. Giwercman A, Rylander L, Hagmar L, Giwercman YL. Ethnic differences in occurrence of TDS – genetics and/or environment? *Int. J. Androl.* 2006;29:291–297.

9. Garner MJ, Turner MC, Ghadirian P, Krewski D. Epidemiology of testicular cancer: an overview. *Int. J. Cancer* 2005;116:331–339.

10. Correa P, Chen VW. Endocrine gland cancer. *Cancer* 1995;75:338–352.

11. Franceschi S, Boyle P, Maisonneuve P, et al. The epidemiology of thyroid carcinoma. *Crit. Rev. Oncol.* 1993;4:25–52.

12. Burke JP, Hay ID, Dignan F, et al. Long-term trends in thyroid carcinoma: a population-based study in Olmsted County, Minnesota, 1935–1999. *Mayo Clin. Proc.* 2005;80:753–758.

13. Davies L, Welch HG. Increasing incidence of thyroid cancer in the United States, 1973–2002. *JAMA* 2006;295:2164–2167.

14. Haselkorn T, Bernstein L, Preston-Martin S, Cozen W, Mack WJ. Descriptive epidemiology of thyroid cancer in Los Angeles County, 1972–1995. *Cancer Causes Control* 2000;11:163–170.

15 Reynolds RM, Weir J, Stockton DL, Brewster DH, Sandeep TC, Strachan MW. Changing trends in incidence and mortality of thyroid cancer in Scotland. *Clin. Endocrinol. (Oxf.)* 2005;62:156–162.

16. Wermers RA, Khosla S, Atkinson EJ, et al. Incidence of primary hyperparathyroidism in Rochester, Minnesota, 1993–2001: an update on the changing epidemiology of the disease. *J. Bone Miner. Res.* 2006;21:171–177.

17. Adami S, Marcocci C, Gatti D. Epidemiology of primary hyperparathyroidism in Europe. *J. Bone Miner. Res.* 2002;17 (Suppl 2):N18–N23.

18. Crocetti E, Buiatti E, Amorosi A. Epidemiology of carcinoid tumours in central Italy. *Eur. J. Epidemiol.* 1997;13:357–359.

19. Hemminki K, Li XJ. Incidence trends and risk factors of carcinoid tumors: a nationwide epidemiologic study from Sweden. *Cancer* 2001;92:2204–2210.

20. Watson RG, Johnston CF, O'Hare MM, et al. The frequency of gastrointestinal endocrine tumours in a well-defined population – Northern Ireland 1970–1985. *Q. J. Med.* 1989;72:647–657.

21. Kloos RT, Gross MD, Francis IR, Korobkin M, Shapiro B. Incidentally discovered adrenal masses. *Endocr. Rev.* 1995;16:460–484.

22. Angeli A, Osella G, Ali A, Terzolo M. Adrenal incidentaloma: an overview of clinical and epidemiological data from the National Italian Study Group. *Horm. Res.* 1997;47:279–283.

23. Andersen GS, Toftdahl DB, Lund JO, Strandgaard S, Nielsen PE. The incidence rate of phaeochromocytoma and Conn's syndrome in Denmark, 1977–1981. *J. Hum. Hypertens.* 1988;2:187–189.

24. Soreide JA, Brabrand K, Thoresen SO. Adrenal cortical carcinoma in Norway, 1970–1984. *World J. Surg.* 1992;16:663–667.

25. Hartley AL, Birch JM, Marsden HB, Reid H, Harris M, Blair V. Adrenal cortical tumours: epidemiological and familial aspects. *Arch. Dis. Child.* 1987;62:683–689.

26. Figueiredo BC, Sandrini R, Zambetti GP, et al. Penetrance of adrenocortical tumours associated with the germline TP53 R337H mutation. *J. Med. Genet.* 2006;43:91–96.

27. Hartley L, Perry-Keene D. Phaeochromocytoma in Queensland – 1970–83. *Aust. N. Z. J. Surg.* 1985;55:471–475.

28. Baguet JP, Hammer L, Mazzuco TL, et al. Circumstances of discovery of phaeochromocytoma: a retrospective study of 41 consecutive patients. *Eur. J. Endocrinol.* 2004;150:681–686.

29. Ezzat S, Asa SL, Couldwell WT, et al. The prevalence of pituitary adenomas – a systematic review. *Cancer* 2004;101:613–619.

30. Gold EB. Epidemiology of pituitary adenomas. *Epidemiol. Rev.* 1981;3:163–183.

31. Aron DC, Howlett TA. Pituitary incidentalomas. *Endocrinol. Metab. Clin. North Am.* 2000;29:205–221.

32. Alexander L, Appleton D, Hall R, Ross WM, Wilkinson R. Epidemiology of acromegaly in the Newcastle region. *Clin. Endocrinol. (Oxf.)* 1980;12:71–79.

33. Etxabe J, Gaztambide S, Latorre P, Vazquez JA. Acromegaly: an epidemiological study. *J. Endocrinol. Invest.* 1993;16:181–187.

34. Mestron A, Webb SM, Astorga R, et al. Epidemiology, clinical characteristics, outcome, morbidity and mortality in acromegaly based on the Spanish Acromegaly Registry (Registro Espanol de Acromegalia, REA). *Eur. J. Endocrinol.* 2004;151:439–446.

35. Etxabe J, Vazquez JA. Morbidity and mortality in Cushing's disease: an epidemiological approach. *Clin. Endocrinol. (Oxf.)* 1994;40:479–484.

3 Inherited Cancers, Genes, and Chromosomes

Emma R. Woodward and Eamonn R. Maher

Key points

- Recognition of patients with inherited endocrine tumors is important in order to reduce morbidity and mortality in affected patients and their relatives.
- Molecular genetic investigations facilitate the management of familial cases by enabling early presymptomatic diagnosis.
- A wide variety of molecular mechanisms may be implicated in endocrine tumor susceptibility but loss of function mutations in tumor suppressor genes are the most frequent.
- Somatic mutations (or epimutations) in inherited cancer genes also often have a key role in the pathogenesis of sporadic tumors.

Introduction

At a cellular level cancer is a genetic (and epigenetic) disease arising from mutations and epigenetic alterations that result in the characteristic features of neoplastic growth: self-sufficiency in growth signals, insensitivity to anti-proliferative signals, resistance to apoptosis, limitless replicative potential, sustained angiogenesis, tissue invasion and metastasis, and genomic instability [1]. Although the vast majority of cancer-associated genetic alterations are non-inherited somatic events, the identification of rare familial endocrine cancer genes has not only enhanced the management of inherited cases but frequently also provided important insights into the molecular pathogenesis of sporadic endocrine tumors. In this chapter we provide an overview of the clinical and molecular aspects of inherited endocrine neoplasia.

Clinical aspects of genetic susceptibility to endocrine tumors

In general about 10% of human cancers are thought to arise in genetically predisposed individuals. However, the exact proportion differs widely between tumor types. Thus familial lung cancer is generally considered to be rare as the vast majority of cases are related to environmental carcinogen exposure (i.e., smoking). In contrast, although traditional dogma maintained that 10% of pheochromocytomas were inherited, molecular genetic studies have revealed a germline mutation in a pheochromocytoma susceptibility gene in up to 24% of sporadic cases [2]. Nevertheless, in most cases the principal indicator of an inherited endocrine

neoplasia is a family history of a specific endocrine tumor, or of different but related tumor types, in two or more individuals. As most endocrine tumors are rare the presence of two endocrine tumors within a family is likely to indicate a genetic susceptibility. This is in contrast to more common non-endocrine cancers (e.g. breast and colorectal) where such clustering might occur as a chance event. Examples of familial endocrine tumor predisposition syndromes and their associated genes are presented in Table 3.1. In Table 3.2 a list of potential genetic causes is provided according to the organ involved. In addition to a family history of benign and malignant tumors, suspicion of a specific familial cancer syndrome should prompt a careful search for other features of the disorder in the proband and possibly affected relatives (e.g., presence of mucosal neuromas or Marfanoid body habitus in multiple endocrine neoplasia (MEN) 2B, cutaneous neurofibromas and café-au-lait patches in neurofibromatosis type 1).

A careful family history informed by knowledge of the inherited patterns of familial endocrine tumor syndromes can also facilitate the recognition of familial cases. This is particularly so when there are unusual patterns of inheritance, for example parent-of-origin effects associated with genomic imprinting. Thus when paternally transmitted, a germline *SDHD* mutation predisposes to head and neck paragangliomas and extra-adrenal pheochromocytoma, but when the mutation is inherited from the mother there is no phenotype [3].

The absence of a family history does not exclude the diagnosis of a familial cancer syndrome. Therefore the presence of an early age at onset and/or multiple tumors in a single individual should always prompt consideration of whether there is an underlying genetic diagnosis, irrespective of family history. In many inherited endocrine tumor susceptibility disorders there is a significant new mutation rate and in most cases the mean age at diagnosis of a tumor will be younger in genetically susceptible individuals than in sporadic cases. Hence, in individuals with early-onset

Clinical Endocrine Oncology, 2nd edition. Edited by Ian D. Hay and John A.H. Wass. © 2008 Blackwell Publishing. ISBN 978-1-4051-4584-8.

tumors, even if there are no other features of genetic susceptibility, molecular genetic testing may be indicated as the identification of a germline mutation in an endocrine neoplasia susceptibility gene is likely to influence the treatment and future management (e.g., tumor surveillance programs) of the proband and their at-risk relatives. Decisions about whether genetic testing should be offered to an individual will depend on a number of factors including the likelihood of a positive result, the cost and complexity of testing (e.g., testing of one or many genes) and the extent to which a specific molecular diagnosis will influence management of the proband and their family. The benefits of testing may be considerable, e.g. the identification of a germline von Hippel–Lindau (*VHL*) mutation in an individual with an apparently isolated pheochromocytoma will prompt a search for other features of VHL disease in the proband and close relatives. As the early detection of VHL-related tumors (e.g., retinal angioma and renal cell carcinoma) reduces morbidity and mortality, and relatives who are found not to carry a mutation detected in the proband can be released from surveillance programs, there is a clear rationale for offering genetic testing to at-risk cases.

Although this clinical scenario differs from that in situations such as Huntington disease in which early diagnosis might not influence clinical management, the implications of a genetic test (e.g., effects on life and health insurance prospects, risks for other family members) differ from those of most routine endocrine investigations and therefore genetic testing should be offered as part of a specific genetic testing protocol through, or in conjunction with, the local Clinical Genetics Service.

Many inherited endocrine neoplasia conditions demonstrate incomplete penetrance (or age-related penetrance) or variable expression such that the familial nature of the disease can be overlooked. (Penetrance = quantitative assessment of proportion of heterozygotes who express phenotype and expression = differences in nature and severity of phenotype between individuals with the same allele [4].) In such cases genetic testing can improve detection of unrecognized familial cases. Thus for MEN 2 (see Chapter 69) the symptomatic clinical disease penetrance is only 59% at age 70 years but as up to 25% of individuals with medullary thyroid carcinoma (MTC) have a germline *RET* mutation, *RET* mutation analysis is recommended for all cases of MTC [5–8].

Table 3.1 Examples of genes associated with major familial endocrine tumor predisposition syndromes, features of the syndromes and function of the gene product (for full details see relevant chapter)

Gene and locus	Syndrome	Features affecting endocrine organs	Non-endocrine features	Function (of gene product)
MEN 1 11q13	MEN 1	*Hyperparathyroidism due to:* Parathyroid adenoma Parathyroid hyperplasia *Gastro-entero-pancreatic tumors:* gastrinoma, glucagonoma, insulinoma, VIP-oma *Anterior pituitary adenoma:* Secretory e.g., prolactin (most commonly) GH, TSH, ACTH or non-secretory *Less common:* Carcinoid Adrenocortical tumor (usually non-functioning)	*Occasionally:* Lipoma Facial angiofibroma	Tumor suppressor gatekeeper Binds promoters of CDK inhibitors (p27^{Kip1} and p18^{Ink4c}) to enable transcriptional activation Interacts with MLL2 to form complex with histone methyltransferase activity Interacts with the serine 5 phosphorylated C terminal domain of RNA pol II and other transcription factors, e.g., c-Jun and NF-κB.
RET 10q11.2	MEN 2A	*Hyperparathyroidism due to:* Parathyroid adenoma Parathyroid hyperplasia Pheochromocytoma MTC Thyroid C cell hyperplasia	*Other features:* Pruritic cutaneous lichen amyloidosis (rare) Hirschsprung disease (rare, depends on mutation)	Proto-oncogene Receptor tyrosine kinase. Activation causes activation of MAPK signaling cascade Attenuates apoptosis of sympathetic neuronal precursor cells during embryogenesis
	MEN 2B	Pheochromocytoma MTC Thyroid C cell hyperplasia	*Other features:* Mucosal neuromas Marfanoid habitus Intestinal ganglioneuromatosis	
	FMTC	MTC Thyroid C-cell hyperplasia		

Table 3.1 (*Continued*)

Gene and locus	Syndrome	Features affecting endocrine organs	Non-endocrine features	Function (of gene product)
VHL 3p25	VHL disease	Pheochromocytoma *Pancreas*: Non-secretory islet cell tumor Benign serous cysts Benign microcystic adenoma Carcinoid (rare)	Clear cell RCC Retinal angioma CNS hemangioblastoma *Other features*: ELST Renal & epididymal cysts	Tumor suppressor gatekeeper Component of E3 ubiquitin ligase complex that targets α-subunits of the HIF transcription factors for ubiquitylation and proteasomal degradation Other functions also e.g., fibronectin matrix assembly, downregulation of JunB causing apoptosis of sympathetic neuronal precursor cells during embryogenesis
PRKAR1A 17q23–q24	Carney complex	Primary pigmented nodular adrenocortical disease Adrenocortical overactivity Pituitary adenoma Thyroid adenoma Thyroid carcinoma (papillary or follicular) Thyroid nodules (mostly follicular adenomas)	*Myxoma*: Cardiac Breast Cutaneous Oropharynx Female genital tract *Pigmented skin lesions*: Lentigines Blue nevi *Other features*: Large-cell calcifying Sertoli cell tumor Schwannoma (psammomatous melanotic schwannoma) Breast ducal adenoma	Tumor suppressor gene gatekeeper Encodes regulatory subunit type 1α of cAMP-dependent PKA. PKA inhibits ERK1/2 cascade of MAPK pathway at level of c-Raf-1
PTEN 10q23.3	Cowden syndrome	*Thyroid*: Goiter Adenoma Carcinoma (mostly follicular)	*Mucocutaneous*: Trichelommomas Palmar–plantar keratoses Papillomatous papules *Breast*: Fibroadenoma Fibrocystic disease Adenocarcinoma *Other*: Hamartomatous polyps GI tract Macrocephaly Uterine leiomyomas Endometrial carcinoma Cerebellar dysplastic gangliocytoma	Tumor suppressor gatekeeper Phosphatase for phosphoinositide-3,4,5-triphosphate Downregulates PI3K/Akt pathway to cause G1 arrest and apoptosis Akt signaling leads to mTOR signaling through inhibition of TSC2 although not clear if mTOR independent function too Nuclear PTEN downregulates MAPK resulting in downregulation of cyclin D1 transcription
SDHD 11q23	Hereditary pheochromocytoma – paraganglioma syndrome	*Paternally inherited due to maternal imprinting*: Parasympathetic paraganglioma Sympathetic paraganglioma		Subunits of mitochondrial respiratory chain complex II (succinate dehydrogenase) Catalyze oxidative dehydrogenation of succinate to fumarate in Krebs' cycle

Table 3.1 (*Continued*)

Gene and locus	Syndrome	Features affecting endocrine organs	Non-endocrine features	Function (of gene product)
SDHC 1q21	Hereditary pheochromocytoma – paraganglioma syndrome	Parasympathetic paraganglioma		SDH inactivation results in build-up of succinate which inhibits:
SDHB 1q34	Hereditary pheochromocytoma – paraganglioma syndrome	Parasympathetic paraganglioma Sympathetic paraganglioma Adrenal pheochromocytoma	RCC (rare)	(i) prolyl hydroxylation of HIFα so pVHL cannot bind causing upregulation of hypoxia-inducible targets (ii) EgIN3-mediated induction of apoptosis of sympathetic neuronal precursor cells during embryogenesis
NF1 17q11.2	Neurofibromatosis type 1	Pheochromocytoma Sympathetic paraganglioma Duodenal carcinoid	Café-au-lait macules Neurofibromas Lisch nodules Axillary/inguinal freckling Optic glioma *Others*: Learning difficulties Macrocephaly	Tumor suppressor gene gatekeeper Ras-GTPase activating protein which regulates mTOR pathway through regulation of TSC2 Other functions also e.g., modulates mesenchymal progenitor cell differentiation into osteoblasts, inhibits downstream signaling by NGF receptor to facilitate normal developmental apoptosis of sympathetic precursor cells
HRPT2 1q31.2	Hyperparathyroidism jaw tumor syndrome	Hyperparathyroidism due to: Parathyroid hyperplasia Parathyroid adenoma Parathyroid carcinoma	Ossifying fibroma mandible/maxilla *Renal*: Hamartoma Wilms tumor Polycystic disease *Uterine pathology*: Adenofibroma Leiomyoma Adenomyosis Endometrial hyperplasia Adenosarcoma	Tumor suppressor gene gatekeeper Component of PAF1 complex Associates with non-phosphorylated and Ser2 & Ser4 phosphorylated forms of RNA polymerase II Interacts with histone methyltransferase complex that methylates histone H3 on lysine 4 which is associated with transcriptional activation Role in Wnt signaling whereby C-terminal region of β catenin recruits N-terminal region of parafibromin (to engage PAF1 complex for transcriptional upregulation of target genes)
AIP 11q12–11q13	PAP	Pituitary adenoma (mostly somatotropinoma, some prolactinoma)		Tumor suppressor gene Binds and stabilizes aryl hydrocarbon receptor (transcription factor) which is main effector of cellular response to environmental toxins. Complex also binds Hsp90 Binds survivin (member of Inhibitor of Apoptosis family). siRNA knockdown of survivin results in destabilization of survivin which lowers the anti-apoptotic threshold

ACTH, adrenocorticotropic hormone; ELST, endolymphatic sac tumor; GH, growth hormone; HIF, hypoxia-inducible factor; MAPK, mitogen-activated protein kinase; MLL2, mixed lineage leukemia 2; NGF, nerve growth factor; NF-κB, nuclear factor κB; PAF1, polymerase-associated factor 1; PAP, pituitary adenoma predisposition; PTEN, phosphatase and tensin homolog deleted on chromosome 10; RCC, renal cell carcinoma; SDH, succinate dehydrogenase; TSH, thyroid-stimulating hormone.

Table 3.2 Genes and familial syndromes associated with endocrine organ pathology

Organ and pathology/clinical manifestation	Gene	Familial syndrome
Thyroid		
Multinodular goiter	PTEN	Cowden syndrome
Papillary carcinoma	PTEN	Cowden syndrome
	APC	FAP
	Unknown	Familial non-medullary thyroid carcinoma
	Unknown ?locus 1q21	Familial papillary thyroid carcinoma with papillary renal neoplasia
C-cell hyperplasia	RET	MEN 2
Medullary carcinoma	RET	MEN 2
Parathyroid		
Parathyroid carcinoma	HRPT-2	HPT-JT
Parathyroid adenoma	MEN 1	MEN 1
	RET	MEN 2A
	HRPT-2	HPT-JT
Parathyroid hyperplasia	MEN 1	MEN 1
	HRPT-2	HPT-JT
	RET	MEN 2A
Adrenal cortex		
Primary pigmented nodular adrenocortical disease	PRKAR1A	Carney complex
Carcinoma	p53	Li–Fraumeni
	Mutation or dysregulation of 11p15.5 imprinted genes (e.g., IGF2 and CDKN1C)	BWS
	MEN 1	MEN 1
Adrenal medulla		
Neuroblastoma	Mutation or dysregulation of 11p15.5 imprinted genes (e.g., IGF2 and CDKN1C)	BWS
Pheochromocytoma	VHL	VHL disease
	RET	MEN 2A, MEN 2B
	NF1	NF1
	SDHB/D	Hereditary pheochromocytoma-paraganglioma syndrome
Paraganglia		
Parasympathetic paraganglioma	SDHD	Hereditary pheochromocytoma-paraganglioma syndrome
	SDHC	
	SDHB	
Sympathetic paraganglioma	SDHD	
	SDHB	
	VHL	
Pituitary		
Adenoma	MEN 1	MEN 1
	PRKAR1A	Carney complex
	AIP	PAP
Endocrine pancreas		
Endocrine tumor	MEN 1	MEN 1
	VHL	VHL disease
Carcinoid	MEN 1	MEN 1
	VHL	VHL disease
	NF1	NF1

BWS, Beckwith–Wiedemann syndrome; FAP, familial adenomatous polyposis; HPT–JT, hyperparathyroidism–jaw tumor syndrome; NF1, neurofibromatosis type 1; PAP, pituitary adenoma predisposition.

The decision to offer genetic testing may also depend on the specific population group involved. Founder mutations may occur in certain ethnic groups. Thus, certain breast cancer susceptibility mutations in *BRCA1* and *BRCA2* are common in the Ashkenazi Jewish population [9–11]. Recently germline mutations in the aryl hydrocarbon receptor interacting protein (AIP) gene were reported in individuals with pituitary adenoma [12]. The mutations were of low penetrance and affected individuals did not display a strong family history of pituitary tumors although, in the northern Finnish population studied, two *AIP* mutations accounted for 16% of all patients diagnosed with a growth hormone-secreting pituitary adenoma (40% of those diagnosed before age 35 years).

Molecular basis of genetic susceptibility to endocrine neoplasia

Epidemiological studies have suggested that four to seven rate-limiting mutational events are required for the transformation of normal cell to cancer cell and the molecular investigation of rare familial cancer syndromes has proved a fruitful strategy to identify genes with critical roles in the pathogenesis of both inherited and sporadic forms of cancer. A classic example of this was Fearon and Vogelstein's model of colorectal tumor development [13]. This paradigm described how colorectal tumorigenesis was characterized by a series of specific molecular events (e.g., mutations in *APC, RAS, DCC, p53*). Tumors arise from the sequential accumulation of mutations each giving rise to a clone of cells with a growth advantage. Generally in colorectal cancer tumorigenesis it is the accumulation of mutations and not the order in which

they occur that is important. However, *APC* tumor suppressor gene mutations (germline *APC* mutations cause the inherited cancer syndrome, familial adenomatous polyposis) occur very early in the transition from normal cell to cancer cell and precede adenoma development. Thus the *APC* gene was designated to have a "gatekeeper" function in view of its critical rate-limiting role in colorectal tumorigenesis development. In contrast to "gatekeeper" genes that directly influence cellular proliferation, "caretaker" cancer susceptibility genes act to maintain the integrity of the genome [14]. Although major familial cancer genes such as *p53, BRCA1, BRCA2* and the mismatch repair genes (*MSH2, MLH1, MSH6, PMS1, PMS2*) can be classed as caretaker genes, many familial endocrine tumor susceptibility genes appear to have a direct influence on cell proliferation (Table 3.2).

Familial cancer gatekeeper genes may be divided into proto-onocogenes and tumor suppressor genes. Many familial endocrine tumor susceptibility syndromes result from loss-of-function mutations in tumor suppressor genes. However, a notable exception is MEN 2 in which specific missense mutations in a single allele cause abnormal activation of the *RET* proto-oncogene [15]. In contrast to the single mutation event required to activate a proto-oncogene, tumor suppressor gene inactivation (e.g. *RB1* or *MEN1*) requires two mutation events (see Fig. 3.1). In familial cases, one mutation is inherited in the germline and the second rate-limiting event is somatic inactivation of the remaining wild-type allele. The nature of the somatic mutation event is variable and may involve chromosome deletion, mitotic recombination, intragenic mutation or epigenetic inactivation by promoter methylation (see Fig. 3.2). Chromosomal loss and mitotic recombination is associated with "loss of heterozygosity" (LOH) at polymorphic DNA markers within the deletion/region of mitotic

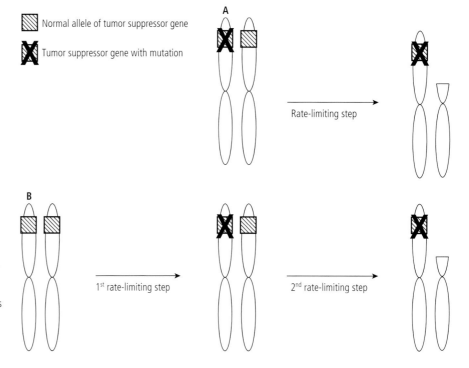

Figure 3.1 In familial cases, individuals inherit a mutation in one copy of the wild-type allele and acquire somatic inactivation (e.g., by partial chromosome deletion) in the remaining copy of the wild-type allele whereas in sporadic cases individuals acquire two separate inactivating events (e.g., by intragenic mutation and then partial chromosome deletion) in each copy of the wild-type allele.

Normal allele of tumor suppressor gene

Tumor suppressor gene with mutation

Rate-limiting step

1st rate-limiting step

2nd rate-limiting step

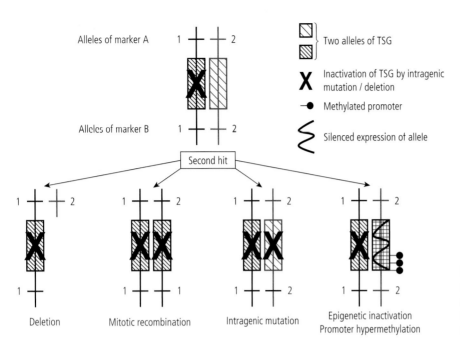

Figure 3.2 Possible mechanisms by which somatic mutation event may occur. Note that allele loss at marker B occurs with deletion and mitotic recombination but not with intragenic mutation or promoter hypermethylation.

recombination segment and LOH has been used to identify candidate regions that may contain tumor suppressor genes.

There is increasing awareness that, in addition to the mechanisms described above, epigenetic events are a major mechanism of tumor suppressor gene inactivation in sporadic cancers [16]. Furthermore, in familial cancer syndromes the second mutational event ("hit") can also be *de novo* promoter methylation.

There are many examples of tumors with a common mechanism of tumorigenesis in familial and sporadic cases. Thus, clear cell renal cell carcinoma (RCC) is a major complication of VHL disease (Chapter 70) and somatic inactivation of the *VHL* tumor suppressor gene is a feature of most sporadic clear cell RCC. However, somatic inactivation of *VHL* is infrequent in sporadic pheochromocytoma. Similarly, somatic mutations of the succinate dehydrogenase subunits B and D genes (*SDHB* and *SDHD*) are rare in sporadic pheochromocytoma. Recently Lee et al. [17] suggested a shared mechanism of tumorigenesis in familial pheochromocytoma susceptibility syndromes (VHL disease, hereditary pheochromocytoma–paraganglioma syndrome, MEN 2 and neurofibromatosis type 1) (see Table 3.1) that provided an explanation for this observation. Loss of pVHL or SDHB/D function results in a failure of the normal developmental apoptosis (triggered by a fall in NGF levels) in sympathetic neuronal progenitor cells. Persisting cells may then (following further mutational and epimutational events) give rise to a pheochromocytoma. This hypothesis predicts that in patients with VHL disease or *SDHB/D* mutations, the timing of the second mutation event is critical – it must take place before the normal developmental culling of the sympathetic neuronal progenitor cells. In patients without an inherited susceptibility to pheochromocytoma it is unlikely that the required two somatic *VHL* (or *SDHB/SDHD*)

mutations would occur prior to the onset of apoptosis. An added complexity in VHL disease is that not all germline *VHL* mutations predispose to pheochromocytoma [18, 19]. The risk of pheochromocytoma with germline deletions, frameshift mutations or missense mutations predicted to disrupt pVHL structural integrity is small, whereas specific missense mutations on the protein surface can be associated with a high risk of pheochromocytoma development. These observations predict that somatic *VHL* mutations in sporadic pheochromocytoma would not only need to occur early in development but would also need to be of a specific type (surface missense substitution), thus further reducing the likelihood of somatic *VHL* mutations being implicated in the pathogenesis of sporadic pheochromocytoma.

The identification of a familial endocrine tumor susceptibility gene generally facilitates clinical management by allowing genetic testing to be instigated. However, the ultimate long-term aim of gene identification is to provide insights into the molecular pathology of the disease and so provide a basis for developing novel approaches to treatment. In many cases, however, identifying the precise function of the gene product has proven to be a slow and difficult process. Many familial cancer gene products have multiple functions (see Table 3.1) and it might be expected that genes for which mutations result in susceptibility to a specific tumor (e.g., pheochromocytoma) might function in a common or related signaling pathway. An example of this is the suggestion that *VHL, SDHB/SDHD, RET* and *NF1* mutations can all impair the cJun/EglN3 developmental apoptosis pathway triggered by NGF withdrawal [17]. In addition, *VHL* and *SDHB/D* inactivation are both reported to cause activation of the hypoxia-inducible factors HIF-1 and HIF-2. This produces a pseudo-hypoxic drive with activation and expression of a wide repertoire of hypoxia-inducible genes implicated in angiogenesis (e.g., vascular endothelial growth factor, VEGF, and platelet-derived growth factor, PDGF), metabolic adaptation (GLUT1, carbonic anhydrase 9), apoptosis (BNip3) and cell proliferation (Cyclin D1, transforming growth factor α). Nevertheless pheochromocytomas from patients with MEN 2 do not show evidence of activation of a hypoxic gene response.

Future directions

The identification of genes involved in the development of a cancer is a key area of cancer research as it provides insights into cellular pathways and the function of the normal gene product. For familial cancer genes there is also the almost immediate benefit that diagnostic testing can be offered to at-risk families. However, in a broader context, the ultimate objective is to use genetic information to develop novel molecularly targeted therapies. Although at present there are relatively few examples of this (e.g., sorafenib and sunitinib in metastatic RCC [small molecule inhibitors of PDGFR and VEGFR], imatinib in Philadelphia chromosome positive chronic myeloid leukemia [small molecule inhibitor of Abl] and trastuzumab in breast cancer [monoclonal antibody with activity against HER-2]), large-scale projects such as the Cancer Genome Project (www.sanger.ac.uk/genetics/CGP/) and The Cancer Genome Anatomy Project (http://cgap.nci.nih. gov/) aim to provide an inventory of the key genetic changes underlying the common human cancers and should facilitate the development of novel therapies. In addition, there is increasing interest in exploiting the potential reversibility of cancer-associated epigenetic alterations with novel epigenetically targeted treatment strategies. Such advances would promise to transform the management of human cancers. We might also speculate that increased knowledge of the molecular pathogenesis of familial endocrine neoplasia syndromes will shift the emphasis from preventative surgery (e.g., thyroidectomy in MEN 2) towards tumor prevention by chemoprophylaxis.

References

1. Hanahan D, Weinberg RA. The hallmarks of cancer. *Cell* 2000;100: 57–70.
2. Neumann HPH, Bausch B, McWhinney SR, et al. for the Freiburg-Warsaw-Columbus Pheochromocytoma Study Group. Germ-line mutations in nonsyndromic pheochromocytoma. *N. Engl. J. Med.* 2002;346:1459–1466.
3. Baysal BE, Ferrell RE, Willett-Brozick JE, et al. Mutations in SDHD, a mitochondrial complex II gene in hereditary paraganglioma. *Science* 2000;287:848–851.
4. Hodgson SV, Maher ER. *A Practical Guide to Human Cancer Genetics.* Cambridge: Cambridge University Press, 1999.
5. Easton DF, Ponder MA, Cummings T, et al. The clinical and screening age-at-onset distribution for the MEN-2 syndrome. *Am. J. Hum. Genet.* 1989;44:208–215.
6. Decker RA, Peacock ML, Borst MJ, Sweet JD, Thompson NW. Progress in genetic screening of multiple endocrine neoplasia type 2A: is calcitonin testing obsolete? *Surgery* 1995;118:257–263.
7. Eng C. RET proto-oncogene in the development of human cancer. *J. Clin. Oncol.* 1999;17:380–393.
8. Brandi ML, Gagel RF, Angelim A, et al. Guidelines for diagnosis and therapy of MEN Type 1 and Type 2. *J. Clin. Endocrinol. Metab.* 2001;86:5658–5671.
9. Struewing JP, Abeliovich D, Peretz T, et al. The carrier frequency of the BRCA1 185delAG mutation is approximately 1 percent in Ashkenazi Jewish individuals. *Nat. Genet.* 1995;11:198–200.
10. Oddoux C, Struewing JP, Clayton CM, et al. The carrier frequency of the BRCA2 6174delT mutation among Ashkenazi Jewish individuals is approximately 1%. *Nat. Genet.* 1996;14:188–190.
11. Roa BB, Boyd AA, Volcik K, Richards CS. Ashkenazi Jewish population frequencies for common mutations in BRCA1 and BRCA2. *Nat. Genet.* 1996;14:185–187.
12. Vierimaa O, Georgitsi M, Lehtonen R, et al. Pituitary adenoma predisposition caused by germline mutations in the AIP gene. *Science* 2006;312:1228–1230.
13. Fearon ER, Vogelstein B. A genetic model for colorectal tumorigenesis. *Cell* 1990;61:759–767.
14. Kinzler KW, Vogelstein B. Cancer-susceptibility genes. Gatekeepers and caretakers. *Nature* 1997;386:761, 763.
15. Santoro M, Carlomngo F, Romano A, et al. Activation of RET as a dominant transforming gene by germline mutations of MEN 2A and MEN 2B. *Science* 1995;267:381–383.
16. Jones PA, Baylin SB. The fundamental role of epigenetic events in cancer. *Nat. Rev. Genet.* 2002;3:415–428.
17. Lee S, Nakamura E, Yang H, et al. Neuronal apoptosis linked to EglN3 prolyl hydroxylase and familial pheochromocytoma genes: developmental culling and cancer. *Cancer Cell* 2005;8:1–13.
18. Crossey PA, Richards FM, Foster K, et al. Identification of intragenic mutations in the von Hippel-Lindau disease tumor suppressor gene and correlation with disease phenotype. *Hum. Mol. Genet.* 1994;3: 1303–1308.
19. Ong KR, Woodward ER, Killick P, Lim C, Macdonald F, Maher ER. Genotype–phenotype correlations in von Hippel–Lindau disease. *Hum. Mutat.* 2007;28:143–149.

4 Hormones, Growth Factors, and Tumor Growth

Andrew G. Renehan

> **Key points**
> - Against a background of an enormous volume of literature and several controversies, there is the emergence of some consensus on the roles of sex steroids and breast cancer risk, as follows: (i) estrogens are important in the development of postmenopausal breast cancer; (ii) the roles of progestins are complex; (iii) hyperandrogenism may have etiological roles in pre- and postmenopausal breast cancers; and (iv) prolactin moderately increases risk of postmenopausal breast cancer.
> - There is strong evidence that estrogens are important in the development of post-menopausal endometrial cancer, and accumulating epidemiological evidence that hyperandrogenism may have etiological roles in pre- and post-menopausal endometrial cancers.
> - Despite conventional wisdom that increased levels of testosterone increase the risk of prostate cancer, experimental studies are inconsistent and epidemiological associations are lacking.
> - There is accumulating epidemiological evidence, supported by experimental observations, that insulin-like growth factor (IGF)-I is relevant to the development of colorectal, prostate, and premenopausal breast cancers.
> - A considerable body of evidence suggests that vitamin D is protective for colorectal and prostate cancers, but there appears to be a threshold effect requiring high dietary intake levels (greater than 500 IU/day).
> - Adipocytokines are a relatively recently studied hormone system, which may modulate tumor formation, and link obesity with cancer.

Introduction

The principal mechanism by which hormones and growth factors are thought to influence cancer risk is their regulation of the balance between cell proliferation, differentiation and apoptosis. The conventional model posits that increased proliferation rates raise the probability that mutations accumulate in proto-oncogenes and tumor suppressor genes. Ultimately, proliferative stimuli may also enhance the progression and metastasize of established tumors. Increasingly, it is recognized that hormones and growth factors influence other hallmarks of cancers, including supporting angiogenesis, increased cell motility and, even initiation (Fig. 4.1). Furthermore, the development of insensitivity to anti-growth factor signals is a key hallmark in progression of some hormone-sensitive tumors and the emergence of resistance to treatment.

This chapter will focus on five broad groups of hormones and growth factors – sex steroids, prolactin, the insulin–insulin-like growth factor (IGF) axis, vitamin D and adipocytokines – relevant to many common adult cancers. Several other growth factor systems may be relevant to tumor development, of which some are summarized at the end of the chapter. Throughout, the emphasis is on the balance of biological and epidemiological evidence, and wherever relevant, clinical implications will be discussed.

Clinical Endocrine Oncology, 2nd edition. Edited by Ian D. Hay and John A.H. Wass. © 2008 Blackwell Publishing. ISBN 978-1-4051-4584-8.

Sex steroids and cancer risk

For the purposes of descriptions, sex steroids and breast cancer risk have been discussed separately – constituting three conventional hypotheses of breast cancer etiology (Table 4.1) – but in practice, these should be considered as a network of inter-relating systems.

Estrogens and breast cancer

Physiology and biology
There is abundant experimental evidence from *in vitro* and animal models that estrogens are mitogenic in normal and neoplastic mammary tissues [1]. At a molecular level, the estrogen receptor (ER) may act as a ligand-dependent transcription factor that binds estrogen in a reversible fashion and with high affinity to the hormone-binding domain. The possible role of estrogens as mutagens in the initiation of breast tumorigenesis has also been evaluated as estrogens may induce direct or indirect free radical-mediated DNA damage, genetic instability, and mutations in cells in culture and *in vivo*. However, even if estrogens can induce genetic damage, the data overall suggest that proliferative effects are likely to be the most important mechanism.

Epidemiology
Most established risk factors for breast cancer (e.g., early menarche, regular menstrual cycles, older age at first full-term birth, nulliparity,

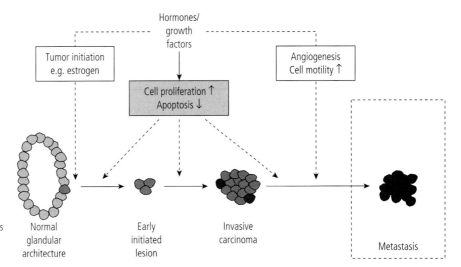

Figure 4.1 Biological mechanisms linking hormones and growth factors with tumor formation and progression.

late menopause, obesity) probably act through estrogen-related pathways, supporting the *unopposed estrogen hypothesis* (Table 4.1). Moreover, there is consistent and strong evidence that increased concentrations of circulating estrogens increase risk of breast

Table 4.1 Three hypotheses of breast cancer development

Unopposed estrogen
This hypothesis stipulates that estrogens stimulate tumor development independently of other hormone, and is supported by the observations that:
- elevated serum concentrations of estrone and estradiol are consistently associated with an increased risk of postmenopausal breast cancer
- factors that increase estrogen exposure (e.g. nulliparity, late age at first birth) are associated with increased breast cancer risk
- factors that decrease estrogen exposure (e.g. multiple births, breast feeding) are associated with reduced breast cancer risk

Estrogen augmented by progesterone
The second major hypothesis posits that breast cancer risk is increased with an elevated exposure to both estrogens and progesterones, and is supported by the observations that:
- increased proliferation rates of breast epithelium occur during the luteal phase of the menstrual cycle, when the ovaries produce both estradiol and progesterone
- combined estrogen–progesterone replacement therapy in post-menopausal women increases breast cancer risk to a greater extent than estrogen alone

Ovarian hyperandrogenism
In the 1960s, Grattarola hypothesized that breast cancer risk is increased among women who have an ovarian androgen excess chronic anovulation, and an associated reduction of luteal-phase progesterone production (later termed the ovarian hyperandrogenism/luteal inadequacy). This hypothesis was based on the observation that breast cancer patients show:
- hyperplasia of the endometrium – a pathognomonic feature of ovarian androgen excess
- chronic anovulation
- progesterone deficiency
The hypothesis is supported by the observation that women with higher plasma or urinary concentrations of testosterone or its urinary metabolites have an increased risk of both pre- and postmenopausal breast cancer

cancer in postmenopausal women. The Endogenous Hormones and Breast Cancer Collaborative Group (EHBCCG) [1], in a pooled analysis of nine prospective studies, showed that postmenopausal breast cancer risk is increased (typically twofold for upper versus lowest quintiles) among women with higher concentrations of circulating sex steroids including dehydroepian-drosterone (DHEA), its sulfate (DHEAS), Δ4-androstenedione, testosterone, estrone, and total estradiol, and decreased concentrations of sex hormone-binding globulin (SHBG) (Table 4.2). The consistency of the associations from earlier studies is borne out in recently reported data from the large European Prospective Investigation into Cancer and Nutrition (EPIC) study [2].

The EPIC study has also reported on the associations of circulating sex hormones and premenopausal breast cancer cases. Whereas previous small-sized cohorts had reported inconsistent findings, EPIC has reported no associations between circulating estrogens and premenopausal breast cancer [3], after adjustment for menstrual cycle changes.

Clinical implications

There is consistent evidence that obesity increases risk of breast cancer in postmenopausal women by approximately 1.5-fold for body mass index (BMI) greater than 30 kg/m^2 compared with less than 25 kg/m^2. This association is partly explained by the increased conversion of androgenic precursors to estradiol through increased aromatase enzyme activity in adipose tissues. Indeed, the EHBCCG analysis demonstrated that the association of BMI with postmenopausal breast cancer risk was almost entirely attributed to the increasing blood levels of estradiol with increasing BMI [1].

Progestins and breast cancer

Physiology and biology

According to the *estrogen augmented by progesterone hypothesis*, the increased risk of breast cancer associated with estrogen is substantially augmented by the addition of progesterone. However,

Table 4.2 Associations of circulating sex steroid concentrations and breast cancer

Studies	Postmenopausal		Premenopausal	
	Cases	RR (95% CIs)*	Cases	RR (95% CIs)†
Estradiol				
EHBCCG	329	2.00 (1.47, 2.71)	–	–
EPIC	261	2.28 (1.61, 3.23)	138‡	1.00 (0.66, 1.52)
Free estradiol				
EHBCCG	189	2.58 (1.76, 3.78)	–	–
EPIC	259	2.13 (1.52, 2.98)	–	–
Non-SHBG estradiol				
EHBCCG	193	2.39 (1.62, 3.54)	–	–
Estrone				
EHBCCG	232	2.19 (1.48, 3.22)	–	–
EPIC	237	2.07 (1.42, 3.02)	138‡	1.16 (0.72, 1.85)
Estrone sulfate				
EHBCCG	129	2.0 (1.26, 3.16)	–	–
Androstenedione				
EHBCCG	193	2.15 (1.44, 3.21)	–	–
EPIC	254	1.69 (1.23, 2.33)	182	1.56 (1.05, 2.32)
DHEA				
EHBCCG	84	2.04 (1.21, 3.45)	–	–
DHEAS				
EHBCCG	295	1.75 (1.26, 2.43)	–	–
EPIC	254	1.69 (1.23, 2.33)	182	1.48 (1.02, 2.14)
Testosterone				
EHBCCG	306	2.22 (1.59, 3.10)	–	–
EPIC	255	1.85 (1.33, 2.57)	181	1.73 (1.16, 2.57)
Free testosterone				
EPIC	255	2.50 (1.76, 3.55)	–	–
Progesterone				
EPIC	–	–	131‡	0.61 (0.38, 0.98)
SHBG				
EHBCCG	223	0.66 (0.43, 1.00)	–	–
EPIC	260	0.61 (0.44, 0.84)	181	0.95 (0.65, 1.40)

Data taken from EHBCCG papers cited in ref. 1, and from refs 2 and 3.

*Based on upper quintile versus referent. The number of cases is breast cancer cases in the upper category.

†Based on upper quartile versus referent. The number of cases is breast cancer cases in the upper category.

‡Based on hormone residuals.

EHBCCG: Endogenous Hormones and Breast Cancer Collaborative Group.

EPIC: European Prospective Investigation into Cancer and Nutrition.

DHEA; dehydroepiandrosterone; DHEAS, dehydroepiandrosterone sulfate; SHBG, sex–hormone binding globulin.

the effect of progesterone on mitogenesis is complex and probably involves several mechanisms [4]. Indeed, progesterone is likely to be neither inherently proliferative nor anti-proliferative and it effects are based on its induction of other growth factors (e.g., epidermal growth factor, EGF, transforming growth factor-α, TGF-α) and proto-oncogenes (e.g., c-fos, c-myc).

Epidemiology

A principal line of evidence advanced in support of the estrogen augmented by progesterone hypothesis is the finding that the proliferation of breast epithelium increases during luteal phase,

reaching a peak 9–10 days after ovulation. However, it has not been established that this peak in proliferative activity is due to progesterone. An alternative hypothesis is that only estrogens stimulate breast epithelial proliferation, but there is a lag of 4–5 days between the estrogen and proliferation peaks. It is well recognized, for instance in endometrial tissues (see below), that the effect of estrogens on proliferation is not direct but through paracrine changes, such as increases in local IGF-I, and this may well also be true for breast. Indeed, in one cohort study (ORDET: 5963 premenopausal women), higher concentrations of mid-luteal progesterone in women with regular menses were associated with a protective effect (relative for upper versus lower tertiles = 0.12, 95% CIs: 0.03, 0.52) [4].

Clinical implications

The main clinical example supporting the estrogen augmented by progesterone hypothesis is that the addition of synthetic progestins to estrogen (both continuous and cyclical) in hormonal replacement therapy (HRT) (see Chapter 84) increases breast cancer risk compared with estrogen alone [5] (Fig. 4.2). However, the increased risk found with the addition of synthetic progestins to estrogen could be due to the progestin used. The progestins used in large randomized trials (namely medroxyprogesterone acetate and 19-nortestosterone derivatives) are endowed with androgenic effects, which may potentiate the proliferative action of estrogens or through hepatocellular effects, decrease insulin sensitivity, decrease levels of SHBG and reverse the reductions in IGF-I induced by oral estrogen [6] – which in turn may be relevant for tumorigenesis.

Androgens and breast cancer

Physiology and biology

There is conflicting experimental evidence regarding the role of androgens in breast cancer development. The conventional wisdom is that androgens inhibit breast growth [7]. Conversely, there are data demonstrating stimulatory proliferative effects on mammary epithelial and breast cancer cells, both *in vitro* and on the growth of experimentally induced mammary tumors in animals [8]. In addition, elevated blood androgen levels may lead indirectly to increased estrogenic exposures to breast tissue because all steroidogenic enzymes necessary for the formation of estrogens from androgenic precursor molecules are present in normal mammary tissues and breast tumors.

Epidemiology

The EHCCBG and EPIC analyses convincingly demonstrate that elevated blood concentrations of androgens are associated with increased risk of breast cancer in both pre- and post-menopausal women (Table 4.2).

Clinical implications

Whereas trials of long-term use of combined estrogen–progesterone have highlighted the enhanced risk of breast cancer, androgens have been postulated to be growth inhibitory for breast tissue, and consequently, testosterone (in combination with estrogen) has been advocated as an alternative HRT approach. The bone stimulatory properties and increased libido may be additional benefits favoring the use of testosterone. While there has been a 500 percent increase in US sales of these preparations in the 10 years following 1993, appropriate patient information on cancer risk and monitoring is recommended [9].

Sex steroids and endometrial cancer

Physiology and biology

During the follicular phase of the menstrual cycle, when the ovaries produce estradiol but virtually no progesterone, epithelial tissue and stromal fibroblasts in the upper two-thirds of the endometrium proliferate. High proliferative rates continue until ovulation, when plasma estradiol levels reach a nadir, and then decline rapidly during the luteal phase of the menstrual cycle, because of the increase in circulating levels of progesterone, which antagonizes the proliferative actions of estrogen. To a great extent, the proliferative actions of estradiol on endometrial tissue are mediated by an increase in the local production (mostly in uterine tissue) of IGF-I. Progesterone diminishes estrogenic action in

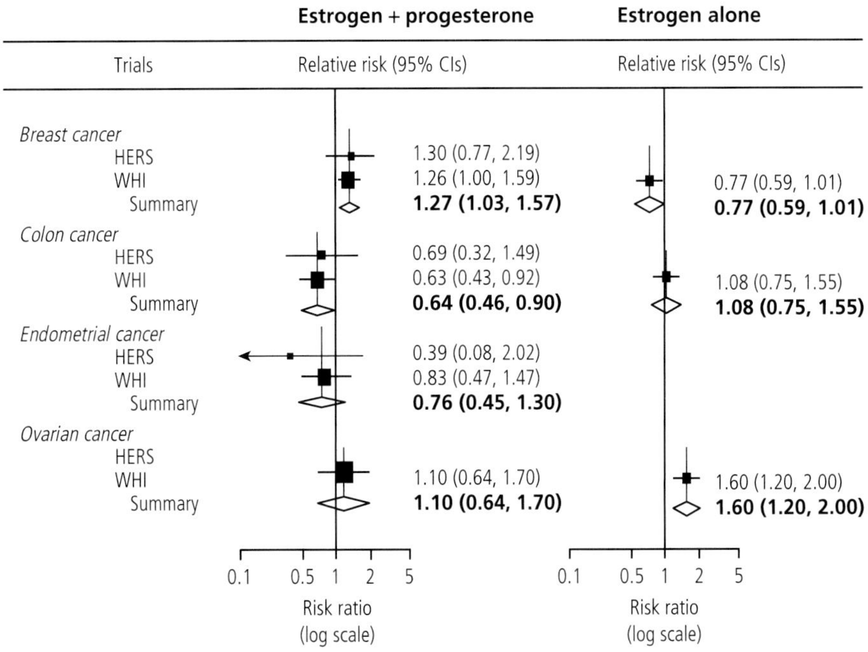

Figure 4.2 Meta-analysis of the two largest HRT randomized trials and risk of main cancers. The Women's Health Initiative (WHI) trial included 27 347 (16 608 with a uterus; 10 739 post hysterectomy) healthy women; the Heart and Estrogen/progestin Replacement Study (HERS) comprised 5526 women with prior coronary heart disease. These data are taken from a variety of papers summarized in ref. 5. Summary estimates generated by random-effect methods in STATA version 8.0 (College Station, TX, USA).

Trials	Estrogen + progesterone Relative risk (95% CIs)	Estrogen alone Relative risk (95% CIs)
Breast cancer		
HERS	1.30 (0.77, 2.19)	
WHI	1.26 (1.00, 1.59)	0.77 (0.59, 1.01)
Summary	**1.27 (1.03, 1.57)**	**0.77 (0.59, 1.01)**
Colon cancer		
HERS	0.69 (0.32, 1.49)	
WHI	0.63 (0.43, 0.92)	1.08 (0.75, 1.55)
Summary	**0.64 (0.46, 0.90)**	**1.08 (0.75, 1.55)**
Endometrial cancer		
HERS	0.39 (0.08, 2.02)	
WHI	0.83 (0.47, 1.47)	
Summary	**0.76 (0.45, 1.30)**	
Ovarian cancer		
HERS		
WHI	1.10 (0.64, 1.70)	1.60 (1.20, 2.00)
Summary	**1.10 (0.64, 1.70)**	**1.60 (1.20, 2.00)**

Risk ratio (log scale)

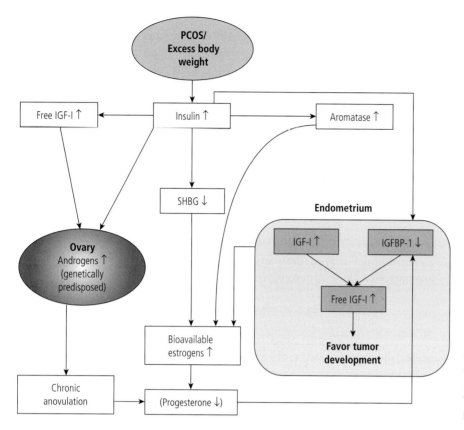

Figure 4.3 Polycystic ovary syndrome (PCOS), obesity and endometrial cancer risk. The examples of increased risk of endometrial cancer in PCOS and obesity share common pathways. SHBG, sex hormone-binding globulin; IGF-I, insulin-like growth factor-I; IGFBP-1, insulin-like growth factor binding protein 1. (Adapted from Calle [11].)

the endometrium by stimulating metabolism of estradiol and inducing the synthesis of IGF binding protein (IGFBP)-1, which inhibits IGF-I action (Fig. 4.3) [10].

Epidemiology

Similar to breast cancer risk, most established risk factors for endometrial cancer (e.g., early menarche, late menopause, obesity) probably act through pathways reflecting greater lifetime exposure to estrogens. Likewise, epidemiological studies have shown that higher levels of plasma estrone and estradiol are associated with increased endometrial cancer risk in post-menopausal women [10]. These relationships may support an "unopposed estrogen" hypothesis for endometrial cancer, but ovarian hyperandrogenism may also be a central mechanism linking lifestyle factors (e.g., obesity: see below) to endometrial cancer risk. Furthermore, epidemiological studies report that elevated plasma androstenedione and testosterone concentrations predict for increased endometrial cancer risk in both pre- and postmenopausal women [10].

Clinical implications

Polycystic ovary syndrome (PCOS) and obesity are associated with an increased risk of endometrial cancer in pre- and post-menopausal women, respectively [11], and share mechanistic pathways that overlap between the estrogen, progesterone, androgen, and IGF systems (Fig. 4.3). PCOS is a complex metabolic syndrome characterized by elevated plasma levels of androstene-

dione, testosterone, and luteinizing hormone. In premenopausal women, ovarian hyperandrogenism probably increases risk by inducing chronic anovulation and progesterone deficiency, decreasing local uterine IGFBP-1 synthesis, which in turn increases bioavailability of IGF-I, favoring tumor formation. While loss of progesterone seems to be the most important physiological risk factor for endometrial cancer development in premenopausal women, in postmenopausal obese women, progesterone synthesis has ceased altogether. Nevertheless, excess weight may continue increasing risk through elevated plasma levels of androgen precursors, and estrogens through the aromatization of the androgens in adipose tissue. In turn, estrogens increase endometrial cell proliferation and inhibit apoptosis, partially by stimulating the local synthesis of IGF-I in endometrial tissue. Additionally, obesity is associated with chronic hyperinsulinemia, which may promote endometrial cancer development by reducing concentrations of SHBG in the blood; this, in turn, increases the levels of bioavailable estrogen that diffuse into endometrial tissue.

Androgens and prostate cancer

Physiology and biology

Conventional medical wisdom decrees that increased levels of testosterone increase the risk of prostate cancer, a belief derived largely from the well-documented regression of prostate cancer following surgical or pharmacological castration. In men, the prostate is the major site of non-testicular production of dihydrotestosterone (DHT), derived primarily through conversion from testosterone by 5α-reductase type 2. In tissue, DHT levels are several times higher than levels of testosterone; by contrast, in serum, levels of DHT are only 10% those of testosterone. In epidemiological studies, serum levels of 5α-androstane-3α, 17β-diol, glucuronide (3α-diol G) are commonly used as an indirect measure of 5α-reductase enzymatic activity, since it is not feasible to measure tissue levels of either testosterone or DHT. In the prostate, DHT binds to the androgen receptor (AR) to form an intracellular DHT–AR complex (testosterone binds with lower affinity), and activates transcription of several genes through binding androgen-response elements, with subsequent induction of DNA synthesis and cell proliferation.

Epidemiology

Despite the above biological evidence, there is an absence of epidemiological data supporting the concept that higher testosterone levels are associated with an increased risk of prostate cancer. Hsing [12] reviewed the evidence from eleven prospective (two cohort; nine nested case–control) studies measuring serum levels of testosterone, DHT and 3α-diol G, and concluded that there was no consistent evidence of association with prostate cancer risk. The same review also described that while many studies report that SHBG is inversely associated with prostate cancer risk, most have not evaluated its independent effect, as levels of SHBG are strongly inversely correlated with levels of free testosterone.

Clinical implications

Clinical trials have shown no increased risk of prostate cancer in hypogonadal men receiving testosterone treatment compared with other hypogonadal men without treatment. However, hypogonadal men have a substantial rate of biopsy-detectable prostate cancer (see Chapter 82), suggesting that low testosterone *per se* has no protective effect against development of prostate cancer.

Prolactin and breast cancer

Physiology and biology

Prolactin is a polypeptide hormone primarily produced in the pituitary gland, important in normal breast development and lactation. During pregnancy, levels of serum prolactin increase in conjunction with estrogens and progesterone, and lead to full lobuloalveolar development of the breasts. Several studies have demonstrated that prolactin mRNA is produced in normal human breast epithelium and that breast cancer cells synthesize appreciate quantities. At least *in vitro*, prolactin may promote cell proliferation and survival, increase cell motility and support tumor vascularization.

Epidemiology

The epidemiologic data on the relationship between circulating prolactin and breast cancer risk are continuing to evolve. In post-menopausal women, most studies have reported a positive association with breast cancer risk, and this association seems strongest for ER+ tumors. Earlier studies in premenopausal women were frequently underpowered and reported no significant association. However, recent data from the Nurses' Health Study cohort II reported a modest increase in breast cancer risk among premenopausal women with higher levels of plasma prolactin ($N = 235$ premenopausal cancers; relative risk = 1.9, 95% CIs: 1.0, 2.3) [13].

Clinical implications

Case reports have suggested that prolactinoma (see Chapter 29), a condition characterized by extremely high prolactin levels, may be associated with increased breast cancer risk. However, a potential confounding issue in these cases is that prolactinomas are frequently associated with hypogonadism, which in turn may counterbalance any increased risk associated with hyperprolactinemia. At a treatment level, past clinical trials aimed at reducing prolactin levels failed to demonstrate effectiveness in the breast cancer treatment as these agents inhibited pituitary prolactin production only. It is now appreciated that prolactin acts locally in breast tissue through prolactin receptor widely expressed in normal and malignant tissues. This receptor system is now an area of active research for targeted anticancer therapy.

Insulin–IGF axis

Insulin and C-peptide

Physiology and biology

Insulin is a two-chain peptide specifically secreted from the pancreatic β cells. Insulin activation of the insulin receptor (IR) triggers intracellular signalling cascades in both the extracellular signal-regulated kinase (ERK) and phosphotidylinositol-3 kinase (PI-3K) pathways, and thus, insulin signalling has the machinery to be mitogenic and anti-apoptotic. Conventionally, however, it is felt that insulin is mitogenic only at supra-physiological levels, and its main proliferative effects are probably mediated through IGF-I receptors [14].

Epidemiology

In cancer epidemiological studies, measurement of serum insulin is highly dependent on the state of fasting, assay characteristics, and genetic factors, and as alternatives, surrogates of insulin secretion (e.g., C-peptide) or of insulin resistance (e.g., HOMA, homeostasis model assessment) are used. Several epidemiological studies have independently linked high circulating levels of serum C-peptide with increased risk of postmenopausal breast cancer, colorectal cancer, and endometrial cancer, consistent with observations that these cancers are also linked with obesity (a hyperinsulinemic state) [14]. Furthermore, insulin resistance is an adverse prognostic factor for breast, colorectal, and prostate cancer-related mortality.

Clinical implications

There is accumulating evidence that type 2 diabetes is associated, independent of obesity, with cancers of the colon, pancreas, kidney and endometrium. Associations are often strongest where the diagnosis of diabetes has been within the 5 years preceding the cancer diagnosis, consistent with the observation that type 2 diabetes is generally characterized by compensatory hyperinsulinemia in its early course. A further dimension is that, at least in the case of colorectal cancer, there is one study in which the use of therapeutic insulin increased the cancer association with type 2 diabetes [15].

Insulin-like growth factors

Physiology and biology

The IGF system is a complex molecular network which includes two ligands (IGF-I and IGF-II), two receptors (IGF-IR and IGF-IIR), six high affinity binding proteins (IGFBP-1 to -6), and several binding protein proteases. IGF-I, IGF-II, and the IGFBPs occur in large quantities in the circulation and are readily measured. The IGF ligands bind IGFBP-3, the main circulating binding protein, to full saturation and together with an acid labile subunit (ALS) form a very stable ternary complex, which does not readily cross compartmental barriers. In terms of cancer risk, studies to date have focused mainly on circulating total IGF-I and IGFBP-3, both of which are growth hormone (GH) dependent, but are also influenced by age, gender, and nutritional status. IGF-I activates the IGF-IR to induce a variety of biological actions that may favor tumor growth including cell proliferation, inhibition of apoptosis, induction of hypoxia-inducible factor (HIF)-1-mediated vascular endothelial growth factor production, induction of tumor-related lymphangiogenesis, and increased cell migration. IGF-I may also regulate cell differentiation, cell size and organization of cellular cytoskeleton, and potentiate the effects of other cell growth stimulants, including estrogens [16].

Epidemiology

Studies in the late 1990s suggested that circulating total IGF-I levels were positively associated, whereas total IGFBP-3 levels were negatively associated, with risk of common cancers including pre-menopausal breast cancer, colorectal cancer, prostate cancer and lung cancer. Subsequent studies and meta-analyses support a relationship between total IGF-I levels and risk of the first three aforementioned malignancies, but reported relationships with IGFBP-3 have been inconsistent [17].

Clinical implications

Obesity is associated with increased risk of several common adult cancers. The molecular mechanisms underlying these associations are not fully understood, but insulin resistance is likely to be important. In its simplest form, the *insulin-cancer hypothesis* postulates that chronic hyperinsulinemia is associated with decreased concentrations of IGF binding proteins 1 and 2, leading to increased availability of free IGF-I with concomitant

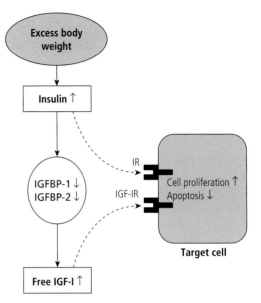

Figure 4.4 Obesity, free IGF-I and cancer risk. Obesity is associated with a state of prolonged hyperinsulinemia, which in turn reduces IGFBP-1 and IGFBP-2 production with resultant increases in the levels of free IGF-I, postulated to be the "bio-active" form of IGF-I. IR, insulin receptor; IGF-IR, insulin-like growth factor-I receptor. (Adapted from Calle [11].)

changes in the cellular environment favoring tumor formation (Fig. 4.4) [11].

Acromegaly (see Chapter 30) is an endocrine disorder characterized by sustained hypersecretion of GH with concomitant elevation of IGF-I, and is associated with a twofold increased risk of colorectal neoplasia [18]. Possible mechanisms underlying this increased risk include direct actions as a consequence of elevated levels of circulating GH and IGF-I and/or other perturbations within the IGF system.

Intimately related to the debate about the IGF system and cancer risk is the potential risk of malignancy in patients receiving GH replacement therapy (see Chapter 81). The scenario of GH therapy in children who have had tumor cranial irradiation previously is well covered but no conclusive evidence presented that tumor recurrence is substantially increased. However, for non-cancer children receiving GH, a UK cohort (N = 1848) study reported an increased incidence and mortality from colorectal cancer in children treated with human pituitary growth hormone (GH) followed up into early adult life [18]. In reality, there were only two cases of colorectal cancer, against an expected incidence of 0.25 cases, and this risk is probably overstated.

Vitamin D

Physiology and biology

In vitro and animal studies indicate that vitamin D may have anti-cancer benefits, including inhibiting progression and metastasis in a wide spectrum of cancers. Supporting an anti-cancer effect of vitamin D is the ability of many cells to convert 25-hydroxyvitamin

D [25(OH)D], the primary circulating form of vitamin D, into 1,25(OH)2D, the most active form of this vitamin.

Epidemiology

Higher rates of total cancer mortality in regions with less UV-B radiation, and among African Americans and obese people, each associated with lower circulating vitamin D, are compatible with a benefit of vitamin D on cancer progression. In addition, poorer survival from cancer in individuals diagnosed in the months when vitamin D levels are lowest suggests a benefit of vitamin D against late stages of carcinogenesis [19].

Clinical implications

The most studied cancer sites are breast, colorectal and prostate. The evidence that higher 25(OH)D levels through increased sunlight exposure or dietary or supplement intake inhibit colorectal carcinogenesis is substantial. However, a key issue that has recently been appreciated is that dietary intakes such as 200–400 IU/day may be too low to exert appreciable benefits, and protection may occur only with higher levels of vitamin D associated with exposure to sunshine.

The biological evidence for an anti-cancer role of 25(OH)D is also strong for prostate cancer, but the epidemiologic data have not been supportive. Some studies suggest that higher circulating 1,25(OH)2D may be more important than 25(OH)D for protection against aggressive, poorly differentiated prostate cancer. Unlike colorectal tumors, prostate cancers lose the ability to hydroxylate 25(OH)D to 1,25(OH)2D, and thus may rely on the circulation as the main source of 1,25(OH)2D.

Adipocytokines

The adipocytokines are biologically active polypeptides that are produced either exclusively or substantially by the adipocytes, which act by endocrine, paracrine, and autocrine mechanisms and may be relevant to tumorigenesis [20]. Leptin, a product of the *ob* gene, is positively associated with obesity and is intrinsically associated with insulin – insulin acts as a positive feedback (IGF-I is a negative regulator) on leptin gene expression, to signal suppression of appetite. Most obese human subjects are leptin-resistant. Leptin binds to the ubiquitous Ob receptor and activates PI3-K and Jak/Stat (Janus kinase/signal transducer and activation of transcription) signalling pathways, critical for cell survival, proliferation and differentiation. Leptin is also pro-angiogenic in both *in vivo* and *in vitro* models. Furthermore, *in vivo* experiments show that calorie restriction significantly decreases tumor growth while concomitantly decreasing circulating leptin levels in rat colon cancer models.

Adiponectin is the most abundant adipocytokine, secreted mainly from visceral adipose tissue, and is inversely related to BMI. It is an important insulin sensitizing agent, with adiponectin-deficient mice being both insulin resistant and diabetes prone. Of importance to tumor development, adiponectin is a negative

regulator of angiogenesis, and in murine models is associated with inhibition of primary tumor growth.

Epidemiology

A variety of case–control and cohort studies have started to emerge addressing the relationships between serum leptin and cancers (prostate and colorectal), and between serum adiponectin and cancers (colorectal, breast and endometrium). The studies to date have been too small to have generalized conclusions, but there have been at least two studies demonstrating that low levels of adiponectin (as it has an inverse relationship with obesity) are significantly associated with endometrial cancer risk.

Clinical implications

Adipocytokines may provide a biological mechanism by which obesity and insulin resistance are causally associated with breast cancer risk and poor prognosis. Both experimental and clinical studies are needed to develop this concept.

Other growth factors

An extensive review of the many other growth factors that may be relevant in cancer is beyond the scope of this chapter, but three specific systems will be summarized.

Vascular endothelial growth factor (VEGF)

Angiogenesis (new blood vessel formation) is a fundamental event in the process of tumor growth and metastatic dissemination, and the VEGF pathway is established as one of the key regulators of this process. The VEGF/VEGF-receptor axis is composed of multiple ligands and receptors with overlapping and distinct ligand–receptor binding specificities, cell-type expression, and function. Activation of this pathway promotes endothelial cell growth, migration, and survival from pre-existing vasculature. Through better understanding of the role of VEGF in promoting tumor angiogenesis, various anti-VEGF/VEGF-receptor therapies have been developed and taken through preclinical studies into everyday oncological practice (e.g., bevacizumab is used in combination with conventional cytotoxic agents for metastatic colorectal cancer).

Epidermal growth factor (EGF)

The importance of EGF is defined by its receptor, a tyrosine kinase which shares considerable homology with the oncogene c-*erb*B2. The EGF receptor (EGFR) is abnormally elevated in many solid tumors, and this in turn is associated with progression and poor prognosis. Multiple mechanisms are involved in the activation of EGFR signaling including production of ligand by tumor and/or stromal cells, high expression of EGFR associated with enhanced sensitivity for EGF-like ligand, and constitutively active EGFR mutations that lead to ligand-independent activation of the receptor. A number of anti-EGFR agents have now been developed and demonstrated to be effective in clinical practice (e.g., gefitinib for non-small cell lung cancer). Whilst these agents induce anti-proliferative cytostatic effects *in vitro*, in several *in vivo* models, anti-EGFR therapies induce tumor regression. This discrepancy suggests that EGFR signaling affects both the tumor and its environment, and it is increasingly emerging that the EGFR receptor is also a key stimulator of angiogenesis. As resistance to anti-EGFR therapy is a clinical problem, these observations have led to the rationale for the development of combined anti-VEGF and anti-EGFR regimens as future anti-cancer approaches [21].

Transforming growth factor beta (TFG-ß)

TGF-β, which bears no structural homology to TGF-α (a tyrosine kinase ligand of the EGF family), comprises three isoforms, TGF-β1, -β2, and -β3. TGF-β1 is most relevant to cancer and was originally shown to be a potent growth inhibitor of epithelial cells through anti-proliferation. Subsequent experiments identified inactivating mutations within the TGF-β1 signalling pathway in cancers, implicating TGF-β1 signalling as a tumor suppressor. However, many human carcinomas (e.g., colon, breast and prostate) overexpress TGF-β1, and this is associated with poor prognosis and increased frequency of metastasis. Similar results have been obtained with tumor cell lines and experimental animal models. Thus, the impact of TGF-β on tumor formation varies in a given circumstance and depends on the cell type involved, the complexity of the TGF-β surface population, the intracellular regulation of the signalling transduction, and the presence of other cytokines. The term *stage specific duality* has emerged to describe this paradigm [22]. Accordingly, the development of specific pharmacological manipulation to prevent or treat cancer through the TGF-β signalling pathway has been difficult.

Acknowledgments

The writings in this chapter represent collaborative studies with many investigators, without whom none of this would have been possible. I would particularly like to thank Professor Stephen M. Shalet for his wisdom, enthusiasm and time in discussing many issues related to the studies presented in this chapter.

References

1. Travis RC, Key TJ. Oestrogen exposure and breast cancer risk. *Breast Cancer Res.* 2003;5:239–247.

2. Kaaks R, Rinaldi S, Key TJ, et al. Postmenopausal serum androgens, oestrogens and breast cancer risk: the European prospective investigation into cancer and nutrition. *Endocr. Relat. Cancer* 2005;12:1071–1082.

3. Kaaks R, Berrino F, Key T, et al. Serum sex steroids in premenopausal women and breast cancer risk within the European Prospective Investigation into Cancer and Nutrition (EPIC). *J. Natl Cancer Inst.* 2005;97:755–765.

4. Campagnoli C, Clavel-Chapelon F, Kaaks R, Peris C, Berrino F. Progestins and progesterone in hormone replacement therapy and the risk of breast cancer. *J. Steroid Biochem. Mol. Biol.* 2005; 96:95–108.

5. Hulley SB, Grady D. The WHI estrogen-alone trial – do things look any better? *JAMA* 2004;291:1769–1771.

6. Renehan AG, Frystyk J, Howell A, et al. The effects of sex steroid replacement therapy on an expanded panel of IGF-related peptides. *Growth Horm IGF Res* 2007;17:210–219.

7. Labrie F, Luu-The V, Labrie C, et al. Endocrine and intracrine sources of androgens in women: inhibition of breast cancer and other roles of androgens and their precursor dehydroepiandrosterone. *Endocr. Rev.* 2003;24:152–182.

8. Liao DJ, Dickson RB. Roles of androgens in the development, growth, and carcinogenesis of the mammary gland. *J. Steroid Biochem. Mol. Biol.* 2002;80:175–189.

9. Rhoden EL, Morgentaler A. Risks of testosterone-replacement therapy and recommendations for monitoring. *N. Engl. J. Med.* 2004;350:482–492.

10. Kaaks R, Lukanova A, Kurzer MS. Obesity, endogenous hormones, and endometrial cancer risk: a synthetic review. *Cancer Epidemiol. Biomarkers Prev.* 2002;11:1531–1543.

11. Calle EE, Kaaks R. Overweight, obesity and cancer: epidemiological evidence and proposed mechanisms. *Nat. Rev. Cancer* 2004;4:579–591.

12. Hsing AW. Hormones and prostate cancer: what's next? *Epidemiol. Rev.* 2001;23:42–58.

13. Tworoger SS, Hankinson SE. Prolactin and breast cancer risk. *Cancer Lett* 2006;66:2476–2482.

14. Renehan AG, Frystyk J, Flyvbjerg A. Obesity and cancer: the role of IGF-I and insulin. *Trends Endocrinol. Metab.* 2006;17:328–336

15. Renehan AG, Shalet SM. Diabetes, insulin therapy, and colorectal cancer. *BMJ* 2005;330:551–552.

16. Pollak MN, Schernhammer ES, Hankinson SE. Insulin-like growth factors and neoplasia. *Nat. Rev. Cancer* 2004;4:505–518.

17. Renehan AG, Zwahlen M, Minder C, O'Dwyer ST, Shalet SM, Egger M. Insulin-like growth factor (IGF)-I, IGF binding protein-3, and cancer risk: systematic review and meta-regression analysis. *Lancet* 2004;363:1346–1353.

18. Renehan AG, O'Connell J, O'Halloran D, et al. Acromegaly and colorectal cancer: a comprehensive review of epidemiology, biological mechanisms, and clinical implications. *Horm. Metab. Res.* 2003;35:712–725.

19. Giovannucci E. The epidemiology of vitamin D and cancer incidence and mortality: a review (United States). *Cancer Causes Control* 2005;16:83–95.

20. Rose DP, Komninou D, Stephenson GD. Obesity, adipocytokines, and insulin resistance in breast cancer. *Obes. Rev.* 2004;5:153–165.

21. van Cruijsen H, Giaccone G, Hoekman K. Epidermal growth factor receptor and angiogenesis: opportunities for combined anticancer strategies. *Int. J. Cancer* 2005;117:883–888.

22. Glick AB. TGFbeta1, back to the future: revisiting its role as a transforming growth factor. *Cancer Biol. Ther.* 2004;3:276–283.

5 Genetic Counseling and Clinical Cancer Genetics

Lucy Side

Key points

- In individuals presenting with a benign or malignant endocrine tumor, an inherited predisposition should be considered because this will have implications for the management of both the patient and their relatives.
- Construction of an accurate three-generation pedigree and recognition of unusual physical phenotypes will facilitate identification of inherited tumor predispositions.
- Predictive genetic testing can identify at-risk individuals in families with an endocrine tumor predisposition and these individuals can be offered screening.
- Where familial conditions manifest in childhood, predictive genetic testing and/or screening can be offered at an age at which complications first present.
- Careful, non-directive genetic counseling is required before offering genetic testing in endocrine tumor predispositions as there are considerable implications for that individual and their family.

Introduction

The majority of cancers, including those of endocrine origin, are sporadic. In general, the risk to relatives is not greatly increased if a single family member is affected with a particular tumor. Nevertheless, a subset of individuals will have an underlying genetic predisposition to developing both benign and malignant tumors. Familial cancer syndromes are characterized by: (i) young age of onset of the primary tumor; (ii) multiple primary tumors in the same individual; (iii) particular types of tumor associated with the condition; and (iv) more than one family member being affected. It is important to recognize these relatively unusual conditions because they will have implications for clinical management of both the patient and their relatives. At-risk individuals can then be identified and offered appropriate screening and early intervention which should be aimed at reducing morbidity and mortality.

Tumor suppressor genes

Most inherited cancer syndromes are caused by mutations in tumor suppressor genes. Tumor suppressor genes encode proteins that play a central role in cellular growth control by regulating diverse processes including signal transduction, cell cycle progression,

Clinical Endocrine Oncology, 2nd edition. Edited by Ian D. Hay and John A.H. Wass. © 2008 Blackwell Publishing. ISBN 978-1-4051-4584-8.

DNA repair and apoptosis [1]. They act in a recessive manner at the cellular level, so that functional inactivation of both alleles is required to deregulate growth. This model was first proposed in 1976 by Knudsen, based on a statistical study of the childhood eye tumor, retinoblastoma. He predicted two "rate-limiting" genetic hits as a prerequisite for developing this tumor in both familial and sporadic cases. This was borne out by molecular studies confirming loss of function mutations in both alleles of the retinoblastoma gene (*RB1*) when the locus was identified. This is a mechanism common to the majority of tumor suppressor genes [1].

Bi-allelic mutations of tumor suppressor genes are found in many sporadic cancers. However, individuals with constitutional mutations of tumor suppressor genes are predisposed to developing a variety of tumors because they have inherited one allele carrying the mutation in every cell. Thus there is a greater chance of the "second hit" occurring in the other allele. This is generally by loss of heterozygosity, whereby there is a somatic deletion encompassing the tumor suppressor and adjacent genes. Other mechanisms include point mutations involving the second allele or, in some cases, imprinting.

A minority of inherited cancer predisposition syndromes are due to mutations in proto-oncogenes. In contrast to tumor suppressor genes, these are activating mutations. The most notable example is the RET proto-oncogene which is mutated in multiple endocrine neoplasia (MEN) type 2. RET encodes a receptor tyrosine kinase and point mutations involving particular codons result in constitutive activation of the receptor and its downstream signalling cascade. As this is a "gain of function" event somatic mutations of the second allele are not generally seen.

Inheritance of cancer predisposition syndromes

Tumor predisposition syndromes, both those due to mutations in proto-oncogenes and tumor suppressors, are generally inherited in an autosomal dominant fashion. Thus an individual inherits a constitutional mutation in one out of the two alleles of the gene. The risk of transmission to offspring is therefore 50:50, or 1 in 2. If a genetic test can be developed for the family it is then possible to use that test to identify individuals at risk before they develop the condition. However, a feature that most dominant conditions share is that of variable expressivity, even within the same family. This is the degree to which the disorder is expressed in an individual and can cause difficulties in genetic counseling. With regard to cancer predisposition, this refers to factors such as age of onset and type of tumor. In addition, non-penetrance may be seen, i.e. individuals who carry a mutation but do not manifest the disorder. Although this is unusual in endocrine cancer predispositions it is important to be cautious in reassuring at-risk individuals that they are unaffected on clinical grounds alone.

Genomic imprinting is seen in the phaeochromocytoma/paraganglioma syndromes due to mutations in the succinate dehydrogenase subunit D (SDHD) gene [2]. Thus, the condition is dominantly inherited, but expression of the disorder is dependent upon the parent of origin of the mutation. In this case, only paternally inherited alleles predispose to tumor development. Autosomal recessive inheritance of tumor predisposition syndromes is the exception, although it does occur.

The role of clinical genetics professionals in the endocrine cancer clinic

Most health professionals are familiar with the term genetic counseling [3]. It encompasses advice and information given to family members where there is a hereditary disorder, concerning their own risk of developing it, likely manifestations, risk to offspring and other relatives, and advice regarding available screening and prevention, including prenatal options. The role may be supportive although genetic counseling would not generally be regarded as psychotherapeutic. One of the central tenets of genetic counseling is that it should be "non-directive." The premise is that the advice given to individuals should enable them to make informed choices for themselves. Thus comments such as "we were told not to have children" should be a thing of the past.

Perhaps the most important contribution of a medical geneticist or genetic counsellor to an endocrine cancer clinic is that they are trained to work with families. This raises a number of different issues compared to the more usual medical scenario of treating an individual patient. Genetics records are generally kept separately as they contain information about a number of individuals; they are kept long term as the information therein may have implications for succeeding generations.

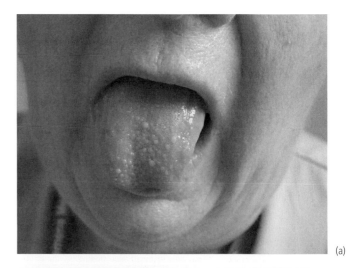

(a)

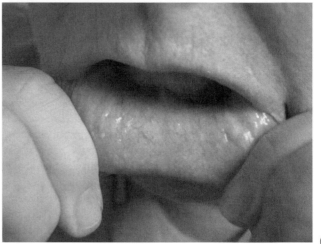

(b)

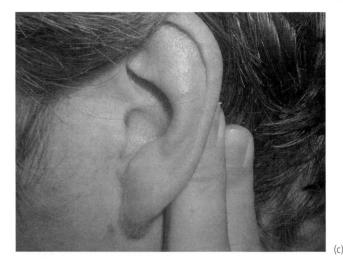

(c)

Figure 5.1 (a–c) Characteristic phenotypic features in Cowden syndrome. This lady presented with bilateral breast cancer aged 40 years. She had macrocephaly (head circumference 62 cm), typical oral mucosal lesions (a and b) and facial trichilemmomas (the pearly white lesions anterior to the pinna). A mutation in the PTEN gene was confirmed. There was a strong family history of breast cancer and thyroid disease.

Accurate recording of a family history may well provide a clue to diagnosis; for example, if a child presents with a pheochromocytoma and there is a family history of brain tumors this might raise the possibility of von Hippel–Lindau (VHL) disease. Recognizing patterns of inheritance may be important; it may be necessary to record a full three-generation pedigree to raise the possibility of an SDHD mutation in a family as the effect of imprinting might lead to apparent non-penetrance. This is not always easy in a busy medical clinic setting but could be carried out by a genetics professional in a joint clinic. In addition, clinical geneticists are trained to recognize unusual phenotypes. For instance, features such as macrocephaly and facial trichilemmomas (benign tumors involving the hair follicle, usually on the face) in a patient with thyroid cancer would be pathognomonic of Cowden syndrome (Fig. 5.1). They can also assist in the clinical application of molecular genetic tests. It is important to remember that a normal gene test in an affected individual does not completely rule out a condition. The majority of techniques routinely used in clinical genetics laboratories are DNA rather than RNA based. They may not detect certain mutations such as those involving the promoter (at the 5′ end of the gene) or intronic mutations giving rise to cryptic splice sites. Likewise, not all genetic alterations are necessarily pathogenic. Finally, geneticists are skilled in counseling unaffected individuals who wish to consider undergoing genetic testing for a hereditary condition. This is termed predictive genetic testing and will be discussed more fully later.

Pedigree drawing

A systematic approach to pedigree drawing is important. Constructing an accurate family tree is the first step in providing genetic advice. Information from both sides of the family should be sought. Although the disorder may be dominantly inherited, this may reveal additional information and go some way toward alleviating anxiety and feelings of guilt in a parent that can sometimes be engendered by a genetic condition. Dates of birth should be recorded rather than ages, and maiden names of women may be helpful in tracking potentially affected relatives. It can be helpful to record addresses of family members. This is because it

may be necessary to verify information from medical records (as patients do not always report this accurately). Cancer registries can be very useful in this regard as they provide accurate records which can be obtained without consent in those deceased, although they do not generally predate the 1970s. Sometimes it may be necessary to obtain consent from living family members to access their medical records. The possibility of non-paternity should be borne in mind when analyzing a pedigree, and although cancer predispositions are generally autosomal dominant, consanguinity should be routinely enquired about as it may alter advice. It may also be important to ask about ethnicity as ancestral or "founder" mutations may be present in certain populations.

Clearly a considerable amount of complex information about family members is required to draw an accurate pedigree and this can be time-consuming. Some cancer genetics services use a questionnaire which is sent out in advance to the patient in order to gather these details. This information can be verified at the consultation. A manually drawn pedigree is usually adequate but there are computerized pedigree drawing programs which can be particularly useful in documenting large families. There are well-recognized symbols for pedigree drawing [4]. The proband is the index affected case in the family (there may be more than one proband) and is generally marked by an arrow, sometimes with the letter "P." Often the individual in the clinic is not the proband, and if they are unaffected are referred to as the consultand. Again, they should be indicated on the pedigree by an arrow, sometimes with the letter "C." A sample pedigree from a MEN 1 family is given in Fig. 5.2.

Risk advice

One of the primary reasons for identifying families with a genetic predisposition to cancer is to give risk estimations to family members. In the first instance there is the risk of carrying the gene. As these conditions are generally dominantly inherited the risk to offspring is 1 in 2. Clearly those family members who do not inherit the gene will have a risk of developing tumors approximating to that of the general population. For those who have inherited the gene, the risk of developing tumors (i.e., the penetrance of the

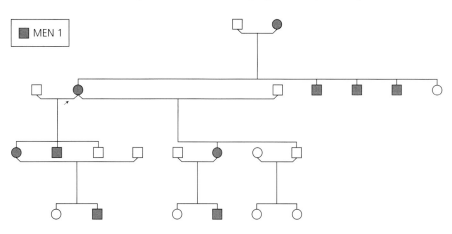

Figure 5.2 A typical pedigree in MEN 1 showing autosomal dominant inheritance.

condition) will generally be available from epidemiological studies. There may be certain genotype-phenotype correlations that need to be considered; for instance, in VHL syndrome the risk of pheochromocytoma may be higher in families with a missense as opposed to a truncating mutation in the VHL gene [5]. MEN 2, MEN 2B, where 95% of cases are due to mutations in codon 918 of RET (M918T), is associated with an earlier onset of medullary thyroid cancer than MEN 2A, where cysteine residues in codons 609, 611, 618, 620, and 634 are generally implicated [6].

If an individual is found to be a gene carrier it may be possible to give accurate advice as to risk, with the caveat that these figures are based on studies rather than being an individual's own personal risk. The question then arises as to how best to express risk so that it is understood by the consultand. Many studies show that family members tend to overestimate their own risk of developing a tumor prior to genetic counseling. However, the results of studies looking at how risk information is conveyed are conflicting; some show a preference for qualitative estimates, i.e., high/moderate/low, whereas others favor numerical risk estimates. The former is more open to different interpretations so current practice tends towards giving quantitative risk figures. It may be useful to do both. Some consultands express a wish not to be given numerical information and it can be helpful to enquire about this.

So if numerical information is to be conveyed, how best to do it? It is useful to give figures both for the risk of developing a tumor versus the chances of not developing it. In terms of tumor risk this may be expressed as: (i) risk per annum; (ii) lifetime risk; (iii) as a fraction or a percentage, e.g. 1 in 5, or 20%; or (iv) age-corrected risk, with the concept that in some conditions an individual may already have "lived through" some of their risk. For instance, in MEN 1 the risk of developing gastrinomas and somatotropinomas is greater in those older than 40 years, whereas insulinomas are commoner under the age of 40 years and one might wish to modify counseling accordingly [7]. Again, it is often helpful to express risk in more than one way numerically. It is also standard practice in clinical genetics to write directly to the patient with this information.

It should also be borne in mind when counseling about risk that different types of penetrance figures exist. In MEN 1 biochemical and clinical penetrance differ. In the study of Trump et al. the percentages of patients who were symptomatic at ages 20, 35, and 50 years were 18%, 52% and 78% respectively whereas in individuals who were screened biochemically percentages at those ages increased to 43%, 85%, and 94% [7].

Principles of predictive genetic testing for endocrine cancer predisposition

Giving accurate and understandable risk advice to individuals with an endocrine tumor predisposition is clearly an important aspect of genetic counseling. Perhaps more challenging is the process of predictive genetic testing; that is, offering unaffected individuals in a family a genetic test to see if they carry the familial mutation. If they do carry the mutation this will have widespread and lifelong implications for a person who is generally healthy at the time of taking the test, not only for their own health but also for the health of their (future) children. It may impinge upon other aspects of their lives such as employment and insurance. It is worth discussing these issues at some length with the consultand so that they can make an informed decision as to whether or not they would wish to proceed with predictive testing. There is considerable evidence from families that they adapt better to an adverse result if some time has gone into preparing for this eventuality [8].

A prerequisite for offering predictive genetic testing should be that a definite pathogenic mutation in the gene for the condition has been identified within the family. Genetic linkage is rarely used now, i.e., polymorphic genetic markers that are closely linked to the disease gene are analyzed in affected family members and used to develop a genetic test. There is a greater chance of error here depending upon the distance of the genetic markers used from the gene locus itself due to the possibility of genetic recombination. In general, testing should not be offered to unaffected individuals if the familial mutation is unknown. In these circumstances a normal genetic test cannot be regarded as completely reassuring. As discussed previously, existing techniques will not detect all mutations so it may be unwise to withdraw screening in these circumstances.

It should also be remembered that a DNA test is not the only type of predictive genetic test. For instance, if an unaffected individual at 50% risk of developing MEN 1 is shown to have an elevated calcium level then it is highly likely that they carry the familial MEN 1 mutation. In essence, this test could also be regarded as a "genetic test." Likewise, examining an at-risk individual can confirm genetic status where there is a definite phenotype associated with the condition. For example, in MEN 2B, the finding of the typical "marfanoid" body habitus or mucosal neuromas [6] would indicate that individual is affected. Consideration should be given to counseling before offering these tests.

Patients should not be directed to undertake genetic testing but allowed to make their own choices. Generally the model that is used follows that used in Huntington disease, a condition where there is probably more experience of the psychological consequences of predictive genetic testing than any other. The issues of testing in endocrine cancer predisposition may be somewhat different to neurodegenerative conditions such as Huntington's in that effective screening and, in the case of MEN 2, effective prophylactic surgery are available. Nevertheless, many of the other issues such as feelings of loss, implications for family dynamics, insurance and possibly employment remain similar. The finding of a mutation should not be a prerequisite for offering screening, and this should be offered to individuals at risk even if they choose not to undergo predictive genetic testing. Certainly, this would be offered to at-risk individuals in families where no mutation could be found.

Sometimes a person at 25% risk of carrying a mutation will request predictive genetic testing, i.e., if a parent who is at 50% risk has chosen not to undertake testing, so their affected status is unknown. In these circumstances efforts should be made to engage with the parent, since a test that shows their offspring to be affected would be in effect testing them without their having solicited the information. This may not be possible in all families in which case the benefits to the individual at 25% risk should be weighed against the potential harms (such as the parent's right "not to know"). Careful counseling is needed before proceeding in these circumstances.

A suggested schedule for predictive genetic testing is given in Table 5.1. Several family members may be present at the first appointment but at the second appointment the consultand should be encouraged to attend with a support person, often a spouse or friend who would not be at risk of carrying the gene. Sometimes it may be appropriate to offer only one appointment before proceeding to a genetic test, in which case it is inadvisable to test more than one individual at the same time. Results should

Table 5.1 A suggested program for predictive genetic testing in endocrine cancer predisposition based on the Huntington disease model [8]

Appointment 1
- Review genetic nature of cancer, mode of inheritance, risks of specific tumors occurring
- Outline the test program and timescale
- Discuss support network and desirability of support person at subsequent appointments
- Discuss the experience of the disease in the family and how it has impacted upon family members, including the consultand. Who else is considering testing?
- Explore family dynamics. Who have they told that they are considering a test?
- Question why they might want a test, e.g., screening/prevention, desire to know, planning for a future family, etc.
- What do they feel is their risk of developing cancer?
- Insurance implications
- Implications of a result showing that they are unaffected, e.g. potential feelings of "survivor" guilt when other family members are affected and they are not
- Implications of a result showing they carry the gene – available screening options, psychological impact, effect on children or possibility of having children
- Schedule next appointment if consultand wishes to proceed

Appointment 2
- Review why they want the test and information given at first appointment
- What difference having the test will make
- Feelings of family, friends
- Timescale and practicalities of testing
- Review potential interventions
- Answer any questions
- Obtain consent for testing and advise them to attend with support for the results appointment

Appointment 3
- Give results
- Discuss ongoing support from genetics team and refer to other health care professionals as appropriate for screening, etc.
- Offer follow-up phone call 1–2 weeks after giving result

be given in person to assess their impact and offer the level of support that may be necessary.

Genetics and insurance

The aim of clinical genetics is to help families with hereditary conditions live and reproduce as normally as possible, without discrimination. The view is that genetic testing should not be required for any type of insurance policy, nor the results of a genetic test need to be disclosed. This has been ratified by the Genetics and Insurance Committee and the Association of British Insurers in the UK and the agreement is in place until 2011, when it will be reviewed. Currently only policies for life insurance above £500 000 (or £300 000 for critical illness cover) require disclosure of the results of an approved genetic test. Nevertheless, insurers can ask for details of family history and may weight policies accordingly [9]. In the USA, the American Society of Clinical Oncology (ASCO) also supports the principle that genetic testing for cancer predispositions should not result in any kind of discrimination with regard to employment and insurance [10]. However, laws governing this issue vary between states and local advice should be sought.

Genetic testing of children

In some circumstances testing may be offered to children who are unable to give fully informed consent. This is appropriate when the onset of the condition may be in childhood and screening or surgery can be offered. However, testing for adult-onset disorders should not generally be offered in childhood [11]. Again, screening can be offered to children at risk even if they or their parents choose to wait before undertaking genetic testing (with the caveat that screening may reveal affected status). According to the Children's Act in the UK parents have a responsibility to act in the best interests of their child. Testing should not generally be carried out to allay parental anxieties or for their "need to know," if a test can be deferred until adulthood because there is no useful medical intervention [11]. In the USA a similar approach has been proposed by the American Society of Human Genetics [12]. In principle testing for endocrine tumor syndromes may be offered at an age at which screening will start. It is beyond the scope of this chapter to discuss detailed screening programs for individual endocrine disorders, but examples are given below (Table 5.2).

Prenatal diagnosis and preimplantation genetic diagnosis for endocrine cancer predisposition

If the familial mutation is known it is possible to offer mutation testing in pregnancy to determine if the fetus is affected. DNA testing can be carried out by chorionic villous sampling at around 11 weeks' gestation or by amniocentesis from around 15 weeks.

Table 5.2 Suggested ages to commence screening and offer predictive genetic testing in endocrine tumor syndromes

Tumor predisposition syndrome	Gene	Suggested screening/prevention	Age (years) screening commences
MEN 1	MEN1	Annual fasting glucose, insulin, Ca^{2+}, PTH, PRL, IGF-1, chromogranin-A; MRI pituitary* (3 yearly), MRI abdo (3 yearly from 20 years)	Consider biochemical screening at 5 years [14]
MEN 2A/Familial medullary thyroid carcinoma (FMTC)	RET	Prophylactic thyroidectomy; annual urine catecholamines, Ca^{2+}, PTH, pentagastrin (8 years)	Before 5 years (thyroidectomy) [14]
MEN 2B	RET	Prophylactic thyroidectomy, annual urine catecholamines, Ca^{2+}, PTH, pentagastrin (8 years)	Before 2 years (thyroidectomy) [14]
Hyperparathyroidism–jaw tumor syndrome (HPT-JT)	HRPT2	Annual Ca^{2+}, PTH	Consider biochemical screening at 10 years
Carney complex	PRKAR1A, 2nd locus on 2p16	Annual echocardiography, urine free cortisol, IGF-1, thyroid exam, consider testicular ultrasound	Echocardiography from birth or at diagnosis
VHL	VHL	Annual direct and indirect ophthalmoscopy, urine catecholamines (10 years), abdominal MRI (15 years), 3 yearly brain MRI (15 years)	Retinal screening at 5 years [18]
Pheochromocytoma/paraganglioma syndromes	SDHB	Annual urine catecholamines, abdominal MRI scans (7 years) and thoracic 3 yearly. MRI neck 3 yearly (20 years)	Annual urine catecholamines from age 5 years [2]
Pheochromocytoma/paraganglioma syndromes	SDHD	Annual urine catecholamines, abdominal MRI scans (7 years) and thoracic 5 yearly. MRI neck 1–2 yearly (20 years)	Annual urine catecholamines from age 5 years [2]
Cowden syndrome	PTEN	Annual thyroid exam, annual mammograms, skin exam (from 30 years)	Thyroid at ~18 years or 5 years younger than earliest cancer in family [19]
Neurofibromatosis type 1 (NF1)	NF1	Annual blood pressure, eye exam incl. visual fields	At diagnosis [20]

MRI, magnetic resonance imaging; PTH, parathyroid hormone; PRL, prolactin; IGF-1, insulin-like growth factor.

Both of these are invasive tests carrying a risk of miscarriage although in future it may be possible to offer non-invasive testing on fetal DNA isolated from maternal blood. Many parents will not choose to undergo prenatal testing unless they would contemplate terminating an affected pregnancy. For the majority of endocrine cancer predispositions, there is no advantage to knowing genetic status at this stage as it would not alter management. The Human Fertilization and Embryo Authority in the UK have recently approved the use of pre-implantation genetic diagnosis in inherited cancer predispositions. Briefly, this is testing of an embryo at the eight-cell stage (usually on DNA extracted from one or two cells) to see if the familial mutation is present. Only embryos not carrying the mutation are implanted into the womb [13]. The chances of carrying a pregnancy successfully to term by this method are around 1 in 5. Both options should be broached as part of genetic counseling so that parents are aware of potential reproductive choices.

Genetic testing in sporadic cancers

Should genetic testing be offered to the proband in apparently sporadic endocrine cancers? In some circumstances this is true. For medullary thyroid cancer, probands should routinely be offered testing for RET mutations. The detection rate for DNA testing in RET is high as these are point mutations at particular codons in the gene. Therefore a normal result in the proband is reassuring for other family members who are at low risk and do not need to be offered screening [14]. If a mutation is found family members can be offered testing and prophylactic thyroidectomy if shown to be mutation carriers. Recent data suggests that up to 25% of sporadic pheochromocytomas are due to an underlying genetic predisposition [15]. Neurofibromatosis type 1 (NF1) may be ruled out on clinical grounds, but DNA testing may be considered for *RET*, *vHL* and *SDHB* and *SDHD* mutations, particularly if the phaeochromocytoma is detected prior to the age of 40 years [15]. With sporadic paragangliomas, testing for SDHB and SDHD may be appropriate. As always, the proband should be counseled as to the implications should a mutation be discovered. The European guidelines for management of MEN 1 advocate testing individuals with isolated parathyroid adenomas for MEN 1 mutations [14]. However the incidence of MEN 1 mutations in these individuals is unknown, so this needs further evaluation. One difficulty with testing in these circumstances (with the possible exception of RET) is that genetic alterations may be found which may or may not be pathogenic – sometimes termed "variants of unknown significance." Usually these are single amino acid changes. It is important to be aware of this as it can cause difficulties in genetic counseling and these variants should not be offered as tests for other family members.

Mosaicism

This means that not all cells of the body carry the mutation and can be difficult to determine clinically. Germline mosaicism refers to one or more gametes being affected, somatic mosaicism that only a part of the body is affected, and gonosomal mosaicism is used where both of the above are present. In practice this means that if a mutation is found on DNA testing in an individual with an apparently sporadic endocrine cancer siblings should also be offered testing because of the possibility of mosaicism, even if both parents do not carry the mutation in blood. In some circumstances parents may also be offered screening if they do not carry the mutation found in their offspring. This is particularly true in VHL, where there is a significant rate of somatic or gonosomal mosaicism estimated to be of the order of 5% [16]. We have also observed gonosomal mosaicism in MEN 1 (R Thakker, personal communication). In conditions with a clinical phenotype such as NF1, mosaicism in parents may be detectable clinically as typical pigmentation affecting only part of the body [17]. This should be looked for, as it may affect reproductive risks.

Genetic registers

Because of the long-term and preventative nature of clinical cancer genetics it may be desirable to develop a register system for the management of families with endocrine cancer predispositions. The register needs to be accurate and regularly updated. It may be used as a patient management tool so that screening is carried out in a timely fashion and patients are not lost to contact. It may be used in genetic counseling so that families are contacted and offered testing when a child reaches an age where screening

would be offered. Families may be contacted if new treatment options become available. Confidentiality is of paramount importance in maintaining genetic registers and consent is advised if a family is to be included [3].

Support groups

Many patients with genetic conditions are very well informed, both from the effect of the disorder in their own family and outside sources such as the internet. However, support groups also provide a useful source of information and, for those interested, contact with other affected individuals, educational meetings and newsletters, often with news about recent research. Information about relevant support groups should form part of the genetic counseling consultation and some examples are given below.

Contact a Family. General information on genetic conditions. http://www.cafamily.org.uk/.
AMEND. The Association for Multiple Endocrine Neoplasia Disorders. http://www.amend.org.uk/
VHL Family Alliance. For von Hippel–Lindau disease. http://www.vhl.org/
Neurofibromatosis Association. http://www.nfauk.org/

References

1. Weinberg RA. Tumour suppressor genes. *Science* 1991;254:1138–1146.
2. Benn DE, Gimenez-Roqueplo A-P, Reilly JR, et al. Clinical presentation and penetrance of pheochromocytoma/paraganglioma syndromes. *J. Clin. Endocrinol. Metab.* 2006;91:827–836.
3. Harper PS. *Practical Genetic Counselling*, 6th edn. Oxford: Oxford University Press, 2004.
4. Bennet RL, Steinhaus KA, Uhrich SB, et al. Recommendations for standardised Human Pedigree Nomenclature. *Am. J. Hum. Genet.* 1995;56:745–752.
5. Ong KR, Woodward ER, Killick P, et al. Genotype phenotype correlations in von Hippel-Lindau disease. *Hum. Mutat.* 2007;28:143–149.
6. Thakker RV. Multiple endocrine neoplasia. *Medicine* 1997;86–88.
7. Trump D, Farren B, Wooding C, et al. Clinical studies of multiple endocrine neoplasia type 1 (MEN1). *Q. J. Med.* 1996;89:653–669.
8. Harper PS, Lim C, Crauford D. Ten years of presymptomatic testing for Huntington's disease: the experience of the UK Huntington's Disease Prediction Consortium. *J. Med. Genet.* 2000;37:567–571.
9. British Society of Human Genetics Statement on Genetics and Life Insurance – May 1998. At http://www.bshg.org.uk/documents/official_docs/Insurance/insuranc.htm
10. ASCO policy statement update: Genetic Testing for Cancer Susceptibility. *J. Clin. Oncol.* 2003;21:2397–2406.
11. Clarke A. The genetic testing of children. Working Party of the Clinical Genetics Society (UK). *J. Med. Genet.* 1994;31:785–797.
12. ASHG/ACMG report. Points to consider: ethical, legal and psycho-social implications of genetic testing in children and adolescents. *Am. J. Hum. Genet.* 1995;57:1233–1241.

13. Braude P, Pickering S, Flinter M, Ogilvie CM. Preimplantation genetic diagnosis. *Nat. Rev. Genet.* 2002;3:941–953.

14. Brandi ML, Gagel RF, Angeli A, et al. Guidelines for diagnosis and therapy of MEN type 1 and type 2. *J. Clin. Endocrinol. Metab.* 2001;86:5658–5671.

15. Neumann HP, Bausch B, McWhinney SR, et al. Germ-line mutations in nonsyndromic pheochromocytoma. *N. Engl. J. Med.* 2002;346: 1459–1466.

16. Sgambati MT, Stolle C, Choyke PL, et al. Mosaicism in von Hippel-Lindau disease: lessons from kindreds with germline mutations identified in offspring with mosaic parents. *Am. J. Hum. Genet.* 2000;66:84–91.

17. Huson SM, Ruggieri M. The clinical and diagnostic implications of mosaicism in the neurofibromatosis. *Neurology* 2001;56:1433–1443.

18. Maher ER, Yates JR, Harries R, et al. Clinical features and natural history of von Hippel-Lindau disease. *Q. J. Med.* 1990;77:1151–1163.

19. Pilarski R, Eng C. Will the real Cowden syndrome please stand up (again)? Expanding mutational and clinical spectra of the PTEN hamartoma tumour syndrome. *J. Med. Genet.* 2004;41:323–326.

20. Ferner R, Huson SM, Thomas N. Guidelines for the diagnosis and management of individuals with Neurofibromatosis 1 (NF1). *J. Med. Gen.* 2007;44:81–88.

6 Prospects for Gene Therapy for Endocrine Malignancies

Christine Spitzweg, Ian D. Hay, and John C. Morris

> **Key points**
> - Gene therapy for endocrine cancer represents a new technology that takes direct advantage of our improved understanding of tumor carcinogenesis at the molecular level.
> - Various gene therapy strategies, including corrective, cytoreductive, antiangiogenic and immunomodulatory gene therapy as well as virus-mediated oncolysis, have shown promising results in follicular cell-derived and medullary thyroid cancer in preclinical studies and therefore represent attractive approaches for future therapy.
> - The sodium iodide symporter (NIS) is one of the most promising suicide genes available for cancer gene therapy that has been studied in a variety of endocrine and endocrine-responsive tumors, including thyroid cancer, prostate, ovarian and breast cancer, neuroendocrine tumors and adrenocortical cancer.
> - Since clinical efficacy of gene therapy is not only determined by the potency of therapeutic genes, but also by the efficiency of vector-mediated gene delivery, the chief challenge facing clinical gene therapy application is the development of safe and efficient gene delivery systems allowing systemic administration.

Cancer gene therapy

Gene therapy for endocrine cancer represents a new technology that, more than any currently available therapy, takes direct advantage of our improved understanding of tumor carcinogenesis at the molecular level. For several reasons gene therapy is particularly attractive for the treatment of endocrine tumors: (1) most endocrine organs are located at easily accessible anatomical sites allowing direct inoculation of the gene transducing vector; (2) for almost all endocrine organs tissue-specific transcriptional control elements (tissue- or tumor-specific promoters) are available, providing a tool for transcriptional targeting of therapeutic genes; (3) endocrine tissues express a variety of tissue-specific surface proteins, such as hormone receptors, that may be used as targets for molecular engineered vectors; (4) the fact that most functions of endocrine organs are either "dispensable" or can be substituted by established hormone replacement therapy allows the clinician to pursue therapeutic strategies, including gene therapy, that might ablate normal as well as malignant endocrine cells.

Cancer gene therapy can be defined as transfer of genetic material to malignant cells for a therapeutic purpose. The term gene therapy encompasses a range of approaches (Fig. 6.1), as follows:

- *Corrective gene therapy*: restoration of the normal function of a deleted or mutated gene (usually a tumor suppressor gene) or negating the effect of a tumor-promoting gene (oncogene).
- *Cytoreductive gene therapy*: delivery of an exogenous gene that causes cell death or allows the application of cytotoxic agents, i.e. a "suicide gene."
- *Immunomodulatory gene therapy*: delivery of genes that enhance immune responses against tumor tissues.
- *Virus-mediated oncolysis*: use of engineered replication-competent viruses that selectively replicate in tumor cells, thereby inducing viral oncolysis.

Gene therapy strategies based on these different approaches have been extensively studied in endocrine malignancies, especially thyroid cancer, but also in other endocrine or endocrine-responsive tumors, including prostate, breast, ovarian and adrenal cancer, as well as neuroendocrine tumors of the gastrointestinal tract. The limiting step for successful clinical application of gene therapy is the development of an efficient and safe gene transfer system. Currently available vectors for gene therapy can be divided into non-viral and viral vectors. While most vectors presently in use are based upon viruses, mainly retro- and adenoviruses, the development of novel non-viral nanoparticles seems to be a promising approach for future systemic gene therapy applications. In the following chapter the most promising gene therapy approaches that have been investigated in thyroid cancer will be summarized, including corrective, cytoreductive and immunomodulatory approaches as well as virus-mediated oncolysis. In addition, the results of a novel cytoreductive gene therapy strategy based on

Clinical Endocrine Oncology, 2nd edition. Edited by Ian D. Hay and John A.H. Wass. © 2008 Blackwell Publishing. ISBN 978-1-4051-4584-8.

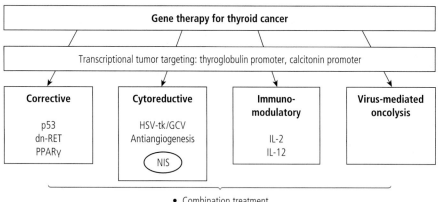

Figure 6.1 Overview of gene therapy approaches for thyroid cancer.

sodium iodide symporter (NIS) gene transfer followed by radioiodine therapy in thyroid cancer and a variety of other endocrine and endocrine-related malignancies will be discussed.

Gene therapy in thyroid cancer

Despite multimodality treatment for thyroid cancer, including surgical resection, radioiodine (^{131}I) therapy, thyroid-stimulating hormone (TSH)-suppressive thyroxine treatment and chemo-/radiotherapy, survival rates have not improved over the last decades, in particular for medullary and anaplastic thyroid cancer. Therefore, development and evaluation of novel treatment strategies, including gene therapy approaches, are urgently needed.

Corrective gene therapy

Restoration of the p53 tumor suppressor gene in follicular cell-derived thyroid cancer

Wild-type (wt)-p53 protein mediates critical cellular responses, including cell cycle arrest and apoptosis, in response to DNA damage. Most poorly differentiated thyroid tumors have lost expression of the normal p53 tumor suppressor gene through inactivating mutations, which seem to be late genetic events associated with loss of differentiation and may be, at least in part, responsible for the aggressive behavior of dedifferentiated tumors. Restoration of wt-p53 expression has recently been investigated in a variety of experimental cancer models including thyroid cancer and has also been tested in first human clinical trials [1–3]. In contrast to other corrective gene therapy approaches, which reveal the central weakness that each cell must be targeted for tumor eradication, one of the advantages of p53 restoration is its association with a bystander effect resulting from an antiangiogenic effect that affects non-transduced neighbor cells. Since *in vivo* transduction efficiency is limited by low levels of vector delivery to tumor cells and by the toxicity of available vector systems, a bystander effect is desirable for any kind of gene therapy strategy, because it reduces the level of transduction efficiency required for a therapeutic response.

Several studies in follicular cell-derived thyroid cancer have demonstrated that viral- and non-viral-mediated p53 re-expression results in apoptosis-induced cell killing *in vitro* and inhibition of tumorigenesis *in vivo*. In addition, wt-p53 expression was shown to sensitize some of the cell lines to the chemotherapeutic effect of doxorubicin, 5-fluorouracil or adriamycin, offering the possibility of combination therapy [1–3]. Further, retrovirally driven p53 restoration in anaplastic thyroid cancer was recently demonstrated to be associated not only with an antitumor effect, but also with a redifferentiating effect allowing the application of therapeutic genes under the control of a thyroid-specific promoter through induction of thyroid-specific gene re-expression, such as thyroglobulin (Tg) [4].

PPARγ overexpression in follicular cell-derived thyroid cancer

Peroxisome proliferator-activated receptor γ (PPARγ) is a nuclear receptor that is involved in a wide range of cellular processes including adipogenesis, insulin sensitization, cell cycle control, apoptosis, and carcinogenesis. PPARγ ligands, such as thiazolidinediones, have been demonstrated to decrease the growth rate of various tumor cell lines in addition to induction of differentiation and apoptosis. A translocation that fuses the thyroid-specific transcription factor PAX8 gene with the PPARγ gene (PAX8/PPARγ fusion gene) has been identified in approximately 50% of follicular thyroid carcinomas and has been further characterized as a novel oncogene that accelerates cell growth and reduces apoptosis through dominant-negative inhibition of wild-type PPARγ [5]. Interestingly, PPARγ gene transfer into follicular cell-derived thyroid cancer cells not only drastically reduced the cell gowth rate but also allowed an additional growth-inhibiting effect by the combined treatment with PPARγ agonists [1], suggesting that PPARγ could be a promising novel target for innovative thyroid cancer treatment, in particular anaplastic thyroid cancer unresponsive to conventional therapy.

Inhibition of oncogenic RET signaling in medullary thyroid cancer

More than 95% of medullary thyroid carcinomas harbor dominant activating mutations in the RET proto-oncogene, which play a central role in the development of medullary thyroid cancer through constitutive activation of RET tyrosine kinase with aberrant downstream signaling and initiation of tumor formation. Inhibition of oncogenic RET signaling by expression of a dominant-negative RET mutant has been investigated as a promising new corrective gene therapy approach in medullary thyroid cancer [6]. These dominant-negative RET mutants inhibit expression of oncogenic RET protein on the cell surface by dimerization with oncogenic RET protein in the endoplasmic reticulum (ER) and disturbing the glycosylation process. Using an adenoviral vector expressing dominant-negative RET under the control of a C-cell specific synthetic calcitonin/calcitonin gene-related peptide promoter, a pronounced shift of endogenous oncogenic RET protein localization from the cell surface to the ER was demonstrated, resulting in strong apoptosis-induced inhibition of cell viability *in vitro* and prolonged survival *in vivo* [6]. However, one of the major drawbacks of this elegant oncogene-inhibiting gene therapy approach in medullary thyroid cancer is its lack of a bystander effect, thus requiring high levels of *in vivo* transduction efficiency, limiting its therapeutic efficacy *in vivo*.

Taken together, corrective gene therapy has shown promising preliminary results in follicular cell-derived and medullary thyroid cancer. However, besides the usual lack of a bystander effect, another serious potential drawback of corrective gene therapy is that correcting a single gene may not be sufficient to achieve a therapeutic effect, considering that the pathogenesis of thyroid cancer is a multi-step process involving sequential accumulation of genetic defects. In the case of p53 gene therapy, this could be compensated by its chemo- and radiosensitizing effect, offering the possibility of a multimodality approach to improve its therapeutic efficacy.

Cytoreductive gene therapy

Suicide gene/prodrug therapy
A common strategy for cytoreductive gene therapy is the use of the suicide gene/prodrug combination of Herpes simplex virus thymidine kinase and ganciclovir. Expression of herpes simplex virus thymidine kinase (HSV-tk) in tumor cells allows phosphorylation of the prodrug ganciclovir (GCV), which then competes with deoxyguanosine triphosphate in the process of DNA polymerization, resulting in DNA synthesis arrest and cell death. Therapeutic efficacy of suicide gene therapy is significantly enhanced by a bystander effect in non-transduced cells resulting from diffusion of phosphorylated GCV to neighboring cells, as well as an antitumor immune response. A therapeutic effect of GVC was demonstrated in follicular cell-derived thyroid carcinoma cell lines following retrovirus- and adenovirus-mediated HSV-tk gene transfer, which was associated with a significant bystander and radiosensitizing effect *in vitro* and *in vivo* in xenografted tumors in nude mice [1–3]. In order to minimize extratumoral toxicity, the tissue-specific thyroglobulin promoter as well as the tumor-specific telomerase reverse transcriptase promoter were successfully applied *in vitro* and *in vivo* to target the HSV-tk gene to Tg-expressing and undifferentiated thyroid carcinoma cells, respectively [1–3].

The effectiveness of the HSV-tk/GCV system has also been demonstrated in medullary thyroid cancer *in vitro* and *in vivo*. To restrict suicide gene expression and toxicity to medullary thyroid cancer cells, C-cell-specific adenoviral HSV-tk gene transfer was performed by introduction of the HSV-tk cDNA into exon 4 of the calcitonin mini gene (exon 3–5) coupled to the calcitonin promoter, thereby taking advantage of C-cell-specific alternative RNA splicing [1–3].

To achieve the ultimate goals of cancer therapy, which are maximal tissue- or tumor-specific cytotoxicity with a minimum of toxic effects in non-malignant cells, as well as elimination of metastatic cancer cells in addition to the local tumor, the application of tissue- or tumor-specific promoters provides a well-established way of transcriptionally targeting therapeutic genes selectively to cancer cells. In the case of thyroid cancer, several tissue-specific promoters, such as the Tg promoter or the calcitonin promoter, are available and have successfully been applied to target therapeutic genes to cancer cells. In the case of the Tg promoter, promoter activity can be enhanced by treatment with histone deacetylase inhibitors and 8-bromo-cAMP, or by application of a tandemly repeated Tg core promoter. In addition, the Cre/loxP system can be used to overcome the weakness of tissue- or tumor-specific promoters, which has successfully been demonstrated for Tg promoter-driven HSV-/tk/GCV therapy [2, 7]. Activity and tissue specificity of the calcitonin promoter were enhanced by combination of a minimal human calcitonin promoter with multiple copies of tissue-specific enhancer elements, and by taking advantage of C-cell-specific RNA splicing as described above [6].

Taken together, *in vivo* as well as *in vivo* experiments in several follicular cell-derived and medullary thyroid cancer cell lines have clearly demonstrated a therapeutic effect of the HSV-tk/GCV strategy, which is enhanced by its bystander effect and the possibility of combination with chemo- or radiotherapy due to its chemo- and radiosensitizing effect, and therefore seems to be a promising therapeutic approach for future therapy of advanced thyroid cancer.

Antiangiogenic gene therapy
Antiangiogenic tumor therapy is emerging as a novel and potentially promising anti-cancer strategy, as angiogenesis is crucial for a tumor to recruit the blood supply that is needed for tumor growth. Angiogenesis is a tightly regulated complex process that involves proangiogenic factors, such as basic fibroblast growth factor and vascular endothelial growth factor (VEGF-1), and antiangiogenic factors, such as angiostatin and endostatin. In follicular thyroid carcinoma cells, both the application of recombinant endostatin and retrovirus-mediated endostatin gene transfer significantly inhibited the growth of xenografts *in vivo* [1–3]. In a more recent study, the antitumor effects of soluble VEGF receptor-1 (sFlt-1) were studied in follicular cell-derived thyroid cancer cells. When a 293 embryonic kidney cell line, that was stably transfected with sFlt-1, was inoculated at a site remote from the xenotransplant tumor, tumor growth was significantly inhibited by the systemic secretion of sFlt-1 [1]. These studies demonstrate

the therapeutic efficacy of antiangiogenic strategies in follicular cell-derived thyroid cancer, which, however, can be limited by the capacity of tumor cells to counteract a single anti-angiogenic agent requiring combination treatment.

Immunomodulatory gene therapy

Many cancers express tumor-associated antigens that can be recognized by the immune system, after they are released from tumor cells physiologically or after cytotoxic therapy, and presented to CD8+ cytotoxic T cells and CD4+ helper T cells in the context of major histocompatibility complex (MHC) class I and II and B7.1/B7.2 co-stimulatory molecules. However, tumors have the capacity to evade the immune system by down-regulation of expression of MHC class I or co-stimulatory molecules, resulting in a poor T-cell response. Mobilization of the immune system by delivery of genes that enhance immunogenicity of tumors and responsiveness of the immune system is associated with a number of advantages, including inherent specificity of the immune system thereby decreasing normal tissue toxicity, a systemic immunogenic effect, signal amplification, and permanent antitumor immunity due to inherent memory of the immune system. Local expression of certain cytokines, such as interferon-γ, tumor necrosis factor-α, interleukin-2 (IL-2) and interleukin-12 (IL-12), is able to elicit an immune response against the tumor by stimulating surrounding immunocompetent cells, targeting cytotoxic T cells and natural killer cells, thereby inducing rejection of tumor cells.

IL-2 has been examined in various studies for genetic immunotherapy of thyroid cancer. In medullary thyroid cancer cells intratumoral injection of an adenovirus harboring the IL-2 gene resulted in tumor regression/stabilization depending on tumor size. The antitumor effect was shown to be dependent on cytotoxic T lymphocyte activity against the tumor, which also prevented tumor growth after reinjection of tumor cells, indicating development of long-term antitumor immunity [3, 7].

An adenovirus carrying two subunits of the murine IL-12 gene showed efficient antitumor activity and development of long-term antitumor immunity after intratumoral injection into tumors derived from rat medullary and follicular cell-derived cancer cells [3, 7]. Interestingly, in rats with two tumors, injection of the adenovirus in one tumor resulted in antitumor activity in the injected as well as non-injected tumor, indicating systemic antitumor immunity [3, 7]. When a modified calcitonin promoter was used to achieve tumor specificity, IL-12 was selectively expressed in rat medullary thyroid carcinoma cells, resulting in a significant therapeutic effect in vivo after intratumoral injection of the adenovirus associated with long-term and systemic antitumor immunity [3, 7].

To further enhance therapeutic efficacy in thyroid cancer, the combination of suicide and immunomodulatory gene therapy has been evaluated by several groups. An adenovirus expressing both HSV-tk and human IL-2 under the control of the calcitonin promoter was shown to have an antitumor effect in rat medullary thyroid tumors after intratumoral injection superior to that of each single vector [3, 7]. In differentiated and anaplastic thyroid carcinoma cells a retroviral vector for combined transfer of the human IL-2 and the HSV-tk gene was employed and showed an enhanced therapeutic effect compared with IL-2 alone with at least 80% tumor volume reduction in xenografted tumors in nude mice and the association with a significant bystander effect [1]. To further optimize this therapeutic approach, a transcriptionally targeted retroviral vector was generated, replacing the viral enhancer with the enhancer sequence of the human Tg gene, which allowed selective transgene expression and cell killing in differentiated thyroid tumor cells [1]. In addition, this combined suicide/cytokine gene therapy strategy was applied in a first pilot study in two patients with end-stage anaplastic thyroid cancer using a retroviral vector carrying the human IL-2 and HSV-tk gene. Although both patients died due to disease progression 6 and 61 days after therapy, this pilot study was able to demonstrate that treatment was safe and well tolerated, resulted in production of T helper type 1 cytokines as shown in tumor biopsies and peripheral blood mononuclear cells, and caused local tumor necrosis after direct intratumoral injection of retroviral vector producer cells followed by GCV application [8].

Based on its association with a systemic and long-term antitumor effect the application of immunomodulatory gene therapy is less affected by the limitations of currently available vector systems and therefore holds great promise for future therapeutic application in thyroid cancer, in particular as part of a multimodality approach.

Virus-mediated oncolysis

Induction of virus-mediated oncolysis by the application of replication-competent adenoviruses may help to circumvent the hurdle of poor transduction efficiency by allowing in vivo viral amplification. The best known example of a replication-competent adenovirus is the E1B-deleted ONYX-015 virus that preferentially replicates in cancer cells lacking functional p53. ONXY-015 was demonstrated to selectively replicate and induce cell death in anaplastic thyroid cancer cell lines, resulting in selective reduction of tumor growth in vivo after local injection of ONYX-015. Further, ONYX-015 treatment acted synergistically with the antineoplastic drugs doxorubicin and paclitaxel, and enhanced radiation induced cell death in human anaplastic thyroid carcinoma cells in vitro and in vivo [1–3]. More recently, a replication-selective adenovirus under the control of a Tg enhancer and promoter fragment was developed that induced oncolysis selectively in Tg-expressing thyroid cancer cells resulting in significant growth inhibition in vivo [9]. These data strongly suggest that with the possibility of tumor- or tissue-specific transcriptional targeting replication-competent adenoviruses may represent a strong tool for the treatment of thyroid cancer, being able to enhance in vivo therapeutic efficacy by the possibility of in vivo viral amplification.

NIS gene therapy

One of the most promising suicide genes available for cancer gene therapy is the NIS. Iodide trapping activity in the thyroid gland

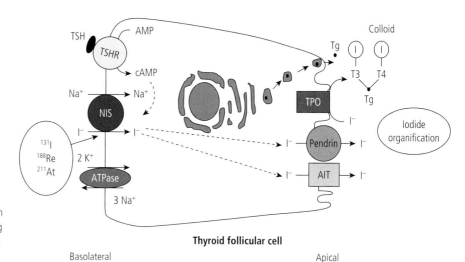

Figure 6.2 Schematic illustration of sodium iodide symporter (NIS)-mediated transport and organification of iodide in the thyroid gland. TSH, thyroid-stimulating hormone; TSHR, TSH receptor; Tg, thyroglobulin; TPO, thyroid peroxidase; AIT, apical iodide transporter.

due to expression of NIS plays a key role in diagnosis and therapy of follicular cell-derived thyroid carcinomas and their metastases. As an intrinsic plasma membrane glycoprotein, NIS mediates the active transport of iodide at the basolateral membrane of thyroid follicular cells (Fig. 6.2) [10]. Functional expression of NIS in papillary and follicular thyroid carcinomas offers the possibility of effective imaging as well as therapeutic destruction of tumors by ^{131}I application contributing greatly to the generally favorable prognosis of patients with differentiated thyroid cancer, where 10-year survival rates of approximately 90–95% are reported. Based upon the highly effective application of radioiodine that has been used for over 60 years in the managment of follicular cell-derived thyroid cancer, cloning and characterization of the NIS gene [11, 12] have paved the way for the development of a novel cytoreductive radioisotope concentrator gene therapy strategy aiming at targeted NIS expression in thyroidal and non-thyroidal cancer cells, making them susceptible to therapeutic destruction by the β-energy emitted by [131]I (Fig. 6.3) [13].

Using various gene delivery techniques, including electroporation, liposomes, adenoviral and retroviral vectors, radioiodine accumulation was induced *in vitro* and *in vivo* in a variety of cancer cell lines by NIS gene delivery [10]. These studies demonstrated that, in contrast to other therapeutic genes, NIS is associated with a number of significant advantages:

1 With application of radioiodine, NIS gene therapy offers the possibility to extend an already established and highly effective anti-cancer strategy with an excellent safety profile to the treatment of other cancer types.

2 NIS gene therapy is associated with a significant bystander effect based on the crossfire effect of the β-emitter ^{131}I with a path length of up to 2.4 mm (0.1 inch).

3 NIS is a normal non-toxic, non-immunogenic human gene and protein.

4 NIS gene transfer allows non-invasive radioiodine imaging to confirm and localize functional NIS expression before proceeding to the application of a therapeutic ^{131}I dose.

NIS gene therapy in thyroid cancer

While in differentiated thyroid cancer functional NIS expression allows effective therapy with radioiodine, patients with poorly differentiated thyroid cancer or patients with medullary thyroid cancer do not benefit from radioiodine therapy due to insufficient or absent radioiodine accumulating activity. In these patients NIS gene transfer could be used to restore or induce radioiodine accumulation, thereby offering the possibility of radioiodine application. Early studies in malignantly transformed rat thyroid cells showed that transfection with rat NIS cDNA is able to restore radioiodine accumulation *in vitro* and *in vivo*, which, however, was not sufficient to allow a therapeutic effect of [131]I (1 mCi) *in vivo* [14]. In contrast, stable transfection of a follicular thyroid carcinoma cell line with the NIS gene was able to re-establish iodide accumulation activity *in vitro* and *in vivo* with significantly increased biological half-life of ^{131}I after thyroid ablation and application of low-iodide diet leading to postponed xenotransplant development after administration of a therapeutic dose of 2 mCi [131]I [15]. In our group, using the calcitonin promoter, tumor-targeted NIS gene transfer was performed in medullary thyroid carcinoma resulting in 84% cell killing after application of a therapeutic ^{131}I dose [16]. In the meanwhile several groups showed induction of perchlorate-sensitive iodide accumulation following NIS transduction in a variety of papillary, follicular and anaplastic thyroid carcinoma cell lines, which, however, was often associated with rapid iodide efflux probably due to low expression levels of Tg, TSH receptor and thyroid peroxidase (TPO), genes involved in iodide organification [17, 18]. In order to limit extratumoral toxicity, the Tg promoter was applied to target NIS expression to thyroid cancer cells and was combined with the Cre/loxP system to compensate for the weakness of the Tg promoter [19].

Thyroid peroxidase catalyzed oxidation and incorporation of trapped iodide into tyrosyl residues along the thyroglobulin backbone in the thyroid gland (a process called iodide organification) increases the retention time of accumulated iodide in the thyroid gland. Due to the lack of a functioning iodide organification

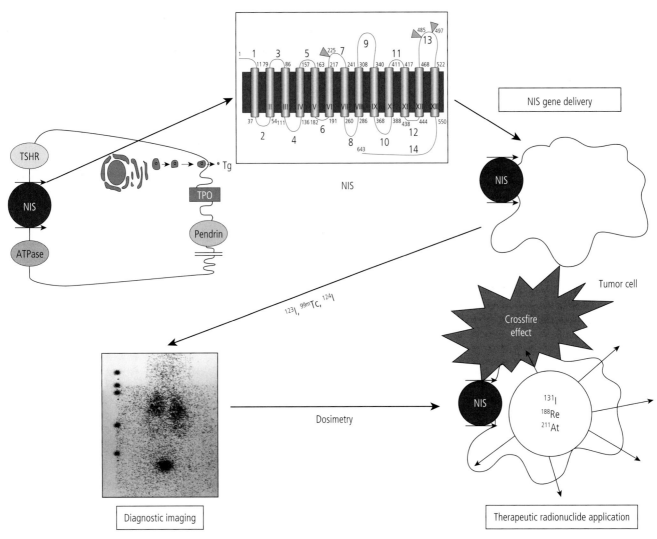

Figure 6.3 Concept of the NIS gene as a novel diagnostic as well as a therapeutic gene.

apparatus, dedifferentiated and medullary thyroid cancer cells, or extrathyroidal cancer cells, are not able to increase intracellular iodide retention after NIS gene transfer, thereby limiting its therapeutic efficacy, which depends on a variety of factors including the amount of trapped radioiodine, the rate of iodide efflux, iodide recirculation and iodide organification. Coupling of NIS and TPO gene transfer may be able to induce iodide organification, thereby enhancing the therapeutic efficiency of NIS gene therapy [10]. In a recent study, TPO and Tg expression was re-established in a NIS-transfected dedifferentiated thyroid cancer cell line by transduction with the thyroid-specific transcription factor TTF-1, which resulted in increased iodide organification and retention *in vitro* and *in vivo* [20].

Other possibilities to increase therapeutic efficacy of NIS gene transfer in non-organifying tumor cells include maximizing iodide uptake by efficient NIS gene transduction, minimizing efflux by blocking iodide efflux mechanisms, or application of alternative radionuclides instead of ^{131}I allowing deposition of higher energy

in a shorter time period. In a very recent study, treatment with substances like 17-AAG (17-(allylamino)-17-demethoxygeldanamycin) and DIDS (4,4′-di-isothiocyanatostilbene-2,2′-disulfonic acid) was demonstrated to be able to significantly decrease iodide efflux out of human anaplastic thyroid cancer cells after NIS transduction, offering the possibility to use these drugs in future clinical applications to enhance therapeutic efficacy of NIS gene transfer [21].

In addition, the high energy α-emitter ^{211}astatine (^{211}At) and the potent β-emitter ^{188}Rhenium (^{188}Re), which are also transported by NIS, have been proposed as alternative radionuclides for application following NIS gene transfer due to their higher energy and shorter half-life, thereby offering the possibility of higher energy deposition in a shorter time period [22, 23]. Petrich et al. demonstrated perchlorate-sensitive accumulation of ^{211}At in papillary and anaplastic thyroid carcinoma cell lines following stable transfection with the NIS gene, resulting in a 14-fold increase of the tumor absorbed dose. These data suggested that application of ^{211}At is able to enhance the therapeutic efficacy of

NIS-based gene therapy, which was confirmed in a recently published *in vivo* study in NIS-transfected papillary thyroid cancer xenografts after fractionated application of ^{211}At [24].

Taken together, these studies show that NIS gene delivery into thyroid cancer cells is capable of restoring or inducing radioiodine accumulation, and might therefore represent an effective strategy to allow application of radioioidine therapy also in dedifferentiated or medullary thyroid cancer that usually lack iodide-accumulating activity.

NIS gene therapy in non-thyroid cancers

Based on the successful application of radioiodine in the treatment of follicular cell-derived thyroid cancer, several investigators have therefore explored the efficacy of NIS gene transfer in non-thyroidal endocrine malignancies.

Prostate cancer

Our group chose prostate cancer as one of the first tumor models to investigate the potential of the NIS gene as novel therapeutic gene. To target NIS expression selectively to prostate cancer cells, the promoters of the prostate-specific antigen (PSA) or probasin, two well-characterized prostate-specific genes, were used [25–27]. Prostate cancer (LNCaP) cells were shown to be selectively killed by accumulated ^{131}I following induction of tissue-specific iodide uptake activity by PSA promoter-directed NIS expression *in vitro* and *in vivo*. A single therapeutic ^{131}I dose of 3 mCi was shown to elicit a dramatic therapeutic response in NIS-transfected LNCaP cell xenografts with an average volume reduction of more than 90% [25, 26]. Further, PSA promoter-driven NIS expression and ^{131}I cytotoxicity were shown to be stimulated by dexamethasone and all-*trans*-retinoic acid, offering the possibility of combination treatment with these substances [28, 29]. As a next crucial step towards therapeutic application of NIS gene delivery followed by radioiodine therapy in prostate cancer patients in a clinical setting, a replication-deficient human adenovirus carrying the human NIS gene linked to the CMV promoter (Ad5-CMV-NIS) was used to perform *in vivo* NIS gene transfer into LNCaP cell tumors. Following intraperitoneal injection of a single therapeutic dose of 3 mCi ^{131}I after adenovirus-mediated intratumoral NIS gene delivery, a therapeutic response with an average volume reduction of more than 80% was achieved [30]. In preparation of the first Phase I clinical trial of adenovirus-mediated NIS gene therapy of prostate cancer, these results were confirmed in a large animal study in which Ad-CMV-NIS was injected into the prostate of male beagle dogs [31]. These data clearly showed the gene therapy and oncology communities for the first time that NIS gene delivery into non-thyroidal non-organifying tumor cells is capable of inducing accumulation of therapeutically effective radioiodine doses, and might therefore represent an effective and potentially curative innovative therapy for extrathyroidal tumors.

Ovarian and breast cancer

The MUC1 promoter was used to target NIS gene expression to ovarian and breast cancer, two of the leading causes of death from gynecological malignances with low survival rates for advanced and recurring disease. MUC1 is a transmembrane glycoprotein that is overexpressed in many tumor types including breast, pancreatic, lung, prostate and ovarian cancer. Using intratumoral injection of a replication-deficient adenovirus which drives NIS expression under the control of the MUC1 promoter, a significant therapeutic effect of ^{131}I was observed in ovarian and breast cancer xenografts in nude mice with tumor volume reduction of up to 83% [32, 33]. In addition, the live attenuated Edmonston B measles virus was developed as a novel replication-competent virus for cancer therapy and has been shown to possess potent antitumor activity in a variety of human malignancies. For treatment of ovarian cancer two measles viruses were developed: one expressing the carcinoembryonic antigen (CEA), which allows monitoring of virus propagation by measurement of CEA levels, and another one expressing NIS, allowing one not only to monitor virus propagation by radioiodine scanning but also to enhance the therapeutic effect of virus-mediated oncolysis by the application of ^{131}I. In addition to the possibility of effective non-invasive monitoring of virotherapy, dual therapy using both of these viruses was demonstrated to be superior to treatment with either virus alone [34].

Neuroendocrine tumors

NIS gene transfer has also been investigated as a novel therapeutic tool in pancreatic neuroendocrine tumor cells using the chromogranin A promoter to achieve tumor-specific NIS gene expression by transcriptional targeting. Induced iodide accumulation was shown to be sufficient to allow a highly significant therapeutic effect of more than 95% in these cell lines [35].

Adrenocortical cancer

Adrenocortical carcinoma is one of the most aggressive tumors in humans, with current treatment options being only complete surgical resection, adjuvant chemotherapy with mitotane, local tumor bed radiation and palliative chemotherapy. We used the adrenocorticotropic hormone (ACTH)-receptor promoter to target the NIS gene to adrenocortical cancer cells to examine the feasibility of radioiodine therapy of adrenocortical cancer following NIS gene transfer. ACTH receptor-mediated NIS gene transfer was able to establish tissue-specific iodide accumulation in adrenocortical cancer cells, resulting in a significant reduction of clone formation in an *in vitro* clonogenic assay after application of ^{131}I [36].

Conclusion

These studies clearly show that cloning of the sodium iodide symporter (NIS) gene has not only revolutionized our understanding of the physiology and pathophysiology of thyroidal iodide accumulation, but has also provided us with a powerful new diagnostic and therapeutic gene, opening exciting new perspectives for cancer therapy.

Since the clinical efficacy of gene therapy is not only determined by the potency of therapeutic genes, but also by the efficiency of vector-mediated gene delivery, the chief challenge facing clinical gene therapy application is the development of a safe and efficient gene delivery system that also allows systemic administration. Currently available vector systems reveal various problems limiting their safety and efficiency, such as significant first-pass effect in the liver, increased toxicity by vector leakage, and neutralization by host immunity, which can only be solved by close collaboration of creative molecular biologists and clinical scientists. However, until a perfectly targeted and safe vector system is developed, the choice of therapeutic gene will be crucially important to compensate for the deficiencies of the currently available vectors. Currently available data, as summarized above, strongly suggest that, with the availability of a variety of potent therapeutic genes, gene therapy holds great promise for future clinical application, at least as part of a multimodality approach.

References

1. Barzon L, Pacenti M, Boscaro M, Palu G. Gene therapy for thyroid cancer. *Exp. Opin. Biol. Ther.* 2004;4:1225–1239.

2. Spitzweg C, Morris JC. Gene therapy for thyroid cancer: current status and future prospects. *Thyroid* 2004;14:424–434.

3. DeGroot LJ, Zhang R. Viral mediated gene therapy for the management of metastatic thyroid carcinoma. *Curr. Drug Targets Immune Endocr. Metabol. Disord.* 2004;4:235–244.

4. Barzon L, Gnatta E, Castagliuolo I, et al. Modulation of retrovirally driven therapeutic genes by mutant TP53 in anaplastic thyroid carcinoma. *Cancer Gene Ther.* 2005;12:381–388.

5. McIver B, Grebe SKG, Eberhardt NL. The PAX8/PPARγ fusion oncogene as a potential therapeutic target in follicular thyroid carcinoma. *Curr. Drug Targets Immune Endocr. Metabol. Disord.* 2004;4:221–234.

6. Drosten M, Pützer BM. Gene therapeutic approaches for medullary thyroid carcinoma treatment. *J. Mol. Med.* 2003;81:411–419.

7. DeGroot LJ, Zhang R. Gene therapy for thyroid cancer: where do we stand? *J. Clin. Endocrinol. Metab.* 2001;86:2923–2928.

8. Barzon L, Pacenti M, Taccaliti A, et al. A pilot study of combined suicide/cytokine gene therapy in two patients with end-stage anaplastic thyroid carcinoma. *J. Clin. Endocrinol. Metab.* 2005;90:2831–2834.

9. Kesmodel S, Prabakaran I, Canter R, Menon C, Molnar-Kimber K, Fraker D. Virus-mediated oncolysis of thyroid cancer by a replication-selective adenovirus driven by a thyroglobulin promoter-enhancer region. *J. Clin. Endocrinol. Metab.* 2005;90:3440–3448.

10. Spitzweg C, Morris JC. The sodium iodide symporter: its pathophysiological and therapeutic implications. *Clin. Endocrinol.* 2002;57:559–574.

11. Dai G, Levy O, Carrasco N. Cloning and characterization of the thyroid iodide transporter. *Nature* 1996;379:458–460.

12. Smanik PA, Liu Q, Furminger TL, et al. Cloning of the human sodium iodide symporter. *Biochem. Biophys. Res. Commun.* 1996;226:339–345.

13. Spitzweg C, Harrington KJ, Pinke LA, Vile RG, Morris JC. The sodium iodide symporter and its potential role in cancer therapy. *J. Clin. Endocrinol. Metab.* 2001;86:3327–3335.

14. Shimura H, Haraguchi K, Myazaki A, Endo T, Onaya T. Iodide uptake and experimental ^{131}I therapy in transplanted undifferentiated thyroid cancer cells expressing the Na$^+$/I$^-$ symporter gene. *Endocrinology* 1997;138:4493–4496.

15. Smit JW, Schroder-Van der Elst JP, Karperien M, et al. Iodide kinetics and experimental (131)I therapy in a xenotransplanted human sodium-iodide symporter-transfected human follicular thyroid carcinoma cell line. *J. Clin. Endocrinol. Metab.* 2002;87:1247–1253.

16. Cengic N, Baker CH, Göke B, Morris JC, Spitzweg C. A novel therapeutic strategy for medullary thyroid cancer based on radioiodine therapy following tissue-specific sodium iodide symporter gene expression. *J. Clin. Endocrinol. Metab.* 2005;90:4457–4464.

17. Petrich T, Knapp WH, Pötter E. Functional activity of human sodium/iodide symporter in tumor cell lines. *Nuklearmedizin* 2003;42:15–18.

18. Lee WW, Lee B, Kim SJ, Jin J, Moon DH, Lee H. Kinetics of iodide uptake and efflux in various human thyroid cancer cells by expressing sodium iodide symporter gene via a recombinant adenovirus. *Oncol. Rep.* 2003;10:845–849.

19. Lin X, Fischer AH, Ryu K-Y, et al. Application of the Cre/loxP system to enhance thyroid-targeted expression of sodium/iodide symporter. *J. Clin. Endocrinol. Metab.* 2004;89:2344–2350.

20. Furuya F, Shimura H, Miyazaki A, et al. Adenovirus-mediated transfer of thyroid transcription factor-1 induces radioiodide organification and retention in thyroid cancer cells. *Endocrinology* 2004;145:5397–5405.

21. Elisei R, Vivaldi A, Ciampi R, et al. Treatment with drugs able to reduce iodine efflux significantly increases the intracellular retention time in thyroid cancer cells stably transfected with sodium iodide symporter (NIS) cDNA. *J. Clin. Endocrinol. Metab.* 2006;91:2389–2395.

22. Dadachova E, Bouzahzah B, Zuckier LS, Pestell RG. Rhenium-188 as an alternative to iodine-131 for treatment of breast tumors expressing the sodium/iodide symporter (NIS). *Nucl. Med. Biol.* 2002;29:13–18.

23. Carlin S, Akabani G, Zalutsky MR. In vitro cytotoxicity of 211At-Astatide and 131I-Iodide to glioma tumor cells expressing the sodium/iodide symporter. *J. Nucl. Med.* 2003;44:1827–1838.

24. Petrich T, Quintanilla-Martinez L, Korkmaz Z, et al. Effective cancer therapy with the α-particle emitter [211-At]Astatine in a mouse model of genetically modified sodium/iodide symporter-expressing tumors. *Clin. Cancer Res.* 2006;12:1342–1348.

25. Spitzweg C, Zhang S, Bergert ER, et al. Prostate-specific antigen (PSA) promoter-driven androgen-inducible expression of sodium iodide symporter in prostate cancer cell lines. *Cancer Res.* 1999;59:2136–2141.

26. Spitzweg C, O'Connor MK, Bergert ER, Tindall DJ, Young CYF, Morris JC. Treatment of prostate cancer by radioiodine therapy after tissue-specific expression of the sodium iodide symporter. *Cancer Res.* 2000;60:6526–6530.

27. Kakinuma H, Bergert ER, Spitzweg C, Matusik RJ, Morris JC. Probasin promoter (ARR2PB) driven, prostate specific expression of h-NIS for targeted radioiodine therapy of prostate cancer. *Cancer Res.* 2003; 63:7840–7844.

28. Spitzweg C, Scholz IV, Bergert ER, et al. Retinoic acid-induced stimulation of sodium iodide symporter (NIS) expression and cytotoxicity of

radioiodine in prostate cancer cells. *Endocrinology* 2003;144:3423–3432.

29. Scholz IV, Cengic N, Göke B, Morris JC, Spitzweg C. Dexamethasone enhances the cytotoxic effect of radioiodine therapy in prostate cancer cells expressing the sodium iodide symporter (NIS). *J. Clin. Endocrinol. Metab.* 2004;89:1108–1116.

30. Spitzweg C, Dietz AB, O'Connor MK, et al. *In vivo* sodium iodide symporter gene therapy of prostate cancer. *Gene Ther.* 2001;8:1524–1531.

31. Dwyer RM, Schatz SM, Bergert ER, et al. A preclinical large animal model of adenovirus-mediated expression of the sodium-iodide symporter for radioiodide imaging and therapy of locally recurrent prostate cancer. *Mol. Ther.* 2005; 12:835–841.

32. Dwyer RM, Bergert ER, O'Connor MK, Gendler SJ, Morris JC. Sodium iodide symporter-mediated radioiodide imaging and therapy of ovarian tumor xenografts in mice. *Gene Ther.* 2005; 13:60–66.

33. Dwyer RM, Bergert ER, O'Connor MK, Gendler SJ, Morris JC. In vivo radioiodide imaging and treatment of breast cancer xenografts after MUC1-driven expression of the sodium iodide symporter. *Clin. Cancer Res.* 2005;11:1483–1489.

34. Hasegawa K, Pham L, O'Connor MK, Federspiel MJ, Russell SJ, Peng K-W. Dual therapy of ovarian cancer using measles viruses expressing carcinoembryonic antigen and sodium iodide symporter. *Clin. Cancer Res.* 2006;12:1868–1875.

35. Schipper ML, Weber A, Behe M, et al. Radioiodide treatment after sodium iodide symporter gene transfer is a highly effective therapy in neuroendocrine tumor cells. *Cancer Res.* 2003;63:1333–1338.

36. Cengic N, Schutz M, Leistner C, et al. Radioiodine therapy of adrenocortical cancer following ACTH-receptor-promoter-driven expression of the sodium iodide symporter. 76th Annual Meeting of the American Thyroid Association, Vancouver, Canada, 2004.

7 Tumor Targeting

Mona Waterhouse and Ashley B. Grossman

> **Key points**
> - Neuroendocrine tumors express specific cell surface markers.
> - Peptide receptor analogs can be used to image neuroendocrine tumors.
> - PET is a useful imaging modality for selected neuroendocrine tumors.
> - Peptide receptor radiation therapy offers targeted therapy for neuroendocrine tumors.
> - Somatostatin analogs can be used in the treatment of acromegaly and carcinoid tumors.

Introduction

Tumors derived from endocrine cells tend to express specific cell surface markers and retain a degree of functional ability, such that they have the capacity to produce polypeptide hormones and biogenic amines. These attributes lend themselves to characterization in terms of a cell surface profile. In this chapter we will outline the modalities available to clinicians to target tumors of the endocrine system: these methods are aimed at localizing sites of primary and secondary tumor involvement at early stages of disease. In addition, they provide a mechanism for targeted therapy and subsequent follow-up of disease response to therapy. The main focus of discussion will be on peptide receptor imaging, positron emission tomography and radionuclide targeted therapy. The references quoted at the beginning of each section refer to review articles for further reading.

Peptide receptor imaging [1–6]

Our knowledge of the number and pattern of regulatory peptide receptors that are over-expressed on tumors of the endocrine system is expanding rapidly. These receptors act as targets for radiolabeled peptides, thus allowing tumor localization and in some instances peptide receptor radiation therapy. The most widely used and clinically important of these receptors are the somatostatin receptors.

Somatostatin receptor targeting

Somatostatin is a peptide which exists in three main forms: a prohormone, a 28 amino-acid peptide and a 14 amino-acid peptide.

There appears to be a predominance of somatostatin 14 in the gastric and pancreatic D cells while the 28 amino-acid peptide is found mainly in the intestinal mucosal cells. The two peptide forms are both biologically active as they contain an identical carboxy terminal sequence.

Somatostatin was first identified by Krulich and McCann in hypothalamic extracts. They named it "the inhibitory factor," and it does indeed act as a regulator of both paracrine and endocrine function throughout the body. In the pituitary it is a physiological regulator of growth hormone (GH) release, and inhibits the secretion of thyroid-stimulating hormone (TSH). Within the gastroduodenal neuroendocrine system it inhibits the action of all glands. Table 7.1 outlines the principal effects of somatostatin.

There are five somatostatin receptors (sstr) identified to date, all being widely distributed throughout the body. They belong to the family of G protein-coupled receptors that exert their effects via actions on various intracellular pathways including:
- inhibition of the adenylyl cyclase-cAMP-protein kinase A pathway
- stimulation of phospholipase A2
- activation of phosphotyrosine phosphatases

Table 7.1 The actions of somatostatin

Pituitary	Inhibits secretion of: TSH, GH
Gastrointestinal tract	Inhibits secretion of gastrin, GIP, motilin, gastric acid, VIP
	Inhibits gastric emptying
	Reduces GI blood flow
	Reduces intestinal absorption
Gallbladder	Inhibits emptying
Pancreas	Inhibits secretion of insulin, glucagon, reduces secretion of pancreatic enzymes

GIP, gastroinhibitory polypeptide; VIP, vasoactive intestinal peptide.

Clinical Endocrine Oncology, 2nd edition. Edited by Ian D. Hay and John A.H. Wass. © 2008 Blackwell Publishing. ISBN 978-1-4051-4584-8.

- MAPK pathway-mediated inhibition of cellular proliferation
- stimulating apoptosis.

These receptors are found in high concentration in somatotroph tumors of the pituitary and neuroendocrine tumors (NET), as well as some adenocarcinomas and lymphomas. There appear to be different patterns of sstr expression depending on the tumor type: ssrt2 is the predominant receptor on 90% of carcinoid tumors and 80% of endocrine pancreatic tumors, whereas somatotroph pituitary tumors express predominantly sstr 2 and sstr 5. Table 7.2 outlines the expression of somatostatin receptors in NET. Both peptide forms of somatostatin bind all five receptors with high affinity. However, somatostatin itself is not a useful peptide to use in imaging as it has a short half-life. Therefore, somatostatin analogs have been produced which are resistant to proteolysis, rendering them longer acting in the circulation. Octreotide and lanreotide are the most widely used somatostatin analogs. They are both cyclic octapeptides which have high affinity for sstr 2 and 5. This makes them ideal candidates for use in radiolabeled peptide scintigraphy to localize NET. In order to be used in scintigraphy, the somatostatin analogs need to be coupled to a radioisotope. Various agents have been used to link octreotide to [111]In. Initially, octreotide was conjugated to DTPA (diethylenetriamine-penta-acetic acid) but more recently DOTA (1,4,7,10 tetra-azacyclododecane-1,4,7,10 tetra-acetic acid) has been used. Scintigraphy with ^{111}In-octreotide has been shown to be superior to that of ^{111}In-lanreotide with a detection rate of all NET of between 67% and 100%. This may well reflect the greater affinity of ^{111}In-octreotide for the sstr 2.

Newer somatostatin analogs have been synthesized, the most promising of which is octreotate. ^{111}In-DTPA-Tyr[3]-octreotate has demonstrated higher tumor uptake than ^{111}In-DTPA-Tyr[3]-octreotide. In addition, better image resolution has been achieved by superimposing ^{111}In-octreotide SPECT (single photon emission computerized tomography) with computerized tomography/magnetic resonance imaging (CT/MRI) slices. However, at present, ^{111}In-octreotide remains the gold standard for scintigraphy.

There are several other peptide receptors which show promise as potential targets for diagnostic nuclear imaging.

Table 7.2 The distribution of somatostatin receptors on neuroendocrine tumors in humans

Tumor	sstr1	sstr2	sstr3	sstr4	sstr5
Somatotroph adenoma		+			+
NFPA		+	+		
Gut carcinoid	+	+			+
Gastrinoma		+		+	+
Insulinoma		+		+	
Glucagonoma		+			
VIPoma	+	+	+	+	+
Paraganglioma		+			
Pheochromocytoma		+			

Cholecystokinin receptors

CCK is a gastrointestinal peptide which acts as a regulator of function in the gastrointestinal (GI) tract. It has also been shown to be a growth factor in the GI tract in health. There are two well-defined receptors, CCK1 and CCKB. CCKB receptor protein has been found in high concentrations in up to 92% of medullary thyroid carcinoma as well as endocrine pancreatic tumors, particularly insulinomas. Members of the gastrin family have shown the highest receptor affinity for the CCKB receptor subtype. Scintigraphy with ^{111}In-DTPA-D-Glu(1) minigastrin has shown great promise. In a study of 75 patients with medullary carcinoma of the thyroid, 43 with known disease and 32 with occult disease, scintigraphy revealed all known disease and at least one lesion in 29 out of the 32 patients with previously occult disease. CCK1 receptors are expressed in neuroendocrine lung and gastroenteropancreatic tumors.

Pituitary adenylate cyclase-activating peptide (PACAP)

PACAP is a peptide that is structurally similar to vasoactive intestinal peptide (VIP). It acts via a G protein-coupled receptor which is found in tumors of the neuronal and endocrine systems. Neuroblastomas, non-functioning pituitary adenomas and somatotroph pituitary adenomas predominantly express the PAC1 receptor. Pheochromocytoma and paragangliomas express PAC2 receptors.

Scanning with radiolabeled VIP has been shown to be equally sensitive to ^{111}In-octreotide in patients with gastro-enteropancreatic (GEP) tumors.

Gastrin releasing peptide (GRP)

GRP is a member of a family of brain–gut peptides which also includes bombesin, a structurally similar peptide. There are four receptor subtypes. GRP has been shown to be synthesized by tumors and stimulate tumor growth. Studies using iodinated bombesin have revealed different receptor expression in neuroendocrine tumors: the BB3 receptor is expressed by bronchial carcinoid tumors, while neuromedin receptors are expressed on ileal carcinoids and GRP receptors on gastrinomas.

Glucagon-like peptide (GLP)

GLP is an incretin hormone which acts to regulate blood glucose levels via the GLP1 receptor. GLP1 receptors are found on pancreatic β-cells and are expressed by insulinomas.

MIBG

MIBG, metaiodobenzylguanidine, is a guanidine derivative that exploits the specific type 1 amine uptake mechanism at the cell membrane. It is subsequently taken up from the cytoplasm and stored within the intracellular storage vesicles. It does not appear to exert any activity at the post-synaptic membrane. MIBG localizes to chromaffin cells, i.e., adrenomedullary tumors, hyperplastic adrenal medulla and healthy adrenal medulla. In addition several other endocrine tumors, including 35% of medullary thyroid carcinomas and ~40% of carcinoid tumors, exhibit this uptake mechanism and can accumulate MIBG. The prolonged storage of MIBG within secretory vesicles permits imaging when conjugated to radiolabeled iodine. Both ^{131}I and ^{123}I can be used to label MIBG. However, the imaging quality achieved with ^{123}I-MIBG has been shown to be superior to ^{131}I-MIBG. ^{123}I-MIBG is 80% sensitive and 90% specific for the visualization of intra-adrenal and extra-adrenal sites of both benign and malignant pheochromocytomas. This compares favorably with both CT and MRI, which are both highly sensitive, detecting some 90–100% of intra-adrenal pheochromocytomas and 90% of extra-adrenal pheochromocytomas. However, these imaging techniques have poor specificity compared to MIBG scintigraphy, especially for intra-adrenal disease, due to the high incidence of incidental and benign adrenal masses. Up to 10% of chromaffin cell tumors do not take up MIBG. In these cases, there may be uptake of ^{111}In-octreotide, especially with malignant disease.

Positron emission tomography [7, 8]

The tracers used for positron emission tomography (PET) imaging reflect the metabolic function of the tumor target. As an imaging modality it offers high sensitivity and the advantage of being able to perform whole-body scans. ^{18}F-deoxyglucose was the first tracer used, and reflects the increased glucose uptake of malignant tumors. However, NET tend to be well differentiated and slow growing. These properties determine the low sensitivity of imaging with ^{18}F-deoxyglucose. However, conventional PET using ^{18}F-labeled deoxyglucose as a tracer is a useful imaging technique in poorly differentiated neuroendocrine tumors that are somatostatin receptor negative.

There is growing experience of using PET with different tracers for targeting NET. Carcinoid tumors exhibit the metabolic pathway which synthesizes 5-hydroxytryptamine (5HT) from 5-hydroxytryptophan (5HTP). These tumors have been targeted by PET using carbon-labelled 5HTP as a tracer. Studies in over 200 patients with carcinoid tumors have shown that [11]C-5HTP PET visualizes over 90% of tumors. In addition, in a smaller study, six out of eight tumors which had not been visualized by conventional radiology or octreotide scanning were localized using PET. Given that ^{111}In-octreotide fails to visualize 10–20% of GEP tumors, there may be a role for PET scanning in these patients.

Octreotide can also be used as a tracer for PET studies. ^{68}Ga-octreotide and ^{64}Cu-TETA-octreotide have been shown to be more sensitive than ^{111}In-octreotide in demonstrating NET.

PET also has a role in defining adrenocortical tumors. CT and MRI scanning are generally the first-line investigations in assessing an adrenocortical mass. CT densitometry can usually differentiate adrenal adenomas from metastases. A density measurement of less than 10 Hounsfield units in a homogeneous mass on unenhanced CT indicates a lipid-rich adenoma. Chemical shift MRI can also distinguish between adrenal adenomas and metastases. However, PET imaging agents can target specific adrenal gland enzymes expressed in tumor cells. ^{11}C-metomidate binds specifically to 11-β-hydroxylase, which is specific to adrenocortical cells. It has proved to be highly sensitive and specific for adrenocortical masses, with no tracer uptake in pheochromocytomas, adrenal metastases or non-adrenal masses. [18]FDG PET can then be used to distinguish between benign and malignant adrenocortical tumors with more than 95% accuracy. [18]FDG PET is also useful in identifying metastases following surgical intervention where conventional imaging is more difficult to interpret.

The final role for PET scanning is in the management of patients with cancers of the thyroid. [18]FDG PET scanning has a defined role in the postoperative management of patients with papillary and follicular thyroid cancer. Radioiodine scintigraphy is the gold standard for diagnostic localization of these carcinomas of the thyroid. Following total thyroidectomy, thyroglobulin levels are used as an extremely sensitive marker for both residual disease and disease recurrence. Unfortunately, between one-third to half of tumor recurrences are not iodine avid either due to small tumor size or tumor dedifferentiation. In the context of thyroglobulin levels above 2 ng/ml or rising levels and negative radioiodine scintigraphy, the imaging techniques available to evaluate the presence of recurrent disease are ultrasound, CT, MRI and PET. CT and MR imaging have the disadvantage of postoperative anatomical distortion leading to low levels of sensitivity. [18]FDG PET scanning has been shown to be between 82% and 95% sensitive and specific for metastatic and recurrent thyroid cancer. It therefore has a role alongside ultrasound and tissue biopsy in diagnosing postoperative residual and recurrent disease. An additional benefit of [18]FDG PET scanning is that prognostic information can be gained from the relative amount of uptake by individual tumors. Poorly differentiated tumors tend to be more metabolically active and therefore take up more substrate than well-differentiated tumors. These tumors tend to be associated with a poor prognosis.

Medullary cancer of the thyroid is often aggressive in nature, presenting with early lymph node metastases. The tumor cells are usually highly metabolically active and are therefore amenable to imaging with [18]FDG PET scanning. Imaging is also possible with both technetium and octreotide. Diagnostic localization of disease is undertaken prior to surgery to allow for maximal disease clearance with the aim of prolonged disease remission.

Targeted tumor therapy

Peptide receptor radiation therapy [9–14]
In appropriately selected patients, peptide receptor radiation therapy (PRRT) offers the clinician a "magic bullet" form of radiotherapy. Using scintigraphy and, where possible, *in vitro* studies of tumor samples, a peptide receptor "fingerprint" can be defined to which the radioligand used for therapy binds with high affinity. In the future it may be possible to target different receptors within the same tumor, thereby increasing the efficacy of treatment. At present, three systems exist for targeted therapy: radiolabeled octreotide, radiolabeled MIBG and radiolabeled CCK-B analogs.

Somatostatin receptor radiotherapy

The somatostatin analogs were the first radiopeptides to be used for targeted radiation therapy of metastatic and inoperable gastro-enteropancreatic NET. In order to be used for radiotherapy, the specific analogs are linked to a radiometal chelator. DTPA is the oldest chelator of octreotide and lanreotide; however, it is not suitable for coupling these analogs to the commercially available β-emitters such as ^{90}Y and ^{177}Lu. ^{111}In-DTPA octreotide emits mainly γ-irradiation, which limits its use as a radionuclide due to its poor tissue penetration. This has been borne out by the results of two studies in a total of 52 patients with metastatic GEP tumors where no patients had complete remission of disease as defined by CT imaging and only two had partial remission of disease. DOTA is a better chelator as it forms stable metal complexes. The DOTA–somatostatin based radiopeptides are ^{90}Y-DOTA-Tyr^3-octreotide (^{90}Y-DOTATOC, ^{90}Y-SMT-487, *OctreoTher*), ^{90}Y-DOTA-lanreotide, and ^{177}Lu-DOTA-Tyr^3-Thre^8-octreotate (^{177}Lu-DOTATATE). Table 7.3 summarizes the differing somatostatin receptor affinity of these agents. They are eliminated by the kidney and renal radiation is minimized by infusing amino acids at the same time as the radionuclide. In addition, transient hepatic damage is seen in those with heavy hepatic tumor burden. Myelosuppression is a problem in those who have bone metastases and also those patients who have been pretreated with chemotherapy. Phase I/II studies using radiolabeled peptides are now in progress, with experience in over 400 patents with neuroendocrine tumors. The treatment rationales used vary between studies. The radiation dose delivered tends to be between 2 and 11 GBq every 4−8 weeks for up to 12 treatments. In general, few patients have had a complete response to therapy. Studies by four groups with ^{90}Y-DOTA-Tyr^3-octreotide in 191 patients with gastro-enteropancreatic neuroendocrine tumors demonstrated complete remissions in 5% of patients and partial remissions in a further 20% of patients Plate 7.1. The structure of DOTA-Tyr^3-octreotate is different to DOTA-Tyr^3-octreotide as the C-terminal threoninol is replaced by threonine. It has a nine-fold increase in the affinity for the sstr 2 compared to DOTA-Tyr^3-octreotide and, when coupled with ^{177}Lu, there is a six- to seven-fold increase in the affinity as compared with yttrium-loaded counterparts. In addition, ^{177}Lu has a lower tissue penetration than ^{90}Y. This is of clinical importance as higher absorbed doses of radiation in tumor compared with normal tissue should be achieved with ^{177}Lu

Table 7.3 The binding affinities of somatostatin analogs for somatostatin receptors [13]

	sstr1	sstr2	sstr3	sstr4	sstr5
Somatostin 14	0.93	0.15	0.56	1.5	0.29
Lanreotide	180	0.54	14	230	17
Octreotide	280	0.38	7.1	+10 000	6.3
SOM230	9.3	1	1.5	+100	0.16

Binding affinities expressed as mean IC$_{50}$ values in nanomoles.

analogs, although this may limit the size of lesions treated. So far, treatment in 76 patients with metastatic gastro-enteropancreatic tumors has resulted in complete remission in 1% and partial remission in 29% of patients. As might have been anticipated, the incidence of side effects from treatment in this group is lower than with other radiopeptides, consisting mainly of mild transient bone marrow suppression.

The results of trials with radiolabeled somatostatin analogs in inoperable and metastatic gastro-enteropancreatic tumors are encouraging in terms of symptom control and tumor regression. However, more work is required to determine the optimum treatment regime for the different somatostatin analogs that are available for PRRT. In addition, gastro-enteropancreatic tumors do not seem to respond homogeneously to this type of therapy. The endocrine pancreatic tumors and gastrointestinal carcinoids tend to have a higher response rate than bronchial carcinoids and NET of unknown origin. It may be that these tumors will be more effectively treated with different peptide receptor analogs in the future.

CCKB receptor radiotherapy

Medullary thyroid carcinoma has been shown to express a high density of CCKB receptors. Scintigraphy with ^{111}In-DTPA-D-Glu(1) minigastrin is a sensitive method for defining patients with CCKB receptor activity. A small study of treatment using ^{90}Y-minigastrin radiotherapy in eight patients with advanced metastatic disease resulted in two partial remissions and stabilization of rapidly progressing disease in four patients. These results are encouraging given the limited treatment options available in this disease.

MIBG therapy

^{131}I-MIBG is used for therapy in patients who show uptake on a diagnostic ^{123}I-MIBG scan. It has been shown to be useful in several neuroendocrine tumors by both reducing tumor size and also hormone production. However, it does not tend to result in complete remission. Therapeutic protocols vary between centers; however, most centers use 100−300 mCi (~3−10 GBq) ^{131}I-MIBG per treatment up to a total radiation dose of 1−1.2 Ci. Hematological toxicity is the main side effect of ^{131}I-MIBG therapy. This is most problematic in patients who have already undergone chemotherapy or who have bone metastases. Those patients with a large burden of liver metastases are also at risk of a transient hepatitis.

Metastatic carcinoid tumors show avidity for MIBG in about 40% of cases. However, there is not always sufficient avidity to go on to therapy. These cases may show somatostatin receptor uptake. There is a very low response rate to chemotherapy in metastatic carcinoids and as such this is reserved as first-line therapy only for aggressive disease. In 1994, the worldwide cumulative data from ^{131}I-MIBG treatment of 52 patients with metastatic carcinoid tumors reported a hormonal response in 15% of patients and a symptomatic response in 65% of patients. To date the results in another 47 patients report a 12.5% hormonal response and a 60%

symptomatic response. Neither data set has reported a reduction in tumor burden.

Medullary thyroid cancer shows avidity for ^{131}I-MIBG in a third of cases: small numbers of patients with metastatic disease have been treated with ^{131}I-MIBG. The worldwide cumulative experience was reported in 1994 for 22 patients of whom 30% had documented objective tumor response and 50% showed a symptomatic response. However, more recent reports in a further 17 patients are less encouraging with only two partial responses and one complete response.

Pheochromocytomas are malignant and metastatic in between 5% and 26% of patients. Following tumor debulking surgery, the treatment options for this group of patients lie between chemotherapy and targeted radiotherapy with ^{131}I-MIBG. The current chemotherapy regimen using a combination of cyclophosphamide, vincristine and dacarbazine has a partial remission rate and hormonal response rate of 50% over 1–2 years.[131]I-MIBG has been used to treat over 100 patients with metastatic pheochromocytoma and paragangliomas. The majority of these patients have shown symptomatic responses with a decrease in catecholamine burden. Stabilization of disease has been seen in 58% of patients with 22% resulting in reduction in tumor bulk. Although these results compare favorably with those from chemotherapy, the tumor response is not as dramatic as one would hope for from targeted therapy. The therapeutic response to ^{131}I-MIBG depends on tumor bulk as well as uptake and retention of MIBG by the tumor. To date, there are no effective means of increasing tumor avidity for ^{131}I-MIBG.

Peptide receptor therapy with somatostatin analogs [15–17]

The somatostatin analogs have an established role in the management of somatotroph pituitary adenomas and secretory neuroendocrine tumors. Once tumor uptake and responsivity to somatostatin has been established, the choice of agent depends very much on patient preference and local clinical expertise. There are two commercially available somatostatin analogs: octreotide and lanreotide. Octreotide is available as a short- and a long-acting formulation while lanreotide comes as a medium- and long-acting formulation. Octreotide has highest affinity for sstr 2 and sstr 5: the affinity for sstr 2 is about 10 times greater than that for sstr 5. It is the shortest-acting of the available somatostatin analog formulations with the GH-suppressive effect lasting 4–6 hours after injection. GH levels tend to rise between doses given every 8 hours. Therefore, a long-acting formulation, octreotide LAR (Sandostatin LAR[TM], Novartis, Basel, Switzerland), has been developed. Octreotide is encapsulated in microspheres of a biodegradable polymer which release the drug slowly following intramuscular injection. Octreotide levels begin to rise over 7–14 days, and plateau for 20–30 days. Thus, typical dosing with octreotide LAR is every 4 weeks. The pharmacological effect of the drug can be manipulated by varying the dose from 10–30 mg per day, and if the drug is till effective at 1 month then longer intervals between injections can be used.

Lanreotide has similar affinities for the somatostatin receptor subtypes as octreotide. It is available for intramuscular or deep subcutaneous administration. Lanreotide SR is encapsulated in microspheres that provide prolonged release over 10–14 days after intramuscular administration. The pharmacological effect is manipulated by changing the dosing interval between every 7, 10, or 14 days. Lanreotide Autogel (Somatuline Autogel[TM], Ipsen, Paris, France) is administered by deep subcutaneous injection. Following injection, the drug congeals into a slow-release aqueous gel. Like octreotide LAR, lanreotide Autogel also has a monthly administration schedule. The pharmacological effect can be manipulated by varying the dose from 60, 90, or 120 mg. There is a rapid burst of lanreotide after injection and then a more maintained level for a month or so. One advantage of this formulation is that self- or partner administration is possible.

Common side effects of treatment with somatostatin analogs include nausea, abdominal cramps, loose stools, steatorrhea and flatulence. These symptoms are dose dependent and usually subside within the first few weeks of treatment. Impaired glucose tolerance and diabetes mellitus have been observed during therapy with somatostatin analogs. A very rare side effect is gastric atony. The risk of developing gallstones and/or gallbladder sludge in patients with metastatic gut NET or malignant islet cell tumors undergoing therapy with somatostatin analogs approaches 50%, but this is rarely symptomatic. The prevalence of somatostatin analog-induced gallstones in acromegalic patients varies geographically. Despite the high incidence of new gallstones in patients receiving somatostatin analogs less than 1% of patients develop acute symptoms requiring cholecystectomy.

Somatostatin analog therapy in acromegaly

The aim of treatment of acromegaly is to decrease GH levels to below 2–2.5 µg/L; at these levels the increased mortality rate associated with GH excess is reverted to normal. The first-line treatment is removal of the pituitary adenoma. However, the outcome of surgery depends on adenoma size, basal GH levels, and surgical expertise. Adenoma size and basal GH levels are inversely correlated to neurosurgical outcome. The surgical cure rate ranges between 80% and 90% for a microadenoma, near 50% for a macroadenoma and far less if the adenoma extends beyond the sella. Unfortunately, at least 60% of patients with acromegaly have a macroadenoma at presentation. The role of somatostatin analogs lies in both primary treatment for patients who are unsuitable for surgery and secondary treatment for patients in whom surgery has not provided a biochemical cure. Again, the response to somatostatin therapy is inversely proportional to the adenoma size and GH level. Studies in patients using both short- and long-acting somatostatin analogs as primary therapy have reported normalization of insulin-like growth factor-1 (IGF-1) in 60–70% of patients. Indeed, one series reported normalization of GH levels in 70% of patients with mainly macroadenomas. This compares well with data from studies looking at somatostatin analogs as secondary therapy. There is also an argument for debulking surgery in order to improve the postoperative efficacy of somatostatin analogs in patients where a curative operation is unlikely. At present, primary therapy is not recommended as sole treatment for acromegaly as the effect of somatostatin analogs on tumor growth is yet to be established. In a recent meta-analysis of the data, Bevan reviewed 921 patients from 36 studies [17]. These patients had all had pituitary imaging performed before and after variable doses of a somatostatin analog for variable lengths of time. In patients with primary therapy, tumor shrinkage occurred in 52% in contrast to 21% of patients with secondary somatostatin analog therapy. More importantly, only 3% of patients exhibited further tumor enlargement over the maximum 3 years of follow-up. This would suggest somatostatin analogs can provide at least effective short-term control of tumor growth. However, until long-term data are available the role of somatostatin analogs in the treatment of acromegaly remains as adjuvant therapy.

Somatostatin analog therapy in NET

Somatostatin analogs can control hypersecretion in NET that express somatostatin receptors. These include functional NET of fore- and mid-gut origin, pancreatic endocrine tumors such as glucagonomas, VIPomas and to a lesser extent gastrinomas and metastatic insulinomas. In about one-third of patients who show progressive disease before somatostatin analog therapy, stable disease is observed after the initiation of treatment. In addition up to half of patients treated with a somatostatin analog will achieve reduction in hormone secretion. Other syndromes where octreotide may provide benefit include ectopic adrenocorticotropic hormone (ACTH) secretion with Cushing syndrome, oncogenic osteomalacia, and hypercalcemia secondary to ectopic parathyroid hormone-related peptide secretion. In patients with ectopic ACTH secretion and Cushing syndrome, octreotide therapy can result in a reduction of ACTH levels in some cases. Unfortunately, this response is unpredictable and there is generally incomplete normalization of ACTH overproduction. NET producing parathyroid hormone-related peptide are usually undifferentiated although some can express somatostatin sst2 receptors. In selected cases a trial with octreotide treatment may improve the clinical and biochemical picture. Although somatostatin analogs may exert some anti-proliferative actions, they are rarely associated with a reduction in tumor bulk by WHO criteria. As such, their role in the treatment of NET remains as adjuvants to surgical resection or chemo/radionucleotide therapy. However, current trials should determine if and to what extent these analogs can have a direct tumoristatic or even tumoricidal effect.

Future directions

The recognition that tumors of the neuroendocrine system express different patterns of peptide receptors has already led to innovations in patient care. There does appear to be a role for combining therapy, thereby targeting different peptide receptors on the same tumor. In addition, newer somatostatin analogs such as SOM 230 (Pesireotide) offer greater affinity to all somatostatin receptors. As our understanding of the regulation of the tumor cell cycle increases, it may also be possible to upregulate peptide receptor expression by tumor cells.

References

1. Krenning EP, Kwekkeboom DJ, de Jong M, Visser TJ, Reubi JC, Bakker WH. Essentials of peptide receptor scintigraphy with emphasis on the somatostatin analog octreotide. *Semin. Oncol.* 1994;21:6–14.
2. Kwekkeboom DJ, Krenning EP. Somatostatin receptor imaging. In *Advances in Oncology: the Expanding Role of Octreotide.* Lamberts SWJ, Dogliotti L (eds) BioScientifica: Bristol, 2002.
3. Reubi JC, Waser B. Concomitant expression of several peptide receptors in neuroendocrine tumours: molecular basis for *in vivo* multireceptor tumour targeting. *Eur. J. Nucl. Med.* 2003;30:781–793.
4. Reubi JC. Neuropeptide receptors in health and disease: the molecular basis for in vivo imaging. *J. Nucl. Med.* 1995;36:1825–1835.
5. Hofland LJ, Lamberts SW. Somatostatin receptor subtype expression in human tumors. *Ann. Oncol.* 2000;12(Suppl 2):S31–S36.
6. Reisine T, Bell GI. Molecular biology of somatostatin receptors. *Endocr. Rev.* 1995;16:427–442.
7. Eriksson B, Bergstrom M, Orlefors H, Sundin A, Oberg K, Langstrom B. Use of PET in neuroendocrine tumors. In vivo applications and in vitro studies. *Q. J. Nucl. Med.* 2000;44:68–76.
8. Pacak K, Eisenhofer G, Goldstein DS. Functional imaging of endocrine tumors: role of positron emission tomography. *Endocr. Rev.* 2004;25:568–580.
9. Reubi JC, Macke HR, Krenning EP. Candidates for peptide receptor radiotherapy today and in the future. *J. Nucl. Med.* 2005;46(Suppl):67S–75S (Suppl).
10. Kaltsas G, Rockall A, Papadogias D, Reznek R, Grossman AB. Recent advances in radiological and radionuclide imaging and therapy of neuroendocrine tumours. *Eur. J. Endocrinol.* 2004;151:15–27.
11. Reubi JC. Peptide receptors as molecular targets for cancer diagnosis and therapy. *Endocr. Rev.* 2003;24:389–427.
12. Kwekkeboom DJ, Mueller-Brand J, Paganelli G, et al. Overview of results of peptide receptor radionuclide therapy with 3 radiolabeled somatostatin analogs. *J. Nucl. Med.* 2005;46(Suppl 1):62S–6S.
13. Kwekkeboom DJ, Kam BL, Bakker WH, et al. Treatment with Lu-177-DOTA-Tyr3-octreotate in patients with somatostatin receptor positive tumors. *J. Nucl. Med.* 2002;43(Suppl):1630–1633.
14. Mukherjee JJ, Kaltsas GA, Islam N, et al. Treatment of metastatic carcinoid tumours, phaeochromocytoma, paraganglioma and medullary carcinoma of the thyroid with (131)I-meta-iodobenzylguanidine (131)ImIBG. *Clin. Endocrinol.* 2001;55:47–60.
15. Öberg K, Kvols L, Caplin M, et al. Consensus report on the use of somatostatin analogs for the management of neuroendocrine tumors of the gastroenteropancreatic system. *Ann. Oncol.* 2004;15:966–973.
16. Lamberts SW, van der Lely AJ, de Herder WW, Hofland LJ. Octreotide. *N. Engl. J. Med.* 1996;334:246–254.
17. Bevan JS. The anti-tumoral effects of somatostatin analog therapy in acromegaly. *J. Clin. Endocrinol. Metab.* 2005;90:1856–1863.

8 Techniques in Radiation Medicine

P. Nicholas Plowman

Key points

- External beam radiotherapy remains an important means of delivering treatment to endocrine tumors.
- Linear accelerators provide a sophisticated means of delivering external beam therapy.
- Gamma Knife radiosurgery is used for small well-delineated tumors within the head and is useful when there are adjacent radio-sensitive tissues.
- Radioisotope therapy is used in the treatment of tumors which avidly and selectively take up a particular isotope. There should also be lengthy retention of the isotope by the tumor cells, e.g., ^{131}I in thyroid cancer and meta-iodobenzylguanidine (MIBG) in malignant pheochromocytoma.

Introduction

Radiation therapy maintains its important role in oncology; its ability to effect durable local control of tumor growth remains critical to successful therapy. For endocrine tumors, where the overall growth rate and rate of metastatic development are often slower than in many commoner cancers, the skilled application of particularly external beam radiotherapy improves overall local control rates; increasing sophistication of dose delivery in the last decade has been an important advance. Whilst external beam radiotherapy is the "backbone" of modern radiation therapy, the use of radio-isotopic therapy is also advancing and this now lends a more "systemic" aspect to radiation therapy. This chapter will explain and review modern methods.

External beam radiotherapy

Simply, for external beam radiotherapy, the patient lies on a bed and a beam is shone at the tumor from an X-ray (or perhaps still in developing countries a ^{60}Co γ ray) source. Both X-rays and cobalt-derived γ rays interact with cells identically as they are both megavoltage photon beams; only the energy of the beams and their collimation into sharp, low penumbra beams vary (of some importance in dosimetry – cobalt being inferior in these areas).

The radiation damage by such external beam treatment occurs instantly and the patient is not radioactive on leaving the treatment room.

The calibration of ionizing radiation delivered to biological tissue is in terms of energy deposited per unit mass of absorbing substance. The unit of radiation dose is the gray; 1 Gy represents 1 J (joule) of ionizing radiation energy absorbed per kilogram of tissue.

"Conventionally fractionated" radiotherapy has evolved over decades, following the original observations that small daily doses of external beam radiation led to a cumulative effect on the tumor but allowed relative sparing of normal tissues – due to normal/homeostatic repair and recovery processes that were lost when cells became neoplastic. "Conventional" fractionation for adults comprises 2 Gy daily fractions, whereas for children this is usually 1.6–1.8 Gy each day. In multiple portal techniques, each portal is treated daily and the minimum tumor isodose is usually chosen for the prescription from computer planning-generated isodosimetric plan; this is the lowest isodose that completely encompasses the tumor volume. In a good plan, the gradient across the tumor should be less than 5%, there should be no "hot spots" outside the tumor volume and the isodoses should "fall off" sharply at the edge of the tumor volume – although not as sharply as in the stereotactic methods (see below).

Developments of technology have allowed the stereotactic mapping of intracranial lesions and the delivery of focal/focused radiation to extremely discrete targets within the head. Unlike most radical radiotherapy treatments to the brain, where conventional fraction sizes are used to spare toxicity to the normal nervous system, these focal radiation techniques allow much larger doses to be delivered as the normal brain surrounding the tumor/target volume receives only a small fraction of the dose, due to the fast falling dose gradient at the periphery of the targeted tumor. Indeed, this can be used to advantage where some tumors will only respond to high-dose fractions (that previously could not safely be given with conventional therapy for fear of radiation morbidity to the surrounding normal brain). In the Gamma Knife system described below, the dose gradient across the field is huge (usually two-fold)

Clinical Endocrine Oncology, 2nd edition. Edited by Ian D. Hay and John A.H. Wass. © 2008 Blackwell Publishing. ISBN 978-1-4051-4584-8.

but in this instance it is viewed as positively advantageous as this allows extra dosage to be deposited in the center of the tumor.

Linear accelerators

Modern linear accelerators (linacs) provide a most sophisticated method of delivering external beam radiotherapy. These machines generate megavoltage X-ray beams that are more penetrating than previous orthovoltage (deep X-ray) or cobalt beams; that is, they give a higher dose of radiation at tumor depth per unit dose delivered on the body surface (entry portal). Furthermore, the beams are skin sparing (deliver maximum dose below rather than at the skin surface) and they are better collimated beams (i.e., less penumbra and side scatter). Linear accelerators are isocentrically mounted such that it is routine to position the tumor at the centre of the arc of rotation of the linear accelerator, which may then rotate to affect the multiple portals all aiming at the target/tumor (isocentric technology).

X-rays are generated when a tungsten target is bombarded by high energy electrons, whose braking energy (as they hit the target) is the *bremsstrahlung* that we call X-rays.

One or more skin entry X-ray portals/fields are used. The advantage of multiple fields (skin entry portals) is that this allows the radiation dose to be concentrated on the pre-mapped tumor by a "cross-fire technique."

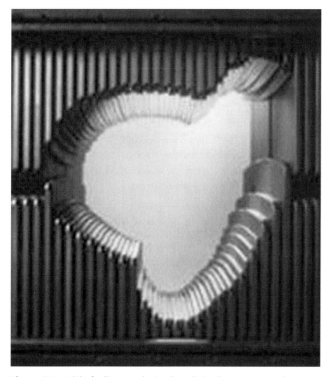

Figure 8.1 Multileaf collimators altering the radiation beam to an irregular shape that conforms to an irregular tumor pattern – a key feature of modern conformal radiotherapy and intensity modulated radiotherapy (IMRT).

Linear accelerator portal/field shaping is effected by defining "jaws" (collimators) working in perpendicular planes to create square or rectangle portals. Multileaf collimation (MLC) or secondary collimators/"jaws" comprise 40–52 finger-like lead processes, which may selectively project into the beam by any predetermined extent to effect much more sophisticated beam shaping than has been hitherto possible. Furthermore, movement of these MLC processes, during a field's exposure, in a technique called intensity modulated radiation therapy (IMRT) [1–3] has allowed a better conformation of dose to target than previously possible (including the ability to produce concavities in a high-dose volume – important in spring e.g. the spinal cord in treating a vertebral tumor) (Fig. 8.1).

Furthermore, the technique of portal imaging ("beam's eye view") allows verification of treatment set-up (i.e. reproducibility of simulated field set-ups) with greater immediacy than the old technique of beam filming. This is critical if beam shaping is, by IMRT or other modern conformal methods, tighter than before.

The major criticism of contemporary IMRT is that there are uncertainties in the anatomic geometry (relative position and shape) of the tumor or organs at risk (OAR) at each treatment episode. The development of methods to check on this reproducibility of set-up and day-to-day accuracy is important and relies on what is called image guided therapy (IGT). In IGT uncertainties in the knowledge of the exact/absolute position of the anatomy at the time of treatment delivery are removed/overcome by acquiring volumetric images of the treatment delivery system itself, and at the time of treatment. There are several approaches currently in operation, the combination of a conventional computerized tomography (CT) scanner or a cone-beam kV – CT with the linear accelerator being the main ones.

Tomotherapy

In tomotherapy (Tomotherapy Inc., Madison, WI, USA), a linear accelerator moves in a helical fashion around the patient, producing a spiral delivery pattern of 6 MV photon therapy. The helically moving linac moves in unison with an MLC (which has two sets of interlaced leaves that move in and out very quickly and continually to modify/modulate the beam during treatment exposure). Furthermore, a CT (MV) detector sub-system is mounted on the same rotating gantry assembly (powered via slip ring technology which also allows for transmission of data). The machine is purpose built to deliver IMRT and to have built-in IGT to verify treatment delivery. The analogy to a marriage between a treatment linear accelerator and a CT is a relevant one – both are spiral technology. Furthermore, the treatment couch upon which the patient is lying, is also moving, guiding the patient slowly through the center of the ring (Fig. 8.2). Thus, every time the rotating linac source comes around, its directing beam is at a slightly different plane – this last needs some further explanation: as the treatment beam rotates around the gantry, the couch, upon which the patient lies, is translated through it. This is parametrized by a

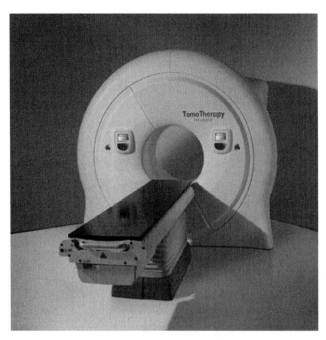

Figure 8.2 Tomotherapy machine. As stated in the text, the patient couch moves through the central "hole" in the machine, which delivers the beam in a helical manner.

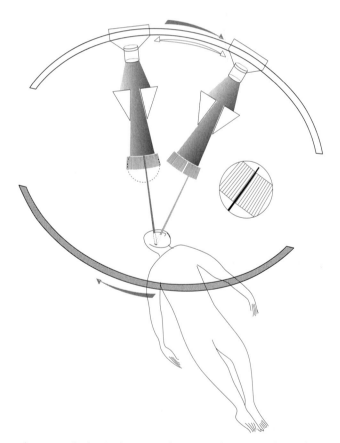

Figure 8.3 This diagram demonstrates the patient, with an intracranial tumor, being treated on a tomotherapy unit. The linac source is rotating as it treats the patient, with different multileaf beam shaping at different positions. On the far side of the patient is the monitoring CT scan detector (shown as the shaded arc in the diagram).

quantity known as the pitch, exactly the same as in a diagnostic CT scanner (except that the pitch – the ratio of patient movement to width of the X-ray beam – is less than unity for each full rotation in the therapy apparatus). The target/tumor volume and critical adjacent normal tissues "split" into voxels; each voxel is irradiated during several gantry rotations or arcs (Fig. 8.3). Factor into this that the MLC will have different configurations during the different segments and it can be immediately appreciated how it is now possible to alter the therapy dose very precisely and intricately, hence achieving extremely good conformity of dose delivery [4].

Gamma knife radiosurgery

Neither a knife nor a surgical technique, this specialist focal method of radiation therapy depends on a pinned stereotactic frame for precise localization; once fitted to the head, the computer software will produce a grid within the confines of the frame (and hence the head), every point having a three-dimensional co-ordinate. The patient is then scanned by MR/CT and the target is delineated. Then the patient is mapped for therapy. The Gamma Knife system (Elekta, Linkoping, Sweden) comprises 201 channels of carefully collimated beams of ^{60}Co radiation, from a hemispherical helmet, all pointing at one central point. By carefully aligning the target, using the three-dimensional co-ordinates within the pinned stereotactic frame, the patient's tumor is irradiated by the 201 beams; if irregular in contour then by several exposures using different co-ordinates. A dose distribution that accurately conforms to the shape of the tumor is thereby created.

Gamma Knife radiosurgery is used for small well-delineated targets/tumors within the head, without infiltrating borders and particularly when there are radiosensitive adjacent normal structures because the dose "fall-off" at the margin of the irradiated target is sharper than by other methods. It is usually employed as a single (high-dose) radiation dose treatment and this has advantages for some tumors that do not readily respond to radiation therapy delivered in conventional sized fractions. There is a growing interest in exploring the use of Gamma Knife therapy as first radiation therapy for pituitary adenoma.

Other focal radiation methods

Proton beams have a focal dose distribution that can be extremely useful, particularly for large targets. Their strength lies in the Bragg peak distribution of dose at the end of the path length of the charged particles; by varying the energy of the protons, it is possible to deliver a huge dose of ionizing radiation at a particular point inside the body.

Usually employing a stereotactic frame that relocates on the upper dentition, linear accelerator-based stereotactic systems have the advantage over Gamma Knife of fractionation, but they are dosimetrically inferior to Gamma Knife and proton therapy (i.e., the beam "fall-off" at the margin of the targeted tumor is less sharp). With the advent of IGT and more sophisticated conventional radiation therapy delivery systems (tomotherapy and IMRT), which themselves approach the accuracy and focal nature of the stereotactic techniques, the place for stereotactic linac therapy is diminishing, although still useful in selected situations.

Cyberknife (Accuray Inc., Sunnyvale, CA, USA) is a compact linear accelerator, emitting circular beams with secondary collimation ranging from 5–60 mm, mounted on a three-dimensional, high precision robotic arm, capable of delivering beam orientations with an accuracy of not worse than 0.2 mm. This linear accelerator is orientated according to information delivered to it via high-resolution image detectors that capture X-ray images and generate digital images of anatomy. These images, which are taken throughout treatment, are compared to the digitally reconstructed radiographs generated from the CT scans used for the initial planning. The imaging system then determines the patient's position and sends commands to the robotic arm for orientating the beam. The Cyberknife is competing with Gamma Knife for stereotactic therapy in the head (although the pinned frame of the Gamma Knife is a better validated technique at present) and seems to have its greatest potential in the spine and body where hitherto stereotactic radiotherapy has not been possible.

Heavy charged beams of protons offer an alternative method of concentrating ionizing radiation on a target by virtue of the Bragg peak phenomenon. Towards the end of their track, charged particles deposit the overwhelming majority of their energy – the Bragg peak of energy deposition. This phenomenon may be harnessed with good effect to deposit therapeutic radiation dosage on exact targets and a new generation of proton therapy machines may allow further exploration of this type of focal radiation therapy in the UK [5].

Radioisotope therapy

Tumor-specific radiopharmaceuticals delivering radiation therapy specifically to tumor cells theoretically meet Ehrlich's objective of "magic bullets" for cancer. Such treatment is systemic, non-invasive and should cause few immediate or long-term side effects. Interestingly, long-term follow-up of patients treated with radioisotope therapy has shown a lower oncogenic potential than for chemotherapy or external beam radiation; is this due to high linear energy transfer (LET) radiation (see below)?

An avid and selective uptake of radioisotope by tumor cells and a lengthy retention of the isotope by these cells are the requirements for successful therapy. The absorbed radiation dose (DB) in grays delivered by a β-emitting radio nuclide can be calculated by the slightly rough and ready equation:

$$DB = 19.9 \times c \times E \times T_{eff}$$

where c is the concentration of isotope measured in megabecquerel per gram (MBq/g) tissue; E is the average β energy

in MeV; and T_{eff} is the effective half-life in days (a composite of physical and biological half-lives).

The activity concentration (or specific activity) within target tissues requires volumetric assessment of the tumor (from palpation or imaging). The effective half-life of the isotope in the tumor and whole body can be determined by several serial quantitative scans.

It must be realized that the requirements of the imaging nuclear medicine physician and the radiation oncologist differ when it comes to selecting radioisotope-labeled pharmaceuticals or monoclonal antibodies. The former requires good quality imaging and is in favor of delivering a relatively high specific activity of a short half-life isotope which is rapidly taken up by the target tissue and, during its short physical half-life, emits a high signal of γ-photons of ideal energy for detection by a γ camera. The radiation oncologist wants an isotope with a high emission of short path length β particles delivering high LET/cytocidal radiation to the tumor cell in which the atom resides plus its neighbors; the γ emission is undesirable. It is for these reasons that in both metaiodobenzylguanadine (MIBG) and monoclonal antibody radioisotope labeling work ^{123}I is used for imaging and ^{131}I for therapy. The only conflict that arises is when, to establish the effective half-life of the labeled substance in the tumor (required to obtain an estimate of absorbed dose), the radiation oncologist needs 48–72 hour data points (difficult for ^{123}I with a physical $T_{1/2}$ of 13.2 hours) in the initial diagnostic/imaging scan. This can be undertaken retrospectively after administration of the therapy by subsequent serial imaging.

Radio-iodine (^{131}I)

The ^{131}I isotope has a physical half-life of 8 days and at disintegration emits β rays (average energy of 0.55 MeV with penetration of approximately 1 mm in soft tissue) and photons (average energy 0.37 MeV).

Between 50% and 80% of differentiated thyroid cancer concentrates radio-iodine. Although Pochin [6] found papillary and follicular cancers equally likely to be iodine avid, other workers found that a lower fraction of papillary cancers as compared to follicular cancers concentrated iodine [7]. Pediatric cancer was more likely (89%) than adult cases (64%) to concentrate ^{131}I in the Villejuif experience, despite a higher percentage of papillary cases in children (M. Tubiana, personal communication, 1985). As the avidity of thyroid cancer for iodine is usually less than that of normal thyroid tissue, a policy of normal thyroid ablation (surgery and ^{131}I) is employed prior to therapy.

Administered activities of 200 mCi (7.4 GBq) are usually prescribed for treatment of metastatic, iodine-avid, differentiated thyroid cancer. Halnan [8] demonstrated that if a tumor concentrated 0.1% activity/g with an effective half-life of 3 days, it would receive an absorbed dose of 6200 cGy from a 7.4 GBq, whilst at the same time the whole body dose would be below 1% of this; indeed the marrow dose is usually of the order of 0.5 cGy/mCi

(0.1 mGy/MBq). If there is a significantly larger uptake and retention in either a normal thyroid remnant or bulky metastatic cancer, the whole body/bone marrow dose is increased up to four- to 10-fold. Renal impairment, leading to reduced iodine excretion and hence increased effective half-life, also increased the whole body dose. Of the complications of repeated therapy dose of ^{131}I, marrow depression and pneumonitis are best documented, the latter being most important in patients presenting with "miliary" lung metastases. Radiation nephritis is a rare risk. Gonadal damage leading to infertility is unusual and Edmonds and Smith [9] could not find evidence to support the concept of reduced fertility, although the calculated dose to the gonads, particularly in some males, is in the range known to cause oligospermia, at least temporarily. Similarly, genetic damage in offspring was not detectable [10]. With regard to late oncogenesis, Edmonds and Smith [9] found a slight excess of acute leukemia (risk one in 100 000 patient-Gray-years) and bladder cancer (risk five in 10 000 patient-Gray-years).

With regard to lower doses of ^{131}I used as therapy for thyrotoxicosis, say 5–15 mCi (185–555 MBq) administered activities, the imperceptible risks with regard to carcinogenesis, leukemogenesis, genetic and fetal damage from huge analyses of more than 100 000 patients are well reviewed by Halnan [11].

Metaiodobenzylguanidine

MIBG, a guanethidine analog, was developed as a radio-iodinated pharmaceutical by Sisson et al. [12] and since then has established itself as an important agent in the imaging and treatment of neural crest tumors. Hoefnagel [13] estimates that 88% of pheochromocytomas, 91% of neuroblastomas, 70% of carcinoid/gut apudomas and 35% of thyroid medullary carcinomas concentrate MIBG. In this author's experience the therapeutically useful avidity percentages are lower, certainly for carcinoid tumors, although it is probably relevant to distinguish gastrointestinal apudomas from atypical carcinoids – the former being less likely to be positive on MIBG scanning – and within the GI tract, those arising from the foregut may have lesser potential to have positive uptake of MIBG than midgut ones.

In an analysis of the dosimetry of 25 children with advanced neuroblastoma treated by therapeutically prescribed activities of 100–200 mCi (3.7–7.4 GBq) of ^{131}I-MIBG following induction chemotherapy, Fielding et al. [14] found red marrow and whole body absorbed doses of the region of 0.1–0.7 mGy/MBq with a mean of approximately 0.35 mGy/MBq (approximately 1 rad/mCi). Obviously, where bone marrow infiltration by neuroblastoma has resisted induction chemotherapy, the bone marrow dose will be higher, as the path length of β rays from ^{131}I is approximately 1 mm in soft tissues.

The mean dose to the bladder in non-catheterized patients was 27 Gy, the dose per unit activity varying from 2.5 to 5.3 mGy/MBq. The liver doses were 1.6–11.3 Gy (0.3–1.9 mGy/MBq). The tumor doses varied widely from 2 to 53 Gy (0.2–16.6 mGy/MBq).

Repeated administration of 150–200 mCi (8 GBq) activities have been delivered with cumulative beneficial effect to malignant pheochromocytoma and neuroblastoma patients, although the optimal scheduling of ^{131}I-MIBG into neuroblastoma therapy is still to be decided. The innovative use is as a first-line treatment to shrink tumors and render them operable [13]. In other tumors, such as metastatic carcinoid, paraganglioma and gastrointestinal apudomas, we have much experience in the slow but assured shrinkage of tumors after successive therapy doses of ^{131}I-MIBG, and it is our first-line therapy option in inoperable apudoma lineage tumors, that are positive in all sites of known disease on tracer dose imaging and where the labeling/mitotic index is not high.

Radioactively labeled somatostatin analogs

Where apudoma cells express somatostatin receptors, ^{111}In-octreotide and ^{111}In-pentreotide have been used in therapeutic dosages and are reported to induce variable responses: partial shrinkage of the tumor, stabilization of disease, clinical and hormonal responses. However, this indium isotope is not perceived to be a useful therapy isotope for all the reasons given above.

[90]Y (β-emitter)-labeled octreotide, octreotate or lanreotide is perceived to be a much better therapeutic isotope but it has proved more difficult to link the isotope to the molecule.

[177]Lu-labelled octreotate, a β- and γ-emitter, used alone, in combination or sequentially with ^{90}Y analogs seems to offer major therapeutic advantages – the field is developing.

Radiolabeled monoclonal antibodies

Diagnostic radioimmunoscintigraphy (RIS) is now a highly developed technique and because tumor deposits show up so well on these static scan pictures, the unwary person is beguiled into thinking that radioimmunotherapy (RIT) should be currently useful for many situations in oncology.

Monoclonal antibodies for both RIS and RIT are gammaglobulin molecules comprising paired heavy and light chains from which, for RIS, antigen-specific Fab fragments are cleaved and may reach tumor cells more easily than the whole antibody molecules; however, the whole antibody molecule often has a greater binding affinity for the tumor, which is more important for RIT. Also relevant is that for RIS, the rapid uptake of a high specific activity but short half-life isotope allows a high signal from the tumor (which swamps the background "noise") to give a good imaging scan. This does not necessarily imply a good potential for RIT, which is more dependent on a sustained, preferential uptake and retention of the monoclonal antibody by the tumor cells, and preferably by all the tumor cells, with retention for days.

Monoclonal antibodies have been tagged as immunotoxins or immunoconjugated with chemotherapy drugs, but radioisotopes have the theoretical advantage in that the complex does not have to be internalized after binding to a cell-surface receptor and there is the real possibility of cell-to-cell crossfire, not applicable to toxins or chemotherapy.

Intravenous administration of monoclonal antibody-directed therapy has to date not been successful. However, such therapy directed towards recurrent cancer, particularly growing in fluid phase or monolayer/bilayers in confined spaces (peritoneum, pleural space, cerebrospinal fluid (CSF)/leptomeninges or intratumor), has generated more interest and appears to hold more potential. However, even this last statement appears optimistic from the data available. Britton et al. [15] reviewed the data on RIT with the, then available, ^{131}I-monoclonal antibodies intraperitoneally for stage III ovarian cancer, reduced to small bulk by prior surgery and chemotherapy. The overall response rate was 18% but these responses were not durable. In the CSF, some slightly better evidence of response exists: using a range of monoclonal antibodies directed at neurectodermal surface antigens and radio-iodinated with ^{131}I, Lashford et al. [16] found a response rate of 11 from 16 patients with leptomeningeal disease from neuroectodermal primaries, but again mainly poorly sustained. The conclusion so far is that single-stage RIT has yet to fulfil its exciting theoretical potential. A two- or three-stage approach using a bifunctional antibody may be more useful in the future.

Intracystic therapy for craniopharyngioma

Recurrent cystic craniopharyngioma represents another area in which unsealed source radioisotope therapy has shown promise. Craniopharyngiomas are difficult to resect completely and often cystic relapse occurs. These cysts may be problematic in that they fill, causing pressure symptoms and, even if treated by a tube drainage (usually to a subcutaneous reservoir), they may require multiple aspirations. The secreted fluid comes from the thin secreting epithelium of the cyst; this has proved sensitive to high-dose β radiation. Baklund [17, 18] described 14 consecutive patients with cystic craniopharyngioma treated with intracystic instillation of the yttrium (^{90}Y). Following diagnostic and volumetric estimation of the cyst (usually by puncture of the cyst and injection of radio-opaque medium prior to X-ray) the cyst was re-punctured to inject ^{90}Y. In the 14 originally reported cases, activity of 0.2– 3.2 mCi, average 1.4 mCi (7.4–118 MBq) was injected into the cyst, although in one case 7.8 mCi (289 MBq), was injected into a large-volume cyst of 45 ml. The activity was calculated (from the volumetric exercise) to deliver a dose of 20 000 rad (200 Gy) to the secretory epithelium of the cyst. Due to the short path length of the β rays, the surrounding brain was spared. Retreatment was safe, if needed. In our own experience, and that of others, the vast majority of the cysts responded by reducing in size and secretion rate and without treatment complications [17–19].

Although other isotopes have been used (e.g. ^{32}P), ^{90}Y is preferred; it has a half-life of 2.67 days (64.1 hours), it is a pure β emitter (maximum energy 2.3 MeV) with a maximum range in biological tissue of 11 mm.

References

1. Boyer AL, Butler EB, DiPetrillo TA, et al. Intensity modulated radiotherapy: current status and issues of interest. *Int. J. Radiat. Oncol. Biol .Phys.* 2001;51:880–914.
2. James HV, Scrase CD, Poynter AJ. Practical experience with intensity modulated radiotherapy. *Br. J. Radiol.* 2004;77:3–14.
3. McNair HA, Adams EJ, Clark CH, Miles EA, Nutting CM. Implementation of IMRT in the Radiotherapy Department. *Br. J. Radiol.* 2003;76:850–856.
4. Beavis AW. Is tomotherapy the future of IMRT? *Br. J. Radiol.* 2004;77:285–295.
5. Jones B. The case for particle therapy. *Br. J. Radiol.* 2006;79:24–31.
6. Pochin EE. Prospects from the treatment of thyroid carcinoma with radioiodine. *Clin. Radiol.* 1967;18:113–135.
7. Simpson EJ, Panzarella T, Carruthers JS, Gospodarowicj HK, Sutcliffe SB. Papillary and follicular thyroid cancer. Impact of treatment in 1578 patients. *Int. J. Radiat.Oncol. Biol. Phys.* 1988;14:1063–1075.
8. Halnan KE. The treatment of thyroid cancer. *Ann. Radiol.* 1977;20: 826–830.
9. Edmonds CJ, Smith T. The long term hazards of the treatment of thyroid cancer with radioiodine. *Br. J. Radiol.* 1986;59:49–51.
10. Arkar SD, Beierwattes EH, Gill SP, Cowley BJ. Subsequent fertility and birth histories of children and adolescents treated with ^{131}I for thyroid cancer. *J. Nucl. Med.* 1976;18:460–464.
11. Halnan KE. Risks from radioiodine treatment of thyrotoxicosis. *Br. Med. J.* 1983;287:1821–1822.
12. Sisson JC, Frager MS, Valk TW, et al. Scintigraphic localisation of phaeochromocytoma. *N. Engl. J. Med.* 1981;305:12–17.
13. Hoefnagel CA. Radionuclide therapy revisited. *Eur. J. Nucl. Med.* 1991;18:408–431.
14. Fielding J, Lashford LS, Lewis I. Dosimetry of ^{131}Iodine metaiodobenzylguanidine for the treatment of resistant neuroblastoma: results of a UK study. *Eur. J. Nucl. Med.* 1991;18:308–315.
15. Britton KE, Mather SJ, Granowska M. Radiolabelled monoclonal antibodies in oncology III radioimmunotherapy. *Nucl. Med. Comm.* 1991;12:333–347.
16. Lashford LS, Davies AG, Richardson RB, et al. A pilot study of ^{131}I-monoclonal antibodies in the therapy of leptomeningeal tumours. *Cancer* 1988;61:199–209.
17. Baklund EO. Studies in craniopharyngioma. III Stereotactic treatment with intracystic yttrium-96. *Acta Chir. Scand.* 1973;139:237–247.
18. Baklund EO, Axelsson B, Bergstrand CG, et al. Treatment of craniopharyngiomas – the stereotactic approach in a ten to twenty three years perspective. *Acta Neurochir. (Wien)* 1989;99:11–19.
19. Blackburn TPD, Doughty D, Plowman PN. Stereotactic intracavitary therapy of recurrent cystic craniopharyngioma by installation of Y-90. *Br. J. Neurosurg.* 1999;13:359–365.

9 Interventional Radiology

Jane Phillips-Hughes and Philip Boardman

> **Key points**
> - Ultrasound and computed tomography are the imaging modalities most commonly used to guide percutaneous biopsy of suspicious lesions.
> - Venous sampling techniques performed under local anaesthetic can be useful in the localization of a number of endocrine tumors, including those of the parathyroid, pituitary, adrenal, and pancreas glands, the liver and duodenum.
> - Neuroendocrine tumor metastases to liver can be treated by arterial embolization, with or without the addition of chemotherapy. Overall 5-year survival rates are said to be 50–60%.
> - Results of radiofrequency ablation of hepatic neuroendocrine metastases are encouraging with relief of hormonal symptoms in around 60–70% cases for a median duration of 10 months.
> - Selective internal radiation therapy involves embolization of tumor with radiolabeled microspheres. Initial results are encouraging but large-scale studies are awaited.

Introduction

Interventional radiology utilizes imaging techniques to guide the placement of devices such as catheters and biopsy needles either to obtain a diagnosis or to provide minimally invasive treatment. Its use in the field of endocrine neoplasia can be either diagnostic or therapeutic.

Image-guided biopsy

Biopsy techniques use image guidance to traverse normal tissue and obtain a sample from the target area of abnormal tissue. Ultrasound guidance is ideal if the target area can be clearly demonstrated along with a suitable path of approach, as it allows the needle insertion to be visualized in real time. Computed tomography (CT) guidance can be used for biopsy of areas that cannot be visualized by ultrasound. Important points to note are as follows:
• The vast majority of biopsies are performed under local anesthetic.
• The platelet count and clotting status should be checked.
• A platelet count of 50 000 or greater and an international normalized ratio (INR) of 1.5 or less are satisfactory.
• When the platelet count is lower or the INR is higher then transfusion of fresh frozen plasma (FFP) ± platelets is recommended prior to biopsy.

Clinical Endocrine Oncology, 2nd edition. Edited by Ian D. Hay and John A.H. Wass. © 2008 Blackwell Publishing. ISBN 978-1-4051-4584-8.

• Fine needle aspiration cytology is generally performed with a 21 or 22 gauge Chiba needle and will provide only cells. However, this is often sufficient to diagnose some types of malignancy, and the risks are low.
• Larger samples are obtained with cutting needles – often referred to as core biopsies. These are typically 1 mm by 20 mm and allow more extensive sub-typing of tumors.

Venous sampling

Parathyroid venous sampling

Primary hyperparathyroidism may be caused by adenoma, hyperplasia or occasionally carcinoma, and causes symptoms associated with hypercalcemia. Several non-invasive diagnostic imaging procedures are available for preoperative localization including neck ultrasound, nuclear medicine scanning (usually with technetium 99m [Tc^{99m}] sestamibi), CT and magnetic resonance imaging (MRI). However, even when these tests are negative, many surgeons will opt for bilateral neck exploration as the next step, with the aim of identifying the hyper-secreting tissue at operation. Surgical resection is the treatment of choice, and cure rates are excellent, approaching 95% in experienced hands. However, a small group of patients re-present with recurrent or ongoing symptoms of hyperparathyroidism and locating the source of excess parathormone (PTH) secretion in this group can present a significant challenge.

Ectopic parathyroid tissue may exist in a number of locations – undescended parathymic, para-esophageal and mediastinal. Occasionally, more than one adenoma may be present. Surgical exploration of all of these areas in search of a small adenoma is a major undertaking, and preoperative localization is desirable.

Selective venous sampling may be performed under local anesthetic, as an outpatient procedure. It involves introducing a 5–7 French catheter via the common femoral vein in the groin and into the various veins in the neck and mediastinum that could potentially drain the site of abnormal hormone production; 4–5 ml of blood are withdrawn from each location.

Samples are labeled and their anatomical source is recorded. They are placed in non-heparinized tubes, on ice, and transported to the laboratory for radioimmune PTH assay.

The parathyroid glands normally drain via the three paired thyroidal veins (superior, middle and inferior). However, in reality there are numerous anatomical variations, and this "text-book" pattern is rarely demonstrated, particularly in patients who have undergone previous surgical exploration of the neck, where a number of veins may have been tied off. A schematic view of the venous anatomy is shown in Fig. 9.1.

Samples should be taken (where possible) from the internal jugular veins cephalad to the superior thyroid veins, all of the thyroidal veins, the subclavian, brachiocephalic (or innominate), azygos, hemiazygos veins, any mediastinal veins identified, the right atrium/inferior vena cava, and in the rare case of malignant hepatic metastases from the hepatic veins. Once the procedure is complete the catheter is withdrawn from the groin and hemostasis is achieved by manual compression of the puncture site for 5 minutes. The patient lies supine for 2 hours and is monitored in a recovery area. If there is no problem, they are then discharged home.

Complications of this procedure are very rare. They include groin hematoma, thrombosis, contrast reaction, arrhythmia and renal failure.

Although it is only minimally invasive, other non-invasive imaging tests are usually performed before selective venous sampling and the latter is reserved for cases where the results are negative or inconclusive.

In a recent review Seehofer et al. [1] compared selective venous sampling (SVS) with other non-invasive preoperative localization tests in patients facing re-operative surgery for recurrent/persistent hyperparathyroidism in a systematic meta-analysis of the interventional literature. The sensitivity of SVS was at least 90%, with no false-positive results. In 31 studies the overall true and false-positive rates respectively were 71% and 9% for SVS, 69% and 7% for Tc^{99m} sestamibi scintigraphy, 54% and 16% for MRI, 55% and 15% for thallium-technetium scintigraphy, 50% and 18% for ultrasound and 45% and 14% for CT. They concluded that Tc^{99m} sestamibi scintigraphy is the non-invasive procedure of choice, with SVS as the gold standard in patients with negative results from non-invasive localization procedures.

Inferior petrosal sinus sampling

A similar technique, whereby samples are taken from the inferior petrosal sinuses, may be used in the differentiation of adrenocorticotropic hormone (ACTH)-dependent (pituitary-dependent) Cushing syndrome from ectopic ACTH syndrome.

Samples are taken from each inferior petrosal sinus and a peripheral vein both before and after administration of corticotropin-releasing hormone, and ratios of central to peripheral ACTH levels are calculated.

Threshold criteria for a pituitary source have been defined as an inferior petrosal sinus to peripheral basal ratio of 2:1 or greater without corticotropin-releasing hormone (CRH) or a ratio of 3:1 or greater after CRH stimulation. Sensitivity after CRH stimulation has been reported as 90% with a specificity of 67% [2]. The simpler technique of internal jugular venous sampling, avoiding the more complex catheterization of the inferior petrosal sinus has been advocated by some, although the results are less sensitive [3]. Transsphenoidal exploration may still prove necessary in cases of unsuccessful sampling where no ectopic source of ACTH can be found.

Adrenal venous sampling

Hypertension secondary to hyperaldosteronism may be caused by an adrenal (Conn) adenoma or hyperplasia. Unilateral disease is amenable to surgical resection. Imaging with CT and MRI is complicated by the fact that improved technology has resulted in very small (e.g., 7 mm) adrenocortical nodules being demonstrated. Not uncommonly these are incidental (i.e., they do not secrete aldosterone). As incidental adrenal adenomas are common and hypertension is common, the picture can sometimes be confusing.

Adrenal venous sampling can therefore be very helpful in distinguishing between a non-functioning adenoma and a functioning

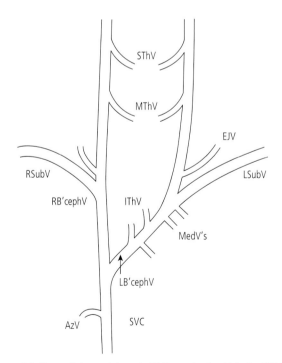

Figure 9.1 Venous drainage of the neck. SThV, superior thyroidal veins; MThV, inferior thyroidal veins; IThV, inferior thyroidal veins; EJV, external jugular vein; RSubV, right subclavian vein; LSubV, left subclavian vein; RB'cephV, right brachiocephalic vein; LB'cephV, left brachiocephalic vein; MedV's, mediastinal veins; AzV, azygos vein; SVC, superior vena cava.

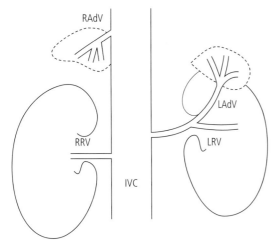

Figure 9.2 Adrenal venous drainage. RAdV, right adrenal vein; RRV, right renal vein; IVC, inferior vena cava; LRV, left renal vein; LAdV, left adrenal vein.

"aldosteronoma," and in localizing or confirming the site of excess aldosterone production prior to adrenalectomy.

A schematic view of the anatomy of adrenal venous drainage is shown in Fig. 9.2. The right adrenal vein usually enters the posterior lateral aspect of the inferior vena cava (IVC) above the upper pole of the kidney at around the level of T12. The short central vein is somewhat difficult to catheterize on occasion, and subtle movements of catheter tip plus a fair degree of perseverance may be required. However, successful catheterization can be achieved in around 90% of cases. In 10% of cases the right adrenal vein drains into the posterior aspect of an hepatic vein, close to the IVC. The left adrenal vein joins the inferior phrenic vein to form the phrenico-adrenal trunk, which enters the left renal vein. It is easier to cannulate.

At the site where adrenal venules join the central adrenal vein the vessel is lacking in musculature, and is thus fragile and susceptible to rupture if, for example, contrast is injected too forcibly. This may lead to adrenal hemorrhage and infarction with subsequent adrenal insufficiency. Hence only limited (0.2–0.5 ml) contrast injection is performed to confirm catheter position – and this after blood has been aspirated if possible to avoid contrast changing the secretory activity of the gland.

To allow for episodic variation in hormone secretion, a number of samples may be taken at 5 minute intervals. ACTH and cortisol levels are measured. Simultaneous sampling from a peripheral vein allows calculation of gradients.

ACTH stimulation may help differentiate between an aldosteronoma and bilateral adrenal hyperplasia. Baseline cortisol and aldosterone levels are taken from each side, and then a 250 µg bolus of ACTH followed by an infusion of 250 µg ACTH in 500 ml N saline is administered over 60 minutes. Repeat samples are taken beginning 15 minutes after the start of the infusion. Samples may be taken simultaneously with two catheters *in situ* or sequentially, moving one catheter from one vein to the other. Carr et al. [4] found the sequential method just as reliable as the simultaneous method.

When an aldosteronoma is present, ACTH stimulation causes a marked rise in cortisol and aldosterone levels of the affected side. The contralateral side shows an increase in cortisol only. With bilateral adrenal hyperplasia the aldosterone and cortisol levels are comparable bilaterally.

Adrenal venous sampling has also on occasion been used in the diagnosis of pheochromocytoma. However, this diagnosis is usually based on the typical clinical presentation combined with increased plasma or urinary catecholamine levels, plus CT/MRI and/or nuclear medicine scan findings. Venous sampling may rarely be helpful in the setting of a positive clinical and biochemical picture, where imaging has failed to identify the tumor.

Venous sampling for islet cell tumors

Islet cell tumors occur in the pancreas and peri-pancreatic tissues and may be functioning (i.e., hormone producing) or non-functioning. Functioning tumors present with symptoms related to hormone excretion and classic clinical symptoms are well recognized, for example in glucagonoma, somatostatinoma, vasoactive polypeptide tumor, gastrinoma and insulinoma. Even very small tumors can produce significant symptoms, and once the clinical diagnosis has been made and elevated hormone levels have been demonstrated by radioimmunoassay, preoperative localization studies are undertaken in the hope that the tumor can be surgically removed. A variety of imaging techniques are available including CT, MRI, endoscopic ultrasound and somatostatin receptor (octreotide) imaging. However, if the tumor remains elusive, or if further information is required in cases where the imaging is inconclusive, then venous sampling techniques with or without arterial stimulation may be required.

Non-functioning tumors tend to be larger at presentation and cause symptoms secondary to the mass effect of a space-occupying lesion; for example, those in the head of pancreas may present with jaundice due to obstruction of the common bile duct. There is no role for venous sampling with non-functioning islet cell tumors.

A thorough knowledge of the arterial and venous anatomy of the hepatic and peri-pancreatic area, plus the many possible congenital variants, is necessary prior to undertaking venous sampling studies. The splenic vein receives blood from the colon via the inferior mesenteric vein, the stomach and body and tail of pancreas via gastric and pancreatic tributaries, and the spleen. The superior mesenteric vein receives blood from the colon via the right and middle colic veins, the ileum and jejunum, plus the head of the pancreas and the duodenum via the gastrocolic trunk. The gastrocolic trunk receives tributaries from the anterior superior and inferior pancreaticoduodenal veins, the right gastroepiploic and colic veins. The splenic vein and the superior mesenteric vein join behind the pancreas to form the portal vein, which runs up to the porta hepatis and divides into left and right branches (Fig. 9.3). Conventional arterial anatomy is shown schematically in Fig. 9.4.

The celiac axis gives rise to the left gastric artery, the splenic artery and the common hepatic artery. The common hepatic artery gives rise to the gastroduodenal artery which in turn gives rise to the superior pancreaticoduodenal artery. The superior mesenteric

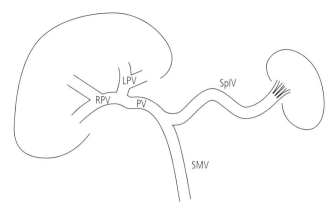

Figure 9.3 Portal venous anatomy. LPV, left portal vein branch; RPV, right portal vein branch; PV, main portal vein; SplV, splenic vein; SMV, superior mesenteric vein.

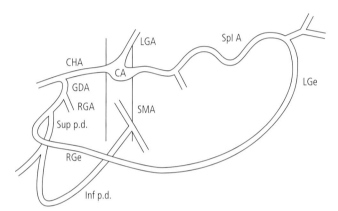

Figure 9.4 Celiac axis and superior mesenteric artery branches. CA, celiac axis; SplA, splenic artery; LGA, left gastric artery; CHA, common hepatic artery; GDA, gastroduodenal artery; RGA, right gastric artery; Sup p.d., superior pancreaticoduodenal artery; Inf p.d., inferior pancreaticoduodenal artery; RGe, right gastroepiploic artery; LGe, left gastroepiploic artery; SMA, superior mesenteric artery.

artery gives rise to the inferior pancreaticoduodenal artery, which anastomoses with the superior branch and supplies the head and uncinate process of the pancreas. The dorsal pancreatic artery may arise from the splenic, hepatic, celiac or superior mesenteric arteries and supplies the whole of the pancreas. In addition, the proximal splenic artery gives rise to the pancreatico-magna artery and the caudal pancreatic artery arises from the distal splenic artery, these two vessels supplying the body and tail of pancreas. However, numerous congenital variations to this standard format may occur and these must be recognized and taken into account.

The commonest reason for performing venous sampling in this territory is for the localization of insulinoma or gastrinoma.

Transhepatic portal venous sampling

Traditional portal venous sampling involves a percutaneous puncture of the portal vein via a transhepatic track, with insertion of a catheter into the splenic vein and then the superior mesenteric vein.

Contrast injections outline the venous anatomy and blood samples are taken from several locations within the splenic vein, the SMV and the portal vein. Each sample is numbered and its exact point of origin is recorded. Simultaneous samples are taken from a catheter in the celiac axis or the aorta or femoral artery. The samples are then sent for radioimmune assay of specific hormones.

Laminar flow in the veins can produce spurious results. Taking a number of samples at each location can counteract this. In addition the arterial samples obtained can be helpful in establishing if there is pulsatile hormone excretion by the tumor influencing the results. Once the hormone levels have been obtained they can be compared with their point of origin on the venogram. Elevations in hormone level should occur in veins close to the tumor site, and in this way tumors can be localized to the body and tail of pancreas, the head and neck of pancreas, and the liver (e.g., metastases).

Whilst achieving good results, the complications of this technique include bleeding and bile leak, and it is now being replaced by newer and less invasive intra-arterial stimulation procedures which do not involve the transhepatic approach.

Hepatic venous sampling with intra-arterial stimulation

This technique involves insertion of a catheter into the right hepatic vein, and a second catheter is placed into the celiac axis and then the superior mesenteric artery. Angiograms are performed to define the arterial anatomy and demonstrate any congenital variations.

In the localization of gastrinoma, 30 units of secretin are injected sequentially into the superior mesenteric artery (SMA), the splenic, gastroduodenal and common hepatic arteries, with blood samples obtained from the hepatic vein and the relevant artery at 20, 40, 60, 90 and 120 s post injection each time. A rise in gastrin levels of over 50% of baseline in the hepatic vein within 30–60 s localizes the tumor to the anatomical territory of that artery. The splenic artery supplies the body and tail of pancreas, the SMA and gastroduodenal artery supply the head of pancreas and duodenum and the hepatic artery supplies any metastases. The sensitivity of this technique for localization of gastrinoma is in the region of 77–89% [5]. Calcium gluconate has also been used as an alternative secretagogue with success [6].

In the localization of insulinoma, arteriography alone may be helpful as these tumors tend to be vascular and may produce a characteristic blush. However, the sensitivity can be increased by performing the previously described intra-arterial stimulation test using injections of calcium gluconate (0.025 µEqCa/kg) in 5 ml normal saline. This test can help differentiate a focal insulinoma from multifocal disease such as islet cell hyperplasia and nesidioblastosis. Hypoglycemia during the procedure can be avoided by intravenous glucose infusion, although regular measurements of blood glucose levels should be performed. Sensitivities for this technique are reported as being between 92% and 100% [5, 7].

Further details of all of the venous sampling techniques can be found in *Venous Interventional Radiology with Clinical Perspectives* [8].

Interventional radiology in the treatment of metastatic neuroendocrine tumors

Introduction

Neuroendocrine tumors (NET) consist of a rare group of carcinomas with the capacity to produce and secrete hormonally active substances. Carcinoid tumors are the most common type. Pancreatic islet cell tumors and medullary carcinoma of the thyroid occur less frequently. NET of gastrointestinal origin have a particular predisposition to metastasize to the liver. The growth of these tumors is frequently indolent leading to their description as "cancers in slow motion" [9]. Despite this, patients often present with incurable metastatic disease and those with the hepatic metastases from carcinoid have a median survival of only 3 years following diagnosis [9].

At least some of the hormonally active products produced are metabolized during the first pass through the liver. Consequently, gastrointestinal tumors with portal venous drainage rarely produce hormonal symptoms until hepatic metastatic disease has developed. Following tumor spread to the liver symptoms may be related to hormone release, pain or tumor bulk.

Symptomatic patients with hormonally active tumors and the presence of type II somatostatin receptors will receive treatment with somatostatin analogs (e.g., octreotide), which has been shown to be both effective and durable. Despite this, many patients can become refractory to such treatment. These patients with NET hepatic metastases present a difficult clinical problem as the role of surgical resection is often limited and systemic chemotherapy has limited effectiveness, particularly in carcinoid tumors. Fewer than 10% of patients will be candidates for hepatic resection. Investigators have reported a 16% response rate to chemotherapy with streptozocin-based regimens [10]. Pooled data from studies utilizing interferon-α suggest a 12% response rate [11]. Islet cell carcinomas are reportedly more responsive to chemotherapy with response in 27–69% of patients. Liver-dominant metastatic disease combined with the relatively indolent clinical course make neuroendocrine metastatic disease attractive for locoregional therapy aimed at reducing tumor bulk, controlling hormonal symptoms or rendering previously unresectable disease resectable. Treatment must be individualized to achieve the therapeutic goal, and take account of other factors including patient performance status, degree of liver dysfunction, portal vein patency and the distribution and extent of disease. Interventional radiological tools available include transarterial embolotherapy, local ablative techniques or selective internal radiation therapy (SIRT).

Transarterial embolization and chemoembolization

Hepatic artery embolization involves the infusion of particles into the tumor feeding vessels, with or without lipiodol, without the addition of chemotherapeutic agents. Chemoembolization combines hepatic artery embolization with simultaneous infusion of a chemotherapeutic drug, followed by particulate embolization. Both techniques have been applied to the treatment of metastatic neuroendocrine tumors.

Neuroendocrine hepatic metastases are typically hypervascular and derive their blood supply primarily from the hepatic artery. This, combined with the liver's dual blood supply (from hepatic artery and portal vein), provides the rationale for the use of a transcatheter arterial embolization (TAE). Established indications include: (i) control of hormonal symptoms, (ii) pain, and (iii) bulk-related symptoms, and in some institutions (iv) rapidly progressive liver disease. Contraindications include complete portal vein occlusion, liver insufficiency and bilio-enteric anastomoses. Involvement of over 50% of the liver parenchyma is used as an exclusion criterion by many and large-volume disease is associated with worse outcomes. Despite this, recent studies [12] have shown that embolization can be used safely in patients with over 75% liver involvement as long as treatment is performed in a staged manner with only a small portion of liver embolized at each session.

The combination of systemic chemotherapy and hepatic arterial occlusion provides greater and more durable disease regression over arterial occlusion alone [13]. As a result many authors favor the addition of chemotherapy to the embolic material (TACE) over TAE. Despite this there is no clear advantage to TACE over bland embolization. A recent study of TAE and TACE attempting to identify the variables affecting outcome [12] has suggested some benefit to the addition of interarterial chemotherapy in patients with islet cell tumors but not carcinoid, although the improvement in survival and imaging response did not reach statistical significance.

Embolization is performed under local anesthetic and is generally well tolerated. It most commonly involves treatment to either right or left hepatic lobe and whole liver treatment is not recommended in view of the high risk of hepatic failure when whole liver embolization is combined with widespread metastatic disease. The increasing use of microcatheters has allowed superselective treatment (Fig. 9.5) of a limited number of large metastases in each lobe simultaneously. In the periprocedural period patients are at risk of the effects of massive hormonal release from the embolized tumor and often require additional treatment with somatostatin analogs during this period. Even patients said to have non-functional tumors may be at risk due to periprocedural hormone release significantly above baseline levels. Treatment with allopurinol is used by some to prevent tumor lysis syndrome.

Many studies have documented the effectiveness of TAE and TACE in NET metastases. Overall 5-year survival post embolization is typically 50–60%. Symptomatic response with symptom-free intervals is achieved in over 90% of patients. Overall mortality is 4–6%. Morbidity includes hepatic abscess and post-embolization syndrome.

It remains unclear whether embolization is best performed early or late in the clinical course of the disease with advocates for both approaches. Good response rates can be achieved by embolization either early or late in the clinical course and the duration of liver metastatic disease before embolization has not been found to affect response rates [12].

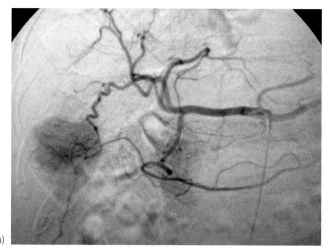

(a)

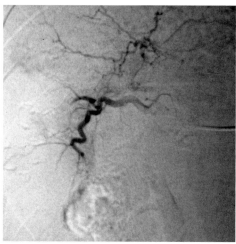

(b)

Figure 9.5 Hepatic metastasis (a) pre- and (b) post-particulate embolization. A large feeding vessel is seen taking origin from the right hepatic artery. Following selective embolization with 355–500 μm PVA there is an avascular area corresponding to the tumor vascular bed.

Cryoablation

Cryotherapy involves tumor ablation by repeated tissue freezing and thawing. The majority of cryosurgery experience has been in the treatment of colorectal liver metastases. However, small numbers of patients with neuroendocrine metastatic disease have been treated in this way, with symptomatic improvement. Siefert et al. [14] treated 13 patients with neuroendocrine liver metastasis using cryosurgery with a significant decrease in hormonal output and complete or partial response in all symptomatic patients. Cryoablation is limited by the relatively large caliber of the cryoprobe, and so the majority of cases have been performed in a surgical setting. Despite the recent introduction of smaller caliber probes cryotherapy has now largely been replaced by radiofrequency ablation.

Percutaneous ethanol injection (PEI)

Although PEI is accepted as less effective in metastatic disease than in treating hepatocellular carcinoma alcohol ablation can be

incorporated into treatment strategies for neuroendocrine metastatic disease. The advent of radiofrequency ablation means that the role of PEI is likely to be small and most commonly used as an adjunct to RFA in difficult cases. Studies have shown good response rates to PEI in small numbers of patients with neuroendocrine hepatic metastases [15], but the technique is limited in its ability to ablate larger tumor volumes. PEI has been used to ablate metastases located adjacent to vital structures (such as colon or central bile ducts) or large vessels vulnerable to a heat sink effect, where radiofrequency ablation may be difficult.

Radiofrequency ablation

Radiofrequency ablation (RFA) is becoming increasingly established as an effective treatment modality in the management of primary and secondary liver malignancy. The technique involves image-guided placement of the radiofrequency electrode within the tumor mass and the application of alternating radiofrequency current to cause ionic agitation which results in tissue heating. This heating causes coagulative necrosis and cell death (Fig. 9.6). Treatments can be performed using a percutaneous approach, laparoscopic guidance or at open laparotomy. The percutaneous approach is least invasive with a lower morbidity and is the most widely used. Ultrasound (US) is the most commonly used imaging guidance and allows real-time visualization of needle placement. However, US is less accurate than contrast-enhanced CT in monitoring the ablation and in difficult cases a combination of the two modalities is often advantageous. Ablation can be performed under conscious sedation or general anesthetic. It is the authors' preference to undertake treatment of metastatic disease under general anesthetic to allow more extensive ablation and in patients with hormonal syndromes management of the potential hormone release is more easily achieved in this setting.

RFA becomes less effective at achieving complete tumor necrosis with increasing tumor size, and in general terms success typically falls off as lesion size increases above 3 cm in diameter. The presence of large vessels adjacent to the tumor also limits the effectiveness of ablation due to the heat sink effect of adjacent flowing blood. Many interventional practices limit the use of radiofrequency ablation for primary and secondary hepatic tumors to patients with less than five lesions, smaller than 5 cm. In metastatic disease this is largely based on the treatment of colorectal metastases and is less relevant in patients with metastatic neuroendocrine tumors. Surgical studies have demonstrated that tumor debulking can improve survival and symptoms, but requires ablation of more than 90% of the tumor burden. A similar approach utilizing RFA for tumor ablation should provide similar benefits.

The largest series of radiofrequency ablation for neuroendocrine metastatic disease involved laparoscopic RFA in 34 patients with 234 tumors [16]. Patients had between 1 and 16 metastases ranging in size from 0.5 to 10 cm; 21% of patients underwent repeat treatment during the 1.6 year follow-up period. Symptoms were improved in 95% with complete relief in 63%. The mean duration of response was 10 months. Local disease recurrence occurred in

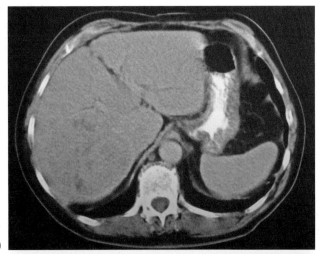

(a)

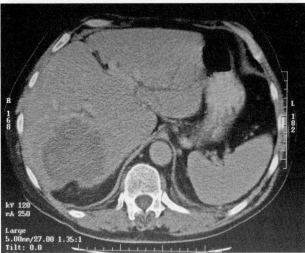

(b)

Figure 9.6 CT demonstrates a large NET metastatic deposit in a patient with carcinoid syndrome (a). Following radiofrequency ablation there is a large area of tumor necrosis (b). Although tumor necrosis is incomplete there was a very good symptomatic response.

of the grounding pads. The worst morbidity is associated with development of a liver abscess within the necrotic ablated tissue and is most commonly managed by percutaneous drainage. This complication is particularly prevalent amongst patients with biliary obstruction or previous bilio-enteric anastomosis and such are relative contraindications. Tumor ablation can be performed in patients with such anastomoses provided they are commenced on a course of rotating antibiotics. Complications are more likely with increasing numbers of needle punctures, larger volumes of tumor necrosis and lesions close to the liver hilum, vessels or adjacent viscera.

Selective internal radiation therapy (SIRT)

There has been recent interest in the use of radiolabeled microspheres for liver-directed therapy with promising results in colorectal liver metastases and hepatocellular carcinoma. Two preparations exist: TheraSphere consists of non-biodegradable glass microspheres, while SIR-spheres utilize resin microspheres. Both products contain yttrium-90 (^{90}Y), a pure β emitter with a mean tissue penetration of 2.5 mm. Most experience has been in the setting of hepatocellular carcinoma or colorectal metastatic disease but both products have been used to treat occasional patients with neuroendocrine metastases. There are significant differences in the use of these materials compared with other hepatic embolotherapy. Meticulous pretreatment angiography and embolization of visceral branches are required to prevent radiation toxicity to the gastrointestinal tract along with preliminary nuclear medicine studies to exclude excessive hepatopulmonary shunting. Despite this the toxicity associated with SIRT appears to be more tolerable than with other hepatic embolization. A small study by McStay et al. [20] has demonstrated the effective use of intra-arterial ^{90}Y-DOTA-lanreotide in patients with extensive hepatic neuroendocrine metastases with partial response and stable disease in 16% and 63% of patients. Larger scale studies are awaited.

Conclusion

Hepatic neuroendocrine metastatic disease poses a unique therapeutic challenge in which interventional radiology has a valuable and increasing role in tumor control and relief of hormonal symptoms.

References

1. Seehofer D, Steinmuller T, Rayes N, et al. Parathyroid hormone venous sampling before reoperative surgery in renal hyperparathyroidism: comparison with non-invasive localisation procedures and review of the literature. *Arch. Surg.* 2004;139:1331–1338.
2. Swearingen B, Katznelson L, Miller K, et al. Diagnostic errors after inferior petrosal sinus sampling. *J. Clin. Endocrinol. Metab.* 2004; 89:3752–3763.

13% of patients (3% of lesions), with the development of new hepatic disease in 28% and new extrahepatic disease in 25%. Local recurrence rates were lower than those reported by the same group for non-neuroendocrine metastatic disease [17], demonstrating the relatively favorable outcome in this group of patients. Others have demonstrated similar promise in smaller numbers of patients. Gillams et al. [18] showed tumor control in 74% of the 19 evaluable patients and relief of hormonal symptoms in 69% of 14 patients with hormone-related symptoms.

A recent literature review [19] containing patients with heterogeneous tumor types has shown that RFA is associated with mortality below 0.5% and morbidity of less than 10%. Needle puncture may result in hemorrhage. Thermal injury can cause thrombosis of the hepatic or portal vein branches, bile duct strictures or injury to adjacent structures such as stomach, duodenum, gallbladder or colon. Skin burns can also occur at the sites

3. Erickson D, Huston J 3rd, Young WF Jr, et al. Internal jugular vein sampling in adrenocorticotropic hormone-dependent Cushing's syndrome: a comparison with inferior petrosal sinus sampling. *Clin. Endocrinol. (Oxf.)* 2004;60:413–419.

4. Carr CE, Cope C, Cohen DL, et al. Comparison of sequential versus simultaneous methods of adrenal venous sampling. *J. Vasc. Interv. Radiol.* 2004;15:1245–1250.

5. Doppman JL, Jenson RT. Localisation of gastropancreatic tumours by angiography. *Ital. J. Gastroenterol. Hepatol.* 1999;31(Suppl 2): 5163–5166.

6. Turner JJ, Wren AM, Jackson JE, et al. Localisation of gastrinomas by selective intra-arterial calcium injection. *Clin. Endocrinol. (Oxf.)* 2002;57:821–825.

7. Brandle M, Pfammatter T, Spinas GA, et al. Assessment of selective arterial calcium stimulation and hepatic venous sampling to localise insulin-secreting tumours. *Clin. Endocrinol. (Oxf.)* 2001;55:357–362.

8. Savader SJ, Trerotola SO (eds). *Venous Interventional Radiology with Clinical Perspectives*, 2nd edn. Basel: Thieme, 2000:569–610.

9. Moertel CG. Karnofsky lecture: an odyssey in the land of small tumours. *J. Clin. Oncol.* 1987;5:1503–1522.

10. Sun W, Lipsitz S, Catalano P, et al. Phase II/III study of doxorubicin with fluorouracil compared with streptozocin with fluorouracil or dacarbazine in the treatment of advanced carcinoid tumours: Eastern Co-operative Oncology Group Study. E1281. *J. Clin. Oncol.* 2005;23:4897–4904.

11. Schnirer II, Yao JC, Ajani JA. Carcinoid: a comprehensive review. *Acta Oncol.* 2003;42:672–692.

12. Gupta S, Johnson MM, Murthy R, et al. Hepatic arterial embolisation and chemoembolisation for the treatment of patients with metastatic neuroendocrine tumours: variables affecting response rates and survival. *Cancer* 2005;104:1590–1602.

13. Moertell CG, Johnson CM, McKusiack MA, et al. The management of patients with advanced carcinoid tumours and islet cell carcinomas. *Ann. Intern. Med.* 1994;120:302–309.

14. Seifert JK, Cozzi PJ, Morris DL. Cryotherapy for neuroendocrine liver metastases. *Semin. Surg. Oncol.* 1998;14:175–183.

15. Livraghi T, Vettori C, Lazzaroni S. Liver metastases: results of percutaneous ethanol injection in 14 patients. *Radiology* 1991;179: 709–712.

16. Berber E, Flesher N, Siperstein AE. Laparoscopic radiofrequency ablation of neuroendocrine liver metastases. *World J. Surg.* 2002; 26:985–990.

17. Siperstein A, Garland A, Engle K, et al. Local recurrence after laparoscopic radiofrequency thermal ablation of the hepatic tumours. *Ann. Surg. Oncol.* 2000;7:106–113.

18. Gillams AR, Cassoni A, Conway G, et al. Radiofrequency ablation of neuroendocrine liver metastases: the Middlesex experience. *Abdom. Imag.* 2005;30:435–441.

19. Mulier S, Mulier P, Ni Y, et al. Complications of radiofrequency coagulation of liver tumours. *Br. J. Surg.* 2002;89:1206–1222.

20. McStay MK, Maudgil D, Williams M, et al. Large-volume liver metastasis from neuroendocrine tumours: hepatic intra-arterial ^{90}Y-DOTA-lanreotide as effective palliative therapy. *Radiology* 2005;237:718–726.

10 Surgical Management of Endocrine Tumors

Gustavo G. Fernandez Ranvier and Orlo H. Clark

Key points

- Thyroid cancers originate from follicular (papillary, follicular and Hurthle cell) or parafollicular/"C cells" (medullary thyroid cancer) and about 95% are well differentiated. Surgical resection is the treatment of choice.
- Preoperative identification and intraoperative finding of a benign parathyroid adenoma with monitoring of intraoperative parathormone levels is successful in >95% of the patients and localization studies (sestamibi scan and ultrasound) allow a focused exploration.
- Surgical resection is recommended in patients with functioning adrenal tumors and for non-functioning lesions that are suspicious for malignancy.
- Insulinoma is the most common islet cell tumor; in 90% of the cases it occurs sporadically and in 10% of the cases it is associated with MEN 1.

Introduction

General and endocrine surgeons have an important role in the management of the endocrine tumors. In the last decade, there have been many changes and advances in the diagnosis, localization and treatment of tumors of the thyroid, parathyroid, adrenal, and endocrine pancreas. As a consequence of these advances and more accurate localization studies, better outcomes have been reached. More advances, however, are necessary, especially for patients with metastatic disease.

In this chapter we will review current information and guidelines for the surgical management of patients with endocrine tumors.

Thyroid tumors

Thyroid cancer is the most common endocrine tumor. It is estimated that there are about 26 000 new cases each year and about 300 000 survivors of thyroid cancer in the United States. It is the most rapidly increasing cancer in women. Tumors of the thyroid gland include a variety of phenotypes: follicular adenomas, differentiated papillary carcinomas (follicular variant, tall, clear and columnar cell and diffuse sclerosing), follicular carcinoma, Hurthle cell carcinoma, medullary carcinoma, poorly differentiated and insular carcinoma and anaplastic tumors. Papillary, follicular and Hurthle cell cancers (differentiated thyroid carcinoma [DTC]) arise from follicular cells and medullary thyroid cancers from the

---

Clinical Endocrine Oncology, 2nd edition. Edited by Ian D. Hay and John A.H. Wass. © 2008 Blackwell Publishing. ISBN 978-1-4051-4584-8.

---

parafollicular cells. Other rare thyroid tumors include lymphoma and secondary metastatic disease to the thyroid, both of which account for about 2% of all thyroid cancers. Fortunately, about 95% of thyroid cancers are well differentiated [1].

Most patients with DTC present with asymptomatic thyroid nodules and some with cervical lymphadenopathy. Approximately 5% of palpable thyroid nodules seen in the adult population are malignant. Today, fine needle aspiration (FNA) and ultrasonography have replaced other tests like scintigraphy with ^{123}I or technetium-99m pertechnetate for the preoperative evaluation of thyroid nodules. The traditional thyroid operation is performed via a Kocher "collar" cervical incision. Other techniques include mini-incisions, pure endoscopic thyroidectomy via different access sites (supraclavicular, axilla, anterior chest and breast approaches) and video-assisted thyroidectomy.

Differentiated thyroid carcinoma

Papillary thyroid carcinoma (PTC) and follicular thyroid carcinoma (FTC) account for approximately 80% and 10% of all thyroid cancers respectively. Surgical resection is the only curative treatment for patients with these DTCs. Patients in whom FNA is positive for PTC can undergo a definitive planned surgical procedure, without the need for frozen section analysis. Because prospective randomized clinical trials have not compared the extent of thyroidectomy that produces the best results for patients considered to have low risk thyroid cancer, controversy persists about whether total or near total (leaving no more than 1 g of thyroid tissue) or thyroid lobectomy is the procedure of choice. Total thyroidectomy is recommended for patients with bilateral thyroid cancers, locally invasive tumors, lymph node or distant metastases, and for all patients when other therapy such as ^{131}I scanning and ablation will be used. In contrast, completion total thyroidectomy would not be recommended by most surgeons when an occult papillary thyroid cancer is identified after a thyroid lobectomy.

Several different scoring systems have been established, such as AMES (age, metastasis, tumor extent and size), AGES (age, tumor grade, tumor extent and size), MACIS (metastasis, age, completeness of surgery, invasion and size), TNM (tumor size, nodal status, distal metastasis) and De Groot (class I: confined to thyroid, class II: nodal metastases, class III: local invasion, class IV: distant metastases); classifications are useful for predicting tumor aggressiveness. Unfortunately, local tumor invasion, and nodal and distal metastases are often only identified postoperatively, which means these scoring systems cannot be used to determine the extent of thyroidectomy.

Papillary thyroid carcinoma is multicentric in about 80% of patients, and bilateral in about 33%; numerous reports document a lower recurrence rate after total thyroidectomy [2]. Total thyroidectomy also makes it possible to use radioactive iodine for scanning and ablative therapy, and blood thyroglobulin levels become a sensitive marker for documenting tumor recurrence or persistence [3]. Lobectomy can be used to treat young patients with small (<1 cm), solitary, well-differentiated papillary thyroid carcinomas with no evidence of nodal or distant spread, or minimally invasive (capsular only) follicular thyroid cancer. The prognosis for these patients is excellent, and complications such as permanent hypoparathyroidism or recurrent laryngeal nerve paralysis are probably somewhat lower than after total thyroidectomy since only one recurrent laryngeal nerve and two parathyroid glands are at risk. Two disadvantages of less than total thyroidectomy is that follow-up monitoring of blood thyroglobulin levels is less sensitive and ^{131}I ablation usually requires completion thyroidectomy for optimal results [4]. Even for low-risk thyroid carcinomas, most studies have shown lower recurrence rates and improved survival after bilateral resection [2]. We therefore favor total or near total thyroidectomy in both low-risk and high-risk patients, when it can be done with a low complication rate.

The current approach for the cervical lymphadenopathy associated with DTC is changing since ultrasonography and blood thyroglobulin testing will be done postoperatively. We recommend preoperative ultrasonography and functional neck dissection with removal of all clinically palpable nodes and any enlarged or abnormal nodes found on ultrasound (Fig. 10.1). Only about 15% of the patients with PTC and lymph node metastasis have contralateral cervical node metastasis; therefore, a contralateral neck dissection is not done unless bilateral lymphadenopathy is evident [1].

Follicular thyroid carcinomas are usually solitary, but may occur in association with benign thyroid disorders, and more frequently, in areas of iodine deficiency. FTCs invade the tumor capsule and the blood vessels within the capsule. The fact that FTC is solitary, together with the inability to obtain a diagnosis by FNA, makes surgical management of these tumors somewhat different than that for PTC. Diagnosis of FTC and of Hurthle cell carcinoma (HCC) is established by permanent histology. About 20% of follicular and Hurthle cell neoplasms by FNA cytology are malignant. Some investigations suggest that patients with large tumors are somewhat more likely to have a malignant tumor. We recommend a diagnostic thyroid lobectomy for these patients and inform them preoperatively that they may need a completion thyroidectomy if the final pathological examination reveals cancer (Fig. 10.1). Because HCCs are more likely to invade regional lymph nodes than are FTCs, preoperative ultrasound is helpful to evaluate for multiple and/or bilateral nodules and abnormal lymph nodes. About 75% of FTCs take up radioactive iodine, whereas 90% of HCCs fail to take up radioactive iodine following total thyroidectomy and most studies document a higher recurrence rate than for FTC [5].

About 30% of patients with papillary thyroid cancer have cervical nodal recurrences noted on physical examination, usually in the ipsilateral central or lateral neck [6]. Palpable and scan-identified recurrent disease should be treated surgically whenever possible. In patients with high thyroglobulin levels after total thyroidectomy in whom no tumor can be identified by ultrasound, magnetic resonance imaging (MRI), computerized tomography (CT) or fluorodeoxyglucose (FDG)–positron emission tomography (PET) scanning, treatment with ^{131}I and post-treatment imaging is recommended.

Unfortunately, about 25% of metastatic thyroid cancers fail to concentrate iodine. In these patients new drug trials may prove helpful. External beam radiation offers only palliative therapy. Chemotherapy is relatively ineffective.

Medullary thyroid cancer

Medullary thyroid carcinoma (MTC) accounts for less than 7% of all thyroid cancers, but for about 14% of thyroid cancer

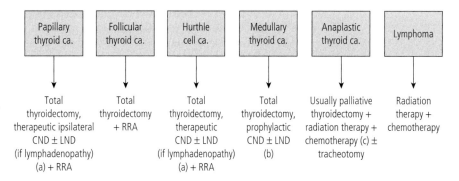

Figure 10.1 Surgical management of thyroid cancer. (a) By physical examination or ultrasound, CT scanning or MR imaging. (b) Some recommend unilateral or bilateral prophylactic LND for tumors over 1.5 cm. (c) Some patients benefit with preoperative radiation therapy and chemotherapy. CND, cervical node dissection; LND, lateral neck dissection; RRA, radioiodine remnant ablation.

deaths. About 75% of patients have sporadic and 25% have familial disease. In sporadic MTC, tumors are usually single and unilateral, and there is no family history of MTC or other related endocrinopathies.

There are three forms of familial MTC: multiple endocrine neoplasia (MEN) 2A and 2B and familial non-MEN MTC (FMTC). In familial MTC the cancers are multifocal, bilateral, associated with C cell hyperplasia and present at an earlier age. About 45% of patients with MEN 2A develop pheochromocytomas and 25% develop primary hyperparathyroidism. Some patients with MEN 2A have lichen planus amyloidosis, and some have Hirschsprung disease. About 50% of patients with MEN 2B develop pheochromocytomas and nearly all patients have mucosal neuromas in the digestive tract. FMTC is generally less aggressive and MEN 2B more aggressive than MEN 2A or sporadic MTC. All patients with MTC should be screened for a *RET* proto-oncogene mutation because 10% of them will have a new mutation so that their children are at risk for MTC.

The primary treatment for MTC patients is total thyroidectomy and central neck dissection (level VI) because of the early involvement of cervical lymph nodes (Fig. 10.1). In children under 6 years of age with a normal thyroid ultrasound and normal calcitonin a prophylactic total thyroidectomy without central neck dissection is recommended. An ipsilateral modified radical neck dissection as well as a bilateral central neck dissection is recommended for all patients with MTC and a primary tumor ≥1.5 cm. Curative surgery is unlikely in patients with MTC when more than six metastatic nodes are present or the nodes are larger than 1 cm. All patients with MEN 2A and 2B should be screened and treated for pheochromocytomas before thyroidectomy or other procedures. Prophylactic thyroidectomy should be performed in early childhood (before age 6) for known *RET* mutation-positive patients and at diagnosis or before age 1 in patients with MEN 2B.

Anaplastic thyroid carcinoma

Anaplastic thyroid carcinoma (ATC) accounts for less than 2% of all thyroid cancers and is one of the most aggressive malignancies; few patients survive more than 6 months. ATC is usually seen in the elderly, most often in women. Patients usually present with a rapidly enlarging neck mass, dysphagia, hoarseness, and dyspnea. The diagnosis can be confirmed by FNA. This tumor is classified as stage IV thyroid carcinoma according to the American Joint Committee on Cancer. Cure is rarely possible because most patients present with local invasion and distant metastases. Young patients and those with completely resectable tumors have a slightly better prognosis.

Surgery is performed in patients with tumors that appear to be resectable or to secure the airway via tracheotomy. Combined radiation therapy and chemotherapy followed by surgical resection appears to benefit some patients (Fig. 10.1) [7].

Lymphoma

Thyroid lymphomas account for 1–2% of all thyroid malignancies and less than 2% of all lymphomas. Most thyroid lymphomas are B-cell lymphomas and occur more often in older women who have a history of Hashimoto's thyroiditis. Thyroid lymphomas can be confused with ATC and MTC, and the surgeon's primary role is to make the diagnosis, often with open biopsy when FNA and/or core needle biopsy is non-specific. Most lymphomas are radiosensitive and chemosensitive. Once diagnosed, the patient is rapidly staged and treated with combined radiation therapy and chemotherapy (Fig. 10.1).

Parathyroid tumors

Hyperparathyroidism (HPT) is a common medical problem occurring in 0.1–0.3% of the general population. About 99% of patients with primary hyperparathyroidism (PHPT) have benign tumors (85% adenomas and 15% hyperplasia or multiple abnormal parathyroid glands), and approximately 1% have parathyroid carcinoma [8]. Benign primary hyperparathyroidism (BPHPT) is more common in women (1 in 500) than in men (1 in 2000), whereas parathyroid carcinoma is equally common in men and women (ratio of 1.04:1), and occurs more frequently in patients with familial hyperparathyroidism and jaw tumor syndrome [9].

Secondary hyperparathyroidism (SHPT) is a common problem in patients with chronic renal failure (CRF), and nearly all patients with chronic renal failure develop some degree of parathyroid hyperplasia. About 5% of these patients will need to be treated surgically. Parathyroid cancer is very rare in patients with SHPT.

Primary hyperparathyroidism

Parathyroidectomy is the only curative treatment for patients with PHPT, and can be performed successfully by experienced surgeons in >95% of patients [10], with a risk of complications of <1%. There is a general consensus that most patients under 50 years of age and all patients with symptomatic PHPT should be treated surgically. However, controversy continues regarding asymptomatic older patients or those with mild symptoms and how "asymptomatic" a patient with PHPT should be in order to have surgery. At a follow-up consensus meeting on asymptomatic hyperparathyroidism at the NIH in 2002, parathyroidectomy was recommended for all patients under 50 and when serum calcium was >1 mg/dl (0.0024 mol) above the normal range, when the 24 h urine calcium was >400 mg, when creatinine clearance was reduced by 30%, when bone mineral density (BMD) by T-score was >2.5 standard deviations below that of sex-matched controls, and in patients for whom medical surveillance was not possible (Fig. 10.2). Parathyroidectomy has been documented to be safe, beneficial and curative in elderly patients [11]. During the past 12 years, improvements in technology have led to a more selective surgical approach to patients with PHPT. Currently, scan-directed focused or unilateral open, radio-guided, video-assisted and videoscopic parathyroidectomy, as well as classic bilateral exploration, are done under general or local anesthesia. Unilateral, focused, and radio-guided techniques are dependent on positive preoperative localizing studies (sestamibi scan with or without single proton emission

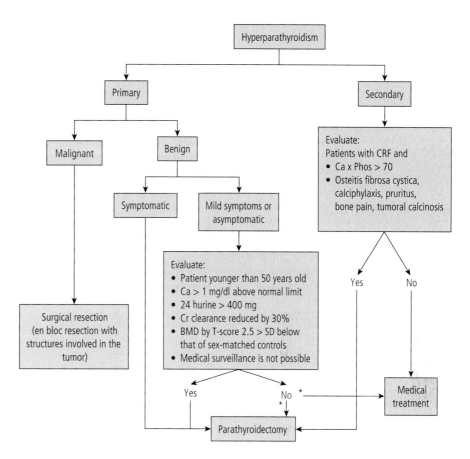

Figure 10.2 Management of parathyroid tumors. BMD, bone mineral density; Ca, calcium; CRF, chronic renal failure; Cr, creatinine; Phos, phosphate. * Controversial.

CT and ultrasound scans). When both studies independently identify the same abnormal gland without the presence of any other suspicious lesion, they have a sensitivity of up to 96% in patients with sporadic PHPT.

Patients with suspected multiglandular or familial disease, those taking lithium, those with coexistent thyroid cancer, clinically significant multinodular goiter or non-localizing studies usually warrant a traditional bilateral approach. This operation offers an excellent visibility of four parathyroid glands and access to most ectopic sites. Intraoperative PTH can be helpful in determining when the abnormal parathyroid gland or glands have been removed but is less accurate in patients with multiple abnormal parathyroid glands.

Secondary hyperparathyroidism

Patients with SHPT and a calcium × phosphorus product >70, osteitis fibrosa cystica, calciphylaxis and symptoms of pruritus and bone pain warrant a neck exploration with subtotal or total parathyroidectomy with parathyroid autotransplantation (Fig. 10.2). Treatment with calcium, vitamin D and phosphate binders and low phosphate diet helps to prevent SHPT. Sensapar and comparable medications are helpful in some of these patients. Localization studies such as sestamibi scans and ultrasound are not essential, but may identify abnormal parathyroid glands and sometimes a hyperplastic parathyroid gland in an ectopic position.

Recurrent/persistent disease

Causes of persistent or recurrent disease are failure to remove an undiscovered abnormal parathyroid gland in the normal position, failure to locate an ectopically situated parathyroid tumor, failure to recognize the presence of chief hyperplasia involving all four parathyroid glands or failure to remove multiple abnormal parathyroid glands, and subtotal resection of a parathyroid tumor, fracturing a parathyroid tumor, causing parathyromatosis, and parathyroid cancer.

Parathyromatosis

Parathyromatosis is a rare cause of persistent or recurrent HPT. It most often occurs as a consequence of seeding during the parathyroid operation or may be secondary to multiple embryological rests of parathyroid tissue. Surgical treatment for parathyromatosis is removal of all gross disease and thyroid lobectomy if the thyroid is involved.

Parathyroid carcinoma

Parathyroid carcinoma is a rare condition that should be considered in the differential diagnosis of patients with profound hypercalcemia ≥14 mg/dL (0.0034 mol) and a palpable neck mass. At operation, parathyroid carcinomas are often scar-like and whitish in color with an irregular surface, in contrast with the smooth surface and dark brown color of a parathyroid adenoma.

When a suspected parathyroid carcinoma involves the thyroid, a thyroid lobectomy should be performed. A therapeutic modified radical neck node dissection is only recommended when lymph node metastases are detected.

Unfortunately many patients with parathyroid carcinoma have an inadequate initial surgical resection, possibly because the tumor is not recognized during the exploration [9]. Frozen section diagnosis is often misleading. Reoperation should be done after localization procedures in patients with persistent hyperparathyroidism and for those whose tumors have positive surgical margins.

Non-functioning parathyroid carcinomas are rare and most patients are diagnosed because they have a neck mass with or without dysphagia or hoarseness. This tumor seems to be more aggressive than its functioning counterpart, perhaps because non-functioning parathyroid carcinoma is diagnosed at a more advanced stage. Complete surgical resection including adjacent tissues is recommended at the initial operation (Fig. 10.2).

Adrenal tumors

Tumors of the adrenal gland are uncommon and may be diagnosed by their associated metabolic conditions (pheochromocytoma, Cushing syndrome, primary hyperaldosteronism and other conditions), localized symptoms (back or abdominal pain), or after abdominal imaging for another clinical indication (incidentaloma).

Today, most functioning and non-functioning adrenal masses are removed laparoscopically (lateral transabdominal, retroperitoneal laparoscopic or trans-abdominal laparoscopic adrenalectomy).

The morbidity for these techniques is similar [12]. Most experts recommend an open procedure for locally invasive cortical carcinomas, those with adjacent nodes and for large pheochromocytomas. In selected patients, the hand-assisted technique is helpful because it provides better exposure for resection but also intraoperative tactile sensation to decrease the risk of tumor rupture. Laparoscopic adrenalectomy is associated with less postoperative pain, shorter hospitalization and more rapid return to normal activities, and better cosmesis.

Incidentaloma

Adrenal incidentalomas are defined as lesions discovered during abdominal imaging when there are no related symptoms and no knowledge of prior adrenal disease. Most incidentalomas are benign non-functioning cortical adenomas (71–86%), but functioning tumors (19–24%) must be ruled out. The differential diagnosis of the functioning tumors includes: adrenocortical carcinoma (5%), pheochromocytoma (5–10%), cortisol-secreting adenoma (5%), aldosteronoma (1%), adrenal metastasis (2.5%) and, less frequently, adrenal cysts and myelolipomas (<1%) [13].

Simple adrenal cysts or myelolipomas can be diagnosed by their appearance on CT scans and only need surgical treatment when they are >8–10 cm or are causing regional symptoms. Observation is recommended for patients with non-functioning, homogeneous adrenal incidentalomas <4 cm. Surgical treatment is recommended for patients with functioning tumors and lesions that are suspicious for malignancy (Fig. 10.3). The overall risk of an incidentaloma being a primary adrenal malignancy is 5%, but the likelihood of malignancy increases with size. In lesions <4 cm the

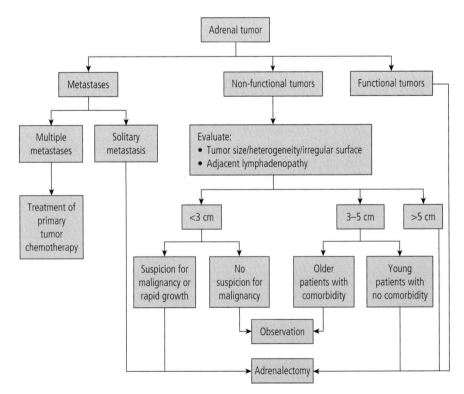

Figure 10.3 Management of adrenal tumors.

risk is 2%, for tumors between 4–6 cm, the risk is 6%, and for lesions >6 cm, the risk is 25%. In 2002, the National Institutes of Health (NIH) recommended the surgical removal of non-functioning adrenal incidentalomas >6 cm; however, other groups prefer resection of these tumors at ≥3 cm [14] (Fig. 10.3). Both CT scans and MRI images often underestimate the size of adrenal tumors by at least 1 cm. Tumors that are heterogeneous have irregular borders or adjacent enlarged lymph nodes are more likely to be malignant, regardless of size. CT scans at 6 and 12 months after diagnosis are recommended for tumors being observed. When no change occurs, the interval between scans can be increased. Enlarging tumors should be removed. Fine needle biopsy is only recommended if a metastatic tumor to the adrenal gland is being considered.

Primary hyperaldosteronism

Primary hyperaldosteronism is caused by an aldosterone-producing adenoma (73%), bilateral adrenal hyperplasia (24%), unilateral primary adrenal hyperplasia (1%), glucocorticoid suppressible hyperaldosteronism (1%), and adrenal cortical carcinoma (1%). Clinical manifestations include hypertension, weakness, muscle cramps, and most patients are hypokalemic. Aldosterone-producing tumors are localized by adrenal spiral CT or MRI, and adrenal vein sampling is indicated to distinguish between unilateral or bilateral disease or when the other tests are equivocal or negative. Most patients with primary hyperaldosteronism and a unilateral adenoma are cured by adrenalectomy.

About 2% of patients with hypertension have an aldosteronoma. Most aldosteronomas are between 0.5 and 2 cm and are encapsulated, making them ideal tumors for laparoscopic resection. Unilateral laparoscopic adrenalectomy is the surgical choice for both aldosteronoma and unilateral hyperplasia. It is important to distinguish between patients with aldosteronomas or unilateral hyperplasia and those with bilateral adrenal hyperplasia, because patients with bilateral hyperplasia should be treated medically whereas those with unilateral disease should be treated surgically. Preoperative preparation of patients for adrenalectomy should include an adequate correction of the hypokalemia and the hypertension. Open adrenalectomy is reserved for large and/or suspected invasive adrenal cortical carcinoma.

Pheochromocytoma

Pheochromocytomas are tumors that arise from chromaffin cells of the adrenal medulla or extra-adrenal chromaffin tissue and secrete catecholamines. These tumors account for approximately 0.1–0.2% of hypertensive patients and present most commonly in the fourth and fifth decades of life. About 10% of pheochromocytomas are malignant, 10% are familial (associated with different syndromes: MEN 2A, MEN 2B, von Hippel–Lindau, neurofibromatosis, tuberous sclerosis, Sturge–Weber, and ataxia–telangiectasia),10% occur in children, 10% are extra-adrenal (paragangliomas), 10% are bilateral and 5–10% present as incidentalomas. The classic triad of episodic headache, palpitations and perspiration is characteristic in these hypertensive patients.

The diagnosis of pheochromocytoma is made by measuring plasma metanephrines or a 24 h urine for catecholamines and creatinine. Most pheochromocytomas are >3 cm at presentation and are localized by CT scans or MRI. Radionuclide scanning with metiodobenzylguanidine (MIBG) helps identify extra-adrenal tumors.

About 40% of extra-adrenal pheochromocytomas or paragangliomas are multicentric and malignant. After the patient undergoes adequate preoperative preparation with alpha blockade and rehydration most pheochromocytomas under 6 cm are removed laparoscopically. Open adrenalectomy is reserved for large, possibly malignant tumors, or those with intra-abdominal metastases that require debulking.

Subtotal adrenalectomy with preservation of some of the adrenocortical tissue is used in some centers for patients with bilateral tumors. Although it is often successful in preserving adrenal function its recurrence rate is about 20%. For recurrent tumors and for metastatic disease, re-resection, radiation therapy, or chemotherapy may provide palliative benefit.

Adrenocortical carcinoma

Adrenocortical carcinoma (ACC) is a rare tumor accounting for 0.2% of all cancers. It occurs most often within the first and second decades or in the fourth and fifth decades of life. About 75% are hormonally functioning. These tumors may secrete excess cortisol (30%), androgens (20%), estrogens (10%) or aldosterone (2%).

Adrenocortical tumors that secrete multiple hormones (35%) are more likely to be malignant [15]. Both CT scans and MR images are useful for evaluating ACC. These tumors are usually larger than 6 cm, heterogeneous (containing hemorrhage and necrosis) and have irregular margins. Locoregional invasion, lymph node and vascular involvement, and distant metastases may be present. Attenuation coefficients >10 HU (Hounsfield units) in adrenal tumors on non-contrast CT can suggest malignancy, but can also be found in a small number of adenomas.

Surgical resection is the only hope for cure. Most agree that the laparoscopic approach is contraindicated for known malignant adrenal tumors and those with local or vascular invasion [13]. Treatment with mitotane is recommended by some for unresectable or incompletely resected ACC. Unfortunately only about 20% of these tumors respond. Both mitotane and ketoconazole can help reduce hormone hypersecretion. Radiation therapy is helpful for bone metastases [15].

Metastatic tumors

Most but not all experts recommend surgical resection of an isolated adrenal metastasis due to metastatic disease [16]. Primary sites include cancers from the lung, breast, kidney, melanoma, and colon. The role of the laparoscopic removal is also controversial, but most studies document that resection margins and survival are the same for open and laparoscopic adrenalectomy for metastatic tumors. It seems that laparoscopic adrenalectomy for adrenal metastasis is safe when preoperative imaging studies demonstrate no evidence of tumor invasion, adjacent lymphadenopathy or extra-adrenal metastases [13] (Fig. 10.3).

Pancreatic neuroendocrine tumors

Neuroendocrine tumors of the pancreas are rare. Most of these tumors are sporadic, but can occur in patients with MEN 1. Approximately 95% of islet cell tumors are insulinomas, gastrinomas or non-functioning tumors. Less commonly found are tumors that produce glucagon, vasoactive intestinal peptide (VIP), somatostatin, adrenocorticotropic hormone (ACTH), parathormone, human pancreatic polypeptide (hPP), histamine or serotonin. The diagnosis of functioning tumors is based on clinically specific findings that depend on the hormone overproduced. Because of the lack of hormone secretion, non-functioning tumors commonly present late in the course of the disease as abdominal masses, jaundice, weight loss, hemorrhage from the tumor, or metastatic disease [17].

Insulinoma

Insulinoma is the most common islet cell tumor. Ninety percent of these tumors are sporadic; of these, 90% are benign, solitary, measure <2 cm, and are evenly distributed throughout the pancreas. In 10% of the cases, insulinomas are associated with MEN 1. In this case, multiple islet cell tumors occur in about 88% of patients.

Once the diagnosis is made and other causes of hypoglycemia are ruled out, attempts should be made to localize the tumor(s). Non-invasive imaging like CT, MRI and ultrasound often fail to demonstrate the tumor but are useful to identify large invasive masses and hepatic metastases. Transgastric endoscopic ultrasound has become the diagnostic modality of choice for tumor localization, especially those in the head of the pancreas, with localization rates of 70–90%. Selective catheterization of the arteries supplying the pancreas with calcium stimulation and hepatic vein sampling (Immamura/Doppman procedure) can also be used to help localize the insulinoma, with localization rates of 90–100%. Preoperative localization is valuable because it can identify tumors that can be removed laparoscopically. Intraoperative ultrasound can also be helpful to determine tumor localization, and the tumor's relationship to the pancreatic duct and vessels.

Although enucleation or spleen-preserving distal pancreatectomy is the treatment of choice for insulinomas, a Whipple procedure may be necessary for tumors over 5 cm in diameter that are situated in the head of the pancreas. Because insulinomas in patients with MEN 1 are usually multicentric and other islet cell tumors are often present, subtotal pancreatic resection with enucleation of tumors from the head of the pancreas is the procedure of choice [17, 18].

Gastrinoma

Gastrinomas are tumors that secrete excessive gastrin and are responsible for a clinical entity of severe acid hypersecretion, peptic ulcer disease and diarrhea known as Zollinger–Ellison syndrome. Eighty percent of gastrinomas are sporadic and 20% familial, associated with MEN 1. The symptoms of gastrinoma can be controlled with H2 blockers and proton pump inhibitors. The most common location of these tumors is in the first and second portions of the duodenum (70%) and in the head of the pancreas, an area known as the "gastrinoma triangle." Eighty-five percent are situated to the right of the superior mesenteric vessels. In patients with MEN 1, the gastrinomas are usually multiple, whereas in sporadic disease, they are usually solitary. In 60% of cases, gastrinomas are malignant and are found to have lymph node, regional or liver metastases during the operative procedure. Somatostatin receptor scintigraphy is the imaging test of choice for localizing primary and metastatic tumors.

The surgical strategy depends upon tumor location, size and presence of metastatic disease. Surgical resection can achieve a cure in 50% of patients with sporadic gastrinomas, but rarely in patients with MEN 1 [19]. The type of operation for sporadic gastrinomas depends on location and includes open or laparoscopic enucleation of single tumors, open operation with enucleation of tumors from the duodenum and head of pancreas, Whipple procedure for large, invasive or multicentric tumors and distal pancreatectomy (spleen preserving) for tumors in the tail of the pancreas. In patients with sporadic or familial disease, duodenotomy and excision of duodenal tumors is essential. In familial cases, systematic periduodenal lymph node dissection should be done. Liver metastasis is associated with a poor prognosis.

References

1. Jossart GH, Clark OH. Well-differentiated thyroid cancer. *Curr. Probl. Surg.* 1994;31:933–1012.
2. Hay ID, Grant CS, Bergstralh EJ, et al. Unilateral total lobectomy: is it sufficient surgical treatment for patients with AMES low-risk papillary thyroid carcinoma? *Surgery* 1998;124:958–964; discussion 964–946.
3. Vini L, Harmer C. Management of thyroid cancer. *Lancet Oncol.* 2002;3:407–414.
4. Phillips AW, Fenwick JD, Mallick UK, et al. The impact of clinical guidelines on surgical management in patients with thyroid cancer. *Clin. Oncol. (R. Coll. Radiol.)* 2003;15:485–459.
5. Grossman RF, Clark OH. Hurthle cell carcinoma. *Cancer Control* 1997;4:13–17.
6. Mazzaferri EL, Kloos RT. Clinical review 128: Current approaches to primary therapy for papillary and follicular thyroid cancer. *J. Clin. Endocrinol. Metab.* 2001;86:1447–1463.
7. Kebebew E, Greenspan FS, Clark OH, et al. Anaplastic thyroid carcinoma. Treatment outcome and prognostic factors. *Cancer* 2005;103:1330–1335.
8. Clark OH. How should patients with primary hyperparathyroidism be treated? *J. Clin. Endocrinol. Metab.* 2003;88:3011–3014.
9. Hundahl SA, Fleming ID, Fremgen AM, et al. Two hundred eighty-six cases of parathyroid carcinoma treated in the US between 1985–1995: a National Cancer Data Base Report. *Cancer* 1999;86:538–544.

10. Clark OH. Surgical treatment of primary hyperparathyroidism. *Adv. Endocrinol. Metab.* 1995;6:1–16.

11. Kebebew E, Duh QY, Clark OH. Parathyroidectomy for primary hyperparathyroidism in octogenarians and nonagenarians: a plea for early surgical referral. *Arch. Surg.* 2003;138:867–871.

12. Duh QY, Siperstein AE, Clark OH, et al. Laparoscopic adrenalectomy. Comparison of the lateral and posterior approaches. *Arch. Surg.* 1996;131:870–875; discussion 875–876.

13. Sturgeon C, Kebebew E. Laparoscopic adrenalectomy for malignancy. *Surg. Clin. North Am.* 2004;84:755–774.

14. Duh QY. Adrenal incidentalomas. *Br. J. Surg.* 2002;89:1347–1349.

15. Shen WT, Sturgeon C, Duh QY. From incidentaloma to adrenocortical carcinoma: the surgical management of adrenal tumors. *J. Surg. Oncol.* 2005;89:186–192.

16. Haigh PI, Essner R, Wardlaw JC, et al. Long-term survival after complete resection of melanoma metastatic to the adrenal gland. *Ann. Surg. Oncol.* 1999;6:633–639.

17. Demeure M. Endocrine tumors of the pancreas. In Clark OH, Duh QY, et al., editors. *Endocrine Tumors: American Cancer Society, atlas of clinical oncology*. Hamilton, Ontario: BC Decker, 2003:177–190.

18. Finlayson E, Clark OH. Surgical treatment of insulinomas. *Surg. Clin. North Am.* 2004;84:775–785.

19. Norton JA. Surgical treatment and prognosis of gastrinoma. *Best Pract. Res. Clin. Gastroenterol.* 2005;19:799–805.

11 Endocrine Tumor Markers

Stefan K.G. Grebe

Key points
- Tumor markers are rarely specific for malignancy.
- Tumor markers are usually better suited for follow-up than diagnosis.
- Tumor marker performance is often impacted dramatically by intrinsic characteristics of a marker, co-existing disease/drug treatment and multiple analytical factors.
- Endocrine tumor markers are often specific for the organ of origin of a tumor.
- Many endocrine tumor markers show considerable overlap between normal or non-neoplastic ranges and tumor-associated ranges.

General principles of tumor marker use in medicine

Endocrine tumor markers are used widely in the diagnosis and follow-up of endocrine neoplasia. There are unique aspects to endocrine tumor markers, but it is useful to consider first some general principles that apply to tumor markers.

Definition and applications [1]

A tumor marker is a substance that is either produced by a tumor itself, or is fashioned by the host in response to the presence of a tumor. Tumor markers might be found in cells, tissues, blood, or other body fluids. Outside of anatomical pathology, where tumor markers are used in subtyping and differential diagnosis of neoplasms in tissue specimens, the term is applied to markers that can be detected in blood or body fluids. Tumor markers are usually measured quantitatively and have many uses in the management of neoplasia:
- Diagnosis
  - Screening
  - Clinical diagnosis
  - Differential diagnosis
- Prognosis
  - Estimating tumor burden
  - Predicting future tumor behavior
- Follow-up
  - Evaluating/monitoring treatment success
  - Detecting progression
  - Detecting recurrence.

Clinical Endocrine Oncology, 2nd edition. Edited by Ian D. Hay and John A.H. Wass. © 2008 Blackwell Publishing. ISBN 978-1-4051-4584-8.

The basic characteristics of a tumor marker and analytical considerations determine its performance within a given category.

Basic characteristics of tumor markers

Most tumor markers are not associated exclusively with the presence of neoplasia, but are also found in other diseases or in healthy individuals. Depending on the degree of overlap between tumor-associated values and concentrations that occur in non-neoplastic disease, this can limit a marker's specificity. Tumor specificity and detection sensitivity determine whether a marker is suitable for screening or early diagnosis. Neoplastic transformation (a few cells) and carcinoma *in situ* ($\sim 10^3$ cells, $\sim 1\,\mu$g tumor mass), the most curable stages of malignancy, are unlikely to ever be detectable by measurement of circulating tumor markers. On the other hand, cure of early clinical disease (10^9–10^{10} malignant cells; ~ 1–10 g tumor mass) might already be uncertain, while a further increase to ~ 0.1–10 kg tumor mass leads to death. The window for screening or early diagnosis lies consequently between $>10^3$ and $<10^9$ tumor cells. The concentration of a tumor marker secreted by such a small neoplasm might be too low (pg/ml to ng/ml) to be distinguishable from background or secretion by non-neoplastic diseases.

The second challenge is tumor localization. A tumor marker might be tumor specific, but not organ specific. This is exemplified by carcinoembryonic antigen (CEA). While serum concentrations of >5 ng/ml are an indicator of possible malignancy, aberrant expression of CEA might be observed in a wide array of malignancies, including cancers of the lung, colon, breast and thyroid C-cells.

With regard to a marker's performance as a prognostic indicator, or for evaluating treatment success and detecting progression or recurrence, the relationship between overall tumor mass and tumor marker concentration has to be linear over a wide range of tumor mass and degrees of tumor differentiation. In addition, the tumor marker half-life should be predictable and, ideally, short. This facilitates early confirmation of cure or recurrence, while variable or very long marker half-lives can make these assessments unreliable.

Analytical considerations [1]

Preanalytical and analytical issues that impact on the performance of tumor marker assays consist of the following:
- coexisting diseases, drug treatment and sample stability
- standardization of assay calibration
- differences between methods
- assay performance stability over time
- assay reproducibility/precision
- susceptibility to assay interference
- unusual sample types.

Co-existing diseases or drug treatment can lead to a greater diagnostic overlap between marker concentrations observed in malignant versus non-malignant conditions. In particular, serum concentrations of peptides or polypeptide markers can be significantly elevated in patients with impaired renal or hepatic function, due to altered metabolism or reduced excretion. Other markers can be falsely elevated in various inflammatory conditions. False-low or negative results can be observed for markers with poor stability, if sample processing or freezing is delayed.

Standardization of assay calibration to a common reference material is very important. In its absence, there can be extreme differences between the results obtained by different assays (Fig. 11.1). An absence of reference standards also impairs manufacturers' ability to produce consistent assay-calibrator lots, thereby contributing to assay lot-to-lot variability.

However, even when a common reference standard is used, significant differences between assays can persist, particularly for immunoassays. This is caused by the large number of possible immunoassay configurations, including: (i) different assay formats (competitive or immunometric); (ii) different antibodies with different antigen affinity/avidity profiles, different cross-reactivity profiles, and different serum lipid and protein interaction profiles; (iii) different antibody concentrations; (iv) different buffer systems; (v) different detection systems; and (vi) different data-reduction methods. Biases between assays can range from none to five-fold. In many cases, the differences between assays exceed the biological variation within a patient. In addition, systematic differences between assays are not necessarily a reliable predictor of the differences that might be observed in an individual patient; some patient samples might show lesser, while other can show much greater than average bias (Fig. 11.1). Consequently, the same assay should always be used for serial testing. When a different assay needs to be used, a new baseline should be established as soon as possible.

Even within the same assay, lot-to-lot variability of ±10% occurs not infrequently, and larger drifts over time or sudden calibration

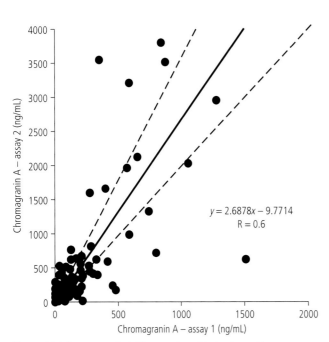

Figure 11.1 Between-method differences that might be observed in some immunoassays. Scatterplot of 91 patient samples tested with two different chromogranin A assays. Passing–Bablok linear fit (solid diagonal line) and 95% confidence intervals of fit (dashed lines) are superimposed. Assay 2 measures approximately 2.7 times higher than assay 1 (see inserted formula of fit). In addition, there are a significant number of individual samples that show even greater discrepancies, some of which are in the opposite direction as predicted by the fit. This is also indicated by the correlation coefficient (R) of only 0.6.

$y = 2.6878x - 9.7714$
$R = 0.6$

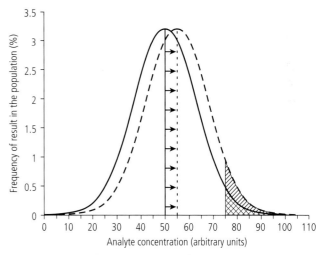

Figure 11.2 Impact of a systematic upward shift on assay performance. The solid Gaussian curve represents the frequency distribution of the concentrations of a hypothetical analyte in a healthy reference population. The mean analyte value (vertical solid line) lies at 50 arbitrary units and the standard deviation (SD) is 12.5 arbitrary units. The upper border of the reference range lies at +2 SD (75 arbitrary units) and approximately 2.275% of the population fall above this cut-off (cross-hatched area under the curve at the right). A systematic 10% shift in the assay would push the entire distribution (dashed curve) to the right (horizontal arrows). This would make a small difference to each individual measurement, e.g. the mean only increases by 5 arbitrary units to 55 arbitrary units (dashed vertical line). However, unless the upper reference range cut-off is adjusted upwards by 10%, the percentage of individuals that would fall above the reference range would approximately double (the diagonal-hatched area represents the additional "cases").

shifts are observed occasionally. The latter are most likely to occur when assays are reformulated, for example when an existing antibody is replaced with a different clone. A systematic shift of just 10% can push a significant proportion of normal individuals outside of reference range boundaries (Fig. 11.2). The impact is less in treatment monitoring or follow-up applications; very few physicians will alter their management based on such a minor change. However, in some patients an assay shift might coincide with biological or assay variability in the same direction, resulting in a large enough change to trigger unwarranted management changes.

In the absence of significant assay shifts or drifts, assay imprecision has the greatest impact on tumor marker performance, in particular in treatment monitoring and follow-up. Assay variability is most often expressed as the coefficient of variation (CV). The CV represents the relative standard deviation (SD) and is derived by dividing the SD of a series of measurements by the mean of the measurements. It is usually multiplied by 100 and expressed as percent CV. A CV of 10% means that the true result is ~95% likely to be within $\pm 2 \times CV$ ($= \pm 20\%$) of the measured value. It is possible for duplicate measurements of the same sample to lie significantly apart within this likelihood distribution. Assuming a normal distribution of analytical and biological variability, the minimal significant (or critical) change (Δ_C) for two measurements can be expressed as $\Delta_C > Z \times 2^{1/2} \times (CV_B^2 + CV_A^2)^{1/2}$, where Z is the Z-score for a given significance level (Table 11.1), and CV_B and CV_A represent biological and analytical CV, respectively. For CV_B and CV_A of 10% each, as are commonly seen in tumor marker tests, the Δ_C for a 95% two-tailed probability that the results of two tests are different becomes: $1.96 \times 2^{1/2} \times (10\%^2 + 10\%^2)^{1/2} = 2.772 \times 200\%^{1/2} = 39.2\%$, a change that is probably larger than most physicians would have guessed.

Intrinsic limitations of assay configurations can also impact tumor marker performance. Competitive immunoassays have a narrow dynamic range, due to their limited antibody concentrations, leading potentially to inaccurate results for very low or very high analyte concentrations. Immunometric assays can sometimes cause false-low/false-normal results due to hooking. Hooking occurs when a large surplus of antigen is present in a sandwich assay.

Both antibodies get saturated independently and can no longer form a sandwich.

Assay interferences include matrix effects, detection signal quenching, cross-reactivity, autoantibody interference, and heterophile antibody interference. Matrix effects represent the impact of abnormal concentrations of serum proteins or lipids on antigen–antibody interactions. For most commercial assays, manufacturers have established cut-offs that are compatible with normal assay functionality, but lipid and protein concentrations of patient samples are often not known to the testing laboratory. By contrast, potential detection signal quenching is most often related to hemolysis or increased bilirubin and can be detected by the associated changes in sample appearance. Cross-reactivity is rarely a problem in modern immunoassays, but interference by autoantibodies or heterophile antibodies remains an issue. Autoantibodies against a tumor marker might impair detection, leading to false-low or false-negative results, but can sometimes also lead to false-high results (Fig. 11.3). Heterophile antibodies are antibodies that can bind to the animal-derived antibodies used in immunoassays. They represent a problem primarily in sandwich assays, where they lead usually to false-positive/false-high results (Fig. 11.4).

Tumor marker measurements are sometimes requested on various body fluids other than blood (e.g., pleural fluid, ascites, cerebrospinal fluid) or biopsy specimens, the rationale being that this might assist in diagnosing malignancy that is missed by cytology. Unfortunately, with rare exceptions, tumor marker measurement in body fluids has limited utility. Assays are optimized for serum or plasma and might fail completely, or generate nonsensical results, in other body fluids. Moreover, even if a valid result is obtained, its interpretation is difficult. There are usually no reference ranges, and marker concentrations in body fluids show often extreme overlap between malignancy and other diseases.

Clinical validation and evidence-based use of tumor marker assays

Early detection of a primary tumor or of tumor progression or recurrence might not ensure an improved outcome. In addition, for malignancies with a high ratio of cases to tumor deaths, such as prostate cancer detected by screening, or small thyroid carcinomas, the benefits to a small proportion of patients can be outweighed by the treatment-related morbidity or mortality inflicted on the majority of patients. Every new tumor marker should therefore be validated clinically. In order to facilitate the objective evaluation of medical tests, criteria have been developed, and adopted by the World Health Organization, for grading the quality of clinical evidence [2]. The American Society of Clinical Oncology (ASCO) has proposed a related set of guidelines, specifically targeted at tumor markers [3]. Both sets of recommendations are in widespread use, with many US professional medical societies endorsing the ASCO recommendations (Table 11.2). Ideally, introduction of a test into clinical practice should be supported by the outcome data of one or more sufficiently powered prospective randomized trials assessing the impact of tumor marker testing versus not testing on cause-specific morbidity and mortality. If there are other

Table 11.1 Z-scores (standard deviation scores) for different probabilities that an observed difference between two measurements is not due to chance

Probability observed difference is not due to chance (%)	Z-score	
	One-tailed	Two-tailed
60	0.25	0.84
70	0.52	1.04
75	0.68	1.15
80	0.84	1.28
85	1.04	1.44
90	1.28	1.65
95	1.65	1.96
99	2.33	2.58

Figure 11.3 Autoantibody interference in immunometric assays. (a) High-avidity auto-antibodies (Auto AB) bind to analyte and prevent detection AB or capture AB from attaching to their respective epitopes. The AB-AG-AB sandwich cannot be formed, resulting in a false-negative result (Auto AB concentration exceeds analyte concentration) or in a false-low result (Auto AB does not exceed analyte concentration). This type of interference is frequently observed in thyroglobulin assays when a sample contains significant concentrations of thyroglobulin autoantibodies. (b) Auto AB either bind to analyte at epitopes distinct from the detection and capture AB epitopes (depicted here) or the Auto AB have low binding avidity and are easily displaced by the detection and capture AB (not shown). There is no interference with accurate analyte detection. However, the Auto AB might prolong *in vivo* analyte half-life, thereby leading to accumulation of analyte, resulting in false-high measurements. The false-high prolactin levels seen in patients with "macro-prolactin," an IgG-prolactin complex, represent an example of this type of Auto AB interference.

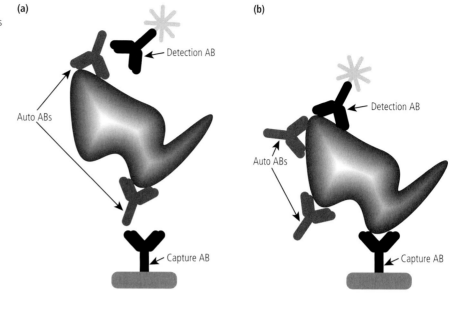

Figure 11.4 Heterophile interference in immunometric assays. (a) In the absence of interfering heterophile antibodies (AB) analyte/antigen (AG) is sandwiched between capture AB and detection AB and can be quantitated accurately. (b) When a sample contains interfering heterophile AB, the most common outcome (>90% of cases) is that the heterophile AB binds to capture and detection AB simultaneously, thereby simulating the presence of AG in its absence (false-positive result), or, if some AG is also present, leading to an overestimation of the true level of AG (false-high result). (c) In rare cases (<10%) heterophile AB might bind only to capture AB (depicted here) or detection AB (not shown), preventing AG from being sandwiched and leading to a false-low or false-negative result.

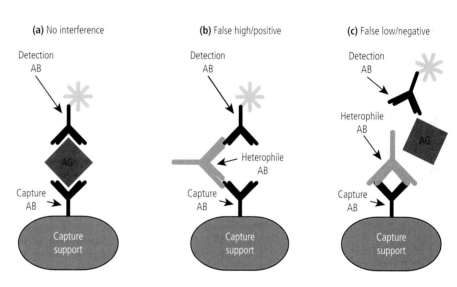

tumor markers that can be used in a given malignancy and that have been validated previously, then a performance comparison of a new marker to the established marker may suffice [4]. While evidence from experimental studies of lesser rigor will also be acceptable in some circumstances, widespread clinical use should be discouraged for those assays that are only supported by descriptive or comparative studies or, worse, expert opinion.

Endocrine tumor markers

Features of endocrine tumor markers and focus of this section

Endocrine tumors can cause severe systemic disease through loss of, or excessive, hormone secretion, even if they are benign.

The secreted hormones are therefore used frequently as tumor markers. This conveys unusual site specificity to endocrine tumor marker testing. However, since hormone levels can show significant biological variability, there is considerable overlap between tumor-associated and tumor-unrelated concentrations. Many dynamic tests have consequently been developed to supplement random or timed hormone measurements. Measurement of organ-specific hormones is also used in follow-up and to monitor treatment success. Examples include prolactin and insulin-like growth factor-1 measurement in prolactinoma and acromegaly, respectively.

Most of the applications of baseline and dynamic measurements of peripheral and tropic hormones as tumor markers are covered in other chapters, devoted to the various endocrine tumors. This chapter will concentrate primarily on endocrine tumor markers

Table 11.2 World Health Organization (WHO) and American Society of Clinical Oncology (ASCO) rankings of evidence for the clinical utility of tumor marker tests*

WHO category	Evidence requirements	ASCO category	Evidence requirements
Ia	Meta-analysis of multiple large prospective randomized controlled trials that include evaluation of marker performance	I	At least one large prospective controlled trial designed specifically to test marker utility
Ib	At least one large prospective randomized controlled trial that includes evaluation of marker performance		*or* Meta-analysis of several level II or III studies
IIa	At least one prospective non-randomized controlled study that includes evaluation of marker performance	II	At least one large prospective controlled trial *not* specifically designed to test marker utility, *but* assessment of marker utility *must* be a pre-defined lower priority objective
IIb	At least one experimental study of some kind that includes evaluation of marker performance	V	Evidence from one or more small pilot studies designed to determine or estimate marker levels in target population(s) ± correlation with other known or investigational markers
III	At least one non-experimental (e.g. observational or descriptive) study, such as cohort studies, comparative studies, retrospective case-analysis, correlative studies, or case–control studies, that includes evaluation of marker performance	III	Pooled evidence from several large retrospective studies *not* necessarily designed to test marker utility
		IV	Pooled evidence from several small retrospective studies *not* necessarily designed to test marker utility
IV	Expert opinion or consensus guidelines about marker performance not based on formal methods of literature analysis	–	–

*The two ranking systems match well, with the exception of ASCO V, which matches WHO IIb, rather than a lower-ranked WHO evidence-category.

that are not considered to be "classic hormones," represent hormone precursors or metabolites, or are not hormones but are endocrine specific. Tables 11.3 and 11.4 list the markers that will be covered. In addition, flowcharts will highlight the clinical use of the makers in diagnosis and follow-up.

Chromogranin A

Granins are located in secretory granules of endocrine and neuroendocrine tissues assisting in the processing and secretion of tissue-specific bioactive secretion products. In addition, granins can undergo cleavage, giving rise to a series of daughter peptides with distinct extracellular functions [5].

Chromogranin A (CG-A) is the best studied granin. Because of its ubiquitous distribution within neuroendocrine tissues, CG-A is a useful diagnostic marker for neuroendocrine neoplasms, including carcinoids, pheochromocytomas, neuroblastomas, medullary thyroid carcinomas (MTC), some pituitary tumors, and functioning or non-functioning islet cell tumors (Table 11.3) [5, 6].

Almost all carcinoids secrete CG-A, often along with modified amines, chiefly serotonin (5-hydroxytryptamine, 5-HT). Serum CG-A measurements are particularly suited for diagnosing hindgut tumors, being elevated in nearly all cases. CG-A is also elevated in 80–90% of patients with symptomatic foregut and midgut tumors (Fig. 11.5). Serum CG-A, and urine 5-hydroxyindole acetic acid (5-HIAA), the major 5-HT metabolite, also provide prognostic

information and are well suited for monitoring treatment success or disease progression, since they increase in proportion to the tumor burden (Fig. 11.6) [6, 7].

False-positive results can be observed due to drugs that stimulate secretion of gastrointestinal neuroendocrine cells, such as proton pump inhibitors. A significant impairment in renal or hepatic function will also lead to artifactual elevations in CG-A, as it is cleared by a combination of hepatic metabolism and renal excretion.

All current CG-A assays are immunoassays. Since there is no universal calibration standard, reference intervals and individual patient results differ significantly between assays and cannot be compared directly (Fig. 11.1). Serial measurements should therefore be performed with the same assay, or, if assays are changed, patients should be re-baselined. Depending on their configuration (competitive or immunometric), these assays can also suffer from other inherent immunoassay vulnerabilities.

Serum, blood and urine 5-HT, and urine 5-HIAA

5-HT is synthesized in enterochromaffin cells (EC) from tryptophan via 5-hydroxytryptophan (5-HTP). On first pass through the liver 50–80% of 5-HT is metabolized, predominantly to 5-HIAA, which is excreted by the kidneys. Ninety percent of the remainder is metabolized in the lungs, also to 5-HIAA. Most of the rest is taken up by platelets, where it remains until release during clotting.

Table 11.3 Summary of main endocrine tumor markers covered in this chapter

Marker	Primary tumor marker use	Other tumor marker uses	Quality of evidence	Comments
Serum chromogranin A (CG-A)	Diagnosis and follow-up of carcinoid tumors	Diagnosis and follow-up of islet cell tumors, pheochromocytoma, neuroblastoma, medullary thyroid carcinoma, pituitary tumors	Primary use: I Secondary uses: II	Best marker for carcinoid diagnosis and useful in follow-up ± 5-HIAA. Interference by drugs. False positive in renal and hepatic failure.
Serotonin (5-HT) in serum/blood	Diagnosis & follow-up of carcinoid		Primary use: IV	Interference by drugs.
5-HT in urine	Diagnosis & follow-up of carcinoid that only produce 5-HTP		Primary use: IV	Interference by drugs and food. Not useful as a serum marker.
5-hydroxyindole acetic acid (5-HIAA) in urine	Diagnosis & follow-up of carcinoid tumors		Primary use: I	Primary follow-up marker for 5-HT producing tumors. Interference by drugs and food.
Fractionated urine & free plasma metanephrines	Diagnosis of pheochromocytoma & paraganglionoma	1. Follow-up of pheochromocytoma & paraganglionoma 2. Diagnosis and follow-up of islet cell tumors & carcinoids	Primary use: I Secondary use 1: II Secondary use 2: V	Best tests for initial diagnosis of pheochromocytoma and paraganglionoma.
Urine & plasma catecholamines	Diagnosis of pheochromocytoma & paraganglionoma	1. Follow-up of pheochromocytoma & paraganglionoma 2. Diagnosis of neuroblastoma	Primary use: I Secondary use 1: II Secondary use 2: IV	Superseded by fractionated metanephrines.
Urine homovanillic acid (HVA), vanillylmandelic acid (VMA)	Diagnosis of neuroblastoma	1. Diagnosis & follow-up of pheochromocytoma & paraganglionoma	Primary use: I Secondary uses: I	Superseded by fractionated metanephrines, except in neuroblastoma.
Calcitonin (CT)	Diagnosis & follow-up of MTC	Diagnosis & follow-up of islet cell tumors and carcinoids	Primary use: I Secondary uses: IV	False positives in renal failure, severe inflammatory conditions and some non-endocrine malignancies. False low results due to instability.
Procalcitonin (ProCT)	Diagnosis & follow-up of MTC		Primary use: V	Superior stability to CT. Limited clinical data.
Thyroglobulin (Tg) in serum	Follow-up of follicular cell-derived thyroid carcinoma	Assess changes in tumor mass	Primary use: I Secondary use: II	Not suited for initial diagnosis. False-low in Tg-AB positive patients.
Tg in non-thyroidal tissues	Diagnosis of lymph node metastases of follicular cell-derived thyroid carcinoma	Diagnosis of other extrathyroidal metastases of follicular cell-derived thyroid carcinoma	Primary use: III Secondary uses: V	No interference by Tg-AB.
Thyroglobulin antibody (Tg-AB) in serum	Assess validity of Tg measurements	Follow-up of follicular cell-derived thyroid carcinoma in Tg-AB positive patients	Primary use: II Secondary use: III	Well supported as a qualitative marker. Few assays sufficiently sensitive.
Tg mRNA in blood	Follow-up of follicular cell-derived thyroid carcinoma in Tg-AB + patients		Primary use: IV	Most of studies suggest very limited clinical utility. Sample instability limits use.

*By ASCO criteria.

EC tumors (carcinoids and, rarely, other neuroectodermal tumors) frequently over-secrete 5-HT (Table 11.3). Measurement of 5-HT in blood, plasma or serum, and measurement of 5-HT and 5-HIAA in urine are therefore useful in the diagnosis and follow-up of carcinoid tumors (Figs 11.5 and 11.6). However, all serotonin-related markers tend to be less sensitive in the initial diagnosis of carcinoid than CG-A, as only midgut tumors (jejunum, ileum, or appendix; ~70% of cases) over-produce 5-HT consistently. Furthermore, levels of 5-HT do not rise until 5-HT secretion exceeds hepatic metabolism. Once this has occurred, often due to hepatic metastases, serum 5-HT, urine 5-HIAA and sometimes urinary 5-HT rise above the reference range, typically by a significant margin. Most patients at this stage have symptoms or signs of excessive circulating 5-HT (and other vasoactive amines or peptides), termed carcinoid syndrome, consisting of (any combination of) flushing, hypertension, diarrhea, bronchoconstriction, or right-sided valvular heart lesions.

5-HIAA is the most widely used and best validated serotonin-related marker, owing to its high concentrations, easy calibrator standardization and linear relationship to EC tumor mass. Their good correlation with tumor mass has made 5-HIAA and CG-A the markers of choice for follow-up and for assessing treatment outcome [6, 7].

By contrast, 5-HT is more difficult to measure, is less stable and displays a non-linear relationship to EC tumor mass; the storage capacity of platelets is exceeded at ~5000 ng/ml and only

Table 11.4 Other endocrine tumor markers – applications in neuroendocrine and other tumors

| Markers[1] | Percentage with marker elevations[2] | | Clinical use and analytical considerations in pancreatic endocrine tumors and carcinoids | Use in other endocrine and non-endocrine tumors |
	Pancreatic endocrine tumors	Carcinoids		
Specific hormones				
ACTH	<1	<10	Differential diagnosis of Cushing syndrome. Secreted primarily by foregut carcinoids. Dynamic testing or selective petrosal sampling required to confirm secretion by neuroendocrine tumor(s). International standard available. Assay agreement[3]: good. Stability[4]: very poor.	Cushing disease. SCLC can secrete extreme amounts.
Gastrin	20–62	~15	Diagnosis and follow-up. Non-pancreatic tumors usually in duodenum. Fasting baseline levels: <100 pg/ml = normal; >1000 pg/ml = gastrinoma (if acid secretion ≥normal). Intermediate levels require secretin testing (post-secretin rise in gastrin >200 pg/ml: ~85% sensitivity and >95% specificity for gastrinoma). No international standard available. Assay agreement[3]: poor. Stability[4]: very poor. False positives: non-fasting, proton pump inhibitors Rx, achlorhydria, renal failure, other neoplasms (see next column). False negatives: sample degradation, gastrin isoforms.	Secreted by some SCLC, but no significant clinical studies/evaluation performed.
GH, GHRH	<1	<1	Diagnosis. Extremely rare. Can not be readily distinguished by biochemical testing from hypothalamic or pituitary disease. Very limited assay availability for GHRH.	GH-secreting pituitary tumors (IGF-1 or glucose suppression testing for diagnosis and follow-up) and (rare) GHRH-secreting hypothalamic tumors.
Glucagon	1–34	–	Diagnosis. Mostly co-secreted in minor quantities with other hormones/markers. Few tumors with predominant glucagon secretion. Tumors might be very small. Non-human (porcine) international standard available. Assay agreement[3]: poor. Stability[4]: poor. False positives: prolonged fasting, liver disease, renal failure.	–
hCG	14–30	0–30	Diagnosis and follow-up. Rarely as high as in germ-cell tumors. International standard available. Assay agreement[3]: average. Stability[3]: good. False positives: pregnancy, menopause, infants <3 months, primary hypogonadism, heterophile antibody interference (relatively common in hCG assays), other neoplasms (see next column).	Well-established marker (diagnosis and follow-up) in male and female germ cell tumors and in trophoblastic tumors.
Insulin	45–75	–	Diagnosis. Tumors almost always in pancreas, but might be very small. Diagnosis based on non-suppressed insulin when blood glucose <40 mg/dl (2.2 mmol/L). Diagnosis might require prolonged fast (72 h) plus ancillary measurement of proinsulin and c-peptide. International standard available. Assay agreement[3]: good. Stability[3]: average. False positives: non-fasting, renal failure, criminal or surreptitious insulin and sulfonylurea administration. False negative/low: (even minor) hemolysis (degraded by red cell enzymes).	–
PTHrP	<1	0–3	Diagnosis. Neuroendocrine tumors are a very rare cause of PTHrP elevation. No international standard available. Limited assay availability. Assay agreement[3]: poor. Stability[3]: very poor. False positives: lactation, mastitis, renal failure, other neoplasms (see next column). False negatives: sample degradation.	Major cause/contributor to hypercalcemia of malignancy, in particular in NSCLC and breast cancer.
Somatostatin	0–21 (most studies <1)	<10 (most studies <1)	Diagnosis. Significant secretion rare. No international standard. Clinical assays not readily available. Assay agreement[3]: poor. Stability[3]: poor	–
VIP	3–23	–	Diagnosis. Mostly co-secreted in minor quantities with other hormones/markers. Few tumors with predominant VIP secretion and related symptoms. Tumors might be very small. No international standard available. Assay agreement[3]: poor. Stability[4]: poor.	–

Table 11.4 (*Continued*) **Chapter 11** Endocrine Tumor Markers

Markers[1]	Percentage with marker elevations[2]		Clinical use and analytical considerations in pancreatic endocrine tumors and carcinoids	Use in other endocrine and non-endocrine tumors
	Pancreatic endocrine tumors	Carcinoids		
Non-specific markers				
α-subunit	0–30	<40	Secondary marker to CG-A and NSE. Rarely elevated when CG-A or NSE are normal. International standard available. Limited assay availability. Assay agreement[3]: average. Stability[4]: good. False positives: pregnancy, menopause, infants <3 months, primary hypogonadism, other neoplasms (see next column).	May be elevated in non-functioning and functioning (gonadotropinoma, thyrotropinoma) pituitary tumors. Large overlap with healthy reference range. Limited clinical validation.
CEA	–	–	Rarely useful and very limited validation in pancreatic endocrine tumors or carcinoids. Useful in MTC and several non-endocrine tumors (see next column). International standard available. Assay agreement[3]: good. Stability[4]: average, but poor tolerance of freeze–thaw cycles. False positives: acute and chronic inflammatory conditions of stomach, small bowel, colon, liver, pancreas, lung, breast, prostate and smoking; other neoplasms (see next column). False negatives: freeze–thaw.	Well-validated complementary marker to CT in MTC diagnosis and follow-up (see main text). Also well-validated and routinely used in multiple other human solid cancers, in particular colon, stomach, esophagus, pancreas and breast. Lesser use in lung, liver and prostate cancer.
NSE	0–74 (most studies <40)	47–66	Diagnosis and follow-up. 2nd most frequently elevated non-specific marker in carcinoids and islet cell tumors after CG-A. No international standard available. Assay agreement[3]: poor. Stability[4]: good. False positives: hemolysis (red cells contain NSE), proton pump inhibitor Rx, hepatic failure, epileptic seizure, brain injury, encephalitis, stroke, rapidly progressive dementia.	Well validated and used clinically in SCLC diagnosis (elevated >50% of cases) and follow-up. Frequently high in neuroblastoma, pheochromocytoma (≥50%), NSCLC, melanoma, seminoma (10–50%), but less well validated.
Neurotensin	21–67	0–17	Diagnosis. Limited clinical validation in carcinoid and pancreatic endocrine tumors. No international standard. Limited assay availability. Assay agreement[3]: poor. Stability[4]: poor. False positives: renal failure, other neoplasms (see next column).	Secreted by some SCLC. Limited clinical validation.
ProGRP	Unknown	Unknown	Very limited clinical data in carcinoids and pancreatic endocrine tumors. However, based on MTC and SCLC, ProGRP is likely to perform on par or better than CG-A and NSE. No international standard available. Limited assay availability (single Japanese vendor). Abbott has recently acquired rights. Stability[4]: good. False positives: early childhood (>10x adult levels at birth, fall to adult levels over 1–2 years), inflammatory lung diseases (particularly fibrosis), renal failure, other neoplasms (see next column).	Relatively new marker (~10 y). Well validated for SCLC diagnosis and follow-up, with excellent clinical performance, superior to NSE. Promising in MTC (elevated >50%) and prostate cancer (predictive of poor prognosis) but limited validation.
PP	<1–74	–	Diagnosis. Traditional marker for "non-functioning" pancreatic endocrine tumors. Limited validation. Diagnostic accuracy <50%. Considered useful when performed in the context of sham feeding, but procedure is poorly standardized and has very limited clinical value. No international standard. Limited assay availability. Assay agreement[3]: poor. Stability[4]: poor. False positives (PP alone): non-fasting, proton pump inhibitors Rx, achlorhydria, renal failure. False positives or negatives (sham feeding and PP): timing, composition, temperature, odor and appearance of meal, timing of blood draws after sham feeding, non-fasting, proton pump inhibitors Rx, achlorhydria, renal failure.	–

ACTH, adrenocorticotropic hormone; CG-A, chromogranin A; GH, growth hormone; GHRH, growth hormone-releasing hormone; hCG, human chorionic gonadotropin; MTC, medullary thyroid carcinoma; NSE, neuron-specific enolase; PP, pancreatic polypeptide; PTH, parathyroid hormone; NSCLC, non-small cell lung carcinoma; SCLC, small cell lung carcinoma; VIP, vasoactive intestinal peptide.

1. CG-A, 5-HT, 5-HIAA, metanephrines/catecholamines and CT have been omitted from this table as they are covered extensively in the main text and Table 11.3. Various other markers that are rarely used and for which there is extremely limited clinical validation (e.g., bombesin, peptide yy, bradykinin) have also been omitted.
2. While many tumors secrete one or two markers preferentially, many also secrete low concentrations of one or several other markers.
3. Assay agreement: poor = systematic bias between assays >40% or $r < 0.7$; average = systematic bias between assays 20–40% or $r = 0.7–0.9$; good = systematic bias between assays <20% or $r > 0.9$.
4. Sample stability: very poor = >20% degradation at 4 °C in <6 h; poor = >20% degradation at 4 °C in <24 h; average = <20% degradation at 4 °C in <24 h; good = <20% degradation at 4 °C in >24 h.

minor further increments occur. Moreover, apparent circulating 5-HT concentrations can vary, depending on the specimen type used. Consistent analytical recovery depends on complete recovery of the platelet 5-HT pool. This is achieved most reliably by using anticoagulated whole blood, or serum from completely clotted specimens (which releases all HT into the serum). Provided these issues are considered, measurement of circulating 5-HT might have superior sensitivity and specificity in the initial diagnosis of carcinoids than 5-HIAA [7].

The value of urinary 5-HT measurement is limited to tumors that produce only 5-HTP rather than 5-HT. In these rare cases,

circulating 5-HT and urinary 5-HIAA are not elevated, but renal conversion of 5-HTP to 5-HT might lead to high urinary 5-HT levels.

Medications that can elevate blood or urine 5-HT or urine 5-HIAA include lithium, monoamine oxidase (MAO) inhibitors, methyldopa, morphine, and reserpine. Some metabolites of nicotine are isomers of 5-HT and can also cause false-positive interference, particularly in urine assays (where metabolites accumulate) performed on heavy smokers. Selective serotonin reuptake inhibitors can deplete platelet serotonin and result in false-low serum/blood 5-HT tests. Serotonin- or tryptophan-rich foods

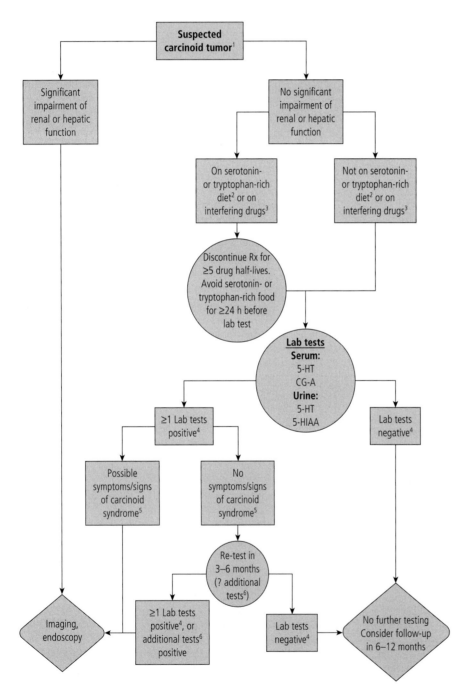

Figure 11.5 Suggested algorithm for tumor marker testing in the diagnostic work-up of suspected carcinoid tumors. 5-HT, serotonin; 5-HIAA, 5-hydroxyindole acetic acid; CG-A, chromogranin A. Notes: 1. Only a minority of carcinoid tumors will present with symptoms or signs of carcinoid syndrome. Most patients present with non-specific gastrointestinal symptoms. 2. See main text for a listing of serotonin- and tryptophan-rich foods. 3. See main text for a listing of drugs that can interfere with accurate CG-A or 5-HT/5-HIAA measurements. 4. At this point, drug and food intake history should be reviewed again. Positive is defined as exceeding the test-specific (rather than a literature-derived) reference range. Negative is defined as falling within the test-specific (rather than a literature-derived) reference range. 5. See main text for a brief discussion of carcinoid syndrome. 6. Additional tests include other specific hormones or non-specific markers that might be elevated in carcinoid tumors. This includes potentially calcitonin or some of the markers listed in Table 11.4.

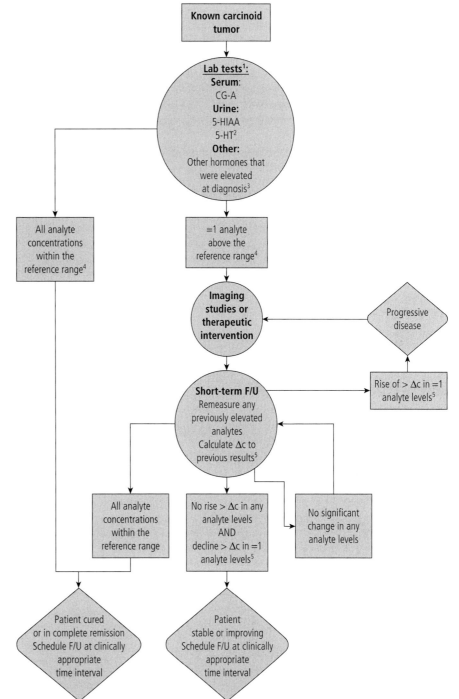

Figure 11.6 Suggested algorithm for tumor marker testing in the follow-up of carcinoid tumors. 5-HT, serotonin; 5-HIAA, 5-hydroxyindole acetic acid; CG-A, chromogranin A. Notes: 1. Consider possible interferences (drugs, food, renal and hepatic function, etc. – see Fig. 11.5, main text and Tables 11.3 and 11.4) before testing and when interpreting test results. 2. The key markers are CG-A and 5-HIAA. Urine 5-HT is only measured if it was elevated at diagnosis. 3. See Fig. 11.5, main text and Table 11.4. 4. At this point, drug and food intake history should be reviewed again. Positive is defined as exceeding the test-specific (rather than a literature-derived) reference range. Negative is defined as falling within the test-specific (rather than a literature-derived) reference range. 5. Δc: minimal significant (critical) change between serial measurements. See main text for details.

(avocado, banana, plum, walnut, pineapple, eggplant, plantain, tomato, hickory nut, kiwi-fruit, date, grapefruit, cantaloupe, and honeydew melon) do not contribute significantly to serum/blood 5-HT measurements, but can elevate platelet-poor plasma 5-HT, urinary 5-HT, and urinary 5-HIAA markedly (up to 10-fold). With assays that are not based on chromatographic methods, interference related to cross-reactivity with various related biogenic amines and drugs can also occur, and immunoassays can suffer from poor comparability between different assays, as well as from

the typical immunoassay problems described in the general tumor marker section.

Plasma and urine metanephrines and catecholamines, and urine homovanillic acid and vanillylmandelic acid

Metanephrine (metadrenaline), normetanephrine (normetadrenaline) and methoxytyramine, collectively referred to as metanephrines, are the 3-methoxy metabolites of epinephrine (adrenaline), norepinephrine (noradrenaline) and dopamine, respectively. Metanephrines are further metabolized to conjugated metanephrines and homovanillic acid (HVA; methoxytyramine) or vanillylmandelic acid (VMA; metanephrine and normetanephrine). The metanephrines are co-secreted with catecholamines by pheochromocytomas and other neural crest tumors. The metabolism of metanephrines is much slower than that of catecholamines, and they are largely resistant to oxidization. Furthermore, secretion of metanephrines is less episodic than that of catecholamines [8].

These characteristics cause sustained elevations of metanephrines in urine and plasma of patients suffering from pheochromocytoma or related tumors [9]. With the exception of neuroblastoma, for which metanephrines have not been sufficiently validated, measurement of HVA, VMA, or catecholamines should therefore be considered obsolete (Table 11.3). Measurements of fractionated plasma free metanephrines or urine fractionated metanephrine approach 100% diagnostic sensitivity in pheochromocytoma and paraganglioma [9]. While both tests have specificities of >90%, urine testing might achieve slightly higher specificity than plasma testing, in particular if hypertensive, rather than normotensive, reference ranges are used [9, 10]. Nearly all patients with pheochromocytoma have plasma or urine normetanephrine levels (>80%), or metanephrine levels (20–40%), of more than twice the upper limit of the normal population reference range. For urine, these disease cut-offs correlate closely with the upper limits of the reference ranges for patients with hypertension of other etiology. Using hypertensive reference ranges therefore reduces the number of false-positive results dramatically. This is particularly important when these tests are used for screening instead of targeted diagnosis, as the prevalence of pheochromocytoma is very low in the general population (<1:100 000).

Following successful treatment, metanephrine levels should return to normal within a few days. Once a post-therapy baseline has been established, any sustained rise is highly suspicious of disease progression in incompletely cured patients, or recurrence in those who were deemed cured.

All testing for metanephrines should be performed by chromatography-based methods, ideally coupled with mass spectroscopy (MS) detection. This allows accurate identification and quantification of the individual metanephrines, and eliminates most interference. However, substances that increase endogenous catecholamine levels can result in borderline elevations of metanephrines, since peripheral catecholamine metabolism makes a small contribution to the circulating metanephrine pool. In particular, MAO inhibitors and catecholamine re-uptake inhibitors (e.g., amphetamines or tricyclic antidepressants), can lead to false high measurements. Renal failure leads to modest increments in metanephrine levels (~1.5-to fourfold), which can vary depending on the timing of the blood draw in relation to dialysis treatment. False-negative tests might be observed in early preclinical disease. This can be seen in asymptomatic patients, who are screened because of known, or suspected, genetic predisposition for paraganglioma or pheochromocytoma. Unlike patients with symptomatic disease, these individuals might have levels just above the upper limit of the normal population reference range, or, rarely, can have normal levels. False-negative results might also occur when treatment with metyrosine, an inhibitor of catecholamine synthesis, has been initiated before biochemical testing. Finally, many fractionated metanephrine assays do not measure methoxytyramine, and can therefore yield false-negative results in rare cases of tumors with exclusive dopamine over-production.

Calcitonin and procalcitonin

Within thyroid C-cells, and, to a very small extent, other neuroendocrine cells in lung, adrenals, and gastrointestinal tract, pre-procalcitonin is expressed and processed to procalcitonin (ProCT) and then calcitonin (CT), which is secreted in response to hypercalcemia. While it inhibits bone resorption, minimizing oscillations in serum calcium, its role in normal human physiology is minimal. Circulating normal concentrations range from undetectable to ~16 pg/ml.

CT is elevated at diagnosis in most patients with sporadic medullary thyroid carcinoma (MTC) and levels parallel tumor burden and predict outcome (Table 11.3) [11, 12]. In patients with familial MTC, FMTC or multiple endocrine neoplasia (MEN) [2], CT levels can be normal during the phase of C-cell hyperplasia or preclinical MTC. In the past, calcium or pentagastrin stimulation testing has been employed in these individuals, but this has been largely superseded by *RET* mutation testing [11]. Calcium stimulation testing, and, where still available, pentagastrin testing, continue to play a role in familial cases without a detectable *RET* mutation, or in sporadic cases, who are incidentally found to have mild to modest CT elevations (<5–10 times upper limit of normal), but no structural thyroid gland abnormalities. Calcium stimulation and (to a lesser degree) pentagastrin testing are unpleasant and potentially risky. Protocols are poorly standardized; intravenous (i.v.) pentagastrin doses are ~0.5 µg/kg body weight (BW), calcium doses are 2–3 mg/kg BW, and the drugs are administered, depending on the protocol used, over 0.1–5 minutes, with samples drawn at baseline and at (variable) multiple further time points over 0.5–10 minutes. Published diagnostic cut-offs range from a more than threefold rise to anywhere between 50 and 300 pg/ml peak CT concentration.

At physiological or modestly elevated levels (as above) CT has a biphasic half-life of <15 min and <40 min, respectively, while at higher concentrations the half-life is prolonged to ~3 h and ~30 h for the rapid and slow components, respectively. Therefore, depending on the pre-surgical CT level, there should be a predictable decline after successful therapy. If CT remains detectable 3–4 weeks after treatment, this indicates either incomplete thyroidectomy or persistent disease [11]. By contrast, most, but not all, patients with undetectable CT can be considered cured (Fig. 11.7).

During long-term follow-up CT levels should stay undetectable in cured patients. Rising levels reflect recurrence or disease progression, with higher CT levels predicting a poorer outcome. However, stable elevations in CT can be compatible with long-term stable disease. It appears therefore that the CT doubling time is a strong and independent predictor of outcome: doubling times

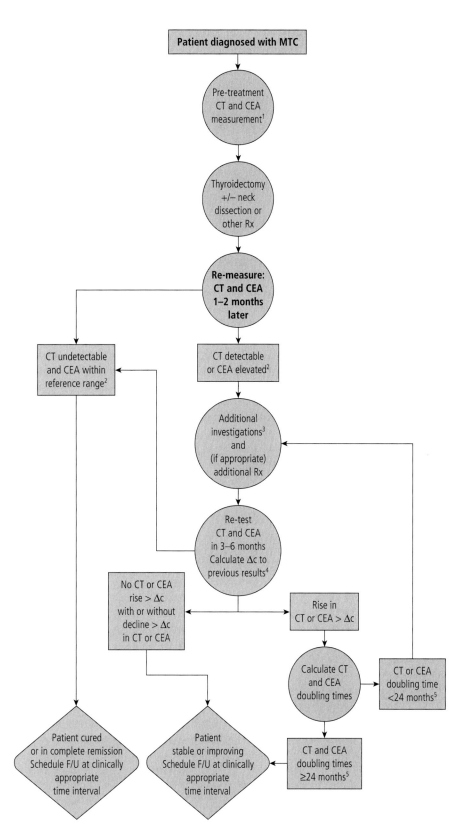

Figure 11.7 Suggested algorithm for tumor marker testing in the follow-up of medullary thyroid carcinoma. CEA, carcinoembryonic antigen; CT, calcitonin; Rx, treatment/therapy. Notes: 1. The pretreatment CT and CEA levels establish a baseline and should be obtained in all patients. Measurements should ideally be taken before any biopsy is performed, or 3–4 weeks after biopsy (but before any treatment). 2. Depending on the pretreatment levels, CT should become undetectable after successful therapy, while CEA should fall within the reference range. Isolated, persistent CEA elevation might also signify the presence of a different, CEA-secreting tumor elsewhere. 3. If additional investigations are negative, then the possibility of heterophile antibody (or rarely autoantibody) interference should be excluded (see main text), before embarking on therapeutic interventions. 4. Δc: minimal significant (critical) change between serial measurements. See main text for details. 5. Doubling times (of CT in particular) of ≥24 months are associated with excellent long-term cause-specific survival rates (see also main text).

of <6 months are associated with cause-specific mortality rates of ~75% and ~90% at 5 and 10 years, respectively, while patients with doubling times >2 years are usually alive at 10-year follow-up (Fig. 11.7) [13].

Comparability between different CT assays remains a problem, despite common calibration to the 2nd WHO International Standard (preparation 89/620). Using the same assay for serial measurements is therefore important. There are also significant differences in detection limit and functional sensitivity between different assays. Correlations between cure and undetectable serum CT levels are much better for more sensitive assays [11].

Neonates, lactating women, patients with renal failure, severe inflammatory conditions, sepsis, hyperparathyroidism and, rarely, active autoimmune thyroiditis can have moderate (as above) serum CT elevations, as can some patients with non-thyroid tumors, in particular islet cell tumors, carcinoids, small cell carcinomas of the lung, and leukemias. In patients with elevated CT levels and no evidence of thyroid nodules, such alternative diagnoses should be considered.

Finally, CT is subject to rapid pre-analytical degradation, potentially resulting in false-low test results. This underappreciated, but not infrequent, problem has prompted evaluation of the CT precursor ProCT, which is more stable and has a longer, concentration-independent, half-life, as an alternative to CT. Early studies suggest that ProCT performs equal or better than CT, but more data need to be accumulated.

Thyroglobulin, thyroglobulin antibodies and thyroglobulin mRNA

Thyroglobulin (Tg) is a large thyroid-specific glycoprotein. Non-iodinated Tg is transported from cytosol to follicular lumen, where thyroid peroxidase catalyzes the iodination of its tyrosine and thyronine residues, followed by intramolecular coupling of pairs of mono- and di-iodotyrosines to thyroxine (T_4) and tri-iodothyronine (T_3). The iodinated Tg is stored in the follicular lumen, forming the colloid. For thyroid hormone release, colloid is reabsorbed and proteolyzed. T_3 and T_4 are secreted into the systemic circulation. Only a very small amount of intact Tg is also secreted. However, rapid disordered growth of thyroid tissue, as may be observed in follicular cell-derived thyroid neoplasms, can result in significant leakage of Tg into the bloodstream. Because of this observation, Tg's organ specificity, and its low circulating concentration in healthy individuals, Tg was investigated more than 30 years ago as a potential thyroid cancer marker. Levels were found to be on average higher in thyroid cancer patients than in normal individuals or patients with non-neoplastic thyroid disease. Unfortunately, there is a large diagnostic overlap. Small thyroid cancers secrete little Tg, while benign hyperplastic growth (diffuse or nodular goiter) and autoimmune follicular destruction (Hashimoto thyroiditis or Graves disease) can result in significant elevations of serum Tg concentration. Serum Tg measurement is therefore not a useful marker for thyroid cancer screening or primary diagnosis. By contrast, measurement of Tg in biopsy needle wash specimens from cervical lymph nodes is a useful adjunct to cytology in the detection of metastatic differentiated thyroid carcinoma at initial presentation or during follow-up [14]. Aspirates from normal lymph nodes are free of Tg, while those from nodal deposits of metastatic thyroid cancer contain Tg, typically >100 ng/ml. However, correlation with serum Tg levels is important, particularly for nodal Tg levels <100 ng/ml, as minor blood contamination can lead to false-positive results if the serum Tg level is very high.

Serum Tg measurement is a good, and almost universally used, marker to assess treatment success and monitor patients for disease progression or recurrence, despite uncertainty as to its impact on patient outcomes (Fig. 11.8). Optimal assessment includes a preoperative Tg measurement as a baseline. Following total thyroidectomy ± radioiodine remnant ablation (RRA), serum Tg levels should fall with a half-life of about 72 h (6–96 h) and become undetectable within ~2 months, if there is no remnant or metastases. Similar rates of decline are observed in patients on T_4 therapy with a small remnant, but Tg might not become completely undetectable; 1 g of thyroid tissue corresponds to serum Tg levels of ~1 ng/ml and ~0.5 ng/ml at normal and suppressed thyroid-stimulating hormone (TSH) levels, respectively. If the size of a remnant can be ascertained, an estimate can be made of the expected Tg concentration in a cured patient [11, 15].

During follow-up, Tg levels should remain low or undetectable in cured patients receiving T_4. A variety of different Tg cut-offs for patients on T_4 have been proffered, ranging from <10 ng/ml down to <0.1 ng/ml. The differences reflect increasing assay sensitivity over time, with newer assays being 5–50-fold more sensitive than older assays, and changing practice patterns, with more complete thyroid removal and increasing rates (and doses) of RRA. Current guidelines suggest to supplement Tg measurements on T_4 with periodic TSH-stimulated Tg levels (T_4 withdrawal or rTSH administration), but acknowledge that <10% of patients with Tg levels of <1 ng/ml on T_4 will show a rise of serum Tg after TSH stimulation above established cut-offs (more than five times the baseline value or >2 ng/ml) [11, 15–17]. More recent data, using the most sensitive of Tg assays, suggest that if 0.1 ng/ml on T_4 is used as a cut-off for cure, and patients with levels between 0.1 and 1 ng/ml are investigated with neck ultrasound, TSH-stimulated Tg testing adds little additional information. Individuals with higher Tg levels on T_4 should probably still be subjected to additional TSH-stimulated Tg testing. In some of these patients diagnostic radioiodine scanning might also have a role; overall, radioiodine scanning is less sensitive than stimulated Tg measurements and should generally be reserved for tumor localization or for post-therapy scanning. Finally, if a patient has Tg levels >1 ng/ml on T_4, but is known to have a relatively large remnant, has no clinical evidence of disease and the Tg levels have been stable over time, stimulated Tg measurement may in some instances also be omitted (Fig. 11.8). Serial Tg measurements should be performed with the same assay if possible, as significant variability persists between different Tg assays (up to two-fold in some patients), despite widespread use of the European calibration standard CRM-457.

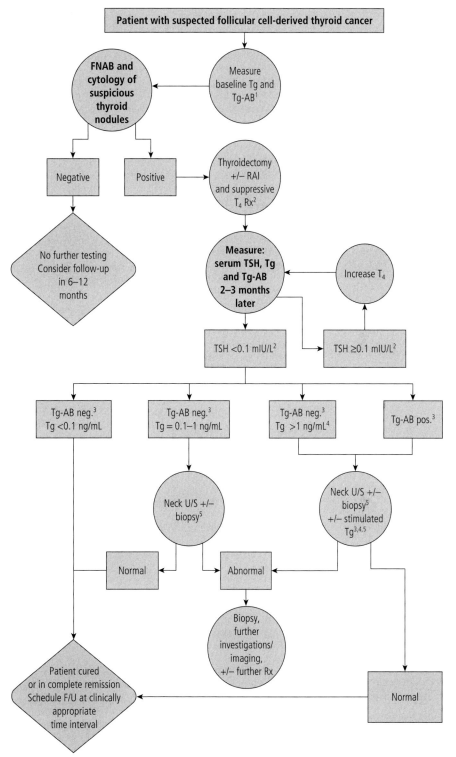

Figure 11.8 Suggested algorithm for tumor marker testing in the follow-up of follicular cell-derived thyroid carcinoma. FNAB, fine needle aspiration biopsy; RRA, radioactive remnant ablation; Rx, treatment/therapy; T$_4$, thyroxine; Tg, thyroglobulin; Tg-AB, thyroglobulin autoantibodies; TSH, thyrotropin/thyroid-stimulating hormone; U/S, ultrasound. Notes: 1.The pretreatment Tg and Tg-AB levels establish a baseline and should be obtained in all patients. Measurements should ideally be taken before any biopsy is performed, or 3–4 weeks after biopsy (but before any treatment). 2. Small thyroid remnants can result in serum Tg levels >1 ng/ml, in the absence of suppressive T$_4$ therapy. 3. Only high-sensitivity Tg-AB assays should be used. Currently, any detectable Tg-AB is considered to potentially cause false-low interference in Tg assays (see main text). The diagnostic accuracy of stimulated Tg measurements in Tg-AB positive patients might be less than in Tg negative patients. Tg-AB positive patients can sometimes be monitored by following Tg-AB levels (with the same assay) serially (see main text). 4. Patients with a known thyroid remnant of ≥2 g are likely to have Tg levels of ≥1 ng/ml (see main text). In selected patients like this, who are clinically stable and have stable Tg levels, stimulated Tg measurements might be omitted (see main text). 5. The majority of recurrences of the most common thyroid cancer, papillary thyroid carcinoma, occur in neck lymph nodes. They are best confirmed by U/S and biopsy of suspicious nodes. Stimulated Tg levels of >2 ng/ml (or a rise by > fivefold in patients with higher baseline levels) are considered abnormal.

The main limitation of Tg in thyroid cancer follow-up is auto-antibodies to Tg (Tg-AB). Depending on the methodology used for their detection, they are found in 15–30% of thyroid cancer patients, about twice the rate observed in the general population. Tg-AB can interfere in Tg assays, leading to false-low results (Fig. 11.3A). There is no consensus about the Tg-AB concentration that might be expected to result in significant Tg-assay interference, and this can vary between different Tg assays, with competitive assays being less susceptible (but also less sensitive) than immunometric assays. Tg-AB assays can also differ significantly from each other, even when standardized to the MRC65/93 standard, and might also exhibit very different detection sensitivities [18]. The recommendation is therefore to regard any detectable Tg-AB as a potential interference. This is probably an over-cautious approach as marked interference is very unlikely at concentrations of <20 mIU/L. However, many clinical decisions are now made on changes in Tg levels of <1 ng/ml. In this setting, even a minor interference could be significant, and low Tg-AB concentrations cannot be ignored universally. Spike recovery studies are sometimes performed, to assess the degree of interference. They can confirm substantial interference, but are an unreliable indicator of mild or modest, but potentially significant, Tg-AB interference [11, 18].

False-high Tg results can be observed in cases of heterophile antibody interference. This might occur in 0.1–2% of Tg measurements, depending on the assay and the patient population. In particular, in patients who have a negative diagnostic or post-therapy radioiodine scan that has been performed due to a Tg elevation, heterophile interference must be suspected strongly. It should also be suspected whenever Tg measurements are higher than expected, based on the clinical picture and previous tests performed. Suspected heterophile antibody interference can be confirmed by re-testing after addition of heterophile blocking reagents, or demonstration of non-linearity of Tg results upon serial sample dilution [19]. Other immunoassay problems, as described in the general section, can also affect Tg assays.

Because of the high prevalence of Tg-AB in thyroid cancer patients there has been interest in using serial measurement of Tg-AB in Tg-AB positive patients as a surrogate marker for Tg. In cured athyrotic patients, Tg-AB become eventually (over 6–18 months) negative. By contrast, rising titers have been correlated to disease progression [11]. Multiple studies have confirmed these findings, and Tg-AB testing as a surrogate maker for Tg has been endorsed in the 2003 US National Academy of Clinical Biochemistry laboratory medicine practice guidelines and the 2006 European thyroid cancer management consensus statement [11, 17]. However, these publications remain vague on the issue of definitive cut-off or action levels, as does the rest of the published literature. In addition, very sensitive and reproducible Tg-AB assays are required; most commercial assays fall short of this ideal. Tg-AB testing remains therefore a qualitative or semi-quantitative tool in thyroid cancer follow-up.

Measurement of circulating Tg mRNA is another potential alternative to Tg measurement in Tg-AB positive patients. While some researchers have found this approach promising when applied under carefully controlled conditions, most investigators have failed to find diagnostic value in Tg mRNA testing [20]. Moreover, RNA is very unstable and can be degraded within minutes, hindering greatly any meaningful use of this methodology in the clinical laboratory.

Other endocrine tumor markers

Many neuroendocrine tumors secrete a variety of other hormones that can cause characteristic clinical syndromes, which are covered in some detail in other chapters. Some of these hormones can also be secreted by certain non-endocrine tumors. Table 11.4 gives an overview of this group of tumor markers and their applications.

There are also a few tumor markers for non-endocrine tumors that are applicable to endocrine tumors. Specifically, CEA is a valuable adjunct marker in patients with MTC. CEA is less commonly elevated than CT (<50% of cases at diagnosis), but might increase later, or remain elevated in cases with secondary decline in CT due to tumor de-differentiation. Levels >3 ng/ml and >5 ng/ml are suspicious in non-smokers and smokers, respectively. Most patients have levels several times above these cut-offs. CEA expression by MTC is also a prognostic marker, indicating a more aggressive tumor, and rising CEA levels correlate with a high risk of cause-specific mortality [11–13]. When measuring CEA in MTC patients, it has to be borne in mind that this marker is not organ specific and elevations could also indicate the presence of a second primary tumor in other organs (Table 11.4). The various problems and limitations of immunoassays also need to be considered in CEA testing and result interpretation.

Novel markers

Several new approaches to tumor marker testing have been explored recently. They center on detection of tumor-specific nucleic acid changes (RNA or DNA) in tissues, blood and body fluids, and identification and simultaneous measurement of multiple potential or confirmed markers by proteomic approaches.

Several RNA-based markers besides Tg mRNA have been explored for thyroid cancer and other endocrine tumors, but none has been shown to be clinically useful at this stage. DNA-based tests might hold greater promise. Single point mutations in oncogenes, such as BRAF V600E, are highly specific targets for minimal residual disease detection, without the preanalytical problems of RNA-based tests. However, clinical utility will have to be demonstrated unequivocally before DNA-based markers can be considered as clinical tools.

Proteomic multiplexing approaches are also promising, the paradigm being that: (i) simultaneous use of multiple markers might offer superior diagnostic accuracy to single markers; (ii) novel markers might be identified and correlated with outcomes; and (iii) proteomic expression patterns in themselves might be indicative of malignancy, even without identification of specific markers. Unfortunately, many obstacles need to be overcome before this potential can be realized: (i) simultaneous measurement of several markers can lead to additive or multiplicative measurement errors, negating the benefits of post-analytical mathematical analysis; (ii) many "novel" markers that have been observed have on further analysis proved to be experimental artifacts or well-known non-specific markers, such as fibrinogen or C-reactive protein; (iii) reliable marker-pattern recognition is dependent on as yet unachievable levels of preanalytical and analytical standardization of proteomic techniques. For these reasons, proteomic tumor markers currently remain elusive.

References

1. Diamanidis EP, Chan DW, Schwartz MK, et al. Part 1: General principles. In: Diamandis EP, Fritsche HA, Lilja H, Chan DW, Schwartz MK (eds). *Tumor Markers – Physiology, Pathobiology, Technology, and Clinical Applications*. Washington, DC, USA: AACC Press, 2002:1–162.

2. Shekelle PG, Woolf SH, Eccles M, Grimshaw J. Clinical guidelines: developing guidelines. *Br. Med. J.* 1999;318:593–696.

3. Hayes DF, Bast RC, Desch CE, et al. Tumor marker utility grading system: a framework to evaluate clinical utility of tumor markers. *J. Natl Cancer Inst.* 1996;88:1456–1466.

4. Lord SJ, Irwig L, Simes J. When is measuring of sensitivity and specificity sufficient to evaluate a diagnostic test, and when do we need randomized trials? *Ann. Intern. Med.* 2006;144:850–855.

5. Taupenot L, Harper KL, O'Connor DT. The chromogranin–secretogranin family. *N. Engl. J. Med.* 2003;384:1134–1149.

6. Lamberts SW, Hofland LJ, Nobels FR. Neuroendocrine tumor markers. *Frontiers Neuroendocrinol.* 2001;22:309–339.

7. Meijer WG, Kema IP, Volmer M, Willemse PH, de Vries EG. Discriminating capacity of indol markers in the diagnosis of carcinoid tumors. *Clin. Chem.* 2000;46:1588–1596.

8. Eisenhofer G, Kopin IJ, Goldstein DS. Catecholamine metabolism: a contemporary view with implications for physiology and medicine. *Pharmacol. Rev.* 2004;56:331–349.

9. Singh RJ. Advances in metanephrine testing for the diagnosis of pheochromocytoma. *Clin. Lab. Med.* 2004;24:85–103.

10. Sawka AM, Jaeschke R, Singh RJ, Young WF, Jr. A comparison of biochemical tests for pheochromocytoma: measurement of fractionated plasma metanephrines compared with the combination of 24-hour urinary metanephrines and catecholamines. *J. Clin. Endocrinol. Metab.* 2003;88:553–558.

11. Baloch Z, Carayon P, Conte-Devolx B, et al. Laboratory medicine practice guidelines. Laboratory support for the diagnosis and monitoring of thyroid disease. *Thyroid* 2003;13:3–126.

12. Leboulleux S, Baudin E, Travagli JP, Schlumberger M. Medullary thyroid carcinoma. *Clin. Endocrinol.* 2004;61:299–310.

13. Barbet J, Campion L, Kraeber-Bodere F, Chatal JF, Group GTES. Prognostic impact of serum calcitonin and carcinoembryonic antigen doubling-times in patients with medullary thyroid carcinoma. *J. Clin. Endocrinol. Metab.* 2005;90:6077–6084.

14. Boi F, Baghino G, Atzeni F, Lai ML, Faa G, Mariotti S. The diagnostic value for differentiated thyroid carcinoma metastases of thyroglobulin (Tg) measurement in washout fluid from fine-needle aspiration biopsy of neck lymph nodes is maintained in the presence of circulating anti-Tg antibodies. *J. Clin. Endocrinol. Metab.* 2006; 91:1364–1369.

15. Mazzaferri EL, Robbins RJ, Spencer CA, et al. A consensus report of the role of serum thyroglobulin as a monitoring method for low-risk patients with papillary thyroid carcinoma. *J. Clin. Endocrinol. Metab.* 2003;88:1433–1441.

16. Cooper DS, Doherty GM, Haugen BR, et al. Management guideline for patients with thyroid nodules and differentiated thyroid cancer. *Thyroid* 2006;16:109–140.

17. Pacini F, Schlumberger M, Dralle H, et al. European consensus for the management of patients with differentiated carcinoma of the follicular epithelium. *Eur. J. Endocrinol.* 2006;154:787–803.

18. Spencer CA, Bergoglio LM, Kazarosyan M, Fatemi S, LoPresti JS. Clinical impact of thyroglobulin (Tg) and Tg autoantibody method differences on the management of patients with differentiated thyroid carcinomas. *J. Clin. Endocrinol. Metab.* 2005;90:5566–5575.

19. Preissner CM, O'Kane DJ, Singh RJ, Morris JC, Grebe SK. Phantoms in the assay tube: heterophile antibody interferences in serum thyroglobulin assays. *J. Clin. Endocrinol. Metab.* 2003;88:3069–3074.

20. Ringel MD. Editorial: Molecular detection of thyroid cancer: differentiating "signal" and "noise" in clinical assays. *J. Clin. Endocrinol. Metab.* 2004;89:29–32.

12 General Management of Cancer Patients

Marcia Hall

> **Key points**
> - The diagnosis of cancer is often a complicated, prolonged process requiring extensive and unpleasant investigations. This is especially true for rarer malignancies such as the endocrine-related tumors.
> - Diagnostic and staging investigations are essential to clarify whether treatment should be aimed at cure or palliation. It must be understood, however, that techniques for staging are never sensitive enough to guarantee that a specific cancer is limited at presentation – hence later "relapses."
> - Good communication with the patient and their family throughout is vital to ensure that the aims and limitations of any therapeutic strategy are understood. It is often important to admit to any limitations in medical knowledge, e.g., with respect to cancer staging.
> - Potential adverse effects of any therapeutic strategies require discussion and preferably written information for patients. Knowledge of possible problems significantly helps patients and their families cope with difficult treatments.
> - Regular review, including documenting current symptoms, diagnostic results, therapy options and the content of discussions with the patient and their family, is essential for the highest quality care of the cancer patient.

Complications of disease

Pain

Pain is the most feared consequence of cancer. It occurs in approximately one third of patients (15% with non-metastatic disease and 60–90% with advanced disease). There are two types of cancer pain.

1 *Acute*: clearly defined temporal onset usually associated with objective physical signs together with signs of increased autonomic nervous system activity. This type of pain is usually self-limiting and readily treatable.

2 *Chronic*: poorly defined onset, usually present for greater than 3 months, with no associated objective clinical signs. This type of pain often results in changes in personality, lifestyle and functioning.

Of cancer pain 70–80% is though to be due to direct tumor involvement (bone, 50%; nerve, 25%; hollow viscus, 15%). Twenty to 30% is thought to be related to cancer therapy and 3–10% to unrelated previous processes, for example rheumatoid arthritis.

Pain symptoms should be clearly identified and documented: somatic (e.g., bony), visceral (e.g., liver metastases), or deafferent (injury to peripheral or central nervous system); assessment must include the degree of functional impairment. Psychosocial factors may be influential and should also be addressed. Verification of the history by another family member may help to prioritize the

Clinical Endocrine Oncology, 2nd edition. Edited by Ian D. Hay and John A.H. Wass. © 2008 Blackwell Publishing. ISBN 978-1-4051-4584-8.

management of multiple complaints. Painful benign conditions may co-exist in patients with cancer and should not be overlooked.

Adequate pain relief usually involves two or more different classes of analgesics (Table 12.1). No additional therapeutic effect exists beyond the maximum tolerated dose of most non-steroidal drugs and each one in this category has a different anti-inflammatory to analgesic ratio. A patient-tailored, pragmatic approach utilizing the many available different opiate doses and preparations is usually the most effective. Helping patients understand how the different preparations of opiates work (quick action versus slow release, etc.) and alerting them to the possible side effects, particularly those to which you might reasonably expect tolerance, is essential. Sedation, nausea (and occasionally vomiting) and heightened dreaming can all occur with the first few doses of opiates. In most patients tolerance to these side effects develops over 48–72 h. However, constipation and a dry mouth remain ongoing adverse effects of opiates. Some opiates, e.g., fentanyl, have a less constipating effect than others but all will require some laxative advice, ranging from general principles such as mobilizing as much as possible and keeping the fluid intake up, to specific laxative prescriptions. A combination of laxatives with different modes of action (e.g., senna and Movicol) is frequently useful; higher than routine recommended doses may be required.

Total pain, as first described by Cicely Saunders, is recognized as pain comprising physical, psychological, emotional, and spiritual elements and this underlines the importance of a multidisciplinary approach to its control. The non-drug treatment of pain includes single fractions of radiotherapy, nerve-stimulating and nerve-blocking techniques as well as a range of psychological

Table 12.1 Pharmacological treatments for pain

Class	Drugs	Indications	Dose/route	Contraindications	Side effects	Interactions
Non-steroidals	Diclofenac	Mild/moderate pain especially if inflammatory component present	50 mg three times daily by mouth/rectally or 75 mg MR twice daily by mouth	Active peptic ulcer Proctitis Aspirin allergy	GI hemorrhage/diarrhea Hematological Headache, edema	Steroids Anticoagulants Digoxin Quinolones
Narcotics Partial agonists	Buprenorphine	Not recommended	60–120 mg four times daily	Severe COPD	Nausea, drowsiness, dizziness, hallucinations, constipation	CNS depressants, MAOIs
Weak opioids	Dihydrocodeine Codeine phosphate Cocodamol (acetaminophen plus codeine)	Moderate / severe pain Severe pain	30–90 mg four times daily i–ii,4–6 hourly max 8 per 24 h	Hepatic failure		
Opioids	Diamorphine Morphine sulfate (Oramorph, sevredol) Morphine sulfate (slow release MST) Fentanyl		Start 5–10 mg s.c. Start 10–30 mg 4 hourly Start 10–30 mg twice daily (Patches) start 12.5 μg per 72 h		Sedation, dry mouth, constipation,	Cimetidine Anticoagulants
Tricyclics	Amitriptyline	Neuropathic pain	10–50 mg max at night 10 day trial	Heart disease	Dizziness, nausea, hyponatremia, blood dyscrasias, severe skin rash	Anticoagulants, oral contraceptives, MAOIs, cimetidine
Anticonvulsants	Carbamazepine Gabapentin	Neuropathic pain (shooting/stinging)	100 mg twice daily increasing slowly (100 mg every 3–4 days) to 200 mg three times daily 200 mg at night for first day increasing by 200 mg per day to max of 1.8 g per day	AV conduction abnormalities, porphyria, agranulocytosis	Headaches, drowsiness	Use lower doses in elderly and renal impairment
Steroids	Dexamethasone	Pain associated with tumor pressure or edema	8–16 mg for 3–5 days then reduce by 2 mg every 2–3 days	Very recent surgery, active peptic ulcer	GI hemorrhage, Mood changes, Prox. myopathy, etc.	Anticoagulants, NSAIDs
Bisphosphonates	Pamidronate Zoledronic acid	Bone pain	60–120 mg 500 ml normal saline over 2 h 2–4 mg in normal saline over 15 min	Osteonecrosis or very recent dental work	Osteonecrosis, renal failure	

COPD, chronic obstructive pulmonary disease; GI, gastrointestinal; MAOI, monoamine oxidase inhibitor; MR, modified release; s.c., subcutaneous.

interventions including relaxation techniques and the teaching of cognitive coping strategies.

Infection

Infections occur commonly in cancer patients, either as a consequence of the underlying malignancy or as a complication of therapy. They may be life threatening. In treating cancer it is important to recognize risk factors contributing to infection and to have a good knowledge of available therapies.

Host defense mechanisms may be compromised by virtue of the malignant disease itself; for example, impaired antibody production in multiple myeloma, altered cellular immunity in lymphomas. The cancer patient is also rendered more vulnerable by cancer treatment. Cytotoxic chemotherapy and radiotherapy deplete granulocyte numbers and produce defects of neutrophil function; corticosteroids diminish phagocytosis and neutrophil migration. As if to add injury to insult, anticancer treatments may also break down some of the physical barriers to pathogenic invasion, such as mucosal and skin reactions. Antibiotic therapy, active or empirical, may induce secondary colonization of these "chinks in the armor," resulting in systemic invasion. Malnutrition exacerbates all the above, adding to the cancer patient's susceptibility.

The febrile response is often significantly diminished in cancer patients, particularly when neutropenic, and fevers may be masked by concomitant steroid or non-steroidal anti-inflammatory drugs (NSAID) treatments. If undetected and untreated, infections may be rapidly fatal. Fifty-five to 70% of febrile episodes in the population have an infective etiology. This incidence is higher in neutropenic patients, where 85–90% of infections are bacterial in origin, although only 30–50% will be positively identified.

Empirical therapy should be considered in non-neutropenic patients after two or three temperature readings greater than 38 °C (100.4 °F). Antibiotics must be commenced in neutropenic (absolute neutrophil count $<1 \times 10^9/mm^3$) patients after a single temperature reading of >37.5 °C (99.4 °F). This reduces mortality from 80% to 10–30%. Bactericidal antibiotics covering Gram-negative bacteria are essential therapy. Standard empirical antibiotics should be tailored for each institution taking into account local microbial isolates, antibiotic resistance patterns and cost. If the response is slow or if organisms are isolated that are not covered, early modifications will be required. Prophylactic antibiotics should be considered for patients undergoing intensive therapy involving long periods of neutropenia; for example, autologous bone marrow transplantation as the major source of infection (85%) is from endogenous flora. Such patients as these are also usually treated with an antiviral agent for the first year after such treatment as this has been shown to reduce the incidence of recurrent herpes infections. Granulocyte colony-stimulating factor (GCSF) has proven a useful adjunct for some, by limiting the period of neutropenia and thus reducing the risk of infections.

Anorexia–cachexia syndrome

Malnutrition is frequently a serious problem in patients with cancer, contributing substantially to the morbidity and mortality from the disease. Approximately one-quarter of cancer patients have lost 10% or more of their premorbid body weight and one third require some form of nutritional support [1]. Clearly, certain tumor types, such as those affecting the gastrointestinal tract, are more commonly associated with significant weight loss and malnutrition. There is often no correlation, however, between tumor extent and weight loss, suggesting influences from many other factors. A complex cytokine cascade, triggered in the host by the tumor, is believed to result in the progressive weight loss, lethargy, weakness and anorexia that characterize cachexia. This abnormal metabolic state may be exacerbated by other tumor-related phenomena such as ectopic hormone production and infective episodes causing hypermetabolism. Abnormalities of taste and smell are common amongst cancer patients, frequently exacerbated by cancer therapy.

The anorexia–cachexia syndrome is notoriously difficult to treat without regression of the underlying cancer. Nevertheless there are numerous strategies that can be considered and tried (Table 12.2). Although corticosteroids have been shown to improve both quality of life and appetite, this adjunct to therapy rarely results in non-fluid weight gain. Progestogens (medroxypro-gesterone acetate 100 mg three times daily) have been shown to have a dose-related effect on appetite and weight, which is secondary to neither fluid retention nor tumor response. Enteral feeding with nutritional supplements can be useful but parenteral feeding should not be undertaken except as a short-term option in the severely malnourished patient expected to respond well to active cancer treatment.

Psychological morbidity

Studies of psychiatric disorders in cancer patients have estimated a prevalence rate of 20–47%. The majority suffer from anxiety and depressive disorders, although other major problems include anticipatory nausea and vomiting, marital and sexual dysfunction. The spectrum of severity is considerable and ranges from mild transient "adjustment reactions" to severe and disabling anxiety and mood disorders. No matter how "understandable" a patient's distress, thorough assessment including a collateral history and appropriate physical investigations should be undertaken if appropriate treatment strategies, both psychological and pharmacological, are to be provided. Many patients will benefit from counseling of a supportive/educational approach, although more specific cognitive behavioral techniques may be needed in severe persistent disorders [2]. Antidepressant medication is generally underprescribed in cancer patients and with the advent of newer agents with fewer side effects (e.g., selective serotonin reuptake inhibitors [SSRIs]) this should be considered if symptoms of anxiety and depression are either of a severe degree or are non-responsive to psychological treatments.

Complications of therapy

Cytotoxic therapy

Cytotoxic agents are renowned for their toxic and plentiful adverse effects. These are often closely related to their very action, killing cells. Malignant cells are targeted by these drugs because, in general, they undergo mitosis faster than normal cells. Clearly this crude warfare will inevitably have some action on other normally dividing cells. One very common and underestimated side effect is lethargy. A patient may feel lethargic as part of their underlying disease but the addition of cytotoxic therapy will invariably exacerbate the situation. The lethargy is particularly profound during episodes of neutropenia. There is no effective remedy for this debilitating condition except to reassure the patients that improvements occur with the resolution of neutropenia. Table 12.3 lists adverse effects common to many cytotoxic treatments and mentions a few problems specific to individual agents, noted in parentheses. Strategies to overcome some of these problems are suggested.

Radiation therapy

Radiation can be used in a number of different ways in the treatment of malignant disease. The most common delivery of radiotherapy is from an external source, targeting an area of cancer – either the primary or a metastasis. If treated in this way, radiotherapy is considered as a local treatment (akin to surgery) and adverse effects are generally confined to the area receiving

Table 12.2 Adverse effects of chemotherapy

System	Adverse effect	Management
Local	Phlebitis	Inject/infuse drug more slowly; resite cannula if persistent. NB Phlebitic drugs, e.g., anthracyclines should, *always* be administered as an infusion or via running saline
	Local tissue necrosis	Irrigate/cold compress/ infiltrate with hydrocortisone
Gastrointestinal	Nausea and vomiting	Emetogenic potential of agents differ:
		Low: e.g., fluoropyrimidines, taxanes, vinca alkaloids, chlorambucil – give domperidone 10–30 mg four times daily as needed
	Stomatitis	Moderate: e.g., cyclophosphamide, methotrexate, doxorubicin – give dexamethasone 8 mg by mouth with chemo plus 2 mg three times daily for 2–3 days
		High: e.g., platinum – give dexamethasone 8 mg by mouth and granisetron 2 mg by mouth with chemo and further 2–3 days dexamethasone $\pm$ granisetron
		NB: TTO rectal preparations of domperidone and prochlorperazine can be useful
		Mouthwash 2–4 hourly e.g., Corsadyl or Difflam (latter contains local anesthetic). For throat mucositis Mucaine is very effective
	Constipation	Very common after 5-HT$_3$ antagonists – give prophylactic laxatives, e.g., Movicol
	Diarrhea	If life threatening, admit to rehydrate. Usually use loperamide or codeine phosphate (occasionally require excessive doses, e.g., 90–120 mg four times daily). Try somatostatin analogs if neuroendocrine related; cyproheptadine for carcinoid
Hematological	Leukopenia	Dose reduction or GCSF support if severe. Consider prophylactic antibiotics if infections are recurrent during chemotherapy
	Thrombocytopenia	Give platelets if $<10 \times 10^3/mm^3$ or active bleeding
	Anemia	Consider erythropoietin 10 000 u s.c. three times per week if platinum-related anemia; otherwise transfuse if symptomatic
Renal	Acute tubular necrosis (platinum)	Check renal function and adjust subsequent doses of platinum
Neurological	Ototoxicity (platinum)	Check high-frequency hearing between repeated doses of cisplatin
	Peripheral neuropathy (vinca alkaloids, platinum compounds or taxanes)	Stop drugs if severe and not improving between doses
Miscellaneous	Alopecia (anthracyclines, cyclophosphamide, taxanes, irinotecan)	Cold cap may reduce amount of hair lost but only suitable with bolus injections
	Hand–foot syndrome (5-Fluoropyrimidines, liposomal doxorubicin)	Trial of pyridoxine 50 mg three times daily, or dose modification
	Cardiotoxicity (anthracyclines)	Do not give in conjunction with trastuzumab. Calculate cumulative doses. Reconsider agent choice if LVEF <50%
	Reduced fertility/sterility	Consider sperm banking if appropriate. Female fertility after breast cancer chemotherapy reduces but extent of reduction related to proximity of patient to "natural menopause"
	Hemorrhagic cystitis (cyclophosphamide or iphosphamide)	Forced diuresis with or without Mesna depending on dose of alkylating agent

treatment. For example, external beam radiotherapy to the thyroid may cause significant mucositis of both the esophagus and trachea as these structures are located just posterior to the organ targeted. Considerable efforts are made to confine and angle the external radiotherapy beams to minimize radiation to unaffected areas. In addition lead shields are used to protect especially vulnerable areas; in the example given above a shield is likely to be employed to protect the spinal cord. Despite the directional beams; however, patients do feel generally more tired following courses of external

beam radiotherapy. Increasing age and lower performance status prior to treatment exacerbate this lethargy.

Radiation can also be delivered systemically using radionuclides conjugated with monoclonal antibodies specific to certain antigen-bearing cancers (e.g., ^{131}I-metaiodobenzylguanidine (^{131}I-MIBG) for carcinoid and other neural crest tumors). Theoretically this controlled targeting should cause few immediate or long-term side effects but the parenteral administration of circulating radionuclides can cause toxicity to the bone marrow, lungs and

Table 12.3 Feeding strategies

Oral diet	
Education	High-calorie foods
	Small meals frequently
	Add supplements, e.g. Ensure, Complan, Build up
	Specific diets may help, e.g. low-fiber/fat/lactose free for short bowel and radiation enteritis
Location	Eat away from bed if possible
	Small portions
	Tastefully presented
Drugs	
Appetite stimulants	Steroids, e.g. dexamethasone 4–8 mg per day
	Progestogens, e.g. medroxyprogesterone acetate 100 mg three times daily
Adequate antiemetics	Regular administration, e.g. 10–30 mg metoclopramide/domperidone four times daily or half hour before meals to counteract early satiety
	Consider cyclizine or levomepromazine 6.25 mg at night
	Only use 5-HT$_3$ antagonists in conjunction with chemotherapy or radiation
Enteral feeding	
Nasogastric	Short-term use
Gastrostomy/jejunostomy	Suitable for long-term feeding
Parenteral feeding	Reserved for patients treated with curative intent

5-HT$_3$, 5-hydroxytryptamine 3 receptors.

heart. Patients receiving these therapeutically are usually isolated for a number of days in specially lead-lined side rooms.

Finally radioactive iodine (I^{131}) is routinely used in the treatment of recurrent thyroid cancers provided that the malignancy is scintigraphically detected and not amenable to surgical removal. Repeated treatments are often required and adverse effects on bone marrow and lungs (pneumonitis) can then be expected.

Biological agents

Although conventional cytotoxic and radiotherapeutic strategies retain the pivotal role in the treatment of cancer, biological therapies are emerging fast as a powerful adjunct, or sole therapy, for some tumor types (Table 12.4) [3]. Those used currently in the management of endocrine-related tumors include somatostatin analogs and α-interferon. Monoclonal antibody agents such as trastuzumab and cetuximab are establishing an important role in breast and GI cancers respectively and undoubtedly further antibody therapies will emerge. In addition to the monoclonal antibodies, treatments targeting the small intracellular molecules downstream of the surface membrane receptors (e.g., tyrosine kinase inhibitors) are beginning to be evaluated in the maintenance of cancer remission.

Recombinant GCSF continues to prove a useful agent in allaying prolonged neutropenia and thus making intensification of cytotoxic therapies possible. It must be emphasized that, with the exception of somatostatin which appears to be relatively non-toxic, biological therapy has the potential to cause serious adverse effects. Examples range from the severe muscle aches experienced by patients after GCSF to the specific cardiac toxicity of trastuzumab and the rare but omnipresent risk of anaphylaxis.

Table 12.4 Common adverse effects with biological agents

Agent	Adverse effect	Observation
Monoclonal antibodies (mostly now humanized with some mouse still used), e.g. Trastuzumab (Herceptin)	Fever, chills, pruritus, arthralgia, rash, myalgia, dyspnea, runny nose, brittle nails	Related to speed of infusion
Bevacizumab (Avastin)	Delayed wound healing, perforation, hemorrhage, hypertension	Longer term problems unknown as yet
Cetuximab	Acneiform rash	
Radionuclide antibody conjugates	^{131}I: neutropenia 25–30 days post treatment ^{90}Y: marrow toxicity	Dose dependent, chelating agents may limit effect
Somatostatin analogs	May worsen hypoglycemia	Suppression of counterregulatory glucagons and growth hormone
Interferons	Fever, chills, fatigue, mood changes, anorexia, autoimmune disorders	Dose dependent Occurs in 19%, 13% thyroid related
Small molecules, e.g. erlotinib, surafinib	Acne-like rash in 88%, diarrhea	Adverse effects occur more prominently in those responding to agent

Quality of life

The good physician knows his patient through and through and his knowledge is bought dearly. Time, sympathy and understanding must be lavishly dispensed but the reward is to be found in that personal bond which forms the greatest satisfaction of the practice of medicine. One of the essential qualities of the clinician is interest in humanity, for "the secret of the care of the patient is in caring for the patient."

(Peabody, 1927: [4])

The general management of the cancer patient requires a multidisciplinary team approach, which is concerned as much with the quality of life as its duration. The modern approach to oncology must include quality of life assessments, increasingly important with the advent of more aggressive, often toxic therapies. Quality of life assessment by doctors is notoriously poor and should always be supplemented by self-reported questionnaires, which patients can complete in a few minutes. The European Organization for Research and Treatment in Cancer (EORTC) questionnaire is a tool regularly used in clinical trials. It is easy to score and measures dimensions such as symptoms of disease, side effects of treatments, physical functioning, psychological distress, social interaction, sexuality, body image, and satisfaction with medical care. It also has modules to make it specifically applicable to individual cancers.

Clearly, improving quality of life is not solely a result of enhanced symptom control; good psychological care invariably reduces the need for hospital admission. A multidisciplinary team approach involving nurses, doctors, psychologists, and social workers is most successful with "professional" psychiatric help when required. The value of peer support, often informally or as self-help groups, should not be underestimated. Cognitive and behavioral psychotherapy, supportive counseling and psychotropic medication need to become an integral part of "orthodox" cancer therapy. It must be emphasized that psychosocial oncology is an area of skilled practice, requiring knowledge of and application of researched, available treatment strategies. It is no longer acceptable to delegate to a "sympathetic ear."

References

1. Shike M, Brennan M. Nutritional support. In Devita V, Hellman S, Rosenberg SA (eds). *Cancer Principles and Practice of Oncology*, 3rd edn. Pennsylvania: Lippincott Company, 1989:2029–2042.
2. Watson M. (ed.) *Cancer Patient Care: Psychosocial Treatment Methods.* Cambridge: BPS Books, 1991.
3. Oberg K. Chemotherapy and biotherapy in neuroendocrine tumors. *Curr. Opin. Oncol.* 1993;5:110–120.
4. Peabody SW. The care of the patient. *JAMA* 1927;88:877–882.

2 Thyroid and Parathyroid Tumors

13 Assessment of Thyroid Neoplasia

Kristien Boelaert, Jayne Franklyn, and Michael Sheppard

> **Key points**
> - Thyroid nodules and goiters are common but few of them harbor malignancy.
> - All patients with thyroid nodules or enlargement should undergo serum TSH measurement.
> - Fine needle aspiration biopsy remains the diagnostic procedure of choice to detect thyroid malignancy.
> - Patients presenting with thyroid enlargement require regular follow-up.
> - Some clinical, biochemical and ultrasonographic characteristics may aid in the prediction of thyroid malignancy.

Introduction

Thyroid enlargement is a common clinical problem. The Framingham study in the US indicated a 5–10% life-time risk of developing a thyroid nodule [1] and the Whickham survey in the north-east of England reported a 15% prevalence of goiters or thyroid nodules [2]. Additionally, high-resolution ultrasound can detect thyroid nodules in 19–67% of individuals with higher frequencies in women and the elderly, even when the gland is normal to palpation [3].

Thyroid cancer is, however, rare, accounting for approximately 1% of all new malignant disease (0.5% of cancers in men and 1.5% in women), although the incidence of thyroid cancer, mainly differentiated carcinomas, is one of the most rapidly increasing [4]. Because of its favorable prognosis, thyroid carcinoma causes an even lower percentage of cancer deaths, reported at 0.21% and 0.3% for men and women respectively [5]. The majority of thyroid cancers are papillary carcinomas (72–85%), with the remainder comprising follicular (10–20%), medullary (1.7–3%), anaplastic (<1%) and other carcinomas (1–4%). Papillary and follicular carcinomas are termed differentiated thyroid cancers [5]. Most patients with thyroid enlargement can be managed conservatively after malignancy is ruled out, the challenge to the clinician being to identify the minority of patients with thyroid cancer who therefore require surgical intervention and additional therapies [3].

Assessment of patients with thyroid enlargement

Most patients with thyroid enlargement need no treatment after biochemical euthyroidism is confirmed and malignancy is excluded [3].

Clinical Endocrine Oncology, 2nd edition. Edited by Ian D. Hay and John A.H. Wass. © 2008 Blackwell Publishing. ISBN 978-1-4051-4584-8.

Clinical evaluation

The history and clinical examination remain the diagnostic cornerstones in evaluating patients with thyroid enlargement and in some cases may be suggestive of thyroid carcinoma [6]. The physical examination should focus on inspection of the neck (including regional lymph nodes) and the upper thorax and palpation of the nodule/goiter to determine its size and nodularity. Notably, there is considerable inter- and intra-observer variation regarding size and morphology of the thyroid [3].

In many cases, however, thyroid glands harboring malignancy are clinically indistinguishable from those that do not and there is substantial variation among practitioners in evaluating nodules, a finding that may explain why an increasing number of thyroid specialists use imaging as part of the evaluation of thyroid nodules [3, 6]. The presence of discomfort in the neck, jaw, or ear and dysphagia, hoarseness or dyspnea can occur in patients with benign thyroid nodules, and particularly in those with large multinodular goiters, but may also indicate thyroid carcinoma. A hard and fixed nodule is suggestive of thyroid carcinoma, as is paralysis of the vocal cords and ipsilateral lymphadenopathy, but these clinical features are absent in the vast majority of patients with this diagnosis [3, 6].

The risk of harboring thyroid cancer is highest in men and in those at the extremes of age [3, 6]. Nodular thyroid disease is 5–10 times more common in females, whereas the rates of thyroid carcinoma are nearly equal in men and women. Therefore the presence of a thyroid nodule in a man is more likely to reflect an underlying carcinoma [3, 6]. In addition, head and neck irradiation in infancy or childhood is associated with subsequent development of carcinoma and epidemiological studies have observed increased rates of childhood papillary thyroid cancer in Belarus and Ukraine following the Chernobyl nuclear reactor accident [3, 6]. Rate of growth is of importance; thyroid carcinomas are generally slow-growing entities and rapid enlargement during thyroid hormone therapy is particularly worrisome [3].

Table 13.1 Factors suggesting the diagnosis of thyroid carcinoma in patients presenting with thyroid enlargement

Rapid tumor growth
Very firm nodules
Fixation to adjacent structures
Vocal cord paralysis
Regional lymphadenopathy
Family history of medullary thyroid cancer (MTC) or multiple endocrine neoplasia (MEN)
Age <20 years or >60 years
Male sex
Solitary nodule
History of head or neck irradiation
Compression symptoms: dysphagia, dysphonia, hoarseness, dyspnea, cough

Overall, when the clinical suspicion of malignancy is high, thyroidectomy should be advocated irrespective of benign cytology, because the likelihood of malignancy is high. Table 13.1 lists clinical criteria suggestive of the diagnosis of thyroid cancer.

Laboratory investigations

Determination of the serum thyrotropin (thyroid-stimulating hormone, TSH) concentration is the test most used by thyroidologists in the evaluation of patients presenting with thyroid enlargement and recent guidelines form the American Thyroid Association (ATA) and British Thyroid Association (BTA) state that serum TSH should be measured in the initial evaluation of a patient with a thyroid nodule [7–10]. If the TSH is below the laboratory reference range, assays for free tri-iodothyronine (fT_3) and free thyroxine (fT_4) are required in order to exclude overt hyperthyroidism (raised free T_4 and free T_3) or "T_3-toxicosis" (raised serum free T_3 alone). Similarly, if TSH is raised then overt hypothyroidism must be excluded (this being indicated by low fT_4 with a raised TSH concentration). Results from surveys have indicated that when TSH levels are within the normal range, subsequent assessment of circulating free thyroid hormone levels is more favored by European physicians when compared with North American thyroidologists [3, 7, 8]. Although virtually all patients with thyroid carcinoma are euthyroid, the presence of a suppressed serum thyrotropin (TSH) level (generally indicative of subclinical or overt thyrotoxicosis) does not rule out the presence of malignancy [3].

Antithyroid peroxidase measurements are measured by more than half of clinicians, but it is notable that thyroid autoantibodies are found in approximately 10% of the population and autoimmunity may co-exist with a thyroid nodule or goiter [3]. The role of routine measurement of serum calcitonin remains controversial. This hormone is a marker of medullary thyroid carcinoma, which accounts for less than 10% of all thyroid cancers and is reported to be elevated in less than 0.5% of all patients with thyroid nodules [3]. Early detection of medullary thyroid cancer is important but due to the presence of heterophilic antibodies, the immunometric calcitonin assay has a high false-positive rate. Again, European

physicians tend to use this assay more routinely that their American counterparts [3, 7, 8], and it seems clear that if the plasma calcitonin level is found to be above 10 pg/ml, this must prompt further investigation. The routine use of measurement of serum thyroglobulin is of little value in the initial laboratory assessment of patients with thyroid enlargement because of marked overlap of measurements in those with benign and malignant disease. Guidelines from the ATA and BTA therefore state that routine measurement of serum thyroglobulin for initial evaluation of thyroid nodules is not recommended [9, 10].

Diagnostic imaging

The number of imaging modalities available to determine size and thyroid gland morphology is growing rapidly. These include ultrasonography, scintigraphy, computerized tomography (CT) scanning, magnetic resonance imaging (MRI) and, most recently, positron emission tomography (PET).

The most widely used form of imaging is ultrasonography, which has many favorable features including detection of non-palpable nodules, estimation of nodule size/goiter volume (e.g., to monitor the effect of therapy) and guidance of fine needle aspiration biopsy (FNAB) [3, 11]. These advantages have led to changes in the attitude of clinicians and 80% of ETA (European Thyroid Association) members and 60% of ATA members now routinely include ultrasonography in the initial management of patients presenting with a goiter [7, 8]. Some ultrasonographic characteristics such as hypoechogenicity, solid nodules, microcalcifications, irregular margins, increased intranodular flow visualized by Doppler, increased ratio of anterior/posterior dimensions in transverse and longitudinal views (more tall than wide) and especially the evidence of invasion or regional lymphadenopathy are associated with increased cancer risk [6]. However, the high sensitivity of this test can also lead to the detection of clinically insignificant nodules resulting in unnecessary work-up and anxiety [3, 11]. Furthermore, the low specificity of findings in most studies disqualifies ultrasound scanning from the differentiation between benign and malignant lesions and it is clearly inferior to FNAB in this setting [3, 11].

Thyroid isotope imaging/scintigraphy has been used for many years and is helpful in the determination of the functionality of thyroid nodules. This technique allows the differentiation between "hot" (functional) and "cold" (non-functional) nodules with the risk of malignancy in cold nodules being reported as high as 8–25%. However, compared with FNAB, this diagnostic tool is significantly less sensitive and specific in distinguishing benign from malignant lesions and has therefore been largely abandoned in routine practice [3, 10].

CT and MRI scanning provide high-resolution three-dimensional imaging of the thyroid gland, but neither of these methods provides advantages over ultrasound scanning in terms of detailed visualization of intrathyroidal structure. Furthermore, these methods have little value in the differentiation between benign and malignant lesions [3]. Newer techniques such as 2-deoxy-2-fluoro-D-glucose (FDG-PET) are more promising in this respect but their use is limited by considerations of cost and accessibility. Tracheal imaging appears to be of limited value in the routine diagnostic work-up of patients presenting with thyroid enlargement although respiratory flow loop determination is helpful in the assessment of patients with large goiters [12].

Overall, FNAB is far superior to any of these diagnostic techniques and remains the current gold standard in the evaluation of patients presenting with thyroid enlargement [3, 7, 8].

FNAB

FNAB provides the most direct and specific information about the pathology of thyroid nodules, has an extremely low complication rate, and is inexpensive, easy to learn and therefore the diagnostic tool preferred by the majority of thyroidologists [7, 8]. Most centers using this procedure have achieved a 35–75% reduction in the number of patients requiring surgery, while at the same time doubling or tripling the malignancy yield at thyroidectomy [13].

The efficacy of this investigative tool has been evaluated in several large series which have confirmed it to be an accurate test in the diagnosis of thyroid cancer, its sensitivity and specificity ranging between 65% and 98% and 72% and 100% respectively [4, 14]. The recent ATA guidelines state that FNAB is the procedure of choice in the evaluation of thyroid nodules [9].

Despite its effectiveness and diagnostic accuracy, the nondiagnostic smear (approximately 15% of all specimens) remains a management dilemma. Although criteria to consider a specimen "adequate" vary among institutions, a commonly accepted definition for a diagnostic sample is one that includes six or more groups of 10–20 well-preserved follicular epithelial cells per group on at least two slides [13]. Inadequate sampling has been cited as the most common cause of false-negative biopsy results but repeat aspiration can augment the accuracy of the procedure [13].

Several studies have demonstrated that ultrasound guidance (UG FNA), compared with palpation guided FNAB, reduces the number of non-diagnostic aspirates thereby increasing its sensitivity and specificity [3, 6]. UG FNA may be necessary for non-palpable or very small thyroid nodules, but there are no studies to demonstrate that the routine use of ultrasonography guidance improves outcome in terms of overall diagnostic rate or long-term outcome from thyroid cancer.

Guidance upon classification of cytological aspirates is provided by the BTA and ATA as displayed in Table 13.2 [9, 10]. The action to be undertaken following cytological diagnosis of fine needle aspirates is also displayed. Cystic nodules that repeatedly yield non-diagnostic aspirates need close observation or surgical excision and if the nodule is solid surgery should be more strongly considered [9]. When cytology is benign but patients belong to a high clinical risk group (see Table 13.1) the decision to proceed to lobectomy may even be made with a benign FNAB diagnosis. This decision might also be made if there are pressure symptoms or rapid growth. In addition, the patient should have the choice to have the lesion removed if they so wish [10]. Indeterminate cytology can be found in 15–30% of FNA specimens. While certain clinical features such as gender or nodule size [15] or cytological features such as presence of atypia [16] can improve the diagnostic accuracy in patients with indeterminate cytology, overall predictive values remain low. Although many molecular markers have been evaluated in the hope of improving diagnostic accuracy for indeterminate specimens, at present none is recommended, because of insufficient data [9].

ATA guidelines state that diagnostic ultrasound should be performed in those patients presenting with multiple thyroid nodules as sonographic characteristics are superior to nodule size in identifying malignancy [9]. It is recommended that aspiration should be performed in the presence of two or more thyroid

Table 13.2 Cytological classification of fine needle aspirates according to BTA and ATA guidance. The action required following cytological diagnosis is also displayed [9, 10]

Type of lesion	BTA diagnostic category	ATA diagnostic category	Required action
Any inadequate specimen	Thy1 non-diagnostic	Non-diagnostic aspirate	Repeat FNAC US-guided FNAB if required Close observation Consider surgery if solid lesion
Nodular goiter or thyroiditis	Thy2 non-neoplastic	Benign cytology	Repeat aspirate after 3–6 months No further diagnostic tests required
Follicular lesions	Thy3 follicular lesions	Indeterminate cytology	Lobectomy or total thyroidectomy Discussion between surgeon and endocrinologist required
Suspicious but not diagnostic of thyroid carcinoma	Thy4 suspicious of malignancy	Indeterminate cytology	Surgical intervention for differentiated tumor Further investigation for anaplastic carcinoma, lymphoma, metastatic tumor
Thyroid carcinoma	Thy5 diagnostic of malignancy	Aspirates diagnostic of malignancy	Surgical intervention for differentiated tumor Further investigation, radiotherapy or chemotherapy for anaplastic carcinoma, lymphoma, metastatic tumor

US, ultrasound.

nodules larger than 1–1.5 cm or suspicious sonographic features. If none of the nodules has a suspicious appearance, the likelihood of malignancy is low and it is reasonable to aspirate the largest nodule(s) only [9].

Micronodules and microcarcinomas

The advent of high-resolution ultrasonography has led to the increasingly frequent discovery of small, asymptomatic and previously unrecognized thyroid nodules. These thyroid incidentalomas are usually smaller that 1.5 cm and are often diagnosed during ultrasonographic evaluation for non-diagnostic neck disorders, posing a management dilemma for the clinician [9, 13]. A recent consensus statement by the Society of Radiologists in Ultrasound on the management of thyroid nodules detected at sonography states that highly suspicious ultrasonographic features such as microcalcifications should prompt a biopsy in nodules 1 cm or larger, other suspicious features such as solid consistency should prompt biopsy at 1.5 cm or larger, while less suspicious appearances such as mixed solid and cystic consistency should be considered for biopsy only if nodules measure 2 cm or larger [17]. These guidelines remain controversial with endocrinologists as it has been reported that patients undergoing surgery for papillary cancers <1.5 cm in size have been found to have distant metastases [18]. Others recommend simple observation for nodules smaller than 1 cm, in the absence of sonographic features of malignancy, and FNAB for larger incidentalomas and those with features suspicious of malignancy [13].

Papillary microcarcinomas are being increasingly diagnosed at earlier stages because of the more widespread use of high-resolution ultrasonography. Most of these subclinical cancers would never become clinically apparent and some studies have shown that in the majority of patients these lesions do not change in size during follow-up [13]. However, others have shown nodal or distant metastasis in patients who underwent thyroidectomy with prophylactic node dissection for papillary microcarcinoma [13].

The management of these incidentalomas remains controversial and clinical as well as sonographic follow-up is generally recommended. FNAB should be performed in rapidly enlarging lesions, as well as in those which exhibit suspicious sonographic features [3, 13].

Follow-up of patients with thyroid enlargement

Thyroid nodules diagnosed cytologically as benign require follow-up because of the finite rate of false-negative aspirates of up to 5% [9, 10]. Easily palpable nodules do not require sonographic monitoring but patients should be followed clinically at 6–18 month intervals. It is recommended by the ATA [9] that all other nodules be followed with serial ultrasound examinations 6–18 months after the initial FNAB. Benign nodules and those revealing inadequate specimens should be re-aspirated after 3–6 months.

If there is evidence for nodule growth, either by palpation or sonographically, repeat FNAB is recommended, possibly under ultrasound guidance [9].

Prediction of thyroid malignancy

Because improvements in imaging modalities have led to increased detection of thyroid nodules, some of which turn out to be microcarcinomas of unclear clinical significance, it is pertinent to establish criteria that select and limit the number of invasive procedures. "Considering the anxiety, costs and potential complications suffered by patients, it is clear that we not only need guidelines that select nodules for further evaluation, but also need tools that allow us to predict which thyroid cancers will remain indolent and which thyroid cancers will become aggressive" [19].

As detailed earlier there are a number of well-established predictors of thyroid malignancy detected by clinical evaluation (Table 13.1). Furthermore, some ultrasonographic characteristics (see earlier) have been shown to reduce the number of thyroid nodules requiring FNAB [19]. We have recently investigated whether a number of clinical and biochemical parameters can predict the likelihood of thyroid malignancy in a consecutive series of 1500 subjects undergoing FNAB [20]. All patients (1304 females and 196 males, mean age 47.8 years) presenting to our center with palpable thyroid enlargement and without overt thyroid dysfunction between 1984 and 2002 were evaluated by FNAB of the thyroid. Patients' demographic details were recorded and goiter type was assessed clinically and classified as diffuse in 183, multinodular in 456 or clinically solitary nodule in 861 cases. Serum TSH concentration at presentation was measured in a sensitive assay in patients presenting after 1988 ($n = 1183$). The final cytological or histological diagnosis was determined after surgery ($n = 553$) or a minimum 2-year clinical follow-up period (mean 9.5 years, range 2–18 years). Serum TSH concentration at presentation was measured in a sensitive assay in patients presenting after 1988 ($n = 1183$) [20].

The overall sensitivity and specificity of FNAB in predicting malignancy in this study were 88% and 84% respectively. In accordance with previous studies (see earlier), male subjects ($n = 196$) presenting with thyroid enlargement had significantly higher rates of malignancy (12.2%) when compared with female patients ($n = 1304$, 7.4%, $p = 0.02$). Significant increases in the prevalence of malignancy ($p = 0.005$) were detected in patients who were aged less than 30 years and in those older than 80 years at presentation. Furthermore, when the goiter type determined clinically at presentation was analyzed, we found the highest rates of malignancy in subjects presenting with a solitary nodule ($n = 861$, 10.8%) compared with those who presented with a diffuse or nodular goiter ($n = 639$, 4.2%, $p < 0.001$). Subsequent binary logistic regression analysis detected significantly increased adjusted odds ratios (AOR) for malignancy in male patients (AOR 1.8, 95%CI 1.04–3.1, $p = 0.04$), those of younger age (AOR 1.1, 95%CI 1.01–1.15,

$p = 0.025$) and those presenting with clinically solitary lesions (AOR 2.53, 95%CI 1.5–4.28, $p = 0.001$) [20].

Interestingly this study also demonstrated, for the first time, that the serum TSH concentration at presentation is an independent predictor of thyroid malignancy. 1183 patients had their serum TSH concentration at presentation measured. The prevalence of malignancy ($n = 182$, 2.8%) was lowest in subjects with serum TSH below the normal range (<0.4 mU/L). Compared with subjects with below normal serum TSH, higher rates of malignancy (3.7%, $p = $ NS) were present in those with serum TSH in the lower tertile of the normal range, i.e., 0.4–0.9 mU/L ($n = 322$). Even higher rates were found in patients with serum TSH 1.0–1.7 mU/L ($n = 336$, 8.3%, $p = 0.02$), compared with TSH <0.4 mU/L, rising to 12.3% ($p = 0.001$ compared with low TSH) for those with serum TSH 1.8–5.5 mU/L (i.e., the highest tertile of the normal range, $n = 316$). The highest prevalences of malignancy (29.6%, $p < 0.001$ compared with low TSH) were evident in those with subclinical hypothyroidism and serum TSH above the normal range (>5.5 mU/L, $n = 27$) [20]. Binary logistic regression analysis simultaneously analyzing gender, age, goiter type and TSH concentration confirmed significantly increased odds ratios for malignancy in males, in those of younger age, in those with solitary nodules and in those with serum TSH >0.9 mU/L.

It is well documented that TSH has a trophic effect on thyroid cancer growth, which is most likely mediated by TSH receptors on tumor cells and furthermore that TSH suppression is an independent predictor of relapse-free survival from differentiated thyroid cancer. We propose that the risk increase associated with serum TSH concentrations in the upper half of the normal range, and even more strikingly in those whose TSH measurements were above normal, may at least in part be mediated by this trophic effect of TSH. An alternative explanation is that patients with lower TSH concentrations were developing autonomous function which is itself associated with lower rates of malignancy [20]. Based on our findings, we propose that simple clinical and biochemical factors can serve as an adjunct to FNAB in predicting risk of thyroid malignancy.

Conclusion

Thyroid nodules and goiters are common clinical entities but only a minority of these will harbor a thyroid carcinoma. Following clinical examination all patients should have their serum TSH measured. Thyroid ultrasound is increasingly used in the assessment of thyroid neoplasia but remains inferior to FNAB in the specific detection of thyroid cancer. When thyroid malignancy is excluded, patients with thyroid nodules require further follow-up and repeat fine needle aspiration biopsy 3–6 months after the initial FNAB is recommended for benign nodules. Several clinical, biochemical and sonographic criteria can serve as an adjunct to cytological diagnosis in the prediction of thyroid malignancy and can help in the identification of patient groups that require earlier surgical referral or more regular follow-up.

References

1. Vander JB, Gaston EA, Dawber TR. The significance of nontoxic thyroid nodules. Final report of a 15-year study of the incidence of thyroid malignancy. *Ann. Intern. Med.* 1968;69:537–540.
2. Tunbridge WM, Evered DC, Hall R, et al. The spectrum of thyroid disease in a community: the Whickham survey. *Clin. Endocrinol. (Oxf.)* 1977;7:481–493.
3. Hegedus L, Bonnema SJ, Bennedbaek FN. Management of simple nodular goiter: current status and future perspectives. *Endocr. Rev.* 2003;24:102–132.
4. Sherman SI. Thyroid carcinoma. *Lancet* 2003;361:501–511.
5. Schneider AB, Ron E. Carcinoma of the follicular epithelium: epidemiology and pathogenesis. In: Braverman LE, Utiger RD (eds). *The Thyroid: A Fundamental and Clinical Text*, 9th edn. Philadelphia, PA: Lippincott, Williams & Wilkins, 2005;889–906.
6. Hegedus L. Clinical practice. The thyroid nodule. *N. Engl. J. Med.* 2004;351:1764–1771.
7. Bennedbaek FN, Perrild H, Hegedus L. Diagnosis and treatment of the solitary thyroid nodule. Results of a European survey. *Clin. Endocrinol. (Oxf.)* 1999;50:357–363.
8. Bennedbaek FN, Hegedus L. Management of the solitary thyroid nodule: results of a North American survey. *J. Clin. Endocrinol. Metab.* 2000;85:2493–2498.
9. Cooper DS, Doherty GM, Haugen BR, et al. Management guidelines for patients with thyroid nodules and differentiated thyroid cancer. *Thyroid* 2006;16:1–33.
10. British Thyroid Association and Royal College of Physicians 2002 Guidelines for the management of thyroid cancer in adults. www.british-thyroid-association.org.
11. Hegedus L. Thyroid ultrasound. *Endocrinol. Metab. Clin. North Am.* 2001;30:339–360.
12. Gittoes NJ, Miller MR, Daykin J, Sheppard MC, Franklyn JA. Upper airways obstruction in 153 consecutive patients presenting with thyroid enlargement. *Br. Med. J.* 1996;312:484.
13. Castro MR, Gharib H. Continuing controversies in the management of thyroid nodules. *Ann. Intern. Med.* 2005;142:926–931.
14. Gharib H, Goellner JR. Fine-needle aspiration biopsy of the thyroid: an appraisal. *Ann. Intern. Med.* 1993;118:282–289.
15. Tuttle RM, Lemar H, Burch HB. Clinical features associated with an increased risk of thyroid malignancy in patients with follicular neoplasia by fine-needle aspiration. *Thyroid* 1998;8:377–383.
16. Kelman AS, Rathan A, Leibowitz J, et al. Thyroid cytology and the risk of malignancy in thyroid nodules: importance of nuclear atypia in indeterminate specimens. *Thyroid* 2001;11:271–277.
17. Frates MC, Benson CB, Charboneau JW, et al. Management of thyroid nodules detected at US: Society of Radiologists in Ultrasound consensus conference statement. *Radiology* 2005;237:794–800.
18. Baskin HJ, Duick DS. The endocrinologists' view of ultrasound guidelines for fine needle aspiration. *Thyroid* 2006; 16:207–208.
19. Ross DS. Predicting thyroid malignancy. *J. Clin. Endocrinol. Metab.* 2006;91:4253–4255.
20. Boelaert K, Horacek J, Holder RL, et al. Serum thyrotropin concentration as a novel predictor of malignancy in thyroid nodules investigated by fine-needle aspiration. *J. Clin. Endocrinol. Metab.* 2006; 91:4295–4301.

14 Thyroid and Parathyroid Imaging

Conor J. Heaney and Gregory A. Wiseman

> **Key points**
> - Ultrasound is the preferred imaging modality in the evaluation of nodular thyroid disease, and facilitates diagnostic fine needle aspiration biopsy.
> - Ultrasound is highly sensitive in detecting postoperative locoregional recurrence of differentiated thyroid carcinoma.
> - Radioiodine is used primarily in the diagnosis of distant metastatic disease in thyroid cancer patients with suspected recurrence.
> - F-18 fluorodeoxyglucose positron emission tomography/computerized tomography and computerized tomography alone can be employed in the staging and restaging of metastatic thyroid cancers that are not iodine-avid.
> - Tc-99m sestamibi parathyroid imaging can localize parathyroid adenomas and help direct surgical resection.

Introduction

Nuclear medicine traditionally has been the principal imaging modality utilized in examination of the thyroid gland. Over the past several decades, however, advances in ultrasound technology have added this very powerful tool, which complements and soon may supersede the role of nuclear medicine in the diagnosis and follow-up of thyroid carcinoma. Initial evaluation and biopsy of the suspicious thyroid nodule may be accurately performed at ultrasound. Ultrasound is also highly sensitive at detecting both local and regional thyroid carcinoma recurrences. Radioiodine imaging is used routinely in the evaluation of distant metastasis in differentiated thyroid carcinoma, whereas computerized tomography (CT) is used in staging locally aggressive malignant thyroid disease and in evaluation of metastatic disease. F-18 fluoro-deoxyglucose (FDG) positron emission tomography (PET)/CT is a newer imaging technique used primarily in evaluation of non-iodine avid metastatic differentiated carcinoma, metastatic medullary thyroid cancer and in staging or follow-up evaluation of anaplastic thyroid carcinoma. [111]In octreotride (somatostatin peptide analog) imaging can also be used for staging radioiodine-negative metastatic thyroid carcinoma or for medullary thyroid carcinoma. Advances in magnetic resonance imaging (MRI), to date, have not yet had a significant impact on the routine management of patients with thyroid diseases, but may occasionally be useful in selected patients.

Clinical Endocrine Oncology, 2nd edition. Edited by Ian D. Hay and John A.H. Wass. © 2008 Blackwell Publishing. ISBN 978-1-4051-4584-8.

Thyroid ultrasound

A thorough ultrasound examination is routinely used for initial thyroid nodule evaluation. The superficial nature of the thyroid lends itself to an exquisite ultrasound examination. A high frequency (8–15 MHz) linear probe is routinely used at our institution which provides optimal spatial resolution. The gland is imaged both transaxially and sagittally. The normal thyroid gland is homogeneous in echotexture. A full examination of the anterior cervical lymph nodes should be performed at the time of thyroid ultrasound. The summary of the ultrasound data can be converted into a graphic "thyroid map" (Fig. 14.1). This is helpful for the

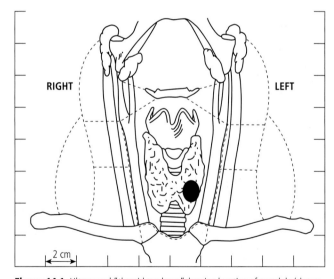

Figure 14.1 Ultrasound "thyroid roadmap" showing location of a nodule (shown here in the left lower lobe) can be helpful in communication with clinicians and in follow up.

clinician as a quick summary of thyroid anatomy, and is also useful when performing follow-up examination.

Approximately 5% of individuals have a palpable thyroid nodule and up to 50% may have a sonographically apparent nodule. The incidence of thyroid carcinoma has been shown to be independent of nodule size and equivalent in the multinodular gland or the solitary thyroid nodule. In addition, carcinoma in the multinodular gland may be present in a non-dominant nodule approximately one-third of the time. The overall incidence of carcinoma in thyroid nodules that are subsequently biopsied approximates 10%, but is dependent on the character of the nodules and the population selected for biopsy [1,2].

A nodule that is entirely cystic has a negligible malignancy risk, and may be assumed to be benign [1]. The vast majority of such nodules prove to be colloid cysts. It is not unusual for these to have some internal hyperechoic foci with comet tail artifacts due to acoustic reverberation (Fig. 14.2). It is presumed that these are due to condensed colloid material within the cyst. These should not be confused with the fine microcalcifications in a thyroid carcinoma which do not have comet tail artifact. The predominantly cystic thyroid nodule (>70% cystic component) has a very low incidence of malignancy (less than 1%). Care must be taken, however, to fully interrogate a cystic thyroid lesion for any additional more ominous signs of malignancy, including thickened nodular wall (Fig. 14.3) with microcalcifications or marked hypervascularity.

Many ultrasound features have been used to characterize the solid thyroid nodule including echogenicity, microcalcifications, irregular margins, incomplete or absent halo, and intranodular vascularity [1]. Although many of these may be more characteristic of malignancy, no single characteristic has a sufficient predictive value to permit discrimination between the benign and malignant solid nodule. Bright echogenic foci within a solid nodule con-

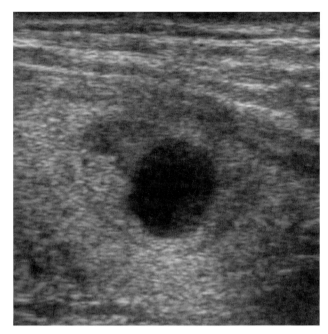

Figure 14.3 A cystic papillary carcinoma is seen on ultrasound with a thickened wall about the central cyst.

sistent with microcalcifications are the most specific feature for malignancy (specificity 85–95%) but have a lower sensitivity. Most thyroid carcinomas are hypoechoic, but the majority of benign nodules are, in fact, also hypoechoic. The combination of individual findings can increase the positive predictive value. Together, a hypoechoic solid nodule with microcalcifications has a positive predictive value of approximately 70%. Nodules which have irregular margins, incomplete or no halo and have significant internal vascularity also have a higher incidence of malignancy. Some ultrasound features are more characteristic of carcinoma subtypes. These features are clearly somewhat academic, as pathology verification by FNA biopsy is necessary to make an accurate cytological diagnosis.

Papillary thyroid carcinoma

Papillary thyroid carcinoma (PTC) is the most common thyroid malignancy. The classic PTC is solid, hypoechoic and may have multiple tiny microcalcifications (Fig. 14.4). The presence of cystic cervical adenopathy or lymph nodes containing microcalcifications is usually diagnostic for metastatic PTC (Fig. 14.5).

Medullary carcinoma

A solid nodule with coarse central shadowing calcifications, although not pathognomonic, is typical of medullary carcinoma (Fig. 14.6). This is non-specific. In fact, because papillary cancer is much more common, this finding is associated most often with papillary cancer.

Follicular adenoma/carcinoma

Follicular thyroid disease is classically an egg-shaped, homogeneously hypoechoic large nodule (Fig. 14.7). This appearance has

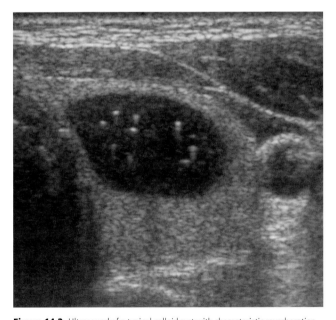

Figure 14.2 Ultrasound of a typical colloid cyst with characteristic reverberation artifacts.

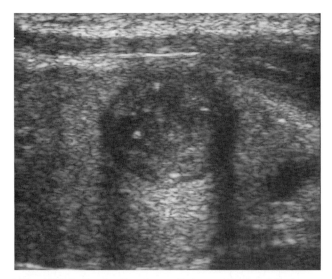

Figure 14.4 Papillary thyroid carcinoma with characteristic microcalcifications.

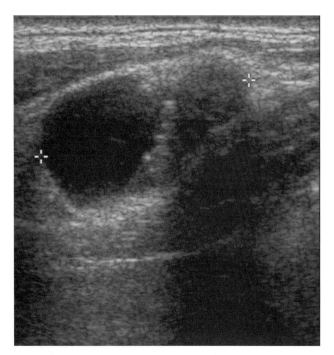

Figure 14.5 Cystic papillary thyroid metastasis to cervical lymph nodes.

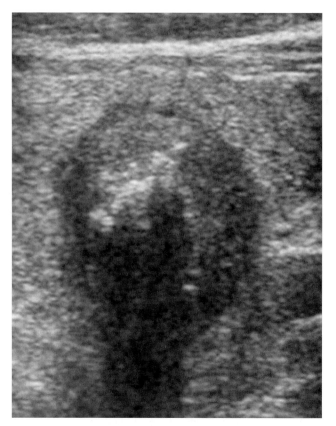

Figure 14.6 Typical appearance of medullary thyroid carcinoma with characteristic coarse central shadowing calcifications.

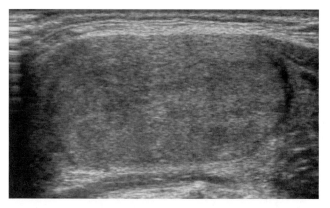

Figure 14.7 Typical egg-shaped appearance of a follicular thyroid neoplasm. Surgical excision is necessary to evaluate for histological evidence of capsular or vascular invasion to differentiate malignant follicular carcinoma from benign follicular adenoma.

been coined the "testicle in the thyroid." In the vast majority of cases these are benign follicular adenomas. The differentiation of follicular adenoma from follicular carcinoma, however, is not possible by thyroid ultrasound or by fine needle aspiration. A surgical excision is necessary to exclude microcapsular invasion.

Anaplastic carcinoma

This rare cancer can have an aggressive ultrasound appearance. It may be very heterogeneous with internal acoustic shadowing.

Thyroid nodule evaluation for malignancy

The fine needle aspirate (FNA) has become standard practice in the evaluation of the "suspicious" thyroid nodule. The near ubiquitous use of FNA has resulted in a decrease in the number of negative surgical excisions. Its use has been associated with an increase in the number of patients being diagnosed with thyroid carcinoma. FNA is very safe when performed by a skilled operator. Ultrasound guidance has been shown to increase the diagnostic yield at FNA. This is particularly true in the case of the complex cystic nodules, where the needle may be directed toward the solid portion. Even in centers performing a large number of thyroid aspirates the non-diagnostic rate approaches 20%. Repeat FNA is indicated with or without core biopsy. The incidence of carcinoma in the non-diagnostic aspirate approaches 10%.

There is significant discussion on which thyroid nodules warrant a biopsy. Some authors contend that the slow growth of most papillary carcinomas and the excellent prognosis in most cases suggests a less aggressive strategy of thyroid intervention. Indeed, with the incidence of sonographically apparent thyroid nodules approaching 50% in the general population and a non-diagnostic aspirate rate of 20%, the indiscriminate FNA of every thyroid nodule would result in a significant thyroidectomy rate for negative disease with significant associated cost and operative morbidity. Several groups have published consensus statements on the appropriate use of FNA in evaluation of the indeterminate thyroid nodule and many of these statements support using a cut-off of 1–1.5 cm for FNA of solid thyroid nodules. Biopsy is recommended for smaller nodules with concerning ultrasound features such as microcalcifications. "Significant" interval growth is concerning and warrants further investigation, though the exact interpretation of "significant" is debated. In the multinodular gland, the dominant nodule may be biopsied and any additional nodules with concerning ultrasound features. Entirely cystic lesions with typical features of a colloid cyst do not warrant biopsy. Predominantly cystic nodules are likely benign but biopsies may be directed to concerning solid portions. For more detail and recommendations concerning management of thyroid nodules reference should be made to the consensus papers [2, 3].

Thyroid scintigraphy

Thyroid scintigraphy relies on differentiating the metabolically active or "hot" nodule from the metabolically inactive or "cold" nodule. Hot nodules are for all practical purposes benign. The "cold" nodule is indeterminate and malignancy must be excluded. The examination previously was used to select patients to biopsy for possible malignancy, but with the use of ultrasound and FNA, it is most appropriately used today in patients who are clinically hyperthyroid, and possibly harbor an autonomous toxic nodule.

There are several nuclear thyroid imaging agents that may be utilized and these are summarized in Table 14.1.

Iodine-131

Radioiodine is taken up by thyroid tissue in a manner identical to normal circulating iodine. Uptake is controlled principally by serum thyroid-stimulating hormone (TSH) levels, which are a function of circulating thyroid hormone, iodine stores and circulating serum iodine levels. Once taken up, the iodine is organified and stored as

Table 14.1 Nuclear thyroid imaging agents

Radionuclide	Energy (keV)	$T_{1/2}$	Emission	Use
TcO4	140	6 h	γ	Diagnosis
^{123}I	159	13 h	γ	Diagnosis
^{131}I	364	8 days	γ and β	Diagnosis and therapy
^{124}I	511	4 days	Positron	Diagnosis

thyroglobulin. ^{131}I has been used for many years for imaging and therapy with its favorable emission spectrum consisting of a high-energy γ emission and a low-energy β emission. This emission spectrum is critical to its dual role as diagnostic and therapeutic agent. Its high-energy γ emission, although far from being ideal, allows for diagnostic imaging. (Newer γ cameras are manufactured with thinner crystals for maximizing spatial resolution. These cameras are insensitive to the higher energy photons emitted by ^{131}I.) The relatively long half-life, however, results in higher radiation doses to the thyroid and the rest of the body, limiting the amount of ^{131}I that can be used for diagnostic purposes. It is generally imaged at 48 h to maximize thyroid tissue sensitivity and decrease background. ^{131}I β emission is ideal as a therapeutic agent in thyroid ablation and treatment of metastatic thyroid carcinoma. These low-energy β particles travel only a short distance (approximately 1 mm) and release all their energy into the tissue. The long half-life of ^{131}I makes the radionuclide easy to store and it can be shipped to many departments even in larger doses. Oral administration is generally preferred with excellent absorption.

Tc-99m pertechnetate

The use of ^{131}I as a diagnostic agent for benign thyroid diseases almost disappeared when technetium pertechnetate was introduced. Pertechnetate is taken up in the thyroid gland, but unlike radioiodine, it is not organified. Therefore, an adenoma can be mistaken for a non-functioning nodule. It is easily manufactured from a molybdenum column, a mainstay in the modern nuclear medicine laboratory. Photon energy of 140 keV makes it ideal for imaging on modern γ cameras. Its uptake and half-life allow for same-day imaging. Unlike radioiodine, it is generally given intravenously, which is somewhat more invasive. It has the disadvantage of moderate background activity. The use of Tc-99m pertechnetate for thyroid nodule evaluation is complicated by the fact that a small minority of nodules will have discordant uptake of Tc-99m pertechnetate compared to radioiodine and may result in misdiagnosis. In addition, no reasonable assessment of overall thyroid activity may be made with Tc-99m pertechnetate.

Iodine-123

^{123}I has far superior imaging characteristics than ^{131}I. Where available, it is generally the preferred thyroid imaging agent. However, the practicalities of its use are complicated by cost and availability. The cyclotron manufacture and the relative short half-life of 13 h require the purchase of unit doses ahead of time, unless there is a cyclotron facility available on site. Generally, it is imaged at 4 h but 24 h images can be obtained and thyroid iodine uptake can be performed. ^{123}I is very useful in quantification of uptake in both the thyroid bed and in metastatic disease to determine stability or change over the interval. Quantification can be useful in ^{131}I administered activity calculation for therapy, such as with extensive lung metastasis.

Iodine-124

Newer thyroid agents include the positron-emitting ^{124}I, which is cyclotron produced. This may be used in PET imaging of the thyroid and in iodine-avid metastasis but remains investigational.

Regardless of the radionuclide used, planar, frontal and oblique views of the thyroid are typically acquired. Pinhole collimation for magnification is preferred. Single photon emission computed tomography (SPECT) acquisition provides data that can be presented in axial, sagittal or coronal slices. SPECT imaging increases the sensitivity of detection for smaller foci of tracer localization. Newer γ cameras have additional CT capabilities for SPECT/CT fusion which may be helpful for further anatomic localization.

A detailed physical thyroid examination should be performed at the time of thyroid imaging to correlate with the scintigraphic findings. It is important to ensure that the palpable nodule correlates with the area of normal/increased ("hot") or decreased ("cold") tracer uptake. Nuclear scintigraphy lends itself best to larger thyroid nodules. It is helpful in the diagnosis of the multinodular gland; however, the resolution of specific nodules within a multinodular gland is suboptimal. It is most useful in the diagnosis of the autonomous functioning thyroid adenoma, where the remainder of the gland is suppressed and the quantification of radioiodine uptake can be useful.

Only a small minority of thyroid nodules are "hot" (approaching 10%). Additional work-up therefore is indicated in a significant majority of cases that are referred to the nuclear lab. It is for these reasons that many find the initial evaluation of the thyroid nodule by nuclear scintigraphy to be incomplete. The role of nuclear medicine in the initial work-up the thyroid nodule has essentially been replaced by high-frequency ultrasound.

Use of imaging for postoperative surveillance in thyroid carcinoma

The majority of thyroid cancer recurrences are in the thyroid bed or in regional lymph nodes within the neck. Ultrasound may be used for routine surveillance of the postoperative thyroid bed and is highly sensitive (95%) for recurrent regional disease. Ultrasound is, however, unsuited for the detection of metastatic disease outside the neck.

In postoperative patients with thyroid cancer suspected of harboring recurrent disease, a whole-body diagnostic radioiodine scan may be usefully performed. Low-dose ^{131}I may be used for this purpose, but the image quality is suboptimal, and there is

theoretical risk for "stunning" of iodine-avid disease, which may decrease the potency of a subsequent treatment dose of ^{131}I. For these reasons, many institutions treat recurrence presumptively with high-dose ^{131}I and obtain thereafter a posttreatment scan for diagnostic purposes. If available, ^{123}I is preferred for the diagnostic scan, as it does not have the same "stunning" properties, since it lacks the low-energy β emission (Fig. 14.8). If diagnostic examinations with either ^{123}I or ^{131}I are performed, and radioiodine treatment is subsequently administered, the patient should be followed with a postablation scan at 1 week, again using the treatment dose as imaging agent, as this is considered to be more sensitive for iodine-avid metastatic disease.

A large dose of non-radioactive iodine can shut down thyroid uptake (trapping of iodine) for several weeks. A common cause is the iodinated agent from a contrast-enhanced CT scan. In a patient on thyroid replacement therapy, thyroid hormone should be held prior to the study as it suppresses the serum TSH. Thyroxine (T_4) replacement medication should be held for 6 weeks, by switching to Cytomel® (T_3) for 4 weeks, and the patient should be off all replacement for 2 weeks prior to radioiodine administration for imaging. Alternatively, thyroid uptake may be stimulated using recombinant human TSH (Thyrogen®) without taking the patient off thyroid replacement. At our institution, the protocol comprises day 1 rhTSH injection, day 2 second rhTSH, day 3 I-123 radioiodine oral administration (111–185 MBq NaI) and day 4 whole-body imaging. This rhTSH technique permits adequate radioiodine uptake without the symptoms associated with T_4 withdrawal. The use of ^{123}I allows for better resolution than ^{131}I, a lower absorbed radiation dose, a lack of thyroid tumor "stunning" by the diagnostic radioiodine and permits tomographic imaging.

Currently, the use of F-18 FDG PET with CT fusion in the evaluation of differentiated thyroid carcinoma is debated. The sensitivity of F-18 FDG PET-CT for the detection of thyroid carcinoma is approximately 50%. It has been shown that incidental focal F-18 FDG uptake in the thyroid (Plate 14.1) carries a risk of malignancy of approximately 35 % [4]. It has been argued that F-18 FDG PET may be useful in non-diagnostic fine needle aspirates. Metastatic differentiated thyroid carcinoma demonstrates highly variable F-18 FDG uptake and metabolism. F-18 FDG PET/CT has been very successful in detecting metastasis in differentiated carcinomas with biochemical recurrence (increased serum thyroglobulin) and negative radioiodine diagnostic whole-body scan [5]. The combination of radioiodine scan and F-18 FDG PET/CT study [6] has a high sensitivity of 89% and a specificity close to 90% (Plate 14.2). F-18 FDG PET/CT has been shown to change management in 44% of patients with differentiated thyroid cancer being evaluated for recurrent disease [7].

In non-iodine avid metastatic disease CT scanning has been the main imaging modality utilized. CT is highly sensitive (70%) in detecting metastasis. F-18 FDG PET/CT has increased specificity, compared to CT alone, in detection of metastasis. ^{111}In Octreoscan® imaging has been used for imaging papillary, follicular and medullary thyroid carcinoma [8,9] to determine if somatostatin receptors are present, thereby indicating possible benefit from somatostatin analog therapy (Plate 14.3). [123]I MIBG imaging has also been used for imaging metastatic medullary thyroid carcinoma.

Parathyroid imaging

The parathyroid glands consist of four pea-shaped glands, two on the left and two on the right. The upper glands are generally located posterior to the upper lobe of the thyroid bilaterally. The lower glands are more variable and may be located anywhere from the posterior thyroid to the mediastinum. Approximately 80% of cases of hyperparathyroidism are caused by a parathyroid adenoma, which is solitary in the vast majority of cases. Parathyroid hyperplasia is a cause of hyperparathyroidism in the other 20% of cases. Rarely, parathyroid carcinoma may be the cause of hyperparathyroidism. The success of the experienced neck surgeon in locating a parathyroid adenoma approximates 95% without preoperative imaging. Preoperative localization of parathyroid adenomas has been shown to decrease postoperative morbidity and actual time spent during surgery. With preoperative localization, a smaller, more directed, surgery can be performed as an outpatient, as opposed to more extensive bilateral neck dissections. Nuclear scintigraphy is routinely used in the work-up of the parathyroid adenoma. Ultrasound can be used in a complementary fashion to the nuclear examination, but is generally limited to parathyroid adenomas in or just posterior to the thyroid.

Modern nuclear imaging of the parathyroid may be performed using a dual-phase technetium sestamibi or dual-agent sestamibi and radioiodine technique. Parathyroid adenomas have been shown to have a slow washout of sestamibi. Normal thyroid will take up sestamibi and will have a more rapid washout. Most institutions utilize the dual-phase examination with early and delayed sestamibi images to detect parathyroid adenoma. These examinations are generally performed with frontal and oblique planar views. Pinhole collimation for magnification is preferred. Imaging through the mediastinum is necessary to exclude ectopic adenomas. SPECT imaging has been shown to increase the sensitivity for adenoma detection by approximately 20%.

The Tc-99m sestamibi/^{123}I dual-agent examination allows simultaneous acquisition of ^{123}I and sestamibi with precise subtraction data. Dual-agent SPECT is also performed through the mediastinum. There is some overlap of sestamibi and iodine emission spectra, and the acquisition windows are narrowed and offset to decrease [123]I (photopeak energy 159 keV) scatter into the Tc-99m (photopeak energy 140 keV) window. [123]I is given orally 2–24 h prior to imaging. Imaging is performed immediately after injection of sestamibi. The sestamibi and iodine are imaged simultaneously. [123]I is taken up by the normal thyroid tissue but not the parathyroid adenoma. Sestamibi is taken up by the normal thyroid and the parathyroid adenoma. A parathyroid adenoma appears as a focus of tracer on the subtracted images with the ^{123}I image subtracted from the Tc-99m sestamibi image (Fig. 14.9). The Tc-99m sestamibi is localized by the thyroid and parathyroid cells with the ^{123}I being taken up only by the thyroid cells. The

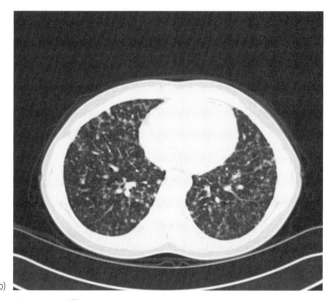

(a)

(b)

Figure 14.8 ^{123}I whole-body scan (a) and CT scan (b) of the same patient with diffuse pulmonary metastasis from papillary thyroid carcinoma.

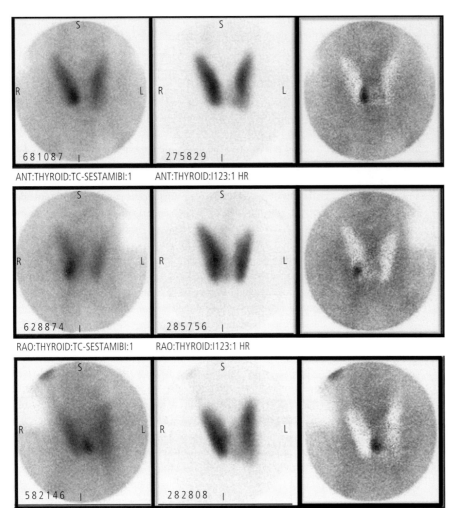

ANT:THYROID:TC-SESTAMIBI:1   ANT:THYROID:I123:1 HR

RAO:THYROID:TC-SESTAMIBI:1   RAO:THYROID:I123:1 HR

Figure 14.9 Parathyroid adenoma demonstrated posterior to the left lower pole of the thyroid on simultaneous acquisition of sestamibi and ^{123}I with subtraction.

subtracted image tracer is generally localized to the abnormal parathyroid tissue. A false-positive finding of Tc-99m sestamibi without ^{123}I uptake (positive on subtraction images) can be seen with hypofunctioning thyroid nodules, in a multinodular thyroid with variable iodine uptake, and in thyroid, parathyroid or metastatic tumors that localize Tc-99m sestamibi but do not have ^{123}I uptake.

At our institution, we have found this examination to have a sensitivity for parathyroid adenomas of approximately 90% and a similar specificity of 90% [10]. Patients who have elevated parathyroid hormone due to a single abnormal parathyroid gland on a preoperative Tc-99m sestamibi/^{123}I uptake scan can undergo a very limited cervical exploration without intraoperative PTH monitoring. In patients undergoing the focused surgery, 97% had normal serum calcium following recovery from surgery [11]. The sensitivity of Tc-99m sestamibi with ^{123}I iodine subtraction is lower in secondary or tertiary hyperparathyroidism, as compared to primary [12]. Most patients had at least one or two hyperplastic glands identified, but not always three or four.

Ultrasound has been used as a complementary examination to nuclear scintigraphy, when using a high-frequency probe (10–15 MHz) and using a technique similar to thyroid ultrasound. The parathyroid adenoma will appear as a homogeneous hypervascular mass posterior to the thyroid (Plate 14.4). It is important to discriminate the parathyroid from a thyroid nodule. Using real-time sonography, by applying slight pressure with the examining probe, the thyroid gland may be seen moving over the parathyroid adenoma. Ultrasound has proven to be quite insensitive for identifying ectopic glands.

References

1. Reading CC, Charboneau JW, Hay ID, Sebo TJ. Sonography of thyroid nodules: a "classic pattern" diagnostic approach. *Ultrasound Q.* 2005;21:157–165.

2. Cooper DS, Doherty GM, Haugen BR, et al. Management guidelines for patients with thyroid nodules and differentiated thyroid cancer. *Thyroid* 2006;16:109–142.

3. Frates MC, Benson CB, Charboneau JW, et al. Management of thyroid nodules detected at US: Society of Radiologists in Ultrasound Consensus Conference statement. *Radiology* 2005;237:794–800.

4. Bogsrud TV, Karantanis D, Nathan MA, et al. The value of quantifying 18F-FDG uptake in thyroid nodules found incidentally on whole-body PET-CT. *Nucl. Med. Commun.* 2007;28:373–381.

5. Stokkel MP, Duchateau CS, Dragoiescu C. The value of FDG-PET in the follow-up of differentiated thyroid cancer: a review of the literature. *Q. J. Nucl. Med. Mol. Imaging* 2006;50:78–87.

6. Iagaru A, Kalinyak JE, McDougall IR. F-18 FDG PET/CT in the management of thyroid cancer. *Clin. Nucl. Med.* 2007;32:690–695.

7. Shammas A, Degirmenci B, Mountz JM, et al. 18F-FDG PET/CT in patients with suspected recurrent or metastatic well-differentiated thyroid cancer. *J. Nucl. Med.* 2007;48:221–226.

8. Stokkel MP, Reigman HI, Verkooijen RB, Smit JW. Indium-111-Octreotide scintigraphy in differentiated thyroid carcinoma metastases that do not respond to treatment with high-dose I-131. *J. Cancer Res. Clin. Oncol.* 2003;129:287–294.

9. Vainas I, Koussis C, Pazaitou-Panayiotou K, et al. Somatostatin receptor expression in vivo and response to somatostatin analog therapy with or without other antineoplastic treatments in advanced medullary thyroid carcinoma. *J. Exp. Clin. Cancer Res.* 2004;23:549–559.

10. Mullan BP. Nuclear medicine imaging of the parathyroid. *Otolaryngol. Clin. North Am.* 2004;37:909–939, xi–xii.

11. Jacobson SR, van Heerden JA, Farley DR, et al. Focused cervical exploration for primary hyperparathyroidism without intraoperative parathyroid hormone monitoring or use of the gamma probe. *World J. Surg.* 2004;28:1127–1131.

12. Pham TH, Sterioff S, Mullan BP, Wiseman GA, Sebo TJ, Grant CS. Sensitivity and utility of parathyroid scintigraphy in patients with primary versus secondary and tertiary hyperparathyroidism. *World J. Surg.* 2006;30:327–332.

15 Pathogenesis of Thyroid Cancer

Jan Zedenius and Theodoros Foukakis

Key points

- The majority of thyroid cancers occur sporadically, but inherited variants exist, in some of which the underlying genetic events are well characterized.
- Radiation exposure is the only well-established risk factor for thyroid carcinogenesis, and specific genetic changes, mainly chromosomal rearrangements, are seen in radiation-induced tumors.
- In papillary thyroid carcinoma, the illegitimate activation of the RET–Ras–Raf–MAPK pathway is evident in the majority of cases.
- Translocations involving peroxisome proliferator-activated receptor γ and *RAS*-activating point mutations are the most common genetic abnormalities described in follicular thyroid carcinoma.
- Activating point mutations of the *RET* proto-oncogene are seen in inherited as well as in some sporadic medullary thyroid carcinomas. Carriers of germ-line *RET* mutations are today usually offered a prophylactic thyroidectomy.
- Mutations in p53, β-catenin, *Ras*, B-Raf and PI3-kinase are often found in anaplastic thyroid carcinomas and in some differentiated carcinomas showing histological signs of de-differentiation or aggressive clinical course.

Pathogenesis of thyroid cancer

Introduction

The rapid advances in cancer research during the last decades have greatly increased our understanding of the pathogenesis of malignancy. It is now well established that cancer is a result of dynamic changes in the genome, whether somatic or inherited. The genes that are altered during the tumorigenic process are generally divided into oncogenes (altered by dominant gain of function mutations) and tumor suppressor genes (altered by recessive loss of function mutations) [1]. More recently the role of genes responsible for the stability of the genome, repair of DNA, formation of blood vessels, as well as the role of genes that promote or inhibit metastasis was recognized. The various genetic changes seen in different tumors essentially target the same regulatory circuits and provide the cancer cells with the same set of functional capabilities: self-sufficiency in growth signals, insensitivity to antigrowth signals, evasion of apoptosis, limitless replicative potential, sustained angiogenesis, and tissue invasion and metastasis [2].

The successive accumulation of genetic defects that ultimately lead to the malignant transformation and then to metastatic potential is sometimes expressed phenotypically, and a multistage evolution to cancer is seen at the cellular or histological level. However, the sequence of benign cell proliferation → dysplasia → malignant tumor → metastatic tumor is very rarely obvious and the pathogenic events in the majority of tumor types are apparently more complex, not necessarily following this simple progression pattern.

Thyroid tumors provide an excellent model for the study of genetic events in carcinogenesis and tumor progression as they show great variation in malignant potential, from benign follicular adenomas (FTA), differentiated papillary thyroid carcinomas (PTC), and follicular thyroid carcinomas (FTC) to highly aggressive anaplastic carcinomas (ATC). Another special feature of the thyroid is the presence, among the follicular thyrocytes, of the parafollicular cells from which the medullary thyroid carcinomas (MTC) arise. Although thyroid cancer is a rare disease, it is relatively well studied, as the patients are in most cases operated upon early and the tumor tissue is often highly homogeneous.

Papillary thyroid carcinoma

PTC is defined as a malignant epithelial tumor showing evidence of follicular cell differentiation and is characterized by distinctive nuclear features. It is the most common type of malignant thyroid neoplasm comprising more than 80% of all thyroid malignancies in areas of sufficient dietary iodine intake. Radiation exposure is a clearly demonstrated etiologic factor of PTC, especially pediatric PTC. PTC develops from the follicular thyrocytes and despite isolated evidence, no certain precursor lesion is identified. PTC is frequently multifocal and the individual foci in these cases often arise as independent tumors [3].

Clinical Endocrine Oncology, 2nd edition. Edited by Ian D. Hay and John A.H. Wass. © 2008 Blackwell Publishing. ISBN 978-1-4051-4584-8.

The genetic alterations leading to PTC development are well characterized. In the majority of cases, illegitimate activation of the *RET-Ras-Raf-MAPK* (MEK-ERK) oncogenic pathway is evident (Fig. 15.1, Table 15.1). The *RET* proto-oncogene, located on chromosome 10q11.2, encodes for a transmembrane receptor tyrosine kinase and is normally expressed in neuroendocrine and neural cells as well as during embryogenesis. *RET* is illegally activated in different human tumors by different mechanisms. As will be discussed later in this chapter, activating point mutations of *RET* are found in medullary thyroid cancer and in multiple endocrine neoplasia type 2 (MEN 2) syndromes. In PTC, chromosomal rearrangements linking the promoter and N-terminal domains of unrelated genes to the C-terminal fragment of RET, designated as *RET/PTC*, are found in 10–40% of cases. Several molecular forms have been identified that differ according to the 5′-partner gene involved in the rearrangement, with *RET/PTC1* and *RET/PTC3*, both resulting from paracentric inversions in chromosome 10, being the most prevalent. Similar chromosomal rearrangements of *TRKA* (*NTRK1*), a tyrosine kinase receptor that functionally interacts with *RET*, are also found in PTC, although at a lower frequency of 3–12%. To date, three fusion partners to *TRKA* have been described. *RET/PTC* fusions are more common in radiation-induced PTCs, as demonstrated by analysis of tumors from Japanese atomic bomb survivors and patients in Ukraine and Belarus after the Chernobyl accident, and indeed, experimental data suggest a direct causative relationship of radiation-induced DNA damage and *RET/PTC* oncogene generation. PTCs harboring *RET/PTC* fusions are generally considered to have a slow clinical course and *RET/PTC* has been detected in occult microcarcinomas and in some studies even in benign nodules and in Hashimoto thyroiditis. It is therefore generally considered as an early, initiating event in papillary carcinogenesis, probably less important for tumor progression and metastasis [4].

The Ras proteins (H-, K- and N-Ras) are small GTPases with a central role in transmitting oncogenic signals from the cell surface to the intracellular signaling network (Fig. 15.1). *RAS* mutations are found in nearly one-third of all human malignancies. In the thyroid, activating point mutations of *RAS* are found at varying frequencies in all tumor subtypes, mainly in follicular tumors. In PTC, *RAS* mutations are recurrently detected, although at a lower frequency (up to 10%) than in FTC. However, a high frequency of *RAS* mutations has been reported in the follicular variant of PTC.

B-Raf belongs to the Raf family of serine/threonine kinases. Although previously known for its role in propagating mitogenic signals from activated growth factor receptors through Ras, B-Raf came into focus as an oncogene when activating mutations (in most cases a V600E substitution) were found in the majority of melanomas and in several other cancer types. Mutation of the *BRAF* gene is the most common alteration in PTC, reported in nearly half of the cases (range 28–83% in different series). In addition to *BRAF* point mutations, a *AKAP9-BRAF* fusion has been reported in radiation-induced PTC. *BRAF* mutations are specific for PTC and some apparently PTC-derived ATC but have not been detected in FTC, MTC or benign thyroid neoplasms. This specificity for PTC, taken with the presence of the mutation in papillary microcarcinomas, clearly indicates a role of *BRAF* in the initiation of PTC tumor formation. On the other hand, the detection of *BRAF* mutations in some ATC and in PTC showing histological evidence of dedifferentiation strongly suggests its importance in tumor progression. Moreover, a correlation between the presence of *BRAF* mutations and aggressive clinical course in PTC has been observed [5].

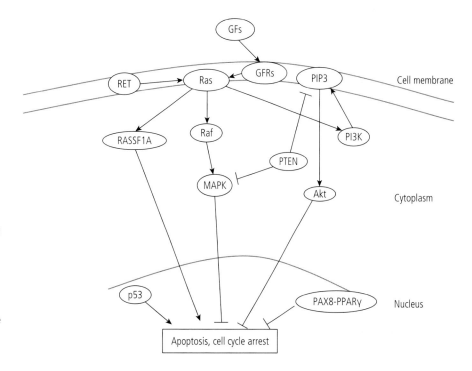

Figure 15.1 The genes and pathways involved in thyroid cancer pathogenesis. The central role for Ras is evident which, although not as frequently mutated as in other human cancers, mediates oncogenic signals from RET and other growth factor receptors (GFR). Furthermore, aberrations in Ras effectors (B-Raf, PI3K, RASSF1A) are the most prevalent genetic defects described in thyroid tumors. PTEN has a dual activity mainly acting as lipid phosphatase antagonizing PI3K but also as protein phosphatase inhibiting the MAPK cascade.

Table 15.1 Genes involved in the pathogenesis of thyroid cancer

Gene	Tumor subtype	Mechanism
RET	PTC	Activation by RET/PTC fusions
	MTC	Activation by point mutations
RAS	FTC, PTC, ATC, FTA	Activation by point mutations
BRAF	PTC, ATC	Activation by point mutations or rarely translocations
PPARγ	FTC, FTA	PAX8–PPARγ fusion, inhibition of wild-type PPARγ
TP53	ATC, PDTC	Inactivation by point mutations and/or deletions
PIK3CA	ATC	Activation by point mutations
PTEN	FTC, PTC, ATC, FTA	Inactivating mutations and/or functional silencing

PDTC, poorly differentiated thyroid carcinoma.

Other genes implicated in PTC, though with a less clear pathogenetic role, include *MET* and *RASSF1A*. *MET* is a gene for a tyrosine kinase receptor that is overexpressed in the majority of PTC but not in other thyroid tumors. *RASSF1A* is a Ras effector with tumor suppressor function. It is located on chromosome 3p21, a common site of deletion or loss of heterozygosity in thyroid cancer, and is often inactivated by promoter methylation in several human cancers. *RASSF1A* promoter methylation is commonly seen in all subtypes of thyroid cancer. Interestingly, in PTC, RASSF1A methylation and *BRAF* mutations are reported to be mutually exclusive events.

As shown in Fig. 15.1, *RET/PTC* (and *TRKA*) rearrangements, *RAS* mutations and *BRAF* mutations/rearrangement act in the same oncogenic pathway, leading to mitogen-activated protein kinase (MAPK) activation. They are essentially non-overlapping, indicating that one mutation in the pathway is sufficient for PTC tumor formation [6]. Novel therapies targeting the different factors of this important oncogenic cascade have been developed and are currently being tested in clinical trials of several cancers, including thyroid (Table 15.1).

Follicular thyroid carcinoma

FTC is derived from the follicular epithelial cell. No certain precursors are known, but at least some FTC may arise from FTA. Several genes, genomic loci and functional pathways have been implicated in the pathogenesis of FTC, which thus appears to be a biologically heterogeneous group of tumors.

Deletions or loss of heterozygosity of the short arm of chromosome 3 and the long arm of chromosome 10 (especially 3p21–25 and 10q22–24, respectively) are the most common numerical chromosomal aberrations in FTC. Recurrent structural chromosomal aberrations involve the peroxisome proliferator-activated receptor γ (*PPARγ*) locus at 3p25. The first fusion oncogene identified in FTC involves the *PAX8* gene, which encodes a paired domain transcription factor essential for thyroid development, and PPARγ, a transcription factor, member of the superfamily of nuclear receptors. Through a translocation between chromosomes 2 and 3, t(2;3)(q13;p25), the 3′ end of *PAX8* is fused in-frame to exon 1 of *PPARγ* [7]. Apparently driven by the promoter of *PAX8*, which is active in the follicular thyrocytes, the *PAX8–PPARγ* fusion gene is abundantly expressed and exerts its oncogenic effects. However, the precise mechanism by which *PAX8–PPARγ* promotes tumorigenesis is not fully understood. A plausible hypothesis described in the initial report and supported by subsequent studies is that PAX8–PPARγ acts by inhibiting wild-type PPARγ transcriptional regulation in a dominant negative manner. The *PAX8–PPARγ* fusion is detected in about 25% (18–63%) of FTC and more rarely in follicular adenomas. It is specific for conventional follicular tumors, as it has not been found in ATC, poorly differentiated FTC, or multinodular hyperplasias and is extremely rare in Hürthle tumors and PTC.

Activating point mutations in *RAS* oncogenes are detected in 20–50% of FTC, most frequently in codon 61 of *N*- and *H-RAS*. The reported prevalence varies greatly depending on the demographics, the history of radiation exposure, the histological variants and the methods used for mutation screening in different studies. The presence of *RAS* mutations in FTA indicates that *RAS* mutations occur early in thyroid tumorigenesis and activated Ras has also been implicated in tumor progression and dedifferentiation, probably by causing genomic instability. Interestingly, *RAS* mutations and *PAX8–PPARγ* fusion are essentially mutually exclusive alterations, indicating the existence of alternative pathways to FTC pathogenesis [8].

In addition to MAPK activation, the Ras/PI3K/Akt pathway plays an important role in follicular thyroid carcinogenesis (Fig. 15.1). Akt is activated in a large proportion of FTC and in animal models Akt activation has been coupled to FTC aggressiveness and metastasis. Accordingly, inactivation of the tumor suppressor phasphate and tensin homolog (PTEN) and activating somatic mutations within the phosphoinositol-3-kinase (PI3K) catalytic subunit, PIK3CA, are mainly seen in undifferentiated carcinomas. The importance of PTEN is indicated by the fact that patients with Cowden disease, characterized by germ-line mutations in *PTEN*, develop follicular thyroid tumors in at least 10% of the cases. Nevertheless, in sporadic FTC, *PTEN* mutations are very rare [9].

The Hürthle cell (oncocytic) carcinomas have previously been considered as FTC variants, yet they appear to be a separate entity, both at the clinical and the molecular level. Hürthle cell carcinomas are generally more unstable genetically than conventional FTC and are characterized by point mutations and deletions in the mitochondrial DNA. Furthermore, germ-line and somatic mutations in *GRIM19*, a dual function gene involved in mitochondrial metabolism and cell death, have been reported in Hürthle cell carcinomas.

Follicular thyroid adenoma

The majority of thyroid tumors are benign adenomas. A multitude of different genetic alterations have been described in FTA. Numerical chromosomal aberrations are commonly encountered, mainly trisomy 7, alone or with other characteristic trisomies.

Structural chromosomal aberrations specific for FTA are recurrently seen in regions 2p21 and 19q13. The *PAX8–PPARγ* translocation, which is characteristic of FTC, is occasionally found also in benign tumors. It is to date still unclear whether FTAs with *PAX8–PPARγ* fusion have an underlying malignant potential. Mutations of the *RAS* oncogenes are detected in a considerable number of FTA, supporting a role of Ras pathways early during thyroid tumorigenesis. On the other hand, aberrations in the *RET* and *BRAF* genes are very rare in adenomas. Mutations in the mitochondrial DNA have been described in Hürthle adenomas. Finally, somatic activating mutations in the *TSHR* gene or in the guanine nucleotide stimulatory factor α subunit (Gsα) are found often and almost exclusively in hyperfunctioning (toxic) adenomas. Taken together with the rarity of cancer developing from toxic adenomas, the activation of the thyroid-stimulating hormone (TSH)-initiated and cAMP-mediated signaling pathway seems to be of minor importance for the development of malignant thyroid tumors [10].

Medullary thyroid carcinoma

It is not always obvious that knowledge of the genetic pathogenesis of a certain tumor is of clinical importance. However, it may be stated that MTC treatment is highly dependent on such knowledge, and MTC is an excellent example of a disease in which the distance between the laboratory bench and the hospital bed has been largely reduced.

The RET proto-oncogene (*RET*) encodes for a receptor tyrosine kinase, whose main ligand is glial cell line-derived neurotropic factor (GDNF). RET activation by GDNF appears to occur via membrane-bound proteins, GFRα1–4, which seem to function as the ligand-binding domain of the ligand–receptor complex. The normal function of RET is only partially known: it is expressed in neural crest-derived tissue, and seems to play a role in kidney and gastrointestinal neuronal development. *RET* is also expressed in tumors of neural crest origin, such as medullary thyroid carcinoma, pheochromocytoma and neuroblastoma.

RET was confirmed to be the gene responsible for multiple endocrine neoplasia (MEN) type 2A, 2B and familial MTC (FMTC) when germ-line mutations were identified in affected patients but not in their unaffected relatives. More than 97% of these activating mutations in MEN 2A and FMTC involve the alteration of one of five cysteine residues (codons 609, 611, 618, 620 or 634) within exon 10 and 11 of *RET*. These missense mutations have been shown to result in RET dimerization at steady state, and hence activation of downstream signal transduction. MEN 2B patients show, instead, a mutation substituting a methionine with a threonine at codon 918 in exon 16 of RET, a highly conserved substrate-recognition site in the catalytic core of the tyrosine kinase. It results in a shift of substrate specificity and involves downstream signaling proteins not normally activated by RET. Several other codons have been described in a subset of MTC families, and *RET* mutation screening must be extended to these if they are not found in the "hot spots" of exons 10 and 11 [11]. Genotype–phenotype correlations have been made using the large number of families in a

RET Consortium analysis. The presence of any mutation in codon 634, for example, correlates significantly with the presence of pheochromocytoma and hyperparathyroidism [12].

As seemingly sporadic MTC prove to be caused by *RET* germline mutations in 5–10% of cases, *RET* mutation screening is advocated also in these patients. This is of utmost importance for the offspring of such patients: once an individual has been identified as a *RET* mutation carrier, prophylactic thyroidectomy is recommended from the age of 5 to 6 years, or in the case of MEN 2B even earlier [13].

A subset of sporadic MTCs have been shown to harbor somatic mutations in *RET*, predominantly in codons 918, 768 and 883. The prevalence of somatic codon 918 *RET* mutations in sporadic MTC varies from 28% to 86%, and has been correlated with a poorer prognosis.

Several other events have been described in MTC, including loss of various genomic regions, indicating putative tumor suppressor genes at these loci. It is logical to search for genetic disruptions along the RET signaling pathway. However, no specific changes in other parts of this chain (ligands, receptor partners, downstream effectors) have been established to play a major role. Still, the Raf-1/MEK/ERK1 signaling pathway seems to play a role; activation of Raf-1 leads to lower production of the typical MTC hormones (calcitonin and chromogranin A) and decreased cell growth, which is in contrast to tumors of non-neuroendocrine origin. Furthermore, the transcription factor human achaete-scute homolog 1 (hASH1) may play a role in the neuroendocrine phenotype of MTC.

Anaplastic thyroid carcinoma

ATC is characterized by its aggressive clinical course: rapid growth, extensive invasion and resistance to treatment. These are also features reflected in the genotype of ATC, leading to disruption of growth control and the apoptotic pathway, and stimulation of invasive and angiogenic components.

The first gene reported to be involved mainly in ATC was the *TP53* gene, sometimes called "the guardian of the genome." *TP53* is the most commonly mutated tumor suppressor gene in human cancer. The *TP53* gene product, p53, binds to nuclear proteins in cells containing mutations and arrests the cells at the G1 phase of the cell cycle. These cells are then allowed to either repair DNA or undergo apoptosis. In ATC, DNA binding sites of p53 are often mutated, leading to decreased activity of p21^{CIP1}, which in turn leads to genomic instability, inability to repair DNA and disruption of apoptosis. Although *TP53* mutations are not exclusive for ATC, other thyroid tumor types display these mutations to a much lesser degree [14]. However, in poorly differentiated thyroid cancers, mutations in *TP53* are found in about one-quarter; this may indicate p53's role in the tumor dedifferentiation progress. Disruption of p53 normal function may indeed be a marker of aggressive tumors, regardless of other histopathological features.

Loss of adhesive properties and ability to invade extracellular matrix characterize the ATC cell, and are reflected by its genotype.

Mutations of the *CTNNB1* gene lead to nuclear localization of its product β-catenin, which contributes to the very low expression of the cell–cell adhesion molecule E-cadherin in ATC. Altered expression of integrins involved in cell-matrix adhesion is also common. The tumor suppressor PTEN (see above) is expressed to a very low degree compared with differentiated cancer, probably leading to loss of fibronectin-mediated cell adhesion.

Fibroblast growth factors (FGF) and their receptors, vascular endothelial growth factors (VEGF) and their receptors, and other angiogenic molecules are grossly overexpressed in ATC, reflecting these tumors' extreme ability to form metastases which may grow extremely rapidly, especially after removal of the primary tumor, supporting the hypothesis of "dormant metastases."

Recently, PI3K was proven to be more often mutated in ATC compared with well-differentiated neoplasms, connecting the pathways from Ras activation and PTEN inactivation in these tumors (Fig. 15.1) [15].

It is sometimes disputed whether or not ATC evolves from dedifferentiation of well-differentiated thyroid cancers. Genetic evidence suggests that many ATC have undergone such dedifferentiation. For example, *BRAF* mutations which are present in PTC but not FTC, are found in at least 10% of all ATC. *RAS* mutations, more prominent in FTC than in PTC, are also found in a rather high proportion of ATC. Interestingly, the fusion oncogenes seen in PTC (*RET/PTC*) and FTC (*PAX8–PPARγ*) respectively have not been found in ATC [16]. This points toward a separate pathway for these tumors, possibly leading to a maintained differentiation state, in contrast to tumors evolved from activating point mutations along the *RAS–RAF–MAPK* pathway, which seem to have the ability to dedifferentiate. The detailed genetic regulation of this obvious difference in clinical behavior is not fully understood. Its clarification may have an impact on development of future medications aimed at hampering this specific pathway in undifferentiated thyroid cancers.

Conclusion

Thyroid cancer is a well-studied disease in terms of its pathogenesis, and both initiating events and the subsequent steps in tumor progression and even dedifferentiation are well described [17]. However, the clinical importance of these discoveries remains to be elucidated to a large degree. However, knowledge of tumor pathogenesis forms the basis for development of novel therapeutic strategies. Several such routes are now used also in clinical trials around the world. One example is tyrosine kinase inhibitors, which are tested for advanced differentiated thyroid carcinomas in which the ordinary treatment, including surgery and adjuvant radioiodine, has failed. Antiangiogenic therapy is also tested in patients with ATC, to whom no truly effective cure can be offered.

All steps in thyroid cancer pathogenesis may be outlined in models including the steps in tumor progression, and many variants have been presented. These reductionist models do not reflect the extremely complex nature of carcinogenesis, yet they offer a practical overview of the different central genetic events in tumor progression (Fig. 15.2). These events can become the targets for more effective and individualized cancer therapy in the future, in situations in which the current established treatment modalities can no longer help our patients.

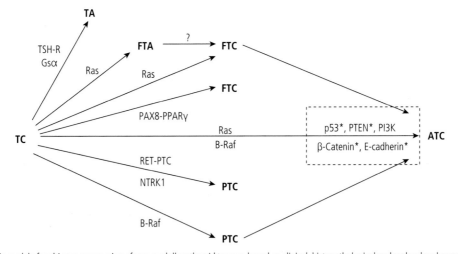

Figure 15.2 A simplistic model of multi-step progression of non-medullary thyroid tumors, based on clinical, histopathological and molecular observations. TC, normal thyrocyte; TA, "toxic adenoma", or "hyperfunctioning nodule"; FTA, follicular thyroid adenoma; FTC, follicular thyroid carcinoma; PTC, papillary thyroid carcinoma; ATC, anaplastic thyroid carcinoma. * Indicates loss of function. Note that the oncogenic effect of PAX8–PPARγ probably is attributed to a dominant negative inhibition of wild-type PPARγ. Accordingly, PAX8–PPARγ is a fusion oncogene, but PPARγ has a tumor-suppressing role in the thyroid. The presence of the two fusion oncogenes PAX8–PPARγ and RET/PTC in FTC and PTC respectively, but not in ATC, could be an indirect sign of a "protective" effect for dedifferentiation. Alternatively, the absence of this in ATC could be attributed to the loss of the chimeric (or rearranged) chromosomes during the process of dedifferentiation. Both scenarios indicate a role of the fusion oncogenes in tumor initiation rather than tumor progression. In addition, some ATC seem to develop from differentiated forms, but evidence of *de novo* ATC formation also exists.

References

1. Strachan T, Read A. *Human Molecular Genetics*, 3rd edition. London: Taylor & Francis, 2003.

2. Hanahan D, Weinberg RA. The hallmarks of cancer. *Cell* 2000;100: 57–70.

3. Shattuck TM, Westra WH, Ladenson PW, Arnold A. Independent clonal origins of distinct tumor foci in multifocal papillary thyroid carcinoma. *N. Engl. J. Med.* 2005;352:2406–2412.

4. Tallini G, Santoro M, Helie M, et al. RET/PTC oncogene activation defines a subset of papillary thyroid carcinomas lacking evidence of progression to poorly differentiated or undifferentiated tumor phenotypes. *Clin. Cancer Res.* 1998;4:287–294.

5. Xing M. BRAF mutation in thyroid cancer. *Endocr. Relat. Cancer* 2005;12:245–262.

6. Fagin JA. Challenging dogma in thyroid cancer molecular genetics – role of RET/PTC and BRAF in tumor initiation. *J. Clin. Endocrinol. Metab.* 2004;89:4264–4266.

7. Kroll TG, Sarraf P, Pecciarini L, et al. PAX8–PPAR gamma1 fusion oncogene in human thyroid carcinoma. *Science* 2000;289:1357–1360.

8. Nikiforova MN, Lynch RA, Biddinger PW, et al. RAS point mutations and PAX8-PPAR gamma rearrangement in thyroid tumors: evidence for distinct molecular pathways in thyroid follicular carcinoma. *J. Clin. Endocrinol. Metab.* 2003;88:2318–2326.

9. Eng C. Role of PTEN, a lipid phosphatase upstream effector of protein kinase B, in epithelial thyroid carcinogenesis. *Ann. N. Y. Acad. Sci.* 2002;968:213–221.

10. Fagin JA. Minireview: branded from the start–distinct oncogenic initiating events may determine tumor fate in the thyroid. *Mol. Endocrinol.* 2002;16:903–911.

11. Kouvaraki MA, Shapiro SE, Perrier ND, et al. RET proto-oncogene: a review and update of genotype-phenotype correlations in hereditary medullary thyroid cancer and associated endocrine tumors. *Thyroid* 2005;15:531–544.

12. Eng C, Clayton D, Schuffenecker I, et al. The relationship between specific RET proto-oncogene mutations and disease phenotype in multiple endocrine neoplasia type 2. International RET mutation consortium analysis. *JAMA* 1996;276:1575–1579.

13. Brandi ML, Gagel RF, Angeli A, et al. Guidelines for diagnosis and therapy of MEN type 1 and type 2. *J. Clin. Endocrinol. Metab.* 2001;86: 5658–5671.

14. Fagin JA, Matsuo K, Karmakar A, Chen DL, Tang SH, Koeffler HP. High prevalence of mutations of the p53 gene in poorly differentiated human thyroid carcinomas. *J. Clin. Invest.* 1993;91:179–184.

15. Garcia-Rostan G, Costa AM, Pereira-Castro I, et al. Mutation of the PIK3CA gene in anaplastic thyroid cancer. *Cancer Res.* 2005;65: 10199–10207.

16. Nikiforov YE. Genetic alterations involved in the transition from well-differentiated to poorly differentiated and anaplastic thyroid carcinomas. *Endocr. Pathol.* 2004;15:319–327.

17. Kondo T, Ezzat S, Asa SL. Pathogenetic mechanisms in thyroid follicular-cell neoplasia. *Nat. Rev. Cancer* 2006;6:292–306.

16 Papillary Thyroid Carcinoma

Ian D. Hay

Key points

- Papillary thyroid carcinoma is the most frequently diagnosed malignancy derived from an endocrine gland.
- Fortunately, with relatively conservative initial therapy, cause-specific mortality approximates 5% at 25 postoperative years.
- Prognostic factors are well recognised, and permit risk stratification soon after surgical pathology is available.
- The majority are cured with adequate initial surgical resection and postoperative thyroid hormone suppressive therapy.
- The high-risk minority should be identified early, and selected for aggressive adjunctive therapy and increased surveillance.
- A minority recur locally or spread distantly, resist ^{131}I/radiation therapy, and could require molecularly targeted therapies.

Pathology and epidemiology

Papillary thyroid carcinoma (PTC) has been defined as "a malignant epithelial tumor showing evidence of follicular cell differentiation and characterized by the formation of papillae and/or a set of distinctive nuclear changes" [1]. PTC is the most common thyroid malignancy and constitutes worldwide 50–90% of differentiated follicular cell-derived thyroid cancers [2]. Papillary thyroid microcarcinoma (PTM) has been defined by the World Health Organization (WHO) as a PTC 1.0 cm or less in diameter [3]. These microcarcinomas are common in population-based autopsy studies, and as incidental findings in carefully examined resected thyroid glands. The incidence rates for clinically diagnosed PTC in the USA approximate 5/100,000 for tumors more than 1 cm in diameter and around 1/100 000 for PTM. By contrast, the reported incidence of PTM in autopsy material from various continents has ranged from 4% to 36% [1].

The nuclei of PTC cells have a distinctive appearance, which in recent years has acquired a diagnostic significance comparable to that of the papillae. Often the preoperative diagnosis of PTC can be made solely on the basis of the characteristic nuclear changes seen in fine needle aspiration (FNA) cytology material (Plate 16.1). In its most typical form, PTC shows a predominance of papillary structures within the tumor. However, the papillae are usually admixed with neoplastic follicles having similar nuclear features. When the lining cells of the neoplastic follicles have the same nuclear features as those seen in typical PTC, and the follicular predominance over the papillae is complete, the tumor is considered a "follicular variant" of PTC [1].

Another subtype of PTC recognized by the WHO is the diffuse sclerosing variant characterized by widespread lymphatic permeation, prominent fibrosis and diffuse involvement of one or both thyroid lobes. The tall cell variant is characterized by well-formed papillae covered by cells that are twice as tall as they are wide. The columnar cell variant differs from other forms of PTC because of the presence of prominent nuclear stratification. The tall and columnar cell variants are considered more aggressive [1]. However, controversy exists regarding outcome in the diffuse sclerosing variant.

Over the past 60 years PTC has represented in the USA more than 80% of all clinically recognized cases of follicular cell-derived carcinomas (FCDC). During that period, the remaining 20% have been made up by almost equal numbers of patients with either follicular thyroid carcinoma or Hurthle cell carcinoma (see Chapter 17 by Shah and Ringel). Recent epidemiological studies would suggest that the proportion of patients with smaller PTC tumors is likely to increase [4], and will soon approximate 90% in most North American practice settings. In Scotland the overall thyroid cancer increase between 1975 and 2000 was primarily caused by an increase in PTC, particularly over the most recent decade [5]. Recent studies from France [6] and the USA [4] have suggested that evolution in clinical practice has been a major factor responsible for the increased PTC incidence. These included improvements in diagnostic practice, with increased use of more sophisticated diagnostic methods such as FNA biopsy of the thyroid and high-resolution ultrasonography.

Presenting features

Although PTC can occur at any age, most diagnoses are made in patients aged between 30 and 50 years (mean age 44 years). Women are more frequently affected (female predominance 60–80%).

Clinical Endocrine Oncology, 2nd edition. Edited by Ian D. Hay and John A.H. Wass. © 2008 Blackwell Publishing. ISBN 978-1-4051-4584-8.

The majority of primary tumors are 1–4 cm in maximum size, the average approximately 2 cm in diameter [2, 7]. Of PTC tumors, 95% are histological grade 1 (of 4); 80% of primary PTC tumors are DNA diploid by flow cytometry [2, 8]. Extrathyroid invasion of adjacent soft tissues by PTC is reported in about 15% (range 5–34%) at primary surgery [2, 7, 9]. At presentation, about one-third of PTC patients have clinical evident lymphadenopathy (2, 7, 10). Microscopic examination of excised neck nodes in adults typically reveals 35–50% involvement, but in children <17 years old nodal involvement may occur in up to 90% [8]. The primary disease is confined to the neck in about 93–99% of PTC patients at diagnosis [2, 8, 10]. Spread to superior mediastinal nodes is usually associated with extensive neck nodal involvement. At the Mayo Clinic in Rochester, during the period of 1940 through 2000, 2512 PTC patients had initial definitive surgical management. In only 4% of primary surgeries was gross residual disease reported due to incomplete tumor excision [10] and during the same period only 2% of patients had distant metastases diagnosed before or within 30 days of primary treatment. Accordingly, based on presenting features, almost all (98%) patients with PTC have disease localized to the neck, which can in 96% be completely excised at the time of primary definitive surgery. Therefore, in most cases of PTC, adequate initial surgery can be potentially curative.

Recurrence and mortality

Three types of tumor recurrence may occur with PTC. These are, in order of frequency: (i) postoperative nodal metastases (NM); (ii) local recurrences (LR); and (iii) postoperative distant metastases (DM). An LR may be defined as "histologically confirmed tumor occurring in the resected thyroid bed, thyroid remnant, or other adjacent tissues of the neck (excluding lymph nodes)" at any time after complete surgical removal of the primary tumor [11]. In our studies at Mayo, we have considered nodal or distant spread to be postoperative if the metastases were discovered within 180 days or 30 days, respectively [2, 7, 10]. We also chose to consider tumor recurrence only as it occurs to patients without initial DM, who had complete surgical resection of their primary tumors.

Figure 16.1, based on 2370 Mayo Clinic patients with disease confined to the neck and having initial complete tumor resection, demonstrates that the most frequent site of tumor recurrence (TR) was in NM, accounting, to date, for 71% of the total number of first postoperative events [10]. At 25 years, as shown in the figure, the rates for NM, LR and DM were 9.8%, 5.5%, and 4.6%. At 40 postoperative years the comparable figures were 10%, 6% and 5%, respectively [10].

Of our 1940–2000 cohort of consecutively treated PTC patients, at latest follow-up in 2002, 106 (4%) had died directly from PTC, and 771 (31%) had died from all causes of mortality [10]. For a comparable population living in the north central United States during that period, the expected number of deaths from all causes would have been 700, an excess of 71 deaths that is highly significant ($p = 0.006$). However, if one considers the survival to death

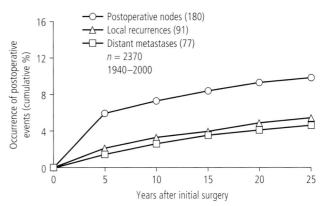

Figure 16.1 Cumulative occurrence during 25 years of postoperative events: metastatic nodes (180 patients), local recurrences (91 patients), or distant metastases (77 patients). Data are based on 2370 PTC patients with disease confined to the neck, who had initial complete tumor resection at Mayo Clinic during 1940 through 2000. (From Hay ID et al. [10], with permission from the American Clinical and Climatological Association.)

from all causes in the potentially surgically cured group of 2370 (having complete surgical resection and presenting with disease localized to the neck), the observed number of deaths was 673, insignificantly different ($p = 0.963$) from the 672 expected [10].

Figure 16.2 illustrates the cause-specific mortality (CSM) and TR rates observed over 25 postoperative years in our total cohort of 2512 patients. CSM rates were 5% at 15, 20, and 25 years. Of those with lethal PTC, approximately 20% died in the first year after diagnosis. By 10 years, 80% of the deaths from PTC had occurred [2, 9, 10]. The TR rates were 8% at 5, and 10% at 10 postoperative years for the subgroup of 2370 who had localized disease which was completely excised. By 25 years the TR rate was 14%, and between 25 and 40 years this figure only rose by one more percent to 15% [10].

Outcome prediction and risk-group stratification

Close scrutiny of the observed rates of recurrence and mortality in PTC reveals that only a small minority (about 15%) of patients are liable to relapse of disease, and even fewer (around 5%) experience a lethal outcome. Those exceptional patients who pursue an aggressive course tend to relapse early, and the rare fatalities usually occur within 5–10 years of diagnosis [7–12]. During the past 20 years many North American centers have used multivariate analyses to identify presenting variables predictive of cause-specific mortality [13–18]. Increasing patient age and presence of extrathyroid invasion have been independent prognostic factors in all these studies [13–18]. The presence of initial DM and increasing size of the primary tumor have also been significant variables in most studies [13, 15–17]. We [2, 7, 13] and others [14] have found that histopathological grade (degree of differentiation) is an independent variable. The completeness of initial tumor resection (postoperative status) has also been relevant in predicting those at

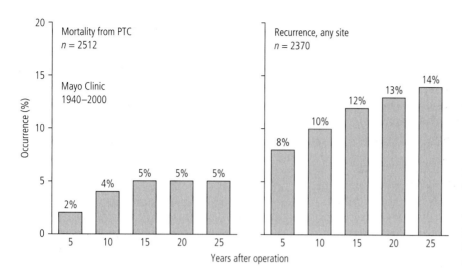

Figure 16.2 Overall outcome of 2512 consecutively treated PTC patients managed at Mayo Clinic during 1940 through 2000, demonstrating 5–25-year rates for (left panel) cause-specific mortality and (right panel) tumor recurrences at any anatomic site. (From Hay ID et al. [10], with permission from the American Clinical and Climatological Association.)

risk of death from PTC [2, 16, 18, 19]. When analyzed by the presence or absence of extrathyroid invasion, the presence of initial neck NM, although very relevant to future nodal recurrence, did not significantly influence cause-specific mortality [2, 7, 18].

In 1987, we devised a simple scoring system to assign patients to prognostic risk groups [13]. The prognostic index was named the AGES score after the five independent variables of patient's age, tumor grade, tumor extent (local invasion, distant metastasis) and tumor size. Using such a scoring system, the "minimal risk" group (AGES score <4) represented 86% of cases, and they experienced a 20-year CSM rate of only 1% [13]. By contrast, the minority (14%) of patients with AGES scores of 4+ (high-risk) had a 20-year CSM of 40%. The development of such a prognostic system was intended to permit more accurate counseling of patients and to aid in the planning of individualized postoperative management programs in PTC [2, 13, 18]. The notion was that the use of such a scheme could allow the "punishment to fit the crime" in terms of PTC management.

Although the AGES scheme had the potential for universal application, many academic centers could not include the differentiation (g) variable because their surgical pathologists would not recognize higher grade PTC tumors [15]. Accordingly, we resolved to define a reliable prognostic scoring system for predicting PTC mortality rates using 15 candidate variables that included, for the first time, completeness of primary tumor resection, but excluded histological grade and nuclear DNA ploidy [18]. Cox model analysis and stepwise variable selection led to a final prognostic model that included five variables abbreviated by metastasis, age, completeness of resection, invasion and size (MACIS).

The final prognostic score was defined as MACIS = 3.1 (if aged 39 years or less) or 0.08 × age (if aged 40 years or more), +0.3 × tumor size (in centimeters), +1 (if locally invasive), +3 (if distant metastases present). In a cohort of 2512 consecutively treated PTC patients the MACIS prognostic scores were <6 in 2099 (84%), 6–6.99 in 215 (9%), 7–7.99 in 84 (3%), and 8+ in 114 (4%). The 25-year CSM rates for these four groups were 1%, 15%, 44% and 63%, respectively. Figure 16.3 illustrates survival to death from

PTC, according to the MACIS low-risk (scores <6) and high-risk (scores 6+) prognostic scheme, for the 2512 patients. At 25 postoperative years, the cause-specific survival rate for the 2099 low-risk patients was 99%, and by 40 years was 98%. Comparable survival rates for the 413 high-risk patients (MACIS scores of 6+) were at 25 years 65%, and at 40 years 63%.

It should be emphasized that the five variables needed for MACIS scoring are readily available after primary operation, and such a prognostic system has the potential for application in any clinical setting with access to conventional chest and skeletal radiography and accurate surgical pathology reporting. The MACIS scoring system can also provide the attending clinician with an accurate tool for counseling the individual patient and can help guide decision making on the intensity of postoperative tumor surveillance and the appropriateness of adjunctive radioiodine therapy. Since the CIS variables need to be verified postoperatively, the scoring system should not be used to decide on the extent of primary thyroid surgery.

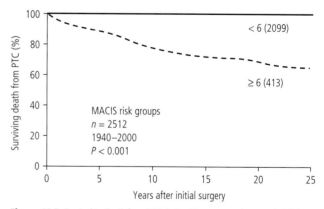

Figure 16.3 Survival to death from PTC during 25 postoperative years in 2512 patients managed during 1940 through 2000, according to MACIS low-risk (scores <6) and MACIS high-risk (scores 6+) prognostic groupings. Numbers in parentheses represent the numbers of patients in each risk group at the time of initial surgery. (From Hay ID et al. [10], with permission from the American Clinical and Climatological Association.)

Extent of primary surgery

The accepted initial treatment of PTC is adequate surgical excision of the primary tumor. However, the extent of thyroid resection remains controversial, with the choice of definitive therapy ranging from unilateral lobectomy through bilateral subtotal lobar resection to near-total or total thyroidectomy [2, 10, 11, 16, 29]. Unfortunately, in many surgical reports where two procedures are compared, only scant attempt is made to match the patient groups with respect to relevant prognostic variables. Accordingly, differences between groups may prove to be primarily due to imbalances in the prognostic factors, rather than to the specific surgical procedure [2, 21]. The field is further confounded because, in recent years, there have been no publications of prospective double-blind randomized controlled trials. Accordingly, the basis of current practice recommendations is largely derived from retrospective analyses of cohorts of FCDC patients either treated at major institutions or documented in cancer registries.

Naturally, I for one freely admit to being biased by the results reported in the series of papers that Mayo Clinic authors have published, in the past two decades on the differences in outcome seen between PTC patients who had either a lobectomy (UL) or bilateral lobar resection (BLR). I am certainly convinced (Fig. 16.4) that BLR results in fewer local recurrences in all PTC patients [2, 3, 7–11, 13, 21], and reduces rates of death from cancer in patients with high-risk disease [2, 10, 13]. I am pleased too that such data have also influenced the American Association of Clinical Endocrinologists (AACE), and the American Association of Endocrine Surgeons (AAES) in the creation of their current practice guidelines [23], and have even found a mention in the latest WHO monograph on thyroid tumour classification [24]. It is my strong belief that if a patient in 2007 has a preoperative FNA diagnosis of PTC,

he or she should expect to be treated with a BLR, either a near-total thyroidectomy or total thyroidectomy, as the preferred primary definitive surgical treatment.

I also believe that, in this setting, a preoperative ultrasound examination of the neck, with identification of metastatic nodes, will allow planning of an appropriate nodal resection at the time of the first neck exploration [25, 26]. If a PTC patient in these times has only a thyroidectomy and no inspection or exploration of the central compartment with sampling of level VI nodes, then I think that patient has been ill served, and has already fallen on only day 1 of their treatment schedule into a "pitfall" [27, 28]. Similarly, if a lateral neck node has been removed at preoperative open biopsy, been shown to be metastatic on a preoperative ultrasound-guided biopsy (USGB), or is found to be pathological at frozen section exam, then the patient deserves to have a modified neck dissection performed under the same anesthetic as the primary definitive thyroidectomy. Pattern recognition, using high-resolution ultrasonography (HRUS), of metastatic nodes takes practice, but is a readily attainable skill, which many AACE, AAES, American Thyroid Association (ATA), European Thyroid Association (ETA) and Endocrine Society members are now rapidly acquiring [29].

Surgeons treating PTC patients should no longer be permitted either to avoid entering the central compartment [30], or to continue performing a safe, but suboptimal, surgical procedure that would be better suited to the management of a benign nodular goiter. Thanks in part to parathyroid autotransplantation, iatrogenic parathyroprivic hypocalcemia is generally avoidable in the surgical management of the routine patient with PTC in 2007. Primary surgery for PTC is routinely elective, and clinicians should choose for their patients an endocrine or head and neck surgeon who is comfortable with intraoperative parathyroid identification, and has an acceptably low rate (<2%) of postoperative permanent hypocalcemia. Radioiodine therapy should certainly

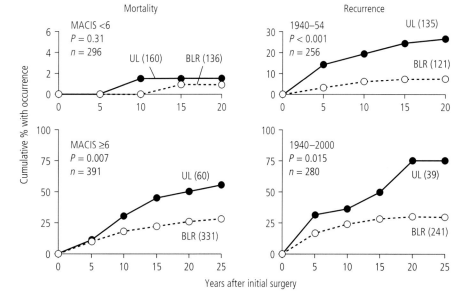

Figure 16.4 Comparison of outcome after either unilateral lobectomy (UL) or bilateral lobar resection (BLR) in MACIS <6 (low-risk) patients treated during 1940–1954 (upper panel) and MACIS 6+ (high-risk) patients (lower panels) during 1940 through 2000. The left panels illustrate CSM in MACIS scores <6 (upper) and 6+ patients (lower). The right panels show comparable rates for TR at any site for each of the two risk groups. (From Hay ID et al. [10], with permission from the American Clinical and Climatological Association.)

not be used in an attempt to overcome the shortcomings of a suboptimal, incomplete excision of PTC at primary surgery [2, 9–11, 20, 31, 32].

Thyroxine suppressive therapy (TST)

It has been traditional in treating PTC patients that, after initial surgery, they will receive relatively high doses of thyroxine (T_4) with the aim of "suppressing" thyroid-stimulating hormone (TSH) secretion. In former days, the goal was to reduce the basal serum TSH enough to allow a "flat thyrotropin-releasing hormone (TRH) test". As more sensitive assays for TSH were developed, this effect was usually achieved by reducing the serum TSH to a level around 0.1 mIU/L. Presently, low-risk patients tend to be treated to a serum TSH in the range between 0.1 and 0.5 mIU/L [26], while the potentially aggressive, "high-risk" minority will be given doses of approximately 2 μg/kg of T_4 to permit the basal TSH to fall below a level of 0.1 mIU/L. There are, to date, no convincing, adequately controlled, long-term studies showing that TR and CSM rates are significantly altered by such careful titration. In "low-risk" PTC patients, the T_4 dose is usually reduced to the lowest dose that will give a TSH in the 0.1 to 0.5 mIU/L range, associated ideally with a free T_4 level within the upper part of the normal range.

Selective use of radioiodine remnant ablation

Clearly, any serious discussion about the role of radioiodine remnant ablation (RRA) in the management of PTC could consume the remainder of the space allocation of this chapter! For much more on this particular topic, the interested reader is directed to a recently published review in the *Journal of Surgical Oncology* [32] and the meta-analysis of Sawka and colleagues published in 2004 in the *Journal of Clinical Endocrinology and Metabolism* [33].

At the Mayo Clinic in Rochester, Minnesota, RRA was performed within 6 months of potentially curative BLR in only 6% of PTC cases during the early 1970s, but by the mid-1980s, perhaps influenced by the encouraging reports of Beierwaltes [34] and Mazzaferri [35], almost 10 times more, or about 60%, were being given RRA (Fig. 16.5). Careful analysis has recently been performed on the 1163 MACIS low-risk (scores <6) PTC patients surgically treated by near-total or total thyroidectomy at Mayo for localized, potentially curable, disease during 1970 through 2000 [10, 32]. These 1163 patients were operated in a standard manner by a small group of specialized Mayo surgeons, who had recognized special expertise in endocrine surgery. The preoperative investigations and the postoperative care were provided by Mayo staff endocrinologists, who also prescribed and monitored the patients' postoperative TST.

Four hundred and ninety-eight (43%) of these low-risk (MACIS scores <6) PTC patients had RRA within 6 months of the surgery that was performed "with curative intent." Those low-risk patients who received RRA during 1970–2000 were more likely

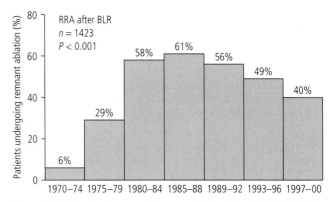

Figure 16.5 Changing frequency of remnant ablation at Mayo Clinic during 1970 through 2000 in 1423 patients, without initial distant metastases, who underwent RRA within 6 months of potentially curative bilateral resection (BLR). (From Hay ID et al. [10], with permission from the American Clinical and Climatological Association.)

to have had positive neck nodes at presentation ($p < 0.001$). Of 636 node-negative patients, 195 (31%) received RRA. However, of 527 node-positive patients, 305 (57%) were ablated.

At 20 postoperative years, the CSM rate for the surgery-alone patients was 0.4%, and for the surgery and RRA group, it was insignificantly different at 0.6% ($p = 0.64$). At 20 years the TR rate was actually significantly higher in the ablated group (14% vs 9%), likely reflecting the tendency to more readily ablate node-positive patients. When the patients were divided by presenting status into 636 node-negative and 527 node-positive cases, as shown in Table 16.1, there were no statistically significant differences in 20-year outcomes (CSM and TR) between those having surgery alone and those who also received postoperative RRA [10, 32].

Of the 1163 low-risk patients in this Mayo-treated cohort, there were at last follow-up no deaths from PTC in the 636 node-negative cases, and only two (0.4%) in the node-positive group. For the node-negative patients (Fig. 16.6), the 20-year TR rates were 3.4% after surgery alone and 4.3% after surgery and RRA ($p = 0.80$).

Table 16.1 Lack of influence of RRA on outcome in 1163 MACIS low-risk (scores < 6) patients (without distant metastases) treated during 1970 through 2000 at Mayo by near-total (NT) or total thyroidectomy (TT)

Low-risk (MACIS < 6)	20-year mortality		20-year recurrence	
1970–2000	NT/TT Alone	NT/TT and RRA	NT/TT Alone	NT/TT and RRA
All patients (1163)	0.4%	0.6%	8.7%	13.6%
p value	$p = 0.64$		$p = 0.008$	
Node-negative (636)	0%	0%	3.4%	4.3%
p value	N/A		$p = 0.80$	
Node-positive (527)	1.2%	0.9%	19.5%	19.9%
p value	$p = 0.99$		$p = 0.66$	

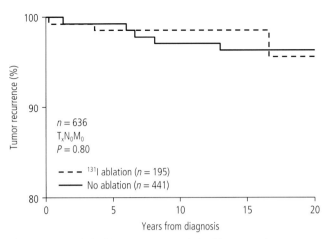

Figure 16.6 Survival to first tumor recurrence during 20 postoperative years in 636 node-negative MACIS low-risk (scores <6) patients treated during 1970–2000. All 636 initially underwent either near-total or total thyroidectomy; 195(31%) additionally had RRA performed. (From Hay ID. *J. Surg. Oncol.* 2006;94:692–700, with permission from John Wiley and Sons.)

For the node-positive group, who clearly had much higher TR rates, the CSM rates at 20 years were 1.2% after surgery alone and 0.9% after RRA ($p = 0.99$). The 20-year TR rates (Fig. 16.7) only differed by 0.4%, being 19.5% for surgery alone and 19.9% for surgery and RRA ($p = 0.66$).

We therefore concluded that RRA did not significantly improve the outcome (either CSM or TR) in low-risk (MACIS <6) patients previously treated by initial near-total or total thyroidectomy. In contrast to many other leading endocrine centers, we at Mayo have since 1994 adopted a selective approach to RRA, and tend to restrict its use only to those few patients with high-risk (MACIS score 6+) PTC or those, now rare, patients who present with a diagnosis of follicular or Hurthle cell thyroid cancer.

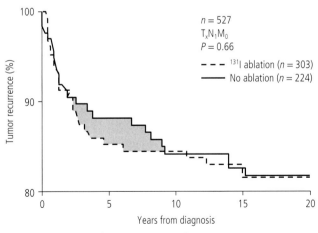

Figure 16.7 Survival to first tumor recurrence during 20 postoperative years in 527 node-positive MACIS low-risk (scores <6) patients treated during 1940–2000. All 527 initially underwent either near-total or total thyroidectomy; 313 (57%) additionally had RRA performed. (From Hay ID. *J. Surg. Oncol.* 2006;94:692–700, with permission from John Wiley and Sons.)

A recent meta-analysis from Canada attempted to define from currently published reports the effectiveness (or not) of RRA for well-differentiated thyroid cancer. These investigators [33] concluded that "the effectiveness of RAI ablation in decreasing recurrence and possible mortality in low-risk patients with well-differentiated thyroid carcinoma, although suspected, cannot be definitively verified by summarizing the current body of observational patient data."

Of further relevance, a recently completed study [36] from Toronto of 729 FCDC patients, treated at Princess Margaret Hospital during 1958 through 1998, found in a multivariate analysis that there was no significant improvement in cause-specific survival with "more aggressive treatment (administration of RAI and/or RT)." Moreover, "in low-risk patients (pTNM/AJCC stage I <45 years) there was no apparent benefit from RAI." As shown in Fig. 16.8, there were no deaths in the 96 patients who did not receive radioactive iodine (RAI), and there was no difference in local recurrence-free rate (LRFR); the 10-year LRFR was 90% with RAI and 85% without RAI ($p = 0.32$). They therefore concluded that "RAI may not be required in young patients under the age of 45 years without distant metastases" [36].

In the United States, the National Thyroid Cancer Treatment Cooperative Study Group (NTCTCSG), now led by Dr Steven Sherman of MD Anderson, was founded in 1986 and has for 21 years maintained a registry contributed to by 11 North American institutions. This registry has prospectively followed a large non-randomized cohort of patients with FCDC, with the object of assessing the effects of initial and longitudinal managements on their outcomes. By June 2001, 2936 such patients were registered. After more than two decades of data entry and very detailed analysis, the NTCTCSG came to the conclusion that "no treatment modality, including radioactive iodine, was associated with altered survival in stage I patients." Moreover, Jonklaas and colleagues [37] "were unable to show any impact, positive or negative, of specific therapies in stage I patients." They concluded that "postoperative RAI therapy does not provide significant benefit in stage I patients, and could even be harmful," and have suggested that "further evaluation of the potential risks and benefits of treatment in stage I patients is, therefore, indicated" [37].

Recently, a European consensus report recommended that "post-surgical use of RAI should be selective, given that uncertainty persists concerning the benefits in decreasing recurrence rates and cause-specific mortality" [38]. This group, derived from 12 European countries, also advised that "remnant ablation should be restricted to patients with incomplete surgical excision or poor prognostic factors for recurrence or death." A more recent consensus publication from Europe, derived from the ETA and the ETA-cancer research network, concluded that the benefits of RRA for low-risk FCDC patients "are controversial and there are still uncertainties as to whether it should be administered to all patients or only to selected patients" [39].

This European consensus report, perhaps leading in the future to a more selective use on the continent for remnant ablation, contrasts with the recommendations of the National Thyroid

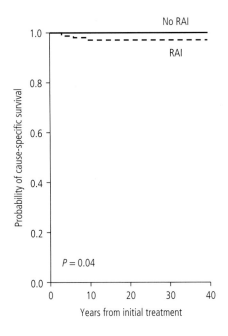
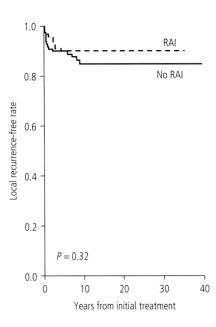

Figure 16.8 Cumulative incidence of cause-specific survival and local recurrence-free rate for AJCC stage I patients under the age of 45. (From Brierley J et al. [36], with permission from Blackwell Publishing.)

Cancer Guidelines Group, formed during 2000 under the auspices of the British Thyroid Association (BTA). This group advised in 2002 that "for most patients with tumors greater than 1 cm in diameter, radioactive iodine ablation of the thyroid remnant should be carried out following total thyroidectomy" [40].

The recently published ATA guidelines have recommended RRA for pTNM/AJCC stage III and IV disease, all patients with stage II disease 45 years or older, and selected patients with stage I disease, "especially those with multifocal disease, nodal metastases, extrathyroidal or vascular invasion, and/or more aggressive histologies" [26]. This relative lack of selection, advised by both the BTA and the ATA, is unfortunate and will likely in future years potentially subject about 70% of PTC patients on both sides of the Atlantic to ^{131}I therapy, that is unlikely either to improve their already excellent prognosis or completely eliminate persistent neck nodal metastases [32]. These proposals should be of particular concern to thyroidologists.

If we consider PTC patients who have undergone an optimal primary surgery (near-total or total thyroidectomy) and at the procedure's end there is no gross residual disease, then at the Mayo Clinic, Rochester, during three decades (1970–1999), only 45% of 1269 such patients received RRA within 6 postoperative months [10, 32]. In 2000, the minority ablated during that year was only 36%. If one applies theoretically the inclusion criteria proposed by the ATA [26] or the BTA [40] to our 1970–2000 cohort of patients, one would see the rates for RRA as outlined in Table 16.2 [41].

Compared to Mayo's past prescribing habits, almost 100% more patients would be ablated currently, if the new guidelines were closely followed. Since neither the Mayo [10, 32] nor the Toronto [36] or NTCTCSG [37] data can demonstrate improvement in either TR or CSM rates with RRA, especially in low-risk

Table 16.2 Actual and proposed rates of RRA after near-total or total thyroidectomy for localized papillary thyroid cancer

	Actual		Proposed	
	Mayo 2000 (**n = 50**)	**1970–1999** (**n = 1269**)	**ATA** (**2006**)	**BTA / RCP** (**2001**)
Ablated	36%	45%	69%	71%
Not ablated	64%	55%	31%	29%

patients, such an escalation of aggressive postoperative adjunctive therapy can hardly be justified [41].

In contrast to other centers, who routinely favor "blind" [131]I administration of large doses with subsequent post-therapy wholebody scans, we at Mayo still prefer in selected "high-risk" PTC cases to perform quantitation of neck uptake of radioiodine with a postoperative whole-body ^{123}I scan. We attempt to customize the administered dose by considering percent RAI neck uptake and distribution of iodine-avid foci, and follow progress with further diagnostic scanning, usually at 3–6 months. We have not been impressed that the information obtained from post-therapy scans regularly provides data that influences subsequent therapy or results in a reassignment of tumor stage [42]. We are, however, impressed that patients with typical ("low-risk") PTC have a very high chance of "cure" after adequate initial surgery and only levothyroxine therapy, and we would caution others that our 25-year cause-specific survival rate of 100% for 636 node-negative "low-risk" (MACIS <6) PTC patients treated by near-total or total thyroidectomy alone cannot be improved by remnant ablation [9, 10].

Long-term surveillance

Like other endocrine tumors, PTC can be followed using a combination of tumor marker measurements and appropriate selective imaging of those anatomical areas most likely to harbor recurrent or metastatic disease. In my own practice, during the last 15 years, when I am pre-scheduling appointments for my returning PTC patients, I arrange routinely for the patient to have drawn at each visit a blood sample for a thyroid "cascade" (screening TSH, followed by a free T_4 only if TSH abnormal) and a serum thyroglobulin (Tg). By the time I see my patients that same day, I know of the adequacy of their T_4 therapy, and I can compare the Tg with previous values in similar conditions (either on or off therapy).

The definition of an "undetectable" serum Tg is presently a moving target, in view of the ongoing development of increasingly sensitive Tg assays. On the other hand, a readily detectable Tg may in certain circumstances trigger further investigation, while in other settings (particularly in the range of 0.1 to 0.5 ng/mL during T_4 suppressive therapy), such a level could be perfectly stable from year to year and may often be rather reassuring. With regards to TSH-stimulated Tg values, I have for more than 20 years measured TSH and Tg off hormone, at the time of whole-body scanning and, until recently, often noted, but largely ignored, the result. To my knowledge, I personally have never in 34 years of practice stopped T_4 or given recombinant human TSH (rhTSH) only for the purpose of determining the level of the resultant Tg increment.

Our endocrine group at Mayo has long contended that a serum Tg level of <0.5ng/mL during thyroxine suppressive therapy (TST), far from being misleading [43], provides reassuring evidence of a lack of clinically relevant tumor recurrence in nearly all patients with low-risk FCDC. Recently, my Mayo Clinic Jacksonville (MCJ) colleagues [44] published a report of 194 FCDC patients with a baseline Tg on TST of <0.1 ng/mL, who underwent rhTSH stimulation and radioiodine scanning. Such patients rarely had levels of stimulated Tg >2ng/mL, and not one of these 194 patients had radioiodine imaging suggestive of locoregional recurrence or distant metastasis. They recommended monitoring low-risk patients with only a T_4-suppressed Tg level and periodic neck ultrasonography, a conclusion also shared by Brazilian authors [45]. As the sensitivity of Tg measurements approaches 0.01 ng/mL, it seems unlikely that in future years we will need to be performing rhTSH stimulation tests [46]. A "positive" biopsy represents proof of disease rediscovery, but a detectable serum Tg may often be misleading and, at most, serves as a possible "surrogate" for tumor recurrence.

In our institution we are using ^{131}I sparingly in "low-risk" PTC, and whole-body radioiodine scans largely to follow effects of therapeutic doses. Like our Italian colleagues [47], we do rely heavily on the skill of our sonographers in identifying or excluding locoregional disease at most of the Mayo visits of our PTC patients. For more than two decades [48] we have used ultrasound to guide biopsies, and in selected refractory cases of PTC we have since 1993 been injecting 95% ethanol to directly ablate, under ultrasound guidance, regional nodal recurrences, when patients are found to have only very limited options for further ^{131}I therapy or surgery [49]. In the long-term surveillance of "low-risk" PTC patients, our attitudes are certainly in accord with those of the 2005 European Consensus Report, which stated that "currently, the most sensitive tool to discover lymph node metastases is neck ultrasonography, which should be performed in all thyroid cancer patients, even if there has been no remnant ablation. In low-risk patients, who have not been ablated (because they have low thyroid bed uptake and undetectable Tg and Tg autoantibodies) follow-up is based on serum Tg determination on L-T_4 plus neck ultrasonography" [38].

Although, indeed, the mainstay of surveillance in PTC would generally be serum Tg levels on TST and high-resolution ultrasonography of the postoperative neck, there are a significant number of PTC patients who do have interfering thyroglobulin autoantibodies, thereby making serial measurements of serum Tg somewhat unreliable. Also, there are many medical centers where diagnostic radiologists may be uncomfortable with the identification of suspicious postoperative intracervical foci of recurrent disease, and perhaps lack experience in performing USGB of these suspicious lesions. In such settings, high-resolution computerized tomographic (CT) scans with reconstructions and magnetic resonance imaging (MRI) can sometimes provide alternative relevant information, but certainly in the USA there is a tendency to consider only the largest neck nodes as being pathological. Often the subtle imaging characteristics of a small, rounded, hypervascular, microcalcified, partially cystic lymph node involved by PTC, which is readily recognizable to an experienced sonographer [50, 51], may go unidentified or be below the detection size limit of the much more expensive imaging modalities. Although, in the pursuit of the source of a detectable basal or TSH-stimulated Tg, a fluorodeoxyglucose (FDG)–positron emission tomographic (PET)/CT fusion scan [52, 53] may sometimes provide novel information with regards to extracervical foci of disease, this technology also yields many "false positives" and may often underascertain the extent of residual microscopic neck nodal disease in recurrent PTC.

In former days, the first line of imaging in postoperative PTC surveillance would have been the neck ultrasound, and if one sought disease outside the neck, a CT of the chest, an isotopic bone scan or a bone MRI would be secondary relevant considerations. Increasingly, despite the drawbacks of its cost (PET = "pretty expensive test"!) and the significant rate (up to 12%) of false-positive foci of FDG uptake [53], the PET/CT fusion scan in our practice at Mayo is certainly taking over as the next logical step in PTC imaging after an ultrasound exam and a CT of the chest. Obviously, the definition provided by the CT used in the fusion studies may not be adequate for a neck or chest surgeon in preoperative planning and, in that particular circumstance, a dedicated higher-resolution CT with thinner "cuts" or an MRI or MR angiogram may be indicated, particularly in the setting of locally invasive recurrent neck disease, superior mediastinal adenopathy or microscopic lung nodules. However, we would certainly agree with our colleagues at Villejuif and Johns Hopkins that "surgery should not be planned solely on the basis of the FDG-PET results, but rather in combination with the serum thyroglobulin level, and, whenever possible, cytological examination and thyroglobulin measurement of FNA biopsy material" [53].

Management of recurrent and metastatic PTC

For the reasons outlined in the section on risk group stratification, it is now generally accepted that more than 85% of patients with PTC present with limited disease and become disease free after initial treatment [54, 55]. This is obviously very encouraging information that clinicians can share with their PTC patients soon after initial diagnosis. Unfortunately, even in 2007, about 10–15% of patients with PTC have persistent or recurrent disease, with less than 5% having distant metastases at initial presentation [56, 57]. In 75% of those with recurrent PTC, the disease is localized in the neck only, most often in regional lymph nodes. Ten-year survival rates after recurrence of neck disease have been reported (55) to range from 49% to 68%, and neck lesions alone can be responsible for a minority of cancer-related deaths [12, 58]. Distant metastases can occur in the lungs (50%), bones (25%), lungs and bones (20%), or at other sites (5%) with 10-year survival rates ranging from 25% to 42% [55–57].

Patients with persistent, recurrent or distantly metastatic PTC represent a highly heterogeneous group with widely differing outcomes. Moreover, as Baudin and Schlumberger [55] have recently stated, "no randomized controlled trials assessing primary treatment or treatment of recurrent disease have been reported, and current practice is based on retrospective studies that are often monocentric and extended over several decades. Until recently, treatment of persistent and recurrent disease has consisted of suppressive thyroid hormone treatment, surgery (when feasible) and radioiodine treatment when radioiodine uptake is present in neoplastic foci".

Neck nodal metastases

NM discovered after apparently successful thyroidectomy probably represent the commonest type of postoperative PTC recurrence seen in clinical practice during 2007, and usually would be found in patients who are "low-risk" PTC with MACIS scores <6 at presentation. Options for treatment typically would range, depending on local expertise, from neck re-exploration with selective neck nodal dissection and postoperative therapeutic radioactive ^{131}I, through external irradiation to targeted therapy such as percutaneous ultrasound-guided ethanol injections [49] or radiofrequency ablation [59]. In many centers, patients with small NM usually undergo ^{131}I treatment, but it is well recognized that on ultrasound "abnormalities can still persist after two to three courses" [55], and in such cases, surgery is generally performed. Such reoperations would include removal of NM in areas that

have already been dissected, in addition to, when indicated by preoperative localization, the complete removal of previously nondissected areas. In skilled hands, morbidity is usually kept to a minimum, and in more than 90% of these patients, no abnormalities persist on neck ultrasound and radioiodine whole-body scans (WBS) after surgery, but increased Tg may still be detected after thyroxine withdrawal or rhTSH in one-third of patients [60].

Many centers take the stance that surgery is indicated if the NM is palpable, its size is 1 cm or more, or the diagnosis is proven by a positive USGB. At Mayo, the vast majority of the low-risk PTC patients who are sent to us because of a detectable Tg without an obvious source are found on careful neck ultrasound to have persistent/recurrent NM, often in a central compartment (level VI) which has never been adequately explored by prior surgeons [27]. Almost invariably, such patients have been given a number of ^{131}I therapeutic doses [23, 26], and have been already shown to be "thyroglobulin positive-scan negative" in terms of their scintigraphic pattern on WBS. In that setting, we would usually re-explore the neck and perform selective nodal dissection [25], particularly in those areas identified as harboring residual disease, as shown by preoperative ultrasound mapping. For reasons outlined below, we are confident that in this setting the rediscovery of such NM, thanks to the sophistication of contemporary detection methods, will not impact an already excellent prognosis.

If such a patient (with prior ^{131}I treatments) has already suffered from complications of surgery (recurrent laryngeal nerve injury) or the NM are tiny (2–5 mm), then rather than commit the patient to another surgery at Mayo we have since 1993 successfully treated with ultrasound-guided ethanol ablation [49] more than 100 pTNM stage I MACIS score <6 PTC patients with biopsy-proven microscopic NM. These patients have invariably been treated elsewhere with multiple incomplete surgeries and repeated doses of apparently ineffective RAI treatments [61]. We at Mayo do not use RFA in the treatment of NM in PTC, and almost never use external irradiation to treat persistent NM in a patient with low-risk PTC.

It should be recognized that most patients with low-risk PTC are prone to have spread of their tumors by lymphatic drainage to regional nodes in the neck and superior mediastinum. This is almost invariably found at presentation, if one looks diligently, in children and adolescents but clearly [7–10] does not influence cause-specific mortality. In MACIS <6 PTC patients, treated at our institution during 1970–2000, no deaths occurred from PTC in 636 patients node negative at presentation, despite a 4% nodal recurrence rate at 20 years [32]. Even more striking, despite having a one in five (20%) chance of NM rediscovery by 20 years, our 527 node-positive low-risk patients still enjoyed a 99% survival, even without the "benefits" of RRA! Although a review published in the *Lancet* in 2007 [55] still states that "neck lesions alone are responsible for a third of cancer-related deaths", such a statistic has in fact no relevance to the rediscovered neck NM of low-risk (MACIS <6) PTC patients. In the same journal, some 21 years before, Schwartz had described these rediscovered NM in low-risk PTC as "benign metastases from thyroid malignancies" [62].

Local recurrences

By contrast, true "LR," as we have defined it [9–11], is a more sinister postoperative event, which can portend a lethal outcome and is most often seen in "high-risk" (MACIS scores 6+) patients aged 60 or older with larger tumors of higher histological grade [2, 7, 11, 13], which are frequently locally invasive at initial presentation [63]. Such recurrences may be located either in the thyroid bed or in adjacent soft tissues and may involve direct invasion of the aerodigestive tract. Therefore, such patients may require staging with endoscopies and various imaging modalities. When disease is limited to the neck, treatment usually includes extensive surgery and, often, is supplemented by postoperative external beam irradiation [64]. It is recognized that "patients older than 40 years, who have poorly differentiated tumors, no radioiodine uptake, large tumor burden, rapidly progressive disease, and high FDG uptake do not normally attain disease-free status after treatment of disease recurrence in the neck" [55]. Such patients with true LR are also much more likely to develop during follow-up DM, which may prove to be fatal. In our own experience of 52 PTC patients with an LR, followed for up to 41 years, 16/20 (80%) who died of PTC also had DM [11]. Interestingly, those LRs that occurred in elderly patients and invaded surrounding structures typically recurred outside the thyroid remnant in the bed of a totally resected lobe or in surrounding tissues of the neck, and probably contributed to a lethal outcome in 4 of our 20 fatal cases. On the other hand, in our series of 963 PTC patients treated during 1946–1975, no patient with an LR limited to the thyroid remnant, who underwent a satisfactory neck re-exploration, subsequently died of PTC [11].

Distant metastases

Spread of tumor to distant sites occurs in much less than 10% of patients with PTC, but DM represents the most frequent cause of PTC-related death [12, 56–58]. ^{131}I is the main treatment modality in a patient with demonstrable iodine avidity, and may be used in association with local treatments such as external beam irradiation or surgery. ^{131}I treatment for lung metastases leads to remission (normal radiographs and absence of residual ^{131}I uptake) in about 45% of patients with radioiodine uptake [57]. Almost all complete responses are attained with cumulative activities of ^{131}I equal to or less than 600 mCi. Few recurrences (7%) and few cancer-related deaths (3%) are seen after remission [57]. Unfortunately, in the case of large bone metastases, treatment also includes surgery, when feasible, and radiotherapy, but remission is rarely achieved. However, local procedures, such as embolization, radiofrequency, cryotherapy or cement injection, and treatment with bisphosphonates can delay tumor progression and palliate symptoms [55]. Currently available treatments provide a complete remission in only about a third of PTC patients with DM [55, 57]. The other two-thirds have a highly variable life expectancy, that cannot often be accurately predicted by available prognostic criteria on an individual basis [55–57]. It is often a clinical challenge to identify, using conventional imaging modalities those patients who may live for many asymptomatic years

with their relatively microscopic lung metastases from that other group of patients with DM, who will have a progressive and potentially life-threatening course. Those patients with progressive disease were in the past considered for conventional cytotoxic chemotherapy, but unfortunately, such therapy has proven to be ineffective for most of these patients [55, 65].

Molecularly targeted treatments

On a more optimistic front, as described in Chapter 15, the past 25 years have seen much progress in our understanding of the pathways involved in thyroid cancer development and progression. Overexpression and/or uncontrolled activation of receptor tyrosine kinases, downstream signaling molecules, and inhibition of programmed cell death (apoptosis) have all been demonstrated to occur in thyroid cancer [65]. Many of the events that initiate thyroid cancer have already been investigated as potential targets for treatment, making "molecularly targeted treatments" an attractive new approach for managing the minority of high-risk PTC patients who tend to pursue a progressive course despite conventional therapy with surgery, TST and radioiodine [55, 65]. There are two main theoretical approaches: the induction of redifferentiation of tumor thyroid tissue, and inhibition of tumor growth by inhibiting cell signaling and angiogenesis [55, 65].

Several methods have recently been used in an attempt to increase the expression of the natrium iodide symporter (NIS). Retinoic acid analogs have been shown to restore radioiodine uptake in only a minority of PTC patients, without a direct effect on tumor growth. As discussed in Chapter 6 by Spitzweg, NIS gene therapy may induce iodine uptake *in vitro* in infected tumor cells and also *in vivo* by direct injection into xenografted tumors. However, retention of radioiodine is short, and the resulting radiation dose quite low. Indeed, increased expression of the NIS gene might not of itself be sufficient to induce meaningful tumor uptake and adequately long retention of radioactive therapeutic iodine [55].

Perhaps there is more early optimism resulting from initial evaluation of compounds that may interfere with signal transduction pathways. The clinical activity of AMG 706, BAY 43-9006, ZD 64-74 and AG-01376 is being presently investigated in phase II trials. These molecules inhibit several targets, including RET tyrosine kinase, vascular endothelial growth factor receptor (VEGFR) 1, VEGFR 2 and VEGFR 3, and have an antiangiogenic effect. BAY 43-9006 also inhibits BRAF kinase. Other targets include membrane receptor kinases, such as those for epidermal growth factor (EGF), platelet-derived growth factor, and c-Met. At present, there are no available reports on the selective inhibition of angiogenesis with antibodies directed against VEGFRs or small molecules targeting specifically the tyrosine kinase of the VEGFR in patients with PTC [55]. The PI3K pathway can be inhibited by several compounds, and an ester analog of rapamycin, with similar antineoplastic properties but reduced immunosuppressive effects, is being tested in a phase I trial for advanced solid tumors, such as PTC [65]. Lastly, agents that destabilize the 90 kDa heat shock chaperone protein, such as 17-*N*-allyl-amino-demethoxy-geldanamycin (17-AAG), can interfere with the MAPK and PI3K pathways, and are being tested in phase I and II trials. At Mayo, this compound is presently being studied, but the necessity for infusions and the frequency of administration do not make this a very attractive prospect for future therapy of patients with progressive disease.

Conclusion

Most patients with PTC can be successfully treated, and others can survive for decades despite persistent disease [66]. Few patients need novel therapeutic modalities, because their disease can be controlled with presently available treatments. However, it is the hope of investigators such as Baudin and Schlumberger [55] that, in the early 21st century, we will soon be seeing the situation that "in most patients, an initiating carcinogenic event can be identified and molecularly targeted treatment can, thus, be given on a rational basis" [55]. As one reflects on this concept during mid-2007, that day may still be quite some time in the future.

For the present, the prospects for the great majority of patients with PTC remain exceedingly bright, and an excellent prognosis can be confidently predicted in low-risk patients after an adequate surgical resection and postoperative TST [9, 10, 32, 41, 66]. For myself, after practicing in the USA for more than 27 years, I have long since come to the conclusion that, when it comes to treating PTC, there are in the American thyroidology community "too many hanging judges"!! I have, during 34 years of practice, tried to pursue the medical dictum of *primum non nocere* and always, in individual PTC patients, attempted to permit "the punishment to fit the crime." In such a "law and order" context, I have always viewed the low-risk PTC patient as having only committed a "misdemeanor" or a "petty offence." In this context, it is my earnest hope: (i) that in the postoperative management of PTC patients the international endocrine community can learn to use RRA more selectively [32], (ii) that in future years we will no longer "worship" serum Tg levels as a surrogate for cancer [43–46], and (iii) that the current nuclear medical exercise of "wiping the scintigraphic slate clean" [31], so ingrained in current practice guidelines [26, 38–41], will soon be a distant memory [10, 32]!

References

1. Rosai J. Papillary carcinoma. *Monogr. Pathol.* 1993; 35: 138–165.
2. Hay ID. Papillary thyroid carcinoma. *Endocrinol. Metabol. Clin. North Am.* 1990;19:545–576.
3. Hay ID, Grant CS, van Heerden JA, et al. Papillary thyroid microcarcinoma: a study of 535 cases observed in a 50-year period. *Surgery* 1992;112:1139–1147.
4. Davies L, Welch HG. Increasing incidence of thyroid cancer in the United States, 1973–2002. *JAMA* 2006;295:2164–2167.
5. Reynolds RM, Weir J, Stockton DL, et al. Changing trends in incidence and mortality of thyroid cancer in Scotland. *Clin. Endocrinol.* 2005;62:156–162.
6. Leenhardt L, Bernier MO, Boin-Pineau MH et al. Advances in diagnostic practices affect thyroid cancer incidence in France. *Eur. J. Endocrinol.* 2004;150:133–139.
7. McConahey WM, Hay ID, Woolner LB, et al. Papillary thyroid carcinoma treated at the Mayo Clinic, 1946 through 1970: initial manifestations, pathologic findings, therapy and outcome. *Mayo Clin. Proc.* 1986;61:978–996.
8. Zimmerman D, Hay ID, Gough IR, et al. Papillary thyroid carcinoma in children and adults: long-term follow-up of 1,039 patients conservatively treated at one institution during three decades. *Surgery* 1988;104:1157–1166.
9. Hay ID, Thompson GB, Grant CS, et al. Papillary thyroid carcinoma managed at the Mayo Clinic during six decades (1940–1999): temporal trends in initial therapy and long-term outcome in 2,444 consecutively treated patients. *World J. Surg.* 2002;26:879–885.
10. Hay ID, McConahey WM, Goellner JR. Managing patients with papillary thyroid carcinoma: insights gained from the Mayo Clinic's experience of treating 2,512 consecutive patients during 1940 through 2000. *Trans. Am. Clin. Climatol. Assoc.* 2002;113:241–260.
11. Grant CS, Hay ID, Gough IR, et al. Local recurrence in papillary thyroid carcinoma: is extent of surgical resection important? *Surgery* 1988;104:954–962.
12. Smith SA, Hay ID, Goellner JR, Ryan JJ, McConahey WM. Mortality from papillary thyroid carcinoma. A case–control study of 56 lethal cases. *Cancer* 1988;62:1381–1388.
13. Hay ID, Grant CS, Taylor WF, McConahey WM. Ipsilateral lobectomy versus bilateral lobar resection in papillary thyroid carcinoma: a retrospective analysis of surgical outcome using a novel prognostic scoring system. *Surgery* 1987;102:1088–1095.
14. Simpson WJ, McKinney SE, Carruthers JS, et al. Papillary and follicular thyroid cancer. Prognostic factors in 1,578 patients. *Am. J. Med.* 1987;83:479–488.
15. Cady B, Rossi R. An expanded view of risk-group definition in differentiated thyroid carcinoma. *Surgery* 1988;104:947–953.
16. DeGroot LJ, Kaplan EL, McCormick M, Straus FH. Natural history, treatment, and course of papillary thyroid carcinoma. *J. Clin. Endocrinol. Metab.* 1990;71:414–424.
17. Shah JP, Loree TR, Dharker D, et al. Prognostic factors in differentiated carcinoma of the thyroid gland. *Am. J. Surg.* 1992;164:658–661.
18. Hay ID, Bergstralh EJ, Goellner Jr, et al. Predicting outcome in papillary thyroid carcinoma: development of a reliable prognostic scoring system in a cohort of 1,779 patients surgically treated at one institution during 1940 through 1989. *Surgery* 1993;114:1050–1058.
19. Kjellman P, Zedenius J, Lundell G, et al. Predictors of outcome in patients with papillary thyroid carcinoma. *Eur. J. Surg. Oncol.* 2006;32:345–352.
20. Grebe SKG, Hay ID. The role of surgery in the management of differentiated thyroid cancer. *J. Endocrinol. Invest.* 1997;20:32–35.
21. Hay ID, Grant CS, Bergstralh EJ, et al. Unilateral total lobectomy: is it sufficient surgical treatment for patients with AMES low-risk papillary thyroid carcinoma? *Surgery* 124;1998:958–966.
22. Hay ID, Bergstralh EJ, Grant CS, et al. Impact of primary surgery on outcome in 300 patients with pTNM stage III papillary thyroid carcinoma treated at one institution from 1940 through 1989. *Surgery* 1999;126:1173–1182.

23. Thyroid Carcinoma Task Force. AACE/AAES medical/surgical guidelines for clinical practice: management of thyroid carcinoma. *Endocr. Pract.* 2001;7:202–220.

24. DeLellis RA, Lloyd RV, Heitz PU, Eng C. *Pathology and Genetics of Tumours of Endocrine Organs. WHO Classification of Tumours.* Lyon, France: IARC Press, 2004.

25. Stulak JM, Grant CS, Farley DR, et al. Value of preoperative ultrasonography in the surgical management of initial and reoperative papillary thyoid cancer. *Arch. Surg.* 2006;141:489–496.

26. Cooper DS, Doherty GM, Haugen BR, et al. Management guidelines for patients with thyroid nodules and differentiated thyroid cancer. *Thyroid* 2006;16:109–142.

27. Sywak M, Cornford L, Roach P, et al. Routine ipsilateral level VI lymphadenectomy reduces postoperative thyroglobulin levels in papillary thyroid cancer. *Surgery* 2006;140:1000–1007.

28. Palazzo FF, Gosnell J, Savio R, et al. Lymphadenectomy for papillary thyroid cancer: Changes in practice over four decades. *EJSO* 2006;32:340–344.

29. Davies T. Personalized thyroid medicine – the time is now. *Thyroid* 2007;17:1.

30. Doherty GM. Invited commentary: routine central neck lymph node dissection for thyroid carcinoma. *Surgery* 2006;124:958–966.

31. Sisson JC. Applying the radioactive eraser: I-131 to ablate normal thyroid tissue in patients from whom thyroid cancer has been resected. *J. Nucl. Med.* 1983;24:743–745.

32. Hay ID. Selective use of radioactive iodine in the postoperative management of patients with papillary and follicular thyroid carcinoma. *J. Surg. Oncol.* 2006;94:692–700.

33. Sawka AM, Thephamongpol K, Brouwers M, et al. Clinical Review 170. A systematic review and metanalysis of the effectiveness of radioactive iodine remnant ablation for well-differentiated thyroid cancer. *J. Clin. Endocrinol. Metab.* 2004;89:3668–3676.

34. Varma VM, Beierwaltes WH, Nofal H, et al. Treatment of thyroid cancer. Death rates after surgery and after surgery followed by sodium iodide I-131. *JAMA* 1970;214:1437–1442.

35. Mazzaferri EL, Young RL, Oertel JE, et al. Papillary thyroid carcinoma: the impact of therapy in 576 patients. *Medicine (Baltimore)* 1977;56:171–196.

36. Brierley J, Tsang R, Panzarella T, Bana N. Prognostic factors and the effect of treatment with radioactive iodine and external beam radiation on patients with differentiated thyroid cancer seen at a single institution over 40 years. *Clin. Endocrinol.* 2005;63:418–427.

37. Jonklaas J, Sarlis N, Litofsky D, et al. Outcomes of patients with differentiated thyroid cancer following initial therapy. *Thyroid* 2006;16:1229–1242.

38. Pacini F, Schlumberger M, Harmer C, et al. Post-surgical use of I-131 in patients with papillary and follicular thyroid cancer and the issue of remnant ablation: a consensus report. *Eur. J. Endocrinol.* 2005;153:651–659.

39. Pacini F, Schlumberger M, Dralle H, et al. European Consensus for the management of patients with differentiated thyroid carcinoma of the follicular epithelium. *Eur. J. Endocrinol.* 2006;154:787–803.

40. British Thyroid Association and the Royal College of Physicians of London. Guidelines for the management of thyroid cancer in adults. London: BTA/RCP, 2002:1–70.

41. Hay ID. Papillary thyroid cancer in the twenty first century: a mid-Atlantic perspective one year after the publication of the American Thyroid Association Clinical Management Guidelines. *Hot Thyroidology* (www.hotthyroidology.com) 2007; March; 1–14.

42. Fatourechi V, Hay ID, Mullan BP. Are post-therapy radioiodine scans informative and do they influence subsequent therapy of patients with differentiated thyroid cancer? *Thyroid* 2000;10:573–577.

43. Mazzaferri EL, Robbins RJ, Spencer CA, et al. A consensus report on the role of serum thyroglobulin as a monitoring method for low-risk patients with papillary thyroid carcinoma. *J. Clin. Endocrinol. Metab.* 2003;88:1433–1441.

44. Smallridge RC, Meek SE, Morgan MA, et al. Monitoring thyroglobulin in a sensitive immunoassay has comparable sensitivity to recombinant human TSH-stimulated thyroglobulin in follow-up of thyroid cancer patients. *J. Clin. Endocrinol. Metab.* 2007; 92: 82–87.

45. Rosario PS, Borges MA, Fagundos FA, et al. Is stimulation of thyroglobulin (Tg) useful in low–risk patients with thyroid carcinoma and undetectable Tg on thyroxin and negative neck ultrasound? *Clin. Endocrinol.* 2005;62:121–125.

46. Fatemi S, Lo Presti JJ. A consensus report on the role of serum Tg as a monitoring method for low-risk patients with papillary thyroid carcinoma. *J. Clin. Endocrinol. Metab.* 2003;88:4507–4510.

47. Torlontanto M, Attard M, Crocetti U, et al. Follow-up of low-risk patients with papillary thyroid cancer. Role of neck ultrasonography in detecting lymph node metastases. *J. Clin. Endocrinol. Metab.* 2004;89:3402–3407.

48. Sutton RT, Reading CC, Charboneau JW, et al. Ultrasound-guided biopsy of neck masses in the postoperative assessment of patients with thyroid malignancy. *Radiology* 1988;168:769–772.

49. Lewis BD, Hay ID, Charboneau JW et al. Percutaneous ethanol injection of cervical lymph nodal metastases in patients with papillary carcinoma. *Am. J. Roentgenol.* 2002;178:699–704.

50. Souza Rosario PW, de Faria S, Bicalho L, et al. Ultrasonographic differentiation between metastatic and benign lymph nodes in patients with papillary thyroid carcinoma. *J. Ultrasound Med.* 2005;24:1385–1389.

51. Leboulleux S, Girard E, Rose M, et al. Ultrasound criteria of malignancy for cervical nodes in patients followed for differentiated thyroid cancer. *J. Clin. Endocrinol. Metab.* 2007 Jul 3 (Epub ahead of print).

52. Joensuu H, Ahonen A. Imaging of thyroid metastases of thyroid carcinoma with flurine-18 fluordeoxyglucose (FDG). *J. Nucl. Med.* 1987;28:910–914.

53. Leboulleux S, Schroeder PR, Schlumberger M, Ladenson. The role of PET in follow-up of patients treated for differentiated epithelial thyroid cancers. *Nat. Clin. Pract. Endocrinol. Metab.* 2007;3:112–121.

54. Schlumberger MJ, Filetti S, Hay ID. Non toxic goiter and thyroid neoplasia. In: Larsen PR, Kronenberg HM, Melmed S, Polonsky KS (eds). *Williams Textbook of Endocrinology*, 10th edition. Philadelphia: WB Saunders Company, 2003:457–490.

55. Baudin E, Schlumberger M. New therapeutic approaches for metastatic thyroid carcinoma. *Lancet Oncol.* 2007;8:148–156.

56. Dinneen S, Valimaki MJ, Bergstralh EJ, et al. Distant metastases in papillary thyroid carcinoma: 100 cases observed at one institution during 5 decades. *J. Clin. Endocrinol. Metab.* 1995;80:2041–2045.

57. Durante C, Haddy N, Baudin E, et al. Long-term outcome of 444 patients with distant metastases from papillary and follicular thyroid carcinoma: benefits and limits of radioiodine therapy. *J. Clin. Endocrinol. Metab.* 2006;91:2892–2899.

58. Carmen F, Eustatia–Rutten A, Corssmit EPM, et al. Survival and death causes in differentiated thyroid carcinoma. *J. Clin. Endocrinol. Metab.* 2006;91:313–319.

59. Monchik JM, Donatini G, Iannuccilli J, Dupuy DE. Radiofrequency ablation and percutaneous ethanol injection treatment for recurrent

local and distant well-differentiated thyroid carcinoma. *Ann. Surg.* 2006;244:296–304.

60. Travagli JP, Cailleux AF, Ricard M, et al. Combination of radio-iodine (I-131) and probe–guide surgery for persistent or recurrent thyroid carcinoma. *J. Clin. Endocrinol. Metab.* 1998; 83:2675–2680.

61. Hay ID, Reading CC, Lee RA, Charboneau JW. Ultrasound-guided percutaneous ethanol injection is an effective long-term solution for persistent neck nodal metastases in pTNM stage I papillary thyroid carcinoma patients apparently resistant to conventional postoperative radioactive iodine therapy. 2006; ETA Abstract book, abstract 038, p 19. http://www.hotthyroidology.com/downloads/abstractbook_hot_thyroidology.pdf

62. Schwartz TB. Benign metastases from thyroid malignancies. *Lancet* 1986;2:733–735.

63. McCaffrey TV, Bergstralh EJ, Hay ID. Locally invasive papillary thyroid carcinoma. *Head Neck* 1994;16:165–172.

64. Morton RP, Ahmad Z. Thyroid cancer invasion of neck structures: epidemiology, evaluation, staging and management. *Curr. Opin. Otolaryngol. Head Neck Surg.* 2007;15:89–94.

65. Braga-Basaria M, Ringel MD. Clinical Review 158. Beyond radio-iodine: a review of potential new therapeutic approaches for thyroid cancer. *J. Clin. Endocrinol. Metab.* 2003;88:1947–1960.

66. Lang BH, Lo CY, Chan WF, Lam YK, Wan KY. Staging systems for papillary thyroid carcinoma. A review and comparison. *Ann. Surg.* 2007;245:366–378.

17 Follicular Thyroid Carcinoma

Manisha H. Shah and Matthew D. Ringel

> **Key points**
> - Benign follicular adenomas are indistinguishable from follicular thyroid carcinomas on fine needle aspiration cytology; thus, thyroid surgery, either lobectomy or total thyroidectomy, is required for diagnosing follicular thyroid carcinoma.
> - Surgery, thyroid stimulating hormone suppressive therapy and ^{131}I therapy are the primary forms of treatment for follicular thyroid carcinoma.
> - Iodine deficiency is the best-described environmental etiology for follicular thyroid carcinoma.
> - While most patients with follicular thyroid carcinoma have an excellent prognosis, novel systemic therapies are being tested in clinical trials for patients with progressive follicular thyroid carcinoma that does not respond to standard therapies.

Introduction

Follicular thyroid carcinoma (FTC) is the second most common follicular cell-derived thyroid cancer (after papillary thyroid carcinoma [PTC]), accounting for approximately 5–15% of all thyroid cancers depending on the population. FTC is typically classified with PTC among the group of differentiated thyroid carcinoma (DTC) that retain features of normal thyroid cells such iodine uptake, thyroid-stimulating hormone (TSH) receptor expression, and thyroglobulin (Tg) production. Thus, many of the treatment paradigms for FTC and PTC are similar and include thyroidectomy and, depending on the stage of the tumor, radioiodine and TSH suppression therapy. However, there are key epidemiological, molecular, and clinicopathological differences between these two types of DTC.

Epidemiology

In the United States between 1992 and 2002, thyroid cancer had among the most rapidly rising incidences of cancer from any organ site (www.seer.cancer.gov). In 2006 alone, the American Cancer Society estimated that approximately 30 180 (22 590 female, 7590 male) new cases of thyroid cancer would be diagnosed in the United States. The incidence of thyroid cancer is also increasing in other parts of the world. For example, between 1960 and 2000, the annual European age-standardized rates of thyroid cancer in Scotland increased from 1.76 to 3.54 per 100 000 for females and from 0.83 to 1.25 per 100 000 in males [1]. This trend in incidence, likely due

Clinical Endocrine Oncology, 2nd edition. Edited by Ian D. Hay and John A.H. Wass. © 2008 Blackwell Publishing. ISBN 978-1-4051-4584-8.

in part to increased use of thyroid ultrasound, is primarily caused by an increase in early-stage DTC (mostly PTC) while the incidences of anaplastic and medullary thyroid cancer have not changed significantly [2].

Similar to PTC, women are approximately 2.5-fold more likely to develop FTC than men and the median age at diagnosis is earlier in women than in men. Interestingly, the median age of diagnosis for FTC appears to be older than PTC for both males and females. The median age at diagnosis is 48 years (compared to 40 years for PTC) for caucasian women and 53 years (compared to 44 years for PTC) for caucasian men [3]. It is also of interest that the proportion of DTC that are FTC appear to be higher in African Americans as compared to caucasians. It has been reported that follicular carcinoma accounts for 15% of all DTC in whites as compared to 34% in African Americans [3]. The etiology for these demographic differences between FTC and PTC is uncertain and requires further study.

Etiology

Chronic iodine deficiency

Epidemiological and animal model studies have demonstrated that iodine deficiency likely plays a role in the development of FTC. For example, chronic dietary iodine deficiency in rats leads to thyroid follicular adenomas (FA) by 12 months and FTC by 18 months [4]. Consistent with these experimental findings, an increased incidence of FTC has been reported in humans living in iodine-deficient areas of the world, likely in part accounting for the marked geographical variations in the relative proportions of FTC and PTC [5]. Moreover, supplementation of dietary iodine results in a decrease in the proportion of thyroid cancers that are FTC [6], further demonstrating a role for iodine deficiency in follicular tumorigenesis. Thus, in comparison to PTC, where radiation is a clear environmental tumor-initiating event; iodine deficiency is the best-described environmental etiology for FTC.

Genetic syndromes

While the vast majority of FTCs are sporadic, there are several uncommon genetic syndromes that increase susceptibility to FTC. Cowden syndrome is an autosomal dominant disorder caused by inactivating mutations in the *PTEN* tumor-suppressor gene on chromosome 10q22–23 that result in constitutive activation of the PI3 kinase signaling cascade [7]. This syndrome is characterized by hamartomas and other tumors of the thyroid, breast, colon, endometrium, and brain. Thyroid follicular neoplasms, both benign and malignant, occur in approximately two-thirds of affected individuals. Carney complex is an autosomal dominant disorder is caused by mutation of the *PRKAR1* gene on chromosome 17q24 in more than half of the analyzed families. It is characterized by myxomas of the soft tissues, skin and mucosal pigmentation (blue nevi), schwannomas, and tumors of the adrenal glands, pituitary, thyroid, and testes [8]. Thyroid gland pathology occurs in approximately 11% of patients and includes adenomatous hyperplasia, cysts, or papillary or follicular carcinoma. Werner syndrome (WS) is a rare autosomal recessive disorder caused by mutations of the *WRN* gene on chromosome 8p11–21 [9] characterized by premature aging, scleroderma-like skin changes, cataracts, subcutaneous calcifications, muscular atrophy, diabetes, and a high incidence of neoplasms. Thyroid cancer (mainly FTC) has been primarily described in individuals of Japanese descent with this disease and it occurs at a young age with male predominance. Interestingly, there is genotype-phenotype correlation as mutations in the C-terminal region of *WRN* correlates with FTC in Japanese patients.

Pathogenesis of non-syndromic forms of FTC

Recent advances in molecular thyroid cancer research have improved our understanding of the pathogenesis of sporadic FTC. As discussed in detail elsewhere in this text and as summarized in Fig. 17.1a, mutations in the gene encoding RAS and rearrangements involving *PPARγ* and *PAX8* are particularly prevalent in FA and FTC suggesting they are early events in FTC development. Whether or not FTC develops from FA is an area of vigorous debate in the literature; however, global gene expression analyses performed by a number of groups have identified differences in the gene expression signatures for FA and FTC [10]. Potential reasons for these expression differences could include differences oncogene signaling and altered regulation of mRNA expression levels through epigenetic and post-transcriptional mechanisms; such has promoter hypermethylation, expression of microRNA or histone modifications. Indeed, alterations in each of these have been demonstrated in FTC [11–13].

In addition to this growing knowledge in FTC pathogenesis, a number of genetic and epigenetic alterations appear to be common in FTCs that are resistant to standard therapies or dedifferentiate.

As summarized in Fig. 17.1b, several of these alterations are common to both aggressive FTC and PTC. Identification of the key molecular events that lead to the development of resistance to standard therapies and anaplastic transformation has been proposed to guide clinical trials for patients with these aggressive FTCs [14].

Pathology

Follicular neoplasms represent a spectrum of tumors characterized by a follicular growth pattern. The accurate diagnosis of FA and FTC poses a challenge even for the most experienced thyroid pathologists. In addition to difficulties distinguishing FA from FTC, accurately diagnosing the follicular variant of PTC (FvPTC) also can be challenging. FvPTC is a histological variant of PTC that has the cytological features of PTC but is characterized by a follicular morphology. It is of interest that this type of PTC has a high frequency of Ras mutations, similar to FA and FTC. Thus, even at the molecular level, there is overlap between FvPTC and FTC. Hurthle cell neoplasms (oxyphil tumor, oncocytoma, mitochondrioma, or Askanazy cell tumor) are considered a variant of FTC according to the World Health Organization (WHO); however, controversy exists regarding their appropriate classification. This group of tumors include Hurthle cell adenomas (HCA), Hurthle cell carcinomas (HCC), and an oncocytic variant of PTC.

FA, FTC and FvPTC usually occur as encapsulated thyroid nodules. The distinction between FA and FTC is based on demonstration of capsular and/or lymphovascular invasion on histological analysis [15] (Table 17.1). The growth pattern of FTC ranges from a well-differentiated pattern with macrofollicular areas to poorly differentiated patterns with areas of solid or nested growth. Unlike PTC, lymphatic metastases are rare in FTC while hematogenous metastases to bone, lungs, brain, and liver are more common. Distant metastases are the principal cause of death from FTC. Up to 25% of patients with FTC develop distant metastases and about 50% of these metastases are present at the time of diagnosis. As in other DTC, immunostains for thyroglobulin (Tg), thyroid transcription factor-1, and cytokeratin (CK)-7 are usually positive in a majority of FTCs while immunostaining for CK-20 is negative in FTC [16].

Based on the type and degree of capsular and vascular invasion, two main types of FTC are recognized: minimally invasive and widely invasive [15] (Table 17.1a). Grossly, the minimally invasive FTC resembles FA; the lesion is well defined and is often encapsulated. The pathological diagnosis of minimally invasive FTC is made when there is microscopic capsular invasion only and often requires examination of multiple histological sections from an individual tumor. Capsular invasion can be limited to or through the capsule into the surrounding thyroid parenchyma. Vascular invasion usually defines non-minimally invasive FTC [17]. Widely invasive FTC is a tumor that is surgically recognized as a cancer due to the extent of invasion grossly obvious in the operating room. Such lesions frequently invade through the thyroid capsule into local structures. Vascular invasion is more typical of more aggressive FTCs and some are characterized by solid, nested,

(a)

Genetic alteration	Well-differentiated thyroid carcinoma	
	Papillary thyroid carcinoma	**Follicular thyroid carcinoma**
RET rearrangement	13–43%	0%
BRAF mutation	29–69%	0%
BRAF rearrangement	1%	Unknown
NTRK1 rearrangement	5–13%	Unknown
Ras mutation	0–21%	40–53%
PPARγ rearrangement	0%	25–63%
CTNNB1 mutation	0%	0%
TP53 mutation	0–5%	0–9%

(b)

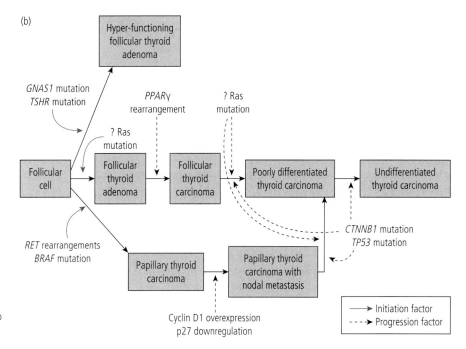

Figure 17.1 Pathogenesis of thyroid cancer. (a) Genetic alterations in differentiated thyroid cancer. Adapted from Kondo [14], with permission from Macmillan Publishers Ltd. (b) Model of multistep thyroid carcinogenesis.

insular, or trabecular growth patterns. Rarely, anaplastic thyroid cancer can be identified in the tumors suggesting that in these cases the anaplastic cancer has arisen from the FTC.

As noted above, FvPTC can be difficult to distinguish from FTC. FvPTC classically presents in two forms: the commonly encountered encapsulated variant that behaves similar to other forms of PTC, and the rare diffuse variant. The latter is mainly seen in young females and extensively involves the thyroid gland. It is usually associated with vascular invasion, extrathyroidal extension, and often distant metastasis to lung and bones.

FA versus FTC

As noted above, preoperative follicular lesion characterization represents an unsolved diagnostic problem in thyroid nodular disease. Although fine needle aspiration (FNA) is the most reliable preoperative diagnostic procedure for thyroid nodules in general, it has inherent limitations in differentiating FA from FTC as this distinction is not based on cytological characteristics. Molecular-based diagnostic strategies are being explored to improve the preoperative diagnosis of FTC by many groups internationally. For example, one recent microarray-based study on surgical samples identified differential expression of cyclin D2, protein convertase 2, and prostate differentiation factor that allowed the accurate molecular classification of FA and FTC. The set of these three genes could differentiate FA from FTC with a sensitivity of 100%, specificity of 95%, and accuracy of 97% [18]. This approach has not yet been applied to FNA samples. Several groups have evaluated the utility of measuring galectin-3 expression to improve the

Table 17.1a Pathological criteria for the diagnosis of follicular carcinoma

Morphological description	Cartoon	Diagnosis
Distinct growth pattern compared with surrounding thyroid parenchyma. No evidence of capsular or vascular invasion		Follicular adenoma
Thickly encapsulated with invasion into the capsule. The focus of invasion is usually mushroom shaped, with a broad base		Minimally invasive follicular carcinoma
Thickly encapsulated with invasion into the capsule and into the surrounding thyroid parenchyma. Tumor is confined to the thyroid and no evidence of vascular invasion		Minimally invasive follicular carcinoma. Tumor is confined to the thyroid
Thickly encapsulated with invasion into the capsular vessel(s) with or without capsular invasion		Angioinvasive follicular carcinoma
Thickly encapsulated nodule with a focus of embedded follicles in the capsule at long axis to the capsule surrounded by hemorrhage and granulation tissue. History of fine needle aspiration		Pseudoinvasion due to fine needle aspiration

Light-shaded area, normal thyroid parenchyma; dark-shaded area, tumor capsule; solid non-shaded area, tumor.
Adapted from LiVolsi [15], with permission from Lippincott Williams & Wilkins.

Table 17.1b TNM staging: American Joint Committee on Cancer (AJCC) stage 2002 classification for thyroid cancer

Primary tumor (T)

Tx	Primary tumor cannot be assessed
T0	Evidence of primary tumor
T1	Tumor 2 cm or less in greatest dimension limited to the thyroid
T2	Tumor more than 2 cm but not more than 4 cm in greatest dimension limited to the thyroid
T3	Tumor more than 4 cm in greatest dimension limited to the thyroid or any tumor with minimal extrathyroidal extension (e.g. extension to sternothyroid muscle or perithyroid soft tissues)
T4a	Tumor of any size extending beyond the thyroid capsule to invade subcutaneous soft tissues, larynx, trachea, esophagus, or recurrent laryngeal nerve
T4b	Tumor invades prevertebral fascia or encases carotid artery or mediastinal vessels

Regional lymph nodes (N)
Regional lymph nodes are the central compartment, lateral cervical, and upper mediastinal lymph nodes

Nx	Regional lymph nodes cannot be assessed
N0	No regional lymph node metastasis
N1	Regional lymph node metastasis
N1a	Metastasis to Level VI (pretracheal, paratracheal, and prelaryngeal/Delphian lymph nodes)
N1b	Metastasis to unilateral, bilateral, or contralateral cervical or superior mediastinal lymph nodes

Metastasis (M)

Mx	Distant metastasis cannot be assessed
M0	No distant metastasis
M1	Distant metastasis

Table 17.1b (*Continued*)

Stage	Age <45 years	Age ≥45 years
Stage I	Any T Any N M0	T1 N0 M0
Stage II	Any T Any N M1	T2 N0 M0
Stage III		T3 N0 M0
		T1 N1a M0
		T2 N1a M0
		T3 N1a M0
Stage IVA		T4a N0 M0
		T4a N1a M0
		T1 N1b M0
		T2 N1b M0
		T3 N1b M0
		T4a N1b M0
Stage IVB		T4b Any N M0
Stage IVC		Any T Any N M1

Used with permission of the American Joint Committee on Cancer (AJCC), Chicago, IL, USA. The original source for this material is the *AJCC Cancer Staging Manual*, 6th edition (2002) published by Springer-New York, www.springeronline.com.

cytological diagnosis. The diagnostic accuracy of preoperative galectin-3 evaluation by immunohistochemistry (IHC) in FA vs FTC was 90% [19]. However, the sensitivity, specificity, positive predictive values, and negative predictive values of galectin-3 staining were 82%, 68%, 75%, and 77%, respectively in another study [20]. IHC for the expression of combinations of proteins, such as galectin-3, fibronectin-1, CITED1, cytokeratin-19, and HBME1, has revealed that co-expression of multiple proteins was seen in 95% of carcinomas and only 5% of adenomas [21]. Furthermore, the detection of human telomerase reverse transcriptase (hTERT) gene expression and telomerase activity in thyroid FNA samples has been identified as a potential diagnostic marker in distinguishing benign and malignant thyroid tumors [22, 23]. Additional research evaluating these markers, and many others, on FNA samples prospectively in the clinical practice setting is needed to determine the true diagnostic accuracy of these methods for the accurate preoperative diagnosis of follicular neoplasias.

Finally, the distinction between FA and FTC also can be challenging in surgical pathology. In addition to the three gene panels noted above, differential expression of p53 (90% of FTC vs 15% of FA), CD44V6 (81% of FTC vs 20% of FA) and CD57 (71% of FTC vs 15% FA) detected by IHC in histological sections may aid in differential diagnosis of FTC vs FA [24].

HCC

Histologically, a Hurthle cell neoplasm is defined as an encapsulated thyroid lesion consisting of at least 75% of Hurthle cells. Hurthle cells are mitochondrion-rich follicular epithelial large polygonal cells with pleomorphic hyperchromatic nuclei and fine granular acidophilic cytoplasm. These cells can be seen in non-tumor benign pathologies, such as Hashimoto thyroiditis, but in these circumstances they do not comprise the majority of the cells in the lesion. Similar to other forms of follicular neoplasia, benign

HCA are not able to be distinguished from HCC based on cellular features, as pleomorphism, hyperchromatism, and atypia are common to both. Thus, like other FTC, the presence of vascular invasion and/or capsular invasion, extrathyroidal tumor spread, and/or metastases is required for the diagnosis of cancer. While hematogenous metastasis to lung, bone brain is observed in 20–30% of FTC as well as HCC, lymph node metastasis are reported to be more common in HCC than other forms of FTC. Despite this higher frequency of nodal metastasis, Finley et al. reported that the molecular profiles of HCA and HCC are more similar to FTC than PTC [25].

Diagnosis

Typically, patients with FTC are asymptomatic, presenting with a palpable lump in the neck noted by a patient or on physical examination, or with a nodule that is incidentally detected by ultrasound. The slow-growing nature of thyroid cancer often leads to delay in obtaining further diagnostic work-up. Clinically and biochemically, most patients are euthyroid and do not have any constitutional symptoms of cancer. Rarely, in patients with advanced stage disease, hoarse voice, dysphagia, hemoptysis, cough, shortness of breath, bone pain or fracture may be present. Patients with bony metastases may develop spinal cord compression requiring urgent diagnostic and/or therapeutic interventions.

Thyroid ultrasound is a critical tool in assessing thyroid nodules as it provides precise size, character, location, and number of nodules. It also makes FNA possible for non-palpable nodules. However, as noted above, follicular lesions are generally indeterminate on FNA, and thyroid surgery is required for a definitive diagnosis. The choice between hemithyroidectomy and total thyroidectomy for patients with follicular lesions on FNA is controversial and is often individualized depending on patient and

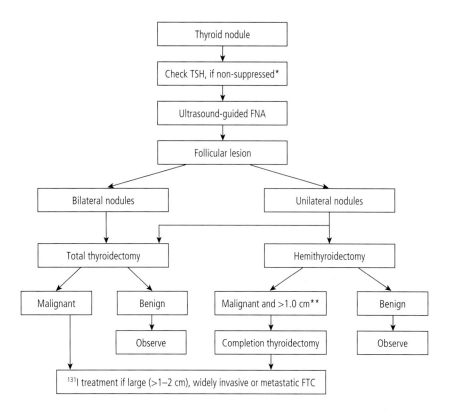

Figure 17.2 Diagnostic algorithm for FTC.
* If TSH is suppressed, perform ^{131}I scan and uptake to determine if nodule is functioning or non-functioning. If non-functioning, proceed with algorithm as above, if functioning, may treat hyperthyroidism and observe the nodule size with ultrasound. ** If FTC is minimally invasive and <1.0 cm, completion thyroidectomy may not be required and the patient can be monitored using ultrasound and Tg levels. LT-$_4$ therapy is administered.

surgeon preferences, the presence or absence of bilateral nodules, and the risks of surgery. As the frequency of FTC in follicular lesions is approximately 15–20%, the patient must be aware of the potential for a second surgery in light of an FTC diagnosis. Conversely, bilateral thyroidectomy in all patients with follicular lesions would expose many patients to increased surgical risk unnecessarily. The effectiveness of intraoperative frozen section for differentiating FA from FTC is variable in the literature and its use to guide intraoperative decisions varies between institutions. A potential diagnostic algorithm for FTC is provided in Fig. 17.2.

The staging work-up for patients with FTC usually includes imaging of the neck using ultrasound; computed tomography (CT) or magnetic resonance imaging (MRI) scan may also be used, particularly in cases where tumors are very large and/or are fixed to local structures or are substernal. Screening for distant metastasis using CT, MRI or positron emission tomography (PET) scanning is typically reserved for high-risk, symptomatic or metastatic FTC cases. Often, distant metastases are identified at the time of radioactive iodine therapy (see below).

Staging and prognostic classification

DTC are among the most curable of all cancers. However, some patients are at high risk of recurrence or even death from their cancer. Among patients with DTC, patients with FTC tend to be older with more advanced stage at the time of diagnosis and have a slightly worse prognosis than patients with PTC. The 10-year survival rates for patients with PTC and FTC were reported as 93% and 85% respectively, in a cohort of 53 856 patients from the National Cancer Data Base in the United States [26]. Similarly, 40-year survival rates for patients with PTC and FTC in 1528 patients treated at the United States Air Force and at the Ohio State University were 94% and 84% respectively [27]. Another study from France reported 10-year survival rates of 80% and 65% for patients with well-differentiated and poorly differentiated FTC respectively [28]. Most of the high-risk patients can be identified at the time of diagnosis using well-established prognostic indicators and staging systems (see below).

Several classification systems such as tumor-node-metastasis (TNM) from the American Joint Committee on Cancer (AJCC), EORTC (age, sex, histological type, extent, metastasis), AMES (age, metastasis, extent, and size), and MACIS (metastasis, age, completeness of resection, invasion, and size) accurately predict cancer-related survival in patients with DTC. In the most widely used TNM staging, all patients younger than 45 years of age with PTC/FTC have stage I or II disease, even those who have distant metastases (Table 17.1b). Older patients (45 years of age or older) with node-negative PTC/FTC are stage I or II while node positives are stage III or IV. Similarly, other prognostic systems include age more than 40 years as a high-risk prognostic factor for cancer-related mortality. It is notable that TNM, EORTC, AMES, and MACIS all provide useful prognostic information about the survival in patients with FTC and a risk stratification schema based on patient and tumor variables has been defined [29]. One retrospective study of 100 FTC patients from the Mayo Clinic reported age greater than 50 years, marked vascular invasion, and metastatic disease at the time of diagnosis as independent predictors of FTC-related mortality. Patients with two or more of these predictors had 5- and 20-year survival rates of 47% and 8%, respectively [30]. In another treatment outcome study 30-year cancer mortality rates were greatest in FTC patients, who were more likely to have adverse prognostic factors: older age, larger tumors, more mediastinal node involvement, and distant metastases [27].

HCC

An individualized treatment approach based on prognostic factors is fundamental for management of HCC given that HCC has an heterogeneous natural history and variable clinical behavior. For early-stage disease, the presence of ≥ 4 foci of vascular invasion has been associated with higher risk of recurrence in encapsulated HCC [31]. The predictors of poor survival reported in various retrospective studies of widely invasive HCC include extrathyroidal extension and nodal metastases [32], older age and larger tumor size [33], and male gender and higher stage of disease [34]. In 56 patients with HCC treated between 1940 and 2000, significant predictors of outcome of HCC were the extent of invasion, size ≥ 4 cm, extrathyroidal extension, and initial nodal or distant metastasis. In this cohort, patients with low-risk cancers did not experience recurrence or die of disease, whereas 73% of high-risk group patients relapsed and 55% died of disease in that time period [35].

Treatment

Due to the long natural history of DTC, no prospective randomized clinical trials exist to guide clinical management. Treatment recommendations are therefore derived from large retrospective cohort studies and are similar for PTC and FTC. Clinical management guidelines for DTC are now offered by a number of organizations, including the American Thyroid Association, the British Thyroid Association, the European Thyroid Association, and the AACE/AAES [36–39]. In general, with the exception of small, minimally invasive FTC, surgery (total or near-total thyroidectomy), TSH suppression therapy, systemic radioactive iodine therapy, and long-term follow-up are the mainstays of management. Multimodality teams including expert pathologists, surgeons, endocrinologists, and nuclear medicine specialists are often involved in management of patients with FTC and traditionally the role of medical oncologists has been peripheral.

Specific sets of principles apply to management of FTC. In patients with FTC:

1 Surgery of the primary tumor is typically performed even in presence of local or distant metastasis.

2 TSH suppressive therapy with LT$_4$ and ^{131}I therapy is utilized for patients with larger or more advanced tumors.

3 A curative goal is realistic in many patients with iodine-avid distant metastasis.

4 Surgery for loco-regional recurrence and ^{131}I therapy for iodine-avid metastatic disease are considered the treatments of choice.

5 Cytotoxic chemotherapy and external beam radiation therapy play secondary roles and are generally used only to palliate the disease.

6 Clinical trials testing novel targeted therapies are good treatment options for patients with iodine-resistant progressive advanced FTC.

7 Long-term follow-up for decades is required for most patients with FTC given that distant metastasis may occasionally be discovered years after initial diagnosis and many patients with distant disease survive for decades.

In general, the above principles also apply for the treatment of patients with HCC. However, given the propensity for HCC to involve regional neck nodes and its relatively low avidity for ^{131}I, a total thyroidectomy with ipsilateral central neck lymphadenectomy has been recommended for patients with HCC with more aggressive resections for individuals with nodal metastasis identified at surgery [40], although performing central neck dissection routinely is controversial. Preoperative mapping of nodes using ultrasound may aid in identifying appropriate compartments for surgery. In comparison to other forms of FTC, HCC is generally believed to be less avid for ^{131}I. The frequency of ^{131}I uptake in HCC reported in the literature varies from <10% to ~50% depending on the study population and perhaps also related to the frequency of iodine deficiency in the region of the center reporting the data. Thus, the use of ^{131}I in patients with HCC is often individualized based on the iodine avidity of the particular tumor.

Surgery

Primary treatment for FTC nearly always includes complete surgical tumor removal. As noted above, follicular neoplasms are usually diagnosed following FNA and thyroid surgery is required for diagnostic purposes in these tumors as 15–20% may be FTC [41]. Based on the intraoperative findings (i.e. gross invasion), the presence or absence of nodules in the opposite lobe, and patient preference, either lobectomy or near-total or total thyroidectomy is performed. With the exception of HCC, lymph node dissection is not routinely performed in patients with FTC due to the low frequency of nodal metastases. If lobectomy is performed and an FTC is diagnosed, a completion thyroidectomy is usually performed with the exception of patients with small, minimally invasive tumors, less than 1 cm in size, although there is considerable debate about the proper size cut-off. Additional reasons to perform completion thyroidectomy in patients with higher risk FTC are to facilitate subsequent use of ^{131}I and to improve the use of serum Tg and imaging for monitoring. Ablation of an entire remnant lobe for early-stage FTC has been reported and can be used for selected cases [42]. The drawbacks of bilateral initial surgery include a greater risk of recurrent laryngeal nerve damage or hypoparathyroidism. These risks should always be discussed with patients prior to devising a treatment strategy following a follicular neoplasm diagnosis on FNA as most patients will ultimately have a benign thyroid nodule.

TSH suppressive therapy

Long-term thyroid hormone replacement therapy is used not only to treat postthyroidectomy hypothyroidism, but also to decrease serum TSH to a level that reduces the risk of TSH-stimulated growth of any remaining thyroid cancer cells while minimizing potential deleterious effects of thyrotoxicosis. The side effects are particularly relevant in older patients with cardiac disease or patients with osteoporosis due to the effects of thyrotoxicosis on the heart and bone. Retrospective cohort studies have suggested an association between the degree of TSH suppression and a lower risk of recurrence for patients with more advanced PTC and FTC [43]. Based on these and other similar data, it has been recommended that the level of TSH for patients with FTC should be individualized based on the presence or absence of disease and risk of recurrence [36, 38]. In general, circulating TSH concentrations are suppressed to <0.1 mIU/L for patients with persistent or high-risk disease or for the first several years after diagnosis for patients with lower risk tumors. It is likely acceptable to reduce the degree of TSH suppression to maintain levels in the detectable but low or low-normal range for patients in complete remission for prolonged periods of time, particularly if they have low-risk primary tumors or are at risk of complications of long-term iatrogenic thyrotoxicosis.

Systemic ^{131}I therapy

^{131}I is one of the key treatment modalities for patients with FTCs, particularly when they are larger than 1–2 cm, widely invasive, and/or metastatic. After initial surgery, ^{131}I is used to destroy residual thyroid tissue (remnant thyroid ablation) and any metastatic tissue that may be present. In addition, remnant ablative ^{131}I improves the ability to detect persistent or progressive thyroid cancer using thyroglobulin monitoring and radioiodine scanning [44]. Due to the outstanding prognosis of patients with early-stage FTCs, especially those small, minimally invasive tumors, adjuvant therapy with ^{131}I is generally not recommended.

An association between reduced recurrence and mortality rates and ^{131}I remnant ablation therapy has been demonstrated in patients with high-risk FTC. For example, in one study that evaluated 82 high-risk FTC patients of which 71% received ^{131}I therapy [45], those treated with ^{131}I had significant improvement in overall mortality [relative risk (RR) 0.17, confidence interval (CI) 0.06–0.47], cancer-specific mortality (RR 0.12, CI 0.04–0.42), progression (RR 0.21, CI 0.08–0.56), and disease-free survival (RR 0.29, CI 0.08–1.01). In this study, it was not possible to clearly define contribution of surgery in the therapeutic benefit noted in the above studies. These data and data from other retrospective studies evaluating the role of ^{131}I in FTC in general support the use of remnant ablation in patients with high-risk FTC. A recent consensus report from a panel of experts from 13 European countries advocated use of remnant ablation therapy in DTC patients (including FTC) with distant metastases, incomplete tumor resection, or complete tumor resection but high-risk histological

features [46]. Probable indications for remnant ablation in this report included patients with tumors >1 cm and with suboptimal surgery (less than total thyroidectomy or no lymph node dissection), with age <16 years, or with unfavorable histology. Doses for remnant ablation for FTC typically are chosen empirically based on the stage of the tumor and generally range from 1.1 to 5.5 GBq (30 to 150 mCi), although dosimetric calculations, if available, are occasionally employed.

TSH stimulation is required prior to diagnostic radioactive WBS or ^{131}I therapy to optimize the transport and retention of radioiodine. Endogenous TSH stimulation (TSH of >30 mIU/L) can be promoted by inducing hypothyroidism by discontinuing LT$_4$ therapy for approximately 5 weeks. Some clinicians prefer to initiate therapy with liothyronine (T$_3$) for the first 2–3 weeks of the LT$_4$ withdrawal followed by withdrawal of T$_3$ for 2 weeks to potentially reduce the duration of hypothyroid symptoms. Administration of exogenous recombinant human thyrotropin (rhTSH) is an alternative method for TSH stimulation that is effective for stimulation of Tg and diagnostic scanning. Advantages of rhTSH are primarily related to avoidance of the symptoms of severe hypothyroidism. However, it is important to recognize that the use of rhTSH for therapeutic administration of ^{131}I is not approved by the Food and Drug Administration in the United States. A recent randomized, controlled, multicenter trial has suggested similar efficacy of remnant ablation following rhTSH administration compared with hypothyroid preparation, although long-term outcomes have not been reported and the number of patients with FTC in this study was small [47]. In addition to TSH stimulation, a low-iodine diet with iodine intake of 50 µg/day is typically prescribed for 2 weeks before therapy.

For patients with FTC treated with ^{131}I for persistent or recurrent/metastatic disease, patients can be treated with empiric fixed doses, or the dose can be determined using whole-body or quantitative tumor dosimetry. Among these, empiric fixed dosing is the most widely employed method with doses most frequently ranging from 3.7 to 7.4 GBq (100 to 200 mCi). Pre- and posttreatment whole body scans (WBS) are generally performed at the time of the ^{131}I therapy, although some investigators no longer perform a pretherapy scan to avoid "stunning" of thyroid cancer tissue with the diagnostic dose. Posttherapy scanning is usually performed 5–10 days after the ^{131}I treatment to localize and confirm the iodine avidity of metastatic foci. Due to the higher dose of ^{131}I given during therapy versus the pretherapy scan, additional metastatic foci are occasionally detected on the posttherapy scan. Occasionally, patients with widely metastatic FTC can develop hyperthyroidism from functional metastases, making endogenous TSH stimulation difficult. These patients often have highly iodine-avid distant metastases [48].

^{131}I therapy is generally well tolerated compared with most forms of cancer therapy. Acute side effects of ^{131}I include sialadenitis, xerostomia, loss of taste, and lacrimal duct stenosis. Chronic or cumulative side effects include damage to salivary glands, gonads, bone marrow, lungs and rarely, secondary malignancies including leukemia, bladder cancer, and others [36]. These side effects, as well as radiation safety precautions, should be discussed in detail with the patient prior to dose administration.

Long-term follow-up

As patients with FTC can occasionally progress or recur years after the initial diagnosis, long-term monitoring is appropriate. This is achieved by serial measurements of TSH-suppressed or -stimulated serum Tg combined with various imaging techniques such as ^{131}I WBS and neck ultrasound. The frequency and intensity of monitoring depend on the risk of recurrence as defined by tumor stage, time since diagnosis, level of differentiation, and response to initial therapy.

Serum Tg measurement is the most sensitive tumor marker for detecting residual FTC and PTC and is valuable for follow-up of persistent metastatic disease. Serum Tg levels are only valid in the absence of potentially interfering anti-Tg antibodies in the serum sample. Thus, anti-Tg antibody levels should be measured on each serum Tg sample. Optimally, serial serum Tg measurement should be measured with a consistent assay. Serum Tg levels should be interpreted in the context of the clinical scenario. For example, levels of serum Tg may not be reflective of tumor burden in patients with poorly differentiated histologies due to reduced Tg production. In addition, rarely, an inappropriately normal or low Tg concentration may be measured due to extremely high serum Tg concentrations ("hook effect"). Despite these caveats, in most FTC patients without measurable anti-Tg antibodies, serum Tg levels have become the most important tool for detecting and monitoring for recurrent FTC.

In general, following initial therapy, serum Tg levels are measured during TSH suppression therapy. If the levels remain detectable after 6–12 months, patients are presumed to have residual thyroid tissue and imaging is performed, most frequently with neck ultrasound, but occasionally with other modalities, such as neck and chest CT scanning, MRI, and PET/CT imaging, if the Tg level is very elevated or the patient has high-risk disease. If CT scans are performed, avoidance of iodinated intravenous contrast is preferable if additional radioactive iodine (RAI) is to be administered. Assessing for distant metastasis is more frequently employed in patients with FTC than PTC due to its greater predilection for distant metastases. For patients with an undetectable Tg on TSH suppression, a TSH-stimulated Tg is generally obtained using rhTSH or LT_4 withdrawal to enhance the sensitivity of Tg measurement. Recent data suggest that such testing may obviate the need for diagnostic ^{131}I WBS. Neck ultrasound is generally also frequently performed by an experienced operator. It is important to note that there is greater reliance on radiographic imaging in patients with anti-Tg antibodies (approximately 15–20% of patients). The loss of detectable anti-Tg antibodies over time has been shown to correlate with reduced tumor burden for DTC; thus following levels of Tg and anti-Tg antibody is generally still a component of monitoring [49]. The frequency of follow-up studies needs to be individualized based on the results of initial testing and the number of years since the initial diagnosis.

Management of advanced disease

As distant metastases are more common in FTC than PTC, systemic ^{131}I therapy using empiric or dosimetrically calculated doses remains the first-line treatment for many patients with metastatic FTC. Multiple doses are sometimes administered over time to achieve a complete remission. Side effects, as described above, may be cumulative, thus patients require close monitoring to assess the risks of additional therapies. Based on the limited short-lasting response rates with potential for significant toxicity, systemic cytotoxic chemotherapy has limited value even in iodine-refractory thyroid cancer. If there is no uptake on the posttherapy WBS, or if the metastases progress in size or number despite demonstrable iodine uptake, clinical trial participation is strongly recommended for such patients (http://www.thyroidtrials.org).

While cervical recurrences are less common in FTC than PTC, surgery remains the treatment of choice for resectable locoregional recurrences when they do occur. This is often performed in combination with ^{131}I if the tissue is iodine avid. [131]I may also be employed alone in these circumstances. Less commonly, external beam radiation therapy or nodal or mass injection with sclerosing agents such as ethanol is employed in individuals with unresectable cervical disease. These therapies are most typically used to stabilize the progressive disease or control locally aggressive or poorly differentiated primary or recurrent tumor masses.

As for all solid malignancies, the presence of distant metastasis in FTC is a poor prognostic factor. However, several factors play a role in defining survival of such patients. A retrospective study in 242 patients with distant metastasis from DTC (36% of patients with FTC in this cohort) identified age 45 years or more, presence of symptoms, site other than lung only or bone only, and no RAI treatment for the metastasis as predictors of poor outcome with 13%, 11%, 16%, and 12% 10-year disease specific survival if one of the factors was present, respectively [50].

Lung and bone metastasis are common in patients with FTC. The size of pulmonary nodules, degree of radioiodine avidity, and pace of progression affect prognosis and the choice of therapy. When iodine avid and when the rate of progression is not rapid, repeated and/or high doses of ^{131}I may be administered in an effort to cure or control the FTC, or patients can be monitored without additional therapy. For symptomatic or rapidly enlarging isolated lesions in bones or the lungs, external beam X-ray therapy, local surgery, and/or embolization are usually recommended for palliation. Bisphosphonates such as pamidronate or zolendronic acid may be used, particularly in patients wtih bone metastases. Brain metastases in patients with FTC are uncommon but the overall survival of such patients is reported to be longer than that noted with other solid tumors (17.4 months), and the majority of patients die of their extracranial disease [51]. Local therapies including surgery, external beam X-ray therapy, and Gamma

Table 17.2 Novel agents in Phase II clinical trials for differentiated thyroid cancer

Class of therapy	Putative targets of the therapy	Name of drugs	Status of Phase II clinical trials in patients with DTC
Antiangiogenic drugs (oral kinase inhibitors)	VEGF receptors, PDGF receptors	AG-013736(axitinib) AMG-706 (motesanib) BAY 43-9006 (sorafenib)	Accrual completed, final results awaited
		GW786034 (pazopanib) SU011248 (sunitinib) ZD6474 (vandetanib)	Accrual to start soon or ongoing
Signaling pathway inhibitors	RAS-RAF-MEK signaling pathway	BAY 43-9006 (sorafenib)	As noted above
		AZD 6244	Accrual to start soon
Histone deacetylase inhibitors	Histone deacetylation	Depsipeptide SAHA (vorinostat)	Accrual completed, final results awaited
Demethylating agents	Methylation	Decitabine	Accrual ongoing
Ansamycin antibiotic	Heat shock protein 90	17-AAG	Accrual ongoing
Proteasome inhibitor	Proteasome	PS-341 (bortezomib)	Accrual ongoing
Cytotoxic chemotherapy	DNA alkylating or antimetabolite	Irofulven and capecitabine	Completed
Cyclo-oxygenase (COX) inhibitor	COX-2	Celecoxib	Completed

Knife radiosurgery appear to control brain metastases in the large majority of DTC patients with metastases to the brain.

Future directions in management of FTC

Novel compounds targeted against molecular pathways involved in DTC initiation and progression are being tested at the preclinical levels and in clinical trials (Table 17.2). It is important to recognize that patients with FTC represent only a small population of the cohort of DTC patients in these studies. In early reports, kinase inhibitors targeting angiogenesis appear to show biological and clinical activity in patients with DTC [52–54]. As knowledge of thyroid cancer biology is rapidly expanding and a plethora of targeted therapies are being developed, these new agents hold great promise for patients with progressive FTC that do not respond to traditional therapy.

References

1. Reynolds RM, Weir J, Stockton DL, Brewster DH, Sandeep TC, Strachan MW. Changing trends in incidence and mortality of thyroid cancer in Scotland. *Clin. Endocrinol. (Oxf.)* 2005;62:156–162.
2. Davies L, Welch HG. Increasing incidence of thyroid cancer in the United States, 1973–2002. *JAMA.* 2006;295:2164–2167.
3. Jossart GH, Clark OH. Well-differentiated thyroid cancer. *Curr. Probl. Surg.* 1994;31:933–1012.
4. Ward JM, Ohshima M. The role of iodine in carcinogenesis. *Adv. Exp. Med. Biol.* 1986;206:529–542.
5. Belfiore A, La Rosa GL, Padova G, Sava L, Ippolito O, Vigneri R. The frequency of cold thyroid nodules and thyroid malignancies in patients from an iodine-deficient area. *Cancer* 1987;60:3096–3102.
6. Huszno B, Szybinski Z, Przybylik-Mazurek E, et al. Influence of iodine deficiency and iodine prophylaxis on thyroid cancer histotypes and incidence in endemic goiter area. *J. Endocrinol. Invest.* 2003;26(2 Suppl):71–76.
7. Nelen MR, Padberg GW, Peeters EA, et al. Localization of the gene for Cowden disease to chromosome 10q22–23. *Nat. Genet.* 1996;13:114–116.
8. Kirschner LS, Carney JA, Pack SD, et al. Mutations of the gene encoding the protein kinase A type I-alpha regulatory subunit in patients with the Carney complex. *Nat. Genet.* 2000;26:89–92.
9. Yu CE, Oshima J, Fu YH, et al. Positional cloning of the Werner's syndrome gene. *Science* 1996;272:258–262.
10. Aldred MA, Ginn-Pease ME, Morrison CD, et al. Caveolin-1 and caveolin-2,together with three bone morphogenetic protein-related genes, may encode novel tumor suppressors down-regulated in sporadic follicular thyroid carcinogenesis. *Cancer Res.* 2003;63:2864–2871.
11. Xing M, Cohen Y, Mambo E, et al. Early occurrence of RASSF1A hypermethylation and its mutual exclusion with BRAF mutation in thyroid tumorigenesis. *Cancer Res.* 2004;64:1664–1668.
12. Xing M, Usadel H, Cohen Y, et al. Methylation of the thyroid-stimulating hormone receptor gene in epithelial thyroid tumors: a marker of malignancy and a cause of gene silencing. *Cancer Res.* 2003;63:2316–2321.

13. Weber F, Teresi RE, Broelsch CE, Frilling A, Eng C. A limited set of human MicroRNA is deregulated in follicular thyroid carcinoma. *J. Clin. Endocrinol. Metab.* 2006;91:3584–3591.

14. Kondo T, Ezzat S, Asa SL. Pathogenetic mechanisms in thyroid follicular–cell neoplasia. *Nat. Rev. Cancer.* 2006;6:292–306.

15. LiVolsi VA, Baloch ZW. Follicular neoplasms of the thyroid: view, biases, and experiences. *Adv. Anat. Pathol.* 2004;11:279–287.

16. Bejarano PA, Nikiforov YE, Swenson ES, Biddinger PW. Thyroid transcription factor-1, thyroglobulin, cytokeratin 7, and cytokeratin 20 in thyroid neoplasms. *Appl. Immunohistochem. Mol. Morphol.* 2000;8:189–194.

17. van Heerden JA, Hay ID, Goellner JR, et al. Follicular thyroid carcinoma with capsular invasion alone: a nonthreatening malignancy. *Surgery* 1992;112:1130–1136; discussion 6–8.

18. Weber F, Shen L, Aldred MA, et al. Genetic classification of benign and malignant thyroid follicular neoplasia based on a three-gene combination. *J. Clin. Endocrinol. Metab.* 2005;90:2512–2521.

19. Saggiorato E, Aversa S, Deandreis D, et al. Galectin-3: presurgical marker of thyroid follicular epithelial cell–derived carcinomas. *J. Endocrinol. Invest.* 2004;27:311–317.

20. Oestreicher-Kedem Y, Halpern M, Roizman P, et al. Diagnostic value of galactin-3 as a marker for malignancy in follicular patterned thyroid lesions. *Head Neck.* 2004;26:960–966.

21. Prasad ML, Pellegata NS, Huang Y, Nagaraja HN, de la Chapelle A, Kloos RT. Galectin-3, fibronectin-1, CITED-1, HBME1 and cytokeratin-19 immunohistochemistry is useful for the differential diagnosis of thyroid tumors. *Mod. Pathol.* 2005;18:48–57.

22. Haugen BR, Nawaz S, Markham N, et al. Telomerase activity in benign and malignant thyroid tumors. *Thyroid* 1997;7:337–342.

23. Liou MJ, Chan EC, Lin JD, Liu FH, Chao TC. Human telomerase reverse transcriptase (hTERT) gene expression in FNA samples from thyroid neoplasms. *Cancer Lett.* 2003;191:223–227.

24. Nasir A, Catalano E, Calafati S, Cantor A, Kaiser HE, Coppola D. Role of p53, CD44V6 and CD57 in differentiating between benign and malignant follicular neoplasms of the thyroid. *In Vivo* 2004;18:189–195.

25. Finley DJ, Zhu B, Fahey TJ, 3rd. Molecular analysis of Hurthle cell neoplasms by gene profiling. *Surgery* 2004;136:1160–1168.

26. Hundahl SA, Fleming ID, Fremgen AM, Menck HR. A National Cancer Data Base report on 53,856 cases of thyroid carcinoma treated in the US, 1985–1995 see comments. *Cancer* 1998;83:2638–2648.

27. Mazzaferri EL, Jhiang SM. Long-term impact of initial surgical and medical therapy on papillary and follicular thyroid cancer. *Am. J. Med.* 1994;97:418–428.

28. Schlumberger MJ. Papillary and follicular thyroid carcinoma. *N. Engl. J. Med.* 1998;338:297–306.

29. Mazzaferri EL, Kloos RT. Clinical review 128: current approaches to primary therapy for papillary and follicular thyroid cancer. *J. Clin. Endocrinol. Metab.* 2001;86:1447–1463.

30. Brennan MD, Bergstralh EJ, van Heerden JA, McConahey WM. Follicular thyroid cancer treated at the Mayo Clinic, 1946 through 1970: initial manifestations, pathologic findings, therapy, and outcome. *Mayo Clin. Proc.* 1991;66:11–22.

31. Ghossein RA, Hiltzik DH, Carlson DL, et al. Prognostic factors of recurrence in encapsulated Hurthle cell carcinoma of the thyroid gland: a clinicopathologic study of 50 cases. *Cancer* 2006;106:1669–1676.

32. Stojadinovic A, Ghossein RA, Hoos A, et al. Hurthle cell carcinoma: a critical histopathologic appraisal. *J. Clin. Oncol.* 2001;19:2616–2625.

33. Lopez-Penabad L, Chiu AC, Hoff AO, et al. Prognostic factors in patients with Hurthle cell neoplasms of the thyroid. *Cancer* 2003;97:1186–1194.

34. Kushchayeva Y, Duh QY, Kebebew E, Clark OH. Prognostic indications for Hurthle cell cancer. *World J. Surg.* 2004;28:1266–1270.

35. Stojadinovic A, Hoos A, Ghossein RA, et al. Hurthle cell carcinoma: a 60-year experience. *Ann. Surg. Oncol.* 2002;9:197–203.

36. Cooper DS, Doherty GM, Haugen BR, et al. Management guidelines for patients with thyroid nodules and differentiated thyroid cancer. *Thyroid* 2006;16:109–142.

37. Guidelines for the management of thyroid cancer in adults. http://wwwbritish–thyroid-associationorg. 2002.

38. Pacini F, Schlumberger M, Dralle H, Elisei R, Smit JW, Wiersinga W. European consensus for the management of patients with differentiated thyroid carcinoma of the follicular epithelium. *Eur. J. Endocrinol.* 2006;154:787–803.

39. American Association of Clinical Endocrinologists and Associazione Medici Endocrinologic medical guidelines for clinical practice for the diagnosis and management of thyroid nodules. *Endocr. Pract.* 2006;12:63–102.

40. Yutan E, Clark OH. Hurthle cell carcinoma. *Curr. Treat. Opt. Oncol.* 2001;2:331–335.

41. Carling T, Udelsman R. Follicular neoplasms of the thyroid: what to recommend. *Thyroid* 2005;15:583–587.

42. Randolph GW, Daniels GH. Radioactive iodine lobe ablation as an alternative to completion thyroidectomy for follicular carcinoma of the thyroid. *Thyroid* 2002;12:989–996.

43. Cooper DS, Specker B, Ho M, et al. Thyrotropin suppression and disease progression in patients with differentiated thyroid cancer: results from the National Thyroid Cancer Treatment Cooperative Registry. *Thyroid* 1998;8:737–744.

44. Woodrum DT, Gauger PG. Role of 131I in the treatment of well differentiated thyroid cancer. *J. Surg. Oncol.* 2005;89:114–121.

45. Taylor T, Specker B, Robbins J, et al. Outcome after treatment of high-risk papillary and non–Hurthle–cell follicular thyroid carcinoma. *Ann. Intern. Med.* 1998;129:622–627.

46. Pacini F, Schlumberger M, Harmer C, et al. Post-surgical use of radioiodine (131I) in patients with papillary and follicular thyroid cancer and the issue of remnant ablation: a consensus report. *Eur. J. Endocrinol.* 2005;153:651–659.

47. Pacini F, Ladenson PW, Schlumberger M, et al. Radioiodine ablation of thyroid remnants after preparation with recombinant human thyrotropin in differentiated thyroid carcinoma: results of an international, randomized, controlled study. *J. Clin. Endocrinol. Metab.* 2006;91:926–932.

48. McLaughlin RP, Scholz DA, McConahey WM, Childs DS, Jr. Metastatic thyroid carcinoma with hyperthyroidism: two cases with functioning metastatic follicular thyroid carcinoma. *Mayo Clin. Proc.* 1970;45:328–335.

49. Spencer CA, Takeuchi M, Kazarosyan M, et al. Serum thyroglobulin autoantibodies: prevalence, influence on serum thyroglobulin measurement, and prognostic significance in patients with differentiated thyroid carcinoma. *J. Clin. Endocrinol. Metab.* 1998;83:1121–1127.

50. Shoup M, Stojadinovic A, Nissan A, et al. Prognostic indicators of outcomes in patients with distant metastases from differentiated thyroid carcinoma. *J. Am. Coll. Surg.* 2003;197:191–197.

51. McWilliams RR, Giannini C, Hay ID, Atkinson JL, Stafford SL, Buckner JC. Management of brain metastases from thyroid carcinoma: a study of 16 pathologically confirmed cases over 25 years. *Cancer* 2003;98:356–362.

52. Kim S, Rosen LS, Cohen EE, et al. A Phase II study of axitinib (AG-013736), a potent inhibitor of VEGFRs, in patients with advanced thyroid cancer. *J. Clin. Oncol.* 2006;(24 No. 18S Abst): 5529.

53. Boughton D, Rosen L, Van Vugt A, et al. Safety and antitumor activity of AMG 706 in patients (pts) with thyroid cancer (TC): a subset analysis from a phase 1 dose-finding study. *J. Clin. Oncol.* 2006;(24 No. 18S Abst):3030.

54. Kloos RT, Ringel MD, Knopp M, et al. Significant clinical and biologic activity of RAF/VEGF-R kinase inhibitor BAY 43-9006 in patients with metastatic papillary thyroid carcinoma (PTC): updated results of a phase II study. *J. Clin. Oncol.* 2006;(24 No. 18S Abst):5534.

18 Anaplastic Thyroid Carcinoma

Richard T. Kloos

Key points
- Anaplastic thyroid cancer is an uncommon, typically lethal malignancy of older adults with no effective systemic therapy.
- The mean survival time is usually around 6 months from diagnosis, an outcome that is typically not altered by treatment.
- Histological confirmation is recommended if the diagnosis is not absolutely certain to exclude tumors with better prognosis or requiring different treatment.
- A few patients with completely resectable disease demonstrate long-term survival.
- Airway patency must be kept in mind throughout the course of the patient's care and those with impending obstruction without imminent death from other sites of disease require a procedure to secure the airway, such as tracheostomy.
- Clinical trials should be given the highest priority at all decision points.

Introduction

Anaplastic thyroid cancer (ATC) is an uncommon, mostly lethal malignancy of older adults with no effective systemic therapy. The mean survival time is around 6 months from diagnosis [1], an outcome that is frequently not altered by treatment. While the usual diagnosis and treatment of ATC should be considered a medical urgency, end of life planning to optimize the quality of the patient's remaining life must also be given a high priority. A few patients with completely resectable disease demonstrate long-term survival.

Epidemiology and tumor characteristics

Wordwide experience

The annual incidence of ATC is about 1–2 cases/million, with the overall incidence being higher in Europe (and areas of endemic goiter) than in the US [2]. From a sample of 53 856 thyroid carcinomas registered in the US between 1985 and 1995 in the National Cancer Data Base, 80% were papillary (PTC), 11% follicular (FTC), 3% Hürthle cell, 3% medullary (MTC), and 2% were undifferentiated/anaplastic [3]. Similar rates and incidence of ATC were reported in Japan and Norway [4, 5]. This percentage may be expected to decrease with the rising diagnosis of incidental differentiated thyroid carcinomas (DTC) [6]. Further, the

Clinical Endocrine Oncology, 2nd edition. Edited by Ian D. Hay and John A.H. Wass. © 2008 Blackwell Publishing. ISBN 978-1-4051-4584-8.

incidence of ATC has been declining worldwide [1], possibly related to reclassification of small cell ATC as lymphoma or undifferentiated MTC, the removal of insular carcinoma as an ATC variant, the decreased incidence of FTC from increased dietary iodine, and the overall earlier diagnosis and treatment of DTC when it is at a lower stage of disease which may eliminate its opportunity to undergo dedifferentiation.

ATC typically presents in the seventh decade of life [1, 7–10], although children with ATC have been reported [8, 11]. Hadar et al. noted that 90% of patients are older than 50 years [12]. The female:male ratio is often between 1.5–2:1 [1, 7–10]. The mean tumor size is usually 6–9 cm [1, 7–9]. The tumor is confined to the thyroid in 0–9% [8–10, 13], lymph node metastases or extrathyroidal extension in the absence of distant metastases are present in 53–64% [8, 9, 13], and distant metastases are present in a quarter to two-thirds of patients [7, 13]. About one-quarter of patients develop distant metastases during the course of their disease [1]. The most common sites of distant metastases in descending order are the lungs (~80%), then bone, skin, and brain (each ~5–15%) [14]. Less common metastatic sites include the heart and abdomen [2, 8–11].

The Ohio State University and Arthur G. James Cancer Hospital experience

ATC has represented 1.4% of the last 1184 patients who underwent all or part of their first course of treatment at this medical center (R.T. Kloos, unpublished data). Women outnumbered men 3:1 and the mean age at diagnosis was 70 years. For non-ATC cases, women outnumbered men 2.6:1 and the mean age at diagnosis was 45 years (Fig. 18.1). Indeed, none of the ATC cases was less than 45 years old and only 25% were less than 60 years old compared to 52% and 79%, respectively, for the non-ATC cases. Twenty-five percent of

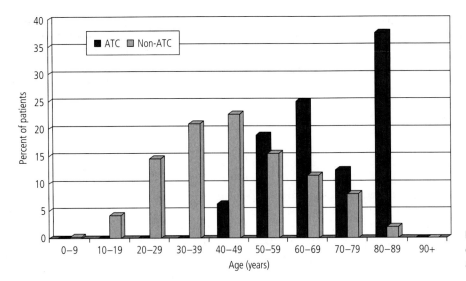

Figure 18.1 Age distribution of the last 1184 consecutive thyroid cancer cases including 16 ATC and 1168 non-ATC cases.

the ATC cases were <7 cm compared to 82% for the non-ATC cases, and 44% of the ATC cases presented with distant metastases compared to only 5% for the non-ATC cases.

Etiology

While it is possible (but not established) that ATC may arise *de novo*, it is generally accepted that ATC may develop from pre existing DTC (PTC or FTC). Indeed, in a study of 161 patients who died from thyroid cancer, 99 had ATC at the time of death while only 62 had this diagnosis at their initial thyroid cancer presentation [15]. About one-quarter to one-half of patients with ATC have a previous or concurrent DTC history [1, 7, 9, 10, 15, 16]. Unique molecular signature events support the idea that ATC may derive from PTC or FTC. For example, PTC initiating BRAF mutations are present in approximately 44% of PTC and are absent in FTC, MTC, and benign neoplasms while they are present in 24% of ATC [17].

Presentation

ATC almost always presents with a rapidly growing fixed and hard neck mass, often with metastatic local lymph nodes appreciable on examination and/or vocal cord paralysis [9, 11]. About one-quarter of cases present as sudden enlargement of a pre-existing thyroid mass or goiter over the previous few weeks or months [7, 9, 13].

Symptoms may reflect rapid growth of the tumor with local invasion and/or compression. Giuffrida and Gharib reported that in a series of 84 consecutive ATC patients, a single nodule was present in 58%, multiple nodules in 36%, bilateral involvement in 24%, and a hard and fixed lesion was present in 75% [2]. The most frequent presenting signs and symptoms included hoarseness (77%), dysphagia (56%), vocal cord paralysis (49%), neck pain (29%), weight loss (24%), dyspnea (19%), and stridor (11%) [2]. Occasionally, thyrotoxicosis from local thyroid destruction is prsent [18]. Tennvall et al. reported that the median duration of symptoms prior to diagnosis was 1.5 months (range 0–8 months) [13].

Cause of death

In a series of 62 patients who presented with ATC and died of their disease, a single specific cause of death could not be identified in 40% because either serious conditions developed simultaneously in multiple organs, or general weakness progressed gradually without specific verified organ failure (cachexia) [15]. In those with a specific cause of death, 35% died from replacement of lung tissue by extensive pulmonary metastases (while 86% had or developed pulmonary metastases), airway obstruction in 16%, tumor-related hemorrhage in 14%, cardiac failure in 11%, 5% from tumor-related pneumonia or disseminated intravascular coagulation from necrotic tumor infection, and 3% from circulatory failure due to vena cava stenosis, cardiac metastases, neutropenic sepsis related to treatment, renal failure, or humoral hypercalcemia of malignancy [15]. The tumor sites mainly responsible for death included both local and distant metastases in 40%, local disease in 34%, distant metastases in 24%, and treatment in 2%.

Diagnosis and histology

ATC histological patterns include giant cell, spindle cell, and squamoid cell [2]. These subtypes frequently co-exist and are not predictive of patient outcome. Areas of necrosis and hemorrhage are common, and mitotic activity is high. Two uncommon ATC variants include the paucicellular variant, which may be confused with Riedel's struma, and a variant including large regions of osteo-sarcomatous differentiation (carcinosarcoma) [11].

Spindled or giant cells, bizarre neoplastic cells that may be multinucleated, or atypical cells with high mitotic activity on fine needle aspiration (FNA) cytology suggest ATC. Histological confirmation is recommended if the diagnosis is not absolutely certain to exclude tumors with better prognoses or that require different therapy including poorly differentiated thyroid cancer, MTC, primary thyroid lymphoma, poorly differentiated metastasis to the thyroid, primary squamous cell carcinoma, and angiomatoid thyroid neoplasms [11]. Tennvall et al. reported that 4% of patients referred for ATC based on FNA cytology were found to have discrepant histological findings at surgery (although they argue that surgical biopsy unnecessarily delays initiation of neoadjuvant chemo-radiation therapy) [13].

ATC usually does not express thyroglobulin, thus this protein cannot be used as a tumor marker for diagnosis or monitoring. Cytokeratin (keratin) may be the most useful immunohistochemical marker, and is present in 40–100% of tumors [2]. Other markers suggesting the epithelial origin of the tumor may be epithelial membrane antigen and carcinoembryonic antigen [2]. Other immunohistochemical markers that may be helpful include vimentin, α-1-chymotrypsin, and desmin [1]. The spindle cell variant may be differentiated from sarcoma with immunostaining to anticytokeratin antibodies [1]. Lymphomas do not have the marked cellular pleomorphism that is typical of ATC, and MTC may be recognized by immunohistochemical staining for neuron-specific enolase, chromogranin, and calcitonin.

Staging and prognostic features

Because of their aggressive behavior, all ATCs are classified as T4 and Stage IV tumors by the *AJCC Cancer Staging Manual*, 6th edition. T4a tumors are intrathyroidal – surgically resectable, while T4b tumors are extrathyroidal – surgically unresectable. Stage IV is subdivided as Stage IVA: T4a, any N, M0; Stage IVB: T4b, any N, M0; and Stage IVC: any T, any N, M1.

In a series of 121 ATC patients, Kim et al. [8] reported that the median survival time was 5.1 months. The overall cause-specific survival was 42% at 6 months, 16% at 12 months, and 9% at 24 months. Multivariate analysis suggested that age less than 60 years, tumor size less than 7 cm, and lesser extent of disease were independent predictors of lower cause-specific mortality. Others have also reported that smaller tumor size (<5–6 cm) is of prognostic importance [19–23]. Hundahl et al. reported that the 1-, 2-, 3-, and 5-year survival rates among 893 undifferentiated/anaplastic carcinomas were 23%, 18%, 15%, and 14%, respectively [3]. Age less than 45 years and small tumor size (and possibly absence of extrathyroidal extension) were more common among those that survived 5 years or more. For example, the 5-year survival rates for those aged <45 years was 55%, while it was 13% for all age groups by decade above age 45 years. Pierie et al. reported that age ≤70 years was an independent predictor of survival [20]. Venkatesh et al. also reported that younger patients survived longer than older patients, and noted that patients presenting

with evidence of only local disease had a median survival of 8 months compared to a median survival of just over 3 months when distant metastases were present [16]. In contrast, however, Haigh et al. found that neither age nor tumor size was associated with survival [7]. Rather, the only variable associated with prolonged survival after multivariate analysis was potentially curative surgery.

Therapy

Treatment options include surgery, external beam radiation therapy (EBRT), tracheostomy, chemotherapy, and investigational clinical trials. The value of these treatment options, and the order and combination in which they are given, must be carefully evaluated in terms of their ability to promote quality of life, to prolong survival, and to reduce tumor-specific mortality. Unfortunately, the data are not convincing that any treatment strategy reduces tumor-specific mortality other than the rare patient cured by surgical resection. Further, it is not clear that survival is prolonged by therapy other than palliative treatments such as those that prevent strangulation. It is impossible to accurately discern the benefits of the many uncontrolled treatment trials because of the potential confounding influences of age, sex [1, 23], tumor size, extent of local invasion and resectability, influence of surgical resection, and the extent of disease. For instance, trials that demonstrate longer survival for patients who respond to EBRT compared to those that do not respond may support the use of EBRT. Alternatively, the response to EBRT may have simply identified less aggressive radiosensitive tumors that were destined to behave less aggressively than their radioresistant counterparts and their improved survival may have been independent of the treatment.

Surgery

Surgical treatment of local disease is currently the best hope for prolonged survival if the tumor is intrathyroidal. Still, some have found that neither the extent of the operation nor the completeness of the tumor resection affects survival [10]. Invasive tumors have a high rate of recurrence which may not be diminished by morbid aggressive surgical resections [7, 9]. However, complete surgical resection is recommended whenever possible if excessive morbidity can be avoided [1]. Lateral neck dissections should be performed only in the setting of complete macroscopic resection. Resections of the larynx, pharynx, and esophagus are generally discouraged [1, 16, 24].

Multimodal or combination therapy

Surgical debulking of local tumor, combined with EBRT and chemotherapy as neoadjuvant (before surgery) or adjuvant (after surgery) therapy, may prevent death from local airway obstruction and at best may slightly prolong survival [1, 2, 10, 25]. Tracheostomy should be performed in patients with impending airway obstruction who are not candidates for local resection or chemo-radiation [1, 15]. Prophylactic tracheostomy in the absence of impending risk to the airway is discouraged [11].

Schlumberger et al. [26] investigated two protocols in 20 ATC patients using different chemotherapy regimens combined with EBRT, with or without surgery. Treatment toxicity was high and a limiting factor. The authors concluded that gross resection of the tumor should be performed whenever possible, and that combined treatment may prevent death from suffocation due to local tumor growth. The authors also concluded that this treatment was effective in terms of survival. However, there was no control group on which to base these conclusions, and the impact of the treatment beyond surgery may be questioned based on historical controls. Of the seven patients in the series with neck disease remaining after surgery, four experienced a best response of a complete remission in the neck, while three had a partial remission. Of the eight patients who did not undergo surgery, one experienced a best response of complete remission in the neck that lasted 8 months, four had a partial remission, and three demonstrated tumor progression. Unfortunately, survival exceeding 20 months was seen in only three patients (15%). Two of these three were among their four patients with no evidence of disease after surgery. These four patients had a mean duration of response of 20 months (range 2–40 months) that may be no different than expected without additional treatment in patients without demonstrable residual disease postoperatively [3, 8, 9]. The third patient to survive more than 20 months was one of four patients with residual disease confined to the neck after surgery. These four patients had an unusually low mean age of 38 years (range 27–42 years) and their mean survival of 10 months (range 4–22 months) may be no different than expected without additional treatment in young patients [3, 8, 9]. The nine patients in this series that had distant metastases at the time of treatment all experienced tumor progression during therapy that resulted in their deaths.

Of additional disappointment is that therapy has not been shown to independently improve overall cause-specific mortality in multivariate analysis that includes patient, tumor, and treatment variables [8, 10]. For example, Kim et al. [8] found that only patient and tumor factors predicted lower cause-specific mortality in a series of 121 ATC patients. In patients with unresectable disease who were considered candidates only for supportive care, palliative EBRT or palliative chemotherapy, the 12-month survival was 3% with a median survival of 2.9 months. As all 11 of their patients who survived longer than 24 months received bilateral surgery with curative intent, they performed a subanalysis of their 71 patients who received this same treatment. The 12-month survival rate in this group of patients was 64% with a median survival of 12.3 months. On multivariate analysis, age less than 60 years, female gender, tumor less than 7 cm, and intrathyroidal disease were identified as independent predictors of lower cause-specific mortality while treatment variables including EBRT and chemotherapy were not. Similarly, others have been unable to clearly demonstrate a benefit of therapy including hyperfractionated EBRT and chemo-radiosensitization [2, 11]. Some have reported improved survival with higher doses of radiotherapy [20, 27],

while others have demonstrated no survival advantage despite an 80% tumor response rate [28]. Aggressive hyperfractionated EBRT protocols that have reported complete or partial local tumor responses have also been associated with high rates of treatment toxicity [29, 30].

In a series of 47 ATC patients, Chang et al. reported that in their patients with unresectable disease median survival was 2–3 months regardless of additional therapies [9]. Their patients who underwent complete tumor resection combined with chemo-radiotherapy had a median survival of 6 months, a difference in survival that was not statistically significant. Thus, regardless of treatment provided, most patients demonstrated rapid disease progression and distant metastases with a mean survival of 4.3 months (range 1–21 months) and no significant difference in survival time was observed between the various types of treatment. No increase in survival was demonstrated with chemotherapy whether it was neoadjuvant or adjuvant. These disappointing results of local and systemic treatment to diminish mortality are consistent with the report of Kitamura et al. who reported that distant metastases were not initially present in 71% of their 62 patients initially diagnosed with ATC who eventually died of their disease [15].

Unlike Chang et al. [9], others have suggested that neoadjuvant chemo-radiotherapy may be superior to adjuvant therapy [1, 14]. Perhaps the most compelling data for neoadjuvant multimodal therapy come from Tennvall et al. who studied 55 patients treated with hyperfractionated (twice daily, 5 days per week) radiotherapy, doxorubicin and, whenever possible, surgery [13]. Patients were not randomized, but rather the three protocols were composed of patients treated at different time periods who received daily radiotherapy doses of 1.0 Gy in protocol A, 1.3 Gy in protocol B, and 1.6 Gy in protocol C. Twenty mg of doxorubicin was administered intravenously weekly starting prior to radiotherapy. Protocols A and B received 30 Gy before surgery and 16 Gy after surgery. Protocol C received the entire 46 Gy before surgery. There was no evidence of local recurrence in 31% of protocol A, 65% of protocol B, and 77% of protocol C. In those that underwent surgery there was no evidence of local recurrence in 56% of protocol A, 79% of protocol B, and 100% of protocol C. While these results are encouraging with regard to local disease control, the overall survival data were sobering in that the median survival was 3.5 months for protocol A, 4.5 months for protocol B, and 2 months for protocol C. Patients surviving >2 years were 13% of protocol A, 12% of protocol B, and 5% of protocol C.

Haigh et al. [7] reported a series of 24 ATC patients with a median survival of 43 months for the eight patients who underwent potentially curative surgery with no residual or minimal residual disease compared to 3 months survival in the 18 patients who underwent palliative surgery ($p = 0.001$). There was no difference in survival between those treated with only chemotherapy and EBRT without surgery (survival 3.3 months) and those who underwent palliative surgery defined as neck surgery in which macroscopic extrathyroidal disease or persistent distant disease remained postoperatively. These findings raise questions about the benefits of surgery for patients whose airway is not an immediate risk, yet who are not candidates for a potentially curable procedure.

Ain et al. evaluated the activity of paclitaxel against ATC [31]. Eleven of 19 patients demonstrated a partial response (nine), complete response (one), or disease stabilization (one) that lasted at least 2 weeks. Responders tended to be younger and female. Disappointingly, the median survival of all 19 evaluable patients was 25 weeks from diagnosis, and 24 weeks from initiation of paclitaxel. Potentially encouraging, however, was that the 10 patients with a partial or complete response to paclitaxel had a median survival of 32 weeks from starting treatment compared to 10 weeks for the others, although this difference was not statistically significant ($p = 0.40$).

Investigational therapies

Dowlati et al. [32] performed a Phase I study of the antiangiogenic prodrug combretastatin A-4 phosphate in patients with various advanced cancers, including three with ATC. One patient with ATC that extended into the mediastinum and palpable nodal involvement had a complete response after eight cycles of therapy and underwent an exploratory neck dissection where no tumor was found. An additional two cycles of treatment were given and he was alive 30 months after treatment. In the treatment cohort, tumor pain occurring shortly after dosing was a unique side effect of the drug, and dynamic contrast-enhanced (DCE) MRI demonstrated a significant decline in gradient peak tumor blood flow consistent with vascular activity.

A preliminary report of an international multicenter two-stage, Phase II trial to evaluate the objective response rate of patients with advanced thyroid cancer included four patients with metastatic ATC. Patients received irofulven intravenously on days 1 and 15 and capecitabine orally on days 1–15 every 28 days. So far, no patient with ATC has demonstrated a response [33]. Similarly, disease stabilization was not demonstrated in patients with metastatic ATC in a Phase II trial of the oral multi-kinase inhibitor Sorafenib [34].

Radioactive iodine and TSH suppression therapy

Radioactive iodine may be considered in patients whose thyroid cancer contains only a minor component of intrathyroidal ATC and was completely resected, although there are no data to demonstrate a benefit. However, ATC does not accumulate ^{131}I and therefore is refractory to this therapy; ^{131}I has no role in the treatment of metastatic ATC. Patients with concomitant DTC typically do not have a better prognosis as they succumb to the anaplastic component of their disease [7, 11].

TSH suppression therapy is an important part of treating metastatic DTC [35]. Conversely, functional TSH receptors are ordinarily absent in ATC and no role for TSH suppressive therapy has been identified.

Author's recommendations

Figure 18.2 suggests a diagnostic and treatment algorithm that is consistent with the guidelines of the National Comprehensive

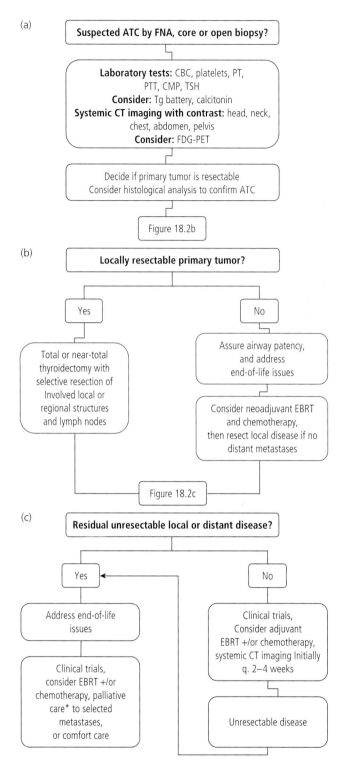

Figure 18.2 Management algorithm for patients based on suspected ATC (a), ability to resect the primary tumor (b), and the presence of unresectable local or distant disease (c). CBC, complete blood count; PT, prothrombin time; PTT, partial thromboplastin time; TSH, thyroid stimulation hormone; Tg battery, thyroglobulin and antithyroglobulin antibody; EBRT, external beam radiation therapy. * May include external beam radiation therapy, surgery, tracheostomy, tracheal stent, radiofrequency ablation, photodynamic therapy, laser thermal ablation, Gamma Knife, tumor embolization.

Cancer Network [36]. Computerized tomography (CT) imaging with contrast of the head, neck, chest, abdomen, and pelvis is suggested to rapidly determine the extent of the tumor, local invasion, and distant metastases. Data regarding the utility of fluorodeoxyglucose–positron emission tomography (FDG-PET) are limited [37], but anecdotal experience suggests a possible beneficial role that includes whole-body screening.

Patients with disease confined to the thyroid should undergo urgent complete tumor resection, generally via near-total or total thyroidectomy. The airway must be kept in mind throughout the course of the patient's care and those with impending obstruction without imminent death from other sites of disease require an urgent procedure to secure the airway, such as tracheostomy. Apart from these two situations, currently available treatment options are largely futile and therefore end-of-life issues and patient comfort must be addressed and a pathway of standard treatment, comfort care, or clinical trials must be selected by a fully informed patient and supportive clinical team. Given the poor impact of all available therapies it is difficult to be dogmatic regarding the necessity of any treatment modality. Clinical trials should be given the highest priority at all decision points.

Locally resectable disease

In the absence of an available clinical trial, patients with local disease that is potentially completely resectable should undergo surgery. If the local tumor is confined to the thyroid and completely resected with no evidence of distant metastases then additional treatment with EBRT and/or chemotherapy (as outlined below) is not mandatory as these patients may be cured, but treatment may be considered (although it may be futile). If the local tumor demonstrated local lymph node metastases and/or extrathyroidal extension yet is completely resected with no evidence of distant metastases then additional chemo-radiation is often considered. Historically, the vast majority of these patients will still have persistent disease as witnessed by eventual local and/or distant recurrent disease and death. If local tumor remains after surgery then it should be resected, or multimodal therapy with chemo-radiation may be elected as discussed below. Operated patients with distant metastases are candidates for additional multimodal therapy, although those with limited residual local disease may not benefit from radiotherapy and may be spared the morbidity of this treatment given their limited survival. Treatment with paclitaxel alone may be offered to these patients [31].

Locally unresectable disease

If after initial staging it is likely that the local disease cannot be completely resected then neoadjuvant radiotherapy and chemotherapy may be instituted. The hyperfractionated radiotherapy protocol C of Tennvall et al. may be combined with doxorubicin as in their study [13], or a regimen of paclitaxel as outlined by Ain et al. [31] may be chosen given its potentially greater efficacy, especially if distant metastases are present (with or without doxorubicin). If after receiving the target dose of radiotherapy the patient has no distant metastases and the local disease is likely resectable

then curative surgery should be attempted if excessive morbidity can be avoided. However, if distant metastases are present after receiving radiotherapy then it is likely that local surgery can be avoided and the airway observed as death is likely to result shortly from distant metastases.

Conclusion

ATC is a rare, lethal disease that has nearly always spread systemically at the time of diagnosis or shortly thereafter. Rare fortunate individuals are diagnosed when the tumor is small and intrathyroidal and are cured by surgical resection. Once the tumor is extrathyroidal the disease is lethal and radical surgery is discouraged. End of life issues should be addressed promptly in all patients and optimal emotional support provided. Currently available treatments may provide limited palliation and possibly prolong survival to a minimal degree. Due to the lack of effective therapies, enrollment in clinical trials is highly encouraged. However, all treatments (conventional and experimental) require commitments of the patient's limited remaining time and are associated with potential treatment-related side effects that may impair their quality of life. Further, it is likely that the patient's functional level and ability to enjoy their remaining time will only deteriorate with time. Thus, decisions to enter into a phase of active treatment or to elect comfort care only should be made in partnership with a fully informed patient.

References

1. Are C, Shaha AR. Anaplastic thyroid carcinoma: biology, pathogenesis, prognostic factors, and treatment approaches. *Ann. Surg. Oncol.* 2006;13:453–464.
2. Giuffrida D, Gharib H. Anaplastic thyroid carcinoma: current diagnosis and treatment. *Ann. Oncol.* 2000;11:1083–1089.
3. Hundahl SA, Fleming ID, Fremgen AM, Menck HR. A National Cancer Data Base report on 53,856 cases of thyroid carcinoma treated in the US, 1985–1995. *Cancer* 1998;83:2638–2648.
4. Akslen LA, Haldorsen T, Thoresen SO, Glattre E. Incidence of thyroid cancer in Norway 1970–1985. Population review on time trend, sex, age, histological type and tumour stage in 2625 cases. *APMIS* 1990;98:549–558.
5. Ezaki H, Ebihara S, Fujimoto Y, et al. Analysis of thyroid carcinoma based on material registered in Japan during 1977–1986 with special reference to predominance of papillary type. *Cancer* 1992;70:808–814.
6. Davies L, Welch HG. Increasing incidence of thyroid cancer in the United States, 1973–2002. *JAMA* 2006;295:2164–2167.
7. Haigh PI, Ituarte PH, Wu HS, et al. Completely resected anaplastic thyroid carcinoma combined with adjuvant chemotherapy and irradiation is associated with prolonged survival. *Cancer* 2001;91:2335–2342.
8. Kim TY, Kim KW, Jung TS, et al. Prognostic factors for Korean patients with anaplastic thyroid carcinoma. *Head Neck* 2007;29:765–772.

9. Chang HS, Nam KH, Chung WY, Park CS. Anaplastic thyroid carcinoma: a therapeutic dilemma. *Yonsei Med. J.* 2005;46:759–764.

10. McIver B, Hay ID, Giuffrida DF, et al. Anaplastic thyroid carcinoma: a 50-year experience at a single institution. *Surgery* 2001;130:1028–1034.

11. Ain KB. Anaplastic thyroid carcinoma: a therapeutic challenge. *Semin. Surg. Oncol.* 1999;16:64–69.

12. Hadar T, Mor C, Shvero J, Levy R, Segal K. Anaplastic carcinoma of the thyroid. *Eur. J. Surg. Oncol.* 1993;19:511–516.

13. Tennvall J, Lundell G, Wahlberg P, et al. Anaplastic thyroid carcinoma: three protocols combining doxorubicin, hyperfractionated radiotherapy and surgery. *Br. J. Cancer* 2002;86:1848–1853.

14. O'Neill JP, O'Neill B, Condron C, Walsh M, Bouchier-Hayes D. Anaplastic (undifferentiated) thyroid cancer: improved insight and therapeutic strategy into a highly aggressive disease. *J. Laryngol. Otol.* 2005;119:585–591.

15. Kitamura Y, Shimizu K, Nagahama M, et al. Immediate causes of death in thyroid carcinoma: clinicopathological analysis of 161 fatal cases. *J. Clin. Endocrinol. Metab.* 1999;84:4043–4049.

16. Venkatesh YS, Ordonez NG, Schultz PN, Hickey RC, Goepfert H, Samaan NA. Anaplastic carcinoma of the thyroid. A clinicopathologic study of 121 cases. *Cancer* 1990;66:321–330.

17. Xing M. BRAF mutation in thyroid cancer. *Endocr. Relat. Cancer* 2005;12:245–262.

18. Kumar V, Blanchon B, Gu X, et al. Anaplastic thyroid cancer and hyperthyroidism. *Endocr. Pathol.* 2005;16:245–250.

19. Sugitani I, Kasai N, Fujimoto Y, Yanagisawa A. Prognostic factors and therapeutic strategy for anaplastic carcinoma of the thyroid. *World J. Surg.* 2001;25:617–622.

20. Pierie JP, Muzikansky A, Gaz RD, Faquin WC, Ott MJ. The effect of surgery and radiotherapy on outcome of anaplastic thyroid carcinoma. *Ann. Surg. Oncol.* 2002;9:57–64.

21. Lo CY, Lam KY, Wan KY. Anaplastic carcinoma of the thyroid. *Am. J. Surg.* 1999;177:337–339.

22. Nel CJ, van Heerden JA, Goellner JR, et al. Anaplastic carcinoma of the thyroid: a clinicopathologic study of 82 cases. *Mayo Clin. Proc.* 1985;60:51–58.

23. Tan RK, Finley RK, III, Driscoll D, Bakamjian V, Hicks WL, Jr., Shedd DP. Anaplastic carcinoma of the thyroid: a 24-year experience. *Head Neck* 1995;17:41–47.

24. Haigh PI. Anaplastic thyroid carcinoma. *Curr. Treat. Options Oncol.* 2000;1:353–357.

25. Heron DE, Karimpour S, Grigsby PW. Anaplastic thyroid carcinoma: comparison of conventional radiotherapy and hyperfractionation chemoradiotherapy in two groups. *Am. J. Clin. Oncol.* 2002;25:442–446.

26. Schlumberger M, Parmentier C, Delisle MJ, Couette JE, Droz JP, Sarrazin D. Combination therapy for anaplastic giant cell thyroid carcinoma. *Cancer* 1991;67:564–566.

27. Levendag PC, De Porre PMZR, Van Putten WLJ. Anaplastic carcinoma of the thyroid gland treated by radiation therapy. *Int. J. Radiat. Oncol. Biol. Phys.* 1993;26:125–128.

28. Shimaoka K, Schoenfeld DA, DeWys WD, Creech RH, DeConti R. A randomized trial of doxorubicin versus doxorubicin plus cisplatin in patients with advanced thyroid carcinoma. *Cancer* 1985;56:2155–2160.

29. Mitchell G, Huddart R, Harmer C. Phase II evaluation of high dose accelerated radiotherapy for anaplastic thyroid carcinoma. *Radiother. Oncol.* 1999;50:33–38.

30. Wong CS, Van Dyk J, Simpson WJ. Myelopathy following hyperfractionated accelerated radiotherapy for anaplastic thyroid carcinoma. *Radiother. Oncol.* 1991;20:3–9.

31. Ain KB, Egorin MJ, DeSimone PA. Treatment of anaplastic thyroid carcinoma with paclitaxel: phase 2 trial using ninety-six-hour infusion. Collaborative Anaplastic Thyroid Cancer Health Intervention Trials (CATCHIT) Group. *Thyroid* 2000;10:587–594.

32. Dowlati A, Robertson K, Cooney M, et al. A phase I pharmacokinetic and translational study of the novel vascular targeting agent combretastatin a–4 phosphate on a single–dose intravenous schedule in patients with advanced cancer. *Cancer Res.* 2002;62:3408–3416.

33. Droz J, Baudin E, Medvedev V, et al. Activity of irofulven (IROF) combined with capecitabine (CAPE) in patients (pts) with advanced thyroid carcinoma: Phase II international multicenter study (preliminary results). *J. Clin. Oncol.* 2006;24:15511. (Meeting Abstracts)

34. Kloos R, Ringel M, Knopp M, et al. Preliminary results of Phase II study of RAF/VEGF-R kinase inhibitor, BAY 43-9006 (Sorafenib), in metastatic thyroid carcinoma. *Thyroid* 2005;5(Suppl 1):22.

35. Cooper DS, Doherty GM, Haugen BR, et al. Management guidelines for patients with thyroid nodules and differentiated thyroid cancer. *Thyroid* 2006;16:109–141.

36. National Comprehensive Cancer Network. Practice Guidelines in Oncology – v.1.2006. accessed 5/23/2006 www.nccn.org/.2006.

37. Khan N, Oriuchi N, Higuchi T, Endo K. Review of fluorine-18-2-fluoro-2-deoxy-D-glucose positron emission tomography (FDG-PET) in the follow-up of medullary and anaplastic thyroid carcinomas. *Cancer Control* 2005;12:254–260.

19 Thyroid Lymphoma

Christopher M. Nutting and Kevin J. Harrington

Key points
- Non-Hodgkin lymphoma of the thyroid is a rare condition which presents with thyroid enlargement associated with cervical lymphadenopathy.
- Diagnosis should be made with fine needle aspiration and a lymph node should be removed for specialist histological examination.
- Treatment usually consists of a combination of cytotoxic chemotherapy and radiation therapy.
- Five-year survival rates for high-grade lesions are in the region of 50–60%, and for some subtypes (localized non-Hodgkin lymphoma of mucosa-associated lymphoid tissue) may approach 95%.

Etiology and pathogenesis

Thyroid lymphoma is an uncommon tumor, representing 2–8% of thyroid malignancies and approximately 1–2% of extranodal lymphomas [1, 2]. It occurs most frequently in elderly females and has been linked to Hashimoto thyroiditis and prior therapeutic irradiation of the thyroid bed. Almost all thyroid lymphomas are thyroid non-Hodgkin lymphoma (NHL), with 70–90% being intermediate grade and the remainder being high grade. Many are considered mucosa-associated lymphoid tissue (MALT) lymphomas and show plasmacytic differentiation and may be associated with similar lesions in other extranodal sites, especially in the gastrointestinal tract or salivary glands. The pathological classification of NHL has undergone significant changes during recent years, which makes comparison of series difficult [3–5]. Most importantly, the identification of NHL of MALT of the thyroid is important, as these tumors have an excellent prognosis if localized to the neck.

Clinical presentation and staging

The majority of thyroid lymphoma present in females aged greater than 55 years with a lump in the neck (Fig. 19.1). Typically the neck mass is large and may be rapidly growing. The differential diagnosis usually lies between thyroid NHL or anaplastic thyroid carcinoma. Local obstructive symptoms (stridor, dysphagia, and dysphonia) are frequently reported. MALT lymphomas may show a more indolent growth pattern. Accurate diagnosis is essential and lymph node excision is recommended to provide an adequate histological sample for sub-typing of lymphoma. Staging should

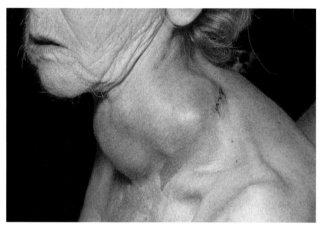

Figure 19.1 Large mass in the neck.

include computerized tomography (CT) scanning of the neck, thorax, abdomen, and pelvis, together with bone marrow aspirate and trephine. The majority of patients present with early-stage disease (Stage IAE or Stage II). Less than 10% present with more advanced Stage III or IV disease (see Table 19.1 for staging). Systemic B symptoms are uncommon, occurring in less than 5% of patients. Up to 30–40% of patients may be hypothyroid at presentation

Table 19.1 Staging of thyroid lymphoma

Stage	Descriptor
IE	Confined to thyroid ("E" denotes extranodal site of origin)
II	Spread of lymphoma to distant nodal site above the diaphragm
III	Involvement of lymph node groups below the diaphragm or spleen
IV	Involvement of other organs, e.g. liver, bone marrow

Suffix "A" is used to indicate asymptomatic patients, "B" indicates the presence of any of the following – drenching night sweats, weight loss >10%, or fever.

Clinical Endocrine Oncology, 2nd edition. Edited by Ian D. Hay and John A.H. Wass. © 2008 Blackwell Publishing. ISBN 978-1-4051-4584-8.

Table 19.2 Summary of patient characteristics for 91 patients with thyroid NHL presenting in the RMH series

Patient characteristic	No.	(%)
Female	77	(85%)
Male	14	(15%)
Stridor	30	(34%)
Dysphonia	28	(33%)
Previous goiter	31	(35%)
Pain	12	(14%)
Neck swelling	87	(98%)
Dysphagia	47	(53%)
Stage I	35	(38%)
Stage II	49	(54%)
Stage III	4	(4%)
Stage IV	3	(3%)

due to untreated Hashimoto disease. Typical characteristics of patients presenting with thyroid NHL are shown in Table 19.2.

Treatment modalities

There exists no universally accepted standard of care for thyroid NHL and a number of controversies exist regarding the roles of surgery, radiotherapy and chemotherapy in the management of this disease [6–8].

Surgery

In the past, thyroid NHL was treated with excision or debulking of disease followed by postoperative radiotherapy [9–12]. More recently, however, the appreciation that thyroid NHL is sensitive to chemotherapy and radiotherapy has resulted in a move towards limited surgical intervention, usually in the form of a diagnostic biopsy followed by definitive radiotherapy and/or chemotherapy.

Radiotherapy

Radiotherapy is a highly active treatment modality in thyroid NHL. After the commencement of radiotherapy rapid resolution of even extensive thyroid NHL can be anticipated. Indeed, in cases of imminent airway obstruction the application of emergency radiotherapy may obviate the need for a tracheostomy. A total radiation dose of 35–40 Gy should be delivered in 20 daily fractions, 5 days a week over a 4-week period. Radiotherapy is usually delivered using parallel-opposed anterior and posterior radiation fields. There is controversy as to whether the radiation fields should be limited to the extent of demonstrable tumor (involved field), or if extended fields including elective nodal groups should be used. Radiotherapy as a single modality is associated with excellent outcomes for localized MALT lymphoma, but in current practice is combined with chemotherapy for higher grade lymphomas, bulky disease or lymphomas of advanced stage.

Chemotherapy

Systemic cytotoxic chemotherapy agents are highly active in the treatment of high-grade NHL, and these can be applied in the treatment of thyroid NHL. Main indications for chemotherapy include bulky disease (>5 cm), high-grade histology, "B" symptoms and advanced stage disease. Chemotherapy is not used as a single modality in the treatment of thyroid NHL, and is usually combined with radiation in a sequential manner with chemotherapy administered for four to six cycles prior to definitive radiotherapy. MALT lymphomas also respond well to cytotoxic chemotherapy, although the excellent outcome of localized MALT lymphoma treated with radiotherapy may suggest that intensive chemotherapy is not required.

Typical regimens for high-grade thyroid NHL comprise cyclophosphamide, vincristine and prednisolone (COP), cyclophosphamide, doxorubicin, vincristine and prednisolone (CHOP), or prednisolone, mitoxantrone, cyclophosphamide, etoposide, bleomycin and vincristine (PMitCEBO). Rapid tumor responses can be obtained, and urgent chemotherapy could be administered as an alternative to radiotherapy to prevent airway complications as described above.

Treatment outcome and prognostic factors

Overall 5-year survival rates for thyroid NHL are in the region of 50–60%. Median relapse-free survival is approximately 3 years. Prognostic factors for overall survival for 91 patients treated at the Royal Marsden Hospital are shown in Table 19.3. Adverse prognostic factors for thyroid NHL include high grade, advanced stage at presentation, extent of surgical procedure (biopsy vs more extensive debulking procedure), extent of radiation field, radiation dose of 40 Gy or more, and the presence of stridor at diagnosis (Fig. 19.2). These factors are shown in a number of series [13–16].

Surgical procedure

Up until the 1980s many patients with thyroid NHL underwent extensive surgical procedures including thyroidectomy and removal of involved cervical nodes. Improvements in preoperative diagnosis, particularly fine needle aspiration techniques, have reduced the number of patients undergoing surgery in modern practice. An analysis of the impact of extent of surgical resection (biopsy alone vs more extensive resection) in the Royal Marsden series revealed a marked change towards less extensive procedures from 1990 onwards. However, the type of surgical procedure performed had a significant impact on the outcome of subsequent radiotherapy as demonstrated in Table 19.3. This may reflect the role of surgery in eliminating clonogens which are resistant to chemotherapy or radiation. Alternatively this observation could be due to interactions between patient selection for surgery and natural history of the disease [16–18].

Radiation field (involved field radiotherapy vs extended field radiotherapy)

In the Royal Marsden series, 72% treated with involved field radiotherapy (IFRT) died of thyroid NHL. The median relapse-free

Table 19.3 Significant independent factors on multivariate analysis of overall survival for 91 patients with thyroid NHL presenting in the RMH series

	Hazard ratio (95% CI)	*p* value
Stage		
I	1	
II	3.74 (1.77–7.92)	
III, IV	6.38 (2.13–19.11)	<0.001
Surgical procedure		
Debulking	1	
Biopsy	3.23 (1.72–6.06)	<0.001
Radiation field		
IFRT	1	
EFRT	0.45 (0.25–0.82)	<0.01

survival was only 10 months and the median overall survival was 21 months. In contrast, only 45% treated with extended field radiotherapy (EFRT) died of thyroid NHL. The median relapse-free survival was 76 months, while the median overall survival had not yet been reached. For IFRT, 52% (20% local alone and 32% combined local and distant) had evidence of locoregional failure at the time of death, compared with only 26% (9% local alone plus 17% local and distant) of patients treated with EFRT. Overall these data support the use of extended field irradiation in terms of local control and survival.

Radiation dose

Radiation doses required to achieve local control of thyroid NHL are in the region of 35–50 Gy. In the Royal Marsden series, survival data were compared for patients who received <40 Gy compared with those who received 40 Gy or more. In this study radiation dose was not significant on multivariate analysis of survival (hazard ratio 0.64, 95% CI: 0.33–1.24, $p = 0.18$), but was significant on multivariate analysis for local control (hazard ratio 0.42, 95% CI: 0.18–0.94, $p = 0.04$). At 5 years, only 26% patients treated at the lower dose level were alive, compared with 56% treated to 40 Gy or more ($p < 0.01$, log rank test). Doses of less

than 20 Gy are associated with low levels of local control [8]. The use of local radiotherapy for Stages IAE and IIAE MALT lymphomas of the thyroid is associated with local control and survival figures in the region of 95% at 5 years (Fig 19.2).

Conclusion

Accurate and timely diagnosis and staging are the key to correct management of thyroid NHL. Most patients will present with bulky, but localized, NHL in the neck and should receive combined modality therapy with chemotherapy followed by irradiation. Careful management of the emergency presentation with airway obstruction may be life saving. The data on extent of surgical resection indicate a significantly improved outcome in patients who underwent a debulking procedure prior to radiotherapy. Despite these observations, it is unlikely that the trend towards performing conservative surgery followed by chemotherapy and radiation will be reversed [15, 18, 19].

The optimum treatment with combination chemotherapy and radiation in high-grade thyroid NHL remains to be defined. However, the generally poor results obtained with radiotherapy alone, even with EFRT, in patients with anything more than Stage I disease provide strong support for the use of chemotherapy as part of the primary treatment. The ability of chemotherapy to "debulk" the tumor prior to starting radiotherapy (in an analogous fashion to surgical debulking) represents a further attraction. Low-grade MALT lymphomas of the thyroid have a very low distant recurrence rate, and a high rate of local control and survival with radiotherapy. Despite this, a review of the published literature suggests that the addition of chemotherapy to radiotherapy may also reduce both distant and overall recurrence for this subtype [20–23].

References

1. Heimann R, Vannineuse A, De Sloover C, Dor P. Malignant lymphomas and undifferentiated small cell carcinoma of the thyroid: a clinicopathological review in the light of the Kiel classification for malignant lymphomas. *Histopathology* 1978;2:201–213.
2. Souhami L, Simpson WJ, Carruthers JS. Malignant lymphoma of the thyroid gland. *Int. J. Radiat. Oncol. Biol. Phys.* 1980;6:1143–1147.
3. Anscombe AM, Wright DH. Primary malignant lymphoma of the thyroid – a tumour of mucosa-associated lymphoid tissue: review of seventy-six cases. *Histopathology* 1985;9:81–97.
4. Kossev P, Livolsi V. Lymphoid lesions of the thyroid: review in light of the revised European-American lymphoma classification and upcoming World Health Organization classification. *Thyroid* 1999;9:1273–1280.
5. Woolner LB, McConahey WM, Beahrs OH, Black BM. Primary malignant lymphoma of the thyroid. Review of forty-six cases. *Am. J. Surg.* 1966;111:502–523.
6. Derringer GA, Thompson LD, Frommelt RA, Bijwaard KE, Heffess CS, Abbondanzo SL. Malignant lymphoma of the thyroid gland: a clinicopathologic study of 108 cases. *Am. J. Surg. Pathol.* 2000;24:623–639.

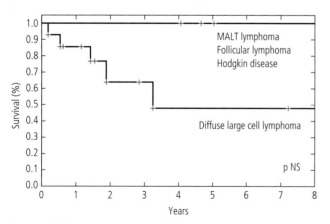

Figure 19.2 Survival curves from thyroid NHL.

7. Ha CS, Shadle KM, Medeiros LJ, et al. Localized non-Hodgkin lymphoma involving the thyroid gland. *Cancer* 2001;91:629–635.

8. Tupchong, Hughes F, Harmer CL. Primary lymphoma of the thyroid: clinical features, prognostic factors, and results of treatment. *Int. J. Radiat. Oncol. Biol. Phys.* 1986; 2:1813–1821.

9. Friedberg MH, Coburn MC, Monchik JM. Role of surgery in stage IE non-Hodgkin's lymphoma of the thyroid. *Surgery* 1994;116:1061–1066.

10. Rasbach DA, Mondschein MS, Harris NL, Kaufman DS, Wang CA. Malignant lymphoma of the thyroid gland: a clinical and pathologic study of twenty cases. *Surgery* 1985;98:1166–1170.

11. Tennvall J, Cavallin-Stahl E, Akerman M. Primary localized non-Hodgkin's lymphoma of the thyroid: a retrospective clinicopathological review. *Eur. J. Surg. Oncol.* 1987;13:297–302.

12. Tsutsui K, Shibamoto Y, Yamabe H, et al. A radiotherapeutic experience for localized extranodal non-Hodgkin's lymphoma: prognostic factors and re-evaluation of treatment modality. *Radiother. Oncol.* 1991;21:83–90.

13. Sasai K, Yamabe H, Haga H, et al. Non-Hodgkin's lymphoma of the thyroid. A clinical study of twenty-two cases. *Acta. Oncol.* 1996;35:457–462.

14. Singer JA. Primary lymphoma of the thyroid. *Am. Surg.* 1998;64:334–337.

15. Wirtzfeld DA, Winston JS, Hicks WL, Loree TR. Clinical presentation and treatment of non-Hodgkin's lymphoma of the thyroid gland. *Ann. Surg. Oncol.* 2001;8:338–341.

16. Harrington KJ, Michaliki VJ, Vini L, et al. Management of non-Hodgkin's lymphoma of the thyroid: the Royal Marsden Hospital experience. *Br. J. Radiol.* 2005;78:405–410.

17. Pyke CM, Grant CS, Habermann TM, et al. Non-Hodgkin's lymphoma of the thyroid: is more than biopsy necessary? *World. J. Surg.* 1992;16:604–609.

18. Tsang RW, Gospodarowicz MK, Sutcliffe SB, Sturgeon JF, Panzarella T, Patterson BJ. Non-Hodgkin's lymphoma of the thyroid gland: prognostic factors and treatment outcome. The Princess Margaret Hospital Lymphoma Group. *Int. J. Radiat. Oncol. Biol. Phys.* 1993;27:599–604.

19. Blair TJ, Evans RG, Buskirk SJ, Banks PM, Earle JD. Radiotherapeutic management of primary thyroid lymphoma. *Int. J. Radiat. Oncol. Biol. Phys.* 1985;11:365–370.

20. Belal AA, Allam A, Kandil A, et al. Primary thyroid lymphoma: a retrospective analysis of prognostic factors and treatment outcome for localized intermediate and high-grade lymphoma. *Am. J. Clin. Oncol.* 2001;24:299–305.

21. Doria R, Jekel JF, Cooper DL. Thyroid lymphoma. The case for combined modality therapy. *Cancer* 1994;73:200–206.

22. Tsang RW, Gospodarowicz MK, Pintilie M, Wells W, Hodgson DC, Sun A. Localized mucosa-associated lymphoid tissue lymphoma treated with radiation therapy has excellent clinical outcome. *J. Clin. Oncol.* 2003;21:4157–4164.

23. Vigliotti A, Kong JS, Fuller LM, Velasquez WS. Thyroid lymphomas stages IE and IIE: comparative results for radiotherapy only, combination chemotherapy only, and mltimodality treatment. *Int. J. Radiat. Oncol. Biol. Phys.* 1986;12:1807–1812.

20 Radiation-induced Thyroid Tumors

David H. Sarne and Arthur Schneider

> **Key points**
> - External radiation exposure before age 20 is associated with the development of thyroid cancer.
> - Radiation doses used to treat benign conditions are associated with an increased risk of thyroid cancer.
> - Radiation doses used to treat childhood malignancies are associated with hypothyroidism and thyroid neoplasia.
> - The relationship between internal radiation exposure from radioactive iodine and thyroid cancer is complex; the Chernobyl accident has led to a marked increase in thyroid cancer among those exposed as children.
> - The risk of thyroid cancer remains elevated for decades, requiring long-term follow-up.

Introduction

The association between external radiation and the development of cancer was first noted in 1950 by Duffy and Fitzgerald who described the link between childhood thyroid cancer and a history of external beam radiation to treat benign conditions [1]. Prospective studies among survivors of the atomic bombs detonated in Japan and children treated for benign conditions in the Rochester, NY, area then confirmed this association [2, 3]. Over time, it has been recognized that the thyroid gland is one of the most sensitive organs to develop neoplasms as a consequence of radiation exposure.

While the use of lower doses of external radiation to treat benign head and neck conditions has been abandoned, many children still have computerized tomography (CT) examinations for a variety of clinical indications and higher doses of radiation continue to be used to treat childhood malignancies. Concerns have also been raised about the risk of thyroid cancer posed by environmental exposures from nuclear testing in the 1950s as well as populations living in proximity to nuclear processing facilities during and shortly after World War II [2]. Finally, the accident at the nuclear power plant in Chernobyl has been followed by a dramatic increase in the number of thyroid cancers in the exposed population [2, 4]. In this chapter, we discuss factors associated with the development of thyroid neoplasms, the risks posed by low- and high-dose therapeutic and environmental exposure, and recommendations for the diagnosis and management of these patients.

Clinical Endocrine Oncology, 2nd edition. Edited by Ian D. Hay and John A.H. Wass. © 2008 Blackwell Publishing. ISBN 978-1-4051-4584-8.

Risk factors for the development of radiation-associated thyroid cancer

Epidemiological studies have confirmed that the major determinant of thyroid cancer risk is the radiation dose to the thyroid [2, 5]. Increasing amounts of thyroid radiation are associated with an increased risk for the development of benign and malignant neoplasms, although there appears to be a leveling off, or even a decline at very high levels (above 30 Gy) [2]. Of greater public health importance is the question of whether there is a threshold level, a level below which there is no risk. From a pooled analysis of several studies, the lowest dose with an observed significant risk is about 10 cGy [2, 5]. It is uncertain as to how the data should be extrapolated below that level, although a linear extrapolation is preferred by most authoritative radiation safety groups. Since almost all studies are retrospective and the thyroid is not often in the direct field of exposure, the dose to the thyroid had to be estimated, making it even more difficult to determine the risk with low-dose exposure. The presence of a dose–response relationship, accounting for other potential risk factors, has provided the strongest evidence supporting the radiation effect. Likewise, the longitudinal cohort studies that have been used to determine these risks are much less susceptible to bias than case control studies. Typical radiation doses to the thyroid and the associated risk for the development of thyroid cancer and hypothyroidism are summarized in Table 20.1.

Across multiple studies and for different types of radiation, there has been an inverse relationship between the age at exposure and the risk of developing thyroid cancer. From the pooled analysis, there was no longer a detectable risk for those exposed after the age of 20 [5]. While the risk may be slightly greater for women as compared to men, the difference is not significant and would not alter the approach to screening or management [2, 3].

Table 20.1 Typical exposure and associated risks

Exposure source	Dose (cGy) to thyroid	Risk for thyroid neoplasia	Risk for hypothyroidism
US Fallout, 1950s for a 10-year-old	2‡	Low	Low*
Residence near Hanford	10–20†	Low	Low*
Residence near Chernobyl	Variable†	Increased	Low*
CT of head – child	0.5–1.5	Low	Low*
^{123}I diagnostic scan	1	Low	Low*
^{131}I diagnostic scan	5	Low	Low*
^{131}I therapy – Graves	1500–2000	Low	High
External beam for enlarged tonsils	10–175	Increased	Low*
External beam for lymphoma	1000–3000	Increased	High

*Not significantly different from unexposed population.
†Dependent on location at time of accident or proximity to plant.
‡Average for US resident born in 1948.

Previously, it was thought that thyroid cancers took at least 10 years to develop after radiation exposure. However, with the availability of more sensitive detection methods and the close surveillance after Chernobyl, cancers were detected as soon as 3 years after the accident [4]. Now, a pressing question is whether the risk disappears with time; that is, does an exposed individual always remain at increased risk? A recently reported follow-up of atomic bomb survivors indicates that the risk persists for decades after exposure [6]. Especially since thyroid cancers are more aggressive in older patients, individuals with a history of radiation exposure must continue to be closely followed.

It is highly likely that genetic factors modify the risk for developing tumors after radiation exposure. Linkage studies have identified candidate loci and/or genes related to radiation susceptibility, with some evidence that this includes thyroid cancer [7]. However, with the exception of uncommon genetic disorders such as ataxia–telangiectasia, no specific genetic risk factors for radiation induced tumors in general, and thyroid cancer specifically, have been confirmed [2].

An important modifying factor, unique to the effect of radiation on the thyroid, is iodine deficiency. The dietary iodine content and the amount of intrathyroidal iodine may alter the effects of both internal and external radiation exposure. The uptake of radioactive iodine into the thyroid is closely correlated with dietary and intrathyroidal iodine levels. The Chernobyl region was an area of relative iodine deficiency. As a result, a larger amount of radioactive iodine would have been taken up by the thyroid, increasing exposure and the risk for developing thyroid cancer [2, 4]. The prompt distribution of iodine to exposed areas of Poland has been credited with the prevention of radiation-induced thyroid cancers. The studies in the Chernobyl area also indicate that iodine deficiency appears to be a risk factor beyond merely increasing the dose. The common denominator for this effect and the effect of age at exposure may be a thyroid with an increased rate of cell division.

There are several other risk factors whose effects remain uncertain. These include differences between internal and external exposure, differences among the different iodine isotopes, and differences when exposure is instantaneous (medical use), over a limited time period (nuclear accident), or extended over a much longer time period (environmental exposure).

Low-dose radiation – diagnostic and therapeutic radioactive iodine

There has been no demonstrated risk for the development of thyroid cancer from the diagnostic use of ^{131}I [2, 3]. The number of children included in the studies of this question, however, has been small. Most reports evaluating the incidence of thyroid cancer after therapeutic ^{131}I for hyperthyroidism have found no increase compared to historical controls [2]. A study of cancer mortality following treatment of hyperthyroidism in adults found an increased risk of death from thyroid cancer, but the absolute number of cases was small and the excess risk was seen in the first few years after treatment [8]. Another large retrospective study also found increased mortality from thyroid disease after ^{131}I but almost all cases occurred in the first year and were thought to relate to hyperthyroidism [9]. All of these studies were retrospective and subject to ascertainment bias.

Low-dose radiation – external radiation for benign conditions

Although radiation was used in the past to treat a number of benign head and neck conditions, the dose to the thyroid (and thus the risk of thyroid cancer) was quite variable. Brachytherapy, the placement of a radioactive source against the skin, was used to treat hemangiomas and those distant from the neck imparted little radiation to the thyroid [3]. Thyroid exposure (and risk) would also have been low for those who had radiation applied to the eustachian tubes using a transnasal applicator rod [3]. External beam radiation for cystic acne produced significant thyroid radiation exposure, but not Grenz ray treatment to the skin [3].

Considering benign conditions, the highest thyroid doses (and greatest risk) would be for infants and children who received external beam radiation to the posterior pharyngeal region to treat the tonsils and adenoids or to the chest to treat an enlarged thymus [2, 3]. For such a child whose thyroid received 100 cGy and developed thyroid cancer, the estimated attributable risk (proportion of cases that would not have occurred in the absence of radiation) is 88% [3].

Low-dose radiation – environmental exposure

Environmental exposure to ^{131}I is largely from the consumption of milk from animals grazing in contaminated pastures. Other than ^{131}I, radioactive isotopes of iodine have short half-lives and are present in the environment only after nuclear reactor accidents or atomic explosions. These short-lived isotopes are much smaller factors at long distances from the site of origin.

Depending on the assumptions used, exposure to radioactive iodine released from atomic testing may have contributed up to 200 000 excess thyroid cancer cases in the United States over the past four decades [10]. Individuals who were residing in certain areas in the United States during the years 1952–1962 may be at greater risk [10]. Since goats concentrate more iodine in their milk, the highest risk would be for those who live in the more heavily exposed areas and drank milk from their own goat. Individual dose estimates for exposure from the atomic tests are available on the internet – http://ntsi131.nci.nih.gov. Even using the worst-case estimates, however, the National Academy of Science advised against routine population screening [10]. Despite intense surveillance, studies of the population residing near the Hanford nuclear facility have failed to find any evidence of any thyroid disease – autoimmune disease, nodules, neoplasm, or cancer [11]. Using cohort analysis of data from the Connecticut Cancer Registry it has been estimated that 9% of the thyroid cancers diagnosed between 1978 and 1980 were attributable to all sources of radiation [3].

In a region of southern China, natural background radiation results in a lifetime thyroid dose of about 14 cGy as compared to a nearby area where the exposure is only 5 cGy. In a screening program of over 2000 women aged 50–65 years who lived in these two regions, there was no difference in the rates of thyroid nodules or cancer [3].

High-dose radiation – external radiation for treatment of malignancies

Radioactive iodine therapy for Graves disease often results in permanent hypothyroidism and has not been associated with the development of thyroid cancer. This observation led to the hypothesis that high-dose radiation leads to cell death rather than neoplastic transformation and the concept that the dose–response relationship for thyroid cancer would diminish at higher doses. With the recognition that the effects of external and internal radiation may differ, this hypothesis has been re-examined. While data pooled from several studies had suggested a leveling off of the risk at 10 Gy [2, 5], a more recent case control study has suggested a fall-off at doses greater than 30 Gy [12].

The relationship between high-dose external radiation to the thyroid and the subsequent development of hypothyroidism is stronger than the association with neoplasia. Most of these patients will present with sub-clinical hypothyroidism – asymptomatic with normal thyroid hormone values and an elevated TSH, unless they also had a partial thyroidectomy [2]. Increasing radiation doses are associated with an increased risk for hypothyroidism [2]. Unlike thyroid neoplasia, older age is not protective. The long-term risk is about 33% for patients who received radiation

for head and neck cancer and about twice that for patients who received radiation for Hodgkin lymphoma. It is unclear if that difference is related to the difference in patient survival after the radiation or to other factors. Most cases occur within the first 3 years after radiation, but patients remain at risk for over 20 years, so long-term follow-up is necessary.

An increased risk for developing thyroid cancer as a second cancer following radiation therapy for Hodgkin lymphoma, non-Hodgkin lymphoma, leukemia, brain tumors, and neuroblastoma has been reported [12–14]. While most series have reported the development of well-differentiated thyroid cancers in patients treated with radiation for other cancers, a few cases with anaplastic carcinoma or thyroid lymphoma have also been reported.

The Late Effects Study Group followed 9170 patients who survived 2 or more years after a diagnosis of childhood cancer [14]. Twenty-three cases of thyroid cancer were diagnosed after a mean follow-up of 5.5 years. This represented a 53-fold increased risk (95% CI; 34–80) compared to the general population [14]. Using case controls, they confirmed a dose–response relationship. In a more recent report, from the Childhood Cancer Survivor Cohort, 69 cases of pathologically confirmed thyroid cancer were detected among 14 054 patients who survived for at least 5 years and were followed for 14–30 years [12]. Using case controls, they noted an increased risk with radiation dose up to 20–29 Gy with an odds ratio of 9.8 (95% CI: 3.2–34.8) but a decreasing risk above 30 Gy [12]. Patients diagnosed before age 10 were at higher risk than those older than 10. Thyroid cancer was more commonly found among patients who had been treated for Hodgkin lymphoma (42% of cases as compared to 19% of the controls). Seventeen (25%) of the thyroid cancers were less than 1 cm at the time of diagnosis; these represented 42% of the tumors in patients who had Hodgkin lymphoma as compared to 17% of those in patients with other primary tumors [12]. This difference in the detection of smaller tumors may have reflected differences in patient follow-up.

One of the criticisms of many of these studies has been the variability in patient follow-up and the potential for ascertainment bias. In a study designed to provide a uniform assessment, Kaplan et al. assessed 95 patients who had received radiotherapy for childhood cancer [13]. Thyroid nodules were palpated in 26 of these patients, and of the 10 patients who had surgery, three had a papillary thyroid carcinoma [13]. Unlike the larger series described above, this one was too small to detect a dose–response relationship.

Radiation from the Chernobyl accident

An increase in the number of thyroid cancers diagnosed in childhood was noted within a few years of the accident at Chernobyl [2, 4]. Unlike those associated with other forms of radiation, these presented with more aggressive features including extrathyroidal extension and lymph node metastases, even when compared to other children with thyroid cancer [2, 4]. The source of the difference in these cases is not known, but it has been suggested that it may reflect either an even younger age at diagnosis or the effects of concomitant iodine deficiency.

Features of radiation-induced thyroid cancer

Unique features that absolutely identify a radiation-induced thyroid cancer, a "radiation signature," have not been found. Since thyroid cancers are common, the inability to determine whether an individual cancer was radiation induced or was spontaneous but discovered during surveillance has limited the ability to completely assess the risks posed by radiation exposure to specific populations. Only the clustering of an unusually high number of cases in an at-risk population (for example, the Michael Reese cohort and people living in the vicinity of the Chernobyl reactor) permits some determination of the population risk and other relevant factors.

As a group, almost all thyroid cancers diagnosed in patients with a history of radiation exposure have been papillary cancers and no other thyroid cancer has occurred with sufficient frequency to prove an association [2, 3]. This has been especially notable in the Chernobyl region, an area of iodine deficiency, where follicular cancers usually occur with a much greater frequency. The solid variant of papillary carcinoma has been reported with increased frequency in the Chernobyl region, but has not been reported in other groups exposed to radiation and does occur in some children without a radiation exposure history [2, 4]. Radiation-induced thyroid cancers are more likely to be multicentric than sporadic ones [2]. In reports from other cohorts with radiation-associated thyroid cancer, no other distinctive histopathological features have been identified. There have been no unusual subtypes or increased evidence of lymphatic involvement, local invasion or distant metastases. The frequency of benign thyroid nodules is also increased in patients with a history of radiation exposure and this poses an obvious challenge in the diagnostic evaluation and follow-up [2, 3]. Patients with a history of external radiation exposure in the head and neck area also have an increased risk for the development of neural, salivary and parathyroid neoplasms [2, 3].

RET is a proto-oncogene which encodes a membrane-bound tyrosine kinase that is not normally expressed in thyroid follicular cells. *RET/PTC* is a rearrangement that results in expression in thyroid cells, localization in the cytoplasm, and constitutive activation of the tyrosine kinase. *RET/PTC* is a common abnormality found in papillary carcinomas (35%) and is even more common in papillary cancers in children and young adults [15]. *RET/PTC* rearrangements have been identified in nearly 60% of thyroid cancers found in children exposed in the Chernobyl region [2, 15].

Different *RET/PTC* rearrangements have been identified. *RET/PTC1* is the form most commonly found in sporadic papillary thyroid carcinomas accounting for 60–70% of *RET/PTC*-positive tumors while only 20–30% are positive for *RET/PTC3* and less than 10% have *RET/PTC2* [15]. In contrast, *RET/PTC3* has been detected in nearly 50% of radiation-associated tumors from the

Table 20.2 Distribution of *RET/PTC* subtypes in papillary thyroid carcinomas with *RET/PTC* translocations*

	Radiation-associated (%)	Sporadic (%)
RET/PTC1	39	60–70
RET/PTC2	1	<10
RET/PTC3	49	20–30
Others	11	–

*Data derived from Nikiforov [15].

Chernobyl region and a number of unique rearrangements have only been found in radiation-associated tumors [15]. The distribution of the most common *RET/PTC* subtypes among *RET/PTC*-positive tumors is summarized in Table 20.2. When Chernobyl cases were separated based on cancer presentation within 10 years of the accident as compared to more than 10 years, the percentages of patients with any form of *RET/PTC* rearrangement, with *RET/PTC3* or with a novel rearrangement were all much higher in the group presenting earlier (66%, 60% and 13% as compared to 46%, 23% and 5%), further supporting the argument that these changes are truly reflective of radiation effects [15]. Elegant experiments from the laboratory of Y. Nikiforov have established that during interphase, alignment of the chromosomes juxtapose the DNA segments that would favor the formation of *RET/PTC3* after DNA damage by ionizing radiation [2, 15].

Frequencies of other mutations associated with sporadic papillary and follicular thyroid cancers have also been examined in radiation-associated cancers. Initial reports of an increased frequency of K-RAS have not been confirmed and no association has been found with H-RAS or N-RAS [15]. A point mutation in BRAF is the most common genetic abnormality in sporadic thyroid carcinomas, but it is rare in radiation-associated tumors [15]. Interestingly, in one radiation-related thyroid cancer, BRAF was activated by a genomic translocation. PAX8-peroxisome proliferator associated receptor-gamma (PPARγ) is a fusion protein found in 25–33% of sporadic follicular cancers. Although there is not a demonstrated association between follicular cancers and radiation, in a small study, three of three follicular cancers from radiation-exposed patients were positive for the PAX8–PPARγ rearrangement [15]. While p53 mutations have been found in radiation-associated tumors (0–20%), the overall low prevalence is not felt to support a major role in the development of thyroid neoplasia after radiation [2, 15].

Diagnostic evaluation of patients with a radiation exposure history

A high-risk patient is a patient who has been exposed before age 20 to radiation from one of the sources listed in Table 20.3. A personal history of other potentially radiation-related neoplasms would increase concern. The history should include information

Table 20.3 Parameters for assessing the risk of thyroid neoplasms after radiation exposure

Exposures associated with an increased risk of thyroid neoplasms
    External radiation for benign conditions before age 20
        Chest/neck radiation for thymic enlargement
        Posterior pharyngeal radiation for tonsillar enlargement
        Head and neck radiation for cystic acne and other indications
    External beam radiation for malignancy before age 20
        Radiation to mediastinum, e.g. for Hodgkin disease
        Head and neck radiation for other malignancies
    Exposure following the Chernobyl accident at a young age
        According to location
        According to precautions, potassium iodide (KI) prophylaxis

Exposure with low or uncertain risk
    Environmental radiation
        Above ground nuclear tests
        Terrestrial sources
    Diagnostic and therapeutic radioactive iodine
    Diagnostic X-rays
    Brachytherapy, including radium-tipped rods

about the radiation exposure and family history of radiation-related head and neck neoplasms. While symptoms related to masses, pain, dysphagia, voice and respiration should be elicited, most thyroid neoplasms are asymptomatic. Patients should also be questioned about tinnitus and decreased hearing (symptoms of an acoustic neuroma) and symptoms associated with hypercalcemia. The physical examination should include a careful examination of the thyroid and cervical nodes as well as the salivary glands.

Only a limited number of laboratory studies are useful in the evaluation of these patients. A serum TSH should be obtained to evaluate thyroid function. While most high-risk patients will maintain normal thyroid function tests, those who received external beam radiation for malignancy are at increased risk for the development of hypothyroidism. Serum calcium should be measured to detect hyperparathyroidism. Parathyroid hormone measurements should be reserved for those whose serum calcium value is borderline or elevated.

Serum thyroglobulin measurements may be useful in these patients [2, 3, 16]. Both an elevated and a rising thyroglobulin level have been associated with an increased risk for a thyroid nodule; however, it cannot discriminate between benign and malignant neoplasms [16]. If not done automatically by the lab, the presence of antibodies to thyroglobulin needs to be assessed as they can interfere with the accurate measurement of thyroglobulin.

Autoimmune thyroid disease is not thought to result from radiation exposure, although this is not completely resolved [2, 6, 17]. Some studies have found that antibodies to thyroid peroxidase are more frequently elevated in patients with a history of radiation exposure; however, this has no utility in the determination of the risk for thyroid cancer. As an increased risk for medullary carcinoma has not been associated with radiation, routine measurements of calcitonin in these patients are not indicated.

Physical examination alone is inadequate for the follow-up of high-risk patients. It is poorly reproducible and many nodules greater than 1.5 cm in size are missed [2, 18, 19]. High-resolution ultrasonography is the modality of choice for evaluating and following these patients. It is able to detect nodules only a few millimeters in size, provides objective measurement which can be followed to assess nodule growth and allows evaluation of blood flow, lymphadenopathy and other features which may provide evidence of the likelihood of benign or malignant disease [2]. As the frequency of small abnormalities is high in the general population, routine thyroid ultrasonography in the general population would not be appropriate, and should be reserved for patients felt to be at substantial risk for radiation-related thyroid neoplasms.

Thyroid scintigraphy is used as an assessment of function, not pathology or anatomy. It is unlikely to detect nodules less than 1 cm and, depending on location and function, may miss even larger abnormalities. It has no role in the routine surveillance of patients with a history of thyroid radiation.

When one or more nodules are found in a patient at risk, fine needle aspiration (FNA) is the method of choice for determining if thyroidectomy is indicated [2, 3]. All nodules larger than 1 cm, all nodules with suspicious features, and all nodules that are increasing in size should be aspirated. If numerous nodules are present, priority should be given to those with suspicious features. The accuracy of FNA in patients with a history of thyroid radiation is comparable to the excellent results in non-irradiated patients [2, 20].

Two studies using palpation by experienced examiners reported the shrinkage or disappearance of nodules in radiated patients treated with suppressive thyroid hormone therapy [2, 3]. Actual measurements by ultrasound were not done. A third study in radiated patients who had already had a benign nodule surgically removed showed that treatment with thyroxine reduced the number of new benign nodules but had no effect on the development of malignant nodules [21]. Given the inability to prevent the development of malignancy and the potential risks, routine thyroid hormone suppressive therapy is not warranted [2]. However, in patients with especially large or enlarging nodules confirmed to be benign by FNA, it may be considered.

As there appears to be an ongoing risk, patients with a history of radiation to the thyroid require lifelong follow-up [2, 3, 6]. Given the usually slow growth of thyroid cancers, it is reasonable to repeat an ultrasound examination every 12–24 months in patients with small, non-suspicious nodules, more often in those with other nodules, and every 3–5 years in patients in whom no nodules had been found [2, 19].

Therapy of patients with thyroid neoplasia and radiation exposure

The general approach to radiation-associated and sporadic papillary cancer should be very similar. Given the high frequency of mulifocality associated with radiation exposure, patients with an FNA result suspicious or diagnostic for papillary cancer should undergo a total thyroidectomy. At the time of surgery, they should undergo appropriate removal of lymph nodes based on the pre-operative ultrasound and the intraoperative findings. In patients without a history of radiation exposure, an indeterminate FNA result suggesting a follicular neoplasm would usually be managed with a lobectomy when the remaining lobe does not have any significant nodules; however, if there is a history of radiation exposure a total thyroidectomy should be considered [2].

Postoperatively, patients with radiation-associated thyroid cancer should have their risk for recurrence and death assessed by one of the multivariate scoring systems, none of which is affected by multifocality or a radiation history [2]. Radioactive iodine ablation and thyroid hormone suppression should be used as they would for other papillary cancers with the same follow-up protocols. In five of six retrospective studies in which standard treatment methods were used, similar outcomes were found for recurrence and death between cancer patients with and without a history of radiation [2]. The exception was the oldest study, which did not match the patients [2].

Conclusion

Patients with a history of radiation to the thyroid should be carefully assessed to determine the level of risk for hypothyroidism and thyroid neoplasia. High-risk patients should be examined, have TSH, calcium and thyroglobulin measured and should undergo thyroid ultrasonography. Subsequent treatment and management should be guided by that initial evaluation. Patients found to have papillary cancer should receive standard treatment. Those without cancer remain at risk and need lifelong follow-up.

References

1. Duffy BJ, Fitzgerald P. Thyroid cancer in childhood and adolescence: A report on twenty-eight cases. *Cancer* 1950;10:1018–1032.
2. Schneider AB, Sarne DH. Long-term risks for thyroid cancer and other neoplasms after exposure to radiation. *Nat. Clin. Pract. Endocrinol. Metab.* 2005;1:82–91.
3. Sarne DH, Schneider AB. External radiation and thyroid neoplasia. *Endocrinol. Metab. Clin. North Am.* 1996;25:181–195.
4. Cardis E, Kesminiene A, Ivanov V, et al. Risk of thyroid cancer after exposure to ^{131}I in childhood. *J. Natl Cancer. Inst.* 2005;97:724–732.
5. Ron E, Lubin JH, Shore RE, et al. Thyroid cancer after exposure to external radiation: a pooled analysis of seven studies. *Radiat. Res.* 1995;141:259–277.
6. Imaizumi M, Usa T, Tominaga T, et al. Radiation dose-response relationships for thyroid nodules and autoimmune thyroid diseases in Hiroshima and Nagasaki atomic bomb survivors 55–58 years after radiation exposure. *JAMA* 2006;295:1011–1022.
7. Mertens AC, Mitby PA, Radloff G, et al. XRCC1 and glutathione-S-transferase gene polymorphisms and susceptibility to radiotherapy-related malignancies in survivors of Hodgkin disease – a report from the childhood cancer survivor study. *Cancer* 2004;101:1463–1472.
8. Ron E, Doody MM, Becker DV, et al. Cancer mortality following treatment for adult hyperthyroidism. *JAMA* 1998;280:347–355.
9. Franklyn JA, Maisonneuve P, Sheppard MC, Betteridge J, Boyle P. Mortality after the treatment of hyperthyroidism with radioactive iodine. *N. Engl. J. Med.* 1998;338:712–718.
10. National Research Council and Institute of Medicine. *Exposure of the American People to Iodine-131 From Nevada Nuclear-bomb Tests: Review of the National Cancer Institute Report and Public Health Implications.* Washington, DC: National Academy Press, 1999.
11. Davis S, Kopecky KJ, Hamilton TE, Onstad L. Thyroid neoplasia, autoimmune thyroiditis, and hypothyroidism in persons exposed to iodine 131 from the Hanford Nuclear Site. *JAMA* 2004;292:2600–2613.
12. Sigurdson AJ, Ronckers CM, Mertens AC, et al. Primary thyroid cancer after a first tumour in childhood (the Childhood Cancer Survivor Study): a nested case-control study. *Lancet* 2005;365:2014–2023.
13. Kaplan MM, Garnick MB, Gelber R, et al. Risk factors for thyroid abnormalities after neck irradiation for childhood cancer. *Am. J. Med.* 1983;74:272–280.
14. Bhatia S, Yasui Y, Robison LL, et al. High risk of subsequent neoplasms continues with extended follow-up of childhood Hodgkin's disease: report from the Late Effects Study Group. *J. Clin. Oncol.* 2003;21:4386–4394.
15. Nikiforov YE. The molecular pathways induced by radiation and leading to thyroid carcinogenesis. In: Farid NR (ed.). *Molecular Basis of Thyroid Cancer.* Boston, MA: Kluwer Academic Publishers, 2004.
16. Schneider AB, Shore-Freedman E, Ryo UY, Bekerman C, Pinsky S. Prospective serum thyroglobulin measurements in assessing the risk of developing thyroid nodules in patients exposed to childhood neck irradiation. *J. Clin. Endocrinol. Metab.* 1985;61:547–550.
17. Tronko MD, Brenner AV, Olijnyk VA, et al. Autoimmune thyroiditis and exposure to iodine 131 in the Ukrainian cohort study of thyroid cancer and other thyroid diseases after the Chernobyl accident: results from the first screening cycle (1998–2000). *J. Clin. Endocrinol. Metab.* 2006;91:4344–4351. Epub 15 Aug 2006.
18. Schneider AB, Bekerman C, Leland J, et al. Thyroid nodules in the follow-up of irradiated individuals: comparison of thyroid ultrasound with scanning and palpation. *J. Clin. Endocrinol. Metab.* 1997;82:4020–4027.
19. Mihailescu DV, Collins BJ, Wilbur A, Malkin J, Schneider AB. Ultrasound-detected thyroid nodules in radiation-exposed patients: changes over time. *Thyroid* 2005;15:127–133.
20. Hatipoglu BA, Gierlowski T, Shore-Freedman E, Recant W, Schneider AB. Fine-needle aspiration of thyroid nodules in radiation-exposed patients. *Thyroid* 2000;10:63–69.
21. Fogelfeld L, Wiviott MBT, Shore-Freedman E, et al. Recurrence of thyroid nodules after surgical removal in patients irradiated in childhood for benign conditions. *N. Engl. J. Med.* 1989;320:835–840.

21 Parathyroid Adenomas and Hyperplasia

Bart L. Clarke

Key points

- Primary hyperparathyroidism is the most common cause of hypercalcemia in ambulatory outpatients.
- Primary hyperparathyroidism is due to a parathyroid adenoma in about 85% of cases, parathyroid hyperplasia in about 15% of cases, and parathyroid carcinoma in less than 1% of cases.
- Parathyroid adenomas and hyperplasia are difficult to distinguish by light microscopic evaluation, but are most easily distinguished by examination at surgery and gland weight.
- Parathyroid hyperplasia does not evolve into parathyroid adenoma or carcinoma over time, and parathyroid adenoma does not evolve into carcinoma over time.
- Parathyroid adenomas and hyperplasia are most often managed surgically when symptomatic, or medically when asymptomatic.

Introduction

Parathyroid adenomas are found in about 85% of patients with primary hyperparathyroidism, whereas parathyroid hyperplasia is found in about 15% of cases of primary hyperparathyroidism, as well as secondary or tertiary hyperparathyroidism. Secondary or tertiary hyperparathyroidism are associated most often with chronic kidney disease. Secondary hyperparathyroidism may also be due to vitamin D deficiency or idiopathic hypercalciuria. This chapter will focus mostly on parathyroid adenomas and hyperplasia occurring in association with primary hyperparathyroidism (Table 21.1).

Table 21.1 Disorders associated with parathyroid adenomas or parathyroid hyperplasia

Parathyroid adenomas	Parathyroid hyperplasia
Primary hyperparathyroidism (85%)	Primary hyperparathyroidism (15%)
Parathyroid cysts (degenerated adenomas)	Secondary hyperparathyroidism
Parathyroid lipoadenomas	Tertiary hyperparathyroidism
Hyperparathyroidism–jaw tumor syndrome	Parathyromatosis
	Familial hypocalciuric hypercalcemia (mild)
	MEN 1 and MEN 2A
Familial isolated primary hyperparathyroidism	Familial isolated primary hyperparathyroidism

Clinical Endocrine Oncology, 2nd edition. Edited by Ian D. Hay and John A.H. Wass. © 2008 Blackwell Publishing. ISBN 978-1-4051-4584-8.

Primary hyperparathyroidism

Primary hyperparathyroidism is the most common cause of adult outpatient hypercalcemia [1]. The incidence of this disorder is estimated to be 1:1000 in men and 2–3:1000 in women, with a much lower incidence in children. Although primary hyperparathyroidism occurs at all ages, it is most common in postmenopausal women in the sixth decade of life. The incidence of primary hyperparathyroidism has been declining in Olmsted County, Minnesota, in the United States, but whether this finding reflects a national or worldwide trend is not yet clear [2]. Restriction of routine measurement of serum calcium in the current health-care environment will likely reduce the number of recognized cases of primary hyperparathyroidism.

Pathogenesis

Primary hyperparathyroidism is caused by inappropriate secretion or oversecretion of parathyroid hormone (PTH) by one or more parathyroid glands. Adult humans have been reported to have four parathyroid glands in 84% of cases, three glands in 1–7% of cases, and five glands in 3–13% of cases, with a range of from 1 to 12 parathyroid glands. Solitary parathyroid adenomas cause primary hyperparathyroidism about 85% of the time, with multiple adenomas found in a small percentage of cases, whereas four-gland hyperplasia is found in about 15% of cases, and parathyroid cancer is discovered in less than 1% of cases.

Most single adenomas represent sporadic disease, whereas four-gland hyperplasia implies a familial disorder, most commonly due to multiple endocrine neoplasia (MEN) type 1 or 2A. Excessive secretion of PTH by an adenoma results from an increased set-point, in which there is loss of feedback control of PTH secretion by extracellular calcium at the cellular level, whereas excessive secretion of PTH by hyperplastic cells is due to an increased number of parathyroid cells with normal calcium set-point.

The cause(s) of sporadic primary hyperparathyroidism is not well understood. Previous exposure to neck irradiation contributes to a small increased risk of developing primary hyperparathyroidism in a small number of cases, usually 20 to 30 years after exposure. More commonly, adenomas represent clonal expansion of a single or several abnormal cells, attributable to a genetic abnormality that results in either stimulation of cell proliferation or loss of inhibition of cell proliferation [3]. A small number of adenomas have been reported with a *PRAD1* (cyclin D1) proto-oncogene rearrangement, in which the *PRAD1* gene is inserted close to enhancer elements of the *PTH* gene. In this situation, parathyroid cell division is stimulated whenever PTH secretion is stimulated. PRAD1 protein expression has been reported to be increased in about 20% of parathyroid adenomas. Up to 17% of parathyroid adenomas have been reported with a mutation in the tumor suppressor *MEN1* (menin) gene. Loss of heterozygosity analysis of parathyroid adenomas has shown several other potential sites for parathyroid oncogenes on chromosomes 16p and 19, and loss of tumor suppressor genes on chromosomes 1p, 1q, 6q, 13q, and other sites. Several recent studies have shown calcium-sensing receptor (CaSR) abnormalities in a small percentage of parathyroid adenomas.

Eucalcemic or "incipient" hyperparathyroidism, where serum calcium is normal but PTH is increased, has recently been described [4]. This condition requires documentation of normal serum 25-hydroxyvitamin D and 24-h urine calcium levels to rule out other causes of secondary physiological hyperparathyroidism, and may be due to an early stage of primary hyperparathyroidism or very mild primary hyperparathyroidism. No genetic analyses have been published of parathyroid glands in this condition, since in most cases surgery is not necessary.

Pathology

Parathyroid adenomas

Parathyroid adenomas are located more commonly in the inferior gland positions. Adenomas are typically red-brown, smooth, oval, encapsulated, and nodular lesions. An adenoma may completely replace normal parathyroid gland structure, and may show areas of hemorrhage or, if large, cystic degeneration. In small adenomas, a visible rim of normal yellow-brown parathyroid tissue may be present. Adenomas typically weigh 300 to several thousand milligrams, with maximum diameter ranging from 1 to 3 cm. Adenomas are typically composed of encapsulated parathyroid chief cells arranged in a delicate capillary network (Plates 21.1 and 21.2). Lobules may rarely be seen, and nodules are sometimes present. Stromal fat is usually absent. About 50% of adenomas have a rim of normal or atrophic parathyroid tissue outside the adenoma capsule. Cells in the rim tend to be smaller and more uniform, with stromal and cytoplasmic fat present in the rim, but absent in the adenoma. Lack of a rim of normal parathyroid tissue does not rule out an adenoma.

In large parathyroid adenomas, areas of fibrosis, hemorrhage, cholesterol clefts, hemosiderin, and calcification may be present. Lymphocytes may occasionally be present. Thymic tissue may be found in association with an adenoma, and adenomas may be embedded within the thymus. Atypical cells may be found in adenomas without malignancy, typically with relatively small, uniform, dark nuclei. Unusual multinucleated cells with dark, crinkled nuclei may be present, probably due to degenerative changes rather than precancerous change. Mitotic activity is usually limited in adenomas. The remaining normal glands in patients with a parathyroid adenoma usually show normal to increased cytoplasmic fat content and normal weight.

Biopsies of visually normal glands at surgery show areas of hypercellularity in about 10% of cases. These hypercellular areas are attributed to microscopic hyperplasia. The cause and significance of these hypercellular areas are still not clear.

Oxyphilic or oncocytic adenomas occur rarely and may be functional, and are typically larger than chief cell adenomas with minimally increased serum calcium levels (Plate 21.3). Double adenomas occur rarely, but some patients diagnosed with double adenomas may in fact have asymmetrical parathyroid hyperplasia.

Parathyroid hyperplasia

Parathyroid hyperplasia is most often due to chief cell hyperplasia, and less commonly due to water clear cell hyperplasia. About 30% of patients with chief cell hyperplasia have isolated familial hyperparathyroidism or a multiple endocrine neoplasia syndrome. All four glands tend to be enlarged equally or, in some cases, asymmetrically. If the glands are asymmetrically enlarged, the inferior parathyroid glands tend to be larger, and occasionally one gland is sufficiently enlarged that it appears to be an adenoma. Individual hyperplastic glands range in weight from 0.15 to 20 g, but most weigh 1–3 g.

Diffuse chief cell hyperplasia typically is associated with solid masses of cells with minimal to no fat. Rare oxyphil cells may be seen. Nodular or pseudoadenomatous hyperplasia is composed of circumscribed nodules of chief cells, transitional cells, or oxyphil cells without fat, with little intervening stromal fat. Hyperplastic glands typically do not have a rim of normal tissue. Atypical cells are only rarely identified, but mitotic figures may occur.

Water clear cell hyperplasia is very rare, and is the only form of hyperparathyroidism associated with larger superior glands than inferior glands. Gland weight is typically greater than 1 g, and usually ranges from 5–10 g. These glands are irregular and have a distinct mahogany color, often with pseudopods and cysts. The glands are composed of sheets of water clear cells without other intervening cells. Most of these glands have no rim of normal parathyroid tissue. Water clear cell hyperplasia is associated with blood group type O.

Clinical manifestations

Most patients with primary hyperparathyroidism have asymptomatic mild hypercalcemia, typically with serum calcium levels less than 1.0 mg/dL (0.25 mmol/L) above the upper end of the normal range of 8.5–10.5 mg/dL (2.13–2.63 mmol/L). Occasional patients may present with severe hypercalcemia, as a form of acute primary hyperparathyroidism or parathyroid crisis.

More severe cases may have classic bone features, including osteitis fibrosa cystica (distal phalangeal subperiosteal bone resorption, distal clavicular resorption, "salt and pepper" skull, bone cysts, and brown tumors of long bones) or osteoporosis, predominantly at cortical sites such as the distal one-third of the radius. In one study [5], fractures were reported to be increased. Bone disease is currently identified in less than 5% of patients with primary hyperparathyroidism.

Renal disease, including calcium-containing kidney stones, nephrocalcinosis, or hypercalciuria, may be found in up to 20% of patients. Hypercalciuria is reported in up to 30% of patients, with a calcium to creatinine clearance ratio of greater than 0.01.

Neuropsychiatric imbalances are often reported, typically manifest as mild fatigue or weakness with subtle cognitive impairment [6]. Associations with peptic ulcer disease and pancreatitis are probably not causally related, unless associated with the MEN syndromes. Mild hypertension, coronary artery and cardiac valvular calcifications, and septal and left ventricular hypertrophy may be detected in some patients with more symptomatic hyperparathyroidism.

Other classic abnormalities of primary hyperparathyroidism, such as gout or pseudogout, anemia, band keratopathy, chondrocalcinosis, or loose teeth due to lamina densa resorption, are virtually never seen in current clinical practice.

Laboratory findings

Patients with primary hyperparathyroidism typically have high-normal or mildly increased serum total calcium and ionized calcium values, with some variation around an upper-normal or mildly increased average value over time. Intraindividual variation in serum calcium measurement is due to normal pulsatile secretion of PTH, variations in dietary or supplemental calcium intake, fluid or acid–base shifts, and other factors. Serum phosphorus is usually low-normal or mildly decreased. Serum total alkaline phosphatase is usually normal or mildly increased. Serum creatinine is usually normal. Intact (whole-molecule) PTH, measured by the older two-site immunoradiometric or immunochemiluminometric assays, or the newer Bio-intact assay, is mildly increased or inappropriately high-normal for the level of serum calcium. No cross-reactivity is present between PTH and PTH-related peptide (PTHrp) in current assays.

Patients treated with thiazides or lithium may have mildly increased serum calcium and PTH levels without primary hyperparathyroidism. To ensure that patients with hypercalcemia who are treated with thiazides or lithium do not have primary hyperparathyroidism, documentation of persistent hypercalcemia and high PTH levels after discontinuation of thiazide or lithium therapy for at least 1–2 months is required, given that there is no other biochemical measurement that reliably distinguishes primary hyperparathyroidism from thiazide- or lithium-induced changes.

Markers of bone turnover may be increased in patients with primary hyperparathyroidism without obvious bone disease, attributable to PTH effects on the skeleton, or possibly to increased interleukin-6 or tumor necrosis factor-α. PTH renal tubular effects may lead to mildly increased serum chloride and decreased bicarbonate. Typically, serum 1,25-dihydroxyvitamin D levels are high-normal or mildly increased, and serum 25-hydroxyvitamin D levels are usually low-normal. Urinary calcium excretion is increased in 25–30% of patients with primary hyperparathyroidism.

Surgical treatment of primary hyperparathyroidism

Surgical intervention is usually recommended for patients with symptomatic primary hyperparathyroidism. Surgical decisions about patients with asymptomatic primary hyperparathyroidism are more difficult. The 1991 US National Institutes of Health Consensus Development Conference [7] recommended surgical management for patients with serum calcium levels >1.0 mg/dL (>0.25 mmol/L) above the upper limit of normal, recognized complications such as nephrolithiasis or overt bone disease, acute primary hyperparathyroidism with life-threatening hypercalcemia, 24-h urinary calcium excretion in excess of 400 mg, distal one-third radial bone density Z-score of less than −2.0, or age younger than 50 years. The 2002 US National Institutes of Health Consensus Development Conference [8] modified these recommendations to advise surgery for patients with serum calcium >1.0 mg/dL (>0.25 mmol/L) above the upper limit of normal, creatinine clearance reduced by 30% or more, recognized complications such as nephrolithiasis or overt bone disease, acute primary hyperparathyroidism with life-threatening hypercalcemia, 24-h urinary calcium excretion greater than 400 mg, bone mineral density T-score below −2.5 at any skeletal site, or age younger than 50 years. Approximately half of patients diagnosed with primary hyperparathyroidism fulfill at least one of these criteria, and of these patients, most are asymptomatic but have high serum or urine calcium levels or low bone density. Patients not requiring surgical treatment generally have stable mild hypercalcemia without progression, although about 27% of patients eventually develop a complication requiring surgery over 10 years of follow-up [9].

Parathyroid surgery is best performed by an experienced surgeon because of the variability in parathyroid gland location. In major medical centers, preoperative localization of parathyroid adenomas before initial neck exploration is often considered unnecessary because of extremely high cure rates (95–98%) with standard neck exploration. However, minimally invasive surgery requires preoperative localization of the abnormal gland(s) to ensure a high success rate [10]. Patient or surgeon interest in minimally invasive parathyroidectomy typically results in use of parathyroid imaging studies, including ultrasonography, ^{99m}Tc-thallium or ^{99m}Tc-sestamibi subtraction scanning, computerized tomography (CT), or magnetic resonance imaging of the neck, before the initial operation. Recent experience has shown that ^{99m}Tc-sestamibi subtraction scanning is capable of detecting about 90% of single parathyroid adenomas before surgery (Fig. 21.1). False-negative and false-positive imaging results, however, are relatively common. During a standard neck exploration, patients

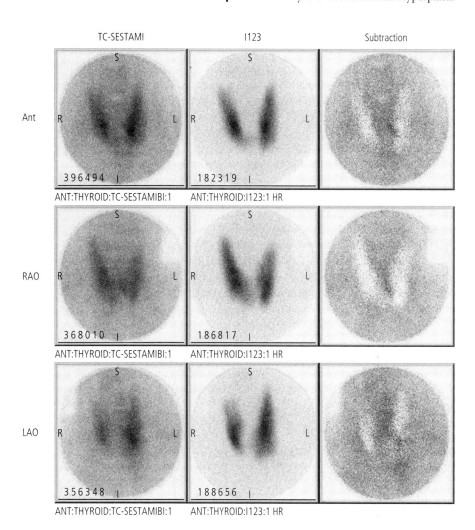

Figure 21.1 Parathyroid ^{123}I–^{99m}Tc sestamibi subtraction scan showing a single left superior parathyroid adenoma.

with single or double adenomas should undergo resection of the tumor(s), with identification of the remaining normal glands. Patients with four-gland hyperplasia should typically undergo removal of three and one-half glands, with one-half gland left *in situ*. The alternative approach of removal of all four parathyroid glands, followed by autotransplantation of part of one gland in the forearm or neck, has become less popular in recent years due to difficulties with resection of recurrent primary hyperparathyroidism from the forearm or neck.

Patients surgically cured of their hyperparathyroidism typically have prompt normalization of their serum calcium level within several hours of surgery, often after a brief period of asymptomatic relative hypocalcemia. Occasional patients may take as long as 24 to 36 h to normalize their serum calcium after surgery. "Hungry bones" syndrome, with rapid skeletal mineral uptake after surgery, may develop in patients with active bone disease or preoperative vitamin D deficiency. Intravenously and orally administered calcium and vitamin D supplementation are often necessary to treat symptomatic hypocalcemia in the days to weeks after surgery with hungry bone syndrome. Potential complications of a parathyroid surgical procedure include hypocalcemia resulting from chronic

hypoparathyroidism, or hoarseness due to recurrent laryngeal nerve damage. In most patients, bone density improves rapidly postoperatively, particularly at the lumbar spine and radius [11].

Reoperation for persistent or recurrent primary hyperparathyroidism is technically more difficult than initial surgery. In patients with persistent primary hyperparathyroidism, hypercalcemia occurs within 6 months after surgery, whereas with recurrent primary hyperparathyroidism, hypercalcemia recurs more than 6 months after surgery. Most surgeons require preoperative imaging to attempt to localize the parathyroid tumor(s) before a second or later operation. Invasive arteriography and selective venous sampling may be helpful to lateralize tumor location, although these are expensive and time-consuming procedures. Confirmation of the diagnosis of primary hyperparathyroidism is necessary before undertaking a second or later operation, primarily to rule out unsuspected familial hypocalciuric hypercalcemia (FHH). Combination CT scan and ^{99m}Tc-sestamibi scan with software superimposition of images (Hawkeye scanning), or intraoperative ^{99m}Tc-sestamibi scan with a handheld γ counter, coupled with rapid intraoperative PTH assay, may be helpful in difficult reoperative cases.

Medical management of primary hyperparathyroidism

Medical options are limited for patients with symptomatic hypercalcemia who are unable or unwilling to undergo surgical treatment [12]. Patients should be encouraged to maintain adequate hydration and remain physically active. Use of thiazides and lithium should be avoided. Dietary calcium intake of 0.8–1.0 g/day is advised to suppress PTH secretion, minimize bone loss, and avoid worsening hypercalcemia or hypercalciuria. Dietary calcium intake of less than 600 mg/day, or vitamin D deficiency, will often exacerbate hyperparathyroidism. Oral or intravenous administration of phosphate should be avoided because of the risk of precipitation of ectopic soft tissue calcification. Estrogen replacement therapy may help normalize serum calcium levels and prevent bone loss in postmenopausal women, although PTH and phosphate levels do not change. Orally administered bisphosphonates may be beneficial, but etidronate and clodronate have not shown long-term benefit. Alendronate, risedronate, raloxifene, and salmon calcitonin administered by nasal spray or injection have not been thoroughly investigated for this indication, although alendronate [13] or raloxifene [14] may help decrease serum calcium levels in the short term. CaSR agonists (calcimimetics) have been shown to decrease serum calcium and maintain normal levels of serum calcium for as long as 3 years [15]. Patients with identifiable tumors on ultrasound studies who do not desire, or are not candidates for, surgical treatment may benefit from alcohol ablation of their tumor under ultrasound guidance. Asymptomatic patients with primary hyperparathyroidism who do not have parathyroidectomy tend to do well, although as many as 27% of these patients may develop progression of disease, defined as development of at least one new indication for surgery over ten years of follow-up [9].

Familial hypocalciuric hypercalcemia (FHH)

Familial hypocalciuric hypercalcemia is an autosomal dominant, highly penetrant disorder characterized by mild to moderate hypercalcemia and relative hypocalciuria since birth [16]. Most kindreds are asymptomatic, but in some patients, mild fatigue, neuropsychiatric imbalances, or polydipsia may develop. Occasional patients have severe pancreatitis or relapsing pancreatitis, and the risk of gallstones, diabetes mellitus, or early myocardial infarction may be increased. No study has yet demonstrated an increased risk for nephrolithiasis, nephrocalcinosis, peptic ulcer disease, low bone mass, or fractures in patients with FHH. Parathyroid glands removed surgically due to lack of appreciation of the diagnosis appear normal or mildly hypercellular.

Families with FHH typically have mildly increased serum total and ionized calcium, mildly decreased serum phosphate, high-normal or mildly increased serum magnesium, normal serum creatinine and creatinine clearance, mildly increased renal calcium and magnesium resorption causing relative hypocalciuria and hypomagnesiuria, renal calcium to creatinine clearance ratio $(ClCa/ClCr = CaU \times CrS/CaS \times CrU)$ of less than 0.01, high-normal

to mildly increased serum PTH and 1,25-dihydroxyvitamin D, and mild parathyroid gland hyperplasia. About 10% of patients with primary hyperparathyroidism may have a ClCa/ClCr ratio of less than 0.01, and about 10% of patients with FHH may have a ratio of greater than 0.01. At least one patient has been reported to have co-existing FHH and idiopathic hypercalciuria, and rare patients have been reported with surgically proven co-existing primary hyperparathyroidism and FHH. Patients with FHH typically have normal X-ray findings, although mild chondrocalcinosis and early vascular calcification may be present. Markers of bone turnover may be mildly increased, but bone density is usually normal and fracture risk is not increased.

Subtotal parathyroidectomy results in transient lowering of serum calcium levels for about 1 week, with recurrence of hypercalcemia within a week, and total parathyroidectomy usually causes the expected chronic hypoparathyroidism in association with hypocalcemia and decreased serum 1,25-dihydroxyvitamin D levels. For these reasons, parathyroidectomy is usually unnecessary and inadvisable in patients with this disorder. Patients with FHH and uncontrollable severe hypercalcemia [>14 mg/dL (>3.5 mmol/L)] or recurrent pancreatitis, however, should consider undergoing total parathyroidectomy without autotransplantation. Several cases of recurrent hypercalcemia have developed after autotransplantation. Diuretics, estrogen, and phosphate therapy have no appreciable effect on serum calcium levels in FHH. There is no evidence that FHH shortens life expectancy, and patients with this disorder have lived into the ninth decade of life.

Pregnancy in an FHH carrier or the spouse of an FHH carrier may result in several outcomes. The affected infant of an FHH mother should have asymptomatic hypercalcemia at birth, whereas the unaffected infant of an FHH mother may have symptomatic hypocalcemia after birth because of suppression of fetal secretion of PTH by maternal-fetal hypercalcemia during pregnancy. The affected infant of an unaffected mother may have severe neonatal hypercalcemia at birth attributable to fetal relative secondary hyperparathyroidism during pregnancy, but this condition should resolve over time to asymptomatic hypercalcemia without neonatal parathyroidectomy.

The prevalence of FHH is unknown but thought to be similar to that for MEN type I, probably accounting for about 2% of cases of asymptomatic hypercalcemia. FHH heterozygotes have virtually 100% penetrance for hypercalcemia at birth, and the degree of hypercalcemia is usually constant within kindreds. Most kindred have mild hypercalcemia in all affected members, but several kindreds with moderate hypercalcemia [serum calcium levels of 12.5–14 mg/dL (3.16–3.5 mmol/L)] have been reported. Germline single allelic inactivating mutations in the calcium-sensing receptor gene (*CASR*) on chromosome 3q13.3–q21 are most commonly found, but in several families, linkages to chromosome 19p or chromosome 19q13 are found, implying heterogeneity in the genetic basis of the disorder. Genetic testing for mutations in the CaSR is available, but current tests may miss up to 25% of the mutations present. Patients with germline double allelic inactivating mutations of the *CASR* gene develop neonatal severe primary hyperparathyroidism, with resultant severe hypercalcemia and massive parathyroid gland hyperplasia, and require total parathyroidectomy.

Familial hyperparathyroidism syndromes

Most cases of primary hyperparathyroidism are sporadic, but about 5–10% of cases represent hereditary forms of hyperparathyroidism. The most common form of heritable primary hyperparathyroidism is MEN 1. Other forms are less common, including MEN 2A, hyperparathyroidism-jaw tumor syndrome, and familial isolated primary hyperparathyroidism.

Multiple endocrine neoplasia (MEN) syndromes

Primary hyperparathyroidism may occur as a manifestation of MEN 1 (Wermer syndrome) or MEN 2A (Sipple syndrome). The most common form of hereditary primary hyperparathyroidism is MEN 1, with an estimated prevalence of 2–3/100 000. MEN 1 may account for 2% of cases of primary hyperparathyroidism. The prevalence of MEN 2A is unknown.

MEN 1 syndrome was initially reported in 1954, with highly penetrant, autosomal dominant inheritance of parathyroid, pancreatic, and anterior pituitary tumors [17]. Primary hyperparathyroidism is present in more than 95% of cases, pancreatic tumors in 30–80% of patients, and anterior pituitary tumors in 15–50% of patients. Other tumors associated with MEN 1 include duodenal gastrinomas, bronchial or thymic carcinoids, gastric enterochromaffin-like tumors, adrenocortical adenomas, lipomas, facial angiofibromas, and truncal collagenomas. Primary hyperparathyroidism in MEN 1 is similar in its initial manifestations to sporadic primary hyperparathyroidism, except that it occurs with equal frequency in men and women and usually manifests in the second to fourth decade of life. The youngest case reported to date was 8 years old. Because patients with primary hyperparathyroidism due to MEN 1 typically have four-gland adenomatous or pseudoadenomatous chief cell hyperplasia, treatment usually involves surgical removal of three and one-half glands or complete parathyroidectomy with autotransplantation in the forearm or neck. Most surgeons prefer to leave about 50 mg of functioning tissue, although recurrent hypercalcemia can develop, and close follow-up is imperative.

Pancreatic tumors secrete gastrin in two-thirds of cases, causing Zollinger–Ellison syndrome, and insulin in one-third of cases, leading to recurrent fasting hypoglycemia. Some pancreatic tumors secrete multiple products, including vasoactive intestinal peptide, prostaglandins, glucagon, pancreatic polypeptide, adrenocorticotropic hormone, or serotonin. Anterior pituitary tumors may secrete prolactin, growth hormone, or adrenocorticotropic hormone, or may be non-secreting. As many as one-third of the patients with MEN 1 may have adrenal enlargement due to a variety of pathological conditions, including diffuse cortical hypertrophy, nodular cortical hypertrophy, cortical hyperplasia, adrenal adenomas, or adrenocortical carcinomas.

MEN 1 syndrome is caused by mutations in the *MEN1* gene located on chromosome 11q13. Various types of mutations have been reported throughout all 10 exons of the gene, without clustering in particular regions of the gene. About 10% of mutations reported are apparently new. The precise function of the menin protein produced is not fully established, although it is thought to function as a tumor suppressor. The risk of developing MEN 1 in siblings of a carrier may be low, but children of a carrier have a 50% risk of inheriting a mutation. MEN 1 may manifest initially in patients as old as 35 years of age, and biochemical screening before manifestation of the disease may not detect all persons who eventually will be affected. First-degree relatives of affected individuals should be screened, however. Genetic testing for MEN 1 has recently become available through a number of laboratories.

MEN 2 is subclassified into MEN 2A, MEN 2B, and familial medullary thyroid carcinoma syndromes. MEN 2A syndrome was initially reported in 1961, with autosomal dominant inheritance of medullary thyroid carcinoma (MTC), bilateral pheochromocytomas, and parathyroid hyperplasia [18]. MTC is diagnosed in greater than 90% of cases, with hypercalcitoninemia produced by C-cell hyperplasia or MTC. Patients typically undergo early total thyroidectomy after detection of either baseline or calcium-stimulated hypercalcitoninemia. Many patients in recognized kindreds are sent for total thyroidectomy once genetic testing confirms presence of a *RET* proto-oncogene mutation on chromosome 10q11.2, even before evidence of baseline or calcium-stimulated hypercalcitoninemia, because of the high likelihood of eventual development of MTC. Germline *RET* mutations are found in more than 90% of MEN 2A families.

Pheochromocytoma may develop in 40–50% of patients with MEN 2A, either before or after MTC is recognized. In these cases, the pheochromocytoma may be unilateral or bilateral, and bilateral adrenalectomy may be advised. Patients with possible MEN 2A should always undergo assessment for pheochromocytoma before total thyroidectomy for MTC, to prevent sudden death from hypertensive crisis during the neck surgical procedure. Patients with MEN 2A die more commonly from metastatic pheochromocytoma than metastatic MTC.

Primary hyperparathyroidism in MEN 2A is usually milder than in MEN 1, and occurs in only about 20% of cases of MEN 2A, but management is similar for all cases because the primary hyperparathyroidism consistently results from four-gland hyperplasia. In some cases only one gland appears to be involved. In some patients with MEN 2A, pruritic, hyperpigmented plaques (known as lichen amyloidosis) develop on the upper back area. This condition is though to be a consequence of dorsal neuropathy, and may serve as an early marker of the disorder.

Hyperparathyroidism–jaw tumor syndrome

The hyperparathyroidism–jaw tumor syndrome was first reported in 1958, and later found to be caused by germline mutations in the *HRPT2* gene on chromosome 1q21–q31 in 60–70% of cases [19]. *HRPT2* germline inactivating mutations cause decreased synthesis of parafibromin, a protein that normally functions as a tumor suppressor. This rare syndrome is characterized by autosomal dominant, highly penetrant, early-onset primary hyperparathyroidism in the first two decades of life with later recurrence, ossifying fibromas of the mandible and maxilla, renal cysts, hamartomas, or Wilms tumors, and uterine tumors. The syndrome frequently is associated with single-gland disease during each episode, separated by periods of normal serum calcium. Parathyroid cancer occurs in 40% of families, and kidney tumors or other abnormalities occur in 46% of families. Hypercalcemia, often severe, develops in late childhood or the teenage years, resulting from solitary enlarged, sometimes cystic, parathyroid adenomas. In patients with untreated hypercalcemia, crippling skeletal disease and early death may ensue. The jaw tumors typically appear in adolescence or young adulthood, and appear as lytic or cystic lesions on X-ray films. Jaw tumors may be small and asymptomatic or large and destructive, and they seem to run a course independent of the hyperparathyroidism. The tumors are composed of woven bone trabeculae in a background of fibrocellular tissue of unknown derivation; they differ substantially from brown tumors by their lack of osteoclasts.

Familial isolated primary hyperparathyroidism

Familial isolated primary hyperparathyroidism distinct from MEN 1, MEN 2A, and the hyperparathyroidism-jaw tumor syndrome may exist [20], although several kindreds initially described with this disorder were later reclassified as MEN 1, familial benign hypercalcemia, or hyperparathyroidism–jaw tumor syndrome based on new manifestations of disease. Genetic mapping in some families with familial isolated primary hyperparathyroidism has shown germline mutations of *MEN1* on chromosome 11q13, *HRPT2* on chromosome 1q21–q31, or *CASR* on chromosome 3q; some of these families may therefore represent allelic variants of these other disorders. Other families, however, do not show such linkages. The existence of multiple genetically distinct forms of familial isolated primary hyperparathyroidism is likely. These patients tend to have aggressive parathyroid disease. *HRPT2* germline mutations may be increased in families with this disorder that develop parathyroid carcinoma.

Conclusion

Parathyroid adenomas and hyperplasia are found in a variety of hyperparathroid disorders. Primary hyperparathyroidism is most frequently due to a single parathyroid adenoma, but may be due to more than one adenoma, or parathyroid hyperplasia. Parathyroid cysts, lipoadenomas, parathyromatosis, or parathyroid carcinomas may also rarely cause primary hyperparathyroidism. Familial hypocalciuric hypercalcemia mimics primary hyperparathyroidism by causing similar biochemical findings, except that urine calcium excretion is lower than expected. About 5–10% of primary hyperparathyroidism is due to germline genetic mutations causing syndromes of MEN 1, MEN 2A, hyperparathyroidism–jaw tumor syndrome, or isolated familial hyperparathyroidism. Most patients with genetic causes of primary hyperparathyroidism have parathyroid hyperplasia. Most patients with significant hyperparathyroidism from whatever cause still require parathyroid surgery, but some patients with asymptomatic primary hyperparathyroidism may be managed conservatively.

References

1. Bilezikian JP, Silverberg SJ. Primary hyperparathyroidism. In: Favus MJ (ed.) *Primer on the Metabolic Bone Diseases and Disorders of Mineral Metabolism*, 6th edn. Washington, DC: American Society for Bone and Mineral Research, 2006;181–184.

2. Wermers RA, Khosla S, Atkinson EJ, et al. Incidence of primary hyperparathyroidism in Rochester, Minnesota, 1993–2001: an update on the changing epidemiology of the disease. *J. Bone Miner. Res.* 2006;21:171–177.

3. Tominaga Y, Takagi H. Molecular genetics of hyperparathyroid disease. *Curr. Opin. Nephrol. Hypertens.* 1996;5:336–341.

4. Silverberg SJ. Bilezikian JP. "Incipient" primary hyperparathyroidism: a "forme fruste" of an old disease. *J. Clin. Endocrinol. Metab.* 2003;88:5348–5352.

5. Khosla S, Melton LJ III, Wermers RA, et al. Primary hyperparathyroidism and the risk of fracture: a population-based study. *J. Bone Miner. Res.* 1999;14:1700–1707.

6. Okamoto T, Gerstein HC, Obara T. Psychiatric symptoms, bone density and non-specific symptoms in patients with mild hypercalcemia due to primary hyperparathyroidism: a systematic overview of the literature. *Endocr. J.* 1997;44:367–374.

7. Consensus Development Conference Panel. Diagnosis and management of asymptomatic primary hyperparathyroidism: Consensus Development Conference Statement. *Ann. Intern. Med.* 1991;114:593–597.

8. Bilezikian JP, Potts JT Jr, El Hajj-Fuleihan G, et al. Summary statement from a workshop on asymptomatic primary hyperparathyroidism: a perspective for the 21st century. *J. Clin. Endocrinol. Metab.* 2002;87:5353–5361.

9. Silverberg SJ, Shane E, Jacobs TP, et al. A 10-year prospective study of primary hyperparathyroidism with or without parathyroid surgery. *N. Engl. J. Med.* 1999;341:1249–1255.

10. Grant CS, Thompson G, Farley D, van Heerden J. Primary hyperparathyroidism surgical management since the introduction of minimally invasive parathyroidectomy: Mayo Clinic experience. *Arch. Surg.* 2005;140:472–478.

11. Silverberg SJ, Gartenberg F, Jacobs TP, et al. Increased bone density after parathyroidectomy in primary hyperparathyroidism. *J. Clin. Endocrinol. Metab.* 1995;80:729–734.

12. Silverberg SJ, Bilezikian JP, Bone HG III, et al. Therapeutic controversies in primary hyperparathyroidism. *J. Clin. Endocrinol. Metab.* 1999;84:2275–2285.

13. Khan AA, Bilezikian JP, Kung AW, et al. Alendronate in primary hyperparathyroidism: a double-blind, randomized, placebo-controlled trial. *J. Clin. Endocrinol. Metab.* 2004;89:3319–3325.

14. Rubin MR, Lee KH, McMahon DJ, Silverberg SJ. Raloxifene lowers serum calcium and markers of bone turnover in postmenopausal women with primary hyperparathyroidism. *J. Clin. Endocrinol. Metab.* 2003;88:1174–1178.

15. Peacock M, Bilezikian JP, Klassen PS, et al. Cinacalcet hydrochloride maintains long-term normocalcemia in patients with primary hyperparathyroidism. *J. Clin. Endocrinol. Metab.* 2005;90:135–141.

16. Marx SJ, Attie MF, Levine MA, et al. The hypocalciuric or benign variant of familial hypercalcemia: clinical and biochemical features in fifteen kindreds. *Medicine* 1981;60:397–412.

17. Bassett JH, Forbes SA, Pannett AA, et al. Characterization of mutations in patients with multiple endocrine neoplasia type 1. *Am. J. Hum. Genet.* 1998;62:232–244.

18. Carney JA. Familial multiple endocrine neoplasia syndromes: components, classification, and nomenclature. *J. Intern. Med.* 1998;243:425–432.

19. Szabo J, Heath B, Hill VM, et al. Hereditary hyperparathyroidism-jaw tumor syndrome: the endocrine tumor gene HRPT2 maps to chromosome 1q21–q31. *Am. J. Hum. Genet.* 1995;56:944–950.

20. Teh BT, Farnebo F, Twigg S, et al. Familial isolated hyperparathyroidism maps to the hyperparathyroidism–jaw tumor locus in 1q21–q32 in a subset of families. *J. Clin. Endocrinol. Metab.* 1998;83:2114–2120.

22 Parathyroid Carcinoma

Göran Åkerström, Per Hellman, and Peyman Björklund

> **Key points**
> - Rare parathyroid carcinoma accounts for 0.4–5% of cases with hyperparathyroidism.
> - Inactivating somatic *HRPT2* gene mutations have been frequently demonstrated in parathyroid carcinoma, often causing decreased expression of the protein product parafibromin.
> - Parathyroid carcinoma should be suspected in hyperparathyroidism patients (with high serum calcium and parathyroid hormone values), if a firm, whitish parathyroid tumor with adhesions to adjacent tissues is detected at surgery.
> - Parathyroid carcinoma should be radically treated by *en bloc* removal of the tumor with the ipsilateral thyroid lobe, overlying strap muscles, surrounding paratracheal fibrolymphatic compartment and other involved tissues.
> - Parathyroid carcinoma is tenacious and reoperation for removal of regional or distant metastases is often needed to facilitate medical treatment of hypercalcemia.
> - Adjuvant radiotherapy may reduce recurrence rate.

Introduction

Parathyroid carcinoma is rare, causing less than 1% of cases with hyperparathyroidism (HPT) in the US and most western European countries [1, 2]. Figures as high as 5% have been reported from Japan, Italy, and developing countries such as India [1–3]. The higher figures may be due to inefficient recognition of common benign HPT, though high rate and remarkably severe symptoms in India have also been related to vitamin D deficiency [3]. Most patients with parathyroid carcinoma have presented at between 40 and 60 years with an average in the mid-50s [4], approximately a decade before the median age of patients with HPT due to parathyroid adenoma [1, 2, 4–7]. Occasional parathyroid carcinomas have occurred in children. Parathyroid carcinoma has been equally frequent in men and women, in contrast to marked female over-representation in HPT due to adenoma.

Etiology

Until recently little has been known about the etiology of parathyroid carcinoma. Prior neck irradiation has been a recognized risk factor for parathyroid adenoma, but has weak association with parathyroid carcinoma [2]. Parathyroid carcinoma has been rarely reported in patients with secondary HPT subjected to long-term hemodialysis [1, 2].

Clinical Endocrine Oncology, 2nd edition. Edited by Ian D. Hay and John A.H. Wass. © 2008 Blackwell Publishing. ISBN 978-1-4051-4584-8.

The risk for parathyroid carcinoma is markedly increased in the familial hyperparathyroidism–jaw tumor (HPT-JT) syndrome, where 10–15% of probands have been diagnosed with malignant parathyroid tumors [2, 5, 6]. Manifestations of this syndrome comprise jaw tumors and kidney lesions including solitary cysts or polycystic renal disease, hamartomas, renal carcinoma and Wilms tumor, and generally benign but typically cystic parathyroid adenomas. Germline mutations in the *HRPT2* gene, encoding parafibromin, have been demonstrated to cause this syndrome [2, 5, 6]. Recently, inactivating somatic *HRPT2* gene mutations were demonstrated in two-thirds of parathyroid carcinomas and associated with absent parafibromin expression in the tumors [2, 5–9]. Germline *HRPT2* mutations were also revealed in patients with apparently sporadic parathyroid carcinoma [8].

Only single cases of parathyroid carcinoma have been reported in patients with the multiple endocrine neoplasia type 1 (MEN 1) or the MEN 2 syndrome, whereas patients with familial isolated HPT may have increased incidence due to inclusion of individuals with the HPT-JT syndrome [2].

Clinical presentation

Patients with parathyroid carcinoma tend to present with more severe hypercalcemia and more marked metabolic disturbance than patients with adenomatous HPT [1, 2, 5, 6, 10]. The carcinoma patients are likely to have severe parathyroid bone disease, with subperiosteal resorption, bone cysts and pronounced osteopenia. They frequently have nephrolithiasis (56%), occasionally concomitant nephrocalcinosis, and often signs of impaired renal function [11]. The severe hypercalcemia may cause general symptoms, anorexia, constipation and abdominal pain, as well as depression, fatigue, weakness and memory disturbance. Polyuria and polydipsia are common. Some patients have recurrent pancreatitis, peptic ulcer disease or anemia. Around 10% present with symptomatic hypercalcemic crisis [1–6]. In contrast to patients with benign HPT, patients with parathyroid carcinoma can often have a palpable neck mass (in 30–50%), and occasionally recurrent laryngeal nerve palsy. At presentation, 15–20% of patients have lymph node metastases, and up to one-third distant metastases, often to lung or bone [7, 10, 12]. Exceptional parathyroid carcinomas are non-functional with normal serum calcium and parathyroid hormone (PTH) and present merely with a large mass in the neck with positive staining for PTH and malignant features [7].

Diagnosis

The carcinoma patients tend to have markedly raised serum calcium values, often above 14 mg/dL (3.5 mmol/L), and unusually high PTH values. The serum levels of alkaline phosphatases are often high and human chorionic gonadotropin α and β subunits may be raised [1, 2, 5–7].

Fine needle aspiration is generally contraindicated with parathyroid carcinoma because of risk for tumor implantation. Intraoperative frozen section may be unreliable and the diagnosis may have to be made by clinical recognition of the gross features at surgery with an adherent, firm, grayish–white parathyroid tumor, with a tendency to invade adjacent neck structures. This is in marked contrast to a benign parathyroid tumor with typical brownish-red color and soft consistency. Parathyroid carcinomas often also have conspicuous size with diameters of around 3 cm or more, and weights between 2 and 10 g or more [1, 2, 5–7].

Imaging modalities used for benign parathyroid disease may visualize parathyroid carcinoma. Ultrasound (US) may show a hypoechoic soft tissue mass with poorly defined margins and possible signs of local invasion, and may also detect lymph node metastases [6, 7]. ^{99m}Tc-sestamibi (MIBI) scanning can identify parathyroid carcinoma and possible metastases [6, 7]. Computed tomography (CT) with contrast enhancement is commonly used to reveal anatomical details of tumor or metastases. Magnetic resonance imaging (MRI) with gadolinium and fat suppression can also localize parathyroid tumors, but is most widely used for visualization of metastases, especially in the liver and bone. Fluorodeoxyglucose–positron emission tomography (FDG-PET) can with high sensitivity reveal metastatic spread.

Histopathology

Typical histopathological findings of parathyroid carcinoma include a thick fibrous capsule and fibrotic bands traversing the tumor, capsular and vascular invasion, and high mitotic activity [1, 2, 5–7, 10] (Fig. 22.1). However, some of these "classic" features may also be present in adenomas, and definite diagnosis of

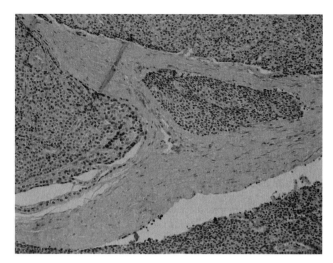

Figure 22.1 Typical but not pathognomonic fibrous banding of parathyroid carcinoma.

carcinoma requires demonstration of vascular invasion, or capsular penetration with growth into adjacent tissue, perineural space invasion, or metastases [13]. Vascular invasion should be in the capsule or in the surrounding tissue rather than within the tumor, and has been present in only 10–15% of carcinoma [2, 13] (Fig. 22.2). Capsular penetration should include growth into adjacent tissues, has been reported in 30–60%, and may lead to obvious tumor invasion in surrounding structures, the thyroid, the esophagus, the trachea, strap muscles or the recurrent laryngeal nerve [13] (Fig. 22.3). Non-penetrating capsular invasion is an unreliable sign not possible to distinguish from cell entrapment in fibrotic areas of degenerated adenomas. Perineural space invasion is uncommon, but a certain criterion of malignancy [2, 7, 13]. In the absence of invasion or metastases a definite diagnosis of parathyroid carcinoma is not possible and the lesion may be named "atypical parathyroid adenoma," implying that the patient has to be followed to exclude recurrence or metastases [1, 2, 6, 7].

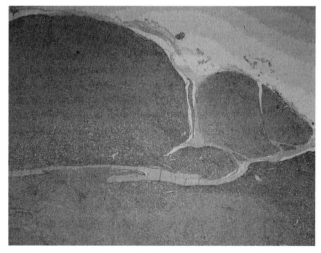

Figure 22.2 Capsular invasion with penetrating growth destroying the tumor capsule in parathyroid carcinoma.

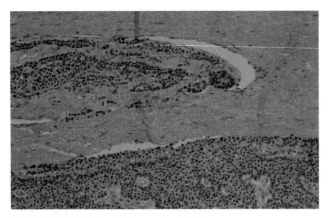

Figure 22.3 Vascular invasion in parathyroid carcinoma.

The thickened tumor capsule and fibrotic bands of the parenchyma, reported in 90% of parathyroid carcinoma, are not pathognomonic, but can be seen also in large adenomas with regressive changes, and around nodules in glands of secondary HPT [1, 2, 6, 7, 13]. Most carcinomas have solid growth pattern, some have a trabecular pattern, whereas follicular, acinar, rosette-like, or spindle cell growths are rare [2, 13]. Chief cells predominate in most parathyroid carcinomas, but occasional tumors are oncocytic, or contain mixtures of cells [13]. High mitotic activity and abnormal mitoses have been proposed as signs of malignancy, but are variable in parathyroid carcinomas, and also common in adenomas and some larger hyperplastic glands [2, 13]. Two-thirds of carcinomas have marked atypia with general nuclear enlargement and macronucleoli as the important signs [13]. Nuclear pleomorphism is common, but also frequent in adenomas [13]. The triad of macronucleoli, greater than 5 mitoses per 50 high-power microscopic fields, and scattered coagulative necroses indicates high risk for malignancy [2, 13].

DNA quantitation cannot distinguish parathyroid adenomas and carcinomas since many adenomas have an aneuploid pattern [13]. Aneuploidy can be associated with worse prognosis in carcinoma, but also aggressive carcinomas are often euploid [1, 7, 13]. Ki67 proliferation index >5% indicates increased risk of malignancy, but overlaps with adenomas and cannot safely distinguish the tumor entities [13]. The higher Ki67 index may reflect worse prognosis in carcinomas and should lead to close follow-up [2, 13].

Parathyroid carcinomas have shown reduced p27 expression, and tissue microarrays have revealed a multiple-marker phenotype (including Ki67, p27, Bcl-2, and mdm2) typical for adenomas, but less specific phenotype in carcinomas [2]. Absent expression of the calcium-sensing receptor has been found in carcinomas with high proliferation index, rarely in adenomas [2, 14]. Immunostaining for the Rb-protein has been absent in parathyroid carcinoma but generally present in adenomas, but this has not been invariably corroborated [1, 2, 9]. Galectin-3, histon-1 family2, amyloid β precursor protein and E-cadherin are suggested markers of parathyroid carcinoma, as is increased telomerase activity. Histological classification of parathyroid carcinoma into low grade (limited local infiltration) and high grade (widespread infiltration) has been proposed, but not convincingly demonstrated to reflect variable clinical aggressiveness [3, 13].

Molecular oncogenesis

Higher fractional allelic loss has been reported in parathyroid carcinomas than in adenomas [15]. Allelic losses of 1q25, 7q13, 10q23, 13q14 and 11p15 have been especially prevalent in carcinomas, and frequently mutated areas have included *HRPT2*, *PTEN*, retinoblastoma (*RB*), *HRAS* and *p53* genes [2, 6, 7, 15]. Common losses on 1p have been more proximal in carcinomas than in adenomas, suggesting presence of two different parathyroid tumor suppressor genes on that chromosome [15]. Combined 1q and 11q losses in one-third of carcinomas have indicated that the *HRPT2* and the *MEN 1* gene may together promote carcinogenesis [14].

Overexpression of the cell cycle regulator cyclin D1 occurs in 20–40% of parathyroid adenomas and up to 90% of parathyroid carcinoma [2, 5]. Loss of heterozygosity (LOH) of chromosome 13q and absent nuclear staining for the RB protein have been demonstrated in parathyroid carcinoma, but rarely found in parathyroid adenomas [2, 5]. *BRCA2*, the gene for familial breast and ovarian cancer syndromes, has close location on chromosome 13q, but sequencing has not revealed mutations of the *RB* or *BRCA2* genes in parathyroid carcinomas. It is possible that other genes with this location or other mechanisms may trigger tumor development [2, 5].

A high rate of somatic *HRPT2* mutations with biallelic inactivation has been revealed in sporadic parathyroid carcinomas. Some patients with apparently sporadic parathyroid carcinoma have carried *HRPT2* germline mutations, possibly representing a phenotypic variant of the HPT-JT syndrome with altered penetrance and without other features of the syndrome [8]. This seems to suggest that patients with apparently sporadic parathyroid carcinoma need to be tested for germline *HRPT2* gene mutations [6–8]. If mutation is identified, clinical features of the HPT-JT syndrome including renal and jaw neoplasia should be evaluated in patients and their families [6–9]. Parafibromin, encoded by the *HRPT2* gene on chromosome 1q25 is a member of the Paf complex with proposed role in transcriptional regulation and with the effect to inhibit cyclin D1 expression. Loss of parafibromin expression verified by immunohistochemistry has been suggested as a remarkably sensitive method to detect parathyroid carcinoma in resected specimens, if rare cystic adenomas of the HPT-JT syndrome, also lacking parafibromin, could be excluded [9]. However, a recent study [16] has shown that parafibromin immunoreactivity has limited diagnostic validity and cannot replace genetic testing or be used as the only discriminator to separate parathyroid adenoma from carcinoma. Positive parafibromin expression indicates benign disease and low risk of malignancy but does not exclude cancer or even presence of *HRPT2* gene mutation [16]. Partial loss or negative staining for parafibromin should motivate genetic analyses of the *HRPT2* gene in blood and tumor tissue from the affected patient. Additional biomarkers for parathyroid malignancy should be sought, possibly within the parafibromin pathways.

Surgery

Parathyroid carcinomas have typical features at surgery with a grayish–white, firm, lobulated, and conspicuously large tumor, surrounded by a dense fibrous capsule that may be adherent to adjacent tissues including the ipsilateral thyroid lobe, the muscularis layer of the esophagus, the trachea, the recurrent laryngeal nerve and the strap muscles [1, 2, 5, 10, 12]. The surgical treatment should consist of radical *en bloc* removal of the tumor together with the ipsilateral thyroid lobe and isthmus, and segmental excision of overlaying strap muscles and removal of the paratracheal fibrolymphatic compartment and other involved soft tissues. If a functioning recurrent laryngeal nerve is involved by tumor it should be resected, but can generally be preserved [6]. Rupture of the glandular capsule has to be avoided since this will cause seeding of tumor cells and multifocal recurrence [7, 10]. Bilateral neck exploration is recommended to exclude presence of additional pathological glands, occasionally reported in association with parathyroid carcinoma [5–7]. Formal lymphadenectomy is only indicated in patients with diagnosed lymph node involvement at presentation, since prophylactic neck dissection has not been shown to improve survival [7, 10, 18].

Radical initial surgery has resulted in a local recurrence rate as low as 10% and improved long-term survival, whereas incomplete resection has caused a local recurrence rate of 59% and high disease-related mortality [2, 5, 7, 10, 11]. Survival analyses have revealed 86% 5-year and 50% 10-year survival rates [4, 10, 18]. Main determinants of prognosis have been early recognition of the malignancy and efficient primary surgery, and adverse prognostic factors include simple parathyroidectomy, nodal or distant metastases at presentation, and non-functional tumor [2, 4–7, 10, 11].

Parathyroid carcinoma is often reported with indolent biology but is markedly tenacious with an overall recurrence rate of 50% [5, 7]. Recurrences have occurred on average 3 years after the initial operation, but sometimes after more than a decade of follow-up [1, 2, 4–7, 10, 11, 18]. A short disease-free interval reflects a poorer prognosis [7].

Surgery is the most effective treatment for recurrence and should always be considered for localized regional tumor [1, 5–7, 10, 18–20]. Cure will not be obtained by reoperation, unless the patient has been subjected to inadequate primary surgery, but even small tumor deposits may cause severe hypercalcemia and significant palliation can be achieved by resection of metastases in neck lymph nodes. Iterative surgery is frequently required, but the period of normocalcemia will become shorter after increased number of reoperations. Surgical removal of distant metastases (in lungs, liver and bone) has less consistent effect, but is recommended when possible, since significant tumor reduction may

facilitate medical treatment of hypercalcemia [1, 5–7, 10, 18–20]. Efforts should be made to localize the site of recurrence and to exclude wide dissemination before reoperation. Palpation and US scanning of the neck may reveal local recurrences while MIBI scanning and/or FDG-PET can verify the site and reveal or exclude distant spread in the chest, abdomen or the skeleton [5, 7, 10, 20].

Initial recurrence is often in cervical lymph nodes, followed by mediastinal nodes, or the lungs; involvement of liver, bone, pleura, pericardium and pancreas occurs at later stages [1, 5–7]. Lymph node metastases should be removed by compartment-oriented, sometimes bilateral, neck dissection, and may involve clearance of mediastinal glands. Lung metastases and other distant metastases may also require iterative surgery for palliation [10, 20].

Radiotherapy

Parathyroid carcinoma was previously not considered a radiosensitive tumor [1, 2]. However, radiation to the neck after surgery for recurrence has appeared to prevent tumor regrowth, and apparent cure of locally invasive parathyroid carcinoma has been reported [7, 21]. Adjuvant radiotherapy has been reported to prolong disease-free interval after primary surgery, and growing consensus suggests that this may offer survival benefits for parathyroid carcinoma [7, 11, 21].

Chemotherapy

Chemotherapy regimens have in general been ineffective in parathyroid carcinoma [1, 7]. A single patient has responded to treatment with dacarbazine, 5-fluorouracil and cyclophosphamide, and some remissions have been reported by a regimen consisting of methotrexate, doxorubicin, phosphoamide and lomustine, but overall results of chemotherapy have been disappointing [1, 7].

Management of hypercalcemia

The prognosis is poor when parathyroid carcinoma has become widely disseminated. Patients usually die of metabolic complications of hypercalcemia rather than from the disseminated tumor growth [5, 7, 10]. Hypercalcemia is treated with hydration by saline infusion and loop diuretics to enhance urinary calcium excretion, combined with agents that interfere with bone resorption [5, 7]. Calcitonin can lower serum calcium but the effect is modest and transient [1, 5, 7]. Bisphosphonates also transiently lower serum calcium, but with longer duration [5, 7]. Mithramycin can inhibit bone resorption, but complete normalization of serum calcium is often not achieved, and treatment should be restricted to life-threatening hypercalcemia unresponsive to bisphosphonates, since risk for severe liver, kidney and bone marrow toxicity increases with number of exposures [1, 2, 5–7]. Gallium nitrate has lowered serum calcium in some patients, but its use is limited by nephrotoxicity [1, 5–7].

Calcimimetics have been reported to have the greatest potential to control serum calcium in patients with parathyroid carcinoma [1, 5–7]. Dendritic cell immunotherapy and immunization with PTH peptides have lowered serum calcium in a few cases [1]. *In vitro* studies have shown apoptotic effect of zidovudine, a telomerase inhibitor used as an antiviral agent, in cultured parathyroid carcinoma cells.

Conclusion

Due to variable diagnostic criteria, and frequently failed recognition and inadequate surgical resection of parathyroid carcinomas even in expert institutions, the outcome has varied between reported patient series [9]. The important aim is to obtain early diagnosis and ensure radical *en bloc* resection of parathyroid carcinoma at the primary operation, and thereby improve survival prospects. Recent demonstration of *HRPT2* mutations in a majority of parathyroid carcinomas can possibly be of value for the histological diagnosis [16]. Positive parafibromin immunoreactivity indicates benign disease but does not exclude parathyroid carcinoma, and still other markers have to be searched for. Hopefully, further molecular characterization of the parafibromin pathway may in the future provide possibilities to diagnose carcinomas and predict a variable prognosis.

Acknowledgment

The authors would like to thank Professor Lars Grimelius for providing the figures.

References

1. Shane E. Clinical review 122. Parathyroid carcinoma. *J. Clin. Endocrinol. Metab.* 2001;86:485–493.
2. DeLellis RA. Parathyroid carcinoma. An overview. *Adv. Anat. Pathol.* 2005;12:53–61.
3. Agarwal G, Prasad KK, Kar DK, et al. Indian primary hyperparathyroidism with parathyroid carcinoma do not differ in clinico-investigative characteristics from those with benign parathyroid pathology. *World J. Surg.* 2006;30:732–742.
4. Hundahl SA, Fleming ID, Fremgen AM, Menck HR. Two hundred eighty-six cases of parathyroid carcinoma treated in the US between 1985–1995: a National Cancer Data Base Report. The American College of Surgeons Commission on Cancer and the American Cancer Society. *Cancer* 1999;86:538–544.
5. Mittendorf EA, McHenry CR. Parathyroid carcinoma. *J. Surg. Oncol.* 2005;89:136–142.
6. Rogers SE, Perrier ND. Parathyroid carcinoma. *Curr. Opin. Oncol.* 2006;18:16–22.
7. Rawat N, Khetan N, Williams DW, Baxter JN. Parathyroid carcinoma. *Br. J. Surg.* 2005;92:1345–1353.
8. Shattuck TM, Valimaki S, Obara T, et al. Somatic and germ–line mutations of the HRTP2 gene in sporadic parathyroid carcinoma. *N. Engl. J. Med.* 2003;349:1722–1729.
9. Tan M–H, Morrison C, Wang P, et al. Loss of parafibromin immunoreactivity is a distinguishing feature of parathyroid carcinoma. *Clin. Cancer Res.* 2004;10:6629–6637.
10. Åkerström G, Juhlin C, Johansson. Parathyroid carcinoma. In: Åkerström G (ed.). *Current Controversies in Parathyroid Operations and Reoperations.* Austin, TX: Landes Company, 1994:201–218.
11. Wynne A, van Heerden J, Carney J, Fitzpatrick LA. Parathyroid carcinoma: clinical and pathological features in 43 patients. *Medicine* 1992;71:197–205.
12. Obara T, Fujimoto Y. Diagnosis and treatment of patients with parathyroid carcinoma: An update and review. *World J. Surg.* 1991;15:738–744.
13. Bondeson L, Grimelius, L, Larsson C, et al. Parathyroid carcinoma. In: DeLellis RA, Lloyd RV, Heitz PU, Eng C (eds). *Pathology and Genetics. Tumours of Endocrine Organs. World Health Organization Classification of Tumours.* Lyon, France: IARC Press, 2004:124–127.
14. Haven CJ, van Puijenbroek M, Karperien M, et al. Differential expression of the calcium sensing receptor and combined loss of chromosomes 1q and 11q in parathyroid carcinoma. *J. Pathol.* 2004;202:86–94.
15. Hunt JL, Carty SE, Yim JH, et al. Allelic loss in parathyroid neoplasia can help characterize malignancy. *Am. J. Surg. Pathol.* 2005;29:1049–1055.
16. Juhlin CC, Villablanca A, Sandelin K, et al. Parafibromin immunoreactivity: its use as an additional diagnostic marker for parathyroid tumor classification. *Endocrine-Related Cancer* 2007;14:501–512.
17. Välimäki S, Forsberg L, Farnebo LO, Larsson C. Distinct target regions for chromosome 1p deletions in parathyroid adenomas and carcinomas. *Int. J. Oncol.* 2002;21:727–735.
18. Sandelin K, Auer G, Bondeson L, et al. Prognostic factors in parathyroid cancer. *World J. Surg.* 1992;16:724–731.
19. Obara T, Okamoto T, Ito Y, et al. Surgical and medical management of patients with pulmonary metastasis from parathyroid carcinoma. *Surgery* 1993;114:1040–1048.
20. Iacobone M, Ruffolo C, Lumachi F, Favia G. Results of iterative surgery for persistent and recurrent parathyroid carcinoma. *Langenbecks Arch Surg* 2005;390:385–390.
21. Munson ND, Foote RL, Northcutt RC, et al. Parathyroid carcinoma: is there a role for adjuvant radiation therapy? *Cancer* 2003;98:2378–2384.

3 Pituitary and Hypothalamic Lesions

23 Molecular Pathogenesis of Pituitary Adenomas

Ines Donangelo and Shlomo Melmed

> **Key points**
> - Pituitary tumors cause significant morbidity by abnormal hormone secretion and compression of regional structures.
> - Pituitary tumor development correlates with alteration in several molecular pathways, including: (1) cell cycle regulators, (2) signaling pathways, (3) angiogenesis, and (4) pituitary transcription factors.
> - The causal role for newly identified genetic imbalances in pituitary tumorigenesis has been tested using transgenic/knockout mouse model approach.
> - The main goal in understanding the pathogenesis of pituitary adenomas is identifying new subcellular signaling pathways for potential use as treatment targets. Gene delivery systems are also probable therapeutical tools.

Introduction

Pituitary adenomas account for ~15% of intracranial tumors, and cause significant morbidity by abnormal hormone secretion and compression of regional structures. Although the pathogenesis of pituitary tumors has been extensively investigated, determinants of initiation and progression of pituitary adenomas are not yet fully understood.

A significant proportion of patients do not achieve optimal control of mass effects and/or hormone hypersecretion despite advances in therapeutic approaches. Decisions on surgical vs. medical treatment of pituitary adenomas depend on the tumor subtype and degree of compression of perisellar structures. Surgical treatment is limited by relatively low cure rates for large, invasive adenomas, and medical therapy is useful only in prolactinomas and growth hormone (GH)-secreting adenomas. No effective medical therapy is currently available for adrenocorticotropic hormone (ACTH)-secreting tumors or clinically non-functioning tumors. Understanding the pathogenesis of pituitary adenomas will likely predict pituitary tumor growth patterns in individual patients, as well as identify new subcellular treatment targets, ultimately decreasing the morbidity and mortality related to these tumor types.

Diverse mechanisms have been described in the pathogenesis of pituitary adenomas, mainly imbalances in cell cycle regulation, signaling pathways, and angiogenesis [1–3]. These molecular changes may be general, or uniquely occur in specific pituitary tumor subtypes, as summarized in Table 23.1. The causal role for selected genetic imbalances for the development of pituitary tumors has also been confirmed in transgenic mouse models (Table 23.2).

Table 23.1 Selected molecular events related to tumorigenesis in human pituitary adenoma subtypes

	NF	GH	PRL	ACTH	TSH
Oncogenes					
Gsp	no	yes		no	
Cyclins	yes	yes	yes	yes	
EGF/EGFR	yes	unclear		unclear	no
GHRHR		yes			
PTTG	yes	yes	yes	yes	
Gal-3	no	no	yes	yes	no
HMGA2	yes		yes		
FGFR	yes	yes	no	yes	
Folate receptor	yes	no	no	no	
Tumour suppressor genes					
RB1	no	yes			
P16INK4a	yes	no			
P27KIP1	yes	yes	yes	yes	yes
MEG3a	yes	yes			
Gadd45-γ	yes	yes	yes		

No, prevalence of genetic imbalance <10% of studied adenomas.
Yes, prevalence of genetic imbalance >10% of studied adenomas.
Unclear, prevalence of genetic imbalance is controversial in different studies.
NF, clinically non-functioning pituitary adenoma; PRL, prolactin.

Clinical Endocrine Oncology, 2nd edition. Edited by Ian D. Hay and John A.H. Wass. © 2008 Blackwell Publishing. ISBN 978-1-4051-4584-8.

Table 23.2 Transgenic mouse models for pituitary tumors

	Hyperplasia/adenoma[b]
Gene overexpression[a]	
CMV.**HMGA1**	GH, PRL
CMV.**HMGA 2**	GH, PRL
Ubiquitin C.**hCG**	PRL
αGSU.**bLH**	Pit1 lineage
GH.**galanin**	GH, PRL
PRL.**galanin**	PRL[c]
PRL.**TGFα**	PRL
αGSU.**PTTG**	LH, GH, TSH
αGSU.**Prop1**	Non-functioning
PRL.**pdt-FGFR4**	PRL
Gene inactivation	
p27/Kip1–/–	ACTH, αMSH
p18/INK4c–/–	ACTH, αMSH
Rb+/–	ACTH, αMSH, αGSU, GH, βTSH
D2R-deficient	PRL
Men1+/–	PRL
PRL–/–	Non-functioning

[a]Genes are listed in bold, and are preceded by the promoter that determines transcriptional control.

[b]Hormone immunoreactivity/secreting profile.

[c]Pituitary hyperplasia, with no tumor formation.

CMV, cytomegalovirus; PRL, prolactin; HMGA, high mobility group A; pdt-FGFR4, pituitary tumor-derived fibroblast growth factor receptor-4; TGFα, transforming growth factor-alpha; Men1, multiple endocrine neoplasia type 1; PTTG, pituitary tumor transforming gene.

Cell cycle regulation

Retinoblastoma susceptibility gene (RB1)

The retinoblastoma susceptibility protein (pRB) encoded by *RB1* regulates the G1 to S phase cell cycle transition. In its active form pRB restrains cell cycle progression by binding E2F, an important transcription factor for the S phase (Fig. 23.1).

Mice with homozygous loss of *Rb1* are non-viable, but mice with heterozygous *Rb1* inactivation develop intermediate lobe pituitary tumors with high penetrance, and less frequently thyroid medullary carcinoma, pheochromocytoma, and anterior lobe pituitary tumors (Table 23.2) [4].

Loss of *RB1* in humans causes retinoblastoma and other tumors such as osteosarcoma; however these patients do not exhibit a predisposition to development of pituitary adenomas. Although aggressive human pituitary tumors exhibit loss of heterozygosity (LOH) of region 13q14 (*RB1* locus), pRB remains expressed suggesting that a tumor suppressor gene other than *RB1* present in the same chromosomal region may be related to pituitary tumor progression. While pRB is detected in most non-functioning pituitary adenomas, 20–25% of GH-secreting adenomas exhibit loss of pRB expression, and this finding does not correlate with tumor

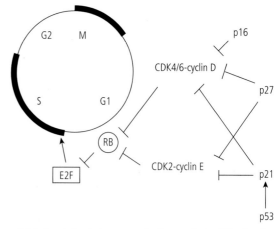

Figure 23.1 Targets for pituitary tumor development in the G1/S cell cycle checkpoint. Active (non-phosphorylated) pRB blocks progression of cell cycle from G1 to S phase by binding E2F. G1 progression and G1/S transition depends on sequential activation of cyclinD-CDK4 or -CDK6 and cyclinE-CDK2 complexes, leading to inactivation (phosphorylation) of pRB and release of E2F. CDK inhibitors (e.g., p16INK4a, p27Kip1, p21cip1) impede activation cyclin-CDK complexes, and are recognized as important tumor suppressor genes. Imbalances in pRB, p16, p27 and cyclins are present in pituitary adenomas, and the disruption of G1/S checkpoint barrier favors unrestrained cell cycle progression and proliferation.

behavior. Silencing of *RB1* expression in these pituitary tumors has been shown to occur due to promoter hypermethylation. Therefore, inactivation of *RB1* may be involved in human pituitary tumor development is a small subset of adenomas.

P16INK4a

The *p16INK4a* gene encodes p16, an inhibitor of the cyclin-dependent kinases CDK4 and CDK6 that favors cell-cycle arrest during G1 phase (Fig. 23.1). Loss of p16 results in phosphorylation (inactivation) of pRB, thus favoring cell cycle progression. Inactivation of p16 by hypermethylation of the *P16INK4a* promoter was detected in non-functioning pituitary tumors and correlates with a larger tumor size. Loss of p16 and pRB in tumors tend to be mutually exclusive, likely because functional pRB is necessary for cell cycle inhibition by p16 and loss of both regulators of the cell cycle would not result in additive growth advantage.

P27KIP1

P27KIP1 encodes p27, a CDK inhibitor, and loss of p27 results in cell cycle progression (Fig. 23.1). p27-null mice develop overall increase in growth, intermediate lobe pituitary tumors, and hyperplasia of hematopoietic organs [5] (Table 23.2). P27 protein is underexpressed in pituitary tumors, particularly in functioning adenomas when compared to non-functioning tumors. Whether p27 expression is further decreased in pituitary carcinomas remains controversial. However, no mutations or abnormal p27 mRNA expression have been detected in pituitary tumor samples, and mechanisms for p27 loss remain unknown.

p53

p53 inhibits cell cycle progression or induces apoptosis. p53 mutations are one of the most common abnormalities found in human cancer; however p53 appears not to play a major role in the pathogenesis of pituitary adenomas. Abnormal expression of p53 has been reported in some but not all pituitary carcinomas.

Cyclins

Cyclins D and E are important in regulation of G1 to S phase cell cycle progression, as cyclin-CDK complexes induce phosphorylation (inactivation) of pRB (Fig. 23.1). Cyclin D expression is increased particularly in non-functioning pituitary adenomas, and in pituitary tumors with aggressive behavior. Cyclin A, B and E are also more abundant in larger, highly proliferative pituitary adenomas [6]. Mechanisms that determine cyclin overexpression are not clear, and their elevated levels may reflect increased cell replication rate.

Signaling pathways

Epidermal growth factor (EGF), epidermal growth factor receptor (EGFR) and erbB-2

EGF has potent mitogenic activity in pituitary cells, and both EGF and its receptor EGFR may be overexpressed in pituitary tumors, particularly in non-functioning adenomas. Correlation between EGF/EGFR expression and aggressive pituitary tumor behavior has been suggested. ErbB-2 is an EGFR related oncoprotein found to be overexpressed in normal pituitary tissue, non-functioning tumors, and a fraction of GH-secreting tumors [7].

Gsα

Activating mutations of the proto-oncogene that encode the α-subunit of Gs protein (gsp) induce constitutive activation of adenylate cyclase. In GH-secreting cells, this oncogene activates growth hormone releasing hormone (GHRH) post-receptor pathways, i.e., cell proliferation and hormone secretion, without requiring ligand binding to the GHRH receptor.

Gsp mutations have been reported in 30–40% of GH-secreting adenomas. No major clinical differences between gsp+ and gsp– pituitary tumors have been identified, such as GH level, age distribution, or cure rate, although adenomas harboring this abnormality tend to be smaller and may be more responsive to medical therapy than gsp-negative tumors [8]. Gsp oncogene has been detected in <10% of non-functioning and ACTH-secreting tumors.

Dopamine receptors

The dopamine 2 receptor (D2R) mediates the inhibitory effect of dopamine on pituitary prolactin synthesis and secretion. D2R-deficient mice exhibit hyperprolactinemia and lactotroph hyperplasia that progresses to pituitary tumor (Table 23.2), suggesting that loss of dopamine inhibition induces murine neoplastic transformation. This finding likely cannot be extrapolated to pituitary

tumor development in humans as D2R mutations have not been identified. Decreased D2R expression has been linked to dopamine agonist resistance in prolactinomas.

Somatostatin receptors

Expression of somatostatin receptors (SST) 1 through 5 has been studied in pituitary adenomas. Although all SST types have been shown positive in all tumor types, SST5 and SST2 are the predominant receptors. Prolactinomas exhibit high SST1 expression compared to other tumor types. SST3 is frequently detected in non-functioning adenomas, while SST4 expression is relatively infrequent in pituitary tumors. In GH-secreting adenomas, SST2 and SST5 expression does not correlate with tumor behavior; however lower SST2 content is observed in adenomas less responsive to somatostatin analog therapy. A germline mutation in the coding sequence of SST5 was reported in a single patient with acromegaly resistant to somatostatin analog therapy, and no mutations have been identified in other SST subtypes. Polymorphisms in the coding (c1044t) and promoter (t-461c) regions of SST5 are associated with lower basal GH and insulin-like growth factor (IGF)-I levels in patients with acromegaly. Nevertheless, these SST2 and SST5 variants do not correlate with responsiveness to somatostatin analog therapy. Therefore, SSTs expression may correlate with responsiveness to medical treatment, but their role in the pathogenesis of pituitary adenomas, if any, remains unlikely.

GHRH receptor

The GHRH receptor (GHRHR) is overexpressed in GH-secreting adenomas compared to normal pituitary tissue. Nevertheless, activating mutations have not been identified in this receptor. The significance of increased expression of GHRHR in the pathogenesis of GH-secreting adenomas is not clear.

Angiogenesis

Vascularization is decreased in pituitary tumors compared to normal tissue, in marked contrast to the pattern observed in other tumor types, such as prostate, breast, stomach, and bladder where cancer development is linked to increased angiogenesis. This unexpected observation may be related to the usual slow growth of pituitary adenomas, i.e., enlargement of this benign tumor with low metabolic demands is likely not limited by the vascularization index. An alternative explanation is that in contrast to the normal gland which is predominantly supplied by the hypothalamo–pituitary portal vein, pituitary adenomas receive a direct systemic blood supply, and the relatively low vascular density in these tumors occurs in parallel to an in-growth of systemic capillaries, with resulting net increase in angiogenesis.

Although microvascular density is decreased in pituitary adenomas compared to normal pituitary tissue, a relationship between vascularization and tumor behavior is apparent, particularly in prolactin (PRL)-secreting tumors which are more vascularized than GH- or follicle-stimulating hormone (FSH)-positive adenomas.

Macroprolactinomas, invasive prolactinomas, or pituitary carcinomas have higher microvascular density compared, respectively, to microprolactinomas, non-invasive prolactinomas, or pituitary adenomas. Conversely, angiogenesis does not increase with tumor size in GH-secreting adenomas. This is consistent with the notion that microprolactinomas may represent a pathological and clinical entity distinct from macroprolactinomas, whereas different-sized GH-secreting adenomas are components of the same disease spectrum [9].

Vascular endothelial growth factor (VEGF)

VEGF is involved in angiogenesis by increasing proliferation and migration of endothelial cells, as well as endothelial permeability and fenestrations. VEGF also functions as an anti-apoptotic factor promoting survival of vessel endothelial cells. VEGF is detected in both the normal pituitary gland and in pituitary adenomas, and its levels correlate with tumor behavior, as VEGF is higher in carcinomas and macroprolactinomas.

VEGF expression is probably under dopaminergic control. Dopamine, signaling through the endothelial cell D2R, can inhibit VEGF action, likely by endocytosis of VEGFR-2. In addition, pituitary glands derived from DR2-knockout female mice have increased VEGF-A expression compared with wild-type mice. Conditioned media derived from D2R(–/–) cells enhanced human umbilical vein cell proliferation. Dopamine agonists such as bromocriptine and cabergoline may therefore inhibit pituitary tumor angiogenesis by blocking VEGF action.

Fibroblast growth factor (FGF)

FGF-2 is an angiogenic factor that stimulates endothelial cell proliferation. Plasma derived from patients harboring pituitary adenomas contains increased FGF-2 levels, and pituitary tumor transforming gene (PTTG)-stimulated increase in FGF induces angiogenesis *in vitro* and *in vivo*. However, it remains to be determined if FGF-2 has a role on pituitary adenoma progression.

Pituitary transcription factors

Expression of transcription factors, such as Prop1, Pit-1 and DAX-1, in pituitary adenomas may reflect the origin of tumor cells, and possibly their level of differentiation. However, whether or not the presence of these transcription factors plays a causal role on the development of human pituitary tumors remains unclear.

Prop-1

Prop-1, or prophet of Pit-1, is a pituitary transcription factor essential for early development and differentiation of GH-, PRL-, thyroid-stimulating hormone (TSH)-, and gonadotropin-secreting cells. Elevated of Prop-1 expression past this developmentalperiod may predispose to tumor formation, as shown in a mouse model with pituitary targeted transgenic Prop-1 overexpresssion (Table 23.2). Long-term exposure to Prop1 induces formation of Rathke's cysts, pituitary hyperplasia and non-functioning

adenomas. In humans, PROP-1 is widely expressed in pituitary adenoma subtypes, and does not correlate with clinical behavior [10].

Pit-1 (POUF-1)

Pit-1 is a transcription factor involved in development and early differentiation of somatotrophs, thyrotrophs, and lactotrophs. In human pituitary adenomas, Pit-1 is expressed in GH-, TSH-, and PRL-secreting tumors. Corticotropinomas are rarely positive for Pit-1. Non-functioning pituitary adenomas can also be positive for Pit-1, especially those expressing the α-subunit, suggesting that this non-functioning tumor subtype arises from an early cell precursor that is both α-subunit and Pit-1 positive [11].

DAX-1

DSS-AHC critical region on the X chromosome, gene 1 (DAX-1) is an orphan nuclear receptor that when mutated causes adrenal hypoplasia congenita with associated hypogonadotropic hypogonadism. DAX-1 expression has been shown in all regions of the hypothalamo–pituitary–adrenal–gonadal axis during development and in adult tissues, suggesting a critical role for DAX-1 in the normal development and function of this axis. DAX-1 is expressed in clinically non-functioning pituitary adenomas of gonadotroph lineage. Non-secreting tumors from mammosomatotropic lineage (adenomas expressing GH, PRL and Pit-1) rarely express DAX-1, emphasizing that clinically non-functioning adenomas are heterogeneous by nature. Prolactinomas and GH-secreting pituitary adenomas are negative for DAX-1.

Miscellaneous

PTTG

Pituitary tumor transforming gene (PTTG) was isolated from the GH4 rat pituitary tumor cell line. PTTG overexpression in mouse NIH-3T3 fibroblasts induces cellular transformation *in vitro* and tumor formation in nude mice. PTTG is present in the normal pituitary gland, and its expression is markedly increased in most human pituitary tumors. PTTG was identified as the index mammalian securin, regulating sister chromatid separation during mitosis, and excess or suppressed PTTG levels result in aneuploidy.

Transgenic mouse models of both PTTG overexpression and inactivation support a causal role for changes in PTTG levels on development of pituitary hyperplasia and hypoplasia, and on conferring tumor growth advantage or tumor growth protection, respectively. Mice with transgenic expression of human PTTG1 to the pituitary gland develop pituitary plurihormonal hyperplasia (Fig. 23.2) [12]. In contrast, global PTTG inactivation results in the opposite trophic effects, i.e. pituitary, pancreatic β-cell, splenic, and testicular hypoplasia. Moreover, Pttg inactivation in Rb+/– mice results in relative protection from pituitary tumor development, and in contrast, targeted pituitary overexpression of PTTG in Rb+/– mice causes increased prevalence of anterior lobe pituitary tumors [13]. These studies support a causal effect of pituitary

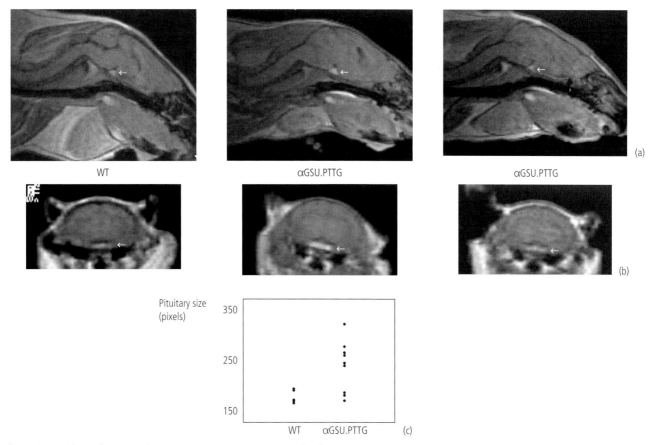

Figure 23.2 Evidence of pituitary enlargement on magnetic resonance images (MRI) in PTTG transgenic mice. Sagittal (a) and coronal (b) MRI images of one wild-type (WT) and two transgenic (αGSU.PTTG) mice. (c) Scattergram depicting pituitary size in total pixels obtained by adding the pituitary area obtained from consecutive sagittal images. (Reproduced from Abbud RA, Mol. Endocrinol. 2005;19:1383–1391, with permission from the Endocrine Society.)

PTTG abundance on tissue trophic status and likelihood of tumor formation.

Several proposed mechanisms may explain the role of PTTG on tumor development. As a securin, PTTG has the critical role of regulating sister chromatid separation during mitosis. Abnormal PTTG levels cause asymmetric sister chromatid separation and aneuploidy. Genomic instability has been associated with cancer and correlates with aggressive neoplasia, including pituitary tumors. In addition, PTTG possesses transactivation ability, and it is shown to activate c-myc transcription and inhibit expression of the cell cycle inhibitor p21. PTTG also induces growth factors expression (FGF and VEGF) and induces angiogenesis [14].

Galectin-3

Galectin-3 (Gal-3) is a β-galactoside binding protein involved in cancer progression and metastasis. It is expressed in ACTH-, PRL-secreting and folliculo-stellate cells in the normal pituitary gland, and ACTH- and PRL-producing pituitary adenomas and carcinomas are positive for Gal-3 [15]. There is a direct correlation between proliferation rate and Gal-3 levels in a pituitary cell line derived from a non functional pituitary tumor (HP75). Gal-3 expression is higher in pituitary carcinomas vs. adenomas, indicating that it may have a role on pituitary tumor progression.

GADD45-γ

Growth arrest- and DNA damage-inducible gene (GADD45-γ) is induced by DNA damage and is involved in growth suppression and apoptosis. It was identified as a candidate tumor suppressor gene for pituitary adenomas by cDNA-representational difference analysis (cDNA-RDA). While expressed in the normal pituitary gland, GADD45-γ is absent in most non-functioning, GH-, and PRL-secreting adenomas, as well as in immortalized pituitary cell lines [16]. Pituitary tumors positive and negative for GADD45-γ do not differ in their clinical parameters. Growth suppression induced by GADD45-γ was shown *in vitro* by decreased colony formation of pituitary derived cell lines in soft agar. Loss of expression in pituitary tumors likely occurs by epigenic changes, i.e., methylation of CpG islands in the GADD45-γ promoter.

MEG3

Maternally expressed gene 3 (MEG3) is a human homolog to mouse Gtl2 involved in fetal and postnatal development. An isoform of this gene that contains an extra exon (MEG3a) has been identified by cDNA-RDA, and is expressed in normal human pituitary, brain and other tissues, but is diminished or absent in pituitary tumors and human cancer cell lines [17]. MEG3a is undetectable in both non-functioning and GH-secreting pituitary adenomas, suggesting that loss of this gene is not specific to a particular pituitary tumor subtype. Introduction of MEG3a in cancer cell lines inhibits proliferation and decreases their ability to form colonies. Hence loss of MEG3a in pituitary adenomas likely confers tumor growth advantage. Hypermethylation of the promoter region is a mechanism for MEG3 silencing in non-functioning pituitary adenomas, and no LOH, deletions, or mutations in this gene have been identified.

High Mobility Group A2 gene

The High Mobility Group A2 gene (*HMGA2*) maps to region 12q14–15 and is a member of the *HMGA* family that includes *HMGA1*. HMGA proteins are involved in regulation of chromatin structure, and HMGA DNA-binding sites have been identified in the functional regions of several gene promoters. The HMGA genes are abundantly expressed during embryogenesis, but not in normal adult tissues. However, they are frequently overexpressed in several neoplasias including thyroid, prostate, cervix, colorectum, and pancreatic carcinomas, and seem to play a critical role in cell transformation. Transgenic overexpression of HMGA1 and HMGA2 in mice causes GH- and PRL-secreting pituitary tumors [18] (Table 23.2). Trisomy of chromosome 12, which harbors *HMGA2*, represents the most frequent cytogenetic alteration in human prolactin-secreting pituitary adenomas, and HMGA2 overexpression was detected in a number of prolactinomas harboring rearrangement of regions 12q14–15. HMGA2 is also expressed in a subset of non-functioning pituitary adenomas; however chromosome 12 polysomy was not detected in this tumor subtype, so alternative mechanisms for overexpression of this gene need to be sought. Recent studies show that HMGA2 tumorigenic effects are mediated by the E2F pathway.

Folate receptor

A cDNA microarray analysis of pituitary adenomas identified that the folate receptor is markedly overexpressed in clinically non-functioning adenomas but not in functional adenomas (ACTH-, GH- and prolactin-secreting adenomas) [19]. The specific overexpression of this receptor was subsequently confirmed by more definite methods. The proper folding and binding of folic acid to this receptor was demonstrated in non-functioning adenomas. Comparison of non-functioning tumor subtypes suggested that the immunohistochemically negative adenomas produce more properly folded folate receptor than non-functioning adenomas that stain positively for anterior pituitary hormones. The significance of these findings remains unclear, but overexpression of functional folate receptor in non-functioning pituitary adenomas may mediate vitamin transport, and potentially facilitate growth of these tumors.

Aryl hydrocarbon receptor interacting protein (AIP) gene

Linkage analysis of three Finnish families with very-low-penetrance susceptibility to GH- and PRL- secreting adenomas provided evidence for linkage in chromosome 11q12–11q13, a region previously implicated in isolated familial somatotropinomas (IFS).

No mutations or altered expression in the multiple endocrine neoplasia (MEN 1) were detected in representative blood samples from this cohort. Mapping of the linked chromosomal region identified AIP, or aryl hydrocarbon receptor interacting protein gene, as the strongest candidate. Three distinct AIP germline mutations have been identified: *Q14X* mutation was detected in members of these Finnish families with pituitary adenoma predisposition, *R304X* mutation was detected in an Italian family with acromegaly, and 16% (7 of 45) of patients with sporadic acromegaly exhibited either *Q14X* or *IVS3-1G>A* AIP mutation. Study of a German and a Turkish family with familial somatotropinomas did not detect mutations in AIP. None of these three specific AIP germline mutations was detected in 66 sporadic pituitary tumors derived from mostly caucasian US patients. Loss of heterozygosity was detected in pituitary adenomas with AIP germline mutations, suggesting that AIP may behave as a tumor suppressor gene. Pituitary expression of AIP in carriers of germline AIP mutations remains to be determined.

Gene therapy for pituitary tumors: perspectives

The major goal of achieving a better understanding of determinants for pituitary tumorigenesis is the expansion of therapeutic options. While management of pituitary tumors is rapidly evolving, current treatment modalities address relieving symptoms, rather than targeting the cause of tumor initiation. The emerging field of gene therapy for the treatment of neoplasias is still at a very early stage, yet results of *in vitro* and preclinical animal models studies are encouraging [20].

The aim of gene therapy is to introduce therapeutic genes into tissues, and this is more efficiently done with viral vectors. A diverse range of viral vector types has been developed, with various degrees of transduction efficiency, stability of transgene expression, and vector associated toxicity and immunogenicity. The ideal gene delivery system should confer efficient delivery and persistent expression of transgene. Transgene expression should be cell-type specific and regulatable. Importantly, the vector should be safe, i.e., no adverse immune response and other cytotoxic reactions should be elicited. Although a "flawless" vector system has not yet been developed, important advances have been achieved in this field. Targeted expression can be performed using cell-type specific promoters, and this is particularly precise in the pituitary gland due to distinct hormone secreting cells subtypes. Transcription regulation can be employed with the tetracycline-dependent regulatory system, where gene expression may be turned "on" or "off" in the presence or absence of an inducer (doxycycline). Novel vectors that do not elicit strong inflammatory response have been generated, allowing for long term transgene expression.

A variety of therapeutic genes has been developed for cancer gene therapy, including: (a) suicide genes (herpes simplex virus thymidine kinase); (b) toxic genes (diphtheria toxin); and (c) tumor suppressor genes (Rb1). (a) Herpes simplex virus thymidine kinase (HSV-TK) is a pro-drug delivery system activated by acyclovir or ganciclovir. It has been shown successful in controlling growth of pituitary cell tumors in nude mice after intratumoral injection. However, HSV-TK/ganciclovir expression driven by the prolactin promoter was not effective in suppressing prolactin levels in a rat model of lactotrope hyperplasia. (b) Cre-mediated activation of diphtheria toxin in GH secreting cells causes significant regression of GH4 somatotropic tumor cells *in vitro* and *in vivo*. Of note, cre-recombinase integrase system confers gene activation only in the presence of a cell type-specific promoter. (c) Rb-deficient mice develop spontaneous pituitary tumors, and adenovirus-mediated Rb1 gene therapy was used in this mouse model. Intratumoral Rb1 cDNA transfer inhibited pituitary tumor growth and prolonged life span of treated mice [20].

Gene therapy will likely be useful for pituitary tumors resistant to conventional treatment or those with tumor recurrence. Gene delivery may potentially be used alone or in combination with current treatments. For instance, intratumoral gene delivery could be used to eliminate non-resectable tumor during neurosurgical intervention. Improvements in vector design and gene therapy technology are required before clinical studies in non-life-threatening diseases such as pituitary adenomas can be implemented. Whether restoring genetic imbalances in individual pituitary tumors will be a useful tool in controlling tumor growth remains to be addressed.

References

1. Melmed S. Mechanisms for pituitary tumorigenesis: the plastic pituitary. *J. Clin. Invest.* 2003;112:1603–1618.
2. Levy A, Lightman S. Molecular defects in the pathogenesis of pituitary tumours. *Front. Neuroendocrinol.* 2003;24:94–127.
3. Scheithauer BW, Gaffey TA, Lloyd RV, et al. Pathobiology of pituitary adenomas and carcinomas. *Neurosurgery* 2006;59:341–353.
4. Jacks T, Fazeli A, Schmitt EM, et al. Effects of an Rb mutation in the mouse. *Nature* 1992;359:295–300.
5. Kiyokawa H, Kineman RD, Manova-Todorova KO, et al. Enhanced growth of mice lacking the cyclin-dependent kinase inhibitor function of p27(Kip1). *Cell* 1996;85:721–732.
6. Jordan S, Lidhar K, Korbonits M, et al. Cyclin D and cyclin E expression in normal and adenomatous pituitary. *Eur J Endocrinol.* 2000;143:R1–R6.
7. Chaidarun SS, Eggo MC, Sheppard MC, et al. Expression of epidermal growth factor (EGF), its receptor, and related oncoprotein (erbB-2) in human pituitary tumors and response to EGF in vitro. *Endocrinology* 1994;135:2012–2021.
8. Spada A, Arosio M, Bochicchio D, et al. Clinical, biochemical, and morphological correlates in patients bearing growth hormone-secreting pituitary tumors with or without constitutively active adenylyl cyclase. *J. Clin. Endocrinol. Metab.* 1990;71:1421–1426.
9. Turner HE, Harris AL, Melmed S, et al. Angiogenesis in endocrine tumors. *Endocr. Rev.* 2003;24:600–632.
10. Cushman LJ, Watkins-Chow DE, Brinkmeier ML, et al. Persistent Prop1 expression delays gonadotrope differentiation and enhances pituitary tumor susceptibility. *Hum. Mol. Genet.* 2001;10:1141–1153.
11. Sanno N, Teramoto A, Matsuno A, et al. In situ hybridization analysis of Pit-1 mRNA and hormonal production in human pituitary adenomas. *Acta Neuropathol. (Berl.).* 1996;91:263–268.
12. Abbud RA, Takumi I, Barker EM, et al. Early multipotential pituitary focal hyperplasia in the alpha–subunit of glycoprotein hormone-driven pituitary tumor-transforming gene transgenic mice. *Mol. Endocrinol.* 2005;19:1383–1391.
13. Donangelo I, Gutman S, Horvath E, et al. Pituitary tumor transforming gene overexpression facilitates pituitary tumor development. *Endocrinology* 2006;147:4781–4791.
14. Heaney AP, Horwitz GA, Wang Z, et al. Early involvement of estrogen-induced pituitary tumor transforming gene and fibroblast growth factor expression in prolactinoma pathogenesis. *Nat. Med.* 1999;5:1317–1321.
15. Riss D, Jin L, Qian X. et al. Differential expression of galactin-3 in pituitary tumors. *Cancer Res.* 2003;63:2251–2255.
16. Zhang X, Sun H, Danila DC, et al. Loss of expression of GADD45 gamma, a growth inhibitory gene, in human pituitary adenomas: implications for tumorigenesis. *J. Clin. Endocrinol. Metab.* 2002;87:1262–1267.
17. Zhang X, Zhou Y, Mehta KR, et al. A pituitary-derived MEG3 isoform functions as a growth suppressor in tumor cells. *J. Clin. Endocrinol. Metab.* 2003;88:5119–5126.
18. Fedele M, Battista S, Kenyon L, et al. Overexpression of the HMGA2 gene in transgenic mice leads to the onset of pituitary adenomas. *Oncogene* 2002;21:3190–3198.
19. Evans CO, Young AN, Brown MR, et al. Novel patterns of gene expression in pituitary adenomas identified by complementary deoxyribonucleic acid microarrays and quantitative reverse transcription–polymerase chain reaction. *J. Clin. Endocrinol. Metab.* 2001;86:3097–3107.
20. Castro M, Goverdhana S, Hu J, et al. Gene therapy for pituitary tumors: from preclinical models to clinical implementation. *Front. Neuroendocrinol.* 2003;24:62–77.

24 Functional Assessment of the Pituitary

John S. Bevan

Key points

- Accurate assessment of pituitary function is essential for patients with pituitary and para-pituitary tumors, both at diagnosis and at intervals after therapies have been applied.
- Despite the development of several other tests, the insulin tolerance test remains the "gold standard" for assessing adrenocorticotropic hormone and growth hormone reserves.
- The short synthetic adrenocorticotropic hormone test may yield false-negative results if used within one month of an acute pituitary insult, but at other times correlates well with the cortisol response to hypoglycemia.
- The combined growth hormone releasing hormone-arginine test is emerging as a useful means of assessing growth hormone reserve in patients for whom hypoglycemia is contraindicated.
- Insulin-like growth factor-1 cannot be used in isolation as a diagnostic test for adult-onset growth hormone deficiency.
- The use of thyrotropin releasing hormone and luteinizing hormone releasing hormone for assessment of pituitary function should be discontinued.

Introduction

The anterior pituitary secretes six hormones – growth hormone (GH), adrenocorticotropic hormone (ACTH), luteinizing hormone (LH), follicle-stimulating hormone (FSH), thyroid-stimulating hormone (TSH) and prolactin (PRL) – all of which are under feedback control by target gland hormones and a complex of hypothalamic regulators. Varying degrees of hypopituitarism may be present at diagnosis in patients with space-occupying pituitary or hypothalamic lesions, or may occur at a later stage, particularly after surgery or radiotherapy. Anterior pituitary failure often evolves in a predictable sequence with early deficiencies in gonadotrophins and GH, followed by ACTH and finally by TSH.

Accurate evaluation of pituitary function is essential, both at diagnosis and at intervals after treatments have been applied. This chapter briefly describes the physiological basis for the various pituitary function tests and examines the evidence base for their clinical application. Some pituitary hormones can be tested using single blood samples (e.g., TSH, together with free T_4) whereas others with more complicated circadian or pulsatile patterns of secretion require dynamic stimulation tests (e.g., ACTH). There is ongoing debate over the best tests for diagnosing ACTH and GH deficiency. Assessment of posterior pituitary failure and the various pituitary hormone hypersecretory syndromes are dealt with elsewhere. The chapter concludes with some practical clinical guidelines

for newly presenting patients, perioperative adrenal management and interval assessments after surgery and radiotherapy.

Hypothalamo–pituitary–adrenal axis

Assessment of the hypothalamo–pituitary–adrenal (HPA) axis, and thus defining a possible need for glucocorticoid replacement therapy, is the most important aspect of anterior pituitary function testing. Two clinical scenarios should be considered. First, the newly presenting patient with a pituitary macro-lesion and symptoms of possible hypoadrenalism (e.g., tiredness, nausea, arthralgia) in whom the clinician wishes to determine whether the symptoms are due to glucocorticoid insufficiency. Second, the patient at *potential* risk of adrenal insufficiency (for instance, after pituitary surgery or radiotherapy) in whom the investigator needs to assess the patient's ability to respond to stress, even in the absence of symptoms of endocrine deficiency.

General considerations

Under normal circumstances, ACTH secretion shows a marked circadian rhythm with highest levels in the early morning and lowest at around midnight. Measurement of the target hormone cortisol is common to all tests of the HPA axis and cortisol has the advantage of being a more stable hormone in serum/plasma than ACTH. It should be remembered that exogenously administered hydrocortisone or prednisolone interferes with the radioimmunoassay determination of endogenous cortisol secretion. Furthermore, dexamethasone – often administered in neurosurgical settings – will render cortisol measurements uninterpretable, both

---

Clinical Endocrine Oncology, 2nd edition. Edited by Ian D. Hay and John A.H. Wass. © 2008 Blackwell Publishing. ISBN 978-1-4051-4584-8.

during treatment and for several days after steroid withdrawal depending on the dose and duration of therapy. Total cortisol levels are significantly raised in patients taking oral estrogens due to an increased production of cortisol-binding globulin (CBG) – if possible, oral estrogens should be discontinued for at least 6 weeks before pituitary adrenal axis testing although, in practice, increments in serum cortisol during dynamic tests may still yield clinically useful information. In the assessment of adrenal function during major stress (such as sepsis or major surgery) the clinician needs to assess what level of cortisol constitutes a "satisfactory" response to the degree of stress. Early studies of cortisol secretion following major abdominal surgery suggested a threshold cortisol level of 580 nmol/L (21 µg/dL), measured using the older fluorimetric assay [1], which probably equates to a figure of 500 nmol/L (18 µg/dL) using modern radioimmunoassays [2]. However, a 26% difference in basal cortisol concentration has been demonstrated using different cortisol immunoassays [3], so knowledge of the local cortisol assay is important, and the clinician should not be overly dependent on absolute cut-off values taken from the literature.

HPA axis tests

Several tests are available to help predict whether the HPA axis is able to respond normally to significant stress including basal serum cortisol, the insulin tolerance test (ITT), the glucagon stimulation test (GST) and the short Synacthen test (SST) standard and low dose versions (Synacthen® [Novartis], tetracosactide [tetracosactrin] =

synthetic ACTH) (Table 24.1). Other tests using CRH or overnight metyrapone are unreliable and not in widespread use. There has been considerable controversy as to whether the more convenient SST can substitute for more complicated tests such as the ITT.

Basal cortisol

Ideally, basal cortisol should be measured between 8 and 9 am since HPA axis activity is maximal at this time. Random cortisol measurements, for example during afternoon clinics, are much less useful and often difficult to interpret. If the basal morning cortisol is less than 100 nmol/L (4 µg/dL) this strongly suggests ACTH deficiency and glucocorticoid replacement should be commenced. If basal cortisol is greater than 450 nmol/L (16 µg/dL) adrenal insufficiency is very unlikely. An intermediate value requires dynamic testing to assess ACTH reserve.

Insulin tolerance test

This test delivers a controlled stressful stimulus to the entire HPA axis by means of insulin-induced hypoglycemia. It has the additional advantage of stimulating GH secretion and is still regarded by many as the "gold standard" test for the evaluation of both ACTH and GH reserves. Whilst the safety of the ITT in children has been questioned, audits of the test performed in adults in specialist endocrine investigation units have shown an acceptably low level of morbidity. Nevertheless, the ITT is labor intensive, requires specialist supervision and is contraindicated in patients

Table 24.1 Dynamic tests of ACTH reserve

Test	Responses	Comments
Insulin tolerance test (ITT) Pre-test morning cortisol, serum potassium and ECG Overnight fast Intravenous bolus of 0.15 U soluble (regular) insulin per kg body weight (higher doses may be required in states of insulin resistance) Nadir glucose should fall to less than 2.2 mmol/L (40 mg/dL) Measure plasma glucose and serum cortisol (and GH, if required) at −15, 0, 30, 60, 90 and 120 minutes	A normal response is a peak cortisol above 500 nmol/L (18 µg/dL) (usually with an increment in excess of 200 nmol/L) (7 µg/dL) Some clinicians prefer to use a more stringent peak cortisol of 550 (20 µg/dL), or even 600 nmol/L (22 µg/dL).	An experienced attendant (doctor or specialist nurse) should be present throughout the test, with 50% dextrose available to reverse severe hypoglycemia The test is contraindicated in patients with a history of ischemic heart disease, cerebrovascular disease or seizures The test should not be performed if morning cortisol is below 100 nmol/L (4 µg/dL) Many clinicians do not perform ITTs in patients over 60 years of age
Synacthen® test (SST) Intravenous bolus of synthetic ACTH (Synacthen®, 250 µg) Measure serum cortisol at 0 and 30 minutes (60 min sampling is not required)	A normal response is a peak cortisol above 500 nmol/L (18 µg/dL) (usually with an increment in excess of 200 nmol/L) (7 µg/dL) Some authors have suggested a peak cortisol of 600 nmol/L (22 µg/dL) above which virtually all patients will have a normal ITT cortisol response [2]	No major side effects Unreliable test of the HPA axis within 1 month of an acute pituitary insult, such as surgery Contraindicated in patients with severe atopy and in pregnant women
Glucagon stimulation test (GST) Subcutaneous injection of 1 mg glucagon (1.5 mg if patient weighs over 90 kg) Measure plasma glucose and serum cortisol (and GH, if required) at −15, 0, 90 and 120, 150, 180, 210 and 240 minutes	A normal response is a peak cortisol above 500 nmol/L (18 µg/dL) (usually with an increment in excess of 200 nmol/L) (7 µg/dL)	Nausea, abdominal cramps and occasional vomiting may occur Impaired responses occur in 10% of normal subjects

with ischemic heart disease or epilepsy. Many endocrinologists avoid its use in patients over the age of 60 years who may have subclinical vascular disease. The standard dose of insulin is 0.15 units per kg body weight, given as an intravenous bolus of soluble insulin. Venous blood glucose should fall to less than 2.2 mmol/L (40 mg/dL); sometimes this target is not achieved and the insulin dose has to be repeated. It is prudent to check a morning cortisol level, serum potassium concentration and resting ECG before performing an ITT. The test should not be performed if the basal cortisol is less than 100 nmol/L (4 µg/dL). Patients with long-standing ACTH deficiency may have low body glycogen stores so it is usual to give a meal and to observe the patient for 2 hours after the test, to ensure complete recovery from the hypoglycemia. Occasionally, severe hypoglycemia requires the administration of intravenous glucose during the ITT; if this occurs, sampling for cortisol and GH should be continued since a more than adequate hypoglycemic stimulus will have been delivered. Most endocrinologists regard a cortisol increment of at least 200 nmol/L (7 µg/dL) together with a peak cortisol level above 500 nmol/L (18 µg/dL) to constitute a normal response. Others prefer to set a more stringent peak cortisol of 550 (20 µg/dL), or even 600 nmol/L (22 µg/dL).

Glucagon stimulation test

This test is a useful method of assessing the HPA and GH axes for patients in whom the ITT is contraindicated. It is used quite widely in the UK [4], but less so in other parts of the world. The test has been studied less intensively than the ITT and SST. The GST uses the same cortisol criteria as those established for the ITT. The ACTH and GH responses to glucagon occur relatively later than during an ITT and blood sampling is carried out every half an hour between 90 and 240 min after the intramuscular injection of 1.0 mg of glucagon. Glucagon may cause nausea, abdominal cramps and occasional vomiting. Some normal individuals fail to mount an ACTH response to glucagon.

Short Synacthen® test

Although initially employed in the investigation of patients with possible primary adrenal failure, Synacthen® stimulation has been used as an "indirect" test of ACTH reserve for the past 30 years. Its sensitivity in this setting depends on the secondary adrenal atrophy that results following ACTH deficiency but it should be recognized that this takes at least 3–4 weeks to develop after an acute pituitary insult, such as pituitary surgery. The standard SST involves the intravenous (more predictable than intramuscular) injection of a pharmacological dose (250 µg) of the ACTH analog. The SST is a simple test, does not require specialist supervision and takes only an hour to complete. Basal and 30 min samples for cortisol are collected. The SST is not a test of GH reserve.

Since the 250 µg dose of Synacthen® provides a supraphysiological stimulus to the adrenals there has been some interest in validating a low-dose (1 µg) test. Normal threshold 30 min values in this version of the SST have been variously documented at between 480 (17 µg/dL) and 600 nmol/L (22 µg/dL), perhaps reflecting the different dilution protocols used and variable adsorption of

Synacthen® to plastic. Until Synacthen® is marketed in 1 µg vials the low-dose test seems to hold little advantage over the standard 250 µg version [5, 6].

There has been much debate as to whether the SST can substitute for the ITT. Hurel et al. [2] compared the standard SST and ITT in 57 normals and 166 patients with hypothalamo-pituitary disease, none of whom were studied within 6 weeks of surgery. For normal subjects, the Mean-2SD cortisol levels were 392 (14 µg/dL) and 519 nmol/L (19 µg/dL) for the 30-min SST value and ITT peak, respectively. Sixty patients failed the ITT but none had a basal cortisol >450 nmol/L (16 µg/dL) and only 10% had a 30-min SST value >600 nmol/L (22 µg/dL). The authors suggested adopting the latter value as a clinically useful SST cut-off, thus reducing the number of ITTs needed to assess ACTH reserve. In a recent survey of UK endocrinologists, Reynolds et al. [7] found that 59% routinely used the SST for postoperative assessment, with the majority using a 30-min cut-off value of 550 nmol/L (20 µg/dL). Several investigators have demonstrated that the SST is unreliable if used in the very early postoperative period. Klose et al. [8] studied 110 patients after transsphenoidal pituitary surgery and of 62 patients with a normal SST (30-min cortisol >500 nmol/L (18 µg/dL)) at one week, 23 subsequently failed a SST during the following 1–3 months. Agha et al. [9] have recently reported long-term follow-up data on 137 patients with borderline SST passes (30-min cortisol levels <15th percentile of normal healthy responses); only two developed clinical or biochemical evidence of adrenocortical insufficiency (in the absence of pituitary surgery or radiotherapy) during mean follow-up of 4.2 years.

Growth hormone–insulin-like growth factor-1 (IGF-1) axis

Normal physiology

GH secretion is pulsatile and its short half-life means that serum GH is undetectable in normal subjects for approximately two-thirds of the day. It therefore follows that GH deficiency cannot be diagnosed by a single blood sample or even multiple sampling. Many of the actions of GH are mediated by IGF-1, especially in muscle, adipose tissue and bone. GH is the most important regulator of IGF-1 production by the liver, particularly in children and young adults, but nutritional status also exerts important influences. GH and IGF-1 levels decrease with age in normal subjects [10].

Provocative tests

When recombinant human GH became available for replacement therapy, accurate tests of GH reserve assumed greater importance. The biochemical diagnosis of GH deficiency depends on the use of pharmacological, provocative tests. As for ACTH, the "gold standard" test is regarded by many to be the ITT, despite the caveats and contraindications discussed above. The criterion for severe GH deficiency is a peak concentration of <3 ng/mL. GH sufficient individuals achieve a peak GH above 7 ng/mL following hypoglycemia, with many young adults attaining peak GH levels

Table 24.2 Provocative tests of GH reserve

Test	Responses	Comments
Insulin tolerance test (ITT) (See Table 24.1)	A normal response is a peak GH above 7 ng/mL Normal young adults usually attain peak GH levels above 15 ng/mL Severe GH deficiency is indicated by peak GH levels below 3 ng/mL	See Table 24.1
Arginine-GHRH test Overnight fast Intravenous bolus of GHRH (1.0 µg/kg body weight) at time 0 Intravenous infusion of L-arginine (30 g in 100 ml sterile water, or in children 0.5 g/kg body weight, up to 30 g maximum) over 30 minutes starting at time 0 Measure serum GH at −15, 0, 30, 60, 90 and 120 minutes	Less established diagnostic values compared with the ITT Mean GH peak in normal subjects is 18 ng/mL [12] Severe GH deficiency is indicated by peak GH levels below 5 ng/mL [12]	Occasional normal subjects fail to respond [12] Significant false-negative rate during the early years after cranial radiotherapy [14] Combined test is better than either agent given alone GHRH may cause facial flushing or a metallic taste Arginine should not be used in patients with significant liver or renal disease
Glucagon stimulation test (GST) (See Table 24.1)	A normal response is a peak GH above 7 ng/mL (20 mU/L) Severe GH deficiency is indicated by peak GH level <3 ng/mL	See Table 24.1

above 15 ng/mL [11]. Many other provocative tests of GH reserve have been developed [11–13] but those used most commonly are summarized in Table 24.2.

Rahim et al. assessed the GH status of young males and found that the most profound GH release was seen during an ITT (mean peak 36 ng/mL, range 9–67) [11]. The next most effective test was the GST (mean peak GH 14 ng/mL, range 4–67), but on an individual basis, two, six and 15 of 18 subjects failed to achieve a peak GH level above 7 ng/mL with glucagon, arginine and clonidine, respectively. Biller et al. reported on the sensitivity and specificity of six tests (ITT, arginine-growth hormone releasing hormone [GHRH], arginine-L-Dopa, arginine, L-Dopa and IGF-1) in normal subjects and patients with minor and major degrees of anterior hypopituitarism [12]. They concluded that the arginine-GHRH test, with 95% sensitivity and 91% specificity at a GH cutoff of 4.1 ng/mL, provided an excellent alternative to the ITT which had 96% sensitivity and 92% specificity at a GH cut-off of 5.1 ng/mL. In this combination test the arginine is presumed to reduce hypothalamic somatostatin secretion whilst the GHRH acts as a pituitary releasing agent. Other investigators have pointed out that hypothalamic dysfunction occurs early whereas somatotroph dysfunction occurs late after radiation damage to the hypothalamo–pituitary axis – this may be responsible for a significant number of false-negative GH responses to arginine-GHRH in the early years after cranial irradiation [14]. It is also important to remember that obesity blunts the GH responses to a variety of stimuli, including arginine-GHRH stimulation, whilst IGF-1 remains normal [15]. In patients with pituitary disease the like-lihood and severity of GH deficiency increase according to the degree of hypopituitarism present [16]. For example, a patient with proven gonadotropin, ACTH and TSH deficiency is likely to have severe GH deficiency and the diagnosis can often be made on the basis of a low IGF-1 level without the need for a GH stimulation test.

IGF-1

Although there is some correlation between the magnitude of GH responses to provocative stimuli and IGF-1 concentration, IGF-1 values become less useful in older subjects because of the age-related decline in GH secretion. Patients with childhood-onset GH deficiency (CO-GHD) have lower IGF-1 levels than those with adult-onset GHD (AO-GHD), even after adjustment for age. In young adults under the age of 40 years with CO-GHD, IGF-1 levels provide a reasonable assessment of GHD. By contrast, individuals over the age of 40 years with AO-GHD frequently have normal IGF-1 levels. In AO-GHD, IGF-1 cannot be used in isolation as a diagnostic test for GHD [10].

Assessment of other pituitary hormones

Hypothalamo–pituitary–thyroid axis

Secondary hypothyroidism is strongly suggested by low levels of free T_4 in association with low, normal or minimally elevated levels of TSH. However, it should be remembered that sick patients with non-endocrine disease ("sick euthyroid") can also exhibit a similar pattern of thyroid function tests. Although used extensively in the past, it is now recognized that dynamic testing using intravenous thyrotropin releasing hormone (TRH) does not provide any additional information for the diagnosis of secondary hypothyroidism. In addition, TRH has been implicated in the precipitation of pituitary apoplexy in some patients with pituitary macroadenomas.

Hypothalamo–pituitary–gonadal axis

Similarly, it is rare for tests other than basal measurements of gonadotropin (LH and FSH) and sex steroid (estradiol and testosterone) levels to be required for assessment of the HPG axis.

Estradiol binds to sex hormone binding globulin (SHBG), levels of which will be raised in women using the oral contraceptive or estrogen hormone replacement therapy. Testosterone in men shows a marked diurnal variation and should be measured at 8–9 am. If relevant, ovulation can be assessed by measuring progesterone during the luteal phase of the menstrual cycle (days 18–25). Dynamic testing with intravenous luteinizing hormone-releasing hormone (LHRH) is no longer used for the diagnosis of secondary hypogonadism.

Prolactin

The syndromes of hyperprolactinemia are discussed elsewhere. However, it is worth noting here that acquired prolactin deficiency (levels consistently below 2 ng/mL (50 mU/L) in a patient not taking prolactin-lowering medication) is associated with severe hypopituitarism and reduced IGF-1 levels [17, 18].

Investigation and management strategies

Initial assessment (baseline tests)

It is important to assess pituitary function at first diagnosis in all patients with space-occupying pituitary or hypothalamic lesions in order to define the need for replacement therapy before tumor treatment and also to audit the effects of surgery and radiotherapy on general pituitary function. A reasonable set of tests would include serum electrolytes, cortisol (at 8–9 am), fT_4, TSH, prolactin, estradiol/testosterone, LH, FSH and IGF-1. If serum cortisol is <450 nmol/L (16 µg/dL) or if GH deficiency is suspected, an ITT may be performed. However, if putting the patient through a preoperative ITT is considered to be excessive, the SST can be used to define baseline HPA axis function.

Perioperative steroid management [19, 20]

The decision to use perioperative glucocorticoids in patients undergoing pituitary surgery can be based on the results of the preoperative screening tests. If the preoperative SST/ITT results are subnormal, the patient should be commenced on hydrocortisone replacement (typically 15–30 mg daily) with an increase to cover surgery and the first 48 h postoperatively. A typical regimen comprises 50 mg hydrocortisone at induction of anesthesia, 50 mg every 8 h for the first day, 20 mg every 8 h for the second day and then a return to regular replacement. In patients with preoperative basal cortisols below 100 nmol/L (4 µg/dL) replacement steroids should be continued, at least until the time of definitive testing 4–6 weeks after surgery. In patients with less severe preoperative deficits and whose surgery has been uncomplicated, hydrocortisone may be withdrawn 48 h after surgery, with sampling for 9 am cortisol on the third to fifth postoperative days. In patients with preoperative basal cortisol above 450 nmol/L (16 µg/dL) and/or a normal SST, no perioperative replacement is necessary, particularly if a selective adenomectomy proves to be possible, and basal

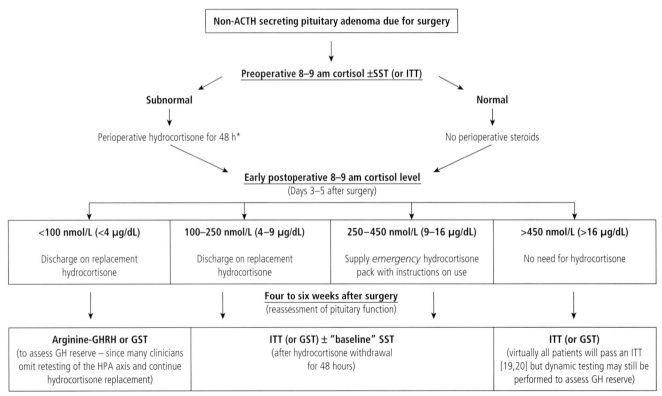

*Unless preoperative basal cortisol <100 nmol/L in which case continue hydrocortisone replacement.

Figure 24.1 Algorithm for perioperative cortisol assessment and therapy.

cortisol sampling should be carried out after surgery, as above (Fig. 24.1).

If the basal postoperative cortisol level is above 450 nmol/L (16 μg/dL) the patient can be safely discharged on no steroid replacement, pending reassessment. If the level is less than 250 nmol/L (9 μg/dL) the patient should be discharged on replacement glucocorticoids. Patients with intermediate cortisol levels between 250 (9 μg/dL) and 450 nmol/L (16 μg/dL) should be provided with an emergency steroid pack together with appropriate education for its use during times of illness or intercurrent stress (Fig. 24.1).

Postoperative pituitary assessment

Many patients are discharged within the first week after transsphenoidal pituitary surgery so it is usually convenient to perform definitive pituitary function testing 4–6 weeks later (Fig. 24.1). This has the advantage of identifying those patients with later recovery of ACTH function. Most patients treated with replacement glucocorticoids since surgery should have therapy withdrawn for at least 48 h prior to definitive testing – physiological hydrocortisone replacement for a few weeks does not suppress the HPA axis. The preferred test is the ITT which assesses the entire HPA axis and also evaluates GH reserve. A GST is acceptable in patients unable to undergo an ITT. Some clinicians elect also to perform a SST at this time point, to establish a postoperative baseline for future testing. Other basal hormones should be measured, as outlined earlier.

Post-radiotherapy endocrine surveillance

Patients are at risk of asymptomatic hypopituitarism after cranial radiotherapy, particularly treatment directed to the pituitary region. There is little information on the optimal frequency for pituitary function testing but endocrine deficits can occur many years after therapy is applied. It is reasonable to undertake the pituitary function tests described earlier, 6 months after completion of radiotherapy to establish a baseline. Thereafter, tests should be repeated at 2-yearly intervals. GH deficiency usually occurs earlier than ACTH deficiency so the more convenient SST can be substituted for the ITT/GST as soon as GH deficiency has been confirmed.

References

1. Plumpton FS, Besser GM. The adrenocortical response to surgery and insulin-induced hypoglycaemia in corticosteroid-treated and normal subjects. *Br. J. Surg.* 1969;56:216–219.
2. Hurel SJ, Thompson CJ, Watson MJ, Baylis PH, Kendall-Taylor P. The short Synacthen and insulin stress tests in the assessment of the hypothalamic-pituitary-adrenal axis. *Clin. Endocrinol.* 1996;44:141–146.
3. Clark PM, Neylon I, Raggatt PR, Sheppard MC, Stewart PM. Defining the normal cortisol response to the short Synacthen test: implications for the investigation of hypothalamic-pituitary disorders. *Clin. Endocrinol.* 1998;49:287–292.
4. Orme SM, Peacey SR, Barth JH, Belchetz PE. Comparison of tests of stress-released cortisol secretion in pituitary disease. *Clin. Endocrinol.* 1996;45:135–140.
5. Arlt W, Allolio B. Adrenal insufficiency. *Lancet* 2003;361:1881–1893.
6. Dorin RI, Qualls CR, Crapo LM. Diagnosis of adrenal insufficiency. *Ann. Intern. Med.* 2003;139:194–206.
7. Reynolds RM, Stewart PM, Seckl JR, Padfield PL. Assessing the HPA axis in patients with pituitary disease: a UK survey. *Clin. Endocrinol.* 2006;64:82–85.
8. Klose M, Lange M, Kosteljanetz M, Poulsgaard L, Feldt-Rasmussen U. Adrenocortical insufficiency after pituitary surgery: an audit of the reliability of the conventional short Synacthen test. *Clin. Endocrinol.* 2005;63:499–505.
9. Agha A, Thompson JW, Clark PM, Holder G, Stewart PM. The long-term predictive accuracy of the short Synacthen (corticotropin) stimulation test for assessment of the hypothalamic–pituitary–adrenal axis. *J. Clin. Endocrinol. Metab.* 2006;91:43–47.
10. Clemmons DR. Clinical utility of measurements of insulin-like growth factor 1. *Nat. Clin. Pract. (Endocrinol. & Metab.)* 2006;2:436–446.
11. Rahim A, Toogood AA, Shalet SM. The assessment of growth hormone status in normal young adult males using a variety of provocative agents. *Clin. Endocrinol.* 1996;45:557–562.
12. Biller BMK, Samuels MH, Zagar A, et al. Sensitivity and specificity of six tests for the diagnosis of adult GH deficiency. *J. Clin. Endocrinol. Metab.* 2002;87:2067–2079.
13. Molitch ME, Clemmons DR, Malozowski S, Merriam GR, Shalet SM, Vance ML. Evaluation and treatment of adult growth hormone deficiency: an Endocrine Society clinical practice guideline. *J. Clin. Endocrinol. Metab.* 2006;91:1621–1634.
14. Darzy KH, Aimaretti G, Weiringa G, Rao Gattamaneni H, Ghigo E, Shalet SM. The usefulness of the combined GHRH and arginine stimulation test in the diagnosis of radiation-induced GH deficiency is dependent on the post-irradiation time interval. *J. Clin. Endocrinol. Metab.* 2003;88:95–102.
15. Bonert VS, Elashoff JD, Barnett P, et al. Body mass index determines evoked GH responsiveness in normal healthy subjects: diagnostic caveat for adult GH deficiency. *J. Clin. Endocrinol. Metab.* 2004;89:3397–3401.
16. Toogood AA, Beardwell CG, Shalet SM. The severity of GH deficiency in adults with pituitary disease is related to the degree of hypopituitarism. *Clin. Endocrinol.* 1995;42:443–444.
17. Mukherjee A, Murray RD, Columb B, Gleeson HK, Shalet SM. Acquired prolactin deficiency indicates severe hypopituitarism in patients with disease of the hypothalamic–pituitary axis. *Clin. Endocrinol.* 2003;59:743–748.
18. Mukherjee A, Ryder WD, Jostel A, Shalet SM. Prolactin deficiency is independently associated with reduced IGF-1 status in severely GH-deficient adults. *J. Clin. Endocrinol. Metab.* 2006;91:2520–2525.
19. Inder WJ, Hunt PJ. Glucocorticoid replacement in pituitary surgery: guidelines for perioperative assessment and management. *J. Clin. Endocrinol. Metab.* 2002;87:2745–2750.
20. Courtney CH, McAllister AS, McCance DR, et al. Comparison of one week 0900h serum cortisol, low and standard dose Synacthen tests with a 4 to 6 week insulin hypoglycaemia test after pituitary surgery in assessing HPA axis. *Clin. Endocrinol.* 2000;53:431–436.

25 Imaging of the Pituitary and Hypothalamus

James V. Byrne

Key points

- Magnetic resonance imaging is the modality of choice, but is unsafe for patients with cardiac pacemakers or metallic corporal implants.
- Computerized tomography or magnetic resonance angiography has replaced conventional catheter angiograms for the localization of the carotid arteries or aneurysms.
- For macroadenomas, imaging should provide a differential diagnosis and accurate tumor localization.
- Postoperative scanning to assess for residual or recurrent tumor should be delayed because acute surgical changes can be confusing.
- Imaging which demonstrates displacement of normal structures helps to identify tumor origins and the formulation of a differential diagnosis.

Introduction

Imaging is an important component in the investigation of patients with suspected pituitary pathology and is often central to monitoring the result of treatment. Magnetic resonance imaging (MRI) is the optimum method with high-quality computerized tomography (CT) an acceptable alternative. The factors that make MRI the modality of first choice are (a) direct multiplanar scanning, (b) lack of ionizing radiation and (c) good anatomical tissue discrimination, without the need for pharmaceutical contrast agents. Assessment of the pituitary gland and hypothalamus is easiest on images obtained in sagittal and coronal planes because they give the best views of the pituitary stalk and the relationships of the gland to adjacent structures, such as the cavernous sinuses, the chiasmatic cistern and the paranasal sinuses. Scanning in the axial plane alone is a poor technique for demonstrating vertical relationships between structures lying between the floor of the third ventricle and sella turcica. Computer-generated reconstructions of axially acquired MRI or CT scan data into the other orthogonal planes or to obtain non-orthogonal oblique views are sometimes useful and can compensate for this limitation of CT.

The only disadvantages of MRI are its relative insensitivity to pathological calcification and lack of signal from corticated bone. CT or even plain film radiography may be required to demonstrate or exclude pathological calcification. In this respect CT is far more sensitive than plain film radiography and the only remaining role for the latter in pituitary imaging is to exclude metallic implants that might be contraindications to MRI. Another

Clinical Endocrine Oncology, 2nd edition. Edited by Ian D. Hay and John A.H. Wass. © 2008 Blackwell Publishing. ISBN 978-1-4051-4584-8.

virtually obsolete imaging method is intra-arterial angiography since MR and CT angiography (MRA, CTA) are capable of identifying the positions of the intracavernous and supraclinoid carotid arteries and differentiating pituitary mass lesions from an intracranial aneurysm. Very rarely the diagnosis of a substantially thrombosed aneurysm requires intra-arterial digital subtraction angiography (IA-DSA). Angiography continues to have a role during catheter navigation for venous sampling in patients being investigated for causes of Cushing syndrome.

MRI techniques

There are an enormous number of potentially useful MRI sequences for imaging the hypothalamic-pituitary axis. It is generally agreed that the structures of the sella region are best imaged using T1-weighted sequences, which produce images with dark cerebrospinal fluid, gray brain and pituitary gland and white fat. Corticated bone returns low signal and appears dark but bone marrow fat returns high signal and therefore appears white. Fast-flowing blood (in arteries) also appears black. The structure of the hypothalamus can be identified but T1-weighted sequences cannot distinguish its nuclei; if, however, phospholipid vesicles are present in the neurohypophysis they are readily apparent as high signal areas (white) [1] (see Fig. 25.1). Areas of bright signal in the stalk and posterior pituitary are evident in up to 50% of T1-weighted scans performed in patients without endocrine disease. Its frequency declines with increasing age [2]. Temporal variations in bright signal from the neurohypophysis and its reduction in patients with diabetes insipidus suggest that it is derived from neurosecretory granules [3]; without the benefit of such a specific chemical change in magnetic property the anterior and posterior lobes of the pituitary gland cannot be readily distinguished.

the consistency of tumors preoperatively [4]. This technique depends on detecting the freedom of intra- and extracellular fluid (water) to diffuse within tissue. Given the large number of potential MRI sequences and imaging protocols available, it is remarkable how consistent most centers are in their choice. This helps in practice to read and compare scans (particularly follow-up scans) performed on different scanners.

The power of MRI to resolve different structures depends on the signal-to-noise ratio (SNR) of the acquired signal. Simply increasing the matrix size of an image, i.e. the number of pixel (or voxel) elements will not improve the SNR though decreasing the pixel size will improve its spatial resolution. To improve the SNR, and spatial resolution, it is necessary to increase the magnet gradient strengths, which are measured in teslas (1 T = 10 000 times the Earth's magnetic field), and to acquire more data by lengthening the scan time [1]. Pituitary MRI is therefore best performance in high field strength imagers using longer sequences [5]. The recent introduction of 3 tesla (3T) imagers into clinical practice is likely to benefit pituitary imaging. It has already been reported to aid diagnosis of cavernous sinus invasion in a study comparing scans obtained at 1.5 T and 3 T [6].

In practice T1-weighted spin echo sequences are performed with repetition times (TR) of 500–600 ms, echo times (TE) of 15 ms and with two or more excitations. Scanning is performed in coronal and sagittal planes using matrix size 256 × 256, to give 3 mm thick contiguous slices. Typically scanning takes 5–8 min at 1.5 T for each sequence. An alternative approach is to use a T1-weighted gradient echo technique with a three-dimensional (3D) Fourier synthesis so that subsequent computer manipulation allows the imaged sample to be viewed in any plane. Some centers perform both sequence types because image clarity is superior in the former but the 3D sequence allows subsequent post-processing, so that the reader can review and clarify any suspicious areas.

Contrast media and enhanced scans

The routine need for intravenous administration of paramagnetic agents, such as gadolinium, is controversial. Injection of gadolinium causes the pituitary gland and stalk to enhance and appear whiter on T1-weighted images. Most tumors and inflammatory lesions also enhance the relative contrast between gland and neoplasm does not increase and they are no more conspicuous. Furthermore, since blood vessels, meninges and the mucosa of the paranasal sinuses enhance, detection of local tumor spread is seldom improved. These agents, like radiographic contrast media used in CT scanning, do not cross the blood–brain barrier. The hypothalamus and optic chiasm do not enhance if the blood–brain barrier is intact. The role of gadolinium-enhanced MRI in the investigation of different pathologies will be considered below.

Dynamic MRI has been used to study the timing of intravenously administered gadolinium uptake by the hypophysis; obtaining single slice images at 20–30 s intervals, Sakamoto et al. [7] demonstrated that the stalk and posterior lobe enhanced 20 s

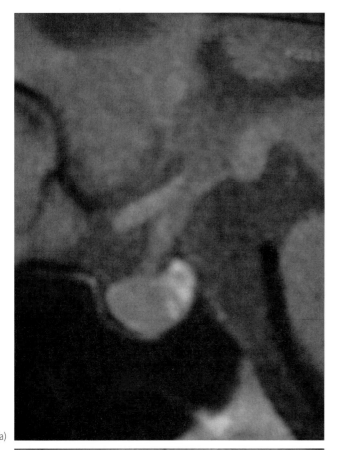

(a)

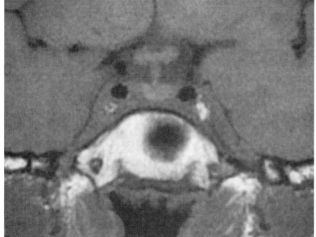

(b)

Figure 25.1 MRI using T1-weighted sequences showing the normal pituitary in sagittal (a) and coronal (b) planes, without administration of gadolinium.

The major alternative sequence choice is to use T2-weighted sequences but generally they add little to the T1-weighted examination because CSF appears white which tends to obscure structures within the chiasmatic and other basal cisterns. The sensitivity of T2-weighted images to changes in cerebral water content is useful in detecting lesions within the brain and therefore the thalamus or hypothalamus. It has recently been suggested that diffusion-weighted imaging can provide information about

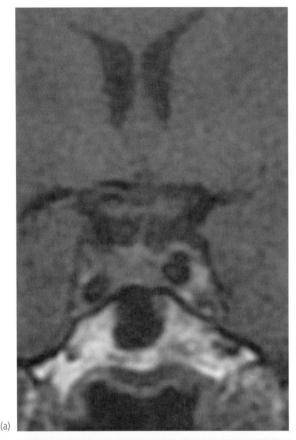

(a)

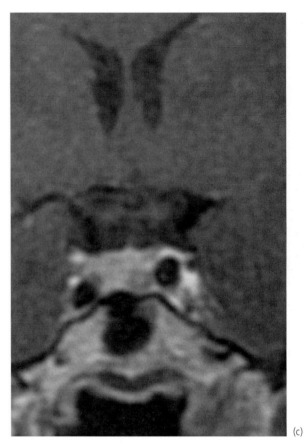

(c)

Figure 25.2 Coronal T1-weighted MRI before (a) and after (b and c) intravenous gadolinium administration. The microadenoma enhances later than normal pituitary gland and is seen as a dark lesion on the enhanced images (b) and (c).

after an intravenous injection and that this extended into the anterior portion of the gland within 80 s. On the basis of different uptake speeds, rapid scanning after injection of contrast media is advocated as a technique to increase the detection rate of microadenomas (Fig. 25.2) using MRI or CT [8].

CT scanning

Apart from its complementary role to MRI for detecting pathological calcification, CT scanning remains the primary imaging modality for the small proportion of patients who are unable to undergo MRI. People who are extremely claustrophobic and those with *in situ* cardiac pacemakers or metal implants such as intracranial aneurysms clips and retained traumatic metallic missile fragments cannot be scanned because of the potential effects of the magnetic field. CT is then used and multi-slice imagers with helical scanning can quickly acquire axial images which can be reformatted into views in the coronal or sagittal planes by computer post-processing (Fig. 25.3). Currently available scanners generally produce images of sufficient quality to demonstrate sella anatomy on unenhanced images but intravenous injection of iodinated contrast media is generally used to improve tissue contrast. It is taken up by the

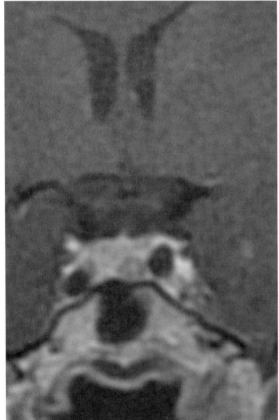

(b)

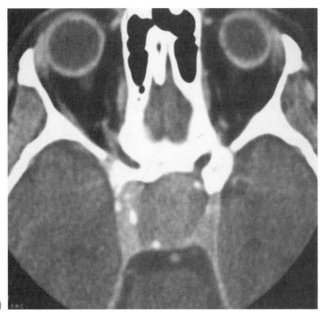

(a)

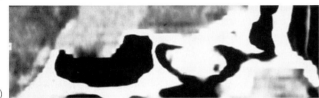

(b)

Figure 25.3 Enhanced CT scan showing a pituitary adenoma, expanding the sella in the axial plane (a) and in the sagittal plane (b) after reformation of the axial data.

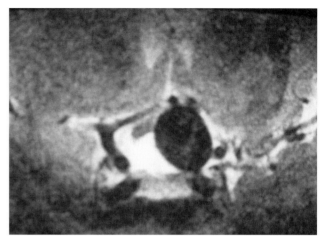

Figure 25.4 T2-weighted coronal MRI showing the intracranial carotid arteries and an aneurysm (arising from the left) and extending into the chiasmatic cistern. Note how the optic chiasm is displaced and the aneurysm dome lies immediately under the anterior cerebral arteries.

hypophysis in the same way as gadolinium. Macroadenoma, craniopharyngioma and tumors of the hypothalamus usually enhance, so the reader compares images before and after enhancement to improve overall diagnostic accuracy. CT, unlike MRI, cannot distinguish blood flow without contrast agents nor intracranial arteries and veins. After contrast enhancement, intradural arteries can be differentiated on CT but similar enhancement levels of arterial and venous blood within the cavernous sinus prevent demonstration of the intracavernous carotid arteries as separate structures. A solution is to perform fast scanning carefully timed to catch the maximum filling of the arteries by contrast media (i.e., first pass technique). This is the basis of CT angiography (CTA) for imaging intracranial arteries. The technique has gained wide acceptance for the detection and depiction of intracranial aneurysms (Fig. 25.4) so it can be used (instead of MR angiography or IA-DSA) to diagnose aneurysms in the sellar region.

The disadvantages of CT over MRI should not be exaggerated. There is a definite concern that an individual undergoing multiple follow-up imagings will be exposed to hazardous levels of ionizing radiation but the accuracy of CT is similar to MRI for diagnosis of macroadenoma [9] and provides virtually all preoperative data for transsphenoidal hypophysectomy, including the bony structure of the ethmoid and sphenoid sinuses, but not an accurate assessment of the position of the carotid arteries. CTA may be able to substitute for preoperative IA-DSA in those situations when

CT raises the possibility of an intrasellar aneurysm [10]. The need for preoperative localization of a pituitary microadenoma will be discussed below.

The history of pituitary imaging unfortunately contains examples of the worst of academic radiology. The analyses of skull radiography of the sella turcica published prior to effective planar scanning are excellent examples of studies performed without proper control groups [11] and the human capacity for self-deception. It remains an imperative, in imaging the patient with endocrine dysfunction, to strike a balance between what is possible and what is needed. To do so requires opinions from physicians of various disciplines and their views synthesized into locally appropriate investigation protocols.

Pituitary macroadenoma

Adenomas larger than 1 cm in maximum diameter are conventionally classified as macroadenomas irrespective of their endocrine characteristics. Imaging for diagnosis is performed to demonstrate the cause of an endocrine disturbance or symptoms/signs of a parasellar mass lesion. It is therefore directed at identifying tumor and its extent. In cases of non-functioning adenoma the differential diagnosis includes other causes of sella region masses (see below). Once a macroadenoma is identified the role of imaging is to accurately localize its extent for surgical or radiotherapy planning and to inform management decisions.

The imaging features are similar, i.e. non-specific, for tumors producing different hormones. On CT adenomas are isodense or hypodense relative to brain tissue and show variable patterns of enhancement after radiographic contrast media administration. On MRI signal return is typically similar to that of brain on both T1-weighted and T2-weighted sequences. Gadolinium administration causes signal change due to shortening of the T_1

recovery time and so vascular areas brighten on the T1-weighted sequence. Cysts or areas of necrosis, where the blood supply is reduced, appear as foci of moderate hypointensity on T1-weighted and hyperintensity on T2-weighted sequences, with heterogeneous enhancement with gadolinium (Fig. 25.5). Features secondary to hemorrhage within cysts, such as layering of hemorrhagic debris, may be helpful in differentiating them from necrosis.

Signal due to hemorrhage can be specific but it depends on the magnetic effects of iron within red blood cells. This changes as the hemoglobin molecule degrades after hemorrhage. In general these changes are best appreciated on T1-weighted MRI, since within days of hemorrhage increased concentrations of methemoglobin (due to red blood cell lysis and breakdown of hemoglobin) causes T_1 recovery time shortening and bright signal on this sequence [13]. The appearance is therefore similar to that seen after gadolinium administration and will only be recognized if prior unenhanced imaging is performed. In the acute period after hemorrhage (less than 3 days) MRI changes are non-specific but acute hemorrhage is hyperdense (i.e., white) on CT. As hematomas liquify in the next 2–3 weeks, their density reduces and they become hypodense on CT. Methemoglobin can persist for months so that chronic hemorrhage is more easily identified on T1-weighted MRI. Its T_1 shortening or paramagnetic effect is simulated by fat and some tumor products secreted by lesions such as craniopharyngioma with which it may be confused.

Physiological bright or hyperintense signal can be seen in the posterior lobe and stalk, as described above. This property of phospholipids is also described as paramagnetic and is due to similar shortening of T_1 recovery time. Less intense areas of bright signal are sometimes evident in tumors of patients without a history suggestive of hemorrhage. Asymptomatic hemorrhage has been confirmed surgically in a small proportion of patients. The scan appearances of tumors in patients presenting acutely with pituitary apoplexy (Fig. 25.6) will reflect the relative extent of hemorrhage and/or necrosis, with gadolinium enhancement evident at the margins of necrotic areas.

There have been attempts to correlate tumor appearances on imaging with hormonal activity. Imaging features such as tumor size, evidence of local invasion, CT density and MRI signal have been correlated with hormone production [12]. MR, which is capable of measuring fundamental chemical characteristics, does not give a hormone-specific image [14], though given the need for and accuracy of biochemical assays and the frequency of mixed hormone adenomas, the need to make the distinction on imaging is debatable. The more important contribution of imaging to patient management is accurate delineation of tumor extent and its effect on adjacent structures.

The preoperative MRI appearances are therefore helpful in directing the surgeon to likely areas of local invasion but do not substitute for operative and histological examinations. Tumor invasion of the cavernous sinus, sphenoid bone and extension into the chiasmatic cistern are evident on MRI (Fig. 25.7). Such behavior has been identified surgically and histologically in all tumor types [15]. Local invasion is evident on surgical examination in 35–40% of tumors [15] but is found nearly twice as frequently on microscopic examination [16]. It is more likely with increasing tumor size [20] and has obvious implications for the patient's prognosis. Scotti et al. [17] studied the MRI features useful in the preoperative diagnosis of cavernous sinus invasion. Encasement of the carotid artery was the most specific sign of cavernous sinus invasion. They correctly identified cavernous sinus involvement in 10 of 11 macroadenomas but in only 2 of 13 microadenomas. Asymmetries of the cavernous sinuses, displacement

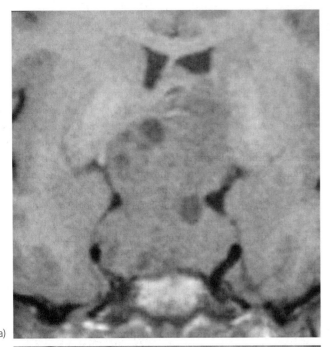

(a)

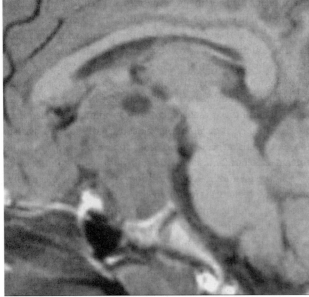

(b)

Figure 25.5 Coronal (a) and sagittal (b) T1-weighted MRI showing a macroadenoma with a large supra-sellar extension with an indistinct superior margin with the left basal ganglia (a), erosion of the floor of the pituitary fossa (b) and discrete cystic areas.

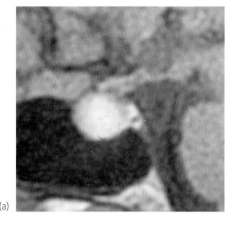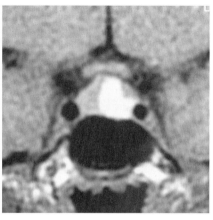

Figure 25.6 Unenhanced T1-weighted MRI of apoplexy in sagittal (a) and coronal (b) planes. The hyperintense signal of hemoglobin breakdown products within the pituitary tumor produces the white areas in the gland.

(a)

(b)

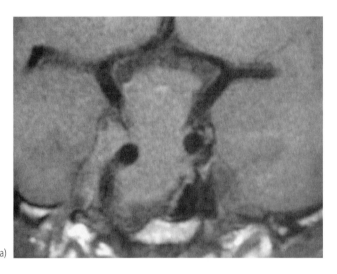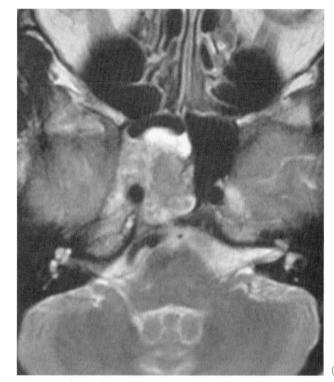

(a)

(b)

Figure 25.7 MRI with coronal T1-weighted (a) and axial T2-weighted (b) images showing a macroadenoma with invasion of the right cavernous sinus. The tumor surrounds the carotid artery and returns more heterogeneous signal on the T2-weighted sequence.

of its lateral wall and of the carotid artery were inconsistent features of invasion. They found an indistinct medial sinus wall an unreliable sign, being common in controls. Administration of gadolinium may be helpful in identifying normal pituitary gland and distinguishing it from tumor.

Postoperative and follow-up scanning

How effective is imaging in defining residual or recurrent tumor after hypophysectomy? The timing of postoperative scanning is important since early post-surgical changes due to local swelling (in the first 1–2 weeks) and surgical packing materials, used in the transsphenoidal exposure, may be confused with residue tumor

[18]. Gel foam packing material returns hypointense or hyperintense signal and enhances after gadolinium administration on early postoperative MRI. Its reabsorption has been shown to take 4–15 months in studies using serial scans [19]. Biological packing materials return mixed signal with fat being hyperintense and muscle isointense on T1-weighted MRI. Re-expansion of the normal pituitary gland and reabsorption of packing material are usually evident on follow-up scans by 3 months after surgery. Early scanning is therefore only useful to investigate possible surgical complications and scanning to identify residual tumor is best delayed for at least 3 months (Fig. 25.8). The signal returned by residual tumor is usually the same as preoperation but gadolinium enhancement is less helpful at distinguishing it from normal gland after operation [18]. In the longer term downward herniation of

the chiasm and optic recess of the third ventricle may be evident but this finding is often difficult to correlate with the severity of any visual symptoms [20].

Demonstration of tumor regression or recurrence relies on comparisons between follow-up scans. The protocol for post-operative follow-up imaging in Oxford is for a baseline study to be obtained 3 months after hypophysectomy followed by interval MRI 12 months and 5 years later. More frequent scans are obtained if the patient's visual fields change or histological examination of the respected tumor suggests local invasiveness. Patients treated medically for functional macroadenomas are also monitored by serial imaging, in combination with biochemical and clinical follow-up assessments. A reduction in the size of prolactin-secreting macroadenomas after treatment with dopamine agonists may be accompanied by hemorrhage and therefore changes in signal returned by the tumor on MRI [21]. This is rarer in growth hormone-secreting tumors following treatment with somatostatin analogs. Reductions in tumor size can be demonstrated within weeks [22] but continued shrinkage has been documented up to 3 years after starting treatment [23]. Early follow-up imaging is therefore useful to document tumor response. A baseline study is obtained when the patient starts treatment and is then repeated 3 and 12 months later. Subsequent imaging is performed in regard to the response to therapy, i.e., data from clinical and biochemical examinations.

Microadenomas

To accurately identify adenomas less than 10 mm in size demands the highest standards of imaging technique and interpretation. In most patients the presence of a microadenoma is assumed from biochemical testing and imaging is undertaken to confirm an intrasellar source and to guide its transsphenoidal excision.

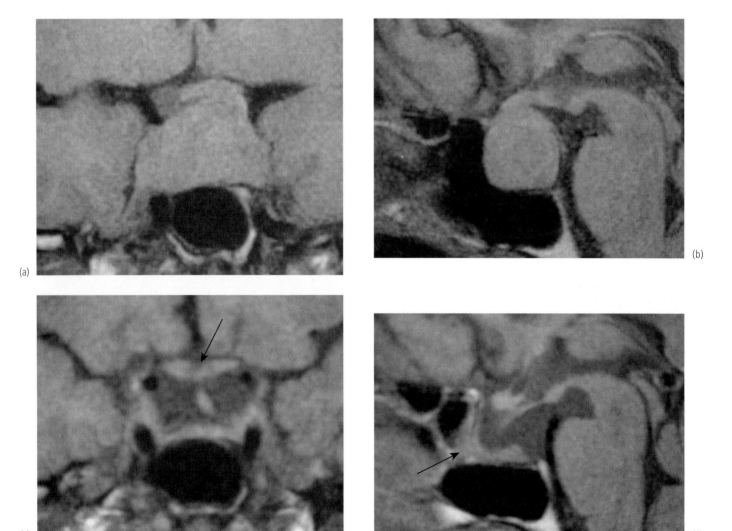

(a)

(b)

(c)

(d)

Figure 25.8 T1-weighted MRI performed before (a and b) and after (c and d) transsphenoidal hypophysectomy. The chiasm has resumed a normal position after tumor removal (arrow – c) and the surgical access into the anterior sella can be seen on the postoperative scan (arrow – d).

Microadenomas show little inherent contrast to normal pituitary tissue on CT and scanning requires intravenous radiographic contrast agents to demonstrate late or non-enhancement of the tumor against a background of normal gland enhancement. On MRI, microadenomas are typically hypointense relative to normal gland on T1-weighted sequences (Fig. 25.9) but may be isointense or hyperintense and the demonstration of pituitary microadenoma remains a major challenge for pituitary imaging.

It is universally accepted that scanning is best performed in the coronal plane and largely accepted that MRI is the modality of choice. Johnson et al. [24] prospectively evaluated CT and MRI in a group of patients with suspected microadenomas and showed that MRI was more accurate. The strength of their conclusion lies in the study's methodology, which was designed to answer the clinical question 'Which modality should be used to investigate the suspected microadenoma patient?'. Most other studies compare detection rates on MRI and CT retrospectively, against

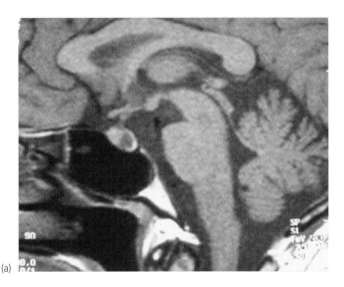

(a)

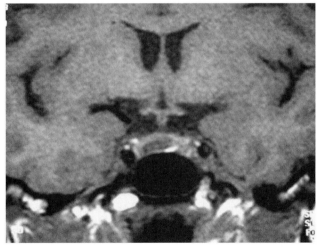

(b)

Figure 25.9 Microadenoma returning hypointense signal on sagittal (a) and coronal (b) T1-weighted MRI. Inherent contrast between adenoma and normal gland means enhancement with gadolinium is not needed to identify the lesion.

surgical or histological diagnoses. However, it is wrong to conclude that CT is markedly inferior to MRI and it continues to have advocates [25] since current scanners are capable of 1.5 mm scan planes and it remains superior to MRI at delineating bone.

The need for high precision scanning has stimulated research to develop better MRI techniques. A coronal T1-weighted sequence with gadolinium performed on 1.5 T imagers has a sensitivity of 80% or better [26]. Typical parameters for a spin-echo sequence are TR 500 ms, TE 25 ms, 3 mm contiguous slice thickness with four excitations which requires 8–9 min scan time. Most centers perform scans in the coronal and sagittal planes before and after gadolinium enhancement. A 3D volume scan has the theoretical advantage of allowing post-processing of images in different planes, higher resolutions and better signal–noise ratios but adds to the overall scan time. Techniques such as 3D-SPGR [25] and 3D-FLASH [27] have demonstrated the utility of this approach. The value of conventional intravenous gadolinium enhancement (i.e., non-dynamic scanning) is controversial since there have been reports of improved sensitivity [28] and the converse [29]. Davis et al. [28] found gadolinium useful when scanning patients at 0.5 Tesla but the benefit is less apparent when scanning on higher field strength imagers [27].

An alternative approach to improve microadenoma detection rates is dynamic MRI. This technique employs rapid sequential imaging to show temporal differences in gadolinium uptake between adenoma and normal gland. In this way microadenomas which enhance shortly after normal gland enhancement can be identified (Fig. 25.2). Early studies showed that normal pituitary enhanced before adenomas [30], and using region of interest analysis, that enhancement of the posterior lobe preceded the anterior lobe [7]. Using faster acquisition times (5–10 s per image), Yuh et al. [31] found that macroadenoma enhanced at the same time as the posterior lobe and before the anterior lobe, suggesting that they have a direct blood supply. Dynamic scanning with various fast imaging techniques has been used to identify microadenomas not detected on conventional MRI [32]. Kucharczyk et al. [32] identified three microadenomas in 18 patients on dynamic imaging which had not been evident on conventional imaging. However, they also reported false-positive results in four of 13 controls. A similar experience was reported by Tabarin et al. [33] for the detection of microadenomas in patients with Cushing disease. Thus the improved sensitivity (67% compared with 52%) enjoyed by dynamic MRI was offset by reduced specificity (80% versus 100%) compared to conventional MRI [33].

The sensitivity of unenhanced high-resolution MRI for pituitary microadenoma is in the order of 60–80%. Conventional scanning with contrast enhancement detects 5–10% more lesions and dynamic scanning a further 5–10% of lesions [34]. Detection rate can thus be improved but at the expense of a higher rate of false positives. The problems associated with imaging at this level are both technical and biological. Technically dynamic MRI demands the maximum of man and machine and both can be frustrated by the occurrence of small coincidental pituitary lesions, so-called incidentalomas [34]. An autopsy study found

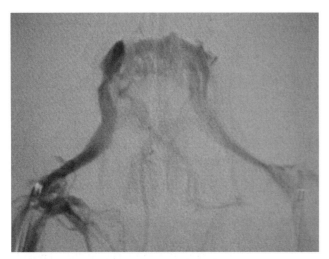

Figure 25.10 Digital subtraction venogram showing the cavernous sinuses, inferior petrosal sinuses and the internal jugular veins. Catheters are placed in the internal jugular veins with their tips at the distal ends of the inferior petrosal sinuses to collect the pituitary venous drainage after CRH stimulation.

asymptomatic small lesions in 27% of normal glands [35] but a more recent report estimated their incidence at only 6% [36]. Chong et al. [37] found focal hypointensities in the pituitary glands of 38% of normal volunteers using unenhanced MRI and Ahmadi et al. [38] found stalk deviation on MRI in 46% of normal subjects. That such "lesions" exist, whatever their incidence, means that we are unlikely to ever achieve 100% specificity rates on imaging alone.

Patients with Cushing syndrome and negative imaging may be further investigated by sampling the venous effluent of the pituitary to differentiate Cushing disease from ectopic sources of adrenocorticotropic hormone. Simultaneous bilateral sampling after stimulation with corticotropin-releasing hormone (CRH) is highly accurate [39] but the test does carry a small risk of neurological complications [40]. The risk of a permanent neurological deficit has been estimated at 0.001% by Doppman [41] and can be minimized by sampling from the internal jugular veins rather than inferior petrosal or cavernous sinuses (Fig. 25.10). The technique is reserved for patients with normal pituitary imaging but the reader should appreciate from the above discussion that there remains a debate over the extent to which imaging is pursued in order to exclude a microadenoma and that protocols vary from center to center [33].

Craniopharyngioma

Craniopharyngiomas arise from remnants of Rathke's pouch. The pouch forms part of the intermediate part of the anterior lobe and pars tuberalis anterior to the pituitary stalk [42]. They represent approximately 3% of all intracranial tumors, with an annual incidence of 0.13 per 100 000 population in the USA [43]. A modest male predominance (1.3:1) has been reported in the

UK but equal incidences between the sexes have been reported in the USA and Finland [43]. The age distribution of patients at diagnosis is highest at 5–15 years with a second peak in late middle age (55–75 years). This bimodal age distribution has been linked to histological tumor variants: an adamantinous type being commoner in children and young adults and a squamous–papillary type in older patients [44]. Approximately 50% of patients present under the age of 20 years and calcification is commoner in younger patients, being demonstrable in 70% of such tumors [45]. Tumors usually are found above the sella, with 5% purely intrasellar, 20% purely suprasellar and 75% both intra- and extrasellar [45]. The 5-year survival reported in one study of their epidemiology was 80% [43].

The imaging appearance of craniopharyngioma depends on how much of the tumor is cystic and how much solid. Typically tumors have a relatively circumscribed outline cystic areas that do not enhance but may have thick enhancing walls and solid elements that do enhance. Calcification patterns vary from solid lumps to popcorn-like foci or less commonly an eggshell pattern lining the wall of a cyst. In addition to calcification these tumors may contain paramagnetic substances which appear white on T1-weighted MRI. Craniopharyngioma cysts contain, variously, cholesterol, triglycerides, methemoglobin and desquamated epithelium. High concentrations of protein or methemoglobin affect the MRI signal and produce the characteristic T1-weighted hyperintensity of a paramagnetic substance.

Imaging protocols therefore need to include both CT and MR scanning, since the former is the most sensitive means of detecting calcification. Craniopharyngiomas on CT, are typically of mixed attenuation, i.e. areas of light and dark, with or without calcification. A typical MRI sequence protocol would include axial T2-weighted, with sagittal and coronal T1-weighted sequences before and after intravenous gadolinium enhancement. The ability of MRI to produce images in multiple planes has simplified the process of assessing the extent of tumors in the suprasellar region and this protocol should provide sufficient data to identify anterior and posterior tumor extent as well as any effect on local structures such as the chiasm and third ventricle. Contrast enhancement with gadolinium improves tumor definition from normal structures [46]. The signal of solid tumor is isointense or hypointense relative to brain on pre-contrast T1-weighted sequences and enhances after gadolinium. On T2-weighted sequences it is usually of mixed hypo- or hyperintensity. Large areas of calcification can be identified as focal areas of hypointensity on both T1-weighted and T2-weighted sequence but axial CT should be performed to show small areas of calcification. Cysts are hyperintense on T2-weighted and hypointense on T1-weighted sequences but if they contain paramagnetic substances, particularly breakdown products of hemoglobin, this pattern may be reversed or they appear hyperintense on both T2-weighted and T1-weighted sequences.

There have been attempts to correlate MRI appearances with histological type. Sartoretti-Schefer et al. [47] compared the scans of 42 patients with histologically proven craniopharyngioma and described typical MRI patterns. The adamantinous types were either mixed solid-cystic or mainly cystic tumors with hyperintense cysts on T1-weighted MRI. The squamous-papillary types were solid or mixed solid-cystic tumors with hypointense cysts on T1-weighted MRI. Imaging features they found to be discriminating were: encasement of vessels, a lobulated shape and hyperintense cyst signal for the former and a round shape, hypointense cysts and a predominantly solid appearance for the latter. Calcification was commoner in the adamantinous tumor but not discriminatory (Fig. 25.11). However, others have not found such imaging features to correlate with the patient's age, or tumor type [48]. Apparently contradictory reports may be due to some series containing high proportions of tumors with mixed histology [48]. Furthermore, the importance of histological type to the patient's prognosis remains controversial [49] and the distinction is not related to the chance of recurrence after surgical excision.

MRI with and without contrast enhancement is the modality of choice for patient follow-up after treatment with surgery and/or radiotherapy. The timing of examinations should be dictated by the extent of surgical resection and clinical findings. MRI may show unsuspected residual tumor elements and early postoperative scanning (i.e., at 3 months) is useful in establishing a baseline for subsequent follow-up imaging [50].

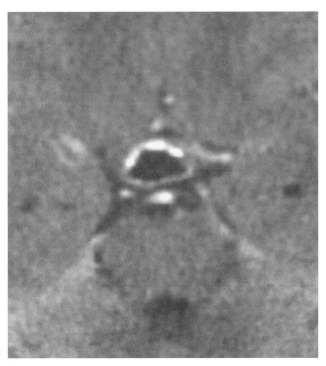

(a)

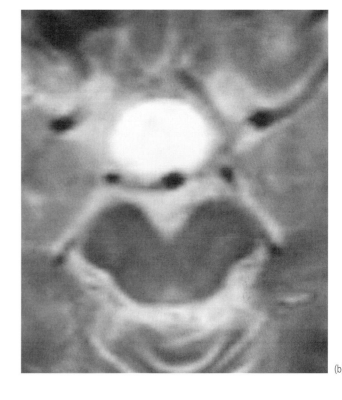

(b)

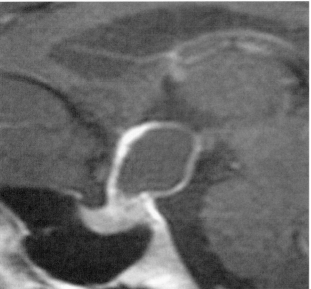

(c)

Figure 25.11 Adamantinomatous craniopharyngioma showing: calcification on CT (a), a large cystic component on axial T2-weighted MRI (b) and a small solid component which enhances on T1-weighted sagittal MRI after gadolinium administration (c).

Rathke's cleft cysts

Symptomatic Rathke's cleft cysts are pathological enlargements of remnant of Rathke's pouch which typically arise between the two lobes of the pituitary. Small intrasellar cysts are benign incidental autopsy findings [51] but enlargement of a cyst within the sella may cause symptoms due to compression of the pituitary gland or, if they expand into the chiasmatic cistern, compression of the anterior optic pathway. Cysts are lined by cuboidal or columnar epithelium and contain a variety of fluid types. At surgery their contents are variously described as "like CSF, motor-oil or a milky fluid" [52].

The imaging characteristics of Rathke's cleft cysts depend on location and content. The appearance can be similar to craniopharyngiomas [53] or suprasellar arachnoid cysts [54]. The CT appearance is typically of a non-calcified intrasellar cystic mass. Demonstrating that they do not contain calcification is helpful in distinguishing them from craniopharyngioma and is an indication for performing CT as well as MRI [53]. On MRI signal returned by the cyst is variable; it may follow that of CSF (i.e., hypointense on T1-weighted and hyperintense on T2-weighted sequences) or have signal characteristic of a protein-rich fluid (i.e., hyperintense on both T1-weighted and T2-weighted sequences) or that of altered hemorrhage (i.e., hyperintense on T1-weighted and hypointense on T2-weighted sequences) [55]. Though the cyst wall does not enhance, administration of intravenous gadolinium is useful in distinguishing them from craniopharyngioma and to show the position of the normal pituitary gland [52] (Fig. 25.12). Cysts in atypical locations may make differentiation from an arachnoid cyst (which also do not enhance) difficult. Rathke's cleft cysts, like craniopharyngioma, have rarely been found in the nasopharynx associated with persistent remnants of the craniopharyngeal duct [56]. Another atypical feature of these cysts is the occasional finding of a central hypo- or isointense focus within the cyst. This is presumed to be due to desquamatized epithelium forming a "waxy nodule" [53]. Preoperative diagnosis is important since simple surgical excision or cyst aspiration is usually curative, unlike craniopharyngioma. Differentiation from cystic craniopharyngiomas, despite the advantages of MRI, can still be difficult, particularly in children [57]. High-quality imaging is therefore mandatory.

Other tumors of the suprasellar and parasellar regions

The preoperative differentiation of pituitary adenomas from other causes of sellar and parasellar tumor masses, relies on imaging. The most common problem in practice, is to distinguish non-functioning pituitary macroadenomas from craniopharyngiomas, meningioma and rarer causes of tumor in this region, since clinical symptoms and signs are unhelpful, with the exceptions of diabetes insipidus, which suggests craniopharyngioma, and precocious puberty which suggests a primary hypothalamic

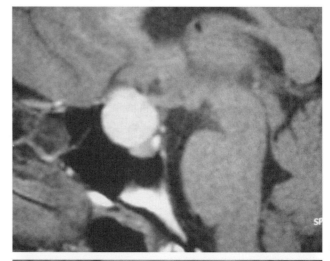

(a)

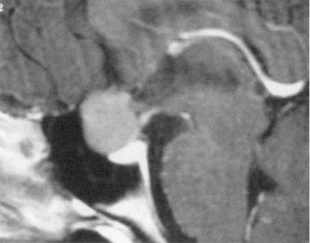

(b)

Figure 25.12 Sagittal T1-weighted MRI before (a) and after (b) gadolinium administration, showing a hyperintense Rathke's cleft cyst expanding the sella and displacing the gland. Note how the posterior lode high signal is masked on (b) after the gland enhances with gadolinium.

lesion (see below). There is a wide gamut of pathologies that may simulate non-functioning pituitary tumor and these are best considered by their effect on the optic chiasm.

Lesions arising above the optic chiasm

Lesions that arise above the chiasm include ependymoma, craniopharyngioma, hemangioblastoma, glioma (usually astrocytoma), hamartoma of the hypothalamus and lipoma. Ependymoma and hemangioblastoma may arise within the anterior part of the third ventricle [58] and Morrison et al. reported five intraventricular craniopharyngiomas in a series of 73 intraventricular tumors [59]. Involvement of the hypothalamus by hamartomas, glioma, teratoma or lipoma causes precocious puberty [42]. Local pressure effects from optic chiasm tumor or an arachnoid cyst may also cause precocious puberty [60]. In children with precocious puberty hypothalamic hamartoma will be the cause in a third of cases though, paradoxically, larger hamartomas are less likely to cause

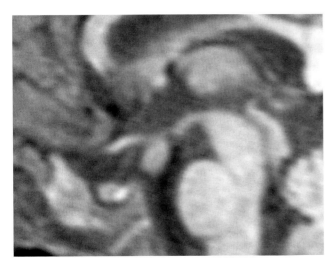

Figure 25.13 Sagittal T1-weighted MRI showing a hamartoma. A nodular mass which is isointense with brain is seen arising from the floor of the third ventricle.

this endocrine disturbance [61]. Unlike other tumors in the region of the hypothalamus, hamartomas are isodense on CT and isointense on MRI relative to gray matter (Fig. 25.13). They also do not calcify or enhance after administration of intravenous contrast media and thereby can usually be distinguished from craniopharyngioma and glioma.

Lesions arising below the optic chiasm

The optic chiasm will be depressed by lesions arising in the floor of the third ventricle but elevated by suprasellar extension of intrasellar or parasellar tumors. The latter include meningioma, aneurysm, schwannoma (particularly of the trigeminal nerve), lymphoma, metastases and tumors arising in bone. These lesions should be considered in the differential diagnosis of pituitary macroadenomas as well as the rare tumors of the neurohypophysis: pilocystic astrocytoma and granular cell tumor, or choristoma. Imaging must distinguish intracranial aneurysm and the possibility of this diagnosis was, prior to MRI, an indication for preoperative IA-DSA. Blood flow in an aneurysm sac should be evident on MRI, which can be supplemented by MR or CT angiography. However, if doubt remains, and rarely this may be the case, intra-arterial angiography should be performed. Meningioma in this region may be parasellar and invade the cavernous sinus or arise from the tuberculum sellae. CT may show calcification but MRI is best at defining tumor extent. Meningiomas typically enhance homogeneously after gadolinium administration. Tumors arising in the sphenoid bone and clivus, such as chordoma, giant cell tumor, chondrosarcoma, or carcinomas arising in the nasopharynx, are associated with bone destruction, calcification and a variable degree of enhancement. They may simulate bone invasion by pituitary macroadenoma. Imaging by both CT and MRI is helpful, since the former will demonstrate bone erosion and the latter the effects of the tumor on adjacent tissues. Intrasellar or suprasellar metastases should always be considered in the differential diagnosis since their CT

and MRI appearance is variable and they can be indistinguishable on imaging from other tumor types.

Lesions arising in the chiasmatic cistern

Finally, tumors may arise in the chiasmatic cistern and simulate suprasellar extension of a macroadenoma. The differential diagnosis includes: optic nerve glioma, meningioma, craniopharyngioma, aneurysm and metastasis. Again MRI has made a substantial contribution to refining the preoperative diagnosis in this region. Its key attribute is its ability to identify the anterior optic pathway and thereby distinguish optic nerve glioma from extra-axial tumor. This largely depends on using T1-weighted coronal images to follow the pathway from optic nerves to tracts. Sumida et al. [62] found that the optic nerves, chiasm and tracts could be visualized in over 84% of patients with pituitary adenoma, craniopharyngioma or Rathke's cleft cyst. The chiasm and tracts could be identified in 85% of 14 patients with meningioma but in only 50% were the optic nerves visible, reflecting the frequent anterior location of this tumor. Contrast media are useful for the identification of meningioma and metastases. Optic nerve glioma involving the chiasm rarely enhances and the imaging diagnosis depends on identifying enlargement of the optic pathway as spread is transneural (Fig. 25.14). Other features of neurofibromatosis type I are evident in a quarter of patients with optic nerve gliomas so imaging should include the whole cranium [63]. Optic nerve and chiasm gliomas are isointense to gray matter on T1-weighted and isointense or hyperintense on T2-weighted sequences. Involvement of the optic tracts and brain parenchyma is identified as hyperintense signal on T2-weighted sequences. Unless tumors are very large it is usually possible to see CSF between the inferior tumor margin and the diaphragma sella and so to exclude suprasellar extension of an intrasellar mass.

Nuclear isotope imaging

Nuclear medicine techniques, such as positron emission tomography (PET) or single-photon emission tomography (SPECT), have been used to obtain *in vivo* characterization of tissue. The presence of octreotide-binding somatostatin receptors in non-functioning adenomas causes them to take up ^{111}In-DTPA-octreotide [64] but meningiomas may also express somatostatin receptors and take up somatostatin receptor-specific isotopes [65]. However, tracers which bind to the enzyme monoamine oxidase β have been used to differentiate meningioma from pituitary adenoma using PET [66] and more recently a D2 dopamine receptor-specific isotope [18F]fluoro-ethyl-spiperone has been reported to differentiate non-functioning adenomas from craniopharyngioma and meningioma [67]. PET using tracers such as [18F] fluorodeoxyglucose and [11C] methionine can be used to study rates of glucose metabolism and protein synthesis. It can be used to assess tumors after treatment by differentiating viable tumor from scar tissue and monitoring pharmacological treatments [68]. However, the current availability of scanners in the UK limits the use of PET to selected patients and research.

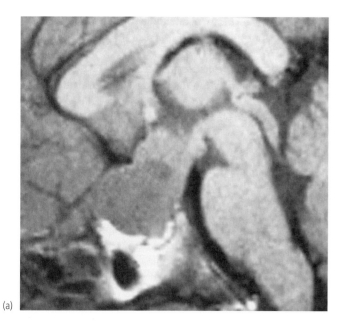

(a)

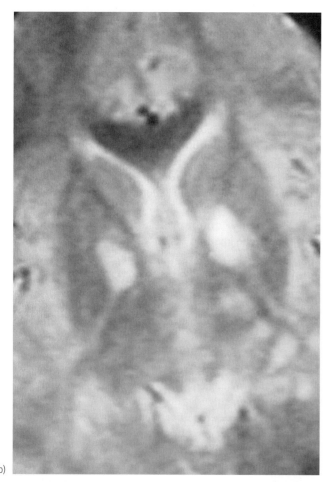

(b)

Figure 25.14 Sagittal T1-weighted (a) and axial T2-weighted (b) MRI showing a mass expanding the pituitary fossa and the chiasmatic cistern. The T2-weighted image at the level of the basal ganglia shows bilateral hyperintense signal due to the spread of this optic nerve glioma.

Inflammatory diseases of the pituitary and chiasmatic cistern

Involvement of the suprasellar region by sarcoidosis, Langerhans cell histiocytosis or tuberculous meningitis may cause endocrine symptoms such as diabetes insipidus and abnormalities on imaging. In Langerhans cell histiocytosis (also called eosinophilic granulomatosis) patients present with diabetes insipidus and bone lesions. The former frequently leads to imaging of the hypothalamic–pituitary axis and MRI typically shows thickening of the pituitary stalk [69]. Normal posterior pituitary high signal is typically absent. The diagnosis may be made by recognition of bone lesions which often occur in the skull, one of the rare situations when plain skull radiographs may be helpful in diagnosis.

Granulomatous leptomeningitis is frequently diagnosed in the chiasmatic cistern because patients present with visual or endocrine symptoms [70]. Sarcoid granulomas may be identified as meningeal masses isodense on CT and isointense on MRI, relative to gray matter. They are best demonstrated on T1-weighted MRI with gadolinium enhancement. Other foci of meningeal enhancement should be sought since it may be necessary to resort to biopsy to confirm the diagnosis [71] and a superficial focus would be more accessible. The differential for pathological meningeal enhancement in the suprasellar region includes metastatic tumor and it is important to keep this possibility in mind. In one report of two patients, initial imaging performed for idiopathic diabetes insipidus was negative, but 1–2 years later, metastatic germinoma was demonstrated in the hypothalamus [72]. Interval imaging and a high degree of suspicion are therefore warranted.

Diffuse enhancement of the pituitary occurs in lymphocytic hypophysitis and other rare forms of hypophysitis on MRI. The gland and in particular the anterior lobe are usually moderately enlarged so hypophysitis is difficult to distinguish from adenoma on imaging alone [73]. This rare form of autoimmune endocrine disease has probably been underdiagnosed in the past because it was mistaken for adenoma or unrecognized prior to MRI being more available [74].

References

1. Kucharczyk W, Lenkinski RE, Kucharczyk J, Henkelman RM. The effect of phospholipid vesicles on the NMR relaxation of water: an explanation for the MR appearance of the neurohypophysis? *AJNR Am. J. Neuroradiol.* 1990;11:693–700.
2. Brooks BS, El Gammal T, Allison JD, Hoffman WH. Frequency and variation of the posterior pituitary bright signal on MR images. *AJNR Am. J. Neuroradiol.* 1989;10:943–948.
3. Mark LP, Haughton VM, Hendrix LE, et al. High-intensity signals within the posterior pituitary fossa: a study with fat-suppression MR techniques. *AJNR Am. J. Neuroradiol.* 1991;12: 529–532.
4. PieralliniA, Caramina F, Falcone C, et al. Pituitary macro adenomas: preoperative evaluation of consistency with diffusion-weighted MR imaging – initial experience. *Radiology* 2006;239:223–231.
5. Scott WA. *Magnetic Resonance Imaging of the Brain and Spine.* Philadelphia, PA: Lippincott-Raven, 1996:59–63.

6. Pinker K, Ba-Ssalamah A, Wolfsberger S, et al. The value of high-field MRI (3T) in the assessment of sellar lesions. *Eur. J. Radiol.* 2005;54:327–334.

7. Sakamoto Y, Takahashi M, Korogi Y, et al. Normal and abnormal pituitary glands: gadopentetate dimeglumine-enhanced MR imaging. *Radiology* 1991;178:441–445.

8. Stadnik T, Srayt D, van Binst A, et al. Pituitary microadenomas: diagnostic serial CT, conventional CT and T1–weighted MR imaging before and after injection of gadolinium. *Eur. J. Radiol.* 1994;18:191–198.

9. Buchfelder M, Nistor R, Fahlbusch R, Huk WJ. The accuracy of CT and MR evaluation of the sella turcica for detection of adrenocorticotropic hormone-secreting adenomas in Cushing disease. *AJNR Am. J. Neuroradiol.* 1992;14:1183–1190.

10. Richmond IL, Newton TH, Wilson CB. Indications for angiography in the preoperative evaluation of patients with prolactin-secreting pituitary adenomas. *J. Neurosurg.* 1980;52:378–380.

11. Moseley I. *Diagnostic Imaging in Neurological Disease.* Edinburgh: Churchill Livingstone, 1986:218–220.

12. Lundin P, Nyman R, Burman P, et al. MRI of pituitary macroadenomas with reference to hormonal activity. *Neuroradiology* 1992;34:43–51.

13. Dooms GC, Uske A, Brant-Zawadzki M, et al. Spin-echo MR imaging of intracranial hemorrhage. *Neuroradiology* 1986;28:132–138.

14. Arnold DL, Emrich JF, Shoubridge EA, et al. Characterization of astrocytomas, meningiomas, and pituitary adenomas by phosphorus magnetic resonance spectroscopy. *J. Neurosurg.* 1991;74:447–453.

15. Scheithauer BW, Kovacs KT, Laws ER, Randall RV. Pathology of invasive pituitary tumors with special reference to functional classification. *J. Neurosurg.* 1986;65:733–744.

16. Selman WR, Laws ER, Scheithauer BW, Carpenter SM. The occurrence of dural invasion in pituitary adenomas. *J. Neurosurg.* 1986;64:402–407.

17. Scotti G, Yu CY, Dillon WP, et al. MR imaging of cavernous sinus involvement by pituitary adenomas. *AJNR Am. J. Neuroradiol.* 1988;9:657–664.

18. Dina TS, Feater SH, Laws ER, Davis DO. MR of the pituitary gland postsurgery: serial MR studies following transspheniodal resection. *AJNR Am. J. Neuroradiol.* 1993;14:763–769.

19. Steiner E, Knosp E, Herold CJ, et al. Pituitary adenomas: findings of postoperative MR imaging. *Radiology* 1992;185:521–527.

20. Kaufman B, Tomsak RL, Kaufman BA, et al. Herniation of the suprasellar visual system and third ventricle into empty sellae: morphologic and clinical considerations. *AJNR Am. J. Neuroradiol.* 1989;10:65–76.

21. Lundin P, Bergström K, Nyman R, et al. Macroprolactinomas: serial MR imaging in long-term bromocriptine therapy. *AJNR Am. J. Neuroradiol.* 1992;13:1279–1291.

22. Lucas-Morante T, Garcia-Uria J, Estrada J, et al. Treatment of invasive growth hormone pituitary adenomas with long–acting somatostatin analog SMS 201–995 before transsphenoidal surgery. *J Neurosurg* 1994;81:10–14.

23. Lundin P, Engström BE, Karlsson FA, Burman P. Long–term octreotide therapy in growth hormone-secreting pituitary adenomas: evaluation with serial MR. *AJNR Am. J. Neuroradiol.* 1997;18:765–772.

24. Johnson MR, Hoare RD, Cox T, et al. The evaluation of patients with a suspected pituitary microadenoma: computer tomography compared to magnetic resonance imaging. *Clin. Endocrinol.* 1992;36:335–338.

25. Wu W, Thuomas KA. Pituitary microadenoma MR appearance and correlation with CT. *Acta Radiol.* 1995;36:529–535.

26. Kucharczyk W, Davis DO, Kelly WM, et al. Pituitary adenomas: high-resolution MR imaging at 1.5T. *Radiology* 1986;161:761–765.

27. Stadnik T, Stevenaert A, Beckers A, et al. Pituitary microadenomas: diagnosis with two- and three-dimensional MR imaging at 1.5T before and after injection of gadolinium. *Radiology* 1990;176:419–428.

28. Davis PC, Hoffman JC, Malko JA, et al. Gadolinium–DTPA and MR imaging of pituitary adenoma: a preliminary report. *AJNR Am. J. Neuroradiol.* 1987;8:817–823.

29. Dwyer AJ, Frank JA, Doppman JL, et al. Pituitary adenomas in patients with Cushing disease: initial experience with Gd–DTPA-enhanced MR imaging. *Radiology* 1987;163:421–426.

30. Miki Y, Matsuo M, Sadahiko N, et al. Pituitary adenomas and normal pituitary tissue: enhancement patterns on gadopentetate-enhanced MR imaging. *Radiology* 1990;177:35–38.

31. Yuh WTC, Fisher DJ, Nguyen HD, et al. Sequential MR enhancement pattern in normal pituitary gland and pituitary adenoma. *AJNR Am. J. Neuroradiol.* 1994;15:101–108.

32. Kucharczyk W, Bishop JE, Plewes DB, et al. Detection of pituitary microadenomas: comparison of dynamic keyhole fast spin-echo, unenhanced, and conventional contrast-enhanced MR imaging. *AJR Am. J. Roentgenol.* 1994;163:671–679.

33. Tabarin A, Laurent F, Catargi B, et al. Comparative evaluation of conventional and dynamic magnetic resonance imaging of the pituitary gland for the diagnosis of Cushing's disease. *Clin. Endocrinol.* 1998;49:293–300.

34. Elster AD. High-resolution, dynamic pituitary MR imaging: standard of care or academic pastime? *AJR Am. J. Roentgenol.* 1994;163:680–682.

35. Burrow G, Wortzman G, Rewcastle N. Microadenomas of the pituitary and abnormal sellar tomograms in an unselected autopsy series. *N. Engl. J. Med.* 1981;301:156.

36. Teramoto A, Hirakawa K, Sanno N, Osamura J. Incidental pituitary lesions in unselected 1000 autopsy specimens. *Radiology* 1994;193:161–164.

37. Chong BW, Kucharczyk W, Singer W, George S. Pituitary gland MR: a comparative study of healthy volunteers and patients with microadenomas. *AJNR Am. J. Neuroradiol.* 1994;15:675–679.

38. Ahmadi H, Larsson EM, Jinkins JR. Normal pituitary gland: coronal MR imaging of infundibular tilt. *Radiology* 1992;171:389–392.

39. Oldfield EH, Doppman JL, Nieman LK, et al. Petrosal sinus sampling with and without corticotrophin–releasing hormone for differential diagnosis of Cushing's syndrome. *N. Engl. J. Med.* 1991;325:897–905.

40. Miller DL, Doppman JL, Peterman SB, et al. Neurologic complications of petrosal sinus sampling. *Radiology* 1993;185:143–147.

41. Doppman JL. There is no simple answer to rare complication of inferior petrosal sinus sampling. *AJNR Am. J. Neuroradiol.* 1999;20:191–192.

42. Taveras JM. *Neuroradiology*, 3rd edn. Baltimore, MD: Williams & Wilkins, 1996:639–641.

43. Bunin GR, Surawicz, TS, Witman PA, et al. The descriptive epidemiology of craniopharyngioma. *J. Neurosurg.* 1998;89:547–551.

44. Adamson TE, Wiestler OD, Kleihues P, Yasargil MG. Correlation of clinical and pathological features in surgically treated craniopharyngiomas. *J. Neurosurg.* 1990;73:12–17.

45. Harwood-Nash DC. Neuroimaging of childhood craniopharyngioma. *Pediatr. Neurosurg.* 1994;21(Suppl 1):2–10.

46. Hald JK, Eldevik OP, Brunberg JA, Chandler WF. Craniopharyngiomas – the utility of contrast medium enhancement for MR imaging at 1.5T. *Acta Radiol.* 1994;35:520–525.

47. Sartoretti-Schefer S, Wichmann W, Aguzzi A, Valavanis A. MR differentiation of adamantinous and squamous–papillary craniopharyngiomas. *AJNR Am. J. Neuroradiol.* 1997;18:77–87.

48. Eldevik OP, Blaivas M, Gabrielsen TO, et al. Craniopharyngioma: radiologic and histologic findings and recurrence. *AJNR Am. J. Neuroradiol.* 1996;17:1427–1439.

49. Petito CK. Craniopharyngiomas: prognostic importance of histologic features. *AJNR Am. J. Neuroradiol.* 1996;17:1441–1442.

50. Hald JK, Eldevik OP, Quint DJ, et al. Pre- and postoperative MR imaging of craniopharyngiomas. *Acta Radiol.* 1996;37:806–812.

51. Shanklin WM. The incidence and distribution of cilia in the human pituitary with a description of micro-follicular cyst derived from Rathke's cleft. *Acta Anat.* 1951;11:361–382.

52. Sumida M, Uozumi T, Mukada K, et al. Rathke cleft cysts: correlation of enhanced MR and surgical findings. *AJNR Am. J. Neuroradiol.* 1994;15:525–532.

53. Kucharczyk W, Peck WW, Kelly WM, et al. Rathke cleft cysts: CT, MR imaging and pathological features. *Radiology* 1987;165:491–495.

54. Onda K, Tanaka K, Takeda N, et al. Symptomatic Rathke's cleft cyst simulating arachnoid cyst. *Neurol. Med. Chir.* 1989;29:1039.

55. Asari S, Ito T, Tsuchida S, Tsutsai T. MR appearance and cyst contents of Rathke's cleft cysts. *J. Comput. Assist. Tomogr.* 1990;14:532–535.

56. Rottenberg GT, Chong WK, Powell M, Kendall BE. Cyst formation of the craniopharyngeal duct. *Clin. Radiol.* 1994;49:126–129.

57. Christophe C, Flamant–Durand J, Hanquinet S, et al. MRI in seven cases of Rathke's cleft cyst in infants and children. *Pediatr. Radiol.* 1993;23:79–82.

58. Black ML, Tien RD, Hesselink JR. Third ventricular hemangioblastoma: MR appearance. *AJNR Am. J. Neuroradiol.* 1991;12:553.

59. Morrison G, Sobel DF, Kelley WM, et al. Intraventricular mass lesions. *Radiology* 1984;153:435–442.

60. Reith KG, Comite F, Dwyer AJ, et al. CT of cerebral abnormalities in precocious puberty. *AJNR Am. J. Neuroradiol.* 1987;8:283–290.

61. Hubbard AM, Egelhoff JC. MR imaging of large hypothalamic hamartomas in two infants. *AJNR Am. J. Neuroradiol.* 1989;10:1277–1279.

62. Sumida M, Arita K, Migita K, et al. Demonstration of the optic pathway in sellar/juxtasellar tumours with visual disturbance on MR imaging. *Acta Neurochir. (Wien)* 1998;140:541–548.

63. Pont MS, Elster AD. Lesions of skin and brain: modern imaging of the neurocutaneous syndromes. *AJR Am. J. Roentgenol.* 1992;158:1193–1203.

64. Krenning EP, Kwekkeboom DJ, Bakker WH, et al. Somatostatin receptor scintigraphy with ^{111}In-DTPA-D-Pne and ^{123}I-Tyr3-octeotride: the Rotterdam experience in more than 1000 patients. *Eur. J. Nucl. Med.* 1993;20:716–721.

65. Lamberts SW, Krenning EP, Renbi JC. The role of somatostatin and its analogs in the diagnosis and treatment of tumours. *Endocr. Rev.* 1991;12:450–482.

66. Bergström M, Muhr C, Jossan S, et al. Differentiation of pituitary adenoma and meningioma: visualization with positron emission tomography and [^{11}C]-L-deprenyl. *Neurosurgery* 1992;30:855–861.

67. Lucignani G, Losa M, Moresco RM, et al. Differentiation of clinically non-functioning pituitary adenomas from meningiomas and craniopharyngiomas by positron emission tomography with [^{18}F]fluoro-ethyl-spiperone. *Eur. J. Nucl. Med.* 1997;24:1149–1155.

68. Muhr C, Bergstrom L, Lundberg PO, et al. Malignant prolactinomas with multiple intracranial metastases studied with positron emission tomography. *Neurosurgery* 1988;22:374–349.

69. Tien RD, Naston TH, McDermott MW, et al. Thickened pituitary stalk on MR images in patients with diabetes insipidus and Langerhans cell histiocytosis. *AJNR Am. J. Neuroradiol.* 1990;11:703–708.

70. Engelken JD, Yuh WTC, Carter KD, Nerad JA. Optic nerve sarcoidosis. MR findings. *AJNR Am. J. Neuroradiol.* 1992;13:228–230.

71. Williams DW III, Elster AD, Kramer SI. Neurosarcoidosis: gadolinium-enhanced MR images. *J. Comput. Assist. Tomogr.* 1990;14:704–707.

72. Appignani B, Landy H, Barnes P. MR in central idiopathic diabetes insipidus in children. *AJNR Am. J. Neuroradiol.* 1993;14:1407–1410.

73. Rivera JA. Lymphocytic hypophysitis: disease spectrum and approach to diagnosis and therapy. *Pituitary* 2006;9:35–45.

74. Bellastella A, Bizzarro A, Coronella C, et al. Lymphocytic hypophysitis: a rare or underdiagnosed disease. *Eur. J. Endocrinol.* 2003;149:363–376.

26 Pathology of Tumors of the Pituitary

Eva Horvath and Kalman Kovacs

Key points

- Benign pituitary adenomas are frequently occurring intracranial neoplasms. By histology, adenomas display variable, but not specific patterns.
- Additional use of immunohistochemistry (hormone content) and electron microscopy (ultrastructural features) permits the morphologic classification of pituitary adenomas and determination their cellular composition.
- In-depth morphologic investigation concluded that three adenoma types arise in yet-uncharacterized cell types.
- In addition to surgery and radiation therapy, medical treatment is available for growth hormone-, prolactin- and thyroid stimulating hormone-producing adenomas. The morphologic effects of medical treatments are discussed.
- The morphologic separation of adenoma types provides useful information helping clinical endocrinologists to select therapeutic modality.

Introduction

The human pituitary gland consists of two major components: the adenohypophysis comprising the hormone-producing cells of the pars anterior, pars intermedia and pars tuberalis; and the neurohypophysis, also called pars nervosa or posterior lobe [1]. In this chapter we deal only with adenohypophysial tumors. In contrast to most mammalian species, the human gland has no anatomically distinct pars intermedia [2]. The exclusively pro-opiomelanocortin (POMC)-producing cells of the pars intermedia are sandwiched between the anterior and posterior lobes in the majority of mammals, whereas in the human they are incorporated within the pars anterior, thereby constituting the pars distalis [3]. The pars tuberalis is a minor upward extension of the adeno-hypophysis attached to the exterior of the lower pituitary stalk.

The unevenly distributed hormone-producing cell types are arranged within evenly sized acini surrounded by a delicate but well-defined reticulin fiber network giving the pituitary its distinct architecture [4, 5].

Pituitary adenomas: general aspects

Adenomas, i.e., benign neoplasms arising in all types of hormone-producing cells of the adenohypophysis, are common, accounting for approximately 15% of intracranial tumors. Adenomas occur as small incidental findings in 5–20% of pituitaries at autopsy [1].

Clinical Endocrine Oncology, 2nd edition. Edited by Ian D. Hay and John A.H. Wass. © 2008 Blackwell Publishing. ISBN 978-1-4051-4584-8.

Regardless of their size, a lack of the normal acinar structure (Plate 26.1a) is evident in every adenoma. Pituitary adenomas are not encapsulated, but, if large enough, the tumors compress the reticulin framework of the surrounding normal gland into a pseudocapsule (Plate 26.1b).

By morphology, the histologic patterns and the tinctorial properties of tumors (acidophilic, basophilic or chromophobic) are largely unrelated to their hormonal function. Demonstration of hormone content (immunohistochemistry), assessment of ultrastructure (electron microscopy), *in situ* hybridization and increasingly popular molecular pathologic techniques are utilized for the functional classification of pituitary adenomas [1, 4–6].

Pituitary tumors may be referred to as microadenomas (less than 10 mm in diameter), or macroadenomas (more than 10 mm in diameter). The growth pattern of these tumors may be expansive, resulting in a slowly growing mass exerting increasing pressure on the surrounding normal gland and the bony sella. In contrast, invasive adenomas spread into the surrounding normal gland, dura or other parasellar structures (sphenoid sinus, cavernous sinus) regardless of their size. Adenomas extending into the suprasellar space may compress or infiltrate the optic chiasm, causing visual disturbances, a frequent clinical manifestation of macroadenomas. Exceptionally large adenomas may grow into the anterior or posterior cranial fossa or downward into the nasopharynx [7–9].

Adenomas associated with hypersecretory syndromes

Adenomas producing growth hormone (GH)

These tumors arise in the most populous GH cells or somatotrophs, which account for approximately 50% of the pars distalis. They are acidophilic by histology and display strong immunoreactivity for GH. Contingents of somatotrophs also express prolactin (PRL) or the alpha subunit of the glycoprotein hormones [4, 5]. Approximately 15% of surgically removed pituitary adenomas represent two forms of GH cell adenoma [1, 4, 5]. Most of these tumors are associated with physical stigmata and clinical signs of acromegaly, whereas tumors in children and adolescents causing gigantism are rare. Although the clinical manifestations and incidence of the two tumor types are similar, there are major differences in their morphology.

The *densely granulated GH cell adenoma* occurs with the same frequency as the sparsely granulated variant and peaks at the same time (in the sixth decade) in both sexes. The tumors display slow, expansive growth resulting in the typical "ballooning of the sella" and may remain intrasellar for several years.

By *histology*, the densely granulated form is strongly acidophilic displaying diffuse or, less frequently, trabecular or sinusoidal pattern. An extensive immunoreactivity for GH (Plate 26.1d) is usually accompanied by similarly strong positivity for alpha subunit [1, 4, 5]. Scattered immunopositivity for PRL and beta-thyroid-stimulating hormone (TSH) is usually unassociated with oversecretion of these hormones. The ultrastructure of adenomatous densely granulated GH cells is similar to that of the normal phenotype featuring well-developed rough endoplasmic reticulum (RER), prominent Golgi complex and numerous large secretory granules mostly in the 350–500 nm range (Fig. 26.1b).

The *sparsely granulated GH cell adenoma* is more common in women, and is also diagnosed earlier, peaking in the fourth decade. The tumors tend to be macroadenomas at the time of diagnosis and are often invasive. Histology detects chromophobic adenomas invariably displaying a diffuse pattern. Nuclear pleomorphism may be evident and adenoma cells frequently harbor a homogenous, spherical juxtanuclear, practically unstained structure. This "fibrous body" is strongly immunopositive for cytokeratin (Plate 26.1e). The striking polka-dot pattern thereby generated is the best histologic marker of the tumor type, since GH immunoreactivity is often scanty. As opposed to the densely granulated type, multiple immunoreactivities for pituitary hormones are rarely noted. The ultrastructural phenotype denoted by the spherical filamentous aggregate of the fibrous body nesting in the concavity of the eccentric crescent-shaped nucleus [6] and scanty, small (less than 250 nm) secretory granules is not seen in the normal gland (Fig. 26.1c).

Morphologic effects of treatment with long-acting somatostatin analogs are neither severe nor consistent [7–9]. Significant shrinkage of cells and marked fibrosis are infrequent. Most common findings are the increase in size and number of secretory granules and/or increased lysosomal activity. The close correlation observed between clinical response and tumor morphology in cases of prolactinomas treated with dopamine agonists is not observed in examples of somatostatin analog treatment.

Additional features and variants

Both types of GH cell adenoma may engage in usually focal, rarely massive production of endocrine amyloid. Approximately 2–3%

of morphologically typical sparsely granulated adenomas are clinically silent, the reason for which is unknown [4, 5]. Rare examples of the sparsely granulated tumors contain variable amounts of nervous tissue (neuron-like cells and neuropil) as a likely result of neuronal differentiation within the adenoma [4, 5].

PRL cell adenoma

PRL cell adenomas derive from PRL cells, or lactotrophs accounting for 10–30% of the cell population. They are scattered throughout the pars distalis with focal accumulation in the posterolateral areas.

The *sparsely granulated PRL cell adenoma* is the most common adenoma type accounting for 27–30% of surgically removed pituitary tumors [1, 4, 5]. It is associated with hyperprolactinemia, primary or secondary amenorrhea and infertility in women. The less specific symptoms in men – decreasing libido and impotence – usually mean delay in diagnosis and development of macroadenomas whereas the majority of tumors in women are small and classified as microadenoma. PRL cell adenoma is most frequent in the third and fourth decades of life in both sexes. However, the incidence of the tumor type is significantly higher in women in their main child bearing years. PRL cell adenomas are associated with wide-ranging biologic behaviors from indolent to highly aggressive, usually not reflected in their morphology. The PRL levels are roughly proportional to the tumor mass. The frequency of the tumor type in autopsy material is around 40% in both sexes.

Histologically, the large majority of PRL cell adenomas are chromophobic with a diffuse pattern. The other two patterns (papillary and the type with abundant hyalinous connective tissue stroma) occur mostly as incidental autopsy findings, suggesting slow growth rate and/or later onset.

Immunostaining demonstrates strong immunopositivity tracing the sacculi of the prominent Golgi apparatus, characteristic of PRL cells (Plate 26.1c). Ultrastructurally the three salient features are: masses of RER, prominent Golgi apparatus and extrusion of the small, sparse secretory granules. The latter is the specific marker of PRL differentiation (Fig. 26.1a) [1, 4–6].

Additional features

While calcification is extremely rare in other adenoma types, an estimated 10–15% of PRL-producing adenomas display varying degrees of calcification. Deposition of endocrine amyloid occurs infrequently.

Morphologic effects of dopamine agonist treatment

Adequate therapeutic response is associated with striking morphologic changes in adenoma cells: the nucleus becomes heterochromatic and the cytoplasm undergoes marked shrinkage due to loss and involution of the hormone-producing apparatus (RER, Golgi complex). PRL immunoreactivity is reduced or lost and, with the exception of granule extrusions, the cells have no

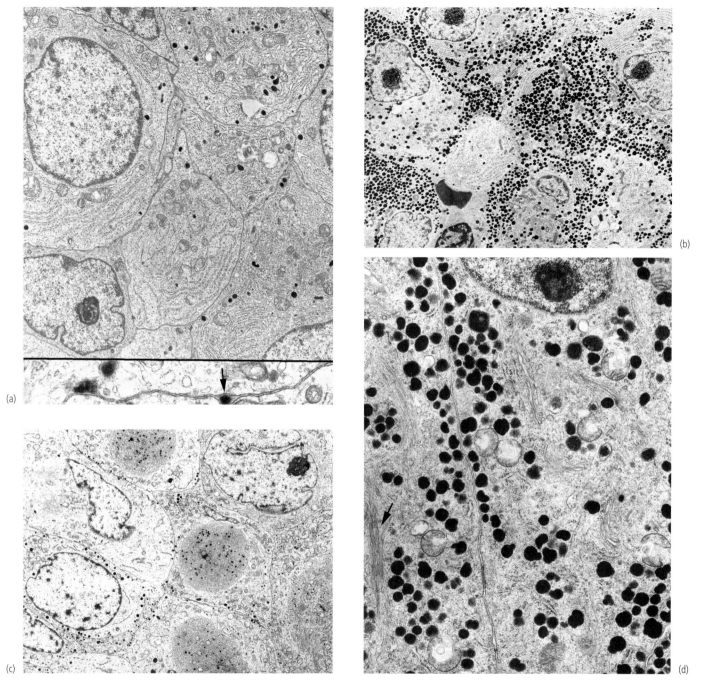

Figure 26.1 (a) Ultrastructure of sparsely granulated PRL cell adenoma displaying abundant RER, prominent Golgi complex and secretory granule extrusions (insert, at foot of image) arrowhead. Magnification ×4300, insert: ×17 000. (b) Densely granulated GH cell adenoma possessing numerous predominantly spherical large secretory granules. Magnification ×4650. (c) Electron microscopy of a sparsely granulated GH cell adenoma. Note fibrous body and scanty, minute secretory granules. Magnification ×4320. (d) The distinguishing ultrastructural features of corticotroph cell adenoma are the unique morphology of secretory granules and bundles of cytokeratin filaments (arrowhead). Magnification x10 200.

ultrastructural markers of PRL differentiation. Effects of treatment with long-acting forms of dopamine agonists can be exceptionally severe. Theoretically the morphologic changes are reversible. However, portions of neoplasms may permanently lose their responsiveness and retain their suppressed features even when treatment is discontinued. Long-term administration of dopamine agonists may also cause varying degrees of fibrosis and calcification [12].

Variants

The densely granulated form of PRL cell adenoma is very rare and clinically behaves similarly to the sparsely granulated variant [4, 5].

Adenomas producing GH and PRL

The *mixed (GH cell–PRL cell) adenoma*, a tumor comprising two distinct cell types, is the most important in this group [1, 4, 5] accounting for an approximate 5% of surgically removed adenomas. The tumors are associated with acromegaly and varying degrees of hyperprolactinemia. They tend to be aggressive and are difficult to treat. Mixed adenomas usually consist of densely granulated GH cells and sparsely granulated PRL cells. Other combinations are rare. Accordingly, they are composed of acidophilic and chromophobic cells immunoreactive for GH and PRL respectively. Alpha subunit positivity is common, as well. By electron microscopy, the cell types constituting mixed adenomas have the features of densely granulated GH cells and sparsely granulated PRL cells as described earlier in this chapter.

The infrequent (2%) mammosomatotroph cell adenoma is monomorphous, i.e., it consists of one cell type displaying markers of both GH and PRL differentiation [1, 4, 5]. Clinically they are associated with acromegaly and variable, usually mild hyperprolactinemia. The acidophilic tumors are immunoreactive for GH and alpha subunit and, to a much lesser extent, for PRL. At the ultrastructural level the densely granulated cells possess unusually large (up to 1000 nm and over) secretory granules and display granule extrusions, a PRL cell marker. The slow-growing mammosomatotroph adenomas show biologic behavior similar to that of densely granulated GH adenomas. They should be considered a morphologic variant of densely granulated GH cell adenoma with no difference in the clinical presentation.

The *acidophil stem cell adenoma* is a rare (2%) monomorphous type with morphologic signs of PRL and GH differentiation [1, 4, 5]. The tumor is associated chiefly with hyperprolactinemia, but the serum PRL levels may be disproportionately low for the size of the tumor. Physical stigmata of acromegaly and significant elevation of GH levels are infrequent. These tumors grow aggressively in young subjects with tendency to invade infrasellar areas. Histology demonstrates chromophobic adenomas with moderate to strong immunoreactivity for PRL. Immunopositivity for GH is weak or negative, but immunostain for cytokeratin reveals the dot-like positivity of fibrous bodies. The striking ultrastructure is characterized by oncocytic change with formation of giant mitochondria, sparse, small secretory granules with extrusion (PRL marker) and fibrous bodies (GH marker).

Adenomas producing ACTH

The source of this adenoma type, the corticotroph or ACTH cell, resides chiefly within the central part (median wedge) of the pituitary. The cells are basophilic, periodic acid–Schiff (PAS) positive and immunoreactive for 1-39 adrenocorticotropic hormone (ACTH) and other POMC peptides. Approximately 10–12% of adenohypophysial cells are immunopositive for POMC peptides, which include a small, but yet undetermined percentage of pars intermedia-derived POMC cells as well.

Corticotroph or ACTH cell adenomas responsible for pituitary-dependent Cushing disease account for 10–12% of surgically removed adenomas. The tumors show marked (4–5:1) female preponderance. The age-related occurrence of corticotroph adenoma is similar in the two sexes, peaking in the last third of the fourth decade. Majority of corticotroph lesions are small microadenomas causing florid Cushing disease [1, 4, 5, 12, 13]. The tumors, often measuring only a few millimeters in diameter, may be too small to conclusively detect by imaging or to clearly identify by the neurosurgeon [14]. Therefore serial sectioning of the biopsied tissue fragments is often needed and it may not result in the demonstration of the tumor in every case.

By histology, corticotroph adenomas are basophilic and PAS positive with a sinusoidal or diffuse pattern [1, 4, 5, 12, 13]. Immunoreactivity can be demonstrated not only for 1-39 ACTH, but for other POMC-derived peptides (beta-endorphin, beta-LPH, CLIP, etc.) as well. Electron microscopy documents densely granulated cells with secretory granules ranging up to 450–500 nm similar to those of normal ACTH cells. The best markers are: (1) the morphology of the secretory granules being spherical as well as notched, drop-shaped and heart-shaped often displaying variable electron density; (2) perinuclear bundles of cytokeratin filaments, characteristic for the human corticotroph (Fig. 26.1d).

In a minority of cases pituitary-dependent Cushing disease is caused by larger tumors. These neoplasms are often associated with a milder form of hypercorticism, but the tumors grow aggressively, often invade and they are frequently macroadenomas at the time of diagnosis [15]. By histology they exhibit variable, often weak PAS positivity and immunoreactivity for ACTH. A few examples of aggressive macroadenomas display immunoreactivity for luteinizing hormone (LH) and/or alpha subunit.

Morphologic features of corticotroph adenomas in cases of Nelson syndrome are similar to those of densely granulated corticotroph adenomas in Cushing disease with few or no cytokeratin filaments.

Variants

Crooke's hyalinization – excessive accumulation of cytokeratin filaments – is the ubiquitous response of the normal human ACTH cell to long-lasting elevations of circulating glucocorticoid levels. Accordingly, Crooke's hyalinization is noted in: (1) non-tumorous corticotrophs adjacent to corticotroph adenomas; (2) in ectopic ACTH/CRH syndrome; (3) in patients with glucocorticoid-secreting adrenocortical tumors; and (4) in subjects treated with pharmacologic doses of glucocorticoids. Crooke's hyalinization is not expected to develop in corticotroph tumors. Yet, a minority of such adenomas contains variable percentage of adenoma cells displaying the alteration [4, 5]. "Crooke's cell adenomas" do not represent an entity and have no clinical correlates. Such tumors may be associated with mild, moderate or severe hypercorticism and with variable biologic behavior.

Adenomas producing thyrotropin (TSH)

A mere 1% of surgically removed adenomas derive in TSH cells or thyrotrophs [4, 5, 16, 17], representing only about 5% of adenohypophysial cells. They reside chiefly within the anterior part of the median wedge. The slightly basophilic, angular thyrotrophs are strongly immunoreactive for TSH and alpha subunit.

TSH adenomas are associated either with hyperthyroidism and inappropriately elevated levels of TSH or they develop in hypothyroid subjects probably preceded by thyrotroph hyperplasia. Inexplicably, some adenomas bearing morphologic characteristics of thyrotroph adenomas occur in euthyroid subjects. At the time of diagnosis, these tumors are often macroadenomas with a tendency to invade. The morphology of the small group of thyrotroph adenomas exhibits surprising diversity. By histology, the adenomas are chromophobic and negative or mildly positive with PAS. They may be highly differentiated, comprising elongate polar cells forming pseudorosettes around vessels. Alternatively, the pattern may be diffuse in some cases with considerable nuclear pleomorphism. Yet another variant is markedly fibrotic. Minute calcifications may be evident as well. Immunoreactivity for TSH is variable; it is often patchy or scattered, rarely extensive. Scattered cells may exhibit immunoreactivity for alpha subunit, GH and PRL. No specific ultrastructural markers exist for the tumors. They are sparsely granulated (granule size: up to 250nm); the secretory granules are often confined to the cell periphery outlining cell contours.

Thyrotroph adenomas possess somatostatin receptors and may show clinical improvement to somatostatin analog therapy [8, 9]. At present no morphologic effects of that treatment are known.

Adenomas unassociated with overt signs of hormone overproduction

Adenomas producing FSH and LH

The number of gonadotrophs producing FSH and/or LH depends on age, sex and hormonal status; it is usually in the 10–20% range. They are scattered throughout the adenohypophysis, are basophilic, PAS positive and strongly immunoreactive for FSH, LH and their alpha subunit.

The incidence of *gonadotroph adenomas* in surgical material is about 10%; they occur with similar frequency in the two sexes [4, 5]. The majority of FSH/LH tumors appear as slow-growing expansive macroadenomas causing local symptoms [10]. Discrepancy between clinical parameters and morphologic signs of gonadotroph differentiation is common; tumors displaying FSH/LH immunoreactivity and signs of high degree of functional differentiation by electron microscopy may be unassociated with

elevated serum FSH/LH levels as shown by currently used hormone assays. The reason for these inconsistencies is unexplained.

Gonadotroph adenomas display significant phenotypic variability [1, 4, 5]. Histology may reveal polar cells forming pseudorosettes around vessels (Plate 26.1f) or a diffuse pattern. Oncocytic change, i.e. undue increase of number and volume density of mitochondria, is frequent. Immunoreactivity for FSH and/or LH is variable, mostly uneven. Alpha subunit, which is a useful clinical indicator, is not a reliable morphologic marker. Electron microscopy documents unique sex-linked dimorphism. Many tumors in both sexes consist of polar cells having small (100–200 nm) secretory granules accumulating in cell processes. The Golgi complex has regular features in tumors of males, whereas it often shows vacuolar transformation (honeycomb Golgi) in females. Adenomas comprising non-polar cells have regular Golgi complex in both sexes.

Null cell adenoma and oncocytoma

These two adenoma types are the morphologic variants of the same tumor [4, 5]. The hormonally inactive adenomas account for approximately 25% of surgically removed tumors. They are twice as common in males, peaking in the sixth decade in both sexes. Most of the tumors are slowly growing expansile macroadenomas causing local symptoms and varying degrees of hypopituitarism [10, 11]. Low-grade hyperprolactinemia may occur ("stalk section effect").

Null cell adenoma is the non-oncocytic form. By histology it is chromophobic with predominantly diffuse pattern. Pseudorosette formation, characteristic of glycoprotein hormone-producing tumors, may also occur. Immunostaining may detect scattered positivity for various pituitary hormones, particularly beta-FSH, beta-LH and alpha subunit, or they may be immunonegative. Electron microscopy documents small cells having poorly developed cytoplasmic organelles and small (100–200 nm) scanty randomly distributed secretory granules, but no markers or cellular derivation.

Oncocytomas always show diffuse pattern by histology. The adenoma cells are larger than null cells and may display acidophilia due to non-specific binding of acidic stains by mitochondria. The pattern of immunoreactivities is the same as seen in null cells. By electron microscopy the sole ultrastructural marker is the extensive accumulation of mitochondria, whereas the other organelles are poorly developed. The secretory granules are sparse, small (100–200 nm) and are often displaced to the cell periphery by the crowding mitochondria.

Uncommon adenoma types

The term *silent adenoma* refers to three types of well-differentiated, morphologically well-characterized adenomas which are unassociated with any known hormonal hypersecretory syndromes and are not derived from any of the known anterior pituitary cell types [1, 4, 5]. Silent adenomas and null cell adenomas are not synonymous, although clinically they cannot be distinguished.

Silent "corticotroph" adenoma subtype 1 (frequency less than 2%) is unassociated with clinical signs and symptoms of Cushing disease. It shows a lesser degree of female preponderance and different age-related occurrence than corticotroph adenomas associated with Cushing disease. The tumors display high propensity for hemorrhage and may present with pituitary apoplexy. By morphology the adenomas have the same basophilia, PAS positivity, ACTH and beta-endorphin immunoreactivity and ultrastructural features as corticotroph tumors associated with Cushing disease.

Silent "corticotroph" adenoma subtype 2 (frequency of 1.5–2.0%) shows marked male preponderance. The tumors appear as non-functioning masses and are usually diagnosed at the macroadenoma stage. Histology reveals chromophobic tumors comprising small cells, which exhibit only modest PAS positivity and scattered immunoreactivity for ACTH and beta-endorphins. Ultrastructurally the small cells possess small to midsize secretory granules (200–400 nm) showing similarity to POMC granules. However, no cytokeratin filaments are present.

The two adenoma types described above probably derive in cells of the pars intermedia, which in the human pituitary are incorporated within the pars distalis [2, 3]. The physiologic function of those cells is unknown.

The silent adenoma subtype 3 (frequency: approx. 2%) is clinically more important owing to its fairly aggressive behavior occurring mainly in young women. The tumor is equally frequent in the two sexes but it has strikingly different age-related distribution. In men, the tumor may occur at any age from the second to the seventh decades. The overwhelming majority of adenomas in women presents between 20 and 40 years peaking in the mid-30s, but occurs infrequently after 40 years of age. It is important to note that silent adenoma subtype 3 consistently mimics PRL cell adenoma in women, being associated with low-grade hyperprolactinemia (usually less than 100 ng/ml) even at the microadenoma stage. The serum PRL levels do not increase proportionally with tumor size. Dopamine agonist treatment is not indicated; it normalizes levels of PRL (probably released from the non-neoplastic pituitary), but it does not cause tumor shrinkage and does not inhibit tumor progression. Some of these tumors possess somatostatin receptors and are responsive to octreotide or lanreotide.

By histology, subtype 3 silent tumors are often acidophilic and may show mild PAS positivity. The large adenoma cells form a diffuse, or lobular pattern. Immunocytochemistry may demonstrate scattered, minor positivity for various adenohypophysial hormones owing to plurihormonal differentiation, but the majority of tumor cells are immunonegative for all known pituitary hormones.

The ultrastructure of adenomas displays features of glycoprotein hormone differentiation and often marked accumulation of smooth endoplasmic reticulum (SER). Owing to unspecific and variable immunoreactivities, electron microscopy is indispensable for diagnosis [18]. The cell derivation of this adenoma type is unknown.

Unclassified plurihormonal adenomas are rare tumors, often with unique ultrastructure [4, 5]. They may consist of one morphologic cell type (monomorphous), or more than one phenotype (plurimorphous). The most common combinations are: GH-TSH-PRL or PRL-TSH.

Pituitary carcinoma

According to the recent WHO classification [19] pituitary carcinoma can be diagnosed only when distant, craniospinal or, less frequently, extracranial metastasis is documented. Such tumors are extremely rare and associated with dire prognosis. The majority of pituitary carcinomas produce either PRL or ACTH. Other types, including those unassociated with signs of hormonal overproduction, are exceptionally rare. Pituitary carcinomas are not accompanied by specific histologic features: enhanced mitotic activity, nuclear and cellular pleomorphism do not necessarily herald malignancy and, vice versa, neoplasms with bland features might give rise to metastasis. Application of the proliferation marker MIB-1 antibody is more useful; carcinomas display nuclear labeling consistently higher than adenomas [20]. Immunoreactivities of pituitary carcinomas follow the pattern of the nonmalignant phenotype, although the degree of immunopositivity may be variably reduced. Relatively few cases have been investigated by electron microscopy revealing significant variability. In some carcinomas enough ultrastructural characteristics are retained to recognize the cell type, whereas other tumors have the appearance of endocrine carcinoma of undetermined origin.

References

1. Kovacs K, Horvath E. *Tumors of the Pituitary Gland*. Washington, DC: Armed Forces Institute of Pathology, 1986.
2. Horvath E, Kovacs K, Lloyd RV. Pars intermedia of the human pituitary revisited: morphologic aspects and frequency of hyperplasia of POMC-peptide immunoreactive cells. *Endocr. Pathol.* 1999;10: 55–64.
3. Horvath E, Kovacs K. Lost and found: the pars intermedia of the human pituitary and its role in the histogenesis of silent "corticotroph" adenomas. In Gaillard RC (ed.). *The ACTH Axis Pathogenesis, Diagnosis and Treatment.* Norwell, MA: Kluwer Academic Publishers, 2003:259–275.
4. Horvath E, Kovacs K. The adenohypophysis. In Kovacs K, Asa SL (eds). *Functional Endocrine Pathology*, 2nd edn., Boston: Blackwell Science, 1998:247–281.
5. Horvath E, Scheithauer BW, Kovacs K, Lloyd RV. Hypothalamus and pituitary. In Graham DI, Lantos PL (eds). *Greenfield's Neuropathology*, Vol 1, 7th edn., New York: Arnold Publishers, 2002:983–1051.
6. Horvath E. Ultrastructural markers in the pathologic diagnosis of pituitary adenomas. *Ultrastruct. Pathol.* 1994;18:171–179.
7. Kovacs K, Stefaneanu L, Horvath E, et al. Effect of dopamine agonist medication on prolactin producing pituitary adenomas. A

morphological study including immunocytochemistry, electron microscopy and in situ hybridization. *Virch. Arch. Pathol. Anat. Histopathol.* 1991;418:439–446.

8. Kovacs K, Horvath E. Effects of medical therapy on pituitary tumors. *Ultrastruct. Pathol.* 2005;29:163–167.

9. Vance ML. Medical treatment of functional pituitary tumors. *Neurosurg. Clin. North Am.* 2003;14:81–87.

10. Selman WR, Laws ER Jr, Scheithauer BW, Carpenter SM. The occurrence of dural invasion in pituitary adenomas. *J. Neurosurg.* 1986;64:402–407.

11. Pernicone PJ, Scheithauer BW. Invasive pituitary adenomas and pituitary carcinomas. In Lloyd RV (ed.). *Surgical Pathology of the Pituitary Gland.* Philadelphia, PA: WB Saunders, 1993:121–36.

12. Lloyd RV, Chandler WF, Mckeever PE, Schteingart DE. The spectrum of ACTH-producing pituitary lesions. *Am. J. Surg. Pathol.* 1986;10:618–626.

13. Saeger W. Surgical pathology of the pituitary in Cushing's disease. *Pathol. Res. Pract.* 1991:187:613–616.

14. Laws Er Jr, Thapar K. Surgical management of pituitary adenomas. *Baillière's Clin. Endocrinol. Metab.* 1995;9:391–405.

15. Thapar K, Kovacs K, Muller PJ. Clinical–pathological correlations of pituitary tumors. *Baillière's Clin. Endocrinol. Metab.* 1995;9:243–270.

16. Greenman Y, Melmed S. Thyrotropin secreting pituitary tumors. In Melmed S (ed.). *The Pituitary.* Cambridge, MA: Blackwell Science, 1995:546–558.

17. Beck-Peccoz P, Brucker-Davis F, Persani L, Smallridge RC, Weintraub BD. Thyrotropin-secreting pituitary tumors. *Endocr. Rev.* 1996;17:610–638.

18. Horvath E, Kovacs K, Smyth HS, Cusimano M, Singer W. Silent adenoma subtype 3 of the pituitary – immunohistochemical and ultrastructural classification: a review of 29 cases. *Ultrastruct. Pathol.* 2005;29:1–14.

19. Scheithauer BW, Kovacs K, Horvath E, et al. Pituitary carcinoma. In DeLellis RA, Lloyd RV, Heitz PU, Eng C (eds). *World Health Organization Classification of Tumours. Pathology and Genetics. Tumours of Endocrine Organs.* Lyon: IARC Press, 2004:36–39.

20. Thapar K, Kovacs K, Scheithauer BW, et al. Proliferative activity and invasiveness among pituitary adenomas and carcinomas. An analysis using the MIB-1 antibody. *Neurosurgery* 1996;38:99–107.

27 Surgery for Pituitary Tumors

Simon A. Cudlip

Key points

- Pituitary tumors account for 10–15% of all intracranial tumors.
- Clinical presentation is due to hormone hypersecretion, hormone undersecretion, mass effect with visual deficit, or as an incidental finding on MRI.
- The aims of surgery are to correct any pituitary hypersecretion, reverse pituitary hormonal hyposecretion, eliminate mass effect and minimize the risk of tumor recurrence.
- Medical therapy is effective for most patients with prolactinoma. For patients with acromegaly, Cushing disease and non-functioning tumors with mass effect, the most effective treatment remains surgery in the vast majority of cases.
- Transsphenoidal surgery is very effective and safe; with the evolution of endoscopic techniques and neuronavigation, the results of pituitary surgery continue to improve.
- All patients having pituitary surgery require long-term follow-up with careful monitoring of pituitary function for deficient hormones, surveillance MRI scans and, in many cases, regular visual assessment.

Introduction

The modern surgical treatment of pituitary tumors is now very much a team effort. The days of surgeons working in isolation have been consigned to the past, and thankfully, we now have a group of specialists involved in the care of patients with pituitary tumors in which the surgeon continues to play an important role.

Pituitary surgery has evolved considerably over the last century; much of this has been due to advances in imaging, and a better understanding of the biology of pituitary tumors. Moreover, there have been considerable changes in the technical nature of pituitary surgery that have made surgery safer and more effective. Many of these changes have been due to advances in investigation, with better selection of patients for surgery and preoperative planning. In addition, there have been major advances in the refinement of both the transsphenoidal approach and craniotomy for pituitary tumors, as well as the development of operative tools such as neuronavigation, intraoperative magnetic resonance imaging (MRI), and endoscopic pituitary surgery. Whilst many of these advances show much promise, they are essentially unproven with respect to the results of surgery. This leaves the most important aspect of pituitary surgery, namely, the subspecialization and experience of the surgeon, and the establishment of a good working relationship with a pituitary endocrinologist.

Clinical Endocrine Oncology, 2nd edition. Edited by Ian D. Hay and John A.H. Wass. © 2008 Blackwell Publishing. ISBN 978-1-4051-4584-8.

The history of pituitary surgery

Interest in pituitary surgery was perhaps initiated by some of the early work by Marie on acromegaly; however, the first operations were performed for reasons of raised intracranial pressure and visual failure and were considered a last resort rather than the first-line treatment of today. Sir Victor Horsley, at what is now the National Hospital for Neurology and Neurosurgery, undertook the first direct surgical approach to a pituitary tumor. The first operation was performed in 1889 when a large tumor was approached via a temporal craniectomy and without illumination or magnification; this was not reported until 1906 [1]. The first report of direct surgical treatment of a pituitary tumor was by F.T. Paul of Liverpool Royal Infirmary in 1893. Paul was advised and encouraged by Horsley, and performed a temporal craniectomy in a young woman with raised intracranial pressure and clinical features of acromegaly. It is not clear whether much of the tumor was removed – indeed the majority of the operation may have been the craniectomy and probable partial temporal lobectomy. The wound never healed and the patient lived for a further 3 months. Over the following two decades Victor Horsley performed a further 10 operations on patients with pituitary tumors with mixed results; he reported two deaths but remained steadfast in his recommendation of surgical treatment. It must be remembered that patients were presenting to Horsley with pituitary tumors at an advanced stage, and most likely large tumors causing mass effect, visual failure and raised intracranial pressure, and at the time there was no real alternative to surgery. A different approach was utilized by Krause in Berlin when a subfrontal approach was used to gain access to the sella in 1904, and a similar approach used to reach the optic canal where a bullet lay lodged in 1908. Krause realized that the subfrontal approach could be used to gain access to the pituitary gland and this principle was modified and utilized by Dandy, Heuer and Frazier. At the turn of the 19th century a craniotomy was a fraught and dangerous procedure with the resultant reported mortality of 50–80%; this led others to seek out a safer means of accessing and operating on pituitary tumors. The transsphenoidal route to the pituitary fossa had been described in cadavers by a number of surgeons and anatomists; however, Herman Schoffler was the first to use this route in a patient in Innsbruck in 1907. The subject was a 30-year-old man who presented with a giant pituitary tumor leading to headaches and visual symptoms. Due to technical limitations, exposure, and more importantly in this approach, illumination of the operative site were limited. Schoffler had arranged preoperative radiographs, which had not suggested a large tumor; this may have played a part in the limited tumor removal. Ten weeks after surgery the patient died of hydrocephalus, and was subsequently found to have a giant tumor compressing the third ventricle. In 1909 Oskar Hirsch demonstrated his lateral endonasal approach to the pituitary on a cadaver [2]. He later asked an anatamopathologist to perform a dissection on the skull-base after he had undertaken his transsphenoidal approach on a cadaver. It was confirmed that the pituitary fossa had been exposed without damage to surrounding structures. Encouraged by this, Hirsch went on to perform a similar operation in a live subject with visual failure in 1910. The operation was performed in five stages spanning 5 weeks, each removing structures approaching the pituitary fossa. All stages were performed under local anesthesia and the patient recovered well with some improvement in vision. This technique later changed as Hirsch incorporated the submucosal dissection of the septum described by Kocher and Killian, performing the first operation of this type on 4 June 1910, and later went on to perform a total of 413 operations of this type. This transnasal/submucosal approach forms the basis for the modern microscopic approach and by coincidence, on exactly the same day but separated by the Atlantic Ocean, Harvey Cushing was performing the first sublabial/submucosal approach to the pituitary. Cushing went on to perform many transsphenoidal operations but eventually became increasingly disillusioned with the transsphenoidal route. It is not clear why Cushing's preference changed – it may have been due to the increasing safety of transcranial surgery. However, from 1929 onwards he operated on patients with pituitary tumors almost exclusively by the transcranial route [3]. Such was Cushing's influence on North American and, to an extent, worldwide neurosurgical practice, that this shift in practice permeated throughout neurosurgery and transsphenoidal surgery fell out of favor.

The surgical lineage keeping transsphenoidal surgery alive took a rather meandering and international route from Boston to Edinburgh, then onto Paris and finally back into the Americas via Montreal. Norman Dott was selected as a Rockefeller Fellow and traveled to the Peter Bent Brigham Hospital in Boston where he spent several months as a surgical fellow working with Cushing. The fellowship was from November 1923 to June 1924 and coincided with Cushing's period of enthusiasm for the transsphenoidal approach. Once back in Edinburgh Dott continued with the transsphenoidal approach, devising new instruments and using a malleable light source rather than a headlight. Dott was visited by Gerard Guiot, the then Chief of Hôpital Foch in Paris, in 1956. Guiot was clearly impressed with the surgical technique he observed and began using the transsphenoidal route once back in Paris [4]. Two refinements he made were the semi-sitting position of the patient, and the use of intraoperative imaging with radiographs confirming entry of the sphenoid and pituitary fossa. The "Foch group" went on to perform 5500 transsphenoidal procedures from 1956 to 1999.

A young Jules Hardy spent time at the Hôpital Foch as part of a year's study in neurophysiology, with the intention of gaining experience in the pioneering functional and stereotactic surgery being performed by Guiot. During this time Hardy was impressed by the results of transsphenoidal surgery, and on returning to Montreal set about introducing the technique. This period coincided with hypophysectomy for metastatic breast cancer, and the introduction of the surgical microscope. The total hypophysectomy was a much more demanding task than a simple tumor debulking, and thus Hardy quickly became very proficient at identifying normal pituitary from tumor. Aided by the vastly enhanced illumination and magnification of the microscope, he introduced the concept of selective microadenoma resection and later went on to to demonstrate surgical cure in pituitary microadenomas using this technique. Hardy also introduced intraoperative televised fluoroscopy and used preoperative angiography routinely principally to exclude vascular lesions such as intrasellar aneurysms. Better preoperative imaging with computerized tomography (CT) scanning and MRI has allowed more accurate planning of surgery, and lower complication rates; however, this surgical technique has remained relatively unchanged until the last decade. Recent advances include the use of intraoperative neuronavigation allowing more accurate identification of the anatomical midline and intraoperative MRI with real-time imaging of pituitary tumors. Further advancement of the transsphenoidal route has led to "extended" transsphenoidal surgery of the suprasellar region pioneered by E.R. Laws and M. Weiss [5], and the application of endoscopic pituitary surgery developed and refined by H. Jho in Pittsburgh and P. Cappabianca in Naples [6, 7]. The tide is changing once again towards a pure endoscopic approach; the merits of this approach are clear but time will tell if the results of surgery can match the transsphenoidal approach.

Indications for surgery

Pituitary apoplexy

The most urgent need for surgical intervention is in cases of pituitary apoplexy, particularly when there is evidence of cranial nerve palsy or acute visual failure. Surgery is aimed at reducing mass effect by removing the hemorrhage and the associated necrotic pituitary tumor. Surgery can be avoided in some cases where the visual apparatus is not affected; this will be discussed later in the chapter.

Progressive mass effect of tumor

A clear indication for surgery in patients with pituitary tumor is correction or prevention of visual deficits. This generally forms the largest single group of patients requiring surgical treatment. Patients presenting with a visual field deficit and reduced visual acuity, and with imaging evidence of a pituitary macroadenoma, require first an urgent endocrine assessment. This will filter out a significant number of patients with prolactin-secreting tumors who are better managed with a dopamine agonist in the first instance; a small proportion of these patients may need surgery if the tumor is resistant to dopamine agonists, or the patient is intolerant of the medication. Occasionally, patients with somatotroph or corticotroph adenomas will also present primarily with symptoms and signs due to tumor mass effect. It is important that these patients have a formal endocrine assessment so that their Cushing disease/acromegaly can be better controlled prior to surgery in order to minimize perioperative risk. Patients with other lesions in this category include craniopharyngioma, Rathke's cleft cyst, pituitary metastasis, intrasellar meningioma and upper third clivus lesions such as chordoma. Endocrine assessment will confirm the diagnosis of a non-functioning tumor in most cases and in cases of pituitary insufficiency will allow preoperative replacement therapy to commence before surgery, thus minimizing perioperative complications.

Normalization of pituitary hypersecretion

The primary treatment of choice in acromegaly and Cushing disease remains transsphenoidal removal of the pituitary adenoma responsible. In many cases the tumor is a microadenoma (<1 cm) and thus a surgical "cure" is possible. In cases of secretory macroadenomas, typically somatotroph adenomas, additional medical therapy or radiotherapy may be required after surgery in order to adequately control hormone levels after surgery. Microprolactinomas causing infertility, amenorrhea and altered bone density, and not suitable for medical therapy, should also be considered suitable for transsphenoidal surgery. Rare tumors include those producing thyroid-stimulating hormone (TSH) and luteinizing hormone (LH)/follicle-stimulating hormone (FSH).

Biopsy of sellar/suprasellar lesion

Where there is doubt over the origin of a pituitary lesion and further treatment hinges on histological diagnosis, a biopsy may be performed. One such example is the enhancing suprasellar lesion seen on MRI with normal serum tumor and inflammatory markers. A biopsy may allow discrimination between inflammatory lesions such as sarcoidosis, histiocytosis X and tuberculosis, and suprasellar tumors such as germinoma or teratoma.

Contraindications to surgery

Contraindications to surgery are rare, and virtually never absolute. The only absolute contraindication to transsphenoidal surgery is an ectatic carotid artery or aneurysm lying within or anterior to the pituitary fossa. A non-pneumatized sphenoid air-sinus can make a pituitary surgeon's life difficult, but with image-guided surgery and angled neurosurgical high-speed drills it is now possible to perform transsphenoidal surgery in these cases.

Relative contraindications include patients with severe systemic disease making general anesthesia more risky. In cases of severe acromegaly, surgery may be made more problematic by co-existent hypertension, diabetes, cardiomyopathy, pulmonary disease, and airway obstruction. In these cases, pretreatment of the acromegaly with somatostatin analogs, and treatment of the other systemic manifestations of acromegaly reduce perioperative complications. Florid Cushing disease also presents increased perioperative risks and thus once again pretreatment may reduce complications. Profound hypopituitarism should also be corrected prior to proceeding with surgery; although cortisol and thyroid replacement leads to only a temporary and short delay, correction of abnormalities of sodium may take slightly longer to correct. In cases where a transsphenoidal operation is deemed not appropriate, the pituitary tumor is best approached via a craniotomy.

Preoperative investigations: general principles

Ascertain the endocrine diagnosis

Any lesion in the vicinity of the hypothalamo–hypophysial axis requires a full endocrine assessment. This allows discrimination between secretory and non-secretory tumors, means that early hormone replacement therapy can be commenced, and establishes the "baseline" pituitary function. Investigations are covered extensively in other chapters but include static and dynamic measures of pituitary function.

Ascertain the anatomical diagnosis

Once the suspicion of a pituitary tumor has been raised, imaging evidence of this should be sought. Historically, this was based on plain skull radiographs, and CT scanning. The gold standard is now high-resolution MR imaging of the pituitary fossa, with and without gadolinium enhancement. Rarely, a conventional angiogram is required in cases of supra- or intrasellar aneurysm; the diagnosis is often obtained with magnetic resonance or CT angiography and planning for embolization performed with a conventional digitally subtracted angiogram. As well as confirming the diagnosis, accurate imaging is crucial in planning surgical treatment. Identification of microadenomas is key in the management of syndromes of hormone overproduction by secretory tumors, both in terms of confirming the diagnosis and allowing a more selective adenomectomy, and can help predict the

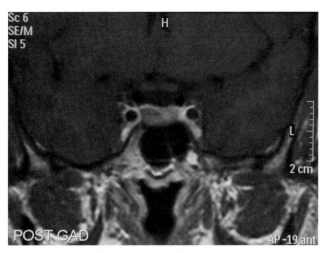

Figure 27.1 Magnified coronal T1-weighted MRI image after intravenous contrast. Right-sided microadenoma is seen with reduced contrast uptake as compared with normal pituitary gland; no cavernous sinus invasion is seen.

Table 27.1 Aims of treatment

Mass effect	Reduction/elimination of mass effect of tumor, in particular compression of the optic pathways
Hormonal	Control of hormone overproduction by pituitary adenoma
Tumor recurrence	Minimize risk of tumor recurrence
Preserve pituitary	Preservation of normal pituitary function
Diagnosis	Obtaining tissue for a definitive histopathological diagnosis

likelihood of a surgical "cure" (Fig. 27.1 and Table 27.1). In cases of macroadenoma, the emphasis is placed upon the relationships of the tumor to surrounding neurovascular structures including the optic nerves and chiasm, the cavernous sinus, sphenoid and clival bones, and in particular the degree of suprasellar extension (Fig. 27.2). Occasionally, in the case of a giant pituitary tumor, or a purely suprasellar lesion such as a craniopharyngioma, a craniotomy is the preferred mode of approach. The anatomy and size of the tumor ultimately determine the surgical approach chosen, and the degree of tumor resection likely to be achieved during surgery.

Minimize the risks of treatment

This includes a careful preoperative assessment, particularly in cases of Cushing disease or acromegaly where there may be significant hypertension, diabetes, cardiac disease, pulmonary disease, narrowing of the airways, or osteoporosis. Full investigation and medical optimization of these conditions are essential before proceeding to surgery. Exceptions to this include pituitary apoplexy or rapid visual failure where the emphasis is placed on rapid surgical decompression of the optic pathways.

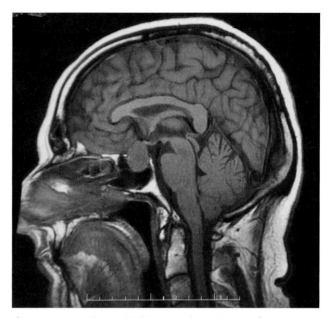

Figure 27.2 Sagittal T1-weighted MRI image showing large non-functioning macroadenoma elevating and compressing optic chiasm, and expanding pituitary fossa.

Choice of surgical approach

The choice of surgical approach is based on many factors (Table 27.2). The most important of these include the size and degree of pneumatization of the sphenoid, the size of the sella and thickness of the bone forming its floor, the degree and configuration of the extension of tumor into the suprasellar compartment, and the location of the carotid arteries in relation to the

Table 27.2 Choice of surgical approaches to the pituitary fossa

Surgical route	Variations
Transsphenoidal route	Endonasal submucosal transseptal/septal pushover approach Direct endonasal approach Sublabial transseptal/septal pushover approach Endoscopic transsphenoidal approach
Extended transsphenoidal approach	
Transcranial approaches	Subfrontal craniotomy Pterional craniotomy Subtemporal craniotomy Orbito-zygomatic craniotomy
Alternative skull-based approaches	Lateral rhinotomy approach Midface degloving approach Transethmoidal and extended transethmoidal approach Transbasal approach of Derome

Table 27.3 Conditions favoring the surgical approach to pituitary tumors

Transsphenoidal approach	Transcranial approach
Lateral, non-tortuous carotid arteries	Tortuous carotids impinging on midline
Probable soft tumor	Known fibrous tumor
Pneumatized sphenoid sinus	Non-pneumatized sphenoid sinus
Expanded sella	Small sella
Little suprasellar extension	Large/multicompartment suprasellar extension

sella. Also, the experience of the surgeon with a particular surgical approach plays an important role. In the case of adenomas, the one feature that cannot be determined preoperatively is the consistency of the tumor. If the tumor is found to be very soft, then it can be possible to remove tumors with large suprasellar extensions transsphenoidally without having to resort to a transcranial approach. This can be aided by the artificial elevation of the intracranial pressure during surgery using the Valsalva maneuver or by giving boluses of saline via a lumbar catheter inserted preoperatively [8]. The rise in intracranial pressure aids prolapse of the tumor from the suprasellar space into the sella, and thus into view. Examples of tumors where the consistency makes a transsphenoidal approach very difficult or impossible include meningiomas and large solid craniopharyngiomas. In the vast majority of cases a transsphenoidal approach is the first-line operation, and if a complete tumor removal is not possible then a transcranial procedure can be performed at a later date. Table 27.3 summarizes the conditions favoring each approach.

Transsphenoidal approaches

There are a number of variations in the transsphenoidal approach to the sella; they all have the same principle, namely the safest and least traumatic route of access to the sella, and the best means of directly visualizing the pituitary gland, its associated structures, and pituitary adenomas. The three main variations of this procedure are the endonasal approach, the sublabial approach and the endoscopic transsphenoidal approach. All of these operations are performed under general anesthesia with an endotracheal tube and cotton throat pack in place. In addition either the lateral part of the thigh or periumbilical region is prepared for harvesting of a fat and/or fascial graft for repair of the sellar region after tumor resection.

The endonasal approach

The patient is positioned with the head elevated and the neck slightly flexed, the surgeon stands at the head of the operating table looking towards the patient's feet. Some surgeons still prefer to stand in the axilla of the patient. In both cases the C-arm of an image-intensifier is placed in position for a lateral skull radiograph during the procedure to check trajectory. The skin of the face and nose is prepared with aqueous chlorhexidine solution, and the nasal cavities sprayed with Moffat's solution (cocaine 2 ml, epinephrine [adrenaline (1:1000)] 1 ml and sodium bicarbonate

2 ml) to reduced mucosal bleeding. The microscope is then used to inspect the nasal mucosa and septum of the right-hand nostril. A linear incision is made in the mucosa overlying the septum in the horizontal plane. This incision is then used to dissect the mucosa from the septum until the junction between cartilaginous and bony septum (perpendicular plate of the ethmoid) is reached. At this point this junction is fractured, allowing submucosal dissection along both sides of the bony septum until the anterior sphenoid is reached (transseptal approach). The mucosa is dissected form the sphenoid and the sphenoid ostia identified. A radiograph is performed to confirm a correct trajectory to the pituitary fossa and a bivalve self-retaining pituitary retractor system placed in the submucosal dissection plane. The sphenoid is then fractured and its anterior wall using bone punches until the pituitary fossa is exposed. Reference to the preoperative imaging must be made to identify the septal arrangement inside the sphenoid air sinus, and its relationship to the midline; the mucosa is usually stripped from the sinus. Anatomic landmarks can now be identified such as the clivus, the carotid eminences either side of the sellar floor, and the anterior cranial fossa. In cases of large tumors the bone of the sellar floor is often expanded and eroded, and it may be possible to fracture the bone with a small blunt hook or even the sucker tip. With a thicker sellar floor bone rongeurs or even a high-speed angle drill may be needed to open the fossa. The bone is removed as widely as possible from one cavernous sinus to the other, the floor is completely removed, and a thin shelf of bone is left superiorly to prevent inadvertent entry into the cerebrospinal fluid (CSF) space via exposed arachnoid. The dura is then opened in a cruciate fashion and the tumor and normal pituitary gland exposed. The pituitary tumor is often visible, and is usually paler in color, and softer than the normal pituitary gland. In cases of large tumors, the pituitary gland may not be seen until the very end of the procedure when the tumor has been removed, and usually consists of a thin rind of compressed gland pushed to the floor, side or posterior part of the fossa. The tumor removal is begun by use of a microdissector to attempt to separate tumor from the normal gland and dura lining the fossa; in some cases it is possible to enucleate the tumor and remove it almost in one piece. The tumor is more commonly removed piecemeal by a combination of micro ring-shaped curettes, and micro-grasping forceps. Use of instruments that are "bayonetted" allows the surgeon to view past the instrument without the surgeon's hands obstructing the view down the microscope. Tumor is cleared from the walls of the cavernous sinus and from the diaphragm until a complete resection is achieved. The diaphragm and thus further suprasellar tumor may be brought into view by raising the intracranial pressure by use of a lumbar drain or a Valsalva maneuver. The sella is reconstructed with some gelfoam if no CSF leak has occurred and the septal mucosal flap reapproximated and held in place with a nasal tampon.

The endoscopic approach

The endoscopic transsphenoidal approach has evolved in recent years, and the two main pioneers in this respect have been Jho and Cappabianca [6, 7]. The favored approach is now an endonasal

Table 27.4 Advantages and disadvantages of endoscopic pituitary surgery

Advantages	Disadvantages
No need for retraction	New skills needed
Reduced postoperative pain	Not intuitive for microscopic surgeon
Better view of sella/sphenoid	Nasal anatomy unfamiliar
Wide angle view allows exploration of cavernous sinus/suprasellar region	2D view
	Learning curve
Allows extended surgical approaches for meningiomas and clivus tumors	Longer procedure
	Optics not as good as microscope
No need for nasal packs	As yet unproven with no randomized controlled studies comparing with conventional procedure

Table 27.5 Complications of transsphenoidal pituitary surgery

Operative mortality	
Meningitis, intracranial haemorrhage, hypothalamic injury	0.5–1%
Major morbidity	
New visual deficit	0.5–1%
Meningitis	0.5–1%
Vascular injury	1%
CSF rhinorrhea (requiring surgical intervention)	2–3%
New cranial nerve palsy	<0.5%
Minor morbidity	
New anterior pituitary deficiency	10–14%
Diabetes insipidus (transient and permanent)	2–3%
Nasal septal perforation	2%
Nasal hemorrhage	1%
Transient cranial nerve palsy	0.5%
Sinusitis	1%

operation using a rigid endoscope to visualize the anatomy, with instruments working alongside the endoscope. Unlike the submucosal approach above a direct endonasal approach is used with the middle turbinate as the landmark for the opening into the sphenoid sinus called the sphenoid ostium. A sphenoidotomy is performed and extended to the contralateral side. The endoscope is then changed for a longer endoscope which is fixed in place with an articulated arm; this frees the surgeon's hands, allowing one hand to hold a dissector and the other a sucker. The operation then proceeds in a very similar fashion to the standard approach. The use of the endoscope allows a more panoramic view of the sphenoid and pituitary fossa (Plate 27.1), and allows the surgeon to see laterally into the cavernous sinus, and into the suprasellar region, which may allow more radical tumor removal. In addition, it is less traumatic due to the fact that no nasal retractor is needed, and thus recovery is claimed to be more rapid. The advantages and disadvantages of the approach are summarized in Table 27.4.

Extended transsphenoidal approach

This technique has been developed in recent years in an attempt to resect larger tumors, and approach tumors arising in the suprasellar space such as craniopharyngioma [5], meningioma, suprasellar germinoma, and pituitary stalk lesions requiring biopsy.

From a technical point of view the exposure often involves division of the superior part of the intercavernous venous sinus; this requires control of the associated venous hemorrhage by pressure, bipolar diathermy or microscopic vascular clips. The extended approach inevitably involves entry into the subarachnoid space with a resultant CSF leak, and thus requires careful repair of this defect to prevent postoperative CSF leak [5, 9].

Complications of transsphenoidal surgery (summarized in Table 27.5)

Overall, transsphenoidal surgery remains one of the safest operations in neurosurgical practice with a reported 30-day mortality of 0.8–1% [10]. One of the commonest complications is CSF leak causing CSF rhinorrhea [10]. This is usually evident during surgery and it is imperative that a meticulous repair of the sella is performed. This usually involves a tissue graft of subcutaneous fat from the abdomen or thigh, sometimes in combination with a layer of grafted fascia. The floor of the pituitary fossa is reconstructed using this material, and if possible the hole in the diaphragm is "buttonholed" using a small piece of the fat graft. The sphenoid air sinus is packed with further fat, and often sealed with tissue glue. After surgery some surgeons prefer to drain CSF via a lumbar catheter for a number of days to allow the repair to seal any leak. Damage to the anterior pituitary is more common where an aggressive resection of tumor is required, especially in cases of Cushing disease and acromegaly. In cases of macroadenoma, anterior pituitary function can be preserved in up to 95% of cases. Patients with preoperative endocrine deficiency only have a 10–15% restoration of these deficiencies after surgery.

Craniotomy for pituitary tumors

Due to the efficacy and safety of the transsphenoidal approach, craniotomy is infrequently needed. The commonest indications include giant pituitary adenomas with multicompartmental extension of the tumor, e.g., extension into the middle and anterior cranial fossa, fibrous pituitary adenoma with failure to resect all of the tumor transsphenoidally, solid craniopharyngioma, and a contraindication to the transsphenoidal approach. The common approaches utilized involve variations on the subfrontal craniotomy with pterional and orbital extensions [11, 12]. The aim of the approach is correct identification and preservation of the optic nerves and chiasm, the carotid arteries and their tributaries, the pituitary stalk, and preservation of the multiple small perforating vessels feeding the optic nerves and chiasm, and the hypothalamus. The tumor is identified under the microscope and internally decompressed by tumor resection. This allows the capsule of the tumor to be collapsed and dissected carefully from the surrounding structures. Plate 27.2 demonstrates the view of the right optic nerve during a pterional craniotomy under magnification.

Complications of craniotomy include those of transsphenoidal surgery with the additions of epilepsy and a slightly higher risk of vascular injury and visual deficit due to the association with operations for larger tumor and the dissection of blood vessels from the chiasm and tumor. In addition there is an increased risk of permanent diabetes insipidus.

Results of surgery

Non-functioning adenomas

The main indication for surgery in these tumors is visual deficit, and in this respect the outcome of surgery is good in the vast majority of patients. Overall, 85–90% of patients gain some improvement in their vision following surgery, with normalization of vision in up to 40% of patients [13]. Factors which tend to predict visual recovery are evidence of optic atrophy, severity of visual field deficit, poor visual acuity, duration of symptoms and increasing age of the patient.

Despite improvements in surgical technique there remains a significant recurrence rate for these tumors, and debate still remains over whether radiotherapy should be given in patients with operated macroadenoma. Studies suggest that the recurrence rate in patients in whom radiotherapy is withheld can be as high as 50% at 10 years; radiotherapy can reduce this rate to 2–3% [14]. Due to the complications of radiotherapy many physicians will now defer radiotherapy if a postoperative MRI scan demonstrates a complete tumor resection. Continued surveillance with MRI can pick up early tumor recurrence before symptoms arise, and based on this either further surgery and / or radiotherapy can be given.

The vast majority of patients retain pituitary function after surgery with up to 95% retaining normal pituitary function after transsphenoidal surgery. However, only 10–16% of patients with established endocrine deficiencies preoperatively have partial or complete restoration of pituitary function after surgery [15].

Cushing disease

In many ways Cushing disease is the most challenging of the pituitary tumors to treat, and this is reflected in the "cure" rates of surgery. Surgery remains the treatment of choice, and it is a realistic proposition to be able to selectively remove the adenoma, cure the hypercortisolemia and maintain normal pituitary function in many cases. Localization of the adenoma plays a key role in the treatment, and this can be difficult as many tumors are only a few millimeters in size. Techniques such as high-resolution MRI and dynamic MRI, together with inferior petrosal venous sampling, have led to better identification of microadenomas prior to surgery. If no tumor is evident prior to surgery the gland must be

inspected sequentially in quadrants during surgery. If no tumor is identified, and fertility is not an issue it may be appropriate to perform a total hypophysectomy. Overall remission rates for microadenomas at first operation are up to 80–90%. For all tumors, including macroadenomas and revision surgery, this falls to 40–50% [16, 17]. Features that predict long-term remission include positive histology for tumor obtained, microadenoma, no cavernous sinus invasion and undetectable early postoperative cortisol levels [18]. Tumor recurrence remains a problem even many years after surgery, with long-term remission figures falling to 60–70%; for this reason follow-up is required for many years [19].

Treatment of recurrent disease can be problematic as results of further surgery are often disappointing. As the morbidity and mortality of repeat surgery continue to fall, and if residual tumor is seen to be accessible to further surgery, then it is often worth performing further transsphenoidal surgery. Ultimately, many of these patients will require adjuvant radiotherapy, given as either conventional or stereotactic radiotherapy. This results in remission in 60–83% of patients at the expense of other endocrinopathies, and a delay in normalization of cortisol levels of up to 3 years.

Acromegaly

Once again surgical resection of the pituitary adenoma remains the treatment of choice. The vast majority of patients will have a tumor suitable for a transsphenoidal approach; rarely, tumors will require a craniotomy. During surgery, the floor of the pituitary fossa is often thickened and thus a high-speed drill with a diamond burr may be needed to open the pituitary fossa and expose the dura. The effectiveness of surgery is related to a number of factors including the size of the tumor, invasion of the cavernous sinus and surrounding structures, and the preoperative GH level. In GH-producing microadenomas with no invasion, the cure rate of surgery as defined by modern criteria is 80–90% [20]. Macroadenomas treated with surgery have a cure rate of 44–56%, largely due to a predilection of these tumors to invade nearby structures, especially the cavernous sinus. Recent data suggest that debulking surgery can allow better control of GH levels with somatostatin analogs, and thus it makes surgery worthwhile even if a cure cannot be realistically expected [21]. Patients who continue to have active acromegaly despite surgery can be managed with somatostatin analogs and radiotherapy if medical management fails to reduce the GH to a level not associated with increased morbidity and mortality.

Prolactinoma

The majority of patients with prolactinoma will be successfully treated with dopamine agonists and will require no surgery. Patients will require surgery in 15–30% of cases with the tumor either not shrinking with treatment, serum prolactin levels remaining high, or patients suffering from side effects of the dopamine agonists to the point of drug intolerance. Other less frequent indications for surgery include the need for repair of a CSF leak due to tumor shrinkage, and tumor necrosis and secondary hemorrhage due to rapid tumor shrinkage and disturbance of tumor blood supply (pituitary apoplexy). Patients requiring surgery for microprolactinoma generally fare well with a remission rate of up to 90% [22, 23]; this can be dependent upon preoperative prolactin levels, though, and a prolactin of over 100 ng/ml in one series was associated with a remission rate of only 50%. Preoperative prolactin is a good indicator of the likelihood of cure of a macroprolactinoma with surgery, with cure rates of tumors with serum prolactin levels over 200 ng/ml only 18–40%. There is some evidence that even if the prolactin cannot be normalized with dopamine analogs preoperatively, some tumor shrinkage can allow an improved cure rate with subsequent surgery. Recurrence rates are estimated at 18% for microprolactinomas and 20% for macroprolactinomas despite initially successful surgery. This phenomenon can be "biological recurrence" with rising serum prolactin, without radiological recurrence. Radiotherapy may be required for patients with residual tumor, and has been shown to be effective in many cases. This is dependent upon residual tumor volume and serum prolactin levels. Primary radiotherapy using stereotactic techniques has been advocated for microadenomas by some workers; this can result in a cure in up to 50%, and an improvement in serum prolactin in 28%.

Pituitary apoplexy

Pituitary apoplexy is a clinical and radiological diagnosis, and is often a medical emergency. As more incidental pituitary tumors are discovered on MRI scans of the brain, asymptomatic, radiological evidence of past apoplexy can be found in up to 10% of macroadenomas.

The clinical features of apoplexy comprise sudden-onset headache, with nausea and vomiting, associated with new visual field defects, reduced visual acuity, and diplopia or ocular palsy due to dysfunction of the IIIrd, IVth, or VIth nerves. In addition, there may be altered level of consciousness, mild pyrexia, neck stiffness, trigeminal nerve dysfunction causing facial numbness, and hypotension due to sudden cortisol deficiency. Rarely, seizures may be the presenting feature due to profound hyponatremia. The differential diagnosis includes subarachnoid hemorrhage and meningitis and therefore it is important to obtain a CT or MRI scan of the brain as soon as the patient has been resuscitated. The diagnosis is usually made on imaging, with acute hemorrhage into a pre-existing macroadenoma, often in association with distortion or compression of the optic chiasm and cavernous sinuses (Plate 27.2). In cases of apoplexy with visual disturbance or other neurological deficit, surgery is usually performed as an emergency procedure. It is imperative that fluid and electrolyte abnormalities are corrected as much as possible prior to surgery, and any hormonal deficiencies corrected. In practice this usually means correction of SIADH-related hyponatremia, administering intravenous hydrocortisone, and often thyroxine. Surgery is then performed as soon as possible with the aim of removing the necrotic tumor and hematoma. The results of surgery in most series suggest an increased mortality of up to 10% compared with less than 1% for routine transsphenoidal surgery, with 80–90% of patients having permanent disturbance in pituitary function needing hormonal replacement [24, 25]. Rates of visual recovery overall are excellent with 80–90% of patients having improved vision after surgery, evidence suggests that the earlier the chiasm is decompressed, the better the visual outcome. In patients with apoplexy without visual deficit or other neurological deficit, there is a case for nonoperative management. This requires careful endocrine assessment and regular follow-up with visual assessment and MRI.

Advances in pituitary surgery

Alongside the many advances made in the medical management and radiotherapy for pituitary tumors, there have been many technological advances in neurosurgery that have led to changes in techniques employed during pituitary surgery.

Perhaps the most significant of these is the development of endoscopic pituitary surgery which has been discussed earlier. In addition, the use of image-guided neurosurgery, otherwise called neuronavigation, has become widespread in neurosurgical practice [26, 27]. This allows real-time navigation during pituitary surgery. Conventionally, fluoroscopy has been used during surgery, and whilst this allows easy identification in the lateral trajectory, the identification of the midline is more problematic. This becomes more important in second-time transsphenoidal surgery where the midline landmarks are obscured, and thus raises the possibility of complications such as carotid injury. Neuronavigation has been shown to be a safe and effective means of guiding the pituitary surgeon to the tumor, and a display on a workstation showing three or four views in differing planes of the surgical approach.

One of the disadvantages of image-guided surgery is that the images being used are usually from the day prior to surgery, and thus cannot give information about the volume of tumor resected. This has led to the use of intraoperative MRI scanners in some centers. These were initially low field MRI scanners, but increasingly higher field scanners are being used to improve the resolution of the images obtained [28, 29]. Whilst this development has much promise, as yet only modest improvements in tumor removal have been obtained in experienced surgical hands.

References

1. Pollock JR, Akinwunmi J, Scaravilli F, et al. Transcranial surgery for pituitary tumors performed by Sir Victor Horsley. *Neurosurgery* 2003;52:914–925; discussion 925–916.

2. Landolt AM. History of pituitary surgery from the technical aspect. *Neurosurg. Clin. North Am.* 2001;12:37–44, vii–viii.

3. Cohen-Gadol AA, Liu JK, Laws ER, Jr. Cushing's first case of transsphenoidal surgery: the launch of the pituitary surgery era. *J. Neurosurg.* 2005;103:570–574.

4. Liu JK, Das K, Weiss MH, et al. The history and evolution of transsphenoidal surgery. *J. Neurosurg.* 2001;95:1083–1096.

5. Couldwell WT, Weiss MH, Rabb C, et al. Variations on the standard transsphenoidal approach to the sellar region, with emphasis on the

extended approaches and parasellar approaches: surgical experience in 105 cases. *Neurosurgery* 2004;55:539–547; discussion 547–550.

6. Cappabianca P, Alfieri A, de Divitiis E. Endoscopic endonasal transsphenoidal approach to the sella: towards functional endoscopic pituitary surgery (FEPS). *Minim. Invasive Neurosurg.* 1998;41:66–73.

7. Jho HD, Carrau RL, Ko Y, et al. Endoscopic pituitary surgery: an early experience. *Surg. Neurol.* 1997;47:213–222; discussion 222–213.

8. Saito K, Kuwayama A, Yamamoto N, et al. The transsphenoidal removal of nonfunctioning pituitary adenomas with suprasellar extensions: the open sella method and intentionally staged operation. *Neurosurgery* 1995;36:668–675; discussion 675–666.

9. Chakrabarti I, Amar AP, Couldwell W, et al. Long-term neurological, visual, and endocrine outcomes following transnasal resection of craniopharyngioma. *J. Neurosurg.* 2005;102:650–657.

10. Ciric I, Ragin A, Baumgartner C, et al. Complications of transsphenoidal surgery: results of a national survey, review of the literature, and personal experience. *Neurosurgery* 1997;40:225–236; discussion 236–227.

11. Couldwell WT. Transsphenoidal and transcranial surgery for pituitary adenomas. *J. Neurooncol.* 2004;69:237–256.

12. Alleyne CH, Jr., Barrow DL, Oyesiku NM. Combined transsphenoidal and pterional craniotomy approach to giant pituitary tumors. *Surg. Neurol.* 2002;57:380–390; discussion 390.

13. Mortini P, Losa M, Barzaghi R, et al. Results of transsphenoidal surgery in a large series of patients with pituitary adenoma. *Neurosurgery* 2005;56:1222–1233; discussion 1233.

14. Turner HE, Stratton IM, Byrne JV, et al. Audit of selected patients with nonfunctioning pituitary adenomas treated without irradiation – a follow-up study. *Clin. Endocrinol. (Oxf.)* 1999;51:281–284.

15. Ebersold MJ, Quast LM, Laws ER, Jr., et al. Long-term results in transsphenoidal removal of nonfunctioning pituitary adenomas. *J. Neurosurg.* 1986;64:713–719.

16. Laws ER, Reitmeyer M, Thapar K, et al. Cushing's disease resulting from pituitary corticotrophic microadenoma. Treatment results from transsphenoidal microsurgery and gamma knife radiosurgery. *Neurochirurgie* 2002;48:294–299.

17. Sheehan JM, Lopes MB, Sheehan JP, et al. Results of transsphenoidal surgery for Cushing's disease in patients with no histologically confirmed tumor. *Neurosurgery* 2000;47:33–36; discussion 37–39.

18. Chee GH, Mathias DB, James RA, et al. Transsphenoidal pituitary surgery in Cushing's disease: can we predict outcome? *Clin. Endocrinol. (Oxf.)* 2001;54:617–626.

19. Yap LB, Turner HE, Adams CB, et al. Undetectable postoperative cortisol does not always predict long–term remission in Cushing's disease: a single centre audit. *Clin. Endocrinol. (Oxf.)* 2002;56:25–31.

20. Krieger MD, Couldwell WT, Weiss MH. Assessment of long-term remission of acromegaly following surgery. *J. Neurosurg.* 2003;98:719–724.

21. Wass J. Debulking of pituitary adenomas improves hormonal control of acromegaly by somatostatin analogues. *Eur. J. Endocrinol.* 2005;152:693–694.

22. Couldwell WT, Weiss MH. Medical and surgical management of microprolactinoma. *Pituitary* 2004;7:31–32.

23. Turner HE, Adams CB, Wass JA. Trans-sphenoidal surgery for microprolactinoma: an acceptable alternative to dopamine agonists? *Eur. J. Endocrinol.* 1999;140:43–47.

24. Semple PL, Webb MK, de Villiers JC, et al. Pituitary apoplexy. *Neurosurgery* 2005;56:65–72; discussion 72–63.

25. Randeva HS, Schoebel J, Byrne J, et al. Classical pituitary apoplexy: clinical features, management and outcome. *Clin. Endocrinol. (Oxf.)* 1999;51:181–188.

26. Sandeman D, Moufid A. Interactive image-guided pituitary surgery. An experience of 101 procedures. *Neurochirurgie* 1998;44:331–338.

27. Jane JA, Jr., Thapar K, Alden TD, et al. Fluoroscopic frameless stereotaxy for transsphenoidal surgery. *Neurosurgery* 2001;48:1302–1307; discussion 1307–1308.

28. Fahlbusch R, Keller B, Ganslandt O, et al. Transsphenoidal surgery in acromegaly investigated by intraoperative high-field magnetic resonance imaging. *Eur. J. Endocrinol.* 2005;153:239–248.

29. Martin CH, Schwartz R, Jolesz F, et al. Transsphenoidal resection of pituitary adenomas in an intraoperative MRI unit. *Pituitary* 1999;2:155–162.

28   Pituitary Radiotherapy

P. Nicholas Plowman

Key points

- Conventionally fractionated radiotherapy remains a useful means of tumor control as well as less frequently controling excessive hormone secretion.
- Focal radiotherapy has been made more possible with the advent of modern MRI imaging.
- Gamma Knife is the best focal radiation technique. Data are needed that show long-term results when compared to conventional irradiation of patients with similar tumors.
- Complications of radiotherapy include visual impairment, late hypopituitarism and radiation oncogenesis.

Radiotherapy today

Introduction

Whilst pituitary radiotherapy remains a highly effective means of durably controlling pituitary adenomas – either in the postoperative setting or primarily for intrafossa tumors – its routine use has reduced in the last decade. Modern surgical series, with almost all cases being operated via the transsphenoidal route, have produced surgical results demonstrating lower numbers of subsequent relapses than had previously been reported; this has impacted on the routine administration of radiotherapy in the postoperative setting.

Prolactinomas

For prolactinomas, the recurrence rate following transsphenoidal surgery has been estimated in some recent series [1] to be approximately 13% at 10 years, with remission assessed by normalization of prolactin (PRL) levels in 87% of patients with microprolactinomas; the pituitary function is preserved in the majority of cases. Whilst these results are superior to some others in terms of low relapse rate, they nevertheless have set the trend towards a lesser routine referral pattern for radiotherapy. Whilst the addition of postoperative radiotherapy might well reduce the recurrence rate well below 5% [2], nevertheless the potential late endocrine sequelae of hypopituitarism following the radiotherapy argue against its routine use – for many patients present with secondary amenorrhea preventing pregnancy and the luteinizing hormone-releasing hormone (LHRH) axis is the most vulnerable after radiation therapy. With adroit use of dopamine agonist

therapy, we now select patients: those with larger tumors and inferior response patterns to dopamine agonists for radiation therapy, or those who want definitive control without long-term commitment to dopamine agonist therapy.

Acromegaly

For acromegaly, transsphenoidal surgery is highly effective in considerably reducing tumor mass and substantially lowering mean growth hormone (GH) levels in the majority of patients, although a surgical cure is rare. Previous considerations for "cure" of acromegaly (mean serum GH, basally or after glucose, of less than 5, 10 or even 20 mU/L [2.5 ng/mL, 5 ng/mL, 10 ng/mL respectively]) have become more strict in the last years, establishing a therapeutic aim for a serum GH below 5 mU/L (<2.5 ng/mL), as residual mean GH levels above 5 mU/L (2.5 ng/mL) were still associated with elevated mortality [3]. More recent consensus has adopted a nadir level of GH less than 2 mU/L (1 ng/mL) [and even 1 mU/L (0.5 ng/mL)] after an oral glucose tolerance test with age-adjusted normalization of the insulin-like growth factor-1 (IGF-1) level [4–6]. Most series report a fall in mean serum GH to less than 5 mU/L (2.5 ng/ml) in approximately 40–60% of all acromegalic patients treated surgically, but this "cure" rate rises to 65% for microadenomas [7, 8]. More recent surgical series [using strict criteria for cure: normalization of IGF-1 levels, random GH <5 mU/L (2.5 ng/mL) and <2 mU/L (1 ng/mL) during oral glucose tolerance test (OGTT)] report improved results with cure rate of 65% for macroadenomas and of 88% for microadenomas, and there is no doubt that when presented with small, discrete somatotroph adenomas, modern surgery can produce excellent results [1, 9]. Hypopituitarism occurs in approximately 25% of such patients.

    External beam radiotherapy has also been used extensively in the treatment of acromegaly and, although it induces a fall in mean serum GH, this may take several years to become fully effective. In our own early series studying 80 patients with advanced disease and very high GH levels at time of conventional radiotherapy,

---

Clinical Endocrine Oncology, 2nd edition. Edited by Ian D. Hay and John A.H. Wass. © 2008 Blackwell Publishing. ISBN 978-1-4051-4584-8.

treated with 45 Gy via a three-field technique, the response rate at 10 years was approximately 70–80%, with levels below 10 mU/L (5 ng/mL) in 90% of patients at this time [10]. In addition, normal pituitary function may be compromised. At 6 years we found that 25% of patients who did not require replacement therapy beforehand now needed some form of therapy, including gonadal steroids (11%), thyroxine (8%) or hydrocortisone (16%). Of course, the series just cited were from an age when patients presented late and surgery was inferior; the current question relates to how "standard" should postoperative radiotherapy be? The answer is not easy and has to balance the quest for normalization of GH levels using the modern criteria outlined above versus the procedure of radiotherapy and its potential sequelae. What is certain is that, used selectively radiotherapy is a safe and powerful tool in acromegaly.

Cushing disease

With Cushing disease, the tumors are usually small and in the best centers immediate "endocrine cure" rates of 75–80% after transsphenoidal surgery are reported [11, 12], although a true cure rate of around 50% is produced when strict criteria are used. In a larger US series including 640 adrenocorticotropic hormone (ACTH)-secreting pituitary adenomas, Laws and Jane [1] achieved remission in 91% of microadenomas but only in 65% for macroadenomas with a recurrence of 12% at 10 years in adults (and higher, of 42% in children). As the normal corticotrophs undergo long-term suppression (histologically demonstrable as Crooke's cell changes), serum cortisol postoperatively should be extremely low and patients will require long-term corticosteroid cover until their own pituitary–adrenal axis recovers. Recurrence appears to be uncommon (3–5%) when patients are "endocrinologically" cured but long-term follow-up is essential.

Where attempted microadenomectomy has not led to a cure, the alternatives are either to re-explore the fossa and perform a total hypophysectomy or to irradiate the pituitary tumor. Radiotherapy of ACTH-secreting tumors, as in the case of other hormonally active pituitary tumors, leads to a gradual fall in ACTH levels over several years and a decrease in requirements for medical therapy [13]. In our series of 22 patients treated with radiotherapy and medical therapy alone, 60% were cured 1–12 years after irradiation, in so far as they have been able to stop all medical treatment [14, 15]. It is particularly efficacious in children [16], where surgery may be hazardous or very difficult, and in whom life-time tumor control implies seven decades of freedom from recurrence.

Non-functioning tumors

Regarding functionless tumors, a number of surveys in the 1990s demonstrated significant recurrence rates, even in those tumors thought to have been completely removed, of the order of 50% at 10 years [17, 18], whereas Laws and Jane [1] reported better results with 16% recurrence at 10 years (but only 6% requiring reoperation), with 83% of patients alive and without evidence of disease. With these data in mind, and having modern magnetic resonance imaging (MRI) scanning facilities at our disposal for annual follow-up, our own postoperative radiation strategy has therefore changed.

For those presenting with the larger tumors, it remains our own policy to recommend external beam radiotherapy in the great majority of patients following surgery, accepting that there will be a gradual increase in hypopituitarism in those patients. Of course, other factors need to be taken into account, such as the age of the patient and presence of pre-existing hormone defects, but generally, by adhering to this policy the rate of recurrence has been less than 5% at 10 years.

In line with other clinicians, our strategy for patients presenting with smaller functionless tumors is less proactive in terms of radiotherapy than 10 years ago. For more patients than previously, we are adopting a "wait and watch" policy for those patients with smaller macroadenomas and those whose operations are deemed to have radically resected the tumor. Another factor allowing such an expectant policy is the capability to serially MR such patients in follow-up. This allows relapses to be picked up early and it is argued (and is probably true) that such early relapses will be as easily controlled by radiotherapy applied at this time rather than irradiating all patients immediately postoperatively.

Methodology

The foregoing discusses: "Who should receive radiotherapy?"; now comes the equally controversial question: "How should radiation be delivered?"

Conventional radiotherapy technique

Conventionally, patients are treated on a linear accelerator with multiple portals of megavoltage X-rays (usually three/two lateral/temporal portals and one anterosuperior) all aiming at the pituitary tumor. The patient is restrained in a purpose-made head cast/shell and each of the three portals is treated daily, such that only the pituitary fossa receives the full (cross-fire) dose. In this manner radiotherapy is concentrated on the pituitary fossa and, using fractionated regimes over 5 weeks, there is a slowly accumulating radiation dose delivered to the disease – typically 45 Gy in 25 fractions over 5 weeks. Such radiotherapy respects all the known factors that allow sparing damage to normal adjacent nervous system (for the adjacent optic chiasm and hypothalamus in particular are vulnerable to radiation and risk to these structures is minimized if the radiation is delivered in small daily fractions/doses) and yet cumulatively effective with regards to tumor control. In our planning session, where the portals are mapped, we target the preoperative volume for large adenomas (except for large prolactinomas that have medically shrunk back into the fossa) plus 0.5 cm "all round;" in small/intrafossa pituitary adenomas, the bony fossa represents the target volume. This type of conventional radiotherapy has a wealth of data supporting its use, its efficacy, and the long-term durability of disease control. It is therefore difficult to eschew. Developments in delivery include enhanced sophistication of linear accelerators (being able to refine the previous rectangular or square portal shapes into "shaped/conformal" portals, bespoke for an individual's tumor shape via multileaf secondary collimators) and new substitute technology such as the tomotherapy machines may indeed reduce the hypothalamic, chiasmal and other adjacent structure dosage, but the plain fact remains that this type of therapy treats the whole fossa and its environs to a relatively high radiation dose equivalent that is only safe to apply because the treatment is given in multiple small (fractionated) doses over 5 weeks, which the adjacent structures tolerate due to this method of delivery.

Results

With regard to results of conventional radiotherapy, Brada et al. [19] found an actuarial progression-free survival of 94% at 5 years and 88% at 10 years after the routine delivery of postoperative radiotherapy to pituitary adenoma patients. Our own data have demonstrated the slow but progressive and durable decline in the secretory product of functioning adenomas following such therapy: acromegaly [20], Cushing/Nelson [14, 15], and prolactinoma [2]; other endocrine data are reviewed above.

Focal radiation therapy

An alternative concept is based on the premise that pituitary adenomas are benign, discrete tumors and that there is no need to treat any "safety margin" around the tumor's boundary (as is necessary in an infiltrative cancer). The argument goes that with a method of focally delivering a very high dose of radiation directly onto the targeted tumor with the dose diminishing rapidly and isotropically at its borders, then one could deliver an obliterative single high dose with relatively little concern for the radiosensitivity of the adjacent structures because the dose has diminished so much by 3–5 mm from the target's boundary that the other structures will not receive more that their single dose tolerance for radiation. This concept was first pioneered in Boston with protons in the 1970s by Kjellberg and Kliman [21]. These workers reported a series of 234 unoperated acromegalic patients so treated and found a 70% decline in the GH levels by 1 year and continued fall over 10 years. In Cushing disease, and studying 175 treated patients, they found complete cure in 21% and an ability to stop all medical therapy in another 20%. These early proton results may not look so good in the modern era but in those days, when imaging was primitive, they sounded a trumpet for the potential of more focal radiation therapy. With the advent of modern MR imaging, definition of targets has improved greatly, facilitating all forms of focal radiation therapy.

Gamma Knife therapy

Gamma Knife therapy (see Chapter 8) represents the most accurate, focused, photon radiation therapy at present. Although early results for pituitary adenoma were not as good as the conventional therapy results and lacked long-term follow-up, nevertheless, with the advent of newer, MR scan-linked planning, the procedure has acquired an accuracy and sophistication that is currently unrivalled as regards pinpointing dose delivery onto small discrete targets and there are emerging good longer term follow-up results. Using a pinned frame (giving accuracy and reproducibility via

rigidity), and with the technology allowing very fast fall-off of the dose at the margin of the mapped target, it is now a good option for selected pituitary adenomas. Interestingly, Landolt first reported that the secretory hormone product levels fell faster after focal (Gamma Knife) radiation therapy than after conventional, fractionated, radiation therapy for pituitary adenoma [22]. Much controversy has developed as to whether "radiosurgery" is as definitively curative as conventional therapy and as to whether it can substitute. In terms of results, there was 17–83% endocrinological "cure" in 314 patients with Cushing disease from different series, with a mean follow-up of 2 years (review by Laws et al. [23]); this percentage was lower (0–36%) in patients with Nelson syndrome, while tumor growth control rate was 82–100% for a mean follow-up of 3 years. In acromegaly, the endocrine remission rates were 20–96% and cure rates of 0–100% in the pooled analysis, demonstrating the current inability to assess this technique. The current author interprets these data as demonstrating largely poor case selection for Gamma Knife therapy; surgeons practising without good radiotherapy facilities are largely damaging the good potential of the Gamma Knife technique by poor case selection.

The present author believes that Gamma Knife therapy represents the current best focal radiation therapy method and, provided the clinician is sure that the entirety of the tumor is imaged and encompassable, then it represents a very good modality of therapy for pituitary adenoma.

Complications of pituitary radiotherapy

With modern radiation methods and techniques, the once-cited risk of brain (especially temporal lobe) necrosis should be close to zero. The three sequelae for consideration are therefore visual impairment, late hypopituitarism and radiation oncogenesis.

Visual impairment

The optic chiasm has long been known to be a particularly radiosensitive structure, and blindness due to chiasmal damage following radiotherapy to tumors in the pituitary region is well documented. However, such a catastrophic event should nowadays be exceedingly rare as the predisposing factors are better understood.

In those cases that have been described, visual deterioration occurs 2–36 months after radiotherapy (rarely later). It tends to progress over days or weeks. The differential diagnosis includes recurrent tumor, arachnoid adhesions around the chiasm or the empty sella syndrome [24]. MRI has been shown to be the most useful diagnostic investigation, particularly using gadolinium enhancement [25].

The pathologic basis of radiation-induced optic chiasmal damage is though to be vascular damage to the chiasmatic blood supply [26]. It is therefore not surprising that the major factors in the radiation prescription predisposing to such damage are the total dose delivered and the dose per fraction. Whilst employing radiotherapy for pituitary adenoma in a dose range of 42–59 Gy in Boston between 1963 and 1973, Harris and Levene [27] found radiation optic neuropathy in four out of the 55 cases, but none in those in whom the daily dose was less than 2.5 Gy per fraction. Aristizabel and co-workers [28] reviewed 122 patients presenting to their institution over a 20-year period who received pituitary radiotherapy. There were four cases of optic neuropathy; all four occurring within a group of 26 patients who had received more than 46 Gy total dose, and all four had received more than 2 Gy per fraction. Several other reports exactly mirror these observations, that larger daily dose fractions put the optic chiasm at much greater risk [29–32]. Jones [33] reviewed 332 cases of pituitary adenoma receiving megavoltage radiotherapy at St Bartholomew's Hospital, all receiving 45 Gy in 25–26 fractions over 35 days (i.e., daily fractions of 1.7–1.8 cGy). With a minimum follow-up of 10 years for all cases, he found no cases of optic chiasmal damage, although in reviewing the literature from other institutions delivering this prescription he found occasional reports of this complication. It is clear that the higher the daily dose and total dose, the more the chiasm is risked.

Anterior pituitary hormone deficiencies have been well documented following radiotherapy to the head and neck when the hypothalamo–pituitary axis falls within the radiation field. The evidence suggests that the hypothalamus is the site of radiation-induced effects. Studies have demonstrated normal serum GH responses to bolus doses of GH-releasing hormone (GHRH), but subnormal GH responses to arginine or insulin-induced hypoglycemia [34]. There have been delayed but present anterior pituitary hormone responses to gonadotropin-releasing hormone (GnRH) and thyrotropin-releasing hormone (TRH). The observation of late hyperprolactinemia following pituitary radiation is interesting, again attributable to a late radiation effect on the hypothalamus [35].

Late hypopituitarism

The total absorbed dose to the hypothalamo–pituitary axis is the major factor in determining the speed of onset, severity and overall incidence of hypopituitarism [36]. Furthermore, the overall incidence of hypopituitarism increases with time after radiation. As expected, the radiation fraction size is another important factor (i.e., the number of treatments in which any total radiation dose is delivered, small numbers of large fractions being proportionately more harmful for any late-responding normal tissue). Thus the Manchester group demonstrated that an increased radiation fraction size and a short treatment course were likely to increase the risk of hypopituitarism for any total radiation dose [37].

The GH axis is most sensitive to these effects of radiation. In conventionally fractionated radiotherapy to children, after a total dose of 27 Gy or more, the serum GH responses to provocative stimuli are blunted. After 24 Gy the serum GH responses to provocative stimuli are often normal but spontaneous secretion of GH is decreased. After 18 Gy there is demonstrable and subtle disturbance of the normal pattern of pulsatile GH secretion, in particular a disturbed GH increase at puberty [38].

Prospective studies in irradiated adult pituitary adenoma patients suggest that following GH deficiency, a deficiency of either gonadotropins or corticotropin is next most likely to occur, and that the TRH–thyroid-stimulating-hormone axis is least likely to be affected. Diabetes insipidus is extremely unusual. The reasons for this "rank order" of radiosensitivity are unknown, but it is interesting that progressive hypopituitarism, often with a non-related pituitary tumor, occurs in the same order.

Lastly, the overall incidence of subsequent hypopituitarism is greater if pituitary function is very abnormal before radiotherapy is delivered, either as a result of the tumor alone or due to both tumor and surgical influences.

All these facts temper the acceptance of exact percentage statistics on the incidence of postradiation hypopituitarism. However, after the application of the St Bartholomew's Hospital radiation prescription to a series of acromegalic patients, 25% of the patients required new endocrine replacement therapy by 5 years after radiotherapy, and the incidence rose further in the next 5-year period [39]. Gonadotropin deficiency occurred before hypoadrenalism, with hypothyroidism being the least common. Feek and colleagues [40] reported that by 10 years after radiotherapy, 47% of patients were hypogonadal, 30% hypoadrenal and 16% hypothyroid. These incidences rose to 70%, 54% and 38%, respectively, when surgery had preceded radiotherapy.

Radiation oncogenesis

Over the last 40 years, instances of sellar fibrosarcoma, osteogenic sarcoma, meningioma and glioma have been reported as anecdotal case reports, illustrating that second tumors can arise in or around the pituitary fossa in the late follow-up of irradiated pituitary tumors. Jones [33] reviewed the world literature on this subject, also researching the incidence of second intracranial tumors in non-irradiated pituitary tumor patients. In the period from 1959 to 1992 there were 30 case reports of parasellar fibrosarcoma following 2–27 years after irradiation and none reported in non-irradiated cases. There were 16 cases of meningioma reported from 1970 to 1992, with latencies of 8–32 cases (median 20 years), but also noteworthy was the incidence of 19 cases of meningioma in non-irradiated pituitary patients. Similarly, from 1983 to 1992 there were 18 cases of glioma reported in a series of irradiated pituitary patients (with a median latency of 9 years), but nine cases of glioma were reported in non-irradiated pituitary patients. From the above data, there are no figures to suggest the denominator (i.e., the total population of irradiated and non-irradiated patients) for these results, from which the risk/incidence could be calculated.

Jones [33] reviewed a personal series of 332 consecutive, irradiated pituitary adenoma patients 7–27 years (median 11 years) postradiation. No case of fibrosarcoma was encountered. There was one case of glioma, but also one in a parallel non-irradiated pituitary adenoma patient. There was no case of meningioma, although there was one meningioma, synchronous with a pituitary adenoma, occurring in a non-irradiated patient. There was one case of nasoethmoidal primitive neuroectodermal tumor. Statistical advice was that for these small index numbers, comparison with general population statistics would be inappropriate.

Brada and colleagues [41] studied 334 pituitary adenoma patients irradiated in the period 1962–1986. They observed five cases of second tumor (two gliomas, two meningiomas, one meningeal sarcoma) and compared this incidence with the population rates in the South Thames region, and concluded that there was a risk of 1.9% for a second tumor by 20 years after radiotherapy. Whether it is relevant to use normal population rates as a comparison is open to question. Bliss and colleagues [42] reviewed the follow-up of 296 irradiated pituitary adenoma patients from Edinburgh (treated 1962) and found only one malignant brain tumor and one meningioma. They concluded no excess risk.

In conclusion, it is possible that there is a risk of second tumor induction with pituitary irradiation and of parasellar fibrosarcoma with high-dose radiation, but whether the true incidence of this late complication is as high as one in 100 is not yet certain.

References

1. Laws ER, Jane JA Jr. Neurosurgical approach to treating pituitary adenomas. *Growth Horm. IGF Res.* 2005;15:S36–41.
2. Tsagarakis S, Grossman AB, Plowman PN, et al. Megavoltage radiotheraopy in the mangement of prolactinomas: long term follow up. *Clin. Endocrinol.* 1991;34:399–406.
3. Bates AS, Van't Hoff W, Jones JM, Clayton RN. An audit of outcome of treatment in acromegaly. *Q.J. Med.* 1993;86:293–300.
4. Giustina A, Barkan A, Casanueva FF, et al. Criteria for cure of acromegaly: a consensus statement. *J. Clin. Endocrinol. Metab.* 2000;85:526–529.
5. Swearingen B, Barker FG, Katznelson L, et al. Long-term mortality after transsphenoidal surgery and adjunctive therapy for acromegaly. *J. Clin. Endocrinol. Metab.* 1998;83:3419–3426.
6. Melmed S, Casanueva F, Cavagnini F, et al. Consensus statement: medical management of acromegaly. *Clin. Endocrinol.* 2005;153:737–740.
7. Wass JAH, Laws ER, Randall RV, Sheline GE. The treatment of acromegaly. *Clin. Endocrinol. Metab.* 1986;15:683–707.
8. Nabarro JDN. Acromegaly. *Clin. Endocrinol.* 1987;26:481–512.
9. Kreutzer J, Vance ML, Lopes MBS, Laws ER. Surgical management of GH-secreting pituitary adenomas: an outcome study using modern remission criteria. *J. Clin. Endocrinol. Metab.* 2001;86:4072–4077.
10. Wass JAH, Plowman PN, Jones AE, Besser GM. The treatment of acromegaly by external pituitary irradiation and drugs. In Tolis G (ed.). *Growth Hormone, Growth Factors and Acromegaly.* New York: Raven Press, 1987:199–206.
11. Fahlbusch R, Buchfelder M, Muller OA. Transsphenoidal surgery for Cushing's disease. *J. R. Soc. Med.* 1986;79:262–269.
12. Swearingen B, Biller BMK, Barker FG, et al. Long-term mortality after transsphenoidal surgery for Cushing's disease. *Ann. Intern. Med.* 1999;130:821–824.
13. Estrada J, Boronat M, Mielgo M, et al. The long–term outcome of pituitary irradiation after unsuccessful transsphenoidal surgery for Cushing's disease. *N. Engl. J. Med.* 1997;336:172–177.
14. Howlett TA, Plowman PN, Wass JA, et al. Megavoltage pituitary irradiation in the management of Cushing's disease and Nelson's syndrome: long term follow up. *Clin. Endocrinol.* 1989;31:309–323.
15. Jenkins PJ, Trainer PJ, Plowman PN, et al. The role of prophylactic pituitary radiotherapy in the long term outcome after adrenalectomy for Cushing's disease. *J. Clin. Endocrinol. Metab.* 1994;79:165–171.
16. Storr HL, Plowman PN, Carroll PV, et al. Clinical and endocrine responses to pituitary radiotherapy in pediatric Cushing's disease: an effective second line treatment. *J. Clin. Endocrinol. Metab.* 2003;88(1):34–37.
17. Gittoes NJL, Bates AS, Tse W, et al. Radiotherapy for non–functioning pituitary tumours. *Clin. Endocrinol.* 1998;48:331–337.
18. Turner HE, Stratton IM, Byrne JV, Adams CBT, Wass JAH. Audit of selected patients with nonfunctioning pituitary adenomas treated without irradiation – a follow-up study. *Clin. Endocrinol.* 1999;51:281–284.
19. Brada M, Rajan B, Traish D, et al. The long-term efficacy of conservative surgery and radiotherapy in the control of pituitary adenomas. *Clin. Endocrinol.* 1993;38:571–578.
20. Cicarelli EC, Orsello SM, Plowman PN, et al. Prolonged lowering of growth hormone after radiotherapy in acromegalic patients followed after 15 years. Advances in the biosciences. In Landholt AM, Heitz PU, Zapf J, Girav del Pozo J (eds). *Advances in the Biosciences.* Oxford: Pergamon Press, 1988:69, 269–272.
21. Kjellberg RN, Kliman B. Life time effectiveness: a system of therapy for pituitary adenomas, emphasisng Bragg peak proton hypophysectomy. In Linfoot JA (ed.). *Recent Advances in the Diagnosis and Treatment of Pituitary Tumors.* New York: Raven Press, 1979:269–286.
22. Landolt AM, Haller D, Lomax N, et al. Stereotactic radiosurgery for recurrent surgically treated acromegaly: a comparison with fractionated radiotherapy. *J. Neurosurg.* 1998;88:1002–1008.
23. Laws ER, Sheehan JP, Sheehan JM, et al. Stereotactic radiosurgery for pituitary adenomas: a review of the literature. *J. Neuro-Oncol.* 2004;69:257–272.
24. Kaufman B, Tomsak RL, Kaufman BA, et al. Herniation of the suprasellar visual system and third ventricle into empty sellae: morphologic and clinical considerations. *Am. J. Neuroradiol.* 1989;10:65–76.
25. Guy J, Mancuso A, Beck B, et al. Radiation induced optic neuropathy: a magnetic resonance imaging study. *J. Neurosurg.* 1991;74:426–432.
26. Hudgins PA, Newman NJ, Dillon WP, et al. Radiation–induced optic neuropathy. Characteristic appearances on gadolinium-enhanced MR. *Am. J. Neuroradiol.* 1989;13:235–238.
27. Harris JR, Levene MB. Visual complications following irradiation for pituitary adenomas and craniopharyngiomas. *Radiology* 1976;120:167–171.
28. Aristizabal S, Caldwell WL, Avila J. The relationship of time–dose fractionation factors to complications in the treatment of pituitary tumours by irradiation. *Int. J. Radiat. Oncol. Biol. Phys.* 1977;2:667–673.
29. Atkinson AB, Allen IV, Gordon DS, et al. Progressive visual failure in acromegaly following external pituitary irradiation. *Clin. Endocrinol.* 1979;10:469–479.
30. Sheline GE. Role of conventional radiotherapy in treatment of functional pituitary tumours. In Linfoot JA (ed.). *Recent Advances in the Diagnosis and Treatment of Pituitary Tumors.* New York: Raven Press, 1979:289–313.
31. Hammer HM. Optic chiasmal radionecrosis. *Trans. Ophthalmol. Soc. UK* 1983;103:208–211.

32. MacLeod AF, Clark DG, Pambakian H, et al. Treatment of acromegaly by external irradiation. *Clin. Endocrinol.* 1989;30:303–314.

33. Jones AJ. Radiation oncogenesis in relation to the treatment of pituitary tumours. *Clin. Endocrinol.* 1991;35:379–397.

34. Blacklay A, Grossman A, Savage M, et al. Cranial irradiation in children with cerebral tumours – evidence for a hypothalamic defect in growth hormone release. *J. Endocrinol.* 1986;108:25–29.

35. Ciccarelli E, Corselllo SM, Plowman PN, et al. Long term effects of radiotherapy for acromegaly on circulating prolactin levels. *Acta Endocrinol.* 1989;121:827–832.

36. Littley MD, Shalet SM, Beardwell CG, et al. Radiation induced hypopituitarism is dose dependent. *Clin. Endocrinol.* 1989;31:363–373.

37. Littley MD, Shalet SM, Beardwell CG, et al. Hypopituitarism following external radiotherapy for pituitary tumours in adults. *Q. J. Med.* 1989;70:145–160.

38. Shalet SM. Radiation and pituitary dysfunction. *N. Engl. J. Med.* 1993;328:131–133.

39. Wass JAH, Plowman PN, Jones AE, Besser GM. The treatment of acromegaly by external pituitary irradiation and drugs. In *International Symposium: Challenges in Hypersecretion: Human Growth Hormone.* New York: Raven Press, 1985.

40. Feek GCM, McLelland J, Seth S, et al. How effective is external pituitary irradiation for growth hormone secreting pituitary tumours? *Clin. Endocrinol.* 1984;20:401–408.

41. Brada A, Ford D, Ashley S, et al. Risk of second brain tumour after conservative surgery and radiotherapy for pituitary adenoma. *Br. Med J.* 1992;304:1343–1346.

42. Bliss P, Kerr GR, Gregor A. Incidence of second brain tumours after pituitary irradiation in Edinburgh 1962–1990. *Clin. Oncol.* 1994;6:36.

29 Prolactinomas

Mary P. Gillam and Mark E. Molitch

Key points

- Prolactinomas are the most common type of pituitary adenoma.
- Laboratory artifacts such as the presence of macroprolactinemia and the "hook effect" can confound the interpretation of prolactin levels.
- The first line of treatment for most prolactinomas is dopamine agonist therapy.
- Prolactinomas that are resistant to medical therapy may require multimodal therapies, including transsphenoidal surgery and/or radiotherapy.
- Pregnancy is a condition that may lead to growth of macroprolactinomas, and requires special monitoring.

Epidemiology

Prolactinomas are the most frequent pituitary tumors. Although older studies report the prevalence of prolactinomas at 100 cases per million adults, recent studies have determined that the prevalence may be up to seven-fold higher than previously estimated [1]. Between the ages of 20 and 50 years, the incidence of prolactinomas is greater in women than in men (10:1). Beyond the age of 50 and in autopsy series, sex-related differences in the prevalence of these tumors are not observed. Microprolactinomas occur more commonly in women, whereas macroprolactinomas occur in equal numbers of women and men. The greater prevalence of microprolactinomas in younger women may reflect the fact that mild hyperprolactinemia results in more apparent clinical consequences in women than in men. However, it is uncertain whether gender-specfic differences in the biological behavior of these tumors also exist. Overall, prolactinomas represent approximately 40–50% of pituitary tumors that come to clinical attention or that are detected in autopsy series. The vast majority of prolactinomas are benign, with fewer than 100 cases of malignant prolactinomas having been reported. Most prolactinomas are sporadic, but familial cases of prolactinomas may occur, usually in association with multiple endocrine neoplasia type 1 or pituitary adenoma predisposition [1].

Pathogenesis

Similar to other subtypes of pituitary adenomas, prolactinomas are monoclonal neoplasms that arise from a single transformed cell

(lactotroph). Candidate genetic alterations involved in the genesis and progression of prolactinomas include the loss of tumor suppressor genes, overexpression of oncogenes, and abnormal expression of proteins that maintain chromosome stability. Alterations in hypothalamic/pituitary growth factors, their receptors, and/or their signaling pathways have also been identified, some of which may play important roles in cellular transformation or clonal expansion. Nonetheless, the extent to which some of these alterations are pathogenetic, contribute to tumor progression, or represent secondary effects that accompany the transformation process, remains an unresolved issue [2]. (See also Chapter 23 for further information.)

Clinical manifestations of prolactinomas

Prolactinomas cause gonadal and sexual dysfunction related to hyperprolactinemia and in larger tumors, may cause neurological symptoms related to tumor expansion [3].

The hallmark symptoms of hyperprolactinemia include amenorrhea (94%) and galactorrhea (up to 85%). Non-puerperal galactorrhea may occur in 5–10% of normally menstruating, normoprolactinemic women, and therefore is suggestive, but not definitive, of hyperprolactinemia. However, when amenorrhea or oligoamenorrhea is associated with galactorrhea, ~75% of these women will have evidence of hyperprolactinemia. Galactorrhea is reported in ~10% of cases in men, and is virtually pathognomonic of a prolactinoma.

Hyperprolactinemia inhibits the pulsatile secretion of gonadotropin-releasing hormone (GnRH), alters the pattern of release of luteinizing hormone (LH) and follicle-stimulating hormone (FSH), and suppresses gonadal steroidogenesis. In women, hyperprolactinemia impairs the positive estrogen feedback effect on gonadotropin secretion and abolishes the ovulatory surge of

Clinical Endocrine Oncology, 2nd edition. Edited by Ian D. Hay and John A.H. Wass. © 2008 Blackwell Publishing. ISBN 978-1-4051-4584-8.

LH. High concentrations of prolactin (PRL) also directly inhibit ovarian production of progesterone and estrogen. Collectively, these hormonal changes result in hypogonadism. In women, hyperprolactinemia usually causes secondary amenorrhea, but it may be associated with primary amenorrhea if the disorder begins before the usual age of puberty. Adolescents with primary amenorrhea due to hyperprolactinemia may present with estrogen deficiency and failure to develop normal secondary sexual characteristics. For unknown reasons, adolescents have a disproportionately high frequency of macroadenomas.

Infertility, which occurs when gonadotropin levels are suppressed with anovulation, may be a presenting feature of some women with prolactinomas. Reduced libido and orgasmic dysfunction are found in most hyperprolactinemic/amenorrheic women; treatment that normalizes PRL levels generally restores normal libido and sexual function.

In men, testosterone levels fall below or into the lower part of the normal reference range, and spermatogenesis is impaired. Sperm counts and motility are decreased, and the percentage of abnormal forms is increased. If there is sufficient normal pituitary tissue, normalization of hyperprolactinemia usually results in a return of normal testosterone levels. Sperm count, volume, and motility return to normal in approximately 80% of men who achieve normal prolactin and testosterone levels with cabergoline therapy [4]. Elevated PRL levels have been detected in 2–25% of males with impotence in various series but only 1–5% of men with infertility exhibit hyperprolactinemia. Testosterone therapy for the treatment of impotence may only become effective once PRL levels are normalized.

In women, hyperprolactinemia is associated with reduced bone mineral density. Whether this effect is mediated indirectly, through estrogen deficiency, or as a direct effect of the hyperprolactinemia is controversial. Correction of the hyperprolactinemia increases bone mass but does not necessarily normalize bone mineral density scores. Studies of hyperprolactinemic women who are not amenorrheic and/or hypoestrogenemic have shown that their bone mineral density is normal, supporting the premise that it is the estrogen deficiency that mediates the reduction in bone density. A similar, androgen-dependent loss of bone density is found in hyperprolactinemic men.

Large macroadenomas can also cause mass effects. Visual field defects occur with compression of the optic chiasm. Ophthalmoplegias are relatively uncommon, being due to invasion of the cavernous sinus with entrapment of cranial nerves III, IV, V_1, V_2, and VI. Local mass effects may also cause hypopituitarism because of direct compression of other pituitary cell types or as a result of hypothalamic dysfunction/stalk disruption. Extrasellar extension in other directions may very rarely cause temporal lobe epilepsy and hydrocephalus. These large, invasive tumors should be differentiated from true carcinomas; a demonstration of metastases distant from the primary tumor is necessary for the latter diagnosis. Rarely, large macroadenomas function as a "cork" at the base of the skull and substantial tumor shrinkage from dopamine agonist therapy can lead to cerebrospinal fluid leaks.

Diagnostic evaluation

Differential diagnosis

A variety of other conditions may cause hyperprolactinemia and must be considered in evaluating the patient with hyperprolactinemia (Table 29.1). Most are due to decreases in dopamine (the PRL inhibitory factor) resulting in modestly elevated PRL levels (25–150 ng/ml). Medications represent the most frequent cause of non-tumoral hyperprolactinemia, the most common being psychotropic medications such as antipsychotic agents, the tricyclic antidepressants, monoamine oxidase inhibitors, serotonin reuptake inhibitors (very rare) and the antihypertensive medications alpha-methyldopa and verapamil [5].

Hyperprolactinemia occurs in most patients with end-stage renal disease and many with lesser degrees of renal insufficiency; concomitant use of medications known to alter hypothalamic dopamine may further increase PRL levels. Primary hypothyroidism is associated with hyperprolactinemia in 10% of cases.

Table 29.1 Differential diagnosis of hyperprolactinemia

Pituitary disease	Prolactinoma
	Somatomammotropinoma
	Plurihormonal adenomas
	Empty sella syndrome
	Lymphocytic hypophysitis
	Non-secreting pituitary adenomas
Hypothalamic disease	Craniopharyngioma, Rathke's cleft cysts
	Meningioma
	Dysgerminoma
	Infiltrative disorders (sarcoidosis, histiocytosis X)
	Neuraxis irradiation
	Pituitary stalk section
Medications	Phenothiazines
	Haloperidol
	Risperdal
	Molinidone
	Monoamine oxidase inhibitors
	Tricyclic antidepressants
	Serotonin reuptake inhibitor
	Reserpine
	Methyldopa
	Metoclopramide
	Cocaine
	Verapamil
Neurogenic	Chest wall lesions
	Spinal cord lesions
	Breast stimulation
Other	Pregnancy
	Hypothyroidism
	Chronic renal failure
	Cirrhosis
	Pseudocyesis
	Adrenal insufficiency
Idiopathic	

Rarely, cases have been reported of hyperprolactinemia occurring with adrenal insufficiency due to the loss of glucocorticoid-mediated repression of PRL gene transcription. Stimulation of afferent neural pathways by chest wall and cervical cord lesions can rarely cause hyperprolactinemia.

Hyperprolactinemia caused by lesions of the hypothalamus and of the pituitary stalk results from interference with dopamine inhibitory effects on the lactotrophs. PRL levels in this situation are typically less than 150 ng/ml. The recognition of this effect is critical for instituting appropriate therapy, as treatment of large non-secreting tumors is surgery, whereas primary treatment of such a prolactinoma would be a dopamine agonist.

There are two laboratory artifacts that can confound the interpretation of PRL levels. Monomeric PRL has a molecular weight of 23 kDa and constitutes up to 95% of adult serum PRL. Macroprolactin is a large antigen–antibody complex of molecular weight greater than 100 kDa. Because it is confined to the vascular space, macroprolactin is believed to have reduced bioavailability. The frequency of this artifact has likely been underestimated in the past. In fact, in one recent study of 2089 hyperprolactinemia samples, macroprolactin accounted for 453 (22%) of the results [6]. The presence of macroprolactinemia should be suspected when a patient's clinical history and/or radiological imaging are incompatible with the reported PRL level. Gel-filtration chromotography is the gold standard method for excluding this condition, but polyethylene glycol precipitation yields results that correlate reasonably well and is the most practical method available. Whether the presence of macroprolactin should be ascertained in all patients with hyperprolactinemia is controversial. Recent guidelines published by the Pituitary Society recommend assessment for macroprolactin in patients with moderately elevated PRL levels and less typical symptoms, such as headaches or diminished libido [3].

The second laboratory artifact, referred to as the "hook effect," occurs less frequently but is important to consider since a misdiagnosis can potentially lead to unnecessary surgery. The "hook effect" can occur when serum PRL levels are extraordinarily high, as found in patients with giant prolactinomas [7]. A two-site immunoradiometric or chemiluminometric assay may produce falsely lowered PRL levels when PRL levels are extremely high due to the large amount of circulating PRL (the antigen), which then saturates the antibody and precludes sandwich formation. To avoid this dilemma, the PRL level should always be re-measured at 1:100 dilution in patients with macroadenomas who have normal to modestly elevated basal PRL levels. If a "hook effect" is present, then PRL levels in the diluted samples will increase dramatically.

When no specific cause is found, and macroprolactinemia has been excluded, the hyperprolactinemia is designated to be idiopathic. In some cases, prolactinomas may be present that are too small to be detected by MRI. In other cases, the hyperprolactinemia presumably results from hypothalamic regulatory dysfunction. In such patients who are followed long-term, PRL levels normalize in about one-third, rise in 10–15%, and remain stable in the remainder. Only about 10% are found to have microadenomas on repeat imaging.

Evaluation

Patient evaluation consists of a careful history and physical examination, serum blood chemistries, thyroid function tests and a pregnancy test [3]. If these are normal, magnetic resonance imaging (MRI) of the hypothalamic–pituitary area is mandatory to evaluate for a mass lesion [3]. This includes patients with even mild PRL elevations. Because MRI studies may detect incidental lesions (including non-secreting tumors, cysts, infarcts), the finding of a "microprolactinoma" on a scan in a patient with elevated PRL levels may not always be a true positive finding [3]. All patients with macroadenomas should undergo an appropriate evaluation for hypopituitarism. Formal visual field testing should be performed in patients whose tumors abut the optic chiasm on MRI [3].

Treatment

The major objectives of treating patients with prolactinomas are: (1) to suppress excessive PRL secretion so as to ameliorate its clinical consequences such as infertility, sexual dysfunction and osteoporosis; (2) to control tumor mass, thereby relieving visual field defects, cranial nerve dysfunction and (where applicable) hypopituitarism; (3) to preserve or improve residual pituitary function; and (4) to prevent disease recurrence or progression.

Asymptomatic patients with microprolactinomas do not have an absolute indication for treatment of their prolactinomas. Significant growth of untreated microprolactinomas occurs in less than 10% of patients. Thus, the treatment of microadenomas should not be instituted merely to prevent further growth. On the other hand, an untreated prolactinoma should be followed closely to determine if it is among the minority that will enlarge. It is very unlikely for a prolactinoma to grow significantly without an increase in serum PRL levels, although this phenomenon has been reported. Therefore, many patients with microadenomas verified by imaging and regular menses may be monitored with periodic measurement of PRL levels. Some clinicians opt to monitor patients with pituitary MRI every few years to verify the absence of tumor growth. If PRL levels rise or symptoms of mass effects develop (such as headaches), then repeat scanning is indicated. A microadenoma with documented evidence of growth demands therapy for the size change alone, as it may be one of the 7% that will grow to be a macroadenoma.

The presence of a macroadenoma already implies that the particular tumor has a propensity for growth. Moreover, most macroprolactinomas are associated with PRL elevations significant enough to elicit symptoms that normally warrant treatment. Therefore, unless there are specific contraindications, therapy is usually advisable for these tumors. Local or diffuse invasion and compression of adjacent structures, such as the stalk or optic chiasm, are additional indications for therapy.

Other indications for therapy are relative, being due to the hyperprolactinemia itself, and include decreased libido, menstrual dysfunction, galactorrhea, infertility, hirsutism, impotence and premature osteoporosis. Estrogen replacement may be an appropriate option for women to prevent osteoporosis. Series of patients with prolactinomas who are treated with oral contraceptives for hypogonadism have not shown substantial risk for tumor enlargement. Individual case reports of tumor enlargement during estrogen therapy have been documented, but whether tumor enlargement in these cases was related to use of estrogen or reflected the natural progression of these particular tumors is not known. Because of this uncertainty, it is advisable to monitor patients who use oral contraceptives carefully with periodic measurement of PRL levels.

The ability to follow patients closely with PRL levels, MRI scans, and bone mineral density studies and the knowledge of the efficacy of various modes of therapy permit a highly individualized approach to managing patients and choosing an ideal form of therapy. For almost all patients, the preferred treatment modality is a dopamine agonist.

Surgery

The primary indications for surgery include failure of medical therapy, defined as inadequate PRL reduction on high doses of dopamine agonists, tumor enlargement despite the use of a dopamine agonist and, in pregnant women, an expanding prolactinoma associated with unstable visual field deficits that do not respond to dopamine agonists.

The transsphenoidal approach represents the standard type of surgery for microprolactinomas and the overwhelming majority of macroprolactinomas. Craniotomy is reserved for tumors which are inaccessible via the transsphenoidal approach. Giant and invasive prolactinomas cannot be cured by surgery, regardless of the surgical technique employed or experience of the neurosurgeon; therefore, if undertaken, the goal of surgery under these circumstances is to debulk with the prospect of improving symptoms related to mass effects. With respect to the standard transsphenoidal approach, preliminary studies suggest that complication rates of the endonasal endoscopic approach may be comparable to, or perhaps slightly lower than, those observed using the traditional operating microscope.

Surgical outcomes are highly dependent upon the expertise and experience of the neurosurgeon, as well as the size of the tumor. Surgical results from 50 published series have been summarized recently [8]. Combining data from all 50 series, 1596/2137 (75%) microadenomas and 755/2226 (34%) macroadenomas were classified as achieving initial surgical remission, i.e., having PRL levels normalized within 1–12 weeks following surgery. Among these series the surgical success rates were highly variable. For macroadenomas, the success rate in large part was dependent on the size of tumors chosen for surgery. In many series, the objective was, appropriately, debulking of a very large tumor

rather than cure and in other series very large tumors were not operated upon.

Data available from the 50 series referred to above show that recurrence rates for microadenomas (147/809 = 18%) and macroadenomas (106/465 = 23%) are similar [8]. Recurrence is most often detected biochemically (hyperprolactinemia), and not necessarily with radiographic documentation of tumor regrowth. Recurrence of the hyperprolactinemia is usually accompanied by sexual/reproductive dysfunction, which thereby serves as an indication for medical therapy to reduce PRL hypersecretion. Overall long-term surgical cure rates, based on the initial remission and recurrence rates cited above, are 61% for those with microadenomas and 26% for macroadenomas. For patients with giant prolactinomas and those with considerable cavernous sinus invasion, the chance for surgical cure is essentially zero.

Complications from transsphenoidal surgery for microadenomas are infrequent, the mortality rate being at most 0.6%, the major morbidity rate being about 3.4% (visual loss 0.1%, stroke/vascular injury 0.2%, meningitis/abscess 0.1% and oculomotor palsy 0.1%) and cerebrospinal fluid (CSF) rhinorrhea occurring in 1.9%. The mortality rate for transsphenoidal surgery for all types of secreting and non-secreting macroadenomas is 0.9%, the major morbidity rate is 6.5% (visual loss 1.5%, stroke/vascular injury 0.6%, meningitis/abscess 0.5% and oculomotor palsy 0.6%), and rate of CSF rhinorrhea is 3.3%. Transient diabetes insipidus is quite common with transsphenoidal surgery for both micro- and macroadenomas and permanent diabetes insipidus occurs in about 1% of surgeries on macroadenomas. Hypopituitarism occurs in greater than 50% of patients with macroadenomas prior to surgery as a result of mass effects. Following surgery, either further worsening or improvement may occur. Surgery involving craniotomy is much more hazardous. Although visual field defects and reduction in visual acuity can be improved in 74% of patients whose macroadenomas abut the optic chiasm, a small number of patients with normal visual fields may have a reduction of vision after surgery due to herniation of the chiasm into an empty sella, direct injury or devascularization of the optic apparatus, fracture of the orbit, postoperative hematoma, or cerebral vasospasm.

Radiotherapy

In most cases, radiotherapy is used after failed transsphenoidal surgery and medical therapy. Approximately 250 patients have been reported who have undergone treatment with conventional radiotherapy alone or after failure of medical and/or surgical therapy, with an overall normalization rate for the entire series of 34% [8]. However, in these patients normal PRL levels were achieved only after many years. Almost 300 patients have been reported who have undergone treatment with single-dose stereotactic radiotherapy alone, or after failure of medical and/or surgical therapy, with an overall normalization rate for the entire series of 31.4% [8]. Only one study reported the outcomes of patients treated with single dose stereotactic radiotherapy as primary therapy for prolactinomas; in this study, the rate of PRL normalization rate was 21% after a median of 2 years [9].

Pituitary adenomas with significant suprasellar extension or those with less than 5 mm clearance between the tumor margin and the optic apparatus are poor candidates for single-dose radiotherapy. On the other hand, tumors with cavernous sinus invasion may be good candidates for single dose radiotherapy, as the cranial nerves in the cavernous sinus are relatively radio-resistant. Fractionated radiotherapy is also preferable to single dose radiotherapy when the tumor volume is so large (>3 cm) that an effective radiation dose cannot be safely delivered in a single session.

The most frequent long-term morbidity of conventional radiotherapy is radiation-induced hypopituitarism, with a cumulative actuarial risk of approximately 50% at 10–20 years. Hypopituitarism is likely secondary to hypothalamic and pituitary damage, although the former is considered of primary importance. In addition, the standardized mortality rate is higher in patients with hypopituitarism that had been treated with radiotherapy for pituitary tumors compared with those who had not received radiotherapy, due primarily to a significant increase in cerebrovascular disease [10]. Additional complications that occur years after radiotherapy include cerebrovascular accidents, optic nerve damage, neurologic dysfunction, and secondary radiation-induced intracranial malignancies.

Following single dose radiotherapy, hypopituitarism appears to occur at rates similar to those for conventional radiotherapy [8]. Cranial neuropathies may occur but are usually transient and radiation necrosis of surrounding brain tissue is very rare. With limited follow-up, there have been no cases of secondary intracranial malignancies reported yet.

Medical therapy

The compounds used in clinical practice to treat prolactinomas are all dopamine agonists. Bromocriptine, pergolide and cabergoline are all ergot derivatives but quinagolide is not. Dopamine agonists inhibit prolactin synthesis and secretion by binding to and activating dopamine D_2 receptors on pituitary lactotrophs. Dopamine agonist treatment causes an involution of the endoplasmic reticulum and Golgi apparatus leading to reduction in the size of individual lactotrophs and also causes perivascular fibrosis and cell necrosis [11, 12]. The issue as to whether dopamine agonists induce apoptosis in lactotrophs is controversial.

Responsiveness to dopamine agonists ranges from complete response at one end of the spectrum to total resistance at the other [11]. In addition, individual prolactinomas may respond variably, such that tumors that respond poorly or incompletely to one dopamine agonist may respond well to another. The concept of dopamine agonist resistance should be distinguished from dopamine agonist intolerance, in which adverse effects of the medication prevent the achievement of an effective response [11].

The molecular mechanisms underlying dopamine agonist resistance are genetically heterogeneous and complex; in some cases, resistance is associated with a reduction in D_2 receptor density on tumorous cells [11].

Bromocriptine

Bromocriptine was the first dopamine agonist introduced into clinical practice. It has a relatively short elimination half-life, so that it is usually taken two or three times daily, although once daily may be effective in some patients. Generally, the therapeutic doses are in the range of 2.5–15 mg/day and most patients are successfully treated with 7.5 mg or less. For microprolactinomas, bromocriptine normalizes serum PRL levels, restores gonadal function, and reduces tumor volume in 80–90% of patients. For macroprolactinomas, bromocriptine normalizes serum PRL levels and reduces tumor volume in about 70% of patients even when given at low doses [8, 12]. Although prolactinomas usually remain sensitive to bromocriptine, this drug does not necessarily "cure" these pituitary adenomas, and the withdrawal of therapy can often result in recurrent hyperprolactinemia.

The major adverse effects of bromocriptine are nausea and vomiting, which tend to occur after the initial dose and with dosage increases, but can be minimized by introducing the drug at a low dosage (0.625 or 1.25 mg/day) at bedtime, taking it with food, and by very gradual dose escalation [8, 12]. Other less common side effects include orthostatic hypotension, vasospasm, cramps, flushing, and nasal congestion. Headache, drowsiness, and psychiatric adverse effects are infrequent. Rarely, in patients with Parkinson's disease treated with very high doses of bromocriptine, pulmonary infiltrates, fibrosis, pleural effusions, pleural thickening and retroperitoneal fibrosis have been described [12]; however, these adverse effects are unlikely to occur at the low doses used for treatment of prolactinomas.

Cabergoline

Cabergoline is a D_2 selective agonist with a long duration of action that permits once or twice weekly administration. The long duration of action stems from its slow elimination from pituitary tissue, its high affinity binding to pituitary dopamine receptors, and extensive enterohepatic recycling. After oral administration, PRL lowering effects are initially detectable at 3 hours and gradually increase so that the prolactin-lowering effect plateaus between 48 and 120 hours [12].

Significant decreases in serum PRL levels occur in as many as 95% of hyperprolactinemic women during chronic cabergoline treatment. In a multi-center, randomized, prospective, 24-week trial conducted in 459 hyperprolactinemic women [13], cabergoline induced normal PRL levels in 83% compared to 59% with bromocriptine; ovulatory cycles or pregnancies were recorded in 72% vs. 52%, and side effects were less frequent, less severe and shorter-lived. A remarkable tumor-shrinking effect of cabergoline has been observed in patients with macroprolactinomas: 12–24 months treatment with cabergoline induced a greater than 20% decrease of baseline tumor size in more than 80% of cases with complete disappearance of tumor mass in 26–36% of cases [14]. Colao et al. showed that 85% of 20 patients resistant to both bromocriptine and quinagolide responded with a normalization of PRL levels and 70% responded with some change in tumor size [15]. Cabergoline treatment is also effective and safe in patients with prolactinomas with onset in childhood or adolescence [16].

About 80–90% of patients who respond to dopamine agonists will do so rapidly and with low doses. However, about 10–15% of patients respond with a step-wise reduction in PRL levels with each increase in dose [17]. Increasing the weekly dose of cabergoline to 7 mg/week permitted recovery of gonadal and sexual function in 30% of those with macroadenomas and all of those with microadenomas [17]. In general, large doses of cabergoline are very well tolerated, as demonstrated by the many studies in which this drug has been used to treat Parkinson disease. As long as adverse effects from higher doses do not develop, dose escalations are reasonable, with the awareness that doses of cabergoline greater than 2.0 mg/week are beyond those recommended in the package insert. However, as noted below, cardiac valvular fibrosis has been reported in patients taking large doses of cabergoline.

Side effects associated with the use of cabergoline are similar to those reported for the other dopamine agonists, but are generally less frequent, less severe, and of shorter duration [8, 12]. The long half-life of cabergoline, which results in a relatively flat plasma drug concentration, may be advantageous with respect to the induction of side effects. Pleuropulmonary inflammatory–fibrotic syndrome has been described in a few patients. Constrictive pericarditis was diagnosed in a patient with Parkinson disease receiving cabergoline therapy at the dose of 10 mg daily [12].

Recently a number of reports have been published describing the occurrence of valvular insufficiency in patients who have been treated with high doses of cabergoline (~4 mg total daily dose) or pergolide for Parkinson disease. Both multivalvular and single mitral valve heart disease have been described [18, 19]. In these cases, the echocardiographic and/or microscopic features resembled those found in valvular disorders associated with ergot alkaloid agents and appetite suppressants. Though causality has not been proven, the similarity of the echocardiographic findings, time course, and partial reversal of symptoms in these cases suggests that the use of the dopamine agonists in high doses may have been responsible for these adverse cardiac effects. Therefore, echocardiographic monitoring should be performed in patients treated with very high doses of cabergoline or pergolide.

Pergolide

Pergolide is approximately 100 times more potent than bromocriptine and suppresses PRL secretion for up to 24 h after a single dose [12, 20], allowing effective control of hyperprolactinemia with once-daily dosing at rates similar to those found with bromocriptine. In a series of 22 patients with macroprolactinomas treated with pergolide reported by Freda et al., PRL levels normalized in 15 patients and approached normal in two others with substantial tumor size reduction also noted [21].

In general, the nature and incidence of most side effects reported with pergolide are similar to those of bromocriptine [12]. Daytime somnolence has been reported at very high doses. As discussed above, cases of pergolide-associated valvular heart disease have been reported in adults with Parkinson disease treated with doses much higher than those used for the treatment of hyperprolactinemia.

Quinagolide

Quinagolide (CV 205-502) is a non-ergot dopamine agonist with similar tolerance and efficacy to bromocriptine and pergolide that can be given once daily. Approximately 50% of patients who are resistant to bromocriptine respond to quinagolide. Its efficacy in reducing tumor size and normalizing PRL levels is similar to that of bromocriptine and pergolide [8, 12].

In a randomized, cross-over study of 20 patients with hyperprolactinemia receiving once-daily quinagolide or twice-weekly cabergoline for 12 weeks, a higher percentage of patients achieved normal PRL levels with cabergoline compared with quinagolide but clinical efficacy, such as amenorrhea, oligomenorrhea, galactorrhea and impotence, was similar as was the occurrence of side effects [22]. Adverse effects are consistent with those reported for other dopamine agonists, although they occur less frequently than with bromocriptine [12].

Dopamine agonist withdrawal

A significant number of patients may achieve remission following withdrawal of cabergoline or bromocriptine. After withdrawal of bromocriptine, remission rates have been reported as high as 20–44%. Importantly, an increase of tumor volume has been found in less than 10% of cases after bromocriptine discontinuation. A more recent retrospective analysis of 131 patients with prolactinomas treated with bromocriptine demonstrated that 26% of patients with microprolactinomas and 16% of patients with macroprolactinomas sustained a normal prolactin level 44 months after drug withdrawal [23].

Following withdrawal of cabergoline, persistent normoprolactinemia has been reported in about one-third of patients in several small studies. A recent prospective analysis of 200 patients treated with cabergoline for 42 months showed that remission of hyperprolactinemia was sustained in 69% of patients with microprolactinomas and 64% of patients with macroprolactinomas 2–5 years after drug withdrawal [24]. In those patients for whom hyperprolactinemia recurred, only 10 women (22.2%) and seven men (38.9%) experienced recurrence of gonadal dysfunction. The patients showing small remnant tumors on MRI at the onset of drug withdrawal had a higher estimated recurrence rate after 5 years compared to those without evident tumor (macroprolactinomas 77.5% vs. 32.6%; microprolactinomas 41.5% vs. 26.2%) [24]. Another recent retrospective study of 89 patients with microprolactinomas treated with bromocriptine or cabergoline showed that 36% maintained normal prolactin levels 1 year following drug withdrawal [25]. In neither of these latter studies was recurrence of hyperprolactinemia associated with regrowth of the tumors.

Two caveats should be kept in mind in interpreting the results of these studies. First, prolactin levels in patients with mild hyperprolactinemia and microprolactinomas can spontaneously normalize without treatment. Therefore, the normalization of prolactin levels in these individuals may or may not be related to effects of prior use of dopamine agonists. Second, follow-up data to assess the long-term efficacy of withdrawal are still limited to 2–5 years. Whether normoprolactinemia can be sustained in these individuals beyond this time period has not been determined. Nevertheless, these results support the concept of periodic treatment withdrawal, especially for patients without demonstrable tumor on MRI during treatment. Following withdrawal, patients should be closely monitored for recurrent hyperprolactinemia and tumor regrowth.

Medical therapy – conclusions

By far, the greatest experience in treating patients with prolactinomas has been with bromocriptine and cabergoline. In head-to-head randomized, prospective comparison studies [13], retrospective analyses [15] and general clinical experience, cabergoline has been shown to be more effective in normalizing PRL levels and more successful in reducing tumor size, while maintaining a more favorable side effect profile. Patients are less likely to be resistant to the therapeutic effects of cabergoline; furthermore, most patients found to be resistant to bromocriptine subsequently respond to cabergoline. Finally, treatment with cabergoline affords a greater chance of obtaining permanent remission and successful withdrawal of medication, compared to treatment with bromocriptine. Thus, in general, cabergoline is preferable to bromocriptine as an initial therapeutic agent. The single exception to a preference for cabergoline may be for treatment of women who wish to become pregnant.

There is much less experience with pergolide and quinagolide in the primary treatment of patients with prolactinomas. However, these drugs appear to have similar efficacy and adverse event profiles compared to bromocriptine. Use of very high doses of pergolide has been associated with organ fibrosis, including cardiac valve fibrosis. Therefore, pergolide should be avoided if high doses are needed. Depending upon pricing in some countries, pergolide may be less expensive than other dopamine agonists and this may factor into its use. Pergolide has been withdrawn by the US Food and Drug Administration because of the cardiac problems discussed above. Quinagolide is currently available in several European countries and in Canada but is not available in the US.

In patients who do not achieve acceptable biochemical or tumor size changes in response to dopamine agonists, transsphenoidal surgery remains an option if the tumor is potentially resectable and an experienced neurosurgeon is available. Radiotherapy may be effective in controlling tumor growth, although its efficacy in restoring PRL levels to normal is limited. If fertility is a major concern, induction of ovulation is possible in hyperprolactinemic patients even without lowering PRL levels, using clomiphene citrate, gonadotropins, and pulsatile GnRH [26].

Pregnancy

Effect of pregnancy on prolactinoma growth

During pregnancy, estrogen stimulates PRL synthesis and secretion, and promotes lactotroph cell hyperplasia, and tumor enlargement during pregnancy has been reported. This enlargement results from both the discontinuation of the dopamine agonist that was responsible for tumor shrinkage and the stimulatory effect of high estrogen levels produced by the placenta [26].

Data on the risk of symptomatic tumor enlargement in pregnant women with prolactinomas, divided according to their status as micro- or macroprolactinomas, have been analyzed [8, 26] (Table 29.2). The risk of symptomatic tumor enlargement for microadenomas is only 2.6% (12/457 pregnancies). Surgical intervention was not required in a single case and therapy with bromocriptine in five individuals was followed by the resolution of their symptoms. Forty-five of 142 pregnancies (31%) in patients with macroadenomas were complicated by symptoms of tumor enlargement (headaches and/or visual disturbances). Surgical intervention was undertaken in 12 of these cases and bromocriptine therapy in 17, leading to resolution of their symptoms. A total of 140 women with macroadenomas have been identified who have undergone surgery or radiation prior to pregnancy. In these individuals, the risk of tumor enlargement was low (2.5%).

Therefore, a patient with a microadenoma treated only with a dopamine agonist pregestationally should be carefully followed throughout pregnancy. Prolactin levels do not always rise during pregnancy in women with prolactinomas, as they do in normal women. Usually PRL levels rise over the first 6–10 weeks after discontinuing bromocriptine and then do not increase further. Prolactin levels may also not rise with tumor enlargement. For these two reasons, periodic assessment of PRL levels is not beneficial. Because of the low incidence of tumor enlargement in microprolactinomas, routine periodic visual field testing is not cost-effective. Visual field testing and MRI scans should be performed, however, in patients who develop visual changes or symptoms of mass effects. If tumor enlargement occurs, reinstitution of a dopamine agonist is often successful in reducing the size; however, persistent visual defects may necessitate transsphenoidal surgery or early delivery [8, 26].

For a woman with a larger macroadenoma that may have suprasellar extension, there is no definitive answer as to the best

Table 29.2 Effect of pregnancy on prolactinomas

	Total no. patients	Symptomatic enlargement	Symptomatic enlargement %
Microadenomas	457	12	2.6
Macroadenomas	142	45	31
Macroadenomas – prior surgery or radiation	140	7	5

therapeutic approach, and the patient should be informed of the risks and benefits of the various therapeutic alternatives and permitted to make a highly individualized decision. Transsphenoidal surgical debulking of the tumor prior to conception should greatly reduce the risk of serious tumor enlargement, but cases with massive tumor expansion during pregnancy even after such surgery have been reported. After surgical debulking, bromocriptine is required to restore normal PRL levels and allow ovulation. Alternatively, the dopamine agonist could be administered continuously throughout gestation but the safety of this approach has not been established. The most common approach is to discontinue the dopamine agonist after pregnancy is confirmed, as done in patients with microadenomas. Careful follow-up with 1–3 monthly visual field testing is warranted. Repeat scanning is reserved for patients with symptoms of tumor enlargement and/or evidence of a developing visual field defect [26].

Should symptomatic tumor enlargement occur with any of these approaches, reinstitution of bromocriptine causes rapid tumor size reduction with no adverse effects on the infant. Any type of surgery during pregnancy results in a 1.5-fold increase in fetal loss in the first trimester and a five-fold increase in fetal loss in the second trimester, although there is no risk of congenital malformations from such surgery [26]. Thus, bromocriptine reinstitution would appear to be preferable to surgical decompression. However, such medical therapy must be very closely monitored, and transsphenoidal surgery or delivery (if the pregnancy is far enough advanced) should be performed if there is no response to bromocriptine and vision is progressively worsening [26].

Effects of dopamine agonists on the fetus

Most patients with prolactinomas that come to clinical attention will require treatment of hyperprolactinemia to ovulate and conceive. Therefore, the fetus is likely to be exposed to these drugs for at least 3–4 weeks of gestation, until a pregnancy test can verify conception and allow discontinuation of the medication.

The use of bromocriptine, when it is taken for only the first few weeks of gestation, has not been associated with an increase in the rates of spontaneous abortions, ectopic pregnancies, trophoblastic disease, multiple pregnancies, or congenital malformations in a very large number of pregnancies [26]. Long-term follow-up studies of 64 children, between the ages of 6 months and 9 years, who were born to mothers who took bromocriptine for a limited duration in early pregnancy, have shown no adverse effects on childhood development [27]. Data available on the effects of giving bromocriptine continuously throughout gestation on fetal/infant development in only about 100 women revealed minor abnormalities in only two infants [26].

Experience with the use of cabergoline in pregnancy is accumulating. Data on exposure of the fetus or embryo during the first several weeks of pregnancy have been reported in just over 350 cases and such use has not shown an increased percentage of spontaneous abortion, premature delivery, multiple pregnancy, or congenital abnormalities [26, 28, 29]. Short-term follow-up studies of 107 infants born to mothers who used cabergoline during pregnancy indicate normal neonatal physical and mental development [29].

Few data are available on the safety of pergolide in pregnancy [26]. In one report, two major and three minor congenital abnormalities were described among 38 pregnancies in women receiving pergolide in pre-marketing studies, but a causal relationship was not definitively established. The manufacturer of pergolide, Eli Lilly & Co., reports limited data on pregnancies in which the fetus was exposed to pergolide, but did find that 7.2% of pregnancy outcomes resulted in spontaneous abortions, 7.2% in minor malformations, 14.3% in intentional abortions, 28.6% in healthy infants, and 43.4% with no information available. This limited information seems sufficient to recommend against the use of pergolide for a woman desiring pregnancy [26].

Quinagolide does not appear to be safe during pregnancy. A review of 176 pregnancies, in which quinagolide was maintained for a median duration of 37 days, reported 24 spontaneous abortions, one ectopic pregnancy, and one stillbirth at 31 weeks of gestation [30]. Furthermore, nine fetal malformations were reported in this group, including spina bifida, trisomy 13, Down syndrome, talipes, cleft lip, arrhinencephaly, and Zellweger syndrome [30].

Thus, bromocriptine has the largest safety database and has a proven safety record for pregnancy. The database for the use of cabergoline in pregnancy is much smaller, but there is no evidence at present indicating that it exerts deleterious effects on pregnant women. The incidence of malformation in their offspring is not greater than in the general population. For the woman who is intolerant to bromocriptine and who is doing well with cabergoline, continuation of cabergoline to facilitate conception is reasonable. The number of abortions and malformations associated with the use of pergolide and quinagolide during pregnancy raises serious concern. Therefore, quinagolide and pergolide should not be used when fertility is desired. If reinstitution of a dopamine agonist is needed later in gestation to control tumor growth, bromocriptine is favored over the other dopamine agonists due to greater experience with this drug in this setting.

Acknowledgment

M.P.G. is supported by NIH grant K08 DK066044.

References

1. Ciccarelli A, Daly AF, Beckers A. The epidemiology of prolactinomas. *Pituitary* 2005;8:3–6.
2. Spada A, Mantovani G, Lania A. Pathogenesis of prolactinomas. *Pituitary* 2005;8:7–15.
3. Casanueva FF, Molitch ME, Schlechte JA, et al. Guidelines of the Pituitary Society for the diagnosis and management of prolactinomas. *Clin. Endocrinol.* 2006;65:265–273.
4. Colao A, Vitale G, Cappabianca P, et al. Outcome of cabergoline treatment in men with prolactinoma: effects of a 24-month treatment

on prolactin levels, tumor mass, recovery of pituitary function, and semen analysis. *J. Clin. Endocrinol. Metab.* 2004;89:1704–1711.

5. Molitch ME. Medication-induced hyperprolactinemia. *Mayo Clin. Proc.* 2005;80:1050–1057.

6. Gibney J, Smith TP, McKenna TJ. The impact on clinical practice of routine screening for macroprolactin. *J. Clin. Endocrinol. Metab.* 2005;90:3927–3932.

7. Schofl C, Schofl-Siegert B, Karstens JH, et al. Falsely low serum prolactin in two cases of invasive macroprolactinoma. *Pituitary* 2002;5:261–265.

8. Gillam MP, Molitch ME, Lombardi G, Colao A. Advances in the treatment of prolactinomas. *Endocr. Rev.* 2006;26:485–534.

9. Pan L, Zhang N, Wang EM, Wang BJ, Dai JZ, Cai PW. Gamma knife radiosurgery as a primary treatment for prolactinomas. *J. Neurosurg.* 2000;93(Suppl 3):10–13.

10. Tomlinson JW, Holden N, Hills RK, et al. Association between premature mortality and hypopituitarism. West Midlands Prospective Hypopituitary Study Group. *Lancet* 2001;357:425–431.

11. Molitch ME. Pharmacologic resistance in prolactinoma patients. *Pituitary* 2005;8:43–52.

12. Colao A, di Sarno A, Pivonello R, di Somma C, Lombardi G. Dopamine receptor agonists for treating prolactinomas. *Exp. Opin. Investig. Drugs.* 2002;11:787–800.

13. Webster J, Piscitelli G, Polli A, et al. The efficacy and tolerability of long-term cabergoline therapy in hyperprolactinaemic disorders: an open, uncontrolled, multicentre study. European Multicentre Cabergoline Study Group. *Clin. Endocrinol. (Oxf.)* 1993;39:323–329.

14. Colao A, Di Sarno A, Landi ML, et al. Long-term and low-dose treatment with cabergoline induces macroprolactinoma shrinkage. *J. Clin. Endocrinol. Metab.* 1997;82:3574–3579.

15. Colao A, Di Sarno A, Sarnacchiaro F, et al. Prolactinomas resistant to standard dopamine agonists respond to chronic cabergoline treatment. *J. Clin. Endocrinol. Metab.* 1997;82:876–883.

16. Gillam MP, Fideleff H, Boquete HR, Molitch ME. Prolactin excess: treatment and toxicity. *Pediatr. Endocrinol. Rev.* 2004;2(Suppl 1):108–114.

17. Di Sarno A, Landi ML, Cappabianca P, et al. Resistance to cabergoline as compared with bromocriptine in hyperprolactinemia: prevalence, clinical definition, and therapeutic strategy. *J. Clin. Endocrinol. Metab.* 2001;86:5256–5261.

18. Schade R, Andersohn F, Suissa S, Haverkamp W, Garbe E. Dopamine agonists and the risk of cardiac-valve regurgitation. *N. Engl. J. Med.* 2007;356:29–38.

19. Zanettini R, Antonini A, Gatto G, et al. Valvular heart disease and the use of dopamine agonists for Parkinson's disease. *N. Engl. J. Med.* 2007;356:39–46.

20. Perryman RL, Rogol AD, Kaiser DL, MacLeod RM, Thorner MO. Pergolide mesylate: its effects on circulating anterior pituitary hormones in man. *J. Clin. Endocrinol. Metab.* 1981;53:772–778.

21. Freda PU, Andreadis CI, Khandji AG, et al. Long-term treatment of prolactin-secreting macroadenomas with pergolide. *J. Clin. Endocrinol. Metab.* 2000;85:8–13.

22. De Luis DA, Becerra A, Lahera M, Botella JI, Valero, Varela C. A randomized cross-over study comparing cabergoline and quinagolide in the treatment of hyperprolactinemic patients. *J. Endocrinol. Invest.* 2000;23:428–434.

23. Passos VQ, Souza JJ, Musolino NR, Bronstein MD. Long-term follow-up of prolactinomas: normoprolactinemia after bromocriptine withdrawal. *J. Clin. Endocrinol. Metab.* 2002;87:3578–3582.

24. Colao A, Di Sarno A, Cappabianca P, di Somma C, Pivonello R, Lombardi G. Withdrawal of long-term cabergoline therapy for tumoral and nontumoral hyperprolactinemia. *N. Engl. J. Med.* 2003;349:2023–2033.

25. Biswas M, Smith J, Jadon D, et al. Long-term remission following withdrawal of dopamine agonist therapy in subjects with microprolactinomas. *Clin. Endocrinol. (Oxf.)* 2005;63:26–31.

26. Molitch ME. Pituitary disorders during pregnancy. *Endocrinol. Metab. Clin. North Am.* 2006;35:99–116.

27. Raymond JP, Goldstein E, Konopka P, Leleu MF, Merceron RE, Loria Y. Follow-up of children born of bromocriptine-treated mothers. *Horm. Res.* 1985;22:239–246.

28. Robert E, Musatti L, Piscitelli G, Ferrari CI. Pregnancy outcome after treatment with the ergot derivative, cabergoline. *Reprod. Toxicol.* 1996;10:333–337.

29. Ricci E, Parazzini F, Motta T, et al. Pregnancy outcome after cabergoline treatment in early weeks of gestation. *Reprod. Toxicol.* 2002;16:791–793.

30. Webster J. A comparative review of the tolerability profiles of dopamine agonists in the treatment of hyperprolactinaemia and inhibition of lactation. *Drug Saf.* 1996;14:228–238.

30 Acromegaly

John A.H. Wass

Key points

- The prevalence of acromegaly is 40–60 cases per million and the annual incidence rate is 4–6 per million.
- The diagnosis is made by measuring growth hormone suppression after oral glucose.
- Acromegaly may be excluded by a basal undetectable growth hormone and a normal insulin-like growth factor 1. Ninety-nine percent of patients have a pituitary adenoma. Growth hormone levels are one of the most important predictors of outcome. Tumor size is also important. High growth hormone levels and large tumors are difficult to cure by any means, including surgery, drugs and radiotherapy.
- Transsphenoidal surgery is the treatment of choice. Microadenomas should be cured in more than 90% and macroadenomas in around 50–60% in good surgical hands. Surgical debulking improves the outcome with somatostatin analog treatment.
- Drug therapy with somatostatin analogs (octreotide or lanreotide) is effective in around 50%. If these drugs are not effective cabergoline should be tried (success rate <20%) and if neither of these two is effective pegvisomant therapy should be advised, together with radiotherapy.

Introduction

The term "acromegaly," introduced by Pierre Marie in 1886, is derived from the Greek *akron* meaning extremity and *megas* meaning great. The typical clinical signs result from prolonged excess growth hormone (GH) and insulin-like growth factor 1 (IGF-1) secretion; the GH excess in more than 99% of cases is due to a functioning pituitary adenoma [1]. Rarer causes of acromegaly result from excess growth hormone-releasing hormone (GHRH) secretion and this may be secondary to the presence of a hypothalamic hamartoma or ganglioneuroma or to ectopic production from carcinoid and other neuroendocrine tumors such as those found in the pancreas, upper gastrointestinal tract or lung.

Recent progress in the understanding of the pathogenesis of pituitary tumors has identified specific gene mutations and chromosome rearrangements [2]. Mutations of the G protein (*gsp* oncogene) occur in 30–40% of GH-secreting adenomas [3] and this is the same defect that is found in a variety of pathological tissues of McCune–Albright syndrome [4]. Rapid development of molecular technology and a greater understanding of tumorigenesis may soon lead to improved diagnosis and treatment for patients with somatotroph adenomas. This chapter describes our current knowledge of the assessment and management of acromegaly.

Clinical Endocrine Oncology, 2nd edition. Edited by Ian D. Hay and John A.H. Wass. © 2008 Blackwell Publishing. ISBN 978-1-4051-4584-8.

Epidemiology

Acromegaly is rare, with an estimated prevalence rate of 40–60 cases per million population. More recent figures suggest that this may be an underestimate and that the true prevalence is 125 per million. Data from the UK suggest an annual incidence rate of four to six per million [5]. Based on these estimates there would be 240 new cases per year in the UK with a population of approximately 60 million.

There is equal frequency of the disease in both sexes. The majority of patients are diagnosed between the ages of 40 and 60 years, although the insidious nature of the disease often contributes to the considerable time lag between onset and diagnosis [6]. Acromegaly during childhood may be more likely to be diagnosed earlier since it also causes the syndrome of gigantism. Typically, acromegaly developing in an older patient is a milder disease with lower GH values and a smaller tumor. Very rarely acromegaly may present as part of a familial endocrine syndrome such as multiple endocrine neoplasia type 1 syndrome (MEN 1).

Clinical presentation

The clinical presentation of acromegaly results either from the general metabolic effects of prolonged excess growth hormone and IGF-1 or from the local effects of an expanding pituitary tumor causing visual loss and hypopituitarism [7]. In addition, hyperprolactinemia, resulting either from direct secretion by the adenoma or from pituitary stalk compression, can contribute to

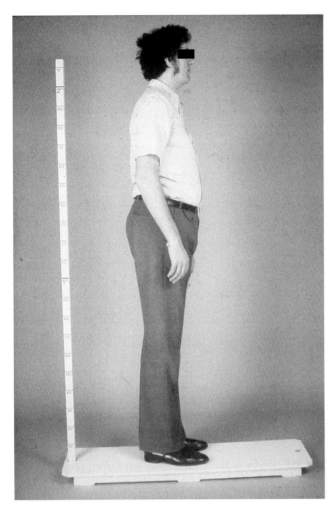

Figure 30.1 An acromegalic giant (height 228 cm) who was found at the age of 27 years, to have a GH-secreting pituitary adenoma, clinical and biochemical evidence of hypogonadotropic hypogonadism and radiological confirmation of unfused epiphyses.

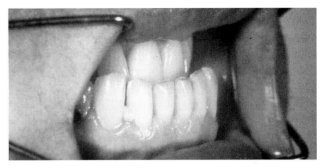

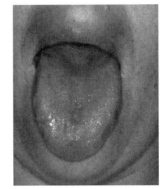 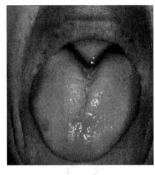

Figure 30.2 An acromegalic patient showing prognathism and a large tongue (normal tongue on the left).

the significant number of patients presenting with galactorrhea, menstrual disturbances and impotence [7].

The coarse acromegalic facial features and enlarged hands and feet remain the most striking of the clinical signs. If the patient is able to produce a series of photographs taken over many years, it may be possible to date the onset of the disease. Occasionally the patient demonstrates an arm span greater than standing height and this suggests the possibility that the disease was manifest during childhood before closure of the epiphyses (Fig. 30.1). In a series of over 400 acromegalic patients at St Bartholomew's Hospital, 2% showed evidence of pituitary gigantism with eunuchoid features.

A typical acromegalic face demonstrates coarse features including deep nasolabial furrows, thick lips, an enlarged nose and frontal bossing. Growth of the mandible causes prognathism and separation of the teeth. Tongue enlargement together with swelling of the nasopharynx and soft tissues of the upper airways contributes to respiratory difficulties, with sleep apnea being prominent amongst the varied list of complications (Fig. 30.2).

The musculoskeletal changes are a cause of significant morbidity in the acromegalic patient. Subtle enlargement of the hands and feet can be recognized by increasing ring and shoe size, whereas more severe changes result in typical spade-like appearances of the hands. Degenerative changes in the joints cause osteoarthritis, particularly of the hips and knees. Changes in the stability of the vertebral column results in kyphoscoliosis (Fig. 30.3). In addition, soft tissue swelling may contribute to neuropathies with carpal tunnel syndrome (40% of patients) a frequent finding at presentation. The combination of these pathologies together with a generalized myopathy is probably a major factor contributing to the weakness and lethargy which are so prominent in this disease.

Chronic excess of GH and IGF-1 is associated with generalized organomegaly. Clinically detectable goiter can be found in 10–20% of patients at presentation. Cardiomegaly, which is well recognized in acromegalic patients, may result directly from GH excess or alternatively be caused by the additional risk factors of hypertension and diabetes mellitus with subsequent ischemic heart disease. The gastrointestinal tract increases in size, usually without symptoms, although there is a well-recognized increased incidence of colonic polyps. The incidence of colonic carcinoma and premalignant polyps is increased in acromegaly.

The local effects of pituitary tumor largely result from expansion within the pituitary fossa, causing hypopituitarism, and from suprasellar extension, causing chiasmal compression with decreased visual acuity, visual field defects and optic atrophy. Exceptionally, these tumors may be large enough to cause hydrocephalus and others which invade the cavernous sinus produce ophthalmoplegia. Headaches are particularly common and are thought to result

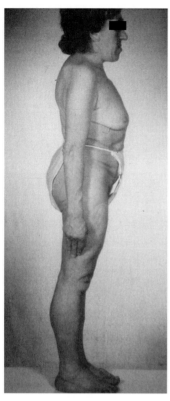

Figure 30.3 A patient with long-standing acromegaly presenting with symptoms and signs of chronic osteoarthritis and a kyphosis.

from dural stretching by the enlarging adenoma. The tumor, by expanding within the fossa, also results in the symptoms and signs of hypogonadism, adrenal insufficiency and hypothyroidism. In a group of 100 patients that we recently studied the prevalence of these conditions at presentation was 28%, 8% and 2% respectively. In addition hyperprolactinemia is found in 30% of patients.

Diagnostic work-up

Confirmation of acromegaly

The physiological fluctuations of GH secretion in both normal and acromegalic subjects makes a random GH estimation often unhelpful as an initial step in the investigation. However, the disease can be excluded if both the GH is undetectable and the IGF-1 is in the normal age-related range. In healthy subjects, basal GH levels are below the sensitivity of most assays (less than 0.1 mU/L) for most of the time, whereas in acromegalic patients the levels are usually significantly higher during the day. However, the definitive test for acromegaly remains the demonstration of failure to suppress the plasma GH to undetectable levels during an oral glucose load (Fig. 30.4). The oral glucose tolerance test is also useful in identifying the significant number of patients with impaired glucose tolerance (40%) and overt diabetes mellitus (20%).

The laboratory diagnosis of acromegaly is also made by measuring a serum IGF-1 level. This reflects the integrated effect of GH on the tissues and has been shown to differentiate between active untreated acromegaly and normal individuals [8]. The long half-life of IGF-1, due mainly to its binding to specific carrier

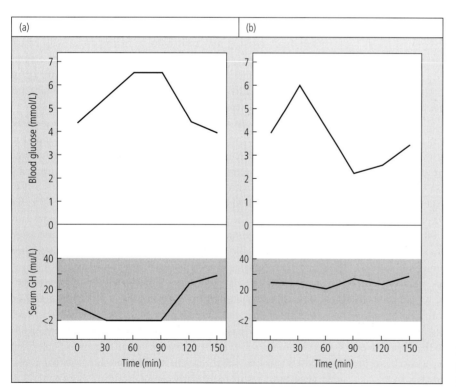

Figure 30.4 Demonstration of the response of the plasma GH to an oral glucose load of 75 g in a normal (a) and acromegalic subject (b).

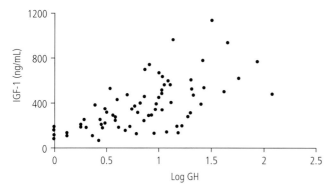

Figure 30.5 The relationship between the serum IGF-1 level and log mean growth hormone (GH) in 73 acromegalic patients.

proteins, excludes the necessity for multiple sampling and this may therefore prove to be a precise and cost-effective test during the initial screening for acromegaly (Fig. 30.5).

Radiological assessment

Magnetic resonance imaging (MRI) may be used to assess the pituitary fossa for the presence of an adenoma. Evidence of a pituitary tumor is found in the majority of cases and macroadenomas with extrasellar extension are found in about one third of cases [7]. Tumors that infiltrate bone and other surrounding structures are well recognized. MRI has been considered particularly helpful by some neurosurgeons in these cases, by delineating which parasellar structures, especially the vascular components, are involved by the tumor (Fig. 30.6).

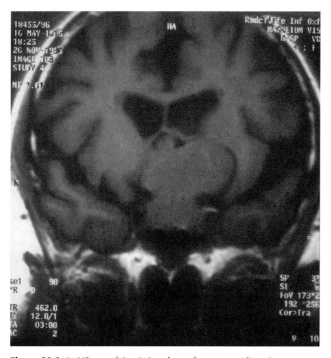

Figure 30.6 An MR scan of the pituitary fossa of an acromegalic patient demonstrating a pituitary tumor invading the parasellar structures.

Visual field testing

The visual fields should be tested by confrontation. In addition, the visual fields should be formally documented using perimetry.

Pituitary function tests

Standard basal pituitary function should be assessed by measuring the serum prolactin and by assessing the pituitary–gonadal axis (luteinizing hormone (LH), follicle-stimulating hormone (FSH), estradiol or testosterone), the pituitary–thyroid axis (the free T_4, thyroid-stimulating hormone, TSH) and the pituitary–adrenal axis (09:00 h serum cortisol). Dynamic testing of the adrenocorticotropic hormone (ACTH) reserve to stress using the insulin tolerance test or synacthen test may also be necessary. Paired early morning plasma and urine osmolarity are necessary to investigate for diabetes insipidus, although in our experience, even with very large pituitary tumors, this is extremely rare and its presence is more likely to indicate hypothalamic disease.

Confirmation of the etiology

Although in more than 99% of patients presenting with acromegaly the cause is a GH-secreting pituitary adenoma, occasionally patients are seen in whom excess GHRH can be demonstrated. A variety of neuroendocrine tumors (gut, pancreas, lung) are known to cause the clinical syndrome of acromegaly by secreting GHRH. A routine chest X-ray is mandatory in all patients and may identify chest lesions, but further investigations, including measuring a serum GHRH level, may be indicated if an obvious pituitary adenoma is not demonstrated by computerized tomography (CT) or MRI scanning. The presence of hypercalcemia or a family history of endocrine neoplasia may also raise the suspicion of MEN 1.

Aims of treatment and definition of cure

Acromegaly, a chronic disease causing significant morbidity, is associated with a mortality of about double the expected rate. Some form of therapy is therefore considered in virtually all patients. The decision of recommending surgery, medical therapy or radiotherapy is influenced by the age and general health of the patient and also whether the pituitary tumor is causing local compressive effects, particularly of the visual pathways. In general, however, the treatment aims are as follows:

- removal of the pituitary tumor to relieve local mass effects;
- relief of symptoms and signs of acromegaly;
- restoration of GH secretion and IGF-1 levels to normal;
- maintenance of normal pituitary function;
- prevention of disease recurrence;
- assessment and treatment of chronic complications.

The most difficult aim and that which has proved difficult to define is the restoration of normal GH secretory dynamics [9]. By international consensus [10] a nadir GH after oral glucose of

<1 mU/L, and a normal age-related IGF-1, currently constitutes biochemical control.

The scientific basis for this is that mean GH levels of <5 mU/L are associated with restoration of the normal body composition of salt and water [11]. Furthermore, a reduction in mortality similar to that of the general population is reported for patients with a mean GH level of <5 mU/L or less [12].

Other studies have confirmed these initial findings [13, 14]. In some but not all studies a normal IGF-1, also predicted mortality [15, 16]. Currently therefore both GH and IGF-1 should be measured to evaluate the biochemical effects of treatment.

Treatment

Transsphenoidal surgery is currently the treatment of first choice for acromegaly. It is associated with a low mortality (<0.5%) and the most serious of the complications, such as cerebrospinal fluid (CSF) leaks and meningitis, are reported to occur in less than 1% of cases [17]. The prevalence of hypopituitarism at presentation is appreciable and although transsphenoidal surgery may cause deterioration of pituitary function (Fig. 30.7), hormone replacement therapy is readily available for long-term treatment. In some individual patients tumor removal by transsphenoidal surgery may even restore to normal previously documented pituitary failure. Selective removal of a pituitary adenoma via the transsphenoidal route limits the development of hypopituitarism and may be guided by MRI images of the sellar region. In the case of focal invasion into the cavernous sinus it may be possible to follow the tumor by endoscopic vision and achieve more total removal of the adenoma [17].

Serial MRI imaging has also been used to investigate a role for preoperative somatostatin analog treatment. GH-secreting adenomas show shrinkage in approximately 80% of cases after several months of octreotide treatment, although the degree of shrinkage is smaller than that of prolactinomas on dopamine agonist therapy. This treatment has not yet been shown to influence the immediate postoperative outcome in terms of GH levels.

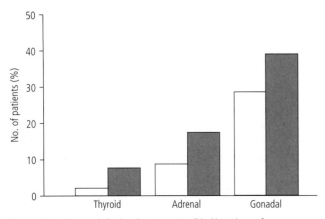

Figure 30.7 The pre- (white) and postoperative (black) incidence of hypopituitarism in 100 acromegalic patients.

Results of transsphenoidal surgery

The outcome of surgery is affected by the preoperative size of the tumor and the preoperative GH levels [18, 19]. Thus with microadenoma, 90% should achieve remission surgically whereas the rate with macroadenoma is much less (55%) [19]. Pretreatment GH levels also affect outcome. Thus if the GH is <20 mU/L preoperatively 65% of patients can achieve a remission surgically in contrast to preoperative GH of >100 mU/L, where only 18% do [18]. Invasion by the tumor of the cavernous sinus adversely affects surgical success rates. Surgical experience is also a key factor in achieving a satisfactory outcome [20].

Medical therapy with somatostatin analogs has been suggested as a first-line treatment. This may be the case in patients unfit for surgery. However, surgical debulking of a tumor that may be incurable surgically improves the responses of GH and IGF-1 to somatostatin analog therapy [21].

Re-emergence of active acromegaly and tumor regrowth following postoperative GH normalization is regarded as a recurrence. Recurrence of elevated GH levels is not common in acromegaly (7% at 5 years) and is less common than the surgical reoccurrence rate after surgery for Cushing disease.

Results of medical therapy

Dopamine agonists inhibit GH release in some acromegalic patients although the biochemical response is highly variable. Significant clinical improvement has been reported following the administration of bromocriptine, lisuride, pergolide, terguride, quinagolide and with the long-acting oral dopamine agonist, cabergoline. It has been demonstrated, however, that GH levels can be reduced to <10 mU/L in only approximately 20% of patients, with IGF-1 levels being restored to normal in only 10% [22]. There are no tests which confidently and consistently predict the dopamine agonist responders.

Octreotide and lanreotide, the long-acting octapeptide analogs of somatostatin, are the first-line medical treatment for acromegaly. Currently available are two long-acting somatostatin preparations, octreotide LAR and lanreotide autogel. They are approximately equally efficacious. They result in normal levels of GH and IGF-1 in approximately 50% of patients. Preoperative GH levels predict subsequent effectiveness of treatment and if the pretreatment GH is <20 mU/L 60% of patients have a successful response, but this is lower (18%) if the GH is >60 mU/L before treatment.

A number of clinical trials using octreotide and lanreotide in the treatment of acromegaly show that a favorable clinical and biochemical response can be maintained for many years. Normalization of IGF-1 levels has been demonstrated in 46% of patients [23]. The administration of a single subcutaneous dose of 100 μg and the subsequent response of the serum GH (<5 mU/L) predicts responsiveness to long-term treatment with octreotide and lanreotide [24].

A decrease in pituitary tumor size during long-term somatostatin analog treatment has been reported in about 80% of patients [25, 26]. However, the tumor shrinkage, in comparison to that of prolactinomas induced by bromocriptine, is much less dramatic and also slower in onset. The main indications for the use of octreotide and lanreotide are in postoperative or postradiotherapy patients in whom the postoperative or postradiotherapy GH levels remain >5 mU/L and as primary treatment in elderly patients.

Acute side effects of somatostatin analog treatment include local effects at the injection site and gastrointestinal symptoms. Approximately 30% of patients note colicky abdominal discomfort and diarrhea at the beginning of treatment, although these symptoms usually settle within 2–3 weeks. The main long-term side effect of chronic somatostatin analog treatment is the increased frequency of gallstones. Gallstones are largely asymptomatic except when treatment with octreotide is stopped, when gallbladder contraction recommences and symptoms may occur.

Pegvisomant is a GH receptor antagonist that effectively reduces IGF-1 to normal in more than 90% of patients. Administrable as a subcutaneous injection daily, it may occasionally be associated with the development of abnormal liver function tests. Tumor enlargement has occurred while on it, but this is probably related to the primary tumor behavior rather than the drug. Pegvisomant is used when somatostatin analogs are ineffective. The two drugs may also be combined to decrease the amount of pegvisomant used and the expense without loss of control of acromegaly [27].

Results of pituitary radiotherapy

Radiotherapy is used less frequently nowadays in the treatment of acromegaly. Either conventional megavoltage radiotherapy or Gamma Knife radiosurgery is used.

Conventional megavoltage radiotherapy has in the past been used either as primary treatment or as an additional alternative following transsphenoidal surgery. Comparisons of published series are hampered by the varying dose regiments used worldwide. Most would now consider that a total dose of 4500 cGy divided into 25 daily fractions of 180 cGy/day is effective in the control of acromegaly and limits the visual complications associated with higher dose schedules. The series at St Bartholomew's Hospital using this dose schedule as treatment for acromegaly demonstrated radiotherapy to be effective after a follow-up period of many years (Table 30.2). The largest fall in serum GH occurs during the first 2 years but the levels of GH continue to fall for many years thereafter. The percentage of patients achieving GH levels of <5 mU/L is cumulative with time and 7 years post-treatment, 86% of patients had achieved this target [28].

Progressive development of hypopituitarism following radiotherapy for acromegaly has been well documented. The prevalence of thyroid, adrenal and gonadal deficiencies 10 years after radiotherapy as sole treatment has been reported in 19%, 38% and 55% of patients respectively [29]. Incidence rates are higher for patients who have undergone prior transsphenoidal surgery.

Table 30.1 Clinical symptoms and signs in 60 patients presenting with acromegaly

Symptoms and signs at presentation	Overall prevalence (%)
Facial change and acral enlargement	100
Excessive sweating	83
Acroparesthesiae	68
Tiredness and lethargy	53
Headaches	53
Arthropathy	37
Goiter	35
Ear, nose, throat or dental problems	32
Congestive cardiac failure/arrhythmia	23
Visual loss or visual field defects	17

Adapted from Lamberts et al. [7].

Table 30.2 Data from the Acromegaly Register showing the percentage of patients achieving a mean growth hormone (GH) of <5 mU/L following radiotherapy [29]

	Years following radiotherapy:			
	0	2	5	7
Patients (%) with GH <5 mU/L	0	18	40	86

Hypopituitarism is dose dependent and favorable results have recently been reported for the treatment of acromegaly using a low radiation dose schedule [30].

Gamma Knife radiosurgery offers irradiation to the pituitary gland via many portals in a one-session treatment. It is not widely available. The fall in GH may be quicker and the hypopituitarism less than with conventional radiotherapy, but more data are required [31].

Conclusion

There is an appreciable morbidity associated with long-standing acromegaly. Approximately 40% of acromegalic patients suffer from hypertension and 20% are diabetic. The incidence of cardiovascular disease is increased, with heart failure, stroke and ventricular arrhythmias well-recognized complications. Respiratory disease is also a major cause of morbidity and mortality. Contributing factors include upper airway obstruction due to hyperplasia of the soft tissues, abnormal small airway function and the development of a progressive thoracic kyphosis. Acromegalic patients often complain of weakness and proximal myopathy; peripheral neuropathy and degenerative joint disease are well-recognized causes. Overall mortality in untreated acromegaly is approximately double that found in the general population. Treatment, whether this is by surgery, medical therapy or radiotherapy, improves mortality. There is now good evidence to support the treatment aim of achieving normal IGF-1 levels and serum GH levels of <5 mU/L since this is associated with a mortality rate similar to the general population [10].

There is a reasonably consistent approach worldwide to the treatment of acromegaly. Transsphenoidal surgery is the treatment of first choice, although in the elderly, medical therapy with somatostatin analogs is an acceptable option. For patients with a raised IGF-1 or GH levels >5 mU/L following surgery the choice lies between medical therapy and reoperation. If somatostatin analog therapy is not successful postoperatively, radiotherapy or Pegvisomant therapy should be considered.

Future prospects

New somatostatin analogs are in trial which through stimulation of somatostatin receptor 5 may be effective in patients resistant to somatostatin analogs at present. Endoscopic surgery may improve results in patients with cavernous sinus disease.

References

1. Barkan AL. Acromegaly; diagnosis and therapy. *Endocrinol. Metab. Clin. North Am.* 1989;18:277–310.
2. Levy A, Lightman SL. The pathogenesis of pituitary adenomas. *Clin. Endodrinol.* 1993;38:559–570.
3. Spada A. G Proteins and hormonal signalling in the aetiology of acromegaly. In Wass JAH (ed.). *Treating Acromegaly.* Bristol: Journal of Endocrinology, 1994:31–37.
4. Levine MA. The McCune–Albright syndrome. The whys and wherefores of abnormal signal transduction. *N. Engl. J. Med.* 1991;325: 1738–1740.
5. Ritchie CM, Atkinson AB, Kennedy AL, et al. Ascertainment and natural history of treated acromegaly in Northern Ireland. *Ulster Med. J.* 1990;59:52–62.
6. Nabarro JDN. Acromegaly. *Clin. Endocrinol.* 1987; 26:481–512.
7. Lamberts SWJ. Acromegaly. In Grossman AG (ed.). *Clinical Endocrinology.* Oxford: Blackwell Scientific Publications, 1992:154–168.
8. Clemmons DR, van Wijk JJ, Ridgeway EC, et al. Evaluation of acromegaly by radioimmunoassay of somatomedin-C. *N. Engl. J. Med.* 1979;301:1138–1142.
9. Sheppard MC. Aims of treatment and definition of cure. In Wass JAH (ed.). *Treating Acromegaly.* Bristol: Journal of Endocrinology, 1994:17–23.
10. Melmed S, Casanueva F, Cavagnini F, et al. Consensus statement: medical management of acromegaly. *Eur. J. Endocrinol.* 2005;153: 737–740.
11. McLellan AR, Connell JMC, Beastall GH, Teasdale G, Davies DL. Growth hormone, body composition and somatomedin C after treatment of acromegaly. *Q. J. Med.* 1988;260:997–1008.
12. Bates AS, Van't Hoff W, Jones JM, Clayton RN. An audit of outcome of treatment in acromegaly. *Q. J. Med.* 1993;86:293–299.
13. Abosch A, Tyrrell JB, Lamborn KR, Hannegan LT, Applebury CB, Wilson CB. Transsphenoidal microsurgery for growth hormone-secreting pituitary adenomas: initial outcome and long-term results. *J. Clin. Endocrinol. Metab.* 1998;83:3411–3418.
14. Swearingen B, Barker FG 2nd, Katznelson L. Long-term mortality after transsphenoidal surgery and adjunctive therapy for acromegaly. *J. Clin. Endocrinol. Metab.* 1998;83:3419–3426.
15. Holdaway IM, Rajasoorya RC, Gamble GD. Factors influencing mortality in acromegaly. *J. Clin. Endocrinol. Metab.* 2004;89:667–674.
16. Ayuk J, Sheppard MC, Bates AS, Stewart PM. Letter re: Monitoring the response to treatment in acromegaly. *J. Clin. Endocrinol. Metab.* 2005;90:4980.
17. Fahlbusch R, Honegger J, Buchfelder M. Surgical management of acromegaly. *Endocrinol. Metab. Clin. North Am.* 1992;3:669–692.
18. Sheaves R, Chew SL, Wass JAH, Grossman A. The dangers of unopposed beta adrenergic blockade in phaeochromocytoma. *Postgrad. Med. J.* 1995;71:58–59.
19. Ahmed S, Elsheikh M, Page RCL, Adams CBT, Wass JAH. Outcome of transsphenoidal surgery for acromegaly and its relationship to surgical experience. *Clin. Endocrinol.* 1999;50:561–567.
20. Wass JAH, Turner HE, Adams CBT. The importance of locating a good pituitary surgeon. *Pituitary* 1999;2:51–54.
21. Colao A, Attanasio R, Pivonello R, et al. Partial surgical removal of growth hormone-secreting pituitary tumors enhances the response to somatostatin analogs in acromegaly. *J. Clin. Endocrinol. Metab.* 2006;91:85–92.
22. Jaffe CA, Barkan AL. Treatment of acromegaly with dopamine agonists. *Endocrinol. Metab. Clin. North Am.* 1992;21:713–735.
23. Vance ML, Harris AG. Long-term treatment of 189 acromegalic patients with the somatostatin analogue, ocreotide: results of the International Multicenter Acromegaly Study Group. *Arch. Intern. Med.* 1991;151:1573–1578.
24. Karavitaki N, Botusan I, Radiant S, Coculescut M, Turner HE, Wass JAH. The value of an acute Octreotide suppression test in predicting longterm responses to depot somatostatin analogues in patients with active acromegaly. *Clin. Endocrinol.* 2005;62:282–288.
25. Colao A, Di Somma C, Cuocolo A, et al. The severity of growth hormone deficiency correlates with the severity of cardiac impairment in 100 adult patients with hypopituitarism: an observational, case–control study. *J. Clin. Endocrinol. Metab.* 2004;89:5998–6004.
26. Bevan JS, Atkin SL, Atkinson AB, et al. Primary medical therapy for acromegaly: an open, prospective, multicenter study of the effects of subcutaneous and intramuscular slow-release octreotide on growth hormone, insulin-like growth factor-I, and tumor size. *J. Clin. Endocrinol. Metab.* 2002;87:4554–4563.
27. Feenstra J, de Herder WW, ten Have SM, et al. Combined therapy with somatostatin analogues and weekly pegvisomant in active acromegaly. *Lancet.* 2005;365:1644–1646. Erratum in: *Lancet* 2005; 365:1620.
28. Jenkins PJ, Bates P, Carson MN, Stewart PM, Wass JA. Conventional pituitary irradiation is effective in lowering serum growth hormone and insulin-like growth factor-I in patients with acromegaly. *J. Clin. Endocrinol. Metab.* 2006;91:1239–1245.
29. Eastman RC, Gordon P, Roth J. Conventional supervoltage irradiation is an effective treatment for acromegaly. *J. Clin. Endocrinol. Metab.* 1979; 48:931–940.
30. Littley MD, Shalet SM, Swindell R, Beardwell CG, Sutton ML. Low-dose pituitary irradiation for acromegaly. *Clin. Endocrinol.* 1990;32:261–270.
31. Nawaz A, Newton D, Sandeman DD, et al. Gammaknife sterotactic radiosurgery for acromegaly. *Endocrine Abstracts* (2004) **7** OC27.

31 Cushing's Disease

John Newell-Price

Key points

- The incidence of Cushing's disease is approximately 3–4 per million, but may be unrecognized in at-risk populations, such as poorly controlled type 2 diabetes.
- Cushing's disease is the commonest form of adrenocorticotropic hormone-dependent Cushing's syndrome, accounts for 70% of all cases of Cushing's syndrome, and is due to a microadenoma of the pituitary in over 90% of cases.
- Diagnosis of Cushing's syndrome is made by measurement of urinary free cortisol, dexamethasone suppression tests, and assessment of midnight plasma, or late night salivary cortisol.
- Diagnosis of Cushing's disease is made by dynamic testing, including corticotropin-releasing hormone-testing, and inferior petrosal sinus sampling. Magnetic resonance imaging pre- and post-contrast is mandatory, but is negative in up to 40% of cases.
- Transsphenoidal surgery remains the mainstay of treatment, but overall long-term remission is only achieved in up to 60–70% of cases, and at the cost of significant hypopituitarism. Laparoscopic bilateral adrenalectomy is being considered at an earlier stage, and even as primary therapy in selected cases.
- By itself long-term adrenal blockade with ketoconazole and metyrapone is not usually effective, and there is no established medical therapy that lowers adrenocorticotropic hormone secretion. New developments are needed in this area.

Introduction

Harvey Cushing originally described the first case of the syndrome that bears his name in 1912. Cushing's disease is the most frequent cause of endogenous Cushing's syndrome, and can be a formidable clinical challenge [1]. It is caused by excess secretion of adrenocorticotropic hormone (ACTH) from a pituitary corticotroph tumor or, much more rarely, hyperplasia of corticotroph cells. The circulating ACTH drives the adrenal gland to synthesize and release excess cortisol, which, over prolonged periods of time, leads to the clinical manifestations of Cushing's syndrome. When presentation is florid diagnosis is usually straightforward, but in modern practice Cushing's syndrome is frequently considered in the absence of the classic signs and achieving diagnosis can be a considerable challenge. Appropriate management of Cushing's disease is dependent on correctly identifying the pituitary as the source of disease, as opposed to the other causes of Cushing's syndrome. Once diagnosis is established a variety of options are available for treatment, but currently the mainstay of therapy remains transsphenoidal surgery. This chapter will review pathophysiology, clinical features, biochemical diagnosis, imaging and management strategies for Cushing's disease, in the context of establishing this diagnosis in a patient presenting with ACTH-dependent Cushing's syndrome.

Clinical Endocrine Oncology, 2nd edition. Edited by Ian D. Hay and John A.H. Wass. © 2008 Blackwell Publishing. ISBN 978-1-4051-4584-8.

Epidemiology and prognosis

The prevalence of Cushing's syndrome has been reported to range from 0.7 to 2.4/million population per year [1], depending on the population studied. New data, however, indicate that Cushing's syndrome is more common than had previously been thought. In studies of obese patients with type 2 diabetes, especially those with poor control and hypertension, there is a reported prevalence of 2–5% [2], even though the diagnosis of Cushing's syndrome was not suspected on the basis of clinical features, but patients' metabolic control improved following intervention for their Cushing's syndrome. If confirmed in further large-scale prospective studies these data suggest that more widespread screening for Cushing's syndrome in such patients is warranted, although it still needs to be proven that control of low-grade cortisol excess is more beneficial than attention to more specific abnormalities of metabolic and cardiovascular risk. In contrast, patients with incompletely controlled clinically obvious Cushing's syndrome of any cause have a five-fold excess mortality.

Causes of ACTH-dependent Cushing's syndrome

Endogenous Cushing's syndrome is more common in women than men and is divided into ACTH-dependent and ACTH-independent (which will not be considered further here) causes (Table 31.1). Overall, ACTH-dependent causes account for approximately 80–85% of cases, and of these 80% are due to

Table 31.1 Etiology of Cushing's syndrome

Cause of Cushing's syndrome	F:M	%
ACTH-dependent		
Cushing's disease	3.5:1♦	70%
Ectopic ACTH syndrome	1:1	10%
Unknown source of ACTH*	5:1	5%
ACTH-independent		
Adrenal adenoma	4:1	10%
Adrenal carcinoma	1:1	5%
Other causes		<2%

♦Male preponderance in children; *Patients may ultimately prove to have Cushing's disease.

pituitary adenomas (Cushing's disease), with the remaining 20% or so due to the ectopic ACTH syndrome. Ectopic ACTH secretion is most common from small cell carcinoma of the lung and bronchial carcinoid tumors, but may also occur with almost any endocrine tumor from many different organs (e.g. pheochromocytoma, pancreatic neuroendocrine tumors, gut carcinoids). Classically, when due to small cell carcinoma of the lung the ectopic ACTH syndrome may have a rapid onset with severe features. In contrast, the clinical phenotype (and some biochemical features) of carcinoid tumors may be indistinguishable from that of Cushing's disease, and this may cause diagnostic difficulty.

Pathogenesis

Cushing's disease is the most common form of endogenous Cushing's syndrome. Relatively little is known about the underlying pathogenesis of these pituitary tumors [3]. In general, corticotroph tumors show particularly low expression of the cyclin-dependent inhibitor, p27 and over-expression of cyclin E and a high Ki-67 expression indicative of a relatively high proliferative activity. The excess of reproductive-aged women may indicate a role of estrogen, and, interestingly, there is a male preponderance in prepubertal Cushing's disease. Corticotroph tumors are usually only a few millimeters in diameter, on average 6 mm, and are larger than 1 cm (macroadenoma) in only 6% of cases.

Corticotroph tumors express the pro-opiomelanocortin gene (*POMC*), the peptide product of which is subsequently cleaved to ACTH. In contrast to the majority of microadenomas, such processing is relatively inefficient in corticotroph macroadenomas, which secrete relatively large amounts of unprocessed *POMC*. Some pituitary macroadenomas are "silent corticotroph adenomas," and may present with tumor mass effects (e.g. optic chiasm compression) alone. The initial absence of Cushingoid features may progress to overt clinical Cushing's syndrome. These tumors can be diagnosed preoperatively, and followed postoperatively, by measuring plasma *POMC*.

Tumors causing Cushing's disease are relatively resistant to the effects of glucocorticoids, but *POMC* expression and ACTH secretion are nevertheless partly reduced by higher doses of

dexamethasone in 80% of cases [4]. Recent data show loss of ACTH receptor expression on corticotrophs, increased inactivation of cortisol by 11β-hydroxysteroid dehydrogenase, and also reduced expression of "bridging protein," which is involved in glucocorticoid feedback. These data partly explain the resistance to glucocorticoids apparent in Cushing's disease. Approximately 90% of tumors express the corticotropin-releasing hormone (CRH)-1 receptor, as evidenced by the release of ACTH in response to exogenously administered CRH. Tumors also express the vasopressin-3 (V3) receptor, and respond to vasopressin and desmopressin *in vitro* and *in vivo*. In the ectopic ACTH syndrome, study of the human DMS-79 cell line, a small cell lung cancer model, has shown that *POMC* is activated by transcription factors distinct from those in the pituitary, including E2F factors [5], that are able to bind the promoter when it is in an unmethylated state [6]. In contrast, carcinoid tumors, which have a more benign behavior, show a molecular phenotype closer to that of pituitary corticotroph tumors.

Clinical features of Cushing's syndrome

Clinical features are variably present in any given patient and are summarized in Table 31.2. Features may vary in a "cyclical fashion," causing diagnostic difficulty. The diagnosis is being increasingly considered in patients with the metabolic syndrome, who may have mild features of slow onset, and this may be a considerable diagnostic challenge [1]. Frequently those with subtler phenotype have Cushing's disease, rather than other causes of Cushing's syndrome, but this is not invariable. The signs that most reliably distinguish Cushing's syndrome from simple obesity are those of protein wasting: the presence of thin skin in the young, easy bruising, and proximal weakness. The sign of proximal weakness is most easily demonstrated by asking the patient to stand

Table 31.2 Clinical features of Cushing's syndrome

Feature	%
Obesity or weight gain	95*
Facial plethora	90
Rounded face	90
Decreased libido	90
Thin skin	85
Decreased linear growth in children	70–80
Menstrual irregularity	80
Hypertension	75
Hirsutism	75
Depression/emotional lability	70
Easy bruising	65
Glucose intolerance	60
Weakness	60
Osteopenia or fracture	50
Nephrolithiasis	50

Based on combined data from [4].
*100% in children [6, 7].

from sitting position without the use of hands: an initial backward movement of the buttocks is present in early myopathy, whilst in more severe cases rising from a chair may not be possible. In children presenting features differ, with obesity and decreased linear growth especially evident. Presentation differs between women and men, with purple striae, muscle atrophy, osteoporosis, and kidney stones being more common in men. Gonadal dysfunction is common in both sexes. The adverse effects of glucocorticoids on bone metabolism are evidenced by decreased bone mineral density, although the exact incidence is unclear and it tends to normalize over time after effective treatment. Bone loss may be more severe in primary adrenal rather than pituitary-dependent Cushing's syndrome. Over 70% of patients with Cushing's syndrome may present with psychiatric symptoms ranging from anxiety to frank psychosis; if present, depression is often agitated in nature. Some degree of psychiatric disturbance often persists following cure of Cushing's syndrome. Impairment in short-term memory and cognition is common and can persist for at least a year following treatment. These effects are associated with a decrease in apparent brain volume that slowly reverses following correction of hypercortisolemia. Patients continue to have impaired quality of life even after resolution of cortisol, and should be counseled regarding this. Cortisol excess predisposes to hypertension and glucose intolerance. Patients with Cushing's syndrome exhibit increased cardiovascular risk, which may not return fully to normal after remission.

Biochemical assessment

In florid cases of Cushing's the diagnosis may be obvious, but biochemical confirmation is still needed. Usually, however, symptoms and signs are less clear. Investigation of Cushing's syndrome is a two-step process. Hypercortisolemia needs to be confirmed and then the cause needs identification. Failure to follow this pathway of diagnosis and then differential diagnosis will result in inappropriate treatment and management.

Biochemical diagnosis of Cushing's syndrome – hypercortisolemia (Fig. 31.1)

No single test is perfect, each having differing sensitivities and specificities, and several tests are usually needed. Investigation should be performed when there is no acute concurrent illness, such as infection or heart failure, as these may cause false-positive results. The three main tests in use are: 24-h urinary free cortisol; the "low-dose" dexamethasone suppression test; and assessment of midnight plasma or late night salivary cortisol. Hypercortisolemia is also found in some patients with depression, alcoholism, anorexia nervosa, and late pregnancy. However, in contrast to true endogenous Cushing's syndrome, the biochemistry improves when the underlying condition has resolved. Establishing a diagnosis of Cushing's syndrome on the rare occasion that it presents in pregnancy is a considerable challenge [7].

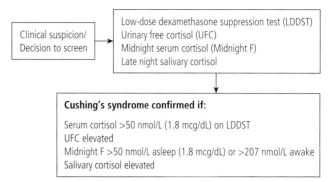

Figure 31.1 Diagnosis of Cushing's syndrome.

Urinary free cortisol (UFC)

Urinary cortisol is a direct assessment of circulating free (biologically active) cortisol. Excess circulating cortisol saturates the cortisol-binding globulin (CBG) and is excreted in urine as free cortisol, and when collected for 24 hours gives an integrated estimation of the level of hypercortisolemia. A single measurement has low sensitivity for patients with intermittent hypercortisolemia, and it is recommend that three 24-h collections are performed [4, 8]. Values four-fold greater than the upper limit of normal are rare except in Cushing's. Specificity is a common problem, since in antibody-based assays the levels of UFC overlap those seen in patients with other causes of hypercortisolemia (see above) [4, 8]. Use of high-performance liquid chromatography (HPLC) and tandem mass spectrometry may improve the diag-nostic accuracy, although substances such as digoxin and carbamazepine may produce peaks in the HPLC assay that give falsely high values [8]. Moreover, if there is renal impairment with a GFR of <30.0 mL/min, or an incomplete collection, the UFC may be falsely low [8]. Review of the collection volume and correction for creatinine concentration may be helpful in assessing whether the collection is complete.

Low-dose dexamethasone suppression tests (LDSST)

Two tests are in common use. In the overnight dexamethasone suppression test, 1 mg of dexamethasone is administered at 23:00 h and serum cortisol measured the next day at 08:00–09:00 h. In the 48-h dexamethasone suppression test, dexamethasone is administered at the dose of 0.5 mg every 6 h for 2 days at 09:00 h, 15:00 h, 21:00 h, and 03:00 h with measurements of serum cortisol at 09:00 h at the start and end of the test. To exclude Cushing's syndrome the serum cortisol value should be less than 50 nmol/L (1.8 µg/dL) following either test [1, 4, 8]. The 48-h test, though more cumbersome, is more specific and with adequate regular instructions can be performed by outpatients. In both tests, caution needs to be exercised if there is potential malabsorption of dexamethasone or if patients are on drugs that increase hepatic clearance of dexamethasone, including carbamazepine, phenytoin, phenobarbital or rifampicin. Patients taking estrogen therapy, or who are pregnant, may have an increase in the CBG. As commercial cortisol assays measure total cortisol, this may give a false-positive result on dexamethasone suppression testing. Oral estrogens need to be stopped for a period of 4–6 weeks so that CBG may return to basal values. Even transdermal estrogens may cause false-positive results and tests should be repeated off transdermal estrogens if positive results are obtained.

One problem with dexamethasone suppression testing is that 3–8% of patients with Cushing's disease retain sensitivity to dexamethasone and show suppression of serum cortisol to <50 nmol/L (1.8 μg/dL) on either test. Additionally, a false-positive rate of up to 30% has been reported in other hospitalized and healthy individuals. Thus, if clinical suspicion remains high, repeated tests and other investigations are indicated.

Midnight plasma cortisol

The normal circadian rhythm of cortisol secretion is lost in patients with Cushing's syndrome. A single sleeping midnight plasma cortisol of <50 nmol/L (1.8 μg/dL) effectively excludes Cushing's syndrome at the time of the test, and this may be particularly helpful. This is one of the harder tests to perform as it requires hospitalization, but it can be of great utility where there has been incomplete suppression on dexamethasone testing. Values >50 nmol/L (1.8 μg/dL) are found in Cushing's syndrome, even those who suppress on dexamethasone [9], but this lacks specificity as patients with acute illness also have values above this level. An awake midnight plasma cortisol of >207 nmol/L (7.5 μg/dL) differentiates between Cushing's and other causes of hypercortisolemia, but may miss mild disease in about 7% [1]. An elevated midnight plasma cortisol does not provide additional information if there is clear lack of suppression on dexamethasone testing.

Late night salivary cortisol

Recent reports have renewed the interest in salivary cortisol for diagnosis of Cushing's syndrome. Salivary cortisol reflects free circulating cortisol and its ease of collection and stability at room temperature make it a highly suitable screening tool for outpatient assessment. The diagnostic ranges vary between reports due to the different assays and the comparison groups used to set cut-off points. The test has a sensitivity and specificity of between 95% and 98%. As the values of salivary cortisol are an order of magnitude lower than serum cortisol, it is essential that the performance of the local assay be known and that the appropriate cut-off point is utilized. The test is of particular use in the assessment of cyclical Cushing's syndrome and in children. It is important to recognize that this test does not have higher diagnostic accuracy than the midnight serum test, but the assays needed are more variable and less available. Indeed, in the UK salivary midnight cortisol in not in widespread use.

Other tests

When doubt remains the dexamethasone-suppressed CRH test and the desmopressin test have been proposed as useful diagnostic tools in cases of doubt. Recent data, however, confirm that the dexamethasone-suppressed CRH test is not more accurate than the 48 h LDDST [10] and its routine application cannot be recommended. In cases of doubt the best option is to repeat the tests at a later date, or seek further opinion.

Establishing the etiology of Cushing's syndrome (Fig. 31.2)

Once a diagnosis of Cushing's syndrome is established the next step is to establish the cause. Investigation will vary depending upon the availability of the biochemical tests and imaging detailed below. The first step is to measure plasma ACTH. Levels consistently below 5 pg/mL indicate ACTH-independent Cushing's syndrome and attention can be turned to imaging the adrenal with computerized tomography (CT). Levels of ACTH persistently above 15 pg/mL almost always reflect ACTH-dependent pathologies and require investigation, as detailed below. The values between these two need cautious interpretation as patients with Cushing's disease and adrenal pathologies may have intermediate values [4, 8, 11]. The plasma should be separated rapidly and stored at −40°C to avoid degradation and a falsely low result. A positive CRH test (see below) clearly demonstrates an ACTH-dependent hypercortisolism in an occasional patient with Cushing's disease with low baseline ACTH plasma levels.

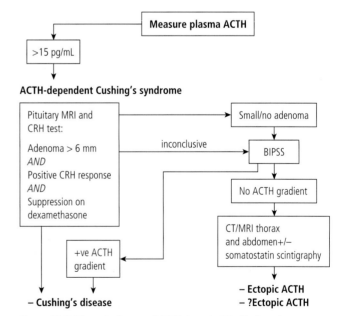

Figure 31.2 Diagnosis of causes of ACTH-dependent Cushing's syndrome. BIPSS: bilateral inferior petrosal sinus sampling.

ACTH-dependent Cushing's syndrome

Overview
Differentiating between pituitary and non-pituitary sites of excess ACTH secretion may be a considerable challenge in clinical endocrinology. Carcinoid tumors may be clinically indistinguishable from Cushing's disease, and are frequently difficult to identify with imaging, especially if radiological (pituitary, thoracic, pancreatic) "incidentalomas" complicate interpretation. As a result, biochemical evaluation rather than imaging is used to differentiate between pituitary and non-pituitary causes. In women with ACTH-dependent Cushing's syndrome, 9 out of 10 cases will be due to Cushing's disease. It is against this pretest likelihood that the performance of any test needs to be judged. The results of CRH and dexamethasone tests, and pituitary magnetic resonance imaging (MRI), should be considered together, and bilateral inferior petrosal sinus sampling (BIPSS) is recommended unless there is a clear diagnosis (see Fig. 31.2 and below).

Plasma potassium
High levels of cortisol may either saturate the 11β-hydroxysteroid dehydrogenase type II enzyme in the kidney, or decrease expression of this enzyme, allowing cortisol to act even more as a mineralocorticoid. The commonest cause of hypokalemia is the ectopic ACTH syndrome, but it is also present in those patients with Cushing's disease with extremely high cortisol production [4].

Dynamic non-invasive tests

High-dose dexamethasone suppression test (HDDST)
The HDDST, 2 mg given every 6 h for 48 h, or a single 8 mg dose, has been in widespread use for many years. The test relies upon the relative sensitivity of pituitary corticotroph adenomas to the effects of glucocorticoids, compared to the resistance exhibited by non-pituitary tumors. Approximately 80% of patients with Cushing's disease will demonstrate suppression of the serum cortisol to a value of <50% of the basal level [4]. This is less than the pretest likelihood of Cushing's disease and, thus, by itself the high-dose dexamethasone suppression test has little diagnostic utility. Moreover, when utilizing the 48-h LDSST, if there has already been the demonstration of suppression of serum cortisol by more than 30%, there is no further advantage to utilizing the HDDST. The continued routine use of the HDDST can no longer be recommended except when BIPSS is not available.

CRH test
Recombinant human or ovine-sequence CRH is administered as an intravenous bolus dose of either 1 μg/kg or more usually 100 μg intravenous. This stimulates corticotroph tumor cells in the pituitary to release ACTH and hence increase serum cortisol concentrations, whilst responses are uncommon in the ectopic ACTH syndrome. The ovine-sequence CRH test has a sensitivity of 93% for Cushing's disease based on ACTH responses at 15 and 30 minutes [12].

Considered in isolation this is only just above the pretest likelihood, at least in women, but is useful information when in context of other tests (see below). An almost identical sensitivity is found for the human-sequence peptide sampling at the same time points [13].

Desmopressin testing
Since the V3 receptor is expressed in pituitary and many ectopic tumors secreting ACTH, the desmopressin test is of limited utility in the differential diagnosis of ACTH-dependent Cushing's syndrome. Similarly, a combined test using CRH and desmopressin has been used, but larger series have suggested that there remains overlap between responses in patients with Cushing's disease and the ectopic ACTH syndrome. Responses to both CRH testing and the HDDST are also more frequently discordant in patients with Cushing's disease secondary to a pituitary macroadenoma.

Invasive testing

BIPSS
If a patient has ACTH-dependent Cushing's syndrome, with responses *both* on dexamethasone suppression *and* CRH testing suggesting pituitary disease, and the pituitary MRI scan shows an isolated lesion of 6 mm or more, most will regard the diagnosis of Cushing's disease to have been made. A major problem is that up to 40% of patients with proven Cushing's disease have normal pituitary MRI scans [11]. In these cases, sampling of the gradient of ACTH from the pituitary to the periphery is the most reliable means for discriminating between pituitary and non-pituitary sources of ACTH. Since the pituitary effluent drains via the cavernous sinuses to the petrosal sinuses and then jugular bulb, there is a gradient of the value of plasma ACTH compared to the simultaneous peripheral sample when there is a central source of ACTH. BIPSS is a highly skilled and invasive technique, requiring placement of catheters in both inferior petrosal sinuses. Catheter position and venous anatomy require confirmation by venography, as non-uniform drainage is not uncommon. The diagnostic accuracy of the test is improved with the administration of CRH. A basal central:peripheral ratio of >2:1 or a CRH-stimulated ratio of >3:1 is consistent with Cushing's disease. The combined data for many series indicate sensitivity and specificity of 94% [14]. Where CRH is unobtainable or too costly, desmopressin offers a reasonable alternative, but few patients with ectopic ACTH secretion have been studied in this way. Small series data have suggested that these false-negative responses can be identified by simultaneous sampling of prolactin to correct values in ACTH. It is possible that false-positive results may be caused by inadequate suppression of the normal corticotrophs; the duration and amount of hypercortisolism should be assessed prior to the test. Pretreatment with cortisol-lowering agents prior to BIPSS is to be strongly discouraged as this increases the likelihood of a false-positive response in a patient with ectopic disease.

In adults, BIPSS is only 70% accurate for lateralization of the source of ACTH within the pituitary gland [4, 8], but in children it may have greater accuracy for this purpose than MRI. Sampling from the cavernous sinuses directly does not improve accuracy.

Internal jugular venous sampling

Sampling from the internal jugular vein has been proposed as a simplified procedure. Direct comparison in the same patients has shown this to be inferior to BIPSS. This test may, however, have utility in centers of limited sampling experience, and BIPSS reserved if the results are negative. It is not in widespread use.

Imaging in suspected Cushing's disease

Adrenal

CT gives the best resolution of adrenal anatomy. In ACTH-dependent Cushing's syndrome nodules may occur and adrenal hyperplasia is not always symmetrical, causing diagnostic confusion with a unilateral primary adrenal cause if the biochemistry is not strictly assessed; in 30% of Cushing's disease the adrenal glands appear normal, whilst in ectopic ACTH the adrenals are virtually always homogeneously enlarged.

Pituitary

Up to 40% of corticotroph adenomas causing Cushing's disease in adults are not visible on MRI scanning [11]. Those that are visible usually fail to enhance following gadolinium on T1-weighted imaging (Fig. 31.3). The use of dynamic MRI, with the administration of intravenous contrast media and rapid sequence acquisition following this, does not improve the overall diagnostic rate. However, spoiled gradient sequences may have greater sensitivity. There is also a 10% rate of pituitary incidentalomas in the normal population, emphasizing the need for careful biochemical discrimination of pituitary from non-pituitary sources of ACTH.

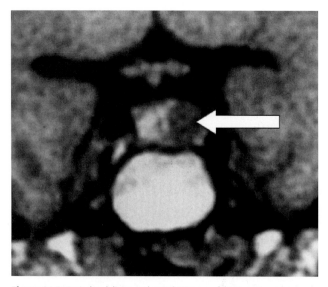

Figure 31.3 Typical gadolinium-enhanced MRI scan of pituitary microadenoma causing Cushing's disease. Note non-enhancement in left sided 6 mm pituitary microadenoma (arrow), with minimal deviation of optic chiasm to the left.

In the absence of a pituitary macroadenoma, an abnormal MRI is not conclusive evidence in favor of Cushing's disease.

Management

Overview

Management is aimed at lowering cortisol levels, removing tumor tissue and causing the least harm to remaining pituitary function. In most cases control of tumor volume is not a priority as the majority have either microadenomas or no visible tumor on MRI. The mainstay of management remains transsphenoidal surgery, but in a given patient it may be necessary to use some or all of the treatments outlined below. Some centers use medical therapy to control hypercortisolemia prior to surgery, and this makes intuitive sense, but there are no published data that this affects overall outcome.

Medical therapies to lower cortisol

Metyrapone, ketoconazole and mitotane may all be used to lower cortisol by directly inhibiting synthesis and secretion in the adrenal gland [1]. Metyrapone and ketoconazole are enzyme inhibitors and have a rapid onset of action, but there is frequent escape of control of hypercortisolism in the face of ACTH over-secretion in Cushing's disease. These agents are not usually effective as the sole long-term treatment of Cushing's disease, and are used mainly either in preparation for surgery, or as adjunctive therapy following surgery and/or pituitary radiotherapy. Doses used for these agents are: metyrapone (500–1000 mg three to four times a day, dose increments every 72 h) and ketoconazole (200–400 mg three times a day, dose increments at 2 to 3 weekly intervals), aiming for a mean plasma cortisol level (five samples over the day) of 5.4–10.9 µg/dL (150–300 mmol/L). Metyrapone causes an increase in steroid androgenic precursors and hirsutism is a major adverse effect in women, whilst this does not occur with ketoconazole. In the UK o,p′DDD (mitotane), an adrenolytic agent, is usually reserved for the treatment of adrenocortical carcinoma. Mitotane acts as an adrenolytic drug, with delayed onset but long-lasting action, but there is no escape phenomenon. Medical therapy may also be used in patients who are unwilling or unfit to undergo surgery. These agents have gastrointestinal side effects, and with ketoconazole hepatocellular dysfunction is not infrequently observed, and rare cases of hepatic failure described. For the acute control of severe hypercortisolemia when the oral route is not available, the short-acting anesthetic agent etomidate can be extremely useful.

New therapies to lower ACTH

Over the past 30 years many agents have been used in an attempt to inhibit the secretion of ACTH by corticotroph tumors, but to date none has been shown to consistently lower plasma ACTH. If a compound were to be developed for the treatment of Cushing's disease with the equivalent efficacy that dopamine agonists have for prolactinomas, this would be a huge step forward.

Recently, there has been renewed interest in the use of agents that might act in this manner. The peroxisome proliferator-activated receptor-γ (PPAR-γ) agonist rosiglitazone reduced ACTH and cortisol levels, and prevented tumor growth, in an animal model of Cushing's disease [15]. While human pituitary corticotroph tumors express PPAR-γ, recent studies in patients with Cushing's disease have, unfortunately, been almost uniformly disappointing. Rosiglitazone achieved only short-term control of cortisol, with later escape [16, 17]. Similarly, the PPAR-γ agonist pioglitazone (at licensed doses) did not affect ACTH levels [18]. Rosiglitazone at 1.5 times the licensed dose did not decrease the high levels of ACTH due to corticotroph tumor progression after bilateral adrenalectomy (Nelson syndrome) despite expression of PPAR-γ in tumor samples [19]. This paradox may be explained by the fact that the action of these compounds in pituitary tumors, at least *in vitro*, may be independent of PPAR-γ expression [20]. Corticotroph tumors may also express the dopamine-2 receptor and short-term administration of cabergoline at a dose of 1–3 mg/week may reduce hypercortisolism in up to 40% of cases [21], but larger studies are needed. The newer somatostatin analog, SOM-230, reduces ACTH secretion in cell culture models and in culture of human corticotroph tumor cells [22], and early data suggest that it appears to lower cortisol levels in some patients with Cushing's disease [23]. Finally, there are preliminary data in an animal model that retinoic acid may cause direct inhibition of ACTH secretion from corticotroph tumors [24].

Surgery

Transsphenoidal surgery

Numerous series, including many within the last 5 years, have reported the results and long-term follow-up following transsphenoidal surgery for Cushing's disease. Transsphenoidal surgery offers the potential for a selective microadenectomy of the causative corticotroph adenoma leaving the remaining pituitary function intact. Taking all series in the world literature together, there is a quoted initial remission rate of 60–80%, but with a relapse rate of up to 20% when followed for many years (Fig. 31.4) [1,25–35]. It is likely that these variations reflect surgical skill as well as the controversy regarding the characterization of remission or continuing disease in the postoperative period. Overall, with careful and prolonged follow-up (10 years) the long-term remission rate is approximately 60%: series suggesting rates higher than this either have shorter follow-up or less stringent criteria for remission. Patients who are hypocortisolemic (low 09:00 h serum cortisol) in the immediate postoperative period require glucocorticoid therapy until the hypothalamic–pituitary–adrenal axis recovers, usually 6–18 months postoperatively. While long-term remission is most likely when postoperative serum cortisol is low [<1.8 μg/dL (<50 nmol/L)], there is no threshold value that fully excludes possible recurrence. Care needs to be taken in the interpretation of postoperative serum cortisol in those patients who have received high-dose perioperative glucocorticoids, as these may suppress the level of cortisol in any remaining corticotroph tumor cells, ostensibly the patient appearing to be in

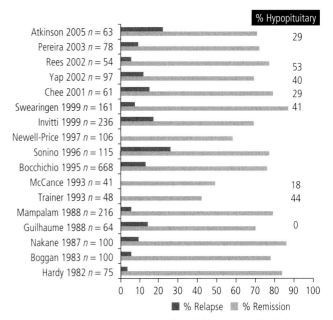

Figure 31.4 Long-term outcome of transsphenoidal surgery for Cushing's disease. Initial remission rates in gray, relapse in black. Note that the lower initial remission rates are frequently associated with less relapse on follow-up. Hypopituitary rates are given in the right-hand column.

remission, but then for the tumor cells to grow slowly and relapse appear years later. Similarly, suppression of serum cortisol on dexamethasone testing in the postoperative period is a poor indicator of long-term remission. Levels of postoperative serum cortisol of 3.6–7.3 μg/dL (100–200 nmol/L) do not necessarily indicate failure of surgery, as some patients may remain in long-term remission. On the other hand levels above 7.3 μg/dL (200 nmol/L) will almost always indicate failure of surgery. If there is clear persistent disease postoperatively, immediate reoperation may be of benefit. There is no agreement as to whether the presence or absence of a microadenoma on MRI makes remission more likely, but remission for macroadenomas is <15%.

On careful endocrine testing some series show that there may be deficiencies of other pituitary hormones in up to 50% of cases. It is important to note that functional deficiencies of growth hormone secondary to hypercortisolemia may remain for 2 years after achieving remission by surgery.

Together, these data emphasize the ongoing need for alternative medical therapies directed against the pituitary.

Adrenal surgery

In any case of ACTH-dependent Cushing's syndrome, total bilateral adrenalectomy induces a rapid resolution of the clinical features. Following surgery, patients require life-long treatment with glucocorticoid and mineralocorticoid. With the low morbidity associated with laparoscopic adrenal surgery, this approach is being considered more frequently, and possibly even as primary therapy in some patients with Cushing's disease, especially when disease is severe or because of patient preference. A major concern

(a)

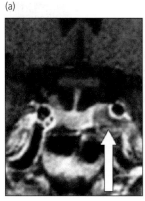

(b)

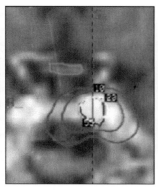

(c)

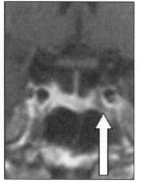

Figure 31.5 Gamma Knife stereotactic radiosurgery for Cushing's disease. (a) Pretreatment the laterally placed tumor (arrow) was inaccessible to surgical approaches. (b) Tumor targeting with Gamma Knife – 50% isodose to the tumor margin is seen, note the margin of safety from the 10% isodose to optic chiasm (outlined). (c) At 2-year follow-up the tumor has shrunk (arrow).

following bilateral adrenalectomy in patients with Cushing's disease is the development of Nelson syndrome: a locally aggressive pituitary tumor that secretes high levels of ACTH, resulting in pigmentation. It remains controversial as to whether the tumor progression is a result of the lack of cortisol feedback following adrenalectomy, or whether the progression reflects corticotroph tumors that were always programmed to behave in an aggressive manner [36]. If no tumor is visible on pituitary MRI at the time of adrenalectomy the likelihood of Nelson syndrome is much less. The tumor itself may be treated with further surgery or radiotherapy. Some advocate pituitary radiotherapy at the time of adrenalectomy to reduce the risk of this syndrome [37], but others have not confirmed this [36].

Fractionated external pituitary radiotherapy

Persisting hypercortisolemia following transsphenoidal surgery may be treated with pituitary radiotherapy. Conventional fractionated radiotherapy is an extremely effective means of treatment but is associated with long-term hypopituitarism [38], and may take many years to be effective, although it tends to be more rapid in children. Whilst waiting for the effect of radiotherapy to happen patients will usually require continued treatment with cortisol-lowering drugs, with regular biochemical assessment.

Stereotactic radiosurgery

More recently, use of stereotactic radiosurgery has been reported [39, 40]. Despite enthusiasm for the "Gamma Knife," recent data show a relapse rate of up to 20% following treatment [41], which does not compare favorably to conventional radiotherapy. It is likely that this poorer outcome reflects case selection. In some circumstances Gamma Knife radiotherapy can be extremely effective, even as primary therapy, and may be more rapid in onset and in efficacy. This depends on absolute confidence in diagnosis, and an anatomically favorable lesion, especially if not approachable by surgery. Such a case treated at our institution is illustrated in Fig. 31.5. This tumor encasing the left cavernous sinus was not treatable by surgery and was confirmed as the source of ACTH by BIPSS. This was treated with Gamma Knife radiosurgery as primary treatment. Within 1 year the patient was hypocortisolemic. By 2 years the HPA axis had shown some recovery. By 3 years

there was a normal circadian rhythm of cortisol (midnight cortisol <1.8 μg/dL [<50 nmol/L]), a normal response of cortisol and GH on an insulin tolerance test (ITT), normal suppression on LDDST and no pituitary deficiency. Now, after over 6 years of follow-up the same clinical picture remains and, as shown in Fig. 31.5, the lesion has shrunk considerably. Except in highly selected cases such as this, Gamma Knife radiosurgery is not yet recommended.

Conclusion

Diagnosis and management of Cushing's syndrome remains a considerable challenge. The underlying pathogenesis of Cushing's disease remains to be elucidated. Given the complexity of diagnosis, differential diagnosis and further management, patients presenting with Cushing's syndrome warrant referral to major centers. The outcome of treatment for Cushing's disease remains disappointing in many patients, and further developments are needed in this area, especially novel approaches to medical therapy to lower ACTH.

References

1. Newell-Price J, Bertagna X, Grossman AB, Nieman LK. Cushing's syndrome. *Lancet* 2006;367:1605–1617.
2. Catargi B, Rigalleau V, Poussin A, et al. Occult Cushing's syndrome in type-2 diabetes. *J. Clin. Endocrinol. Metab.* 2003;88:5808–5813.
3. Dahia PL, Grossman AB. The molecular pathogenesis of corticotroph tumors. *Endocr. Rev.* 1999;20:136–155.
4. Newell-Price J, Trainer P, Besser M, Grossman A. The diagnosis and differential diagnosis of Cushing's syndrome and pseudo-Cushing's states. *Endocr. Rev.* 1998;19:647–672.
5. Picon A, Bertagna X, de Keyzer Y. Analysis of the human proopiomelanocortin gene promoter in a small cell lung carcinoma cell line reveals an unusual role for E2F transcription factors. *Oncogene* 1999;18:2627–2633.
6. Newell-Price J, King P, Clark AJ. The CpG island promoter of the human proopiomelanocortin gene is methylated in nonexpressing normal tissue and tumors and represses expression. *Mol. Endocrinol.* 2001;15:338–348.

7. Lindsay JR, Nieman LK. The hypothalamic–pituitary–adrenal axis in pregnancy: challenges in disease detection and treatment. *Endocr. Rev.* 2005.

8. Arnaldi G, Angeli A, Atkinson AB, et al. Diagnosis and complications of Cushing's syndrome: a consensus statement. *J. Clin. Endocrinol. Metab.* 2003;88:5593–5602.

9. Newell-Price J, Trainer P, Perry L, Wass J, Grossman A, Besser M. A single sleeping midnight cortisol has 100% sensitivity for the diagnosis of Cushing's syndrome. *Clin. Endocrinol. (Oxf.)* 1995;43:545–550.

10. Martin NM, Dhillo WS, Banerjee A, et al. Comparison of the dexamethasone-suppressed corticotropin-releasing hormone test and low-dose dexamethasone suppression test in the diagnosis of Cushing's syndrome. *J. Clin. Endocrinol. Metab.* 2006;91:2582–2586.

11. Invitti C, Pecori Giraldi F, de Martin M, Cavagnini F. Diagnosis and management of Cushing's syndrome: results of an Italian multicentre study. Study Group of the Italian Society of Endocrinology on the Pathophysiology of the Hypothalamic-Pituitary-Adrenal Axis. *J. Clin. Endocrinol. Metab.* 1999;84:440–448.

12. Nieman LK, Oldfield EH, Wesley R, Chrousos GP, Loriaux DL, Cutler GB, Jr. A simplified morning ovine corticotropin-releasing hormone stimulation test for the differential diagnosis of adrenocorticotropin-dependent Cushing's syndrome. *J. Clin. Endocrinol. Metab.* 1993;77:1308–1312.

13. Newell-Price J, Morris DG, Drake WM, et al. Optimal response criteria for the human CRH test in the differential diagnosis of ACTH-dependent Cushing's syndrome. *J. Clin. Endocrinol. Metab.* 2002;87:1640–1645.

14. Lindsay JR, Nieman LK. Differential diagnosis and imaging in Cushing's syndrome. *Endocrinol. Metab. Clin. North Am.* 2005;34:403–421, x.

15. Heaney AP, Fernando M, Yong WH, Melmed S. Functional PPAR-gamma receptor is a novel therapeutic target for ACTH-secreting pituitary adenomas. *Nat. Med.* 2002;8:1281–1287.

16. Cannavo S, Arosio M, Almoto B, Dall'Asta C, Ambrosi B. Effectiveness of long-term rosiglitazone administration in patients with Cushing's disease. *Clin. Endocrinol. (Oxf.)* 2005;63:118–119.

17. Ambrosi B, Dall'Asta C, Cannavo S, et al. Effects of chronic administration of PPAR-gamma ligand rosiglitazone in Cushing's disease. *Eur. J. Endocrinol.* 2004;151:173–178.

18. Suri D, Weiss RE. Effect of pioglitazone on adrenocorticotropic hormone and cortisol secretion in Cushing's disease. *J. Clin. Endocrinol. Metab.* 2005;90:1340–1346.

19. Munir A, Song, F, Ince P, Ross R, Newell-Price J. A pilot study of prolonged high dose rosiglitazone therapy (12 mg/day) in Nelson's syndrome. Society for Endocrinology 194th Annual Meeting. 2004.

20. Emery MN, Leontiou C, Bonner SE, et al. PPAR-gamma expression in pituitary tumours and the functional activity of the glitazones: evidence that any anti-proliferative effect of the glitazones is independent of the PPAR-gamma receptor. *Clin. Endocrinol. (Oxf.)* 2006;65:389–395.

21. Pivonello R, Ferone D, de Herder WW, et al. Dopamine receptor expression and function in corticotroph pituitary tumors. *J. Clin. Endocrinol. Metab.* 2004;89:2452–2462.

22. Hofland LJ, van der Hoek J, Feelders R, et al. The multi-ligand somatostatin analogue SOM230 inhibits ACTH secretion by cultured human corticotroph adenomas via somatostatin receptor type 5. *Eur. J. Endocrinol.* 2005;152:645–654.

23. Boscaro M, Atkinson A, Bertherat J, Petersenn S, Glusman JE, Tran LL. SOM230 Cushing's Disease Study Group. Early data on the efficacy and safety of the novel multi-ligand somatostatin analog, SOM230, in patients with Cushings disease. ENDO 2005. San Diego, CA, USA, 2005.

24. Paez-Pereda M, Kovalovsky D, Hopfner U, et al. Retinoic acid prevents experimental Cushing syndrome. *J. Clin. Invest.* 2001;108:1123–1131.

25. Swearingen B, Biller BM, Barker FG II, et al. Long-term mortality after transsphenoidal surgery for Cushing disease. *Ann. Intern. Med.* 1999;130:821–824.

26. Invitti C, Pecori Giraldi F, de Martin M, et al. Diagnosis and management of Cushing's syndrome: results of an Italian multicentre study. Study Group of the Italian Society of Endocrinology on the Pathophysiology of the Hypothalamic-Pituitary-Adrenal Axis. *J. Clin. Endocrinol. Metab.* 1999;84:440–448.

27. Sonino N, Zielezny M, Fava GA, et al. Risk factors and long-term outcome in pituitary-dependent Cushing's disease. *J. Clin. Endocrinol. Metab.* 1996;81:2647–2652.

28. Bochicchio D, Losa M, Buchfelder M. Factors influencing the immediate and late outcome of Cushing's disease treated by transsphenoidal surgery: a retrospective study by the European Cushing's Disease Survey Group. *J. Clin. Endocrinol. Metab.* 1995;80:3114–3120.

29. McCance DR, Gordon DS, Fannin TF, et al. Assessment of endocrine function after transsphenoidal surgery for Cushing's disease. *Clin. Endocrinol. (Oxf).* 1993;38(1):79–86.

30. Mampalam TJ, Tyrrell JB, Wilson CB. Transsphenoidal microsurgery for Cushing disease. A report of 216 cases. *Ann. Intern. Med.* 1988;109:487–493.

31. Guilhaume B, Bertagna X, Thomsen M, et al. Transsphenoidal pituitary surgery for the treatment of Cushing's disease: results in 64 patients and long term follow-up studies. *J. Clin. Endocrinol. Metab.* 1988;66:1056–1064.

32. Nakane T, Kuwayama A, Watanabe M, et al. Long term results of transsphenoidal adenomectomy in patients with Cushing's disease. *Neurosurgery* 1987;21:218–222.

33. Boggan JE, Tyrrell JB, Wilson CB. Transsphenoidal microsurgical management of Cushing's disease. Report of 100 cases. *J. Neurosurg.* 1983;59:195–200.

34. Hardy J. Presidential address: XVII Canadian Congress of Neurological Sciences. Cushing's disease: 50 years later. *Can. J. Neurol. Sci.* 1982;9:375–380.

35. Newell-Price JDC, Norris J, Afshar F, et al. Transsphenoidal hypophysectomy in Cushing's disease ± results and follow-up in 103 patients. *J. Endocrinol.* 1997;152:72.

36. Assié G, Bahurel H, Coste J, et al. Corticotroph tumor progression after adrenalectomy in Cushing's Disease: a reappraisal of Nelson's Syndrome. *J. Clin. Endocrinol. Metab.* 2007;92:172–179.

37. Jenkins PJ, Trainer PJ, Plowman PN, et al. The long-term outcome after adrenalectomy and prophylactic pituitary radiotherapy in adrenocorticotropin-dependent Cushing's syndrome. *J. Clin. Endocrinol. Metab.* 1995;80:165–171.

38. Estrada J, Boronat M, Mielgo M, et al. The long-term outcome of pituitary irradiation after unsuccessful transsphenoidal surgery in Cushing's disease. *N. Engl. J. Med.* 1997;336:172–177.

39. Devin JK, Allen GS, Cmelak AJ, Duggan DM, Blevins LS. The efficacy of linear accelerator radiosurgery in the management of patients with Cushing's disease. *Stereotact. Funct. Neurosurg.* 2004;82:254–262.

40. Sheehan JM, Vance ML, Sheehan JP, Ellegala DB, Laws ER Jr. Radiosurgery for Cushing's disease after failed transsphenoidal surgery. *J. Neurosurg.* 2000;93:738–742.

41. Vance ML, Chernavvsky DR, Steiner L, Laws ER. OR9-4. Relapse of Cushings disease after successful Gamma Knife treatment. Endocrine Society 87th Annual Meeting, June 4–7, 2005, San Diego, CA.

32 Non-functioning Pituitary Adenomas and Gonadotropinomas

Maarten O. van Aken, Aart Jan van der Lelij, and Steven W.J. Lamberts

---

Key points

- Non-functioning pituitary adenomas are frequently from gonadotroph origin, but they rarely secrete intact gonadotropins leading to a clinical syndrome.
- To differentiate a non-functioning pituitary adenoma from other intra- or parasellar lesions, a thorough work-up should be performed, including pituitary hormone measurements, evaluation of visual fields and magnetic resonance imaging.
- Transsphenoidal surgery is the primary treatment of large non-functioning pituitary adenoma with visual field disturbances.
- If a significant tumor remnant still exists, especially when accompanied with suprasellar extension, pituitary radiation therapy should be considered. In other cases, a policy of wait and see with sequential magnetic resonance imaging can be followed.
- Efficacy of medical therapies for non-functioning pituitary adenoma has been disappointing. In selected cases, treatment with dopamine agonists such as cabergoline has, however, been shown to be effective.

Introduction

All pituitary adenomas without apparent hypersecretion of pituitary hormones with clinical activity are gathered under the definition of non-functioning pituitary adenomas (NFPA). Most patients present late in the course of their disease when the tumor causes mass-related signs and symptoms. Furthermore, some NFPA present themselves as pituitary incidentalomas. The majority of NFPA are derived from proliferation of gonadotroph cells [1]. However, pure gonadotropinomas secreting intact molecules of follicle-stimulating hormone (FSH) or luteinizing hormone (LH) are rarely encountered and usually do not result in a recognizable clinical syndrome. Therefore, the diagnostic and therapeutic approach of gonadotropinomas is similar to that of NFPA.

In the following paragraphs, the multidisciplinary management of NFPA and gonadotropinomas, their diagnosis and therapeutic approaches are discussed.

Epidemiology

Pituitary adenomas are the most frequent type of intracerebral tumors (10%), and are found in 10–20% of subjects at autopsy

[2]. Non-functioning pituitary tumors make up about one third of all pituitary tumors. The incidence of NFPAs amounts to 7–9 new cases/million [3]. Pure gonadotropinomas secreting intact gonadotropins comprise less than 15% of all NFPA, mostly secreting FSH [4].

With the increasing use of (brain) imaging, pituitary incidentalomas are more frequently encountered. Magnetic resonance imaging (MRI) reveals abnormalities of greater than 3 mm in 10% of pituitaries [3]. These incidentalomas are usually non-functioning microadenomas.

Pathology and pathogenesis

NFPAs exhibit a marked heterogeneity of neoplastic pituitary cell types. The majority of tumors are presumably from gonadotroph origin, as shown by positive immunostaining for at least one glycoprotein hormone subunit in over 85% of cases [5, 6]. However, *in vivo* they are rarely associated with increased levels of dimeric LH or FSH. Increased levels of bio-inactive free subunits (free α-subunit mainly, LH-β subunit more rarely) are more frequently encountered, but are generally modest. A pathological classification distinguishes null cell adenomas and oncocytic adenomas, although these subtypes show a similar clinical behavior [7]. This is not the case for so-called silent corticotroph adenomas. These are pituitary adenomas that present as NFPA, but show positive immunoreactivity for ACTH. These adenomas are known for their more aggressive clinical course, especially when they show recurrence of growth after initial treatment [8].

Clinical Endocrine Oncology, 2nd edition. Edited by Ian D. Hay and John A.H. Wass. © 2008 Blackwell Publishing. ISBN 978-1-4051-4584-8.

A number of factors that might stimulate pituitary tumorigenesis have been studied, including the role of activation of specific oncogenes (Ras oncogene, c-myc oncogene, pituitary tumor transforming gene [PTTG]) or the inactivation of tumor suppressor genes (p53-gene, retinoblastoma (Rb) tumor suppressor gene, nm23) [9]. However, at present it is unclear whether the over- or underexpression of these factors may in fact be epiphenomena rather than etiologic molecules, especially as many of these factors are induced only after cells are transformed.

Several hereditary syndromes (multiple endocrine neoplasia [MEN] 1 syndrome, Carney complex, McCune–Albright syndrome) are associated with pituitary tumors, although the majority of these tumors are actively secreting pituitary hormones, especially growth hormone, prolactin and adrenocorticotropic hormone (ACTH). Recently, several cases of non-MEN 1/Carney complex familial isolated pituitary adenomas (FIPA) were described, including 28 NFPA. This could possibly represent a new hereditary endocrine syndrome, requiring further genetic characterization [10].

Apart from genetic alterations, humoral factors are likely involved in pituitary tumor pathogenesis, such as the presence of gonadotropin-releasing hormone (GnRH) in human pituitary adenomas, which might act as a paracrine/autocrine factor to induce a gonadotroph adenoma [11].

Clinical presentation

The main symptomatology problems raised by NFPA are mass effect problems, responsible for optic chiasm compression or deficient hormone secretion resulting from compression of normal anterior pituitary cells.

Visual field disturbance

Not infrequently, visual field abnormalities are the first clinical symptoms in a patient with a NFPA. Suprasellar extension of a pituitary mass can lead to compression of the optic chiasm. Due to the topographic orientation of the nerve fibers in the optical tract, the temporal visual fields (i.e. the innervation of the nasal part of the retina) will usually be compromised first, eventually leading to bitemporal hemianopia. However, depending on the tumor extent relative to the anatomy of the optic chiasm, other types of visual deficits can be seen. With progressive compression of the optical tract, visual accuracy can be reduced as well.

Hypopituitarism

The mass effect of a NFPA can result in damage to and dysfunction of the normal anterior pituitary cells, leading to hypopituitarism. Usually, pituitary hormone deficiency occurs following a specific pattern, with growth hormone (GH) deficiency as the most frequent event, followed by gonadotropin, adrenocorticotropin and thyrotropin deficiency. This order of events might be explained by a different threshold of vulnerability of the specific pituitary cell types. Alternatively, the topographic orientation of the pituitary cells in relation to the vascular supply could render the somatotropic and gonadotropic cells more susceptible to increased pressure in the sellar region.

The clinical manifestations of hypopituitarism are variable, often insidious in onset and dependent on the degree of hormone deficiency [12]. In secondary hormone deficiencies, for example thyrotropin deficiency, some basal hormone secretion can be preserved, resulting in a less severe clinical phenotype compared with primary hypothyroidism. Corticotropin deficiency is less evident than primary adrenal deficiency, since in most cases mineralocorticoid secretion remains intact. During intercurrent illnesses or surgical procedures, however, corticotropin secretion may not increase appropriately, in which case life-threatening adrenal crisis may develop.

In men with recent-onset hypogonadism, physical examination is usually normal, while diminished facial and body hair, gynecomastia and small, soft testes are features of long-standing hypogonadism. Anemia can also occur due to diminished erythropoiesis associated with hypogonadism. In premenopausal women, secondary amenorrhea is a common feature.

GH deficiency is associated with diminished exercise tolerance, an increased (central) body fat and premature atherosclerosis. These physical limitations, in combination with decreased social functioning, lead to a decreased quality of life in patients with severe growth hormone deficiency. In partial growth hormone deficiency, however, these features are often less severe.

Mild hyperprolactinemia (up to three times the upper limit of normal) is common in patients with hypopituitarism, due to the interference of a pituitary mass with dopaminergic inhibition of prolactin secretion or due to a macroprolactinoma. Galactorrhea may occur, but more frequently hypogonadism is observed, due to the effect of raised prolactin levels on normal pulsatile gonadotropin secretion.

Cranial nerves

Lateral extension of a pituitary mass can lead to compression of several cranial nerves (III, IV, and VI) that travel through the region of the cavernous sinus, located at both sides of the sellar region. Clinical signs include ophthalmoplegia and ptosis.

Headache is also frequently presented in patients with macroadenomas, probably induced by the mass effect of a macroadenoma, demonstrated by resolution of headache after successful transsphenoidal decompression.

Gonadotropin excess

In those rare cases with intact gonadotropin secretion, usually no recognizable clinical syndrome develops. There have been several case reports documenting a FSH-secreting pituitary adenoma, resulting in an ovarian hyperstimulation syndrome in premenopausal women and intact LH secretion causing supranormal testosterone secretion [13, 14].

Apoplexy

Finally, acute hemorrhage within a NFPA may lead to a clinical presentation of pituitary apoplexy, characterized by severe acute headache, often accompanied by nausea and vomiting. Following this event, sudden deterioration of visual fields can occur, as a result of expansion of the sellar mass caused by the intralesional bleeding. Pituitary apoplexy should be managed as a medical emergency, with prompt hospitalization and evaluation.

Diagnosis

Because many patients with NFPA lack a specific serum hormone marker, it may be difficult to distinguish these tumors from other intra- and suprasellar non-pituitary masses that may mimic pituitary adenomas in their clinical, endocrinological and radiographic presentation. The differential diagnosis of these lesions includes craniopharyngiomas, meningiomas, arachnoid cysts, granulomatous diseases, gliomas, aneurysm, metastatic tumors, and lymphocytic hypophysitis. Differentiation between these options can be important, as their management is not always the same. However, a definite diagnosis can often only be made after transsphenoidal surgery, as specific clinical, biochemical or radiological markers are lacking.

The work-up (Fig. 32.1) will start with a thorough medical history, focusing on visual field abnormalities and signs of hypopituitarism. Information on the duration of symptoms may provide an estimate of the time-course of the development of a pituitary mass. During physical examination, visual fields and ocular movement can be evaluated, as well as signs of hypopituitarism.

Subsequently, endocrine function can be evaluated, starting with basal hormone levels, followed by, when indicated, specific stimulatory tests. Any pituitary hormone deficiency should be treated accordingly, with the exception of growth hormone deficiency, which is usually evaluated and treated several months after transsphenoidal surgery.

Measurement of serum α-subunits can be performed, either in basal state or after the administration of thyrotropin-releasing hormone (TRH). However, these tests have shown insufficient sensitivity and specificity for the differentiation between NFPA and non-endocrine pituitary tumors [15].

Ophthalmologic evaluation, to determine visual accuracy and visual fields, is mandatory. If cranial nerve palsies are present further neurological evaluation can be performed.

For imaging of a pituitary mass, MRI is the most specific and sensitive technique, allowing detailed determination of extension to the optic chiasm and other structures adjacent to the sella and also differentiation from other lesions in the pituitary region [16]. In addition, using magnetic resonance angiography, an aberrant anatomy of the circle of Willis can be detected, which can be important for subsequent pituitary surgery.

Computerized tomography (CT) can be applied to detect calcifications within a sellar mass, which is suggestive of a craniopharyngioma.

Neurotransmitter-receptor ligand imaging by single photon emission CT (SPECT) with ^{123}I-epidepride and/or ^{111}In-DTPA-octreotide characterizes the dopamine D2 and somatostatin

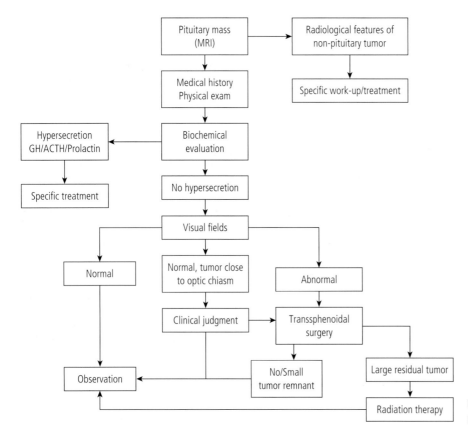

Figure 32.1 Work-up for patients presenting with a pituitary mass.

receptor status of pituitary adenomas, respectively. In selected cases, these techniques may be used for the differential diagnosis of pituitary tumors and primary parasellar lesions with presentations in the sellar region.

Finally, positron emission tomography (PET) might be of use in the work-up of patients with a pituitary mass, but large clinical studies are still lacking.

Management

Observation

The strategy of observation only for patients with incidentally discovered pituitary adenomas may be appropriate, provided that the tumor is well delimited, small, has no extension with risk of neurological or visual chiasm compression, and that a meticulous hormonal work-up has ruled out the possibility of a minimal hormonal hypersecretion. In these cases regular follow-up by MRI is mandatory in order to detect possible NFPA enlargement that could lead to surgical intervention. In addition, medical treatment with a dopamine agonist can be tried in an attempt to achieve stabilization or even shrinkage of the pituitary adenoma (see below).

Surgery

Transsphenoidal surgery is the primary treatment of a NFPA with visual field disturbances. In experienced hands, it is a safe and

effective technique that has recently been refined by the introduction of endoscopic pituitary surgery. Fig. 32.2 shows the MRI scans of a patient with a NFPA before and 3 months after transsphenoidal surgery, resulting in decompression of the optical tract and an empty sella. After surgical relief of the mass effect of a NFPA, vision improves in 70% of patients with preoperative visual field defects. Pre-existing hypopituitarism may also improve in a substantial number of patients, although in case of pre-existing panhypopituitarism this will only rarely be the case [17]. Postoperative complications are cerebrospinal fluid leakage, meningitis and diabetes insipidus.

Given the success rate of transsphenoidal surgery, transfrontal surgery is rarely indicated and is associated with a much higher morbidity and mortality rate. Exceptions are giant macroadenomas where the bulk of the tumor extents suprasellarly.

Radiation therapy

The role of pituitary radiation therapy (RT) in the management of NFPA remains controversial. After transsphenoidal surgery, not unusually adenoma remnants will be present in the sellar region. Observational studies suggest that RT is effective in preventing the regrowth of residual adenoma tissue following initial surgical debulking. For clinical decision making, the risk of regrowth of these tumor remnants and possible complications of pituitary RT are the main issues.

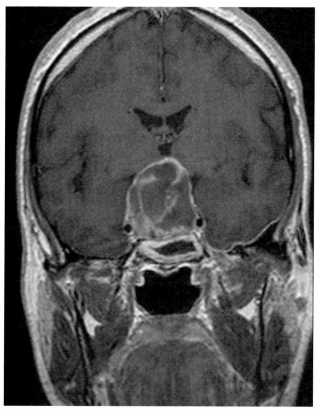 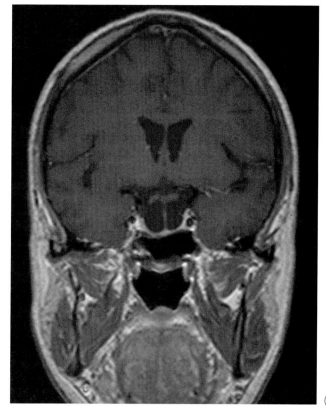

(a) (b)

Figure 32.2 (a) MRI of a patient with NFPA, with signs of previous intraperitoneal haemorrhage. (b) The same patient, 3 months after transsphenoidal surgery. No residual adenomatous tissue can be identified and the optical tract is clearly visible.

There are conflicting data on the risk of regrowth of tumor remnants in the absence of pituitary RT. Initial series after the introduction of transsphenoidal surgery showed tumor regrowth in up to 75% of subjects, probably related to poor surgical techniques [18]. More recent studies have reported that without RT, approximately 10–30% of tumors may show recurrence within 5–20 years after what was considered a successful surgical resection. At present, there are no reliable clinical, pathological or molecular parameters that predict the likelihood of tumor regrowth.

Potential complications of pituitary RT are hypopituitarism and its associated excess mortality, the risk of second brain tumors, damage to the optic chiasm and neuropsychological changes [18].

A pragmatic approach can be adopted, based on the initial postoperative MRI scan [19]. If there is a significant tumor remnant, especially extending above the sella, RT may be considered. In other cases a policy of observation with sequential MRI scanning can be followed. In case of a silent corticotroph adenoma, RT can be considered even with small postoperative tumor remnants, to prevent the recurrence of an aggressive pituitary tumor.

Medical therapy of NFPA

NFPA can express functional dopamine D2 receptors. Therapy with dopamine agonists may, therefore, result in a reduction of tumor size in some NFPA patients. Indeed, some patients with NFPA show dramatic tumor shrinkage with dopamine agonist therapy, especially with cabergoline. However, in most studies the response to dopamine agonists has been disappointing, with stabilization or tumor shrinkage in less than 10% of subjects. The heterogeneity of responses to treatment has been attributed to the different pattern and level of expression of dopamine receptor subtypes in the individual tumors, as well as to possible alterations in the signal transduction pathway. No useful clinical test currently exists which can predict the response to dopaminergic treatment in a NFPA patient, including ^{123}I-epidepride dopamine D2 receptor imaging.

Somatostatin receptor subtypes 2, 3 and 5 have been identified on human NFPA. *In vitro*, incubation of adenoma cells with octreotide resulted in mild inhibition of gonadotropin or α-subunit release [20]. However, *in vivo*, long-term treatment with high doses of octreotide did not result in substantial tumor size reduction, despite improvement of visual field defects in a substantial number of patients [21, 22]. Whether new somatostatin analogs (e.g. SOM230 which is a multiligand agonist) will improve these results is presently unknown.

Long-term administration of GnRH agonists to normal persons downregulates gonadotropin-releasing hormone receptors on normal gonadotroph cells and decreases gonadotropin secretion. In patients with gonadotroph adenomas, however, these agonists produce either agonist effects or no effect on hormone secretion, with no effect on adenoma size [14]. Similarly, GnRH antagonists have not proven effective.

The nuclear hormone receptor peroxisome proliferator-activated receptor-γ (PPAR-γ) was shown to be present on pituitary adenomas [23]. *In vitro*, PPAR-γ agonists induced cell cycle arrest and apoptosis in murine gonadotroph pituitary tumor cells, and suppressed *in vitro* hormone secretion.

However, clinical results, especially in ACTH-secreting pituitary adenomas, have been disappointing, possibly explained by the very high *in vitro* concentrations that cannot be used *in vivo*.

In summary, novel pharmacological treatments have not proven successful, and transsphenoidal surgery is still the primary treatment for large, symptomatic NFPA.

Conclusion

For the multidisciplinary management of patients with NFPA, endocrinologists, radiologists, clinical chemists, neurosurgeons, pathologists and radiotherapists are involved. From several studies it appears that in patients with NFPA, even after successful treatment, quality of life is considerably reduced. Optimization of diagnostic, therapeutic and prognostic tools could lead to further improvement of care for these patients.

References

1. Snyder PJ. Gonadotroph cell pituitary adenomas. *Endocrinol. Metab Clin. North Am.* 1987;16:755–764.
2. Suhardja AS, Kovacs KT, Rutka JT. Molecular pathogenesis of pituitary adenomas: a review. *Acta Neurochir. (Wien).* 1999;141:729–736.
3. Clayton RN. Sporadic pituitary tumours: from epidemiology to use of databases. *Baillière's Best. Pract. Res. Clin. Endocrinol. Metab.* 1999;13:451–460.
4. Hanson PL, Aylwin SJ, Monson JP, Burrin JM. FSH secretion predominates in vivo and in vitro in patients with non-functioning pituitary adenomas. *Eur. J. Endocrinol.* 2005;152:363–370.
5. Kovacs K. The pathology of clinically non-functioning pituitary adenomas. *Pathol. Res. Pract.* 1991;187:571–573.
6. Melmed S. Pathogenesis of pituitary tumors. *Endocrinol. Metab Clin. North Am.* 1999;28:1–12, v.
7. Kovacs K, Scheithauer BW, Horvath E, Lloyd RV. The World Health Organization classification of adenohypophysial neoplasms. A proposed five-tier scheme. *Cancer* 1996;78:502–510.
8. Bradley KJ, Wass JA, Turner HE. Non-functioning pituitary adenomas with positive immunoreactivity for ACTH behave more aggressively than ACTH immunonegative tumours but do not recur more frequently. *Clin. Endocrinol. (Oxf.)* 2003;58:59–64.
9. Heaney AP, Melmed S. New pituitary oncogenes. *Endocr. Relat. Cancer* 2000;7:3–15.
10. Daly AF, Jaffrain-Rea ML, Ciccarelli A, et al. Clinical characterization of familial isolated pituitary adenomas. *J. Clin. Endocrinol. Metab.* 2006;91:3316–3323.
11. Miller GM, Alexander JM, Klibanski A. Gonadotropin-releasing hormone messenger RNA expression in gonadotroph tumors and normal human pituitary. *J. Clin. Endocrinol. Metab.* 1996;81:80–83.
12. van Aken MO, Lamberts SW. Diagnosis and treatment of hypopituitarism: an update. *Pituitary* 2005;8:183–191.
13. Shimon I, Rubinek T, Bar-Hava I, et al. Ovarian hyperstimulation without elevated serum estradiol associated with pure follicle–stimulating

hormone-secreting pituitary adenoma. *J. Clin. Endocrinol. Metab.* 2001;86:3635–3640.

14. Snyder PJ. Extensive personal experience: gonadotroph adenomas. *J. Clin. Endocrinol. Metab.* 1995;80:1059–1061.

15. Nobels FR, Kwekkeboom DJ, Coopmans W, et al. A comparison between the diagnostic value of gonadotropins, alpha-subunit, and chromogranin-A and their response to thyrotropin-releasing hormone in clinically nonfunctioning, alpha-subunit-secreting, and gonadotroph pituitary adenomas. *J. Clin. Endocrinol. Metab.* 1993;77:784–789.

16. De Herder WW, Lamberts SW. Imaging of pituitary tumours. *Baillière's Clin. Endocrinol. Metab.* 1995;9:367–389.

17. Arafah BM, Prunty D, Ybarra J, Hlavin ML, Selman WR. The dominant role of increased intrasellar pressure in the pathogenesis of hypopituitarism, hyperprolactinemia, and headaches in patients with pituitary adenomas. *J. Clin. Endocrinol. Metab.* 2000;85:1789–1793.

18. Boelaert K, Gittoes NJ. Radiotherapy for non-functioning pituitary adenomas. *Eur. J. Endocrinol.* 2001;144:569–575.

19. Gittoes NJ. Radiotherapy for non-functioning pituitary tumors – when and under what circumstances? *Pituitary* 2003;6:103–108.

20. de Bruin TW, Kwekkeboom DJ, Van't Verlaat JW, et al. Clinically nonfunctioning pituitary adenoma and octreotide response to long term high dose treatment, and studies in vitro. *J. Clin. Endocrinol. Metab.* 1992;75:1310–1317.

21. Lamberts SW, van der Lely AJ, De Herder WW, Hofland LJ. Octreotide. *N. Engl. J. Med.* 1996;334:246–254.

22. Hofland LJ, Lamberts SW. Somatostatin receptors in pituitary function, diagnosis and therapy. *Front. Horm. Res.* 2004;32:235–252.

23. Heaney AP, Fernando M, Melmed S. PPAR-gamma receptor ligands: novel therapy for pituitary adenomas. *J. Clin. Invest.* 2003;111:1381–1388.

33 Thyrotropinomas

Paolo Beck-Peccoz and Luca Persani

> **Key points**
> - Thyrotropinomas are a rare cause of hyperthyroidism. Somatic mutations of thyroid hormone receptors, increased expression of basic fibroblast growth factor and loss of heterozygosity and particular polymorphisms of somatostatin receptor type 5 are involved in tumor pathogenesis.
> - Ultrasensitive thyroid stimulating hormone assays allow a clear distinction between patients with primary hyperthyroidism (Graves disease or toxic nodular goiter) and those with thyrotropinoma or pituitary resistance to thyroid hormone.
> - Failure to recognize the presence of a thyrotropinoma may result in dramatic consequences, such as improper thyroid ablation that may cause the pituitary tumor volume to further expand.

Introduction

Thyrotropinomas are rare pituitary adenomas and an even more rare cause of hyperthyroidism. The biochemical features are quite characteristic, as the levels of circulating free thyroid hormones (fT_4 and fT_3) are elevated in the presence of normal/high serum thyroid-stimulating hormone (TSH) concentrations. TSH secretion from the tumor is autonomous and thus refractory to the negative feedback of thyroid hormones ("inappropriate TSH secretion") and TSH itself is responsible for the hyperstimulation of the thyroid gland and the consequent hypersecretion of thyroid hormones (Fig. 33.1) [1, 2]. Therefore, this entity can be appropriately classified as a form of "central hyperthyroidism." The first case of thyrotropinoma was documented in 1960 by measuring serum TSH levels with a bioassay [3]. In 1970, Hamilton et al. [4] reported the first case of thyrotropinoma proved by measuring TSH by radioimmunoassay (RIA). The routine use of ultrasensitive immunometric assays for TSH measurement greatly improved the diagnostic work-up of hyperthyroid patients, allowing the recognition of the cases with unsuppressed TSH secretion. As a consequence, thyrotropinomas are now more often diagnosed earlier, before the stage of macroadenoma, and an increased number of patients with normal or elevated TSH levels in the presence of high free thyroid hormone concentrations have been recognized [2]. Since these biochemical features are shared with patients with resistance to thyroid hormones (RTH), particularly the "selective" pituitary form of RTH (PRTH), a correct differential diagnosis between the two disorders is mandatory [1, 2, 5].

Clinical Endocrine Oncology, 2nd edition. Edited by Ian D. Hay and John A.H. Wass. © 2008 Blackwell Publishing. ISBN 978-1-4051-4584-8.

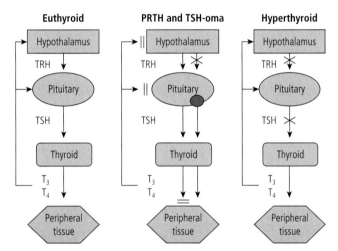

Figure 33.1 Schematic representation of hypothalamic–pituitary–thyroid axis in patients with "inappropriate secretion of TSH," i.e. thyrotropinoma and pituitary resistance to thyroid hormone (PRTH), as compared to that present in euthyroid subjects and in patients with "primary" hyperthyroidism. Note that thyrotropin-releasing hormone and TSH secretions are inhibited in patients with primary hyperthyroidism. In thyrotropinomas, TSH secretion is autonomous and insensible to thyroid hormone feedback mechanism, TRH secretion is blocked, goiter is the rule and hyperthyroidism is present at the peripheral tissue level. In PRTH, TRH and TSH secretions are not inhibited due to resistance to thyroid hormone action, which is also present at the level of some peripheral tissue, with the exception of PRTH where the resistance appears less potent in some tissues, mainly myocardium (tachycardia) and bone (osteopenia).

Failure to recognize these different diseases may result in dramatic consequences, such as incorrect thyroid ablation in patients with central hyperthyroidism or unnecessary pituitary surgery in those with RTH. Conversely, early diagnosis and correct treatment of thyrotropinomas may prevent the occurrence of neurological and endocrine complications, such as headache, visual field defects and hypopituitarism, and should improve the rate of cure.

Pathogenesis and molecular studies

The molecular mechanisms leading to the formation of thyrotropinomas are presently unknown, as is true for other types of pituitary adenomas. Inactivation analysis of the X-chromosome demonstrated that most pituitary adenomas, including the small number of thyrotropinomas investigated, derive from the clonal expansion of a single initially transformed cell. Accordingly, the general principles of tumorigenesis, that assume the presence of a transforming event providing gain of proliferative function followed by secondary mutations or alterations favoring tumor progression, presumably also apply to thyrotropinomas.

A large number of candidate genes, including common protooncogenes and tumor suppressor genes as well as pituitary-specific genes, have been screened for mutations able to confer growth advantage to pituitary cells. In analogy with the other pituitary adenomas, no mutations in oncogenes commonly activated in human cancer, particularly *Ras*, have been reported in thyrotropinomas. In contrast with growth hormone (GH)-secreting adenomas in which the oncogene *gsp* in frequently present, none of the thyrotropinoma screened has been shown to express activating mutations of genes encoding for G protein subunits, such as αs, αq, α11 or αi2, or for the thyrotropin-releasing hormone (TRH) receptor [6]. In consideration of the crucial role that the transcription factor Pit-1 plays in cell differentiation and prolactin (PRL), GH and TSH gene expression, Pit-1 gene has been screened for mutations in 14 thyrotropinomas and found to be wild type [2]. By contrast, as it occurs in GH-omas, Pit-1 was demonstrated to be overexpressed also in thyrotropinomas, though the proliferative potential of this finding remains to be elucidated.

In addition to activating mutations or overexpression of protooncogenes, tumors may originate from the loss of genes with antiproliferative action. As far as the loss of antioncogenes is concerned, no loss of p53 was found in one thyrotropinoma studied, while the loss of retinoblastoma gene (Rb) was not investigated in thyrotropinomas. Another candidate gene is *menin*, the gene responsible for the multiple endocrine neoplasia type 1 (MEN 1). In fact, 3–30% of sporadic pituitary adenomas show loss of heterozygosity (LOH) on 11q13, where *menin* is located, and LOH on this chromosome seems to be associated with the transition from the non-invasive to the invasive phenotype. A recent screening study carried out on 13 thyrotropinomas using polymorphic markers on 11q13 showed LOH in three, but none of them showed a *menin* mutation after sequence analysis [2]. Interestingly, hyperthyroidism due to thyrotropinomas has been reported in five cases within a familial setting of MEN 1 syndrome.

Finally, the extreme refractoriness of neoplastic thyrotrophs to the inhibitory action of thyroid hormones led to a search for alterations in thyroid hormone receptor (TR) function. Absence of TRα1, TRα2 and TRβ1 expression was reported in one thyrotropinoma, but aberrant alternative splicing of TRβ2 mRNA encoding TRβ variant lacking T_3 binding activity was recently shown as a mechanism for impaired T_3-dependent negative regulation of both TSHβ and glycoprotein hormone α-subunit (α-GSU) in tumoral tissue [7]. Moreover, recent data suggest that somatic mutations of TRβ may be responsible for the defect in negative regulation of TSH secretion in some thyrotropinomas [8].

Finally, LOH and particular polymorphisms at the somatostatin receptor type 5 gene locus seem to be associated with an aggressive phenotype and resistance to somatostatin analog treatment, possibly due to lack of somatostatin-induced inhibition of TSH secretion [9]. Moreover, overexpression of basic fibroblast growth factor by some thyrotropinomas suggests the possibility that it may play a role in the development of fibrosis and tumor cell proliferation of this unusual type of pituitary neoplasm [10].

Diagnostic procedures

In patients with thyrotropinoma, signs and symptoms of hyperthyroidism are frequently associated with those related to tumor expansion, such as headache and visual field defects [1, 11, 12]. In the past, about one third of patients had been diagnosed as having a primary hyperthyroidism (Graves disease or toxic goiter) and thus mistakenly treated with thyroid ablation (thyroidectomy and/or radioiodine). Clinical features of hyperthyroidism are usually milder than expected owing to the levels of circulating thyroid hormones, probably due to the longstanding duration of the disease. In patients with mixed TSH/GH adenoma, hyperthyroid features can be overshadowed by those of acromegaly, thus emphasizing the importance of systematic measurement of TSH and fT_4 in patients with pituitary tumor.

The presence of goiter is the rule, even in patients with previous partial thyroidectomy, since thyroid residue may regrow as a consequence of the continuous TSH hyperstimulation [11, 12]. Occurrence of uni- or multinodular goiter is frequent (about 72% of reported cases), but progression towards functional autonomy seems to be rare [1, 12]. Also rare appears to be the presence of differentiated thyroid carcinomas [2].

Disorders of the gonadal axis are not rare, with menstrual disorders present in all patients with mixed TSH/PRL adenomas and in one third of the pure thyrotropinomas. Central hypogonadism, delayed puberty and decreased libido were also found in a number of males with thyrotropinomas and/or mixed TSH/follicle-stimulating hormone (FSH) adenomas. As a consequence of tumor suprasellar extension or invasiveness, signs and symptoms of expanding tumor mass are predominant in many patients. Partial or total hypopituitarism was seen in about 25% of patients, headache reported in about 20% and visual field defects in about a half.

As far as the biochemical findings are concerned, along with the elevated levels of fT_4 and fT_3 in the presence of measurable TSH concentrations, a unbalanced hypersecretion of circulating free glycoprotein hormone α-subunit (α-GSU) levels and elevated α-GSU/TSH molar ratio were detected in more than 80% of patients with documented thyrotropinoma [1, 11, 13]. Moreover, measurements of several parameters of peripheral thyroid hormone action have been proposed to quantify the degree of tissue hyperthyroidism [2]. In particular, liver (sex hormone-binding globulin, SHBG) and bone (carboxyterminal cross-linked telopeptide of type I collagen, ICTP) parameters have been successfully used to differentiate hyperthyroid patients with thyrotropinoma from those with PRTH [1, 14]. In fact, as it occurs in the common forms of hyperthyroidism, patients with thyrotropinoma have high SHBG and ICTP levels, while they are into the normal range in patients with hyperthyroidism due to PRTH (Table 33.1).

Both stimulatory and inhibitory tests had been proposed for the diagnosis of thyrotropinoma. Classically, the T_3 suppression test has been used to assess the presence of a thyrotropinoma. A complete inhibition of TSH secretion after T_3 suppression test (80–100 µg/day per 8–10 days) has never been recorded in patients with thyrotropinoma (Table 33.1). In patients with previous thyroid ablation, T_3 suppression seems to be the most sensitive and specific test in assessing the presence of a thyrotropinoma [1, 11, 12]. Indeed, this test is strictly contraindicated in elderly patients or in those with coronary heart disease. Therefore, the

Table 33.1 Differential diagnosis between thyrotropinomas and pituitary resistance to thyroid hormones (PRTH)

Parameter	Thyrotropinomas	PRTH	Significance (*p*)
Female/male ratio	1.3	1.4	NS
Familial cases (%)	0	84	<0.0001
TSH (mU/L)	2.7 ± 0.6	2.2 ± 0.3	NS
FT_4 (pmol/L)	40.0 ± 4.2	29.5 ± 2.5	NS
FT_3 (pmol/L)	14.5 ± 1.4	11.7 ± 1.0	NS
SHBG (nmol/L)[a]	113 ± 17	62 ± 4	<0.0001
Presence of lesion at CT scan or MRI (%)	98	6	<0.0001
High α-GSU levels (%)	65	3	<0.0001
High α-GSU/TSH m.r. (%)	81	2	<0.0001
Abnormal TSH response to T_3 suppression test (%)[b]	100	100	NS
Blunted TSH response to TRH test (%)	94	4	<0.0001

Only patients with intact thyroid were taken into account. Data are obtained from patients followed at our Institute (36 thyrotropinomas and 27 PRTH) and are expressed as mean ± SE.

[a]SHBG: sex-hormone binding globulin, measured as a parameter of thyroid hormone action at the peripheral tissue level.

[b]Werner's test (80–100 µg T_3 for 8–10 days). Quantitatively normal responses to T_3, i.e. complete inhibition of both basal and TRH-stimulated TSH levels, have never been recorded in either group of patients. Nonetheless, the majority of patients with PRTH shows a qualitatively normal TSH response to T_3 suppression test.

TRH test has been widely used in the work-up of these adenomas. In the vast majority of patients, TSH and α-GSU levels do not increase after TRH injection (Table 33.1). In patients with hyperthyroidism, discrepancies between TSH and α-GSU responses to TRH are pathognomonic of thyrotropinomas co-secreting other pituitary hormones [13].

The majority of thyrotropinomas maintain the sensitivity to native somatostatin and its analogs [15–18]. Indeed, administration of native neuropeptide or its analogs (octreotide and lanreotide) induces a reduction of TSH levels in the majority of cases and these tests may be predictive of the efficacy of long-term treatment. Recently, we have chronically treated a series of patients with thyrotropinomas or PRTH with long-acting somatostatin analogs documenting a marked decrease of fT_4 and fT_3 levels in all patients but one with tumor, while patients with PRTH did not respond at all. Thus, administration of long-acting somatostatin analogs for at least 2 months can be useful in the differential diagnosis in problematic cases of central hyperthyroidism [19]. Nevertheless, since none of these tests is of clear-cut diagnostic value, it is recommended to use both T_3 suppression and TRH tests whenever possible, because the combination of their results increases the specificity and sensitivity of the diagnostic work-up [1, 11, 12].

Finally, nuclear magnetic resonance imaging (MRI) is nowadays the preferred tool for the visualization of a thyrotropinoma. High-resolution computerized tomography (CT) is the alternative investigation in the case of contraindications, such as patients with pacemakers. Most thyrotropinomas were diagnosed at the stage of macroadenomas with frequent suprasellar extension or sphenoidal sinus invasion. Microadenomas are now reported with increasing frequency, accounting for about 15% of all recorded cases in both clinical and surgical series. Recently, pituitary scintigraphy with radiolabeled octreotide (octreoscan) has been shown to successfully localize thyrotropinomas expressing somatostatin receptors [20]. However, the specificity of octreoscan is low, since positive scans can be seen in the case of a pituitary mass of different types, either secreting or non-secreting. Such a procedure may be useful in the recognition of the possible ectopic localization of a thyrotropinoma, as two cases of thyrotropinomas were recently found in the nasopharyngeal region.

Differential diagnosis

In a patient with signs and symptoms of hyperthyroidism, the presence of elevated TSH and detectable TSH levels rules out primary hyperthyroidism (Fig. 33.1). Once the existence of central hyperthyroidism is confirmed and the presence of methodological interferences excluded [1], several diagnostic steps have to be carried out to differentiate a thyrotropinoma from RTH, particularly PRTH. Indeed, the possible presence of neurological signs and symptoms (e.g. visual defects and headache) or clinical features of concomitant hypersecretion of other pituitary hormones (acromegaly, amenorrhea/galactorrhea) points to the presence of

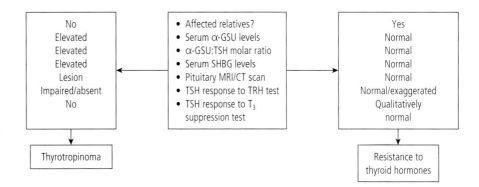

Figure 33.2 Main clinical and biochemical parameters useful in the differential diagnosis between thyrotropinomas and resistance to thyroid hormone action. α-GSU, pituitary glycoprotein hormone α-subunit; SHBG, sex hormone-binding globulin; TRH, thyrotropin-releasing hormone.

a thyrotropinoma. Furthermore, the presence of alterations of the pituitary gland at MRI or CT scan strongly supports the diagnosis of a thyrotropinoma. Nevertheless, the differential diagnosis with PRTH may be difficult when the pituitary adenoma is very small, or in the case of confusing lesions, such as ectopic tumors, empty sella or pituitary incidentalomas, the latter lesion being frequently found in the general population [19]. In these cases, elevated α-GSU concentrations or high α-GSU:TSH molar ratio and TSH unresponsiveness to TRH stimulation or to T_3 suppression tests, or both, favor the presence of a thyrotropinoma (Fig. 33.2). Moreover, the finding of similar biochemical data in family relatives definitely points to the presence of RTH, as familial cases of thyrotropinomas have not been documented (Fig. 33.2). Finally, an apparent association between thyrotropinoma and RTH has been recently reported and somatic mutations in the thyroid-hormone receptor have been found in some tumors [8]; thus the occurrence of thyrotropinoma in patients with RTH should be carefully considered.

Treatment of thyrotropinomas

Surgery and irradiation

Removal of the pituitary tumor and restoration of euthyroidism are the primary goals of thyrotropinoma treatment. Therefore, the first therapeutic approach to thyrotropinomas should be the transsphenoidal or subfrontal adenomectomy, the choice of the route depending on the tumor volume and its suprasellar extension. This may be particularly difficult because of the marked fibrosis of these tumors, possibly related to high expression of basic fibroblast growth factor [10]. In addition, these tumors may be locally invasive involving the cavernous sinus, internal carotid artery or optic chiasm, thus rendering complete resection of the tumor either impractical or dangerous. Antithyroid drugs (methimazole or propylthiouracil, 20–30 and 200–300 mg/day, respectively) or octreotide (100 μg subcutaneously, twice or three times daily) along with propranolol (80–120 mg/day orally) can be administered in order to restore euthyroidism before surgery. However, they may obscure the immediate postoperative course of TSH secretion, which is expected to be totally inhibited if the tumor removal was completely achieved, and therefore a useful criterion

to assess definitive cure of the disease may be lost [21]. If surgery is contraindicated or declined, pituitary radiotherapy (no less than 45 Gy fractionated at 2 Gy per day or 10–25 Gy in a single dose if a stereotactic Gamma Unit is available) should be considered. A successful experience of an invasive thyrotropinoma associated with an unruptured aneurysm treated by two-stage operation and Gamma Knife has been recently reported [22].

Table 33.2 shows the general outcome after surgery alone or combined with radiotherapy, data being collected from 211 patients reported in the literature. Normalization of thyroid hormone circulating levels and apparent complete removal of tumor mass were observed in 38% of patients who may therefore be considered apparently cured (follow-up ranged from 2 to 121 months). An additional 28% of patients were judged improved, as normalization of thyroid hormone circulating levels was achieved in all, though there was no complete removal of the adenoma. Together these findings indicate that more than two thirds of thyrotropinomas are under control with surgery and/or irradiation. In the remaining patients, TSH hypersecretion was unchanged after the above treatments, a fact that undoubtedly reflects the large size and the invasiveness of the tumor. Previous thyroid ablation or antithyroid drug treatments did not significantly affect the results of surgery and/or radiotherapy. Postsurgical deaths were reported in few cases. Because of the possible iatrogenic hypopituitarism, evaluation of other pituitary functions, particularly adrenocorticotropic hormone (ACTH) secretion, should be

Table 33.2 Results of pituitary surgery and/or irradiation in the treatment of thyrotropinomas (data from the literature)

Treatment	No.	Apparently cured[a] (%)	Improved[b] (%)	Unchanged (%)
Pituitary surgery alone	154	38	28	34
Pituitary surgery and/or irradiation	57	37	32	31

[a]Normalization of thyroid hormone circulating levels with complete removal of tumor mass.
[b]Normalization of thyroid hormone circulating levels without complete removal of tumor mass.

carefully undertaken soon after surgery and checked again every year, especially in patients treated by radiotherapy. In addition, in the case of surgical cure, postoperative TSH is undetectable and may remain low for many weeks or months, causing central hypothyroidism. A permanent central hypothyroidism may occur due to either compression by the tumor or surgical damage of the normal thyrotrophs. Thus, transient or permanent L-T$_4$ replacement therapy may be necessary. Finally, in a few patients total thyroidectomy was performed after pituitary surgery failure, as the patients were at risk of thyroid storm.

Medical treatment

Although earlier diagnosis has improved the surgical cure rate of thyrotropinomas, at least one out of three patients requires medical therapy in order to control the hyperthyroidism. The rationale for medical treatment is based on *in vitro* studies. In fact, somatostatin (SRIH) binding experiments indicate that almost all thyrotropinomas express a variable number of SRIH receptors, the highest SRIH-binding site densities being found in mixed GH/TSH adenomas [15]. Since somatostatin analogs are highly effective in reducing TSH secretion by neoplastic thyrotrophs [1, 11, 12, 16–19], the inhibitory pathway mediated by somatostatin receptors appears to be intact in such adenomas. Consistently, there is a good correlation between SRIH-binding capacity and maximal biological response, as quantified by inhibition of TSH secretion and *in vivo* restoration of euthyroid state [15]. The presence of dopamine receptors in thyrotropinomas was the rationale for therapeutic trials with dopaminergic agonists, such as bromocriptine and cabergoline. Several studies have shown a large heterogeneity of TSH responses to dopaminergic agents either in primary cultures or *in vivo*, the best results having been achieved in mixed TSH/PRL adenomas [2]. Effects of these two inhibitory agents should now be re-evaluated in light of the demonstration of possible heterodimerization of somatostatin receptor type 5 and dopamine D2 receptor [23].

Today, the medical treatment of thyrotropinomas rests on long-acting somatostatin analogs, such as octreotide LAR or lanreotide SR or lanreotide Autogel [1, 11, 12, 16–19]. Treatment with these analogs leads to a reduction of TSH and α-GSU secretion in almost all cases, with restoration of the euthyroid state in the majority of them (Table 33.3). Circulating thyroid hormone levels normalized in 96% of patients not previously thyroidectomized. Goiter size was significantly reduced by somatostatin analog therapy in 20% of cases. Vision improvement was documented in 68% of patients and pituitary tumor mass shrinkage occurred in about 40% of them. Resistance to somatostatin analog treatment, true escape of TSH secretion from the inhibitory effects of the drugs or discontinuation of treatment due to side effects was documented in a minority of cases. Of interest are the findings of octreotide treatment in pregnant women that was effective in restoring euthyroidism in the mother and had no side effects on development and thyroid function of the fetuses. Moreover, in almost all patients with mixed TSH/GH hypersecretion, signs and symptoms of acromegaly concomitantly disappeared. Patients

Table 33.3 Results of the treatment with somatostatin analogs (octreotide LAR or lanreotide SR or lanreotide Autogel) in 121 patients with thyrotropinoma recorded in the literature as of June, 2005

TSH reduction (>50% vs. basal)	90%	Vision improvement	68%
α-GSU reduction	93%	Tumor mass shrinkage	40%
TSH and α-GSU normalization	75%	True escape	10%
Thyroid hormone normalization	96%	Resistance (long-term studies)	4%
Goiter size reduction	20%	Discontinuation of therapy due to side effects	7%

on octreotide have to be carefully monitored, as untoward side effects, such as cholelithiasis and carbohydrate intolerance, may become manifest. The administered dose should be tailored for each patient, depending on therapeutic response and tolerance (including gastrointestinal side effects). The tolerance is usually very good, as gastrointestinal side effects are transient with long-acting analogs. The marked somatostatin-induced suppression of TSH secretion and consequent biochemical hypothyroidism seen in some patients may require L-T$_4$ substitution. Finally, no data have been reported on somatostatin analog treatment of thyrotropinomas in patients who underwent thyroid ablation by thyroidectomy or radioiodine. Since aggressive and invasive macroadenomas are more frequently found in these patients [1], it is mandatory to treat them in order to block further growth of pituitary tumor mass.

In conclusion, whether somatostatin analog treatment may be an alternative to surgery and/or irradiation in patients with thyrotropinoma still remains to be established. However, the therapeutic success of both octreotide and lanreotide administration is quite high, approaching 95% of treated patients. Somatostatin analogs may, therefore, represent a useful tool for long-term treatment of such rare pituitary tumors.

References

1. Beck-Peccoz P, Brucker-Davis F, Persani L, Smallridge RC, Weintraub BD. Thyrotropin-secreting pituitary tumors. *Endocr. Rev.* 1996;17:610–638.
2. Beck-Peccoz P, Persani L. Thyrotropin-secreting pituitary adenomas. In Thyroid Disease Manager. http://www.thyroidmanager.org/
3. Jailer JW, Holub DA. Remission of Graves' disease following radiotherapy of a pituitary neoplasm. *Am. J. Med.* 1960;28:497–500.
4. Hamilton C, Adams LC, Maloof F. Hyperthyroidism due to thyrotropin-producing pituitary chromophobe adenoma. *N. Engl. J. Med.* 1970;283:1077–1080.
5. Refetoff S, Weiss RE, Usala SJ. The syndromes of resistance to thyroid hormone. *Endocr. Rev.* 1993;14:348–399.
6. Dong Q, Brucker-Davis F, Weintraub BD, et al. Screening of candidate oncogenes in human thyrotroph tumors: absence of activating

mutations of the Gαq, Gα11, Gαs, or thyrotropin-releasing hormone receptor genes. *J. Clin. Endocrinol. Metab.* 1996;81:1134–1140.

7. Ando S, Sarlis NJ, Krishnan J, et al. Aberrant alternative splicing of thyroid hormone receptor in a TSH-secreting pituitary tumor is a mechanism for hormone resistance. *Mol Endocrinol.* 2001;15: 1529–1538.

8. Ando S, Sarlis NJ, Oldfield EH, Yen PM. Somatic mutation of TRbeta can cause a defect in negative regulation of TSH in a TSH-secreting pituitary tumor. *J. Clin. Endocrinol. Metab.* 2001;86:5572–5576.

9. Filopanti M, Ballare E, Lania AG, et al. Loss of heterozygosity at the SS receptor type 5 locus in human GH- and TSH-secreting pituitary adenomas. *J. Endocrinol. Invest.* 2004;27:937–942.

10. Ezzat S, Horvath E, Kovacs K, Smyth HS, Singer W, Asa SL. Basic fibroblast growth factor expression by two prolactin and thyrotropin-producing pituitary adenomas. *Endocr. Pathol.* 1995;6:125–134.

11. Brucker-Davis F, Oldfield EH, Skarulis MC, Doppman JL, Weintraub BD. Thyrotropin-secreting pituitary tumors: diagnostic criteria, thyroid hormone sensitivity, and treatment outcome in 25 patients followed at the National Institutes of Health. *J. Clin. Endocrinol. Metab.* 1999;84:476–486.

12. Socin HV, Chanson P, Delemer B, et al. The changing spectrum of TSH-secreting pituitary adenomas: diagnosis and management in 43 patients. *Eur. J. Endocrinol.* 2003;148:433–442.

13. Terzolo M, Orlandi F, Bassetti M, et al. Hyperthyroidism due to a pituitary adenoma composed of two different cell types, one secreting alpha-subunit alone and another cosecreting alpha-subunit and thyrotropin. *J. Clin. Endocrinol. Metab.* 1991;72:415–421.

14. Persani L, Preziati D, Matthews CH, et al. Serum levels of carboxy-terminal cross-linked telopeptide of type I collagen (ICTP) in the differential diagnosis of the syndromes of inappropriate secretion of TSH. *Clin. Endocrinol. (Oxf.)* 1997;47:207–214.

15. Bertherat J, Brue T, Enjalbert A, et al. Somatostatin receptors on thyrotropin-secreting pituitary adenomas: comparison with the inhibitory effects of octreotide upon *in vivo* and *in vitro* hormonal secretions. *J. Clin. Endocrinol. Metab.* 1992;75:540–546.

16. Gancel A, Vuillermet P, Legrand A, Catus F, Thomas F, Kuhn JM. Effects of a slow-release formulation of the new somatostatin analogue lanreotide in TSH-secreting pituitary adenomas. *Clin. Endocrinol.* 1994;40:421–428.

17. Chanson P, Weintraub BD, Harris AG. Octreotide therapy for thyroid stimulating-secreting pituitary adenomas. A follow-up of 52 patients. *Ann. Intern. Med.* 1993;119:236–240.

18. Kuhn JM, Arlot S, Lefebvre H, et al. Evaluation of the treatment of thyrotropin-secreting pituitary adenomas with a slow release formulation of the somatostatin analog lanreotide. *J. Clin. Endocrinol. Metab.* 2000;85:1487–1491.

19. Mannavola D, Persani L, Vannucchi G, et al. Different response to chronic somatostatin analogues in patients with central hyperthyroidism. *Clin. Endocrinol. (Oxf.)* 2005;62:176–181.

20. Losa M, Magnani P, Mortini P, et al. Indium-111 pentetreotide single-photon emission tomography in patients with TSH-secreting pituitary adenomas: correlation with the effect of a single administration of octreotide on serum TSH levels. *Eur. J. Nucl. Med.* 1997;24: 728–731.

21. Losa M, Giovanelli M, Persani L, Mortini P, Faglia G, Beck-Peccoz P. Criteria of cure and follow-up of central hyperthyroidism due to thyrotropin-secreting pituitary adenomas. *J. Clin. Endocrinol. Metab.* 1996;81:3086–3090.

22. Ohki M, Sato K, Tuchiya D, et al. A case of TSH-secreting pituitary adenoma associated with an unruptured aneurysm: successful treatment by two-stage operation and gamma knife. *No To Shinkei* 1999;51:895–899.

23. Rocheville M, Lange DC, Kumar U, Patel SC, Patel RC, Patel YC. Receptors for dopamine and somatostatin: formation of hetero-oligomers with enhanced functional activity. *Science* 2000;288:154–157.

34 Pituitary Carcinoma

Olaf Ansorge

Key points

- Pituitary carcinoma is currently defined as a neoplasm of adenohypophyseal endocrine cells with cerebrospinal or systemic dissemination.
- Pituitary carcinoma is very rare (~0.2% of operated pituitary neoplasms), affects adults of either sex, and is not associated with specific risk factors.
- Most pituitary carcinomas develop from recurrent endocrinologically functioning invasive macroadenomas with a highly variable lag period.
- There are currently no clinical or laboratory criteria that allow reliable identification of pituitary carcinoma while still in the premetastatic phase.
- The predictive value of the recently introduced category of "atypical pituitary adenoma," characterized by high proliferative activity and p53 oncoprotein overexpression, remains to be established.
- The prognosis of pituitary carcinoma is very poor despite multimodal treatment.

Definition and introduction

A pituitary carcinoma is defined as a *tumor of adenohypophyseal endocrine cells with evidence of cerebrospinal or systemic metastasis* [1]. This restrictive definition is clinically unsatisfactory, because it precludes early detection and treatment. The current terminology reflects the lack of specific biological and clinical markers that clearly distinguish benign from malignant adenohypophyseal neoplasms while they are still confined to the sellar region. However, as outlined below, such markers are beginning to become available. Fortunately, pituitary carcinomas are very rare; however, this contributes to the relative lack of data concerning their clinicopathological characteristics and treatment options. Approximately 150 cases have been documented in the medical literature, mostly as single case reports or small series; these have been recently reviewed [2–4].

Incidence, epidemiology and risk factors

Pituitary carcinomas account for approximately 0.2% of all operated pituitary tumors [5]. They occur with almost equal frequency in males and females. Most patients are in their fifth or sixth decade when the diagnosis is made; however, the age range is very

wide (third to eighth decade) [5, 6]. Pituitary carcinomas occur sporadically; individuals with inherited endocrine tumor syndromes such as multiple endocrine neoplasia type 1 (MEN 1) or Carney complex do not carry a higher risk. There is also no evidence that exposure to specific carcinogens or irradiation contributes to pituitary carcinoma development. The large majority (~75–80%) of pituitary carcinomas are endocrinologically functional [1, 2, 7] (Table 34.1). Most produce adrenocorticotropin (ACTH) or prolactin (PRL). Somatotroph tumors are underrepresented among carcinomas relative to their overall frequency among patients with functioning adenomas. Thyrotroph carcinomas are extremely rare. Approximately 20% of carcinomas are clinically non-functioning, comprising silent ACTH, gonadotroph or,

Table 34.1 Hormonal profile of 139 pituitary carcinomas as reported by Ragel and Couldwell in 2004 [7]

Hormonal subtype	Number of cases (%)
Corticotroph	59 (42)
Lactotroph	46 (33)
Somatotroph	9 (6)
Gonadotroph	7 (5)
Thyrotroph	1 (1)
Hormone-negative*	17 (12)

*Note that this likely represents an overestimation since immunostaining for pituitary hormones and testing of PRL serum levels were not routinely carried out before the 1970s. Other authors report slightly different figures relating to their case series (see text), with a higher percentage of lactotroph carcinomas.

Clinical Endocrine Oncology, 2nd edition. Edited by Ian D. Hay and John A.H. Wass. © 2008 Blackwell Publishing. ISBN 978-1-4051-4584-8.

rarely, null cell tumors [1]. Among patients with ACTH expressing pituitary carcinomas, those whose initial sellar tumors were macroadenomas associated with previous bilateral adrenalectomy (Nelson syndrome), apparently no endocrine hormonal excess, or Crooke's hyaline change in tumor cells, may have been at greater risk of malignant progression then patients with classic Cushing microadenoma [6, 8–10]. However, reliable clinical, morphological or molecular parameters are currently not available to predict the risk of pituitary carcinoma in individual patients (see below).

Clinical presentation and diagnostic investigations

Clinical features of pituitary carcinoma depend on the pattern of metastatic dissemination and hormones secreted by the tumor cells. A history of previous sellar adenoma, with or without multiple recurrences or locally invasive features, is usually present. It is crucial to obtain this history because in the absence of any obvious symptoms of hormone excess the presentation of pituitary carcinoma is indistinguishable from that of any other metastatic carcinoma of unknown origin.

The interval between documentation of precursor adenoma and carcinoma is highly variable (4 months to 18 years) and appears to be significantly shorter in PRL-producing tumors (~5 years) than corticotrophin-expressing ones (~10 years) [5]. The clinical pattern before the diagnosis of pituitary carcinoma is made can be very variable [3]. For example, patients may suffer from multiple sellar recurrences of an invasive pituitary adenoma treated by repeated surgery or radiotherapy, followed after many years by distant metastases. Or, less commonly, patients with a newly diagnosed invasive macroadenoma may present after a brief interval with evidence of disseminated disease before or at the same time as sellar recurrence. *De novo* pituitary carcinoma, i.e. the presentation with metastatic disease without a previously known intrasellar lesion, is exceedingly rare. By definition, *in situ* pituitary carcinoma currently does not exist.

The great majority of pituitary carcinomas that have been described since sensitive methods for pituitary hormone detection have become available are endocrinologically functional. Cushing disease (47%) or symptoms and signs of hyperprolactinemia (40%) are the most commonly found endocrinological manifestations associated with pituitary carcinoma (see [5]). Acromegaly, hyperthyroidism, or no clinical evidence of hormone excess is much less common. In patients with clear evidence of a sellar lesion, pituitary hormone excess and metastatic disease of unknown origin, pituitary carcinoma should be suspected, particularly if the level of secreted hormone is very high in relation to the size of the (residual) sellar mass.

Although clearly not specific, the pattern of metastatic disease may point to the pituitary as the primary site if liver, lymph node, lung or bone metastases are associated with lesions within the neuraxis and sella. However, simultaneous systemic and neuraxial dissemination occurs only in the minority (~13%) of pituitary carcinomas [5]. It has been suggested that metastases limited to the craniospinal axis are more common in corticotroph than lactotroph pituitary carcinomas [4].

Magnetic resonance imaging (for parenchymal metastases), computer-assisted tomography or plain X-ray (for bone metastases) should be combined with imaging of the sellar region to establish the extent of disease (Plate. 34.1); however, a formal staging protocol does not exist. The sellar component is usually an invasive macroadenoma of Hardy grade 3 or 4 [9]. Metastatic lesions may be small and only vaguely contrast enhancing. Scintigraphy with radiolabeled somatostatin analogs or other tracers, or positron emission tomography with 18-fluor-labeled deoxyglucose may also aid in the detection of metastases (see [3]). However, there is currently no imaging modality that specifically distinguishes metastatic deposits of pituitary origin from those of other cancers. The diagnosis rests therefore on the immunohistological or ultrastructural demonstration of endocrine pituitary differentiation of the metastatic deposit following biopsy or autopsy (Plate 34.1). Ideally, this should be matched with tissue from the sellar tumor.

Pathology, pathogenesis and predictors of carcinoma development

The macroscopic pathology of pituitary carcinoma is not diagnostic. The sellar component consists generally of a locally invasive tumor indistinguishable from corresponding non-metastatic adenomas. Local invasion typically involves dura mater, bone, or the cavernous sinus. Brain invasion contiguous with the sellar component may also be present; whether this in itself is sufficient for the diagnosis of carcinoma remains controversial. Appearances of the metastatic deposits may range from well-circumscribed nodules superficially attached to spinal nerve roots to infiltrative space-occupying lesions of any organ system. Clinically silent metastases may be discovered at autopsy.

Routine light microscopy generally reveals sheets of tumor cells with neuroendocrine features, sometimes remarkably similar in cytology to those of benign intrasellar adenomas that never progress to carcinoma (e.g. [11]). Classic histological features of carcinomas arising from other tissues, such as infiltrative growth, cytological or nuclear atypia, mitoses or necrosis, may be partially or completely lacking in both the primary sellar as well as metastatic pituitary tumor. This has led to the suggestion that a proportion of pituitary "carcinomas," i.e. those disseminated only in the subarachnoid space, represent mere "seedlings" of benign adenoma tissue resulting from repeated sellar surgery. However, the poor survival of these patients argues against this hypothesis. Furthermore, successive biopsies from patients who suffer several intrasellar tumor recurrences before the manifestation of metastatic disease may show clearly increased cytological atypia with each recurrence [6]. Generic neuroendocrine differentiation of the carcinoma should be confirmed by immunohistochemistry for vesicle-associated proteins synaptophysin or chromogranin, while positive staining for a pituitary hormone establishes the definitive diagnosis.

The observation of increasing atypia in premetastatic sellar adenoma recurrences in some patients and the extreme rarity of *de novo* metastatic pituitary carcinoma suggest a stepwise adenoma–carcinoma sequence of pathogenesis rather than direct carcinogenic transformation of normal adenohypophyseial cells [9]. One study, however, found evidence of distinct clonality in a corticotroph carcinoma metastasis compared with its sellar precursor lesions [12]. The molecular pathogenesis of pituitary adenomas is complex and may vary between adenoma subtypes (see Chapter 23). Molecular progression to carcinoma may not be uniform either. It is therefore not surprising that in this rare entity no consistent genetic or molecular signature of pituitary carcinoma has emerged so far. Comparative genomic hybridization, a technique allowing genome-wide detection of chromosomal imbalances, has shown that there are more aberrations in metastatic than primary tumors, principally consisting of gains on chromosomes 5, 7p, 13q, and 14q [13]. A pilot study of oligonucleotide array gene expression profiling found that 29% of 15 000 studied genes differentially expressed between a corticotroph carcinoma and a group of four adenomas [14]. Specific genetic changes such as *H-RAS* oncogene point mutations [15] and gene amplification or over-expression of epidermal growth factor receptor (EGFR) and phospho-EGFR [16] or HER-2/neu [11] have been reported in a handful of cases. Interestingly, mutations in the tumor suppressor gene *TP53*, the most commonly mutated gene in human cancers, are rarely present in pituitary adenomas or carcinomas. However, immunocytochemical evidence of nuclear p53 overexpression (which may occur independently of *TP53* mutations) has been found to be significantly more frequent in pituitary carcinomas compared with invasive non-metastatic adenomas, while it is absent in non-invasive tumors [17]. Its expression is also generally higher in metastases than corresponding primary tumors, but p53 negative carcinomas do occur [11]. Expression of Ki67 (a nucleoprotein upregulated in all phases of the cell cycle except G0 and detected with antibody clone MIB-1) as a marker of increased proliferative activity is higher in p53-positive than p53-negative tumors and invasive than non-invasive adenomas [17]. Correspondingly, it is also higher in metastases than their respective "premetastatic" sellar lesions [9]. Therefore, both p53 overexpression and Ki67 labeling by MIB-1 antibody of more than 3% of tumor cell nuclei, together with the presence of an "elevated" mitotic count, have been introduced as criteria for the diagnosis of "atypical pituitary adenoma" in the 2004 World Health Organization classification of pituitary tumors. Whether this constellation truly helps to identify *in situ* precursor tumors of pituitary carcinomas remains to be established in prospective studies [9].

Prognosis and treatment

Since the presence of metastasis is currently the *sine qua non* of pituitary carcinoma diagnosis, it is not surprising that the prognosis is very poor. In a series of 15 patients, the mean survival was 2 years with two thirds of patients dying within 1 year of discovery of metastases [5]. Patients with systemic metastases had a poorer prognosis than those with disease limited to the neuraxis (12 vs 30 months). It has also been suggested that patients whose tumors express ACTH fare worse than those with tumors of other subtypes (see [3]). Rare patients may survive for decades [18]. Morbidity and mortality generally are determined by the complications of invasive tumor growth rather than the effects of uncontrollable hormone excess.

There is no consensus about the best treatment for pituitary carcinomas. Systematic trials have not been conducted because of the rarity of the condition. Repeated surgical debulking of the sellar lesion and of accessible metastases appears to be the commonest approach and may reduce the symptoms of local mass effect as well as hormone excess. The latter may also be treated pharmacologically according to the same principles that apply to the specific hormone hypersecretion syndromes associated with non-metastatic pituitary tumors. However, pharmacoresistance, particularly of PRL-producing carcinomas to dopamine agonists, is common. Surgery may be followed by adjuvant radiotherapy, usually in the form of external beam irradiation, but also more focussed as stereotactic or Gamma Knife radiosurgery (see [3]). Systemic cytotoxic therapy with lomustine and 5-fluorouracil has been tried with little success in several patients [19]. However, chemotherapy with temozolomide achieved a remarkable remission in a patient with PRL-producing carcinoma [20]. This approach may warrant further study in other patients. More pathophysiologically targeted therapies with somatostatin agonists or α-interferon have so far been of little value (see [3]).

Conclusion

Pituitary carcinomas are rare neoplasms of adenohypophyseal endocrine cells whose current classification is clinically unsatisfactory because early (*in situ*) detection is not possible. Since most arise from known sellar precursor adenomas, the best hope of identifying useful biomarkers of predictive value would rest with pooling of precursor and carcinoma tissue for comprehensive molecular profiling. The designation of "atypical adenoma" based on p53 overexpression and high Ki67/MIB-1 tumor cell labeling represents a step in the right direction but its predictive value needs to be firmly established. The main clinical pitfall in making the diagnosis of pituitary carcinoma is not suspecting the pituitary as a primary site in patients with metastatic disease of unknown origin and a history of adenoma that may have been treated many years previously. Once the diagnosis is considered, evidence of pituitary hormone excess should be sought, and systemic and neuraxial imaging performed. The definitive diagnosis requires confirmation of endocrine pituitary differentiation of the metastasis. Most patients with pituitary carcinoma die within a year of diagnosis. Treatment relies mostly on surgery and management of hormone excess, with a limited role for radio- and chemotherapy. The potential of temozolomide in pituitary carcinomas, however, may warrant further study.

References

1. Scheithauer BW, Kovacs K, Horvath E, et al. Pituitary carcinoma. In DeLellis RA, Lloyd RV, Heitz PU, Eng C (eds). *Tumours of Endocrine Organs*. World Health Organization Classification of Tumours. Lyon: IARCPress, 2004:36–39.
2. Lopes MB, Scheithauer BW, Schiff D. Pituitary carcinoma: diagnosis and treatment. *Endocrine* 2005;28:115–121.
3. Kaltsas GA, Nomikos P, Kontogeorgos G, Buchfelder M, Grossman AB. Clinical review: diagnosis and management of pituitary carcinomas. *J. Clin. Endocrinol. Metab.* 2005;90:3089–3099.
4. Scheithauer BW, Kurtkaya-Yapicier O, Kovacs KT, Young WF, Jr, Lloyd RV. Pituitary carcinoma: a clinicopathological review. *Neurosurgery* 2005;56:1066–1074.
5. Pernicone PJ, Scheithauer BW, Sebo TJ, et al. Pituitary carcinoma: a clinicopathologic study of 15 cases. *Cancer* 1997;79:804–812.
6. Gaffey TA, Scheithauer BW, Lloyd RV, et al. Corticotroph carcinoma of the pituitary: a clinicopathological study. Report of four cases. *J. Neurosurg.* 2002;96:352–360.
7. Ragel BT, Couldwell WT. Pituitary carcinoma: a review of the literature. *Neurosurg. Focus* 2004;16:E7.
8. Roncaroli F, Scheithauer BW, Young WF, et al. Silent corticotroph carcinoma of the adenohypophysis: a report of five cases. *Am. J. Surg. Pathol.* 2003;27:477–486.
9. Scheithauer BW, Gaffey TA, Lloyd RV, et al. Pathobiology of pituitary adenomas and carcinomas. *Neurosurgery* 2006;59:341–353.
10. George DH, Scheithauer BW, Kovacs K, et al. Crooke's cell adenoma of the pituitary: an aggressive variant of corticotroph adenoma. *Am. J. Surg. Pathol.* 2003;27:1330–1336.
11. Roncaroli F, Nose V, Scheithauer BW, et al. Gonadotropic pituitary carcinoma: HER-2/neu expression and gene amplification. Report of two cases. *J. Neurosurg.* 2003;99:402–408.
12. Zahedi A, Booth GL, Smyth HS, et al. Distinct clonal composition of primary and metastatic adrencorticotrophic hormone-producing pituitary carcinoma. *Clin. Endocrinol. (Oxf.)* 2001;55:549–556.
13. Rickert CH, Scheithauer BW, Paulus W. Chromosomal aberrations in pituitary carcinoma metastases. *Acta Neuropathol. (Berl.)* 2001;102:117–120.
14. Ruebel KH, Leontovich AA, Jin L, et al. Patterns of gene expression in pituitary carcinomas and adenomas analyzed by high-density oligonucleotide arrays, reverse transcriptase-quantitative PCR, and protein expression. *Endocrine* 2006;29:435–444.
15. Pei L, Melmed S, Scheithauer B, Kovacs K, Prager D. H-ras mutations in human pituitary carcinoma metastases. *J. Clin. Endocrinol. Metab.* 1994;78:842–846.
16. Onguru O, Scheithauer BW, Kovacs K, et al. Analysis of epidermal growth factor receptor and activated epidermal growth factor receptor expression in pituitary adenomas and carcinomas. *Mod. Pathol.* 2004;17:772–780.
17. Thapar K, Scheithauer BW, Kovacs K, Pernicone PJ, Laws ER Jr. p53 expression in pituitary adenomas and carcinomas: correlation with invasiveness and tumor growth fractions. *Neurosurgery* 1996;38:763–770.
18. Landman RE, Horwith M, Peterson RE, Khandji AG, Wardlaw SL. Long-term survival with ACTH-secreting carcinoma of the pituitary: a case report and review of the literature. *J. Clin. Endocrinol. Metab.* 2002;87:3084–3089.
19. Kaltsas GA, Mukherjee JJ, Plowman PN, Monson JP, Grossman AB, Besser GM. The role of cytotoxic chemotherapy in the management of aggressive and malignant pituitary tumors. *J. Clin. Endocrinol. Metab.* 1998;83:4233–4238.
20. Lim S, Shahinian H, Maya MM, Yong W, Heaney AP. Temozolomide: a novel treatment for pituitary carcinoma. *Lancet Oncol.* 2006;7:518–520.

35 Pituitary Incidentalomas

Karin Bradley

Key points

- Pituitary incidentalomas are predominantly asymptomatic microadenomas detected coincidentally following imaging for another clinical indication.
- The prevalence of pituitary incidentalomas is increasing with advances in neuroradiology and more frequent brain imaging in modern medical practice.
- Alternative intrasellar or parasellar diagnoses must be carefully excluded.
- Subclinical hormone hypersecretion from pituitary incidentalomas may have long-term clinical consequences.
- Current management of pituitary incidentalomas is controversial and is most appropriately carried out in a specialist center with a multidisciplinary team including an endocrinologist, endocrine specialist nurses, a neuroradiologist and a neurosurgeon.
- The majority of asymptomatic pituitary incidentalomas <10 mm appear to follow a benign course.

Definition

Pituitary "incidentalomas" are defined as tumors of the pituitary that are essentially diagnosed serendipitously as a consequence of computerized tomography (CT) or magnetic resonance imaging (MRI) imaging carried out for another clinical indication (Fig. 35.1). To confirm the diagnosis the patient should be asymptomatic and exhibit no overt clinical features consistent with pituitary-dependent disease.

Incidence

The incidence and prevalence of these lesions are hard to define but are definitely increasing with the more widespread use of and improvements in modern imaging techniques. Autopsy series have highlighted a prevalence for pituitary adenomas, that were silent during life, of between 3% and 27% [1, 2], whereas imaging studies have proposed that approximately 4–20% of the adult population may harbor a pituitary incidentaloma [2, 3]. The vast majority of these lesions are microadenomas, <10 mm, although a few of the imaging studies have detected incidental macroadenomas, >10 mm, in up to ~30–50% of cases [1, 4, 5]. Of note, however, many of these patients with macroadenomas were actually demonstrated to have visual field defects or partial hypopituitarism at presentation and consequently do not represent such a conundrum regarding management (Fig. 35.2). Reassuringly, the

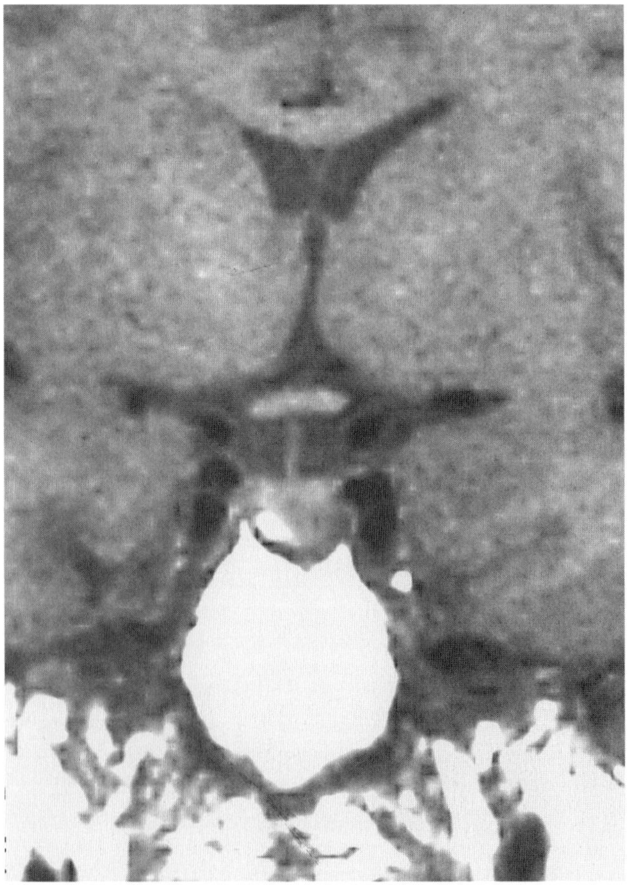

Figure 35.1 Coronal MRI section demonstrating a left-sided pituitary microadenoma identified coincidentally, in an asymptomatic 70-year-old woman, after brain imaging was carried out for an unrelated clinical indication.

Clinical Endocrine Oncology, 2nd edition. Edited by Ian D. Hay and John A.H. Wass. © 2008 Blackwell Publishing. ISBN 978-1-4051-4584-8.

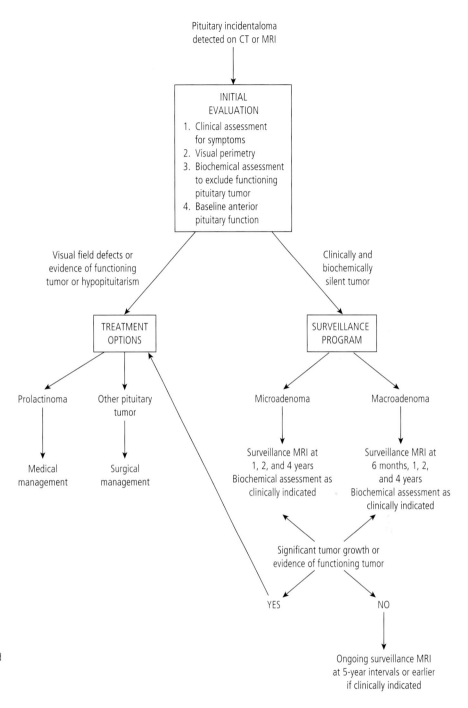

Figure 35.2 Schematic diagram detailing suggested evaluation, management and surveillance guidelines for pituitary incidentalomas.

post mortem studies identified almost exclusively microadenomas, suggesting that either progression from a microadenoma to a macroadenoma is relatively rare and/or that nearly all patients with macroadenomas present with symptoms during life [3].

Alternative diagnoses

It should be highlighted that although the commonest intrasellar mass is a pituitary adenoma, and it is generally accepted in the

literature that the term pituitary incidentaloma refers specifically to this pathology, other potential intrasellar and parasellar lesions must first be considered and excluded. These alternative diagnoses are numerous but include craniopharyngiomas, Rathke cleft cysts, meningiomas, gliomas, hamartomas, pituitary metastases, and inflammatory masses such as sarcoidosis, tuberculosis, or lymphocytic hypophysitis [3, 6]. A diagnosis other than a pituitary adenoma essentially rests on the radiological findings and becomes more likely if the mass is >10 mm in diameter. Consequently, because the natural history and management of these lesions varies considerably, all patients should ideally be initially assessed in a multidisciplinary setting with input from an endocrinologist, a neuroradiologist, and a pituitary neurosurgeon; a biopsy may be required in order to enable an appropriate management plan to be devised on an individual patient basis. However, once this small subgroup of patients is excluded, the majority of individuals diagnosed with a pituitary incidentaloma will have an underlying pituitary adenoma.

Presentation

Although the concept of a pituitary incidentaloma has been recognized in the literature for a number of decades it has only become a significant clinical problem for endocrinologists in recent years with the increasing use of modern neuroradiology modalities. Limited data are available regarding the natural history of these lesions, although based on the known presentation and progression of clinically significant pituitary adenomas there are obviously the theoretical concerns of tumor growth and hormone hypersecretion. It is well recognized that tumor growth, although rarely truly malignant, may be very destructive due to damage to local structures including the optic chiasm, cavernous sinus invasion or the development of hormone deficiencies secondary to compression of normal pituitary endocrine tissue. States of hormone excess as a consequence of pituitary tumor hypersecretion typically lead to well-characterized clinical syndromes with significant associated morbidity and mortality. Diagnosis of these syndromes, such as Cushing disease and acromegaly, have been refined over time but increasingly it is being proposed that these diseases may actually represent a spectrum where the actual diagnostic cut-off is somewhat arbitrary and more subtle "subclinical" states may also confer a degree of increased risk. For example, patients with subclinical Cushing disease might experience a worsening in glycemic control and hypertension sufficient to influence long-term cardiovascular morbidity and mortality. There is no clear consensus on the management of these subclinical states and currently any studies on the follow-up of so-called pituitary incidentalomas will clearly be influenced by these subgroups. If increasing evidence suggests a higher risk of adverse events for these patients then it is likely that they will be redefined as a separate entity and managed appropriately.

Evaluation

Following a radiological diagnosis of a pituitary incidentaloma in an asymptomatic individual, the first priority is to evaluate the patient carefully to exclude subtle clinical or biochemical effects of the tumor, which may be appropriately treated surgically or medically (Fig. 35.2). However, if careful assessment confirms a clinically and biochemically silent tumor then management becomes more controversial. Macroadenomas, by virtue of their size, have already demonstrated their capacity to proliferate and

enlarge and a number of studies have confirmed that up to ~30% of clinically and biochemically silent pituitary incidentalomas >10 mm will exhibit further significant increases in size when monitored radiologically over relatively short time periods [1, 4, 5]. Consequently, if surveillance rather than treatment is the initial management decision, then these lesions must be carefully and frequently reassessed to ensure that treatment intervention precedes any significant adverse effects (Fig. 35.2). Patients with macroadenomas managed conservatively must especially be counseled about the rare but potentially serious complication of pituitary apoplexy [7], especially in an era with ever-increasing therapeutic anticoagulation and antiplatelet treatments for the prevention of cardiovascular morbidity and mortality. In contrast, there are numerous studies providing evidence that the majority of microadenomas do not enlarge and that radiological surveillance is an acceptable strategy in these patients [4, 8]. However, the mean follow-up in the majority of studies is relatively short at 2.7–8.0 years [1, 4, 5, 7, 8] and complications including tumor enlargement and slowly progressive hormonal hypersecretion have been described [3, 4] and consequently most endocrinologists would advocate ongoing surveillance for these patients. Long term, in patients with stable non-progressive lesions the intervals between monitoring may be extended but discharging patients from any surveillance is controversial since regrowth has been described in a few cases even after many years of tumor quiescence [9].

Management

As a consequence of the lack of evidence, current management of clinically and biochemically silent pituitary incidentalomas varies widely between specialist centers and between different countries and this was nicely illustrated in a survey of endocrinologists from the UK and USA carried out in 1997 [10]. Two hypothetical scenarios involving a 5 mm pituitary incidentaloma in a 25-year-old woman and a 15 mm pituitary incidentaloma in a middle-aged man were utilized. In both cases UK endocrinologists carried out significantly more biochemical tests at initial assessment than their US colleagues but were less likely to obtain a follow-up scan and the intervals between repeat imaging were longer [10]. With an increasing prevalence of pituitary incidentalomas, these differing approaches clearly have financial implications and a cost-effective and safe approach needs to be identified, ideally with further prospective studies. One US study has attempted to assess both the financial cost and the clinical implications of four differing approaches to the management of pituitary incidentalomas [11]. These included expectant management where no assessment was carried out if the patient remained asymptomatic, prolactin screening, a panel of anterior pituitary function tests or repeat MRI imaging at 6 and 12 months. Based on QALYs (quality-adjusted life-years) a single test for prolactin was the most cost-effective strategy [11], but clearly this approach entails a significant degree of clinical risk and is not widespread current practice. To ensure that the management of pituitary incidentalomas is clinically effective and cost effective it may be viewed using the same criteria which are applied when assessing the feasibility of any disease-screening program in a particular population, albeit in this case an unintentional screening program. For example, the condition must have a recognized presymptomatic phase which is both easily detectable and treatable, the diagnostic tests must be acceptable to patients, the condition must progress such that adverse outcomes are reasonably frequent and not as easily treatable as in the presymptomatic phase and an infrastructure must be in place for counseling these patients. For pituitary incidentalomas the answers to some of these questions are outstanding and only as increasing evidence accumulates will clearer guidelines be devised. In the interim, Fig. 35.2 provides a proposed management strategy based on the combined evidence available to date.

References

1. Feldkamp J, Santen R, Harms E, Aulich A, Modder U, Scherbaum WA. Incidentally discovered pituitary lesions: high frequency of macroadenomas and hormone-secreting adenomas – results of a prospective study. *Clin. Endocrinol. (Oxf.)* 1999;51:109–13.
2. Hall WA, Luciano MG, Doppman JL, Patronas NJ, Oldfield EH. Pituitary magnetic resonance imaging in normal human volunteers: occult adenomas in the general population. *Ann. Intern. Med.* 1994;120:817–820.
3. Molitch ME. Clinical review 65. Evaluation and treatment of the patient with a pituitary incidentaloma. *J. Clin. Endocrinol. Metab.* 1995;80:3–6.
4. Reincke M, Allolio B, Saeger W, Menzel J, Winkelmann W. The "incidentaloma" of the pituitary gland. Is neurosurgery required? *JAMA* 1990;263:2772–2776.
5. Donovan LE, Corenblum B. The natural history of the pituitary incidentaloma. *Arch. Intern. Med.* 1995;155:181–183.
6. Teramoto A, Hirakawa K, Sanno N, Osamura Y. Incidental pituitary lesions in 1000 unselected autopsy specimens. *Radiology* 1994;193:161–164.
7. Nishizawa S, Ohta S, Yokoyama T, Uemura K. Therapeutic strategy for incidentally found pituitary tumors ("pituitary incidentalomas"). *Neurosurgery* 1998;43:1344–1348; discussion 1348–1350.
8. Sanno N, Oyama K, Tahara S, Teramoto A, Kato Y. A survey of pituitary incidentaloma in Japan. *Eur. J. Endocrinol.* 2003;149:123–127.
9. Frohman L, Kupersmith MJ, Warren F. The pituitary incidentaloma beyond the first year of follow-up. *JAMA* 1990;264:2387.
10. Howlett TA, Como J, Aron DC. Management of pituitary incidentalomas. A survey of British and American endocrinologists. *Endocrinol. Metab. Clin. North Am.* 2000;29:223–230, xi.
11. King JT Jr., Justice AC, Aron DC. Management of incidental pituitary microadenomas: a cost-effectiveness analysis. *J. Clin. Endocrinol. Metab.* 1997;82:3625–3632.

36 Craniopharyngioma

Niki Karavitaki

Key points

- Craniopharyngiomas are epithelial tumors with an annual incidence of 0.13/100 000 and peak incidence rates between the ages of 5–14 and 50–74 years. Two primary pathological subtypes have been recognized: the adamantinomatous and the papillary (transitional or mixed forms have also been described).
- They may exert pressure effects on various brain structures resulting in multiple clinical features (neurological, visual, hypothalamo–pituitary).
- A suprasellar component is found in 94–95% and calcification in 45–57% of cases. They can be purely/mainly cystic in 46–64%, purely/mainly solid in 18–39% and mixed in 8–36%.
- If gross total surgical removal cannot safely be achieved, adjuvant external beam irradiation improves the local control rates significantly (10-year recurrence rates: gross total removal 0–62%, partial/subtotal 25–100%, partial/subtotal + radiotherapy 0–23%). There are no consistent data on other predictors of recurrence.
- They are associated with significant long-term morbidity (mainly endocrine, visual, hypothalamic, neurobehavioral/cognitive), compromising normal psychosocial integration and the quality of life. Mortality rates three to six times higher than that of the general population have been reported. Survival is negatively affected by recurrence.

Epidemiology

Craniopharyngiomas are epithelial tumors arising along the path of the craniopharyngeal duct (the canal connecting the stomodeal ectoderm with the evaginated Rathke's pouch). They have an overall incidence of 0.13 per 100 000 person-years and they account for 2–5% of all the primary intracranial neoplasms (5.6–15% of the intracranial tumors in children). They may be diagnosed at any age with peak incidence rates between 5–14 and 50–74 years [1].

Pathogenesis and pathology

Their pathogenesis has not been clarified. Two theories have been suggested: neoplastic transformation of embryonic squamous cell rests of the involuted craniopharyngeal duct or metaplasia of adenohypophyseal cells in the pituitary stalk or gland [1].

Craniopharyngiomas are grade I tumors (WHO classification). Histologically, two primary subtypes have been recognized, the adamantinomatous and the papillary, but transitional or mixed forms have also been described [1, 2]. The adamantinomatous is

Clinical Endocrine Oncology, 2nd edition. Edited by Ian D. Hay and John A.H. Wass. © 2008 Blackwell Publishing. ISBN 978-1-4051-4584-8.

the most frequently reported and may be diagnosed at all ages. Macroscopically, it shows cystic and/or solid components, necrotic debris, fibrous tissue and calcification. The liquid within the cysts ranges from "machinery oil" to shimmering cholesterol-laden fluid, and it is mostly composed of desquamated squamous epithelial cells, rich in membrane lipids and cytoskeleton keratin. The borders often merge into a peripheral zone of dense reactive gliosis, which may lead to the misdiagnosis of a glioma. Furthermore, the margins are frequently sharp and irregular, posing significant difficulties in the manipulation of the surgical planes and the preservation of critical structures. The epithelium is composed of a palisaded basal layer of small cells, an intermediate one with loose aggregates of stellate cells (stellate reticulum), and a top layer of abruptly enlarged, flattened and keratinized to flat plate-like squamous cells (Fig. 36.1). The flat squamous epithelial cells may be desquamated in distinctive stacked clusters forming characteristic nodules of "wet" keratin, and the keratinous debris often elicits an inflammatory and foreign body giant cell reaction [1–4]. The papillary subtype has been almost exclusively found in adult patients. Macroscopically, it is usually solid or mixed, calcification is rarely seen and the cyst content is mostly viscous and yellow. Infiltration of adjacent brain tissue is less frequent than in the adamantinomatous type. Microscopically, it is composed of mature squamous epithelium forming pseudopapillae and an anastomosing fibrovascular stroma, which includes a small number of chronic inflammatory cells (Fig. 36.2). The differential diagnosis between a papillary craniopharyngioma and

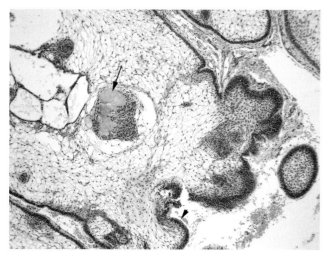

Figure 36.1 Adamantinomatous craniopharyngioma. The epithelium consists of palisaded basal layer of cells (arrowhead), the intermediate stellate reticulum, and a layer of flattened, keratinized squamous cells. Nodules of "wet" keratin are characteristic (arrow) (HE ×20). (Reproduced from Karavitaki N et al. [1], with permission from The Endocrine Society.)

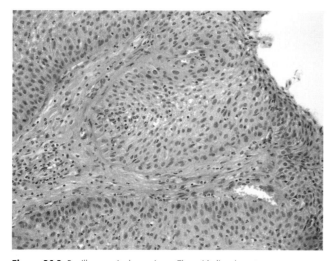

Figure 36.2 Papillary craniopharyngioma. The epithelium is mature squamous forming pseudopapillae (HE ×10). (Reproduced from Karavitaki N et al. [1], with permission from The Endocrine Society.)

a Rathke's cleft cyst may be occasionally perplexing, due to the squamous differentiation that the epithelial lining of the Rathke's cysts may undergo [1, 2, 4].

Clinical, hormonal and imaging features at presentation

Most of the craniopharyngiomas are detected in the sellar/parasellar region; rare ectopic locations have also been described, such as the pineal gland, the cerebellopontine angle or completely within the third ventricle. A suprasellar component has been reported in 94–95% of the cases (purely suprasellar 20–41%, both supra- and intrasellar 53–75%, purely intrasellar 5–6%), and extension into the anterior or middle or posterior fossa in nearly 30% of them [1, 3, 5].

Craniopharyngiomas may exert pressure effects to various brain structures resulting in multiple clinical features (neurological, visual, hypothalamo–pituitary); headaches, nausea/vomiting, visual disturbances, growth failure (in children), and hypogonadism (in adults) are the most frequently described. A substantial number of patients present with compromised hypothalamo–pituitary function; reported rates for pituitary hormone deficits include 35–95% for growth hormone (GH), 38–82% for follicle-stimulating hormone (FSH)/luteinizing hormone (LH), 21–62% for adreno-corticotropic hormone (ACTH), 21–42% for thyroid-stimulating hormone (TSH), and 6–38% for antidiuretic hormone (ADH) [1, 3, 5, 6].

Useful imaging tools for the diagnosis of craniopharyngiomas include plain skull X-rays, computerized tomography (CT), magnetic resonance imaging (MRI) and occasionally, cerebral angiography. Plain skull X-rays, although seldom used nowadays, may show calcification and abnormal sella [1]. CT is helpful for the evaluation of the bony anatomy, the identification of calcifications and the discrimination of the solid and the cystic components (the cystic fluid is hypodense and the solid portions, as well as the cyst capsule, show enhancement following contrast administration) [1]. MRI is particularly important for the top-ographic and structural analysis of the tumor. A solid lesion appears as iso- or hypointense relative to the brain on precontrast T1-weighted images, shows enhancement following gadolinium administration and is usually of mixed hypo- or hyperintensity on T2-weighted sequences. Large amounts of calcification may be visualized as areas of low signal on both T1- and T2-weighted images. A cystic element is usually hypointense on T1- and hyper-intense on T2-weighted sequences (Fig. 36.3). On T1-weighted images a thin peripheral contrast-enhancing rim of the cyst is demonstrated. Protein, cholesterol, and methemoglobin may cause high signal on T1-weighted images, while very concentrated protein, calcification and various blood products may be associated with low T2-weighted signal [1].

The size of craniopharyngiomas has been reported as >4 cm in 14–20% of cases, 2–4 cm in 58–76% and <2 cm in 4–28% [1, 7]. Their consistency is purely or predominantly cystic in 46–64%, purely or predominantly solid in 18–39% and mixed in 8–36% [1, 5, 7]. Calcification has been shown in 45–57% and is probably more common in children (78–100%) [1, 3, 6, 7]. Hydrocephalus has been reported in 20–38% and is probably more frequent in childhood populations (41–54%) [1, 5, 6, 8]. There is no agree-ment on the radiological features discriminating the two histolo-gical subtypes [1]. The differential diagnosis includes a number of sellar or parasellar lesions, including Rathke's cleft cyst, dermoid cyst, epidermoid cyst, pituitary adenoma, germinoma, hamar-toma, suprasellar aneurysm, arachnoid cyst, suprasellar abscess, glioma, meningioma, sacroidosis, tuberculosis and Langerhans cell histiocytosis [1].

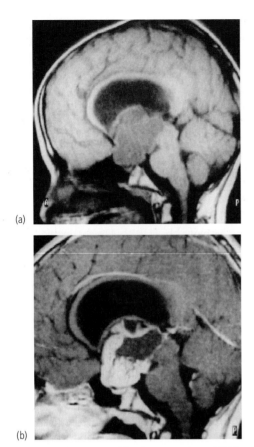

(a)

(b)

Figure 36.3 Sagittal non-contrast (a) and contrast-enhanced (b) T1-weighted MRIs demonstrating a hypointense suprasellar tumor with peripherally enhancing cystic areas and an inhomogeneously enhancing solid tumor part. (Reproduced from Sartoretti-Schefer et al., *Am. J. Neuroradiol.* 1997;18:77–87, with permission from the American Society of Neuroradiology.)

Treatment

Surgical removal alone or combined with external beam irradiation

Surgery alone or combined with adjuvant external beam irradiation is currently one of the most widely used first therapeutic approaches for these tumors. Craniopharyngiomas remain challenging tumors, even in the era of modern neurosurgery. This is mainly attributed to their sharp, irregular borders and to their tendency to adhere to vital neurovascular structures, making surgical manipulations potentially hazardous to vital brain areas. Consequently, the attempted degree of excision has been a subject of long-standing debate. The extent of resection depends on the size (achieved in 0% of lesions >4 cm) and location (particularly difficult for retrochiasmatic or within the third ventricle) of the tumor, the presence of hydrocephalus, of >10% calcification and of brain invasion, as well as on the experience, the individual judgment during the operation and the general treatment policy (aggressive or not) adopted by each neurosurgeon. Notably, in various large series radical surgery has been accomplished in

18–84% of the cases [1, 5, 7, 8]. The advances in neuroimaging, microsurgical techniques, perioperative care and hormone replacement therapy have significantly improved the perioperative mortality, which in recent reports ranges between 1.7% and 5.4% for the primary operations. Although not widely accepted, procedures resulting in radical excision may carry substantial perioperative morbidity and mortality [1, 5–8].

Recurrence may arise even from small islets of craniopharyngioma cells in the gliotic brain adjacent to the tumor. The mean interval for their diagnosis following various primary treatment modalities ranges between 1 and 4.3 years [1, 5, 9]. Series with radiological confirmation of the radicality of resection show that the recurrence rates following gross total removal range between 0% and 62% at 10 years follow-up. These are significantly lower than those reported after partial or subtotal resection (25–100% at 10 years follow-up). In cases of limited surgery, adjuvant radiotherapy significantly improves the local control rates (recurrence rates 10–63% at 10 years follow-up). Notably, studies with statistical comparisons of the recurrences detected after gross total removal or combination of surgery and radiotherapy have not provided consistent results. Finally, radiotherapy alone provides 10-year recurrence rates ranging between 0% and 23% [1, 5–10]. In cases of predominantly cystic tumors, fluid aspiration provides relief of the obstructive manifestations and facilitates the consecutive removal of the solid tumor portion; the latter should not be delayed for more than a few weeks, due to the significant risk of cyst refilling (reported in up to 81% of the cases at a median period of 10 months) [5, 7]. The interpretation of the data on the effectiveness of each therapeutic modality has to be done with caution, since the published studies are retrospective, non-randomized and often specialty biased. The growth rate of craniopharyngiomas varies considerably and reliable clinical, radiological and pathological criteria predicting their behavior are lacking. Thus, apart from the significant impact of the treatment modality, attempts to identify other prognostic factors (age group at diagnosis, sex, imaging features, pathological subtypes) have not provided consistent data [1].

The management of recurrent tumors remains difficult, as scarring/adhesions from previous operations or irradiation decrease the chances of successful excision. In such cases, total removal is achieved in a substantially lower rate when compared with primary surgery (0–25%) and is associated with increased perioperative morbidity and mortality (10.5–24%), suggesting that for many recurrent lesions palliative surgery is the most realistic target [1, 5, 7]. The beneficial effect of radiotherapy (preceded or not by second surgery) in recurrent lesions has been clearly shown [1, 5].

Other treatment options

Intracavitary irradiation (brachytherapy) is a minimally invasive treatment modality, which involves stereotactically guided instillation of β-emitting isotopes into cystic craniopharyngiomas, thereby delivering a higher radiation dose to the cyst lining than the one offered by external beam radiotherapy. Its beneficial effect is achieved through destruction of the secretory epithelial lining leading to elimination of the fluid production and cyst shrinkage. Based on studies with the largest series of patients and with relatively long follow-up periods, brachytherapy seems to offer a good prospect for the reduction or stabilization of cystic craniopharyngiomas. This effect combined with its reported low surgical morbidity and mortality render this management option attractive for predominantly cystic tumors, and particularly the monocystic ones. Still, the most beneficial isotope and the impact on the quality of survival and long-term morbidity remain to be assessed [1, 11].

A small number of reports have shown that the intracystic installation of the antineoplastic agent bleomycin may be an effective therapy for some cystic tumors. Direct leakage of the drug to surrounding tissues during the installation procedure, diffusion though the cyst wall or high drug dose have been associated with various toxic (hypothalamic damage, blindness, hearing loss, ischemic attacks, peritumoral edema) or even fatal effects. The value of this treatment option in tumor control or even in the delaying of potentially harmful surgery and/or radiotherapy, as well as the optimal protocol and the clear-cut criteria predicting the long-term outcome, remain to be established in large series with appropriate follow-up [1, 12].

Stereotactic radiosurgery delivers a single fraction of high-dose ionizing radiation on precisely mapped targets, keeping the exposure of adjacent structures to a minimum. Tumor volume and close attachment to critical structures are limiting factors for its application. Based on a small number of reports, which cover relatively short follow-up periods, it achieves tumor control in a substantial number of patients with small volume lesions. It may be particularly useful for well-defined residual disease following surgery or for the treatment of small solid recurrent tumors, particularly after failure of conventional radiotherapy. In cases of large cystic portions multimodality approaches with instillation of radioisotopes or bleomycin may provide further benefits. Studies with long-term follow-up evaluating the optimal marginal dose, its role in the prevention of tumor growth and its effects on the neurocognitive and neuroendocrine functions are needed [1, 13].

Stereotactic radiotherapy combines the accurate focal dose delivery of stereotactic radiosurgery with the radiobiological advantages of fractionation. The data on its usefulness for the management of craniopharyngiomas are limited, but the largest series published so far provides promising results [14].

Systemic chemotherapy has been offered in a limited number of patients mainly with aggressive tumors, with relative success [1]. Its application remains rather experimental and its value, particularly in the treatment of aggressive tumors, remains to be established.

Long-term morbidity and mortality

Craniopharyngiomas are associated with significant long-term morbidity mainly involving endocrine, visual, hypothalamic, neurobehavioral and cognitive sequelae, which compromise normal psychosocial integration and the quality of living. These complications are attributed to the damage of critical structures by the primary or recurrent tumor and/or to the adverse effects of the therapeutic interventions. Notably, the severity of radiation-induced late toxicity is affected by the total and per fraction doses, the volume of the exposed normal tissue and the young age in childhood populations [1].

In studies with variable follow-up periods and after different treatment modalities, the rates of individual hormone deficits range between 88–100% for GH, 80–95% for FSH/LH, 55–88% for ACTH, 39–95% for TSH and 25–86% for ADH. Apart from symptomatic diabetes insipidus, which is probably more common in surgically treated patients, the long-term endocrine morbidity is not affected by the type of tumor therapy [1, 5, 10]. The phenomenon of growth without GH has been reported in some children with craniopharyngioma (normal or even accelerated linear growth, despite their untreated GH deficiency), but its pathophysiological mechanism has not been clarified. GH replacement does not seem to increase the risk of tumor recurrence [1, 5, 15].

Compromised vision has been reported in up to 62.5% of the patients treated by surgery alone or combined with radiotherapy during observation period of 10 years [6].

Hypothalamic damage may result in hyperphagia and uncontrollable obesity, disorders of thirst and water/electrolyte balance, behavioral and cognitive impairment, loss of temperature control and disorders in the sleep pattern [1, 5, 6, 8, 10]. Among those, obesity is the most frequent, reported in 26–61% of the patients treated by surgery alone or combined with radiotherapy. It is a consequence of the disruption of the mechanisms controlling satiety, hunger and energy balance and it often results in devastating metabolic and psychosocial complications [1, 5, 6, 10]. Factors associated with significant hypothalamic morbidity have been proposed to be young age at presentation in children, manifestations of hypothalamic disturbance at diagnosis, hypothalamic invasion, tumor height greater than 3.5 cm from the midline, attempts to remove adherent tumor from the region of the hypothalamus, multiple operations for recurrence and hypothalamic radiation doses >51 Gy [1].

The compromised neuropsychological and cognitive function in patients with craniopharyngioma contributes significantly to poor academic and work performance, disrupted family and social relationships and impaired quality of life [1]. Duff et al. [6], in a series of 121 patients treated by surgery with or without adjuvant radiotherapy and followed up for a mean period of 10 years, found that 40% of them had poor outcome (the assessment was based on motor and visual deficits, dependence for activities of daily living, Karnofsky Performance Scale, school and work status, debilitating psychological or emotional problems). De Vile et al. [8], in a series of 75 children treated by surgery alone or combined with radiotherapy and followed up for a mean period of 6.4 years, demonstrated that 40% of them had IQ <80. There is no consensus on the therapeutic option with the least unfavorable impact on the neurobehavioral outcome, necessitating prospective studies with formal neuropsychological testing and specific behavioral assessment before and after any intervention [1]. Such data will be particularly important for the young children, in whom the uncertainties of whether delaying irradiation is a reasonable policy, and whether the neurotoxicity of the recurrent disease and the subsequent surgery is higher than the one associated with irradiation offered to prevent relapse, need to be answered.

Further rare long-term irradiation-attributed morbidities include vasculopathy and second brain tumors [1].

The overall mortality rates of patients with craniopharyngioma have been reported to be three to six times higher than that of the general population; in studies published during the last decade, the survival rates range between 80% and 91% at 5 years and 83% and 92.7% at 10 years [1, 5, 7]. Apart from the deaths directly attributed to the tumor (pressure effects to critical structures) and to the surgical interventions, the risk of cardio-/cerebrovascular

and respiratory mortality is increased [1, 5, 7, 10, 16]. It has also been suggested that in childhood populations the hypoadrenalism and the associated hypoglycemia, as well as the metabolic consequences of ADH deficiency and absent thirst, may contribute to the excessive mortality [1, 17]. The impact of tumor recurrence on the long-term mortality is widely accepted and the 10-year survival rates in such cases range between 29% and 70% (depending on the subsequent treatment modalities) [1, 5].

Treatment algorithm

Based on the significant literature available, the proposed treatment algorithm is shown in Fig. 36.4 [1]. Surgical removal is suggested

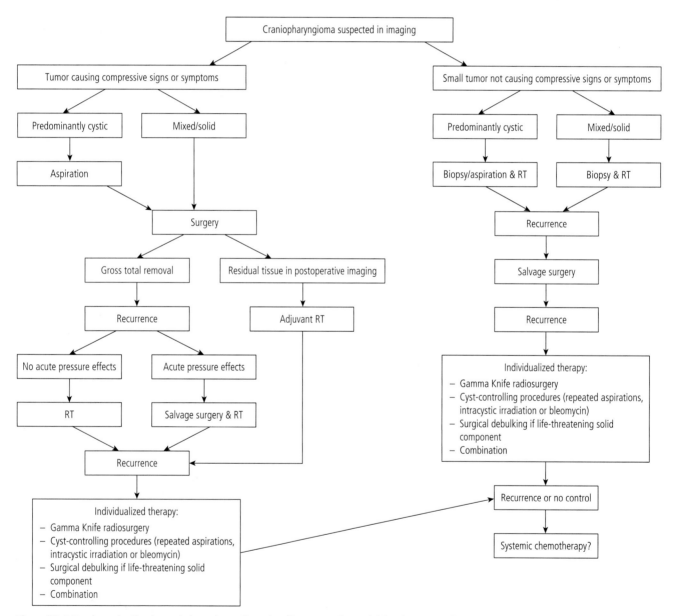

Figure 36. 4 Treatment algorithm for craniopharyngiomas. (Reproduced from Karavitaki N et al. [1], with permission from The Endocrine Society.)

for all tumors resulting in compressive signs or symptoms (if a predominantly cystic lesion, the resection may be facilitated by previous aspiration of the cyst fluid). Gross total removal is a reasonable target, provided it is performed by an experienced neurosurgeon and hazardous manipulations to vital brain structures are avoided. In cases of residual tumor following primary surgery, postoperative irradiation is recommended; this is because of the high risk of relapse and its negative impact on morbidity and mortality. Although this strategy may be debated for young children, the radiation toxicity to the developing brain needs to be balanced with the consequences of a recurrent mass and subsequent possible multiple surgical procedures. In small tumors not causing pressure effects (visual, neurological, hypothalamic), radiotherapy (preceded by biopsy for confirmation of the diagnosis) is an attractive option avoiding the risks of surgery. In predominantly cystic tumors, previous aspiration of the fluid may decrease the adverse sequelae of possible cyst enlargement during irradiation.

The treatment of recurrent disease depends on the previous interventions and the severity of the clinical picture. In recurrent lesions not previously irradiated, radiotherapy provides satisfactory local control rates. Taking into account the high morbidity and mortality of a second surgery, such an intervention is advocated only in cases of acute pressure effects. The treatment of further recurrence should be individualized and options include Gamma Knife radiosurgery, cyst-controlling procedures, surgical debulking (for significant solid life-threatening component), and systemic chemotherapy [1].

References

1. Karavitaki N, Cudlip S, Adams CBT, Wass JAH. Craniopharyngiomas. *Endocr. Rev.* 2006;27:371–397.
2. Crotty TB, Scheithauer BW, Young WF, et al. Papillary craniopharyngioma: a clinico-pathological study of 48 cases. *J. Neurosurg.* 1995;83:206–214.
3. Petito CK, De Girolami U, Earle K. Craniopharyngiomas. A clinical and pathological review. *Cancer* 1976;37:1944–1952.
4. Miller DC. Pathology of craniopharyngiomas: clinical import of pathological findings. *Pediatr. Neurosurg.* 1994;21(Suppl 1):11–17.
5. Karavitaki N, Brufani C, Warner JT, et al. Craniopharyngiomas in children and adults: systematic analysis of 121 cases with long-term follow-up. *Clin. Endocrinol.* 2005;62:397–409.
6. Duff JM, Meyer FB, Ilstrup DM, Laws ERJr, Scleck CD, Scheithauer BW. Long-term outcomes for surgically resected craniopharyngiomas. *Neurosurgery* 2000;46:291–305.
7. Fahlbush R, Honegger J, Paulus W, Huk W, Buchfelder M. Surgical treatment of craniopharyngiomas: experience with 168 patients. *J. Neurosurg.* 1999;90:237–250.
8. De Vile CJ, Grant DB, Kendall BE, et al. Management of childhood craniopharyngioma: can the morbidity of radical surgery be predicted? *J. Neurosurg.* 1996;85:73–81.
9. Rajan B, Ashley S, Gorman C, et al. Craniopharyngioma – long-term results following limited surgery and radiotherapy. *Radiat. Oncol.* 1993;26:1–10.
10. Hetelekidis S, Barnes PD, Tao ML, et al. 20-year experience in childhood craniopharyngioma. *Int. J. Radiat. Oncol. Biol. Phys.* 1993;27:189–195.
11. Hasegawa T, Kondzilka D, Hadjipanayis CG, Lunsford LD. Management of cystic craniopharyngiomas with phosphorus-32 intracavitary irradiation. *Neurosurgery* 2004;54:813–822.
12. Hader WJ, Steinbok P, Hukin J, Fryer C. Intratumoral therapy with bleomycin for cystic craniopharyngiomas in children. *Pediatr. Neurosurg.* 2000;33:211–218.
13. Chung WY, Pan DHC, Shiau CY, WY G, Wang LW. Gamma knife radiosurgery for craniopharyngiomas. *J. Neurosurg.* 2000;93(Suppl 3):47–56.
14. Schulz-Ertner D, Frank C, Herfarth KK, Rhein B, Wannemacher M, Debus J. Fractionated stereotactic radiotherapy for craniopharyngiomas. *Int. J. Radiat. Oncol. Phys.* 2002;54:114–120.
15. Karavitaki N, Warner JT, Marland A, et al. GH replacement does not increase the risk of recurrence in patients with craniopharyngioma. *Clin. Endocrinol.* 2006;64:556–560.
16. Tomlinson JW, Holden N, Hills RK, et al. and the West Midlands Prospective Hypopituitary Study Group. Association between premature mortality and hypopituitarism. *Lancet* 2001;357:425–431.
17. De Vile CJ, Grant DB, Hayward RD, Stanhope R. Growth and endocrine sequelae of craniopharyngioma. *Arch. Dis. Child.* 1996;75:108–114.

37 Benign Cysts: Rathke's Cleft Cysts, Mucoceles, Arachnoid Cysts, and Dermoid and Epidermoid Cysts

Niki Karavitaki

Key points

- Rathke's cleft cysts are benign, rarely symptomatic, cystic sellar and/or parasellar lesions; their recurrence rate following surgical intervention (mostly evacuation and biopsy) range between 8% and 33%.
- Mucoceles of the sphenoid sinus are very rare, benign, cystic lesions resulting from chronic obstruction of the sinus; marsupialization by partial removal of its walls prevents relapse and complications in most of the cases.
- Arachnoid cysts are benign, mostly supratentorial, intra-arachnoidal cysts filled with clear cerebrospinal fluid and accounting for 1% of all intracranial lesions; their optimal management is still a subject of debate.
- Dermoid cysts are rare, benign lesions, most commonly found in the midline sellar, parasellar or frontonasal areas; radical surgical resection, when possible, is generally curative.
- Epidermoid cysts are benign, cystic lesions representing 0.2–1.8% of all primary intracranial tumors and usually detected in the paramidline area; surgical intervention in most cases offers good results.

Rathke's cleft cysts

Rathke's cleft cysts are common benign sellar and/or suprasellar lesions found in 13–33% of routine autopsies [1, 2]. The symptomatic cases are rare [3].

The pathogenetic mechanisms implicated in the formation of Rathke's cleft cysts have not been fully clarified. According to the prevailing hypothesis, they arise from remnants of the Rathke's pouch [4, 5], a structure apparent during the third week of gestation and formed by the infolding of simple ciliated columnar epithelium lining the roof of the stomodeum. Rathke's pouch extends cranially to form the craniopharyngeal duct; its anterior and posterior walls give rise to the anterior and intermediate lobes of the pituitary gland, respectively. The obliteration of the craniopharyngeal duct is associated with the involution of Rathke's pouch. Failure of obliteration of the lumen results in the development of a cyst between the pars distalis and the pars nervosa [4, 6]. It has been proposed that the craniopharyngiomas and the Rathke's cleft cysts may represent a continuum of ectodermally derived epithelial masses [7].

Rathke's cleft cysts are smoothly marginated cysts with size usually ranging between a few millimeters to 1–2 cm. Cases with cyst size up to 45–50 mm have also been described. Their contents vary from clear cerebrospinal fluid CSF-like fluid to thick mucoid (made of cholesterol and protein) material [1, 3, 8, 9]. They are lined by single or pseudostratified cuboidal or columnar epithelium, with or without cilia, and with goblet cells. Squamous metaplasia (making them occasionally indistinguishable from craniopharyngiomas) with cholesterol clefts and eosinophilic amorphous material, macrophages and lymphocytes have also been reported [7, 8, 10]. Intracystic nodules of mucinous material may also be present [1].

The presenting manifestations are the result of compression to adjacent structures. The most frequent ones include headaches (49–81%), hypopituitarism of varying degrees (24–88%), hyperprolactinemia (19–77%), visual disturbance (38–47%), and diabetes insipidus (11%) [2, 8, 10, 11]. Rarely, aseptic meningitis or hemorrhage into the cyst may occur [12]. Notably, spontaneous resolution has been reported [8].

The imaging features of Rathke's cleft cysts are highly variable and the neuroimaging diagnosis may be difficult. Forty percent are completely intrasellar, whereas 60% have some suprasellar extension. The entirely suprasellar ones are rare [1, 8]. On computerized tomography (CT), the cyst density may be hypodense, isodense or mixed [3, 8]. On magnetic resonance imaging (MRI), they have a

---

Clinical Endocrine Oncology, 2nd edition. Edited by Ian D. Hay and John A.H. Wass. © 2008 Blackwell Publishing. ISBN 978-1-4051-4584-8.

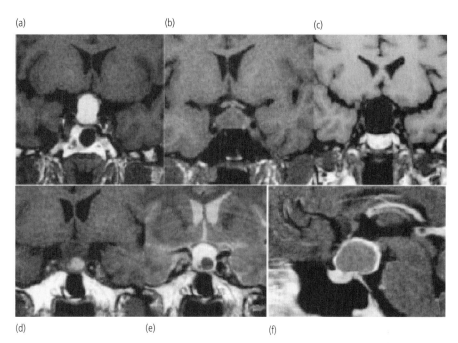

Figure 37.1 T1-weighted coronal (a–e) and gadolinium contrast-enhanced sagittal (f) MRI of Rathke's cleft cysts. Although MR intensity of the cysts is variable, it is homogeneous apart from a waxy nodule, demonstrated as a T1-high (d) and T2-low (e) signal intensity mass within the cyst. (f) Entirely suprasellar Rathke's cleft cyst with distinct rim enhancement. (Reproduced from Nishioka H et al. [8], with permission from Blackwell Publishing.)

variable T1 signal (hyper-, hypo- or isointense) depending on their biochemical content. It has been proposed that on T1 images, approximately half are hyperintense and half hypointense, whereas on T2 images, 70% are hyperintense and 30% iso- or hypointense. Cysts with high protein concentration show high T1 signal intensity and usually have a low intracystic water content leading to T2 signal decrease [1, 8, 13] (Fig. 37.1). Rim enhancement has been reported in a small number of cases [2,10]. It has been attributed to changes due to squamous metaplasia, inflammation or deposition of hemosiderin or cholesterol crystals in the cyst wall [10]. Rim enhancement has also been shown in cases in which a circumscribed area of pituitary tissue is peripheral to the cyst [10]. Small intracystic nodules corresponding to proteinaceous concentrations may be demonstrated presenting with lower T2 and higher T1 signal intensity than the rest of the cyst. The nodules do not enhance and are virtually pathognomonic for the Rathke's cleft cysts [1, 13]. The differential diagnosis includes craniopharyngiomas (typically showing calcification, may be multilobulated or with an irregular shape or rim enhancement, demonstrating heterogeneous or strong homogeneous enhancement, as well as solid-enhancing nodules in the cyst), cystic pituitary adenoma or other non-neoplastic cysts [1].

Symptomatic cases are managed by surgery. Apart from the rare entirely suprasellar cyst requiring a transcranial approach, most patients are treated transsphenoidally [2]. The endocrine prognosis after the operation remains poor, as the reversal of pituitary deficits is not common; progressive inflammation of the pituitary gland has been proposed as one of the causes [2, 8]. The risk of recurrence following (in most series) evacuation and biopsy ranges between 8% and 33% [2, 3, 10, 11, 14]. Although not widely accepted, the extent of removal (gross total vs partial) may predict relapse [2].

Mucoceles of the sphenoid sinus

Mucoceles of the sphenoid sinus are very rare, benign, cystic lesions lined by a secretory pseudostratified columnar epithelium. They result from chronic obstruction of the sinus leading to the accumulation and dehydration of the secretions and their protein contents. The cause of the obstruction is not clear; prior sinus disease, allergic history, trauma or surgery of the sphenoid sinus have been implicated [15, 16]. The clinical manifestations depend on the degree of involvement of the adjacent structures and include headache, decrease in visual acuity, oculomotor palsies, exophthalmos, trigeminal nerve hypoesthesia, and pituitary insufficiency [15, 17]. On CT, they appear as well-encapsulated, non-enhancing cystic masses. A suggestive feature may be erosion of the walls of the sphenoid bone. On MRI, they are expansive, well-delineated masses with a homogeneously hyperintense T1 (attributed to the high protein content) and T2 signal. They show no enhancement [13, 15] (Fig. 37.2). The differential diagnosis includes skull base tumors. The treatment ranges from incision and drainage to total excision of the cyst. The access to the sphenoid sinus can be achieved by several routes; craniotomy is very rarely required and the sphenoid can be usually approached by transseptal routes or by endoscopic techniques [15]. Marsupialization by partial removal of the anterior and inferior walls of the mucocele with an endoscopic endonasal approach is probably the treatment of choice, preventing relapse and complications in most of the cases [18].

Arachnoid cysts

These are benign, intra-arachnoidal, space-occupying lesions filled with clear cerebrospinal fluid and not communicating with

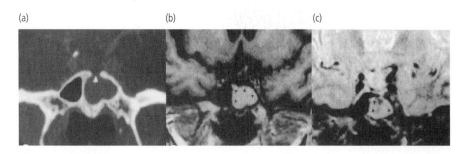

Figure 37.2 Mucocele of the sphenoid sinus. (a) CT showing opacification of the left sphenoid sinus. There is also a bone defect related to previous pituitary surgery (arrowhead). (b) Coronal T1-weighted MRI demonstrating heterogeneous increased signal from a mucocele (arrowheads); the signal intensity is increased along the sinus border. (c) Coronal T2-weighted MRI showing heterogeneous signal intensities within a sphenoid sinus mass (arrowheads). (Reproduced from Herman P et al. [17], with permission from the Annals Publishing Company.)

the ventricular system. They account for 1% of all intracranial lesions and are most often diagnosed in the first two decades of life [1]. Most are supratentorial. Five to 60% are found in the middle cranial fossa, anterior to the temporal lobes. Other locations include the suprasellar cistern, posterior fossa, within the interhemispheric fissure, over the cerebral convexity, in the choroidal fissure, cisterna magna, quadrigeminal cistern and in the vermian fissures [1]. Arachnoid cysts are usually congenital, but they may also arise after infection, trauma and hemorrhage [19]. The precise mechanism for the formation is not known. They tend to be unilocular, smoothly marginated expansible lesions that are molded by the surrounding structures [1]. Microscopically, the cyst wall consists of vascular collagenous membrane lined by flattened arachnoid cells [1].

Symptomatic patients present with hydrocephalus, visual impairment, endocrine dysfunction and syndromes resulting from brain stem compression [19, 20]. On imaging, they typically appear as sharply demarcated extra-axial cysts, with no identifiable internal architecture and no enhancing. The cyst has the same signal intensity as CSF in all sequences (Fig. 37.3). Occasionally, hemorrhage, high protein content or lack of flow within the cyst may complicate the MRI appearance [1]. The differential diagnosis

includes epidermoid cyst, chronic subdural hematoma and porencephalic cyst [1]. Their rare occurrence has limited the experience of any single center and the optimal management is still a subject of debate. Symptomatic patients have been treated with stereotactic aspiration, cyst fenestration, cystoperitoneal shunting, microsurgical excision and endoscopic ventriculocystostomy or ventriculocisternostomy. Even with the newer neuroendoscopic techniques, treatment is not always successful and the complications may be significant [20, 21]. The natural history of the asymptomatic arachnoid cysts is unknown, but a number of case reports have described spontaneous resolution [20].

Dermoid cysts

Dermoid cysts are rare (accounting for less than 0.5% of primary intracranial tumors), benign lesions most commonly found in the midline sellar, parasellar or frontonasal areas. Other locations include the midline in the posterior fossa, where they occur either as vermian lesions or within the fourth ventricle. They arise from the inclusion of ectodermally committed cells at the time of neural tube closure (third to fifth week of embryogenesis). The cyst is a

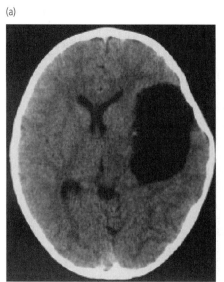 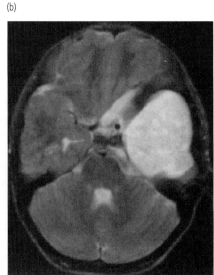

Figure 37.3 (a) Axial CT section and (b) axial T2-weighted MRI showing a large middle cranial fossa arachnoid cyst. (Reproduced from Williams SM et al. [29], with permission from the British Institute of Radiology.)

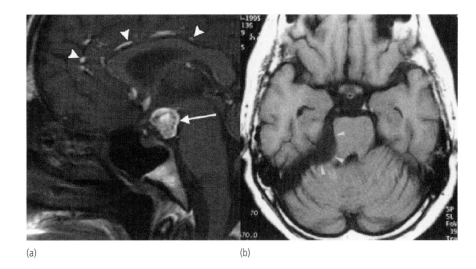

(a)　　　　　　　　　　　　　　(b)

Figure 37.4 (a) Ruptured dermoid cyst; sagittal T1-weighted image shows a large heterogeneously hyperintense suprasellar dermoid cyst (arrow) and multiple subarachnoid foci of high signal intensity consistent with fat accumulations (arrowheads). (Reproduced from Bonneville F et al. [13], with permission from the Radiological Society of North America.) (b) Epidermoid tumor in the right cerebellopontine angle cistern; on T1-weighted MR image the tumor (arrowheads) is nearly isointense with CSF. (Reproduced from Ikushima I et al. [30], with permission from the American Society of Neuroradiology.)

well-defined, lobulated, "pearly" mass of variable size containing thick, foul-smelling, yellow material attributed to the secretion of sebaceous glands and desquamated epithelium. Hair or teeth may also be present. The capsule is made of keratinized squamous epithelium supported by collagen and often has plaques of calcification. In thicker parts, the lining is supplemented with dermis containing hair follicles, sebaceous and apocrine glands. Dermoid cysts may increase in size by means of glandular secretion and epithelial desquamation [1]. The presenting manifestations are attributed to local mass effect [22]. They may rarely rupture spontaneously in the subarachnoid space, causing headache, seizures, sensory or motor hemisyndrome, or aseptic meningitis [23]. Malignant transformation has also been reported with poor prognosis [24]. On CT imaging, they are usually rounded, well-circumscribed, extremely hypodense lesions with a Hounsfield unit of −20 to −140, in keeping with their lipid content. Peripheral capsular calcification is frequent. Enhancement after contrast administration is rare [22]. On T1-weighted images non-ruptured cysts appear hyperintense with no enhancement. On T2-weighted images the signal intensity is heterogeneous varying from hypo- to hyperintense [13]. In case of rupture, they present with the pathognomonic features of T1-hyperintense speckles in the cortical sulci and a fat–fluid level in the ventricles [13] (Fig. 37.4a). Extensive pial enhancement can result from chemical meningitis. The differential diagnosis includes an epidermoid cyst, craniopharyngioma, teratoma, or lipoma [13]. Radical surgical resection, when achievable, is generally curative [25].

Epidermoid cysts

These are benign, cystic lesions representing 0.2–1.8% of all primary intracranial tumors [26]. They arise from the inclusion of ectodermal epithelial tissue into the neural tube during the fifth and sixth weeks of fetal life. They are usually detected in the paramidline area and the cerebellopontine angle is the most common location (40–61% of all intracranial epidermoids) [26].

They can also be found in the fourth ventricle (17%), in the sellar/parasellar regions (10–15%) or less commonly in the cerebral hemispheres or brainstem [1]. Ten per cent are extradural, located in the skull or spine [1]. Macroscopically, they have an irregular cauliflower-like outer surface that grows to encase vessels and nerves. The cyst content includes a soft, waxy or flaky keratohyalin material resulting from the desquamation of its wall [1]. They are lined by squamous epithelium with a linear keratohyalin granule layer [7]. They are slow-growing lesions with most of them being asymptomatic. Occasionally, they may be associated with mass effects, cranial neuropathy, seizures or (in case of rupture) with granulomatous meningitis. Malignant transformation has also been reported with poor prognosis [27]. On CT scans, they appear as well-defined hypoattenuated masses resembling CSF and not enhancing. Calcification may be detected in 10–25% of the cases. On T1- and T2-weighted MRI sections, they are typically isointense or slightly hyperintense to CSF (Fig. 37.4b). Most do not enhance, although some minimal rim enhancement is found in approximately 25% of them [1]. The differential diagnosis includes arachnoid and dermoid cyst, neurocysticercosis and cystic neoplasm [1]. Surgical treatment offers good results [26, 28].

References

1. Osborn AG, Preece MT. Intracranial cysts: radiologic-pathologic correlation and imaging approach. *Radiology* 2006;239:650–664.
2. Kim JE, Kim JH, Kim OL, et al. Surgical treatment of symptomatic Rathke cleft cysts: clinical features and results with special attention to recurrence. *J. Neurosurg.* 2004;100:33–40.
3. Mukkherjee JJ, Islam N, Kaltsas G, et al. Clinical, radiological and pathological features of patients with Rathke's cleft cysts: tumours that may recur. *J. Clin. Endocrinol. Metab.* 1997;82:2357–2362.
4. Fager CA, Carter H. Intrasellar epithelial cysts. *J. Neurosurg.* 1966;24: 77–81.
5. Shanklin WM. The histogenesis and histology of an integumentary type of epithelium in the human hypophysis. *Anat. Rec.* 1951;109:217–231.

6. Kunwar S, Wilson CB. Cysts, hamartomas and vascular tumours. In Wass JAH, Shalet SM (eds). *Oxford Textbook of Endocrinology and Diabetes.* Oxford: Oxford University Press, 2002:225–230.

7. Harrison MJ, Morgello S, Post KD. Epithelial cystic lesions of the sellar and parasellar region: a continuum of ectodermal derivatives? *J. Neurosurg.* 1994;80:1018–1025.

8. Nishioka H, Haraoka J, Izawa H, Ikeda Y. Magnetic resonance imaging, clinical manifestations, and management of Rathke's cleft. *Clin. Endocrinol.* 2006;64:184–188.

9. Tominaga J, Higano S, Takahashi S. Characteristics of Rathke's cleft cyst in MR imaging. *Magn. Res. Med. Sci.* 2003;2:1–8.

10. Billeci D, Marton E, Tripodi M, Orvieto E, Longatti P. Symptomatic Rathke's cleft cysts: a radiological, surgical and pathological review. *Pituitary* 2005;7:131–137.

11. Shin JL, Asa SL, Woodhouse LJ, Smyth HS, Ezzat S. Cystic lesions of the pituitary: clinicopathological features distinguishing craniopharyngioma, Rathke's cleft cyst, and arachnoid cyst. *J. Clin. Endocrinol. Metab.* 1999;84:3972–3982.

12. Steinberg GK, Koenig GH, Golden JB. Symptomatic Rathke's cleft cysts. Report of two cases. *J. Neurosurg.* 1982;56:290–295.

13. Bonneville F, Cattin F, Marsot-Dupuch K, Dormont D, Bonneville JF, Chiras J. T1 signal hyperintensity in the sellar region: spectrum of findings. *RadioGraphics* 2006;26:93–113.

14. Cohan P, Fouland A, Esposito F, Martin NA, Kelly DF. Symptomatic Rathke's cleft cysts: a report of 24 cases. *J. Endocrinol. Invest.* 2004;S 27:943–948.

15. Buchinsky FJ, Gennarelli TA, Strome SE, Deschler DG, Hayden RE. Sphenoid sinus mucocele: a rare complication of transsphenoidal hypophysectomy. *Ear Nose Throat J.* 2001;80:886–888.

16. Iqbal J, Kanaan I, Ahmed M, al Homsi M. Neurosurgical aspects of sphenoid sinus mucocele. *Br. J. Neurosurg.* 1998;12:527–530.

17. Herman P, Lot G, Guichard JP, Marianowski R, Assayag M, Tran Ba Huy P. Mucocele of the sphenoid sinus: a late complication of transsphenoidal pituitary surgery. *Ann. Otol. Rhinol. Laryngol.* 1998;107:765–768.

18. Moriyama H, Hesaka H, Tachibana T, Honda Y. Mucoceles of ethmoid and sphenoid sinus with visual disturbance. *Arch. Otolaryngol. Head Neck Surg.* 1992;118:142–146.

19. Mohn A, Schoof E, Fahlbusch R, Wenzel D, Dorr HG. The endocrine spectrum of arachnoid cysts in childhood. *Pediatr. Neurosurg.* 1999;31:316–321.

20. Dodd RL, Barnes PD, Huhn SL. Spontaneous resolution of prepontine arachnoid cyst. *Pediatr. Neurosurg.* 2002;37:152–157.

21. Fewel ME, Levy ML, McComb JG. Surgical treatment of 95 children with 102 intracranial arachnoid cysts. *Pediatr. Neurosurg.* 1996;25:165–173.

22. Brown JY, Morokoff AP, Mitchell PJ, Gonzales MF. Unusual imaging appearance of an intracranial dermoid cyst. *Am. J. Neuroradiol.* 2001;22:1970–1972.

23. Stendel R, Pietila TA, Lehmann K, Kurth R, Suess O, Brock M. Ruptured intracranial dermoid cysts. *Surg. Neurol.* 2002;57:391–398.

24. Sanghera P, El Modir A, Simon J. Malignant transformation within a dermoid cyst: a case report and literature review. *Arch. Gynecol. Obstet.* 2006;274:178–180.

25. Caldarelli M, Massimi L, Kondageski C, Di Rocco C. Intracranial midline dermoid and epidermoid cysts in children. *J. Neurosurg.* 2004;100:473–480.

26. Liu P, Saida Y, Yoshioka H, Itai Y. MR imaging of epidermoids at the cerebellopontine angle. *Magn. Res. Med. Sci.* 2003;2:109–115.

27. Michael LM, Moss T, Madhu T, Coakham HB. Malignant transformation of posterior fossa epidermoid cyst. *Br. J. Neurosurg.* 2006;19:505–510.

28. Yamakawa K, Shitara N, Genka S, Manaka S, Takakura K. Clinical course and surgical prognosis of 33 cases of intracranial epidermoid tumours. *Neurosurgery* 1989;24:568–573.

29. Williams SM, Dean AM. A new lump. *Br. J. Radiol.* 2002;75:489–490.

30. Ikushima I, Korogi Y, Hirai T, et al. MR of epidermoids with a variety of pulse sequences. *Am. J. Neuroradiol.* 1997;18:1359–1363.

38 Hypothalamic Hamartomas and Gangliocytomas

Lawrence A. Frohman

Key points

- Hamartomas are hypothalamic developmental nodules associated with gelastic seizures and/or precocious puberty.
- Seizures cannot be managed medically and surgical excision of the hamartoma is the preferred therapy.
- Precocious puberty can be effectively and safely treated by long-acting gonadotropin-releasing hormone agonists.
- Pituitary gangliocytomas are rare, slowly growing tumors frequently associated with pituitary adenomas and hormone hypersecretory syndromes.
- Growth hormone-secreting adenomas are associated with more than half of all reported pituitary gangliocytomas and are likely caused by growth hormone-releasing hormone secretion from the tumor.

Introduction

Hamartomas and gangliocytomas are two rare disorders of the hypothalamic–pituitary region associated with disturbances in neuroendocrine function. Although the terms have occasionally been used interchangeably, clear distinctions exist between the two. There are differences in their pathogenesis (gangliocytomas are neoplasms while hamartomas are developmental abnormalities), spectra of endocrine and non-endocrine clinical syndromes, age of onset, and therapy. This warrants consideration as two separate entities.

Hamartomas

The term hamartoma is derived from *hamartia* (Greek: error/mistake) and was first used to describe non-neoplastic developmental nodules resembling hypothalamic gray matter, but in ectopic locations. They usually occur as 10–30 mm round or ovoid masses but can range from 5 to 50 mm in diameter (Fig. 38.1). Hamartomas may occur within the hypothalamus or may be attached to it by a pedunculated stalk. Rarely, they may be located in the interpeduncular or prepontine cistern without direct connection to the hypothalamus [1, 2].

Hamartomas are composed of mature neurons intermingled with glial cells. The neuronal component is generally similar

to that within the ventral hypothalamus. Although dysplastic neurons and moderate glial cellularity may be present, neoplastic features are absent. Both myelinated and non-myelinated fibers are present and some fiber bundles terminate on hypothalamic nuclei. Ependymal cells may also be present, suggesting a developmental diverticulum from the third ventricle. Neuroendocrine cells containing neurosecretory granules, blood vessels with fenestrated capillary endothelium, and double basement membranes have been observed on ultrastructural studies.

The prevalence of hypothalamic hamartomas has been estimated at 1:50 000 to 1:100 000 from clinical studies [3]. However, a 10% incidence of small (1–1.5 mm) hamartomatous nodules has been reported in a consecutive autopsy series [4], suggesting that symptomatic hamartomas may represent the clinical extreme of a common developmental variant. Hamartomas show no gender, racial or familial predilection and, with one exception, no genetic abnormalities have been identified.

The exception is the association with the Pallister–Hall syndrome, which consists of hypothalamic hamartomas, polydactyly, imperforate anus, various visceral anomalies, holoprosencephaly, impaired olfactory bulb and tract development, hypopituitarism, and craniofacial and renal anomalies [5]. Although initially believed to be a lethal disease, some patients have prolonged survival and a few experience seizures. The syndrome is associated with frameshift mutations on the *GLI3* gene, located on chromosome 7p14.1. *GLI3* codes for a zinc-finger transcription factor that acts both as a transcriptional activator and repressor of downstream targets in the sonic hedgehog pathway during development. Mutations in the same gene are also associated with the Greig cerebropolysyndactyly syndrome, which does not include hypothalamic hamartomas. Detailed molecular-clinical correlations

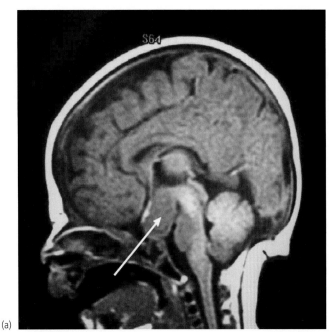

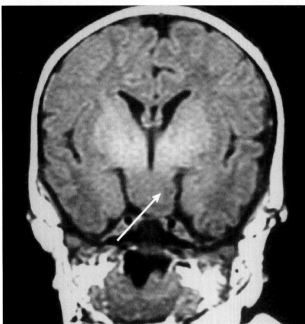

Figure 38.1 Coronal (a) and sagittal (b) MRIs of an intrahypothalamic hamartoma (arrow) in a 2-week-old infant. (Courtesy of Dr. Andrew Poznansky, Children's Hospital, Chicago, IL, USA.)

have shown a robust genotype-phenotype correlation for *GLI3* mutations, suggesting that the two allelic disorders are pathogenetically distinct [6]. *GLI3* mutations, while important for the Pallister–Hall syndrome, do not appear to be responsible for the development of hamartomas since mice with targeted mutations of the gene regions associated with the Pallister–Hall syndrome do not develop hamartomas despite exhibiting the other manifestations of the syndrome [7].

Clinical manifestations

Most patients with hamartomas present with seizures and/or precocious puberty. Slightly more than 60% of patients present with seizures, a similar percentage have precocious puberty, and about 25% have both. The characteristics of the hamartomas and their location differ between the subgroups associated with seizures and those with precocious puberty.

Seizures

Most patients exhibit seizures during infancy (some as early as the first day of life) with half occurring by the end of the first year. However, in some, the first occurrence may not occur until adolescence. The initial seizures in >90% are *gelastic* (Greek: laughter/mirth) seizures, consisting of daily stereotypic attacks of laughter. They are initially unassociated with loss of consciousness but, with time, may exhibit various autonomic disturbances, epigastric aura, crying, motor symptoms and altered states of consciousness and may progress to focal and generalized seizure activity, developmental delays, and impaired cognition. These features are seen in about 50% of patients by 7 years of age. Patients may show emotional instability, agitation, aggression, antisocial behaviors, speech retardation, learning impairment, and anxiety and mood disorders. In many this has resulted in institutionalization. The neurological and behavioral disturbances are generally related to the size of the hamartoma. In nearly all patients with seizures, hamartomas are 10 mm or greater in diameter [8]. A more benign form of gelastic seizures without subsequent deterioration may be seen in patients with smaller (5–6 mm) hamartomas. The hamartomas in all patients with isolated seizures and in most with combined seizures and precocious puberty are intrahypothalamic in location and often involve the third ventricle. Seizures are more commonly seen in males (67%) than in females (22%).

The pathogenesis of the seizures is not entirely clear. Because the EEG features and seizure characteristics resemble partial complex seizures originating in the temporal and/or frontal lobes, the possibility of an associated cortical dysgenesis has been considered. However, cortical resections have failed to control seizures. The possibility of mechanical compression of the hypothalamus has been considered because of the association of seizures with larger hamartomas, but comparably sized parahypothalamic tumors are unassociated with seizures. Deep electrode recordings suggest that the seizures are due to discharges from the hamartoma itself and electrical stimulation of the hamartoma elicits gelastic seizures. An alternative explanation, that the cellular dysplasia may be responsible, is possible, but the association with the intrahypothalamic location of the hamartoma argues for the importance of aberrant conductivity from the nodule itself, as does the improvement or cessation of seizures subsequent to surgical removal, stereotactic irradiation, or radiofrequency lesioning. There are abundant neuronal network connections between the hamartomas and the diencephalon and propagation of the ictal activity originating in the hamartoma may result in epileptogenic activity in the frontal or temporal lobes. The recurrent excitatory damage may then cause the progressive cognitive deterioration observed in patients with hamartomas.

Central precocious puberty

Hypothalamic hamartomas are seen in 14–36% of patients with organic central precocious puberty [9]. The first clinical manifestations are seen before 2 years of age in >80% of patients and occasionally during the first year. Although the definition of precocious puberty varies in the literature, it is generally characterized by the presence of breast development (≥Tanner stage B2) before the age of 8 years in girls and by pubic hair development and/or testicular enlargement to ≥3 ml before the age of 9 years in boys in association with pubertal levels of pituitary–gonadal hormones. Other manifestations include deepening of the voice and penile enlargement in males, and increased skeletal and muscular development, bone age advancement, and adolescent behavioral changes in both sexes. Gonadotropin responses to gonadotropin-releasing hormone (GnRH) stimulation are typical of those seen in puberty. Hamartomas in patients with precocious puberty are frequently pedunculated, most often in a parahypothalamic location, and infrequently involve the third ventricle. The frequency of precocious puberty in hypothalamic hamartomas varies considerably in different series, from 33% to 85%, most likely as a result of selection bias.

The pathogenesis of hypothalamic hamartoma-associated precocious puberty is also controversial. Some hamartomas have shown GnRH-containing neurons, which have been proposed to activate pituitary gonadotrophs. In others, GnRH neurons have not been detected, though astroglial cells containing transforming growth factor-α (TGF-α) have been found. TGF-α has been hypothesized to stimulate GnRH release at the time of physiological puberty. Another hypothesis has been that of inhibition of hypothalamic neuronal tracts that are normally inhibitory to GnRH secretion due to hypothalamic compression by the hamartoma. In addition, hypothalamic hamartomas have been reported to produce several other neuropeptides, including corticotropin-releasing hormone (CRH), met-enkephalin, growth hormone (GH), β-endorphin, oxytocin, somatostatin, and thyroid-stimulating hormone (TSH) [10].

Diagnosis

The diagnosis of seizure-associated hypothalamic hamartomas is usually made during the work-up for the seizure disorder and magnetic resonance imaging (MRI) examination provides the definitive evidence. In contrast, the work-up of children with precocious puberty has gone through various evolutionary states. Initially, clinical characterization (i.e. age of onset, degree of sexual development, gender, body mass index [BMI]) was used in an attempt to distinguish those children with idiopathic central precocious puberty from those with organic lesions. Since only 5–10% of girls with central precocious puberty have occult intracranial lesions, algorithms have been developed in an attempt to avoid imaging studies in all children. Although the peak luteinizing hormone (LH) response to GnRH has been used as the

"gold standard" to demonstrate the central origin of precocious puberty, it has not been particularly useful in identifying those children with hypothalamic lesions [11]. Neither has there been agreement on the use of a particular algorithm that can exclude the presence of a hamartoma. Consequently, MRI is now considered the most reliable technique to establish or exclude the diagnosis [9, 12]. Because of the greater frequency of organic lesions in boys with precocious puberty, MRI evaluation should be routinely performed.

Therapy

The therapy of hypothalamic hamartomas is dependent on the associated syndrome.

Seizures

In patient with gelastic seizures, medical therapy with antiepileptic agents is almost invariably unsuccessful. Surgical intervention targeted at the frontal, temporal, or occipital cortex provides only minimal relief of seizure activity. Therefore, therapy should be directed at the hamartoma itself. Improvement in seizure activity is dependent on the extent of removal of the hamartoma. In recent series, more than 50% of the hamartomas have been totally removed. Gelastic seizures generally subside shortly after hamartoma removal while other types of seizure activity, EEG abnormalities, cognitive function and behavioral abnormalities usually improve with time [13].

Radiotherapy using Gamma Knife surgery has also been reported to control seizure activity, though with a mean interval to seizure reduction of 9 months [14]. Although no serious complications have been observed, the effects of hypothalamic irradiation, particularly in young children, remain to be fully determined. Stereotactic radiofrequency thermocoagulation has been reported in a handful of cases, though the results are variable and the procedure has not gained many adherents.

Precocious puberty

The recognition that pulsatile GnRH was required for stimulation of LH and follicle-stimulating hormone (FSH) release by gonadotrophs and that continuous exposure led to receptor downregulation and inhibition of LH and FSH release led to the use of long-acting GnRH agonists for treatment of central precocious puberty. The drugs have proven effective in suppressing pituitary gonadal function in practically all patients. The drugs are well tolerated and there is full reversal of the hormone suppression upon discontinuation of therapy. There are no long-term sequelae of treatment and fertility appears to be unimpaired [15]. The treatment of patients with hypothalamic hamartoma-associated precocious puberty does not differ from those without hamartomas. Hamartoma size does not increase on treatment and may occasionally decrease.

Prior to the availability of hormonal treatment, surgical removal of the hamartoma was the only available therapy. Although high rates of success were reported in some series, many children still required GnRH agonist therapy. In children with both seizures and precocious puberty, the use of medical therapy for suppression of precocious puberty has not been helpful in reducing or eliminating the seizure activity. Therefore, surgery and other forms of ablative therapy are reserved for patients manifesting both precocious puberty and seizures.

Gangliocytomas

Gangliocytomas are rare, ganglion cell-containing tumors of the pituitary. They are histologically benign neoplasms consisting entirely or primarily of neoplastic or binucleate ganglion cells with varying amounts of fibrillary neurophil-like structures. They have also been called ganglioneuromas or neural choristomas (tumor-like growths of heterotopic tissue). Together with gangliogliomas they have been termed "ganglion cell tumors" but can be interdistinguished by the presence of neoplastic glial elements. Gangliocytomas contain either no glial elements or only reactive astrocytes. The infrequent presence of glial fibrillary acidic protein (GFAP) staining helps to distinguish between these two tumors. Macroscopically, gangliocytomas appear as firm, lobulated gray tumors, commonly containing cysts or calcifications that are well demarcated from the surrounding brain or pituitary.

Ganglion cell tumors constitute from 0.4% to 3.8% of all brain tumors and are most commonly found in the spinal cord, cerebral hemispheres, and brain stem [16]. Their occurrence in other loci, including the sellar region, is a rarity. They can be distinguished from hamartomas by the presence of tumoral or binucleate ganglion cells, infrequent (<20%) connections to the hypothalamus, symptom onset during adult life, and occasional increases in size when followed by observation alone.

Fewer than 100 patients with intrasellar gangliocytomas have been reported to date (Table 38.1). Nearly 80% are associated with pituitary hormone hypersecretory syndromes and among those a hormonally active pituitary tumor is present in 80%. The most frequently found syndrome is acromegaly, occurring in more than half (59%) of reported patients, followed by Cushing disease in 8%, Isolated case reports of prolactinomas have also been published. In some of the patients with hypersecretory

Table 38.1 Reported cases of pituitary gangliocytomas

	Total cases no. (% of total)	Associated with pituitary adenoma
Acromegaly	54 (59)	48
Prolactinoma	5 (5)	5
Mixed GH-prolactin	6 (7)	3
Cushing disease	7 (8)	5
Non-secreting	19 (21)	11
Excessive ADH secretion	1 (1)	0
Total	92 (100)	72

Cases prior to 1995 compiled in [21].

syndromes, no adenoma has been observed, though corticotroph hyperplasia has been described in two Cushing disease-associated tumors. Pituitary tumors were described in 3 of the 11 patients without evidence of a hormonal excess syndrome. Some of these tumors have exhibited positive immunocytochemical staining for pituitary hormones but were clinically "silent."

Pathogenesis

Three conflicting hypotheses have been advanced to explain the pathogenesis of these tumors [17]. The first is that gangliocytomas arise from a proliferation of heterotopic hypothalamic-like neurons within the sella [18, 19]. Such neurons have been reported to show the presence of immunoreactive GH-releasing hormone and CRH in nearly all reported cases and it is assumed that surrounding pituitary cells of the appropriate type (i.e. somatotrophs and corticotrophs) are stimulated to proliferate and undergo neoplastic transformation by endocrine and/or paracrine mechanisms. Ultrastructural studies have identified secretory granules both in neuronal perikarya and axonal processes, which interdigitate with sparsely granulated adenomatous somatotrophs and/or corticotrophs. The most likely mechanism of action appears to be paracrine, rather than endocrine, because of the failure to detect elevated levels of the hypothalamic releasing hormone in peripheral circulation, as occurs with ectopic hormone secretion from peripheral locations [20, 21]. Although a limitation of this hypothesis is its failure to explain the absence of somatotroph (or corticotroph) hyperplasia seen in other forms of ectopic hormone-associated somatotroph proliferation in man and experimental animals, it remains the most likely explanation at the present time. It is also interesting to speculate that yet undefined substances produced by some gangliocytomas may exert a role in the pathogenesis of prolactinomas and/or nonfunctioning pituitary adenomas.

A second hypothesis suggests that the gangliocytoma is the result of differentiation of neuronal components from within the sparsely granulated adenoma, where neuronal-like processes have been observed in GH-cell adenomas [22]. However, this hypothesis fails to explain those gangliocytomas that do not have associated pituitary adenomas.

A third hypothesis explains the neuronal and adenohypophyseal components as originating form embryonal rests that contain cells with features intermediary between neuronal and pituitary cells. While such cells have been identified in the neuronal components of the tumors, they have yet to be observed in the normal pituitary gland.

Clinical and laboratory findings

The overall experience is that the clinical features of patients with gangliocytomas with associated pituitary adenomas, irrespective of the associated endocrine hypersecretory disorder, cannot be distinguished from those with solitary pituitary adenomas, on the basis of routine or even sophisticated endocrine testing. Similarly, the findings on CT and MRI are indistinguishable from the more commonly seen pituitary adenomas. In contrast to similar tumors in other locations, pituitary gangliocytomas are hyperdense and show contrast enhancement on CT and rarely contain calcifications. The neuronal and pituitary adenoma components are not separable on MRI, but appear as a single homogeneous intrasellar mass. This explains the fact that the diagnosis is invariably made by the pathologist, either at or after the time of surgery.

Therapy

The pituitary adenomas tend to be sparsely granulated and are almost always macroadenomas. Until recently, surgical treatment was usually recommended for such tumors and the results have been similar to those with isolated pituitary adenomas. However, with the routine use of dopaminergic agonists for the primary treatment of prolactinomas and the increasing interest of somatostatin analogs for the primary treatment of some somatotropinomas, it is likely that some patients with mixed gangliocytoma–adenoma will be initially treated medically. It is not currently known how such tumors may respond, though it is likely that there will be less overall reduction in tumor size than in isolated pituitary adenomas. In particular, gangliocytomas associated with prolactinomas would be expected to show less tumor reduction, though this remains speculative in the absence of reported results in the literature. Since gangliocytomas are slowly growing tumors, a conservative approach to their management would appear to have merit.

References

1. Arita K, Kurisu K, Kiura Y, Iida K, Otsubo H. Hypothalamic hamartoma. *Neurol. Med. Chir. (Tokyo)* 2005;45:221–231.
2. Nguyen D, Singh S, Zaatreh M, et al. Hypothalamic hamartomas: seven cases and review of the literature. *Epilepsy Behav.* 2003;4:246–258.
3. Weissenberger AA, Dell ML, Liow K, et al. Aggression and psychiatric comorbidity in children with hypothalamic hamartomas and their unaffected siblings. *J. Am. Acad. Child. Adolesc. Psychiatry* 2001;40: 696–703.
4. Sherwin RP, Grassi JE, Sommers SC. Hamartomatous malformation of the posterolateral hypothalamus. *Lab. Invest.* 1962;2:89–97.
5. Hall JG, Pallister PD, Clarren SK, et al. Congenital hypothalamic hamartoblastoma, hypopituitarism, imperforate anus and postaxial polydactyly – a new syndrome? Part I: clinical, causal, and pathogenetic considerations. *Am. J. Med. Genet.* 1980;7:47–74.
6. Johnston JJ, Olivos-Glander I, Killoran C, et al. Molecular and clinical analyses of Greig cephalopolysyndactyly and Pallister–Hall syndromes: robust phenotype prediction from the type and position of *GLI3* mutations. *Am. J. Hum. Genet.* 2005;76:609–622.
7. Bose J, Grotewold L, Ruther U. Pallister–Hall syndrome phenotype in mice mutant for *Gli3*. *Hum. Mol. Genet.* 2002;11:1129–1135.
8. Jung H, Neumaier PE, Hauffa BP, Partsch CJ, Dammann O. Association of morphological characteristics with precocious puberty and/or gelastic seizures in hypothalamic hamartoma. *J. Clin. Endocrinol. Metab.* 2003;88:4590–4595.
9. Chemaitilly W, Trivin C, Adan L, et al. Central precocious puberty: clinical and laboratory features. *Clin. Endocrinol.* 2003;54:289–294.
10. Jung H, Parent AS, Ojeda SR. Hypothalamic hamartoma: a paradigm/model for studying the onset of puberty. *Endocr. Dev.* 2005;8: 81–93.
11. Ng SM, Kumar Y, Cody D, Smith C, Didi M. The gonadotrophins response to GnRH test is not a predictor of neurological lesion in girls with central precocious puberty. *J. Pediatr. Endocrinol. Metab.* 2005;18:849–852.
12. Chalumeau M, Hadjiathanasiou CG, Ng SM, et al. Selecting girls with precocious puberty for brain imaging: validation of European evidence-based diagnosis rule. *J. Pediatr.* 2003;143:445–450.
13. Freeman JL, Harvey AS, Rosenfeld JV, et al. Generalized epilepsy in hypothalamic hamartoma: evolution and postoperative resolution. *Neurology* 2003;60:762–767.
14. Regis J, Bartolomei F, de Toffol B, et al. Gamma knife surgery for epilepsy related to hypothalamic hamartomas. *Neurosurgery* 2000; 47:1343–1351.
15. Partsch CJ, Heger S, Sippell WG. Management and outcome of central precocious puberty. *Clin. Endocrinol. (Oxf.)* 2002;56:129–148.
16. Miller DC, Lang FF, Epstein FJ. Central nervous system gangliogliomas. Part 1: Pathology. *J. Neurosurg.* 1993;79:859–866.
17. Towfighi J, Salam MM, McLendon RE, Powers S, Page RB. Ganglion cell-containing tumors of the pituitary gland. *Arch. Pathol. Lab. Med.* 1996;120:369–377.
18. Saeger W, Puchner MJ, Ludecke DK. Combined sellar gangliocytoma and pituitary adenoma in acromegaly or Cushing's disease. A report of 3 cases. *Virchows Arch.* 1994;425:93–99.
19. Asa SL, Scheithauer BW, Bilbao JM, et al. A case for hypothalamic acromegaly: a clinicopathological study of six patients with hypothalamic gangliocytomas producing growth hormone releasing factor. *J. Clin. Endocrinol. Metab.* 1984;58:796–803.
20. Frohman LA. Growth hormone releasing factor – a neuroendocrine perspective. *J. Lab. Clin. Med.* 1984;103:819–832.
21. Puchner MJ, Ludecke DK, Saeger W, Riedel M, Asa SL. Gangliocytomas of the sellar region – a review. *Exp. Clin. Endocrinol. Diabetes* 1995;103:129–149.
22. Horvath E, Kovacs K, Scheithauer BW, Lloyd RV, Smyth HS. Pituitary adenoma with neuronal choristoma (PANCH): composite lesion or lineage infidelity? *Ultrastruct. Pathol.* 1994;18:565–574.

39 Cranial Ependymoma

Silvia Hofer and Michael Brada

> **Key points**
> - Ependymomas are currently discerned by histopathological criteria and proliferation markers.
> - Intracranial ependymomas are currently best treated by radical local therapies (surgery and radiotherapy).
> - The incidence of iatrogenic endocrinopathies is declining due to more localized treatment.
> - Genomic profiling is on the verge of recognizing distinct subgroups that exhibit different prognosis and needs for therapy.

Introduction

Ependymomas are tumors of the ependymal cells lining ventricular surfaces in the spinal and cranial locations. Intracranial ependymomas principally occur in the posterior fossa and are typically tumors of childhood and adolescence. They account for 9% of primary brain tumors in the first decade of life, 4% in the second and third decades and only 1% beyond the age of 30. This contrasts with ependymomas of the spinal cord, which commonly present in middle life and comprise 13% of primary spinal cord tumors.

Intracranial ependymomas can originate in relation to any part of the ventricular system but occur twice as frequently in infratentorial than supratentorial locations, arising from the roof, floor or lateral recesses of the fourth ventricle. Supratentorial ependymomas originate from the lining of the third and lateral ventricles. Ependymomas may be found away from the ventricular system within the cerebral hemispheres, probably arising from remnants of the central canal of the spinal cord.

Pathology

The World Health Organization (WHO) classification [1] distinguishes four main ependymoma variants. These are graded according to degree of anaplasia: ependymoma (WHO grade II), anaplastic ependymoma (WHO grade III), myxopapillary ependymoma (WHO grade 1) and subependymoma (WHO grade I).

WHO grade II ependymomas are solid, cystic or papillary masses, apparently demarcated from the adjacent neural tissue. They are usually located with the ventricular system in the posterior fossa and may block cerebrospinal fluid (CSF) pathways. Tumor cells are frequently aligned around a small central lumen described as rosettes or clusters or as pseudorosettes if they surround a blood vessel. Ependymal lesions may contain areas of myxoid degeneration, hemorrhage, non-palisading foci of necrosis, calcification and occasionally focal cartilage and bone formation. The majority are glial fibrillary acid protein (GFAP) positive and express S100 protein and vimentin with frequent epithelial membrane antigen (EMA) positivity. Expression of nestin, a neurodevelopmental intermediate filament protein, has also been reported. Grade II ependymomas show limited proliferation, with a mean growth fraction <3% on Ki-67 antibody staining.

The presence of increased cellularity and high mitotic activity, pleomorphism (giant cell formation), multiple nuclei, microvascular proliferation, pseudopalisading necrosis and perivascular rosettes are histological features of *anaplastic ependymoma* (WHO grade III). Anaplastic ependymomas tend to remain demarcated, with occasional evidence of invasion and subarachnoid dissemination. The immunohistochemical profile resembles grade II ependymoma, with reduced GAFP expression.

Myxopapillary ependymomas (WHO grade I) are slowly growing tumors, almost exclusively located in the lower spinal canal around the conus, cauda equina and filum terminale and most frequently present in young adults. They consist of mucocystic cells with papillary arrangement around vascular networks and very low mitotic activity.

Subependymoma (WHO grade I) is considered a separate tumor entity. It is a slow-growing tumor typically attached to a ventricular wall of the fourth ventricle, septum pellucidum, or cervical cord, composed of subependymal glial tumor cell clusters embedded in a dense fibrillary background matrix. The tumors are usually found incidentally as asymptomatic lesions although they may cause ventricular obstruction.

The prognostic significance of morphological features and grading of ependymomas is not clear, but proliferation characteristics,

Clinical Endocrine Oncology, 2nd edition. Edited by Ian D. Hay and John A.H. Wass. © 2008 Blackwell Publishing. ISBN 978-1-4051-4584-8.

determined by MIB-1 (Ki-67) labelling index, are considered to have an independent influence on prognosis [2].

Molecular and cellular genetics

The most common abnormality, occurring in 50% of spinal ependymomas, is loss of 22q [3]. Mutation on 22q12, the NF2 tumor suppressor gene locus, is also seen in spinal cord ependymomas. Gain of 1q25 tends to occur more frequently in posterior fossa ependymomas in children, and this is associated with more aggressive behavior and higher recurrence rate [3, 4]. Gains at 5p15.33 covering hTERT (human telomere reverse transcriptase, the catalytic subunit of telomerase) and overexpression of epidermal growth factor receptor (EGFR) protein are also associated with adverse prognosis [4, 5], with possible separation of intracranial grade II ependymomas into two subgroups. SV40 sequences have been found in childhood ependymomas [6].

Diagnosis

Presenting features of ependymoma vary with the location of the tumor. They include classic features of intracranial tumors with raised intracranial pressure especially in the presence of hydrocephalus, focal neurological deficits and seizures. Vomiting in posterior fossa tumors may be due to increased intracranial pressure or due to tumor infiltration of the area postrema in the floor of the fourth ventricle. Extension of the tumor into the cervical subarachnoid space may cause nuchal rigidity, neck pain, torticollis and head tilt.

On computerized tomography (CT) and magnetic resonance imaging (MRI), ependymomas are usually well demarcated, partly solid and partly cystic heterogeneously enhancing tumors. In the posterior fossa, they tend to fill the fourth ventricle and are difficult to distinguish from medulloblastoma. The tumor may extend through the foramen of Luschka into the cerebellopontine angle or through the foramen magnum into the cervical spinal canal. While in the supratentorial location the proximity and attachment to the ventricular surfaces suggest the diagnosis, in other locations it is not possible to differentiate ependymoma from other gliomas.

The propensity for leptomeningeal spread is less than initially reported. CSF seeding occurs in 6% of patients at diagnosis and is more common in grade III than grade II tumors. Even though the incidence is low, spinal MRI is considered part of the initial staging investigations. CSF cytology is unreliable either as a marker of the presence of disseminated disease at diagnosis or as a predictor of future CSF spread and does not currently play a role in staging.

Treatment

There are few prospective studies which provide reliable information on the value of different management strategies. Nevertheless radical local treatment is considered the most important component of therapy with surgery the mainstay of initial treatment. The aim of primary surgery is to achieve complete tumor removal as the extent of resection is a significant predictor of outcome [7–10, 13, 14, 16]. Image-guided surgery aided by modern imaging techniques and ultrasound and neurophysiological monitoring may allow for more radical and safer resection. The principal surgical challenge is how to deal with the attachment of the tumor to the floor of the fourth ventricle where an attempt at radical removal carries significant morbidity, in the form of lower cranial nerve dysfunction [9].

Early postoperative imaging is considered important to assess the extent of residual disease. In the presence of visible and resectable disease reoperation is recommended to remove the tumor residue. In patients with hydrocephalus due to a fourth ventricular ependymoma, preoperative shunting may be avoided as tumor removal usually leads to restoration of normal drainage.

Postoperative irradiation has been offered to patients with residual grade II and III ependymomas after surgery. The policy of adjuvant radiotherapy is based on retrospective studies which report better outcome in patients who received irradiation and this also includes patients following apparently complete excision. With greater reliance of perspective MRI imaging, the increasing tendency is to avoid radiotherapy in patients with documented complete strenuous removal, reserving radiotherapy for patients with unresectable residual disease. Historically, patients with ependymoma, particularly those with grade III tumors, were offered craniospinal irradiation to prevent CSF seeding. As the incidence of developing cranial or spinal metastases is low (7%) and there is little evidence that prophylactic irradiation alters the risk of CSF seeding, craniospinal irradiation is no longer recommended [11]. The principal cause of failure is recurrence at the primary site [11] and the treatment is confined to the site of residual tumor and local region at risk of recurrence. Modern radiotherapy employs conformal techniques and is given to a dose of 50–60 Gy (at ≤1.8 Gy per fraction). Chemotherapy has been used as adjuvant treatment with the aim of improving prognosis. A prospective study of adjuvant platinum-containing chemotherapy in 55 children with anaplastic ependymomas showed no improvement compared to historical controls [12].

Because of late effects of radiation in young children (<3 years of age), chemotherapy is used to avoid or defer radiotherapy. The 2-year progression-free survival following platinum-containing chemotherapy alone is 40%. Deferring radiotherapy until evidence of progression did not seem to compromise survival in some studies, particularly in patients without residual disease after surgery [10, 13, 14]. It is not clear if this represents the efficacy of chemotherapy or is simply a reflection of good disease control with radical surgery alone. Other studies indicate compromised survival even after intensive chemotherapy, particularly inpatients following incomplete resection and grade III tumors [15] and this suggests that chemotherapy is of limited benefit in achieving local disease control. An ongoing prospective trial (ACNS 0121, www.nci.nih.gov/clinicaltrials) aims to assess the value of gross total resection alone in grade II tumors avoiding local radiotherapy.

Summary of management and prognosis

Localized low-grade tumors in accessible locations should be radically excised providing surgical morbidity is considered acceptable. In the presence of residual tumor patients are offered radical local radiotherapy. Following imaging-confirmed complete excision the options include adjuvant local radiotherapy or surveillance.

The 10-year survival of patients receiving adjuvant radiotherapy following apparent complete excision of low-grade ependymoma is of the order of 80%, compared to 50% in patients with incompletely excised tumors. Patients with localized high-grade tumors are offered local radiotherapy regardless of the extent of excision. The respective 5- and 10-year survival probabilities are 40% and 30% [16, 17].

Patients with disseminated disease at initial diagnosis receive craniospinal irradiation after debulking surgery with a boost of radiation to the primary and metastatic sites to doses to central nervous system tolerance.

Local relapse is the principal cause of failure [10, 15]. Although second-line treatment is unlikely to be curative, patients should be considered for repeat surgery, which can achieve long-term remission, particularly in patients with indolent tumors.

Stereotactic radiosurgery or fractionated stereotactic radiotherapy can also achieve local tumor control in patients with unresectable residual or recurrent ependymoma [18, 19]. These techniques are being investigated as a component of initial management. Chemotherapy has shown modest benefits in patients with recurrent ependymoma after failure of local treatment [20].

Endocrine implications

Ependymomas rarely occur in the third ventricle in the proximity of the hypothalamic pituitary axis and hypothalamic dysfunction at presentation is therefore uncommon. Children and adults treated with whole brain or craniospinal axis irradiation have frequent endocrine dysfunction, regardless of the site of primary disease [22, 23].

The incidence of endocrinopathy is reported in up to 90% of children treated before the age of 3, and this compares with 68% incidence after local radiotherapy and 26% after surgery alone [21]. The incidence of hypopituitarism after craniospinal axis radiotherapy is in the region of 40% [23]. The principal determinant of the speed of onset and the incidence and severity of anterior pituitary hormone deficiency is the total dose of radiation delivered to the hypothalamo–pituitary region [23, 24].

Following craniospinal irradiation, early detection of growth hormone deficiency identifies patients at risk for other pituitary deficiencies. Annual clinical and biochemical testing should be part of routine follow-up in this group of patients [22, 23].

The current policy of local treatment alone, avoiding wide field irradiation, is likely to reduce the incidence of pituitary dysfunction and routine monitoring may not be necessary in adults. Nevertheless, it should continue in children regardless of the extent of irradiation.

References

1. Kleihues P, Cavanee WK. Ependymal tumors. In Kleihues P, Cavanee WK (eds). *World Health Organization Classification of Tumours of the Nervous System.* Lyon: IARC/WHO, 2000:71–80.
2. Kurt E, Zheng P, Hop W, et al. Identification of relevant prognostic histopathologic features in 69 intracranial ependymomas, excluding myxopapillary ependymomas and subependymomas. *Cancer* 2006;106:388–395.
3. Carter M, Nicholson J, Ross F, et al. Genetic abnormalities detected in ependymomas by comparative genomic hybridisation. *Br. J. Cancer* 2002;86:929–939.
4. Mendrzyk F, Korshunov A, Benner A, et al. Identification of gains on 1q and epidermal growth factor receptor overexpression as independent prognostic markers in intracranial ependymoma. *Clin. Cancer Res.* 2006;12:270–279.
5. Tabori U, Ma J, Carter M, et al. Human telomere reverse transcriptase expression predicts progression and survival in pediatric intracranial ependymoma. *J. Clin. Oncol.* 2006;24;1522–1528.
6. Bergsagel DJ, Finegold MJ, Butel JS, et al. DNA sequences similar to those of simian virus 40 in ependymomas and choroid plexus tumors of childhood. *N. Engl. J. Med.* 1992;326:988–993.
7. Perilongo G, Massimino M, Sotti G, et al. Analysis of prognostic factors in a restrospective review of 92 children with ependymoma: Italian Pediatric Neuro-Oncology Group. *Med. Pediatr. Oncol.* 1997;29:79–85.
8. Nazar GB, Hoffmann HJ, Becker LE, et al. Infratentorial ependymomas in childhood: prognostic factors and treatment. *J. Neurosurg.* 1990;72:408–417.
9. Epstein FJ, Goh KYC. Ependymomas of the posterior fossa. In Kaye AH, Black PM (eds). *Operative Neurosurgery.* London: Churchill Livingstone, 2000:429–436.
10. Geyer JR, Sposto R, Jennings M, et al. Multiagent chemotherapy and deferred radiotherapy in infants with malignant brain tumors: A report from a children's cancer group. *J. Clin. Oncol.* 2005;23:7621–7631.
11. Vanuytsel L, Brada M. The role of prophylactic spinal irradiation in localised intracranial ependymoma. *Int. J. Radiat. Oncol. Biol. Phys.* 1991;21:825–830.
12. Timmermann B, Kortmann RD, Kühl J, et al. Combined postoperative irradiation and chemotherapy for anaplastic ependymomas in childhood: results of the German prospective trials HIT 88/89 and HIT 91. *Int. J. Radiat. Oncol. Biol. Phys.* 2000;46:287–295.
13. Duffner PK, Horowitz ME, Krischer JP, et al. Postoperative chemotherapy and delayed radiation in children less than three years of age with malignant brain tumours. *N. Engl. J. Med.* 1993;328:1725–1731.
14. Grill J, Deley ML, Gambarelli D, et al. Postoperative chemotherapy without irradiation for ependymomas in children under 5 years of age: a multicenter trial of the French Society of Pediatric Oncology. *J. Clin. Oncol.* 2001;19:1288–1296.

15. Timmermann B, Kortmann RD, Kühl J, et al. Role of radiotherapy in anaplastic ependymoma in children under age of 3 years: Results of the prospective German brain tumor trials HIT-SKK 87 and 92. *Radiother. Oncol.* 2005;77:278–285.

16. Vanuytsel L, Bessel EM, Ashley SE, et al. Intracranial ependymoma: long term results of a policy of surgery and radiotherapy. *Int. J. Radiat. Oncol. Biol. Phys.* 1992;23:313–319.

17. Mansur DB, Perry A, Rajaram V, et al. Postoperative radiation therapy for grade II and III intracranial ependymoma. *Int. J. Radiat. Oncol. Biol. Phys.* 2005;61:387–391.

18. Hodgson DC, Goumnerova LC, Loeffler JS, et al. Radiosurgery in the management of pediatric brain tumors. *Int. J. Radiat. Oncol. Biol. Phys.* 2001;50:929–935.

19. Lo SS, Abdulrahman R, DesRosiers PM, et al. The role of Gamma Knife radiosurgery in the management of unresectable gross disease or gross residual disease after surgery in ependymoma. *J. Neuro-Oncol.* 2006;76:51–56.

20. Merchant TE, Fouladi M. Ependymoma: new therapeutic approaches including radiation and chemotherapy. *J. Neuro-Oncol.* 2005;75:287–299.

21. Fouladi M, Gilger E, Kocak M, et al. Intellectual and functional outcome of children 3 years old or younger who have CNS malignancies. *J. Clin. Oncol.* 2005;23:7152–7160.

22. Constine LS, Woolf PD, Cann D, et al. Hypothalamic–pituitary dysfunction after radiation for brain tumors. *N. Engl. J. Med.* 1993;328:87–94.

23. Agha A, Sherlock M, Brennan S, et al. Hypothalamic-pituitary dysfunction after irradiation of nonpituitary brain tumors in adults. *J. Clin. Endocrinol. Metab.* 2005;90:6355–6360.

24. Littley MD, Shalet SM, Beardwell CG, et al. Radiation-induced hyppituitarism is dose-dependent. *Clin. Endocrinol.* 1989;31:363–373.

40 Perisellar Tumors including Chordoma, Optic Nerve Glioma, Meningioma, Hemangiopericytoma, and Glomus Tumors

David Choi and Alan Crockard

> **Key points**
> - The differential diagnosis of perisellar tumors is large, but most are either benign or slowly growing malignant tumors.
> - Surgical excision is usually the most effective primary treatment.
> - Approaches to the skull base are often difficult with significant morbidity, and an initial biopsy may aid surgical decision making.
> - Radiotherapy and chemotherapy are often required as adjunctive treatment.
> - Radiological surveillance is required after primary treatment.

Introduction

The pituitary fossa, or sella turcica, is a depression in the sphenoid bone which contains the pituitary gland. The gland is covered by a dural layer, the diaphragma sellae, and above this lies the supraclinoid parts of the carotid arteries on both sides, the optic nerves, chiasm and tracts, and the pituitary stalk in the midline. Lateral to the sella are the cavernous sinuses, containing the intracavernous parts of the carotid arteries, sympathetic nerve fibers, and VIth cranial nerve, with the IIIrd, IVth and ophthalmic division of the Vth nerves in the dura of the lateral walls of the sinuses.

Anterior to the sella is the tuberculum sellae and planum sphenoidale, sphenoid and ethmoid air sinuses, and posteriorly lie the posterior clinoids, clivus, and interpeduncular cistern containing the IIIrd and IVth cranial nerves. The sphenoid sinus and clivus continue inferiorly.

Tumors may arise from a multitude of structures and tissues in the perisellar region (Table 40.1). They may present with headache, visual disturbance or cranial nerve palsy depending on the exact location of the tumor and effect on neighboring structures.

Chordoma

Etiology

Most of the bones of the skull base are preformed in cartilage and then undergo enchondral ossification, although the orbital roof

Table 40.1 Differential diagnosis of perisellar masses

Chordoma
Chondrosarcoma
Meningioma
Hemangiopericytoma
Optic nerve glioma
Glomus tumor
Pituitary adenoma
Epidermoid tumor
Dermoid tumor
Arachnoid cyst
Craniopharyngioma
Cavernous angioma
Rathke's cyst
Metastasis
Germ cell tumors
Aneurysm
Histiocytosis
Tuberculoma
Sarcoidosis

and greater wings of the sphenoid form from intramembranous ossification. The notochord is a temporary longitudinal structure which orchestrates segmentation of the developing embryo and induces the formation of the vertebral column. It provides the template for spinal development by co-ordinating the production of numerous signaling molecules from the neural tube and somites, initiated by the production of the protein product of a gene called *sonic hedgehog* from the notochord. *Sonic hedgehog* induces differentiation in the ventral and lateral neural tube as well as sclerotome differentiation in the somites. In the human,

Clinical Endocrine Oncology, 2nd edition. Edited by Ian D. Hay and John A.H. Wass. © 2008 Blackwell Publishing. ISBN 978-1-4051-4584-8.

the notochord develops from day 17 from cells originating from the primitive pit, initially as a notochordal process. This process grows longitudinally and is flanked on both sides by the paraxial mesoderm. The ectoderm and mesoderm overlying the notochord form the neural plate and central nervous system. The notochordal tract begins within the developing sphenoid cartilage, exits posteriorly and proceeds caudad in front of the basisphenoid between it and the pharynx, and continues into the developing alar ligament and odontoid process and on through the vertebral bodies and discs, as far as the coccyx. By week 10, however, the notochord has degenerated although remnants of it persist in the nucleus pulposus of the cartilaginous disks.

Chordomas arise from persistent rests of notochordal remnants, and are largely restricted to the axial skeleton, commonly in the clivus and sacrum, and were probably first described by Virchow in 1857 [1]. They account for 1–8% of primary malignant bone tumors and 20% of those arising in the spine [2]. The overall incidence in Europeans is 0.5 per million [3]. Skull base chordomas typically occur in caucasians of 30–50 years old, with a roughly equal sex distribution, whereas spinal tumors tend to occur slightly later, and more commonly in males. Most chordomas arise in the sacrum (50%), with 35% occurring at the skull base, and 15% in other parts of the spine.

Presentation

Chordomas may present with headaches, cranial nerve palsies, diplopia, brainstem dysfunction or as an incidental finding on magnetic resonance imaging (MRI). They are slow growing and locally invasive, resulting in symptoms and signs when neighboring structures are affected, often after many years of growth. The facial and abducens nerves are the most commonly affected, followed by the glossopharyngeal and the vagus nerves [4].

Radiology

Investigation includes computerized tomography (CT) scans with bone windows and soft tissue algorithms, magnetic resonance imaging (MRI) scan with and without gadolinium, and in some cases angiography or magnetic resonance angiography (MRA) if the vertebrobasilar or internal carotid arteries are closely related to the tumor.

On CT, chordomas are most often midline and centered on the clivus, with bone destruction and an isodense or hypodense soft tissue mass. Islands of bone may be seen within the tumor, and should be distinguished from areas of tumor calcification, which is more common in chondrosarcomas and craniopharyngiomas.

T1-weighted MRI shows isointense regions of solid tumor, but images are usually heterogeneous due to cystic and hemorrhagic areas, and bony sequestra within the tumor (Fig. 40.1). T2-weighted images show bright hyperintensity.

Pathology

Histologically, chordomas can be conventional, chondroid and dedifferentiated. Conventional tumors are soft, pale gray, and well demarcated from adjacent tissues. Nests and cords of malignant

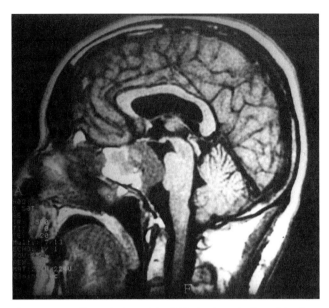

Figure 40.1 Midline sagittal T1-weighted MRI, showing a chordoma of the clivus.

cells are seen in a mucoid matrix. The neoplastic cells have multiple cytoplasmic vacuoles giving them a bubbly or "physaliphorous" appearance. Chondroid chordomas contain areas that resemble low-grade chondrosarcomas, and are associated with a better prognosis than the conventional type, leading some to consider them as a subgroup of chondrosarcomas rather than chordomas. The dedifferentiated type is the rarest, and morphologically resembles a high-grade sarcoma, with an equally poor prognosis.

Chordomas rarely metastasize, but are usually slow growing and locally infiltrative. The rate of local recurrence is high, and seeding within a resection cavity or superficial tissues is common after surgery.

Treatment

Primary treatment is by surgical resection, most often by a midline transoral or transfacial approach [5].

Radiation treatment may be given as an adjunct, either using intensity modulated radiotherapy or, more effectively, proton beam irradiation [6]. Chordomas are relatively radioresistant to standard fractionated radiotherapy.

Protons are produced by ionizing hydrogen and may be accelerated in a cyclotron to produce a beam. These protons exhibit the Bragg peak effect, whereby more energy is released after traveling a certain distance through a tissue. Thus, an increased radiation effect can be given at the depth of the tumor. For irradiation of larger tumors the beam energy is modulated and superimposed to spread out the Bragg peak. Heavy carbon beams may also be used to the same effect, but the major limiting factor for this and proton beam therapy is that the technique is only available in a few centers.

Stereotactic radiosurgery is a third option which may be used for small tumors less than 3 cm in diameter, when surgical resection would be difficult or declined by the patient [7].

Prognosis

Prognosis depends largely on age, tumor size, location, and resectability. In one series after surgery and radiotherapy, 5-year recurrence-free survival was 65% [8].

Chondrosarcoma

Chondrosarcomas are the second most common primary bone malignancy. They occur most commonly in middle-aged patients with a slight female preponderance, are usually situated in the clivus and, more rarely, the spine. Chondrosarcomas probably arise from primitive mesenchymal cells or embryonal rests from the cartilaginous matrix of the skull base, rather than the noto-chord. They are not usually midline, unlike chordomas, and are found most commonly in the middle cranial fossa, arising from the spheno-occipital or the petro-occipital synchondroses, but may also be found in the posterior or anterior fossa floors. They are three times more common in men, and may be associated with other bone disorders such as Paget disease.

Radiology

CT and MRI are the investigations of choice, revealing adjacent bone destruction, and calcification is more common than in chordomas, occurring in around half of chondrosarcomas [9]. The tumor itself is heterogenous in signal intensity and contrast enhancement, similar to a chordoma, but usually not in the midline (Fig. 40.2).

Pathology

Conventional chondrosarcomas consist of hyaline and myxoid regions of neoplastic cartilage, and sometimes contain vacuolated cells which may be confused with the physaliphorous cells of a chordoma. They are macroscopically bulky gray tumors with heterogeneous consistency and infiltrate local bone and soft tissues. They may be graded from 1 to 4 according to the degree of cellularity, pleomorphism and mitotic activity, but most chondrosarcomas of the skull base are of low grade and are associated with a relatively good prognosis [10]. Dedifferentiated and mesenchymal chondrosarcomas have a poorer prognosis.

Prognosis

After local excision and proton beam radiation, the 5-year recurrence-free survival is 90–100% [8]. As with chordomas, most patients die from local recurrence.

Meningioma

Etiology

Meningiomas arise from arachnoid cells or their precursor cells, usually located at the arachnoid granulations of the dura. However, they may occur also at sites which are distant from the dura, such as the trigone of the lateral ventricle.

Many genetic and environmental factors have been associated with meningiomas. Most meningiomas have monosomy of chromosome 22 and a genetic predisposition is also seen in type II neurofibromatosis. Environmental factors which have been implicated include papova- and herpes viruses, radiation treatment for intracranial tumors or tinea capitis in the past and hormonal influences. Meningiomas are more common in females and after menopause, may increase in size during pregnancy, show a positive correlation with breast carcinoma, and may show androgen receptor or somatostatin receptor positivity. Meningiomas

(a)

(b)

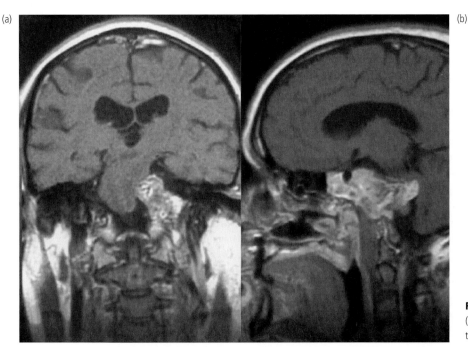

Figure 40.2 T1-weighted coronal (a) and sagittal (b) MRI scans of a chondrosarcoma, showing a typical tumor on the left side.

account for 20% of intracranial tumors, and of these about 3–4% are perisellar, arising from the tuberculum sellae, cavernous sinus, diaphragma sella, or planum sphenoidale.

Presentation

Perisellar meningiomas usually present with visual disturbance due to chiasmatic compression, or ocular palsies due to involvement of cranial nerves in and around the cavernous sinus. Occasionally impaired sense of smell, trigeminal nerve or pituitary dysfunction may be the presenting feature. Endocrine imbalances, however, are uncommon compared to pituitary adenomas.

Radiology

On CT scan, meningiomas are isodense, and enhance uniformly with contrast. They may contain regions of calcification, and have a dural attachment with a dural tail blending into neighboring dura which also may be thickened. Meningiomas can invade bone or cause local hyperostosis. MRI scanning reveals more detail in the perisellar region, without the beam-hardening artefacts of a CT scan. MRI characteristics are similar to CT, with iso- or hypointensity and homogeneous gadolinium uptake (Fig. 40.3). Around the cavernous sinus, meningiomas tend to compress and narrow the carotid arteries, encircling them, as distinct from chordomas which tend to displace the vessels. The pituitary fossa is usually normal in size, compared to the expanded fossa of a pituitary adenoma, and meningiomas demonstrate bright early enhancement with contrast as distinct from the poor early enhancement of adenomas.

Pathology

Meningiomas are usually benign tumors, and can have meningothelial, fibroblastic, transitional, or psammomatous features. More aggressive tumors (WHO grade II) include atypical, clear cell, and chordoid meningiomas, and malignant tumors (WHO grade III) consist of rhabdoid, papillary, and anaplastic subtypes.

Treatment

The optimal treatment is a complete resection including removal of the dural attachment and any involved underlying bone [11]. However, this is not usually possible for tumors around the cavernous sinus and pituitary fossa, unlike convexity meningiomas. A grade II Simpson resection (with diathermy of the dural origin) is more usual in the perisellar region, using an operating microscope, loop diathermy and ultrasonic aspirator.

With large vascular tumors, preoperative endovascular embolization of the feeding arteries may make resection easier.

Postoperative radiotherapy should be considered if there is evidence of cellular atypia, malignancy, or for recurrent benign tumors that are difficult to resect. Radiation planning must take into consideration the close proximity of the pituitary gland, optic chiasm, cranial nerves and brainstem, which are susceptible to radiation damage.

Prognosis

Recurrence rates are influenced greatly by the extent of surgical resection [12], which is determined by the site of attachment, relation to intracranial structures, and age of the patient. Benign tumors with extensive brain "invasion" have a higher recurrence rate [13]. Malignant features are associated with a worse prognosis, with a median survival of 2 years from diagnosis in one study [14].

Hemangiopericytoma

Etiology

In the past, hemangiopericytomas have been classified with meningiomas, but are now considered a separate entity. They arise from meningeal capillary pericytes rather than arachnoidal cells, and are more vascular and histologically aggressive than meningiomas. They occur slightly more often in males, and in younger

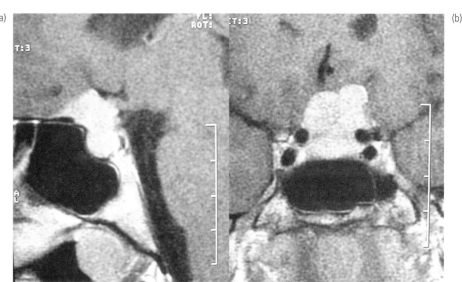

(a)   (b)

Figure 40.3 Sagittal (a) and coronal (b) T1-weighted MRI with gadolinium enhancement of a planum sphenoidale meningioma.

age groups (30–40 years) than meningiomas [15]. Perisellar hemangiopericytomas are very rare and account for less than 0.01% of all intracranial tumors [16].

Radiology

They are more commonly solitary durally based falcine or parasagittal lesions, and are occasionally found in the suprasellar and perisellar regions. CT and MRI characteristics are very similar to those of meningiomas, but hemangiopericytomas are more likely to invade and destroy adjacent bone without hyperostosis, are less likely to be calcified, and have a rich dural and cortical blood supply with flow voids in the tumor.

Pathology

Histologically, hemangiopericytomas are vascular tumors consisting of vascular channels ensheathed by tumor cells, producing the appearance of "staghorn" clefts or sinusoids with dense surrounding reticulin staining. They have more malignant potential than meningiomas, corresponding with WHO grade II and III tumors, and a higher rate of local recurrence and distant metastasis [15].

Treatment

Surgical resection is the principal treatment, with postoperative radiotherapy due to the high risk of recurrence. The exact surgical approach depends on the location and direction of growth of the tumor.

Prognosis

Due to the rarity of perisellar hemangiopericytomas there are insufficient data for the prediction of long-term outcome. For all hemangiopericytomas, the 5-year recurrence rate is 65% [15], but this is likely to be higher in perisellar tumors because incomplete resection is more common in this region.

Optic nerve and hypothalamic gliomas

Etiology

Optic nerve and hypothalamic gliomas may occur sporadically in children, or up to a third may be in association with neurofibromatosis type 1 (NF1). They account for 1% of all intracranial tumors, and 10–15% of supratentorial tumors in children.

Presentation

They usually present with slowly progressive visual loss. Hypothalamic tumors may present primarily with pituitary imbalance, obesity, diabetes insipidus, precocious puberty, or with obstructive hydrocephalus. Intraorbital tumors may present with proptosis.

Radiology

Pilocytic astrocytomas in this region are well circumscribed, solid, contrast-enhancing lesions, usually without calcification. The optic nerve sheath restricts growth in a longitudinal direction along the course of the nerve, producing a fusiform appearance.

Pathology

The majority of optic nerve gliomas are low-grade pilocytic astrocytomas, which may be bilateral in NF1. They may also extend into, or originate from, the chiasm and hypothalamus. Histological examination reveals a mass of bipolar cells with hair-like extremities and Rosenthal fibers, interspersed with loose-textured microcystic areas. Although pilocytic astrocytomas may contain areas of nuclear pleomorphism, microvascular proliferation and meningeal infiltration, they are considered WHO grade I benign tumors. Tumor cells are found diffusely related to neurons, contrasting with the well-circumscribed appearance of the commoner cerebellar pilocytic astrocytomas. Malignant transformation is rare, but is heralded by multiple mitoses per high power field and palisading necrosis.

Treatment

Initial treatment is by radiological observation, since most optic nerve gliomas are very slowly growing or may regress, although a biopsy may be performed if the diagnosis is in doubt. Progressive optic nerve gliomas extending into the orbit are best treated by surgical resection with sacrifice of ipsilateral residual eyesight, whereas extension into the chiasm is treated by radiotherapy. Exophytic optic nerve tumors, or progressive tumors confined to the nerve may be treated surgically to prevent spread to the chiasm and contralateral optic nerve. Chemotherapy may be used for patients with progressive disease who are too young for radiation treatment.

Prognosis

Optic nerve gliomas may remain static for years, and some may actually regress spontaneously. Patients with NF1 have a better prognosis and tumor progression is rarely seen after 6 years of age in this group. After radiation treatment, progression-free survival was seen in 72% of patients at 5 years in one study [17]. Results for radiation treatment of hypothalamic gliomas are comparable: in one study, radiological improvement was seen in 46%, and progression in 54% of patients after radiotherapy. In the same study, chemotherapy provided tumor control in 30%, and partial resection was associated with improvement in 25%. The overall 5-year survival was 93% [18].

Glomus tumors

Etiology

Glomus tumors (also known as paragangliomas or chemodectomas) are usually benign encapsulated tumors, occurring in one in a million people, more commonly in females of the fifth decade. They arise from neural crest cells which are destined to become autonomic ganglia or paraganglia, which are small 0.5–1.5 mm bodies found along branches of the glossopharyngeal and vagus nerves. Tumors may occur around the jugular bulb, middle ear, vagus nerve, or cauda equina. More rarely involved are the sellar region and cerebellopontine angle, and outwith the nervous system they may arise in the retroperitoneal and mediastinal regions, and from the carotid body, thyroid and adrenal glands.

Glomus tumors are usually sporadically occurring, although carotid body tumors may show familial clustering, and other glomus tumors are sometimes associated with multiple endocrine neoplasia syndromes 2A and 2B, von Hippel–Lindau syndrome, and neurofibromatosis.

Jugulotympanic tumors tend to occur more commonly in females, with a peak in the fifth decade.

Presentation

Glomus jugulare tumors may extend into the cranial cavity to produce multiple lower cranial nerve palsies. Glomus tympanicum tumors present with progressive hearing loss, facial palsy, and a feeling of fullness or pounding in the ear. Occasionally they may secrete catecholamines resulting in hypertension, palpitations, sweating and anxiety although most do not have significant endocrine activity. Sellar tumors may present with endocrine or visual disturbance, mimicking a pituitary adenoma [18].

Radiology

Glomus tumors are homogeneously enhancing isodense masses on CT, and iso- or hypointense on T1-weighted MRI with strong gadolinium enhancement, and hyperintense on T2-weighted images. Angiography should be performed, including the external carotid system to look at the feeding vessels and patency of the draining sinuses prior to surgery.

Pathology

The tumor is usually well differentiated, and resembles autonomic ganglia, with nests of chief cells surrounded by rims of sustentacular cells.

Treatment

Surgical extirpation is the primary treatment, with radiation treatment as an adjunct. Endovascular embolization aids the resection of these often vascular tumors. In a meta-analysis of surgical treatment, it was possible to completely resect glomus jugulare tumors in 88% of patients [19]. Fractionated radiotherapy and stereotactic radiosurgery may be used alone for tumor control in patients who would not tolerate or choose not to have surgery.

Prognosis

The recurrence rate after excision of glomus jugulare tumors was 3.1% in one study, with a mean time to recurrence of 83 months [19]. The behavior and prognosis of sellar tumors are similar to those of invasive pituitary adenomas or meningiomas [20], and are largely dependent on the extent of surgical removal.

Miscellaneous perisellar tumors

Other perisellar masses which are covered elsewhere include pituitary adenoma (Chapters 25–35), craniopharyngioma (Chapter 36), epidermoid, dermoid, arachnoid, and Rathke's cysts (Chapter 37), cavernous hemangioma (Chapter 42), histiocytosis (Chapter 43) and sarcoidosis (Chapter 44).

Metastatic tumors including lymphoma and leukemia may also occur in the pituitary fossa or cavernous sinus region.

Germ cell tumors, particularly germinomas, may arise from the midline in the suprasellar cisterns of teenage patients, whereas non-germinomatous germ cell tumors tend to occur in the pineal region. After histological diagnosis, germinomas are treated by radiotherapy, with chemotherapy as an adjunct.

Tuberculosis should always be considered in susceptible ethnic groups, a history of travel to endemic areas, and in the immunocompromised.

For the surgeon, it is important to remember that a large aneurysm of the terminal internal carotid or basilar arteries may mimic a perisellar or suprasellar tumor, with potentially fatal consequences if a resection is attempted.

Surgery

The aim of surgery is to obtain a histological diagnosis, and to excise the tumor. Removal of the tumor will relieve pressure on adjacent neurological structures, and increase patient survival. *En bloc* resection is not usually possible in the perisellar region due to the complex anatomy, delicate neighboring structures, and deep narrow exposures, and therefore maximal debulking of the tumor is the usual objective, supplemented by adjunctive radiation treatment. The approach will be determined by the size and location of the tumor, direction of growth, tumor origin, nerves and vessels encroached upon, and the experience or preference of individual surgeons (Fig. 40.4). A combination of approaches at different stages is often required for larger tumors.

Local tumor recurrence is often the cause of death in these patients, and therefore good surgical excision is key to improving outcomes. Occasionally a tumor may be observed radiologically, for example, a small asymptomatic perisellar meningioma in an elderly patient, or a tumor in the cavernous sinus which is intimately related to nerves and vessels. A biopsy, however, may be required to facilitate effective treatment decisions. For most perisellar tumors surgery is the treatment of choice.

Anterior approaches to the clivus

• *Subfrontal approaches.* A unilateral or bilateral frontal craniotomy allows access to the anterior cranial fossa floor and suprasellar regions. Removal of the fronto-orbital nasal bar allows exposure of the perisellar regions via the ethmoid and sphenoid sinuses (Fig. 40.4a).
• *Transsphenoidal approaches.* Endonasal or endoscopic techniques are useful for approaching pathology in the sphenoid sinus and pituitary fossa, and are covered in detail in Chapter 27 (Fig. 40.4g).
• *Transethmoidal approaches.* Midline suprasellar and sphenoidal pathology can be excised by this route (Fig. 40.4f).

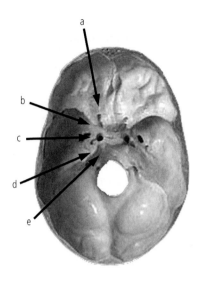

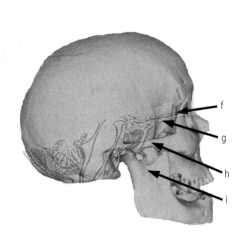

Figure 40.4 Diagram of approaches to the perisellar region. (a) Subfrontal; (b) pterional; (c) subtemporal; (d) translabyrinthine; (e) retrosigmoid suboccipital; (f) transethmoidal; (g) transnasal; (h) transmaxillary; (i) transoral.

• *Transmaxillary approaches*. The upper clivus may be exposed through the nasal cavity and maxillary sinus with a midface-degloving approach. For a more extensive exposure the maxilla may be divided and each half displaced laterally: the "open-door maxillotomy", which is effectively an extended transoral technique (Fig. 40.4h).

• *Transoral surgery*. The midline lower clivus, atlas and axis vertebrae may be approached through the mouth. After transoral surgery the craniocervical junction may become unstable, and often posterior fixation is required (Fig. 40.4i).

Anterolateral approaches to the clivus

• *Fronto-pterional craniotomy*. Dissection of the Sylvian fissure allows access to the top of the clivus and cavernous sinus (Fig. 40.4b).

• *Subtemporal approach*. The superior half of the clivus may be approached via a middle cranial fossa craniotomy, sometimes supplemented by a zygomatic osteotomy, looking over the anterior petrous temporal bone and posterior cavernous sinus.

For lower exposures a petrosectomy may be performed (Fig. 40.4c).

Posterolateral approaches to the clivus

• *Translabyrinthine* and *transcochlear* approaches involve a posterior petrosectomy and provide exposure of the petrous apex, cerebellopontine angle, and lateral aspect of the mid-clivus (Fig. 40.4d).

• *Retrosigmoid suboccipital* approach. This may be used to access the cerebellopontine angle and petroclival junction, and can be combined with a supratentorial approach by ligation and division of the transverse and superior petrosal sinuses (Fig. 40.4e).

References

1. Stewart MJ. Malignant sacrococcygeal chordoma. *J. Pathol. Bacteriol.* 1922;25:40–62.

2. Rosenberg AE. Pathology of chordoma and chondrosarcoma of the axial skeleton. In Harsh G (ed.). *Chordomas and Chondrosarcomas of the Skull Base and Spine.* New York: Thieme Medical Publishers, 2003:8–15.

3. Ericksson B. Chordomas. *Acta Orthop. Scand.* 1987;52:49–58.

4. Weber AL, Liebsch NJ, Sanchez R, et al. Chordomas of the skull base: radiologic and clinical evaluation. *Neuroimaging Clin. North Am.* 1995;4:515–527.

5. Watkins L, Khudados ES, Kaleoglu M, et al. Skull base chordomas: a review of 38 patients, 1958–88. *Br. J. Neurosurg.* 1993;7:241–248.

6. Castro JR, Collier M, Petti PL, et al. Charged particle radiotherapy for lesions encircling the brainstem or spinal cord. *Int. J. Radiat. Oncol. Biol. Phys.* 1989;17:477–484.

7. Kondziolka D, Lunsford LD, Flickinger JC. The role of radiosurgery in the management of chordoma and chondrosarcoma of the skull base. *Neurosurgery* 1991;29:38–46.

8. Gay E, Sekhar LN, Rubinstein E, et al. Chordomas and chondrosarcomas of the cranial base: results and follow-up of 60 patients. *Neurosurgery* 1995;36:887–897.

9. Bahr AL, Gayler BW. Cranial chondrosarcomas: a report of four cases and review of the literature. *Radiology* 1977;124:151–156.

10. Barnes L. Pathobiology of selected tumours of the base of the skull. *Skull Base Surg.* 1991;1:207–216.

11. Samii M, Tatagiba M, Monteiro ML. Meningiomas involving the parasellar region. *Acta Neurochir. Suppl.* 1996;65:63–65.

12. Jaaskelainen J, Haltia M, Laasonen E, et al. The growth rate of intracranial meningiomas and its relation to histology. An analysis of 43 patients. *Surg. Neurol.* 1985;24:165–172.

13. Perry A, Stafford SL, Scheithauer BW, et al. Meningioma grading: an analysis of histologic parameters. *Am. J. Surg. Pathol.* 1997;21:1455–1465.

14. Perry A, Scheithauer BW, Stafford SL, et al. "Malignancy" in meningiomas: a clinicopathologic study of 116 patients, with grading implications. *Cancer* 1999;85:2046–2056.

15. Guthrie BL, Ebersold MJ, Scheithauer BW, et al. Meningeal hemangiopericytoma: histopathological features, treatment, and long-term follow-up of 44 cases. *Neurosurgery* 1989;25:514–522.

16. Morrison DA, Bibby K. Sellar and suprasellar hemangiopericytoma mimicking pituitary adenoma. *Arch. Ophthalmol.* 1997;115:1201–1203.

17. Combs SE, Schulz-Ertner D, Moschos D, et al. Fractionated stereotactic radiotherapy of optic pathway gliomas: tolerance and long-term outcome. *Int. J. Radiat. Oncol. Biol. Phys.* 2005;62:814–819.

18. Scheithauer BW, Parameswaran A, Burdick B. Intrasellar paraganglioma: report of a case in a sibship of von Hippel-Lindau disease. *Neurosurgery* 1996;38:395–399.

19. Gottfried ON, Liu JK, Couldwell WT. Comparison of radiosurgery and conventional surgery for the treatment of glomus jugulare tumors. *Neurosurg. Focus* 2004;17:22–30.

20. Rodriguez LA, Edwards MS, Levin VA. Management of hypothalamic gliomas in children: an analysis of 33 cases. *Neurosurgery* 1990;26:242–246.

41 Pineal Tumors: Germinomas and Non-germinomatous Germ Cell Tumors

Frank Saran and Sharon Peoples

Key points

- Primary germ cell tumors of the central nervous system are rare neoplasms usually arising in the pineal or/and suprasellar region. They primarily affect children and adolescents, with 75% of patients less than 20 years of age at diagnosis.
- Germ cell tumors can present with a combination of symptoms such as obstructive hydrocephalus as well as endocrine, visual and focal neurological deficits.
- Germ cell tumors can be associated with the secretion of tumor markers such as alpha fetoprotein and β human chorionic gonadotropin (secreting non-germinomatous germ cell tumors). Germinomas have a tendency to spread subependymally whilst secreting non-germinomatous germ cell tumors primarily metastasize through the cerebrospinal fluid.
- Treatment strategies are stage- and risk-adapted. Pure germinomas are usually treated by primary radiotherapy with long-term survival rates in excess of 90%. Secreting non-germinomatous germ cell tumors are best treated by a combination of cisplatinum-based chemotherapy and radiotherapy with overall survival rates in the range of 50–65%.
- Current clinical trials in germinomas are aiming to maintain the high cure rates whilst trying to minimize the late sequelae while in secreting non-germinomatous germ cell tumors the primary aim remains improving survival.

Introduction

Intracranial germ cell tumors (GCT) are rare tumors of the central nervous system. GCT account for 1–3% of all intracranial neoplasms and commonly arise in midline structures adjacent to the third ventricle. The most common regions involved are the pineal (~45%) and suprasellar (~35%) areas [1] (Fig. 41.1). In rare cases the basal ganglia and non-midline structures can be involved (~5%). In around 15% of cases concurrent lesions are detected in both the pineal gland and either the suprasellar, cavernous sinus, optic chiasm or wall of third ventricle (Fig. 40.2). These tumors are termed bifocal or multiple midline GCT and in Europe are considered as localized disease while the same patient diagnosed in the States would be classified as metastatic [2]. GCT have a tendency to spread through the cerebrospinal fluid (CSF) and approximately 5–10% of patients present with either microscopic or macroscopic metastatic disease in the CSF at time of diagnosis.

Incidence

There is a marked geographical variation in the incidence of GCT. In the West they constitute only 0.5% to 3% of all primary

intracranial neoplasms and approximately 3% to 5% of tumors in children and adolescents. In contrast, in Japan GCT account for 2% to 5% of all primary intracranial neoplasms but up to 15% of all pediatric brain tumors [1, 3]. The peak age of onset is in the second decade and only 10% of cases are diagnosed after the age of 20 years.

GCT are more common found in males with a male to female ratio of 2:1. In female patients GCT occur more frequently in the suprasellar region whereas in male patients GCT more regularly affect the pineal gland.

Histology

GCT are a heterogeneous group of tumors and knowledge of the histological subtype is important in terms of treatment and prognosis. It is thought that GCT arise from primordial germ cells that became misplaced when migrating to the gonadal fold. Tumors composed of cells resembling the cells in earlier stages of embryogenesis are considered more malignant than those resembling cells in later stages. Each stage of embryonic development gives rise to a different histological subtype of GCT. Choriocarcinomas arise from the trophoblast, yolk sac tumors from the yolk sac endoderm, embryonal carcinomas from pluripotential stem cells, teratomas from embryonic differentiated cells and germinomas arise from primordial cells [4].

Clinical Endocrine Oncology, 2nd edition. Edited by Ian D. Hay and John A.H. Wass. © 2008 Blackwell Publishing. ISBN 978-1-4051-4584-8.

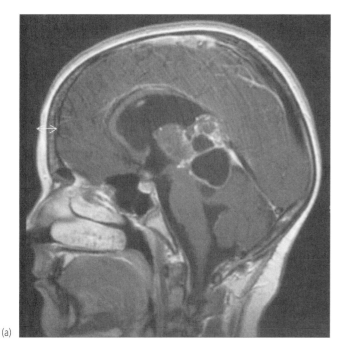

(a)

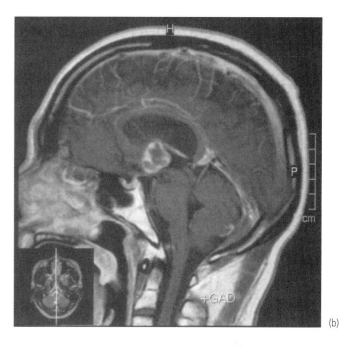

(b)

Figure 41.1 (a) T1-weighted sagittal postcontrast magnetic resonance image of a patient with a partially solid, partly cystic mass in the pineal region and obstructive hydrocephalus due to compression of the aquaeductus cerebri. The patient underwent a third ventriculostomy and biopsy of the mass. Histopathology was consistent with a mature teratoma. (b) T1-weighted sagittal postcontrast magnetic resonance image of a patient with a centrally necrotic contrast-enhancing mass in the suprasellar region. Examination of serum tumor markers revealed a isolated pathological elevation of αFP and no histopathological verification was required. Staging indicated a localized yolk sac tumor and the patient was treated with cisplatinum-based chemotherapy followed by involved field irradiation.

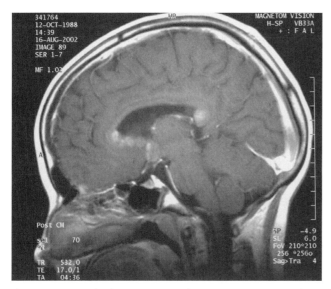

Figure 41.2 T1-weighted postcontrast sagittal magnetic resonance image of a patient with metastatic germinoma. The image demonstrates both disease in the pineal and suprasellar area as well as multiple maximally 1 cm metastases attached to the ventricular surface. Germinomas typical spread along the subependymal lining prior to establishing spinal metastases via dissemination through the CSF.

The WHO classification divides GCT into subtypes depending on the final differentiated cell. With regard to their management they are divided into three major subgroups: pure germinomas, secreting (malignant) non-germinomatous germ cell tumors (NGGCT) and teratomas. NGGCT include choriocarcinomas, yolk sac tumors, embryonal carcinoma and mixed tumors. Outcome differs depending on the histological subtype and extent of disease at diagnosis [5].

Pure germinomas are histologically identical to their gonadal counterparts (seminomas) and represent approximately 40–50% of all intracranial GCT. Classically they consist of large uniform cells with clear cytoplasm. Syncytiotrophoblastic cells can be present and may secrete low levels of β human chorionic gonadotropin (β-HCG). Despite this germinomas are often referred to as non-secreting germ cell tumors if the β-HCG levels are ≤50 IU/L. The evidence on whether such a component is associated with a worse outcome is controversial [6, 7].

There remains debate regarding the classification of germinomas which demonstrate elevated β-HCG levels. In Europe and more recently in the US elevations above 50 IU/L are perceived not to be consistent with a pure germinoma and are classified and treated as secreting NGGCT. This view is not shared by the Japanese GCT working group which allocates a patient with an elevated β-HCG and histopathological diagnosis of a germinoma an intermediate risk with a separate treatment strategy. This three tier classification is currently not mirrored in the risk-adapted therapeutic strategies of SIOP and COG who only recognize a two-tier classification: germinomas (low risk) and secreting NGGCT (high risk).

NGGCT are usually mixed tumors. Most tumors harbor yolk sac elements which secrete alpha fetoprotein (αFP) (Table 41.1).

Table 41.1 Secretion of tumor markers by histological subtype

Tumor markers	Germinoma	Teratoma	Yolk sac tumor	Choriocarcinoma	Embryonal carcinoma
β-HCG	+/−	−	−	+++	+/−
αFP	−	−	+++	−	+/−

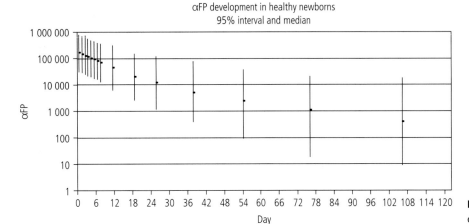

Figure 41.3 Nomogram showing how the level of αFP falls naturally after birth.

In view of this they are often referred to as secreting NGGCT or simplified as secreting germ cell tumors. αFP is normally synthesized by yolk sac endoderm, fetal hepatocytes and embryonal intestinal epithelium and is therefore present in the serum of normal infants up to 8 months old. Outside this age group the presence of an elevated serum αFP (≥25 ng/mL) is diagnostic of a secreting GCT. If the diagnosis of GCT is suspected in an infant serum αFP has to be adjusted for age according to accepted nomograms (Fig. 41.3).

Pure choriocarcinomas are rare and are composed of cytotrophoblast, syncytiotrophoblast, ectatic vessels and areas of hemorrhagic necrosis. The syncytiotrophoblasts secrete high levels of HCG and can give rise to clinical symptoms such as gynecomastia (Table 41.1).

Mature teratomas are histologically benign tumors and are derived from ecto-, meso- and endoderm. As a consequence they may contain ectopic normal tissue such as bone, cartilage, hair and teeth. Immature teratomas are composed of fetal-like tissue in a mitotically active stroma.

Clinical presentation

Presenting symptoms and signs depend on the anatomical site of the tumor and the age of the patient.

Pineal tumors

The classic symptom of pineal tumors is Parinaud syndrome (paralysis of upward gaze, headache and impaired pupillary con-

striction to light with preservation of accommodation). This is due to tumor compression on the quadrigeminal plate interrupting fibers running from the cerebral cortex to the superior caliculi and oculomotor nuclei. In addition tumors in this location frequently compress the Sylvian aqueduct leading to obstructive hydrocephalus indicated by symptoms of raised intracranial pressure (diurnal headache, vomiting and lethargy).

Suprasellar tumors

The commonest presenting symptoms of suprasellar tumors are obstructive hydrocephalus, endocrine deficiencies and visual field defects. The close proximity of the tumor to the hypothalamo–pituitary axis can lead to diabetes insipidus (DI) being an early presenting symptom, sometimes preceding the development of a radiological detectable mass and is present in around 85% of patients. This isolated endocrine deficit develops into panhypopituitarism with increasing tumor growth. In our experience in children with germ cell tumors diabetes insipidus is often associated with hypothalamic osmoreceptor dysregulation affecting their thirst sensation. These children have an inappropriate thirst threshold with sensation of thirst when plasma osmolality is in the low or below normal range when in normal circumstances thirst is suppressed, opposite to adipsia where there is no thirst stimulation despite high plasma osmolality. The clinical implication of the association of DI and this osmoreceptor dysregulation is that thirst is not reduced after the administration of desmopressin, and therefore patients tend to develop hyponatremia if their fluid intake is not supervised after desmopressin administration. Low doses of desmopressin are usually well tolerated but at the expense of an increased daily fluid intake. Other symptoms of hypothalamic damage include anorexia or weight gain, somnolence, mood swings, disrupted sleep pattern and failure to thrive. Diabetes insipidus or other symptoms associated with a suprasellar location seen in apparently isolated pineal tumors are frequently associated with bifocal germinomas. Other endocrine symptoms include delay or arrested or precocious puberty. This latter symptom is nearly exclusively seen in male patients [8] and is predominantly associated with choriocarcinomas. The mechanism is felt to be related to the excess production of HCG which is secreted by these tumors and mimics luteinizing hormone, simulating testosterone secretion by testicular Leydig cells. In girls the absence of excess follicle-stimulating hormone (FSH) protects to a certain extent against this symptom. Early involvement of endocrinologists in the management of these patients is vital and their "real time" input is required in most patients at all stages during treatment (preoperative, perioperative, during chemo- and radiotherapy and follow-up).

Due to the spatial proximity of suprasellar tumors to the optic chiasm patients can present with either a visual field defect or reduced visual acuity. Hemiparesis or other focal neurological deficits are first presenting symptoms if the tumor arises in atypical (non-midline) structures such as the basal ganglia.

Investigations

When a primary CNS GCT is suspected the first radiological investigation should be magnetic resonance imaging (MRI) with intravenous contrast. The classic appearance of a germinoma on MRI is an iso- or hyperdense, well-defined lesion that uniformly enhances with contrast. Calcification or low density lesions consistent with fat or cystic areas are suggestive of a NGGCT although calcifications are more likely to be identified on a computerized tomography scan (CT). In addition, MRI of the head can detect macroscopic leptomeningeal or intraventricular seeding. In view of the propensity of GCT to spread through the CSF, imaging the whole craniospinal axis with MRI is required to detect macroscopic spinal disease.

If there is evidence of raised intracranial pressure a sample of ventricular CSF may be analyzed at the time of surgery. After relief or in the absence of an obstructive hydrocephalus a lumbar puncture has to be performed to obtain CSF for cytology. To avoid false-positive results a CSF analysis for cytology should be performed after a minimum of 14 days after the last surgical intervention. The CSF must also be examined for tumor markers: αFP and β-HCG. If previous tumor marker sampling was negative paired serum samples for αFP and β-HCG must be requested.

Analysis of levels of tumor markers in the CSF differentiates tumors into either secreting or non-secreting germ cell tumors. In the presence of a typical clinical presentation, neuroimaging and positive tumor markers, it is acceptable practice to commence therapy in the absence of a tissue diagnosis [7]. In the absence of positive tumor markers and a suspected diagnosis of NGGCT, it is mandatory to obtain a histopathological diagnosis as there are a number of differential diagnoses influencing management decisions and prognosis. The differential diagnosis of a pineal mass includes pinealoblastoma, pineocytoma, glioma and benign cysts. In the suprasellar region the differential diagnosis includes predominantly craniopharyngioma, Rathke's pouch cysts and astrocytomas of optic pathways and hypothalamus/third ventricle.

Treatment

Given the rarity of the disease and the complexity of management, patients with suspected or verified CNS GCT should be referred to a supraregional specialist center with experience in treating these tumors. It is strongly recommended that children are treated in an age-appropriate environment under the care of a pediatric oncologist. The age limit between pediatric, adolescent, and adult services may vary from country to country. In the UK patients less than 16 years of age are exclusively treated in a center affiliated with the Children's Cancer and Leukaemia Group (CCLG) formerly known as the United Kingdom Children's Cancer Study Group (UKCCSG) [7]. A multidisciplinary approach is required with a team including the pediatric oncologist, pediatric neurosurgeon, neuropathologist, pediatric radiotherapist, pediatric endocrinologist, pediatric ophthalmologist, pediatric neuropsychologist, pediatric anesthetist, specialist nurses in the hospital and community, play therapist, physiotherapist, occupational therapist, and social worker. Patients should be preferentially treated according to current national or international trial protocols (e.g. SIOP, COG).

The presence of an obstructive hydrocephalus represents a medical emergency and is neurosurgically addressed. Under these conditions most frequently an endoscopic third ventriculostomy is performed or in selected cases a ventriculoperitoneal (VP) shunt inserted with or without a prior external ventricular drainage (EVD). If the patient required emergency relief of a hydrocephalus, pathological verification should preferentially be obtained in a two-step procedure. Historically in the absence of elevated serum tumor markers, the inherent radiosensitivity of germinomas was utilized as a diagnostic tool. If a germinoma was suspected radiologically an empirical dose of 20 Gy was given to the visible tumor. If repeat imaging demonstrated a significant regression of the mass the diagnosis of germinoma was assumed. The patient proceeded then to receive craniospinal irradiation without histopathological diagnosis. Significant improvements in neurosurgical techniques and postoperative care have led to very low morbidity and mortality associated with stereotactic biopsies and other neurosurgical procedures [8]. Therefore in today's practice a radiosensitive test is no longer acceptable and it is mandatory to obtain a tissue diagnosis as the "radiosensitivity test" is unspecific and could, for example, be false-positive for pineoblastomas.

Germinomas

Surgery

In the absence of preoperatively elevated serum tumor markers, tissue for histopathological diagnosis should be obtained via an elective procedure of an open or stereotactic biopsy. Endoscopic third ventriculostomy enables neurosurgeons to inspect the ventricles and can in some cases visualize plaques on the walls of the ventricles not visible on MRI. When biopsied these plaques are consistent with germinomatous ventricular spread. The prognostic significance of this remains unclear when treated with wide field radiotherapy. There is no advantage in attempting a gross total resection in intracranial germinomas as it does not alter management or outcome but can be associated with significant surgical-related morbidity [9]. Radical surgery is reserved for the very few patients with a significant residual mass following completion of treatment which usually represents a mature teratoma component on histopathological assessment.

Radiotherapy

Pure germinomas are extremely radiosensitive and 5-year survival rates of up to 95% have been reported with radiotherapy alone [2, 10]. Historically the gold standard treatment for germinomas has been craniospinal radiotherapy followed by a boost to the primary site (Plate 41.1). The pattern of relapse in localized germinomas is dominated by ventricular recurrences and it is unusual to develop an isolated spinal cord relapse. A recent literature review confirmed that there is good evidence that in completely staged patients with localized germinomas irradiation of the ventricles followed by a boost to the primary tumor area gives equivalent long-term control rates compared to wide field radiotherapy with craniospinal radiotherapy [11]. Originally the craniospinal axis was treated to a dose of 30 to 35 Gy followed by a boost of 10 to 20 Gy in 6 to 12 fractions to the primary site. Over the last two decades consecutive studies have demonstrated that a reduction of the dose to the craniospinal axis to 24 Gy is equivalent with respect to long-term disease-free survival [12, 13]. In addition there was no loss of local control when reducing the primary tumor dose from 50–54 Gy to 40 Gy. The use of three-dimensional planning and conformal radiotherapy in conjunction with reduced volumes is likely to minimize the amount of normal tissue irradiated to high doses of radiotherapy and thus will reduce late sequelae.

There is some evidence suggesting that the primary tumor dose can be lowered when combined multiagent chemotherapy has achieved a complete response [5, 15]. However, there is controversy over what volume requires treatment in patients with bifocal tumors [16]. In Europe these tumors are regarded as localized disease whilst in the States these patients are treated in accordance with strategies designed for primary metastatic disease.

There is currently no controversy over the volume that should be treated in patients with evidence of metastatic disease. In germinoma CSF positive disease is a risk factor for spinal seeding but does not predict for recurrence when treated with craniospinal radiotherapy [3, 14]. Long-term control in excess of 85–90% at 5 years is achieved even in the presence of widespread macroscopic metastatic disease if craniospinal irradiation to dose levels of 24–30 Gy and boosts to all sites of macroscopic disease up to a dose of 40–45 Gy are given.

Chemotherapy

Germinomas are inherently chemosensitive and radiotherapeutic strategies in very young children are associated with noticeable late morbidity [16]. Thus the pediatric oncology community has focused on developing chemotherapeutic strategies for germinomas. Despite being chemosensitive only a limited number of patients are chemocurable and most patients require salvage treatment including radiotherapy [17]. In addition, this comes at the expense of significant morbidity and mortality not associated with radiotherapy alone. Yet it might be anticipated that with continuing improvements in research and supportive care as well as the availability of novel chemotherapeutic agents some of the current shortcomings may be overcome in the future. At present chemotherapy is successfully used in combined modality treatment approaches in patients with localized disease [18]. This aims to reduce the volume and/or the dose of radiotherapy with a reduction of late morbidity associated with radiotherapy in very young children. There is no proven benefit of the use of chemotherapy with respect to survival in patients with metastatic disease at diagnosis. The backbone of most reported multiagent chemotherapy protocols is platinum derivates (particularly carboplatinum), epipodophyllotoxins (etoposide), alkylating agents (e.g. cyclophosphamide, ifosfamide) and/or antibiotics (bleomycin) [19]. The commonest chemotherapy morbidities are short term but can be life threatening. These include hematological morbidities with the risk of bleeding and infection (particularly neutropenic sepsis), renal and hearing impairment, hemorrhagic cystitis, electrolyte disturbances and infertility, to name a few. Patients with known DI should not be treated in a center without access to or active involvement of a tertiary endocrinologist. While recurrences are rare they are potentially salvageable by further chemo- and/or radiotherapy.

Teratomas

The actual incidence of teratomas of the CNS is unclear as there are no available cancer registry data available. Only a few observational studies are published with very few patients per series. Clinically it is helpful to distinguish between mature or differentiated teratomas as opposed to immature teratomas. Mature teratomas are neither chemo- nor radiosensitive and therefore complete surgical resection is the treatment of choice if feasible. If a surgical complete resection is achieved cure rates are in the order of 90% at 10 years.

Macroscopic complete surgical resection is also the treatment of choice for immature teratomas. Reported survival rates at 10 years are in the order of 70–75% [5, 10]. In case of an incomplete resection an initial watch and wait policy should be adopted. Chemo- or radiotherapy along with the recommendations for NGGCT can be considered with or without repeat surgery at the time of progression based on anecdotal reports of clinical responses.

Secreting NGGCT

Surgery

In patients for whom the clinical and radiological appearances are consistent with a primary CNS GCT and there is evidence of pathologically elevated tumor markers (e.g., either serum or CSF) a histopathological verification of the diagnosis is not mandatory [20]. However, surgical intervention is required in patients presenting with acute hydrocephalus. There is no proven benefit of debulking surgery at the time of diagnosis but it carries a risk of peri- and postoperative morbidity [20]. Therefore, surgery is reserved for the removal of any large residual mass (usually consisting only of mature teratoma elements) after completion of chemotherapy or radiotherapy as patients with radiological residual disease have a higher relapse rate. Surgery is also indicated if the imaging demonstrates progressive disease during chemotherapy even when the tumor is biochemically responding (i.e. normalization of tumor markers [growing teratoma syndrome]).

Chemotherapy

Historically, surgery followed by radiotherapy alone was associated with a disappointing survival rate of less than 25% [21]. The emergence of platinum-based chemotherapy in the 1960s has substantially improved the survival of these patients and forms the cornerstone of current therapies with 5-year survival rates in the range of 50–65%. Although complete responses to chemotherapy have been documented, these are only rarely sustained without further treatment [13, 22, 23]. Induction chemotherapy is based on similar agents as used for germinomas. At present the consensus is that multiagent chemotherapy is mandatory as induction treatment. Cisplatinum has proved to be superior to carboplatinum in this setting and forms the backbone of all current treatment strategies. In addition, the dose intensity is noticeably higher for secreting NGGCT compared to germinomas. Acute and long-term morbidity of chemotherapy is in line with those mentioned for germinoma. By the nature of the need for hyperhydration when using cisplatinum or ifosfamide it is even more pivotal to seek advice from an endocrinologist at an early stage, particularly in patients with DI.

Based on a recently presented analysis of the data of the SIOP CNS GCT 96 study, patients with a pretreatment αFP level in excess of 1000 ng/mL have a significantly worse outcome (~35% 5-year survival) and may benefit from an intensified treatment strategy. The study employed four cycles of cisplatin, etoposide and ifosfamide chemotherapy with response rates approaching 100% and in European pediatric oncology is perceived as the gold standard. The full publication of this largest ever performed prospective study in CNS GCT is awaited. Regular monitoring of αFP levels during chemotherapy is important as the fall in αFP is constant when plotted on a semi-logarithmic scale. Deviation from the predicted speed of decline or a rise at the end of first-line chemotherapy predicts poor outcome with all such patients dying within a year from diagnosis.

Radiotherapy

Although NGGCT are less radiosensitive than their germinoma counterparts, radiotherapy represents an essential component of the curative treatment approach. There is good evidence of a dose–response relationship with radiation doses equal to or in excess of 50 Gy giving improved tumor control. In Europe patients with localized secreting tumors receive focal irradiation while craniospinal irradiation (dose range 30–35 Gy) followed by a boost (≥50 Gy to the primary and 45 Gy to spinal metastases) is limited to patients with proven metastatic disease (e.g. positive CSF cytology [M1] or macroscopic metastases [M2–3]) (Plate 41.2). In contrast most American series favor the use of craniospinal irradiation for all patients with secreting NGGCT regardless of stage. Analysis of the pattern of recurrence of patients with secreting NGGCT treated within the SIOP CNS GCT 96 study was not suggestive that an increase in the radiation volume to craniospinal irradiation followed by a boost in patients with localized disease could have reduced the risk of recurrence. The pattern of relapse was predominantly local and no different from patients treated with craniospinal irradiation (F. Saran, personal communication). Anecdotally, the use of radiosurgery (i.e. the delivery of a high-dose, single fraction of radiotherapy) particularly for residual disease has been reported. At present this is regarded as experimental and does not form part of a standard first-line treatment strategy. As the presence of residual radiological disease represents a risk factor for recurrence, the primary aim remains the macroscopic complete excision of any residual disease during or after first-line therapy. Recurrences of NGGCTs are only rarely salvageable by further treatment.

Follow-up

Close follow-up is recommended for all GCT. Baseline imaging should be performed on all patients once the acute effects of treatment have settled and at regular time intervals for 5 years after completion of treatment. At each consultation, the patient's history needs to be taken, clinical examination performed and tumor markers checked. It has been reported that non-secreting GCT have exceptionally recurred as secreting NGGCT although this is most likely in patients with incomplete staging at the time of first diagnosis.

In addition, patients with visual or endocrine deficits at diagnosis must undergo regular ophthalmological and endocrinological assessments. Most patients will become growth hormone (GH) deficient within 12–24 months after completion of radiotherapy even when not deficient at diagnosis. There is no evidence to suggest that GH replacement should be withheld for fear of inducing a recurrence. Regular adjustments are required to adapt to developing and growing patients as well as monitoring for other progressive endocrine deficits. Patients with DI and/or panhypopituitarism require lifelong monitoring. Atypical (non-midline) tumors presenting with focal neurological deficits can benefit from neurophysiological rehabilitation.

Over time the focus of follow-up shifts to monitoring for tumor- and treatment-related late sequelae. In patients where the limbic system has been disrupted (memory and concentration impairment) a neuropsychological assessment is beneficial to assess the patient's strength and weaknesses and facilitate posttreatment rehabilitation. This also helps in defining the educational needs of patients still in full-time education. Neurocognitive late sequelae include decreased IQ and reduced attention and memory spans and processing speeds. Neurosurgery and chemotherapy can lead to an effect on perceptual and motor skills [24]. However, radiotherapy-associated cognitive impairment is associated with higher doses of radiotherapy and young age (approximately under 8–10 years) at the time of treatment. However, there is no evidence to suggest that adolescent and adult patients experience a clinically relevant neurocognitive decline when treated with radiotherapy alone [24].

Depending on treatment modality other potential long-term toxicities need to be considered. Cisplatin can cause ototoxicity – as does radiotherapy albeit at a lower risk – and renal impairment. The use of bleomycin is associated with pulmonary fibrosis. Alkylating agents such as ifosfamide and cyclophosphamide can lead to infertility as may spinal radiotherapy if the radiation beam passes through the ovaries. In prepubertal patients radiotherapy of the spine leads to age- and dose-dependent spinal growth retardation. The younger the patient at time of radiotherapy, the more pronounced the effect on growth and cognitive function. Both radiotherapy and chemotherapy carry an increased risk of inducing second malignant neoplasms and thus warrant life-long monitoring although best practice of organizing long-term follow-up is not defined.

Conclusion

Intracranial GCT are rare primary CNS tumors that occur predominantly in children and adolescents. Treatment should preferentially be given under the auspices of a comprehensive cancer center with expertise in pediatric and/or adolescent oncology with "real-time" access to tertiary endocrinological services. In order to select the appropriate stage- and risk-adapted treatment strategy, patients must be adequately staged with MRI imaging of the whole craniospinal axis, serum and CSF tumor markers, CSF cytology and histopathological verification if required.

Prognosis for patients with both localized and metastatic germinomas is excellent with cure rates exceeding 90% at 5 years when using either radiotherapy only or a combined modality approach. Ongoing clinical trials are attempting to define the role of chemotherapy and reduce late sequelae.

Benign and immature teratomas are best treated with a primary surgical resection.

For secreting non-germinomatous germ cell tumors prognosis has improved with the addition of cisplatin-based chemotherapy to radiotherapy. However, the best 5-year survival rates remain around 50–65%.

Due to the rarity of these tumors participation in national and international studies should be encouraged to improve outcome, reduce late sequelae and increase our understanding of the tumor biology.

References

1. Jennings MT, Gelman R, Hochberg F. Intracranial germ cell tumors: natural history and pathogenesis. *J. Neurosurg.* 1985;63:155–167.
2. Sawamura Y, Shirato H, Ikeda J, et al. Induction chemotherapy followed by reduced-volume radiation therapy for newly diagnosed central nervous system germinoma. *J. Neurosurg.* 1998;88:166–172.
3. Brada M, Rajan B. Spinal seeding in cranial germinoma. *Br. J. Cancer* 1990;61:339–340.
4. Diez B, Balmaceda C, Matsutani M, et al. Germ cell tumors of the CNS in children: recent advances in therapy. *Child's Nerv. Syst.* 1999;15:578–585.
5. Matsutani M, Sano K, Takakura K, et al. Primary intracranial germ cell tumors: a clinical analysis of 153 histologically verified cases. *J. Neurosurg.* 1997;86:446–455.
6. Yoshida J, Sugita K, Kobayashi T, et al. Prognosis of intracranial germ cell tumors: effectiveness of chemotherapy with cisplatin and etoposide (CDDP and VP–16). *Acta Neurochir.* (Wien) 1993;120:111–117.
7. Shibamoto Y, Takahashi M, Sasai K. Prognosis of intracranial germinoma with syncytiotrophoblastic giant cells treated by radiation therapy. *Int. J. Radiat. Oncol. Phys.* 1997;37:505–510.
8. Starzyk J, Starzyk B, Bartnik-Mikuta AJ. Gonadotrophin releasing hormone – independent precocious puberty in a 5 year old girl with suprasellar germ cell tumor secreting beta-HCG and alpha-fetoprotein. *Pediatr. Endocrinol. Metab.* 2001;6:789–796.
9. Shibamoto Y, Abe M, Yamashita J, et al. Treatment result of intracranial germinoma as a function of the irradiated volume. *Int. J. Radiat. Oncol. Biol. Phys.* 1998;15:285–290.
10. Sano K. So-called germ cell tumors: are they really of germ cell origin? *Br. J. Neurosurg.* 1995;9:391–401.
11. Rogers SJ, Mosleh-Shirazi MA, Saran FH. Radiotherapy of localized intracranial germinoma: time to sever historical ties? *Lancet Oncol.* 2005;6:509–519.
12. Bamberg M, Kortmann RD, Calaminus G, et al. Radiation therapy for intracranial germinoma: results of the German cooperative prospective trials MAKEI 83/86/89. *J. Clin. Oncol.* 1999;17:2585–2592.
13. Calaminus G, Bamberg M, Baranzelli MC, et al. Intracranial germ cell tumors: a comprehensive update of the European data. *Neuropediatrics* 1994;25:26–32.
14. Shibamoto Y, Oda Y, Yamashita J, et al. The role of cerebrospinal fluid cytology in radiotherapy planning for intracranial germinoma. *Int. J. Radiat. Oncol. Biol. Phys.* 1994;29:1089–1094.
15. Buckner JC, Peethambaram PP, Smithson WA. Phase II trial of primary chemotherapy followed by reduced-dose radiation for CNS germ-cell tumors. *J. Clin. Oncol.* 1999;17:933–940.
16. Lester L, Saran F, Hargrave D, et al. Germinoma with synchronous lesion in the pineal and suprasellar regions – a case based update. *Childs Nerv. Syst.* 2006;22:1513–1518.

17. Balmaceda C, Heller G, Rosenblum M, et al. Chemotherapy without irradiation – a novel approach for newly diagnosed CNS germ cell tumors: results of an international cooperative trial. The First International Central Nervous System Germ Cell Tumor Study. *J. Clin. Oncol.* 1996;14:2908–2915.

18. Alapetite C, Ricardi U, Saran F, et al. Whole ventricular irradiation in combination with chemotherapy in intracranial germinomas: the consensus of the SIOP CNS GCT study group. *Med. Pediatr. Oncol.* 2002;39:248.

19. Weiner HL, Pietanza MC, Balmaceda C, et al. Chemotherapy without irradiation for newly-diagnosed CNS germ cell tumors: long-term follow-up and quality of life on an international cooperative trial. *J. Neurosurg.* 1999;90:421A.

20. Nicholson JC, Punt J, Hale J, et al. Germ Cell Tuumour Working Groups of the United Kingdom Children's Cancer Study Group (UKCCSG) and International Society of Pediatric Oncology (SIOP). Neurosurgical management of pediatric germ cell tumors of the central nervous system – a multi-disciplinary approach for the new millennium. *Br. J. Neurosurg.* 2002;16:93–95.

21. Hooda BS, Finaly JL. Recent advances in the diagnosis and treatment of central nervous system germ cell tumors. *Curr. Opin. Neurol.* 1999;12:693–696.

22. Kida Y, Kobayashi T, Yoshida J, et al. Chemotherapy with cisplatin in AFP–secreting germ-cell tumors of the central nervous system. *J. Neurosurg.* 1985;65:470–475.

23. Baranzelli MC, Patte C, Bouffet E, et al. An attempt to treat pediatric intracranial alpha FP and beta-HCG secreting germ cell tumors with chemotherapy alone. SFOP experience with 18 cases. Societe Francaise d'Oncologie Pediatrique. *J. Neuro-oncol.* 1998;37:229–239.

24. Sands SA, Kellie SJ, Davidow AL, et al. Long-term quality of life and neuropsychologic functioning for patients with CNS germ-cell tumors: from the First International CNS Germ-Cell Tumor study. *J. Neuro-oncol.* 2001;3:174–183.

42 Cavernous Sinus Hemangiomas

Mark E. Linskey

Key points

- Cavernous sinus hemangiomas are benign neoplasms arising within the dural confines of the cavernous sinus that only secondarily involve the sella turcica.
- They are distinguishable from 67–80% of meningiomas by hyperintensity on T2-weighted magnetic resonance images and from most cranial nerve schwannomas by characteristic vascular blush on angiography and absence of skull base neural foramen enlargement.
- Since the dura of the medial wall of the cavernous sinus separates the tumor from the pituitary gland, hormonal assessment is usually normal with rare cases demonstrating mild prolactin elevations from stalk dysinhibition, occasionally leading to amenorrhea and/or galactorrhea.
- Surgical resection is curative but requires specialized skull base microsurgical techniques, and is fraught with danger from intraoperative blood loss. The VIth cranial nerve is least likely to be spared since it will be usually be found within the substance of the tumor mass.
- Stereotactic radiosurgery is emerging as an important alternative to microsurgical resection with theoretical advantages over fractionated radiotherapy and promising early results.

Introduction

Intracranial extradural cavernous hemangiomas are benign, well-demarcated true neoplasms that arise within cranial dural venous sinuses. While they have been reported to arise in the petrosal sinus, the torcula heterophili, and the posterior sagittal sinus, the most common point of origin is the cavernous sinus [1, 2]. Cavernous sinus hemangiomas are rare tumors, accounting for <3% of benign cavernous sinus tumors referred to a major cranial base microsurgery referral center in the US [3]. Indeed, in the 48 years between 1943 and 1991, only 53 cases of cavernous sinus hemangioma were published [3]. Since that time, this type of lesion has become increasingly recognized. Our own extensive Medline search in March of 2006 revealed 114 additional reported cases over the subsequent 14 years (total, approximately 167 cases now reported). The largest two series of patients reported (*n* = 24 and *n* = 13) come from China and India, respectively [4, 5].

As a cavernous sinus hemangioma develops (Figs 42.1 and 42.2), it acquires its blood supply directly from the intracavernous segment of the internal carotid artery (ICA). As it enlarges it develops a pseudocapsule and begins to push the dura of the medial, superior, and lateral walls inward, upwards, and outwards. When it gets

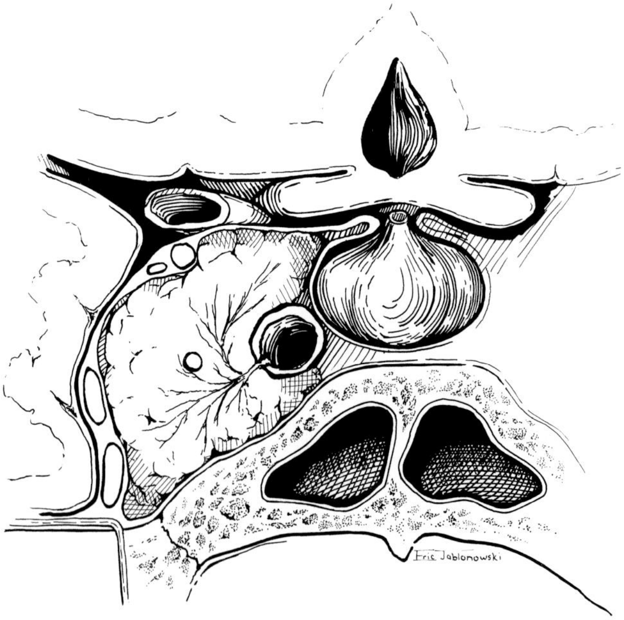

Figure 42.1 Artist's conception of the anatomy of a small cavernous sinus hemangioma still confined to the cavernous sinus examined in coronal cross-section. The tumor bulges the walls of the cavernous sinus superiorly and laterally with lateral displacement of the temporal lobe. Tumor blood supply is derived from the intracavernous ICA and the tumor displaces the ICA medially. Cranial nerve VI lies within the tumor substance, whereas cranial nerves III, IV, V1 and V2 remain separate from the tumor within the dura of the lateral wall of the cavernous sinus. (Reproduced from Linskey ME [3], with permission from Lippincott Williams & Wilkins.)

Clinical Endocrine Oncology, 2nd edition. Edited by Ian D. Hay and John A.H. Wass. © 2008 Blackwell Publishing. ISBN 978-1-4051-4584-8.

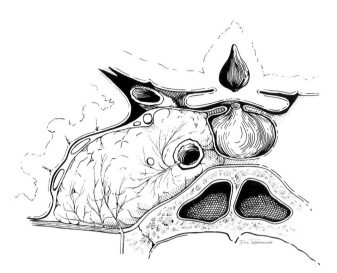

Figure 42.2 Artist's conception of the anatomy of a large cavernous sinus hemangioma examined in coronal cross-section (cf. Fig. 42.1). The tumor has grown medially encasing the intracavernous ICA and displacing the pituitary gland within the sella turcica. The supraclinoid ICA is displaced superiorly. Laterally, the tumor has dissected between the two layers of the middle cranial fossa dura displacing the temporal lobe superiorly and laterally. Additional tumor blood supply is now derived from the middle meningeal artery. Cranial nerve VI lies within the tumor substance, whereas CNs III, IV, V1 and V2 remain separate from the tumor stretched over its lateral surface within the overlying dura. (Reproduced from Linskey ME [3], with permission from Lippincott Williams & Wilkins.)

large enough, it begins to push its way between the two layers of dura lining the floor of the middle cranial fossa, where it may pick up additional blood supply from the middle meningeal and accessory middle meningeal arteries. The tumor does not invade the ICA, but eventually comes to encase it by encircling pseudopod extensions, much like a "hotdog in a bun." Cranial nerves III, IV and V all course within the lateral wall of the cavernous sinus and thus will always be found stretched over the lateral tumor surface with an anatomic potential plane between the tumor pseudocapsule and the lateral cavernous sinus wall. Because cranial nerve VI is the only nerve that actually truly runs through the cavernous sinus (lateral to the ICA), it will most often be found within the substance of the hemangioma, and is thus the most difficult to preserve with surgery. With time and continued growth, the tumor can extend medially into the sella turcica or contralateral cavernous sinus, superiorly into the suprasellar space, or anteriorly into the orbital apex via the superior orbital fissure.

Clinical presentation

Patient demographic characteristics

Cavernous sinus hemangiomas have an overwhelming predilection for women. Ninety-four percent of the 39 cases reported from 1948–1991 arose in women [3], and this observation has remained consistent since. The neoplasm also appears to be more common in Asian–Oceanian cultures (China, Japan, Korea, and

India with largest series and with >70% of reported world cases), although it has been reported in Europe, North America, South America, Asia Minor, and Australia as well. Median age at diagnosis is 44 years with a range of 22–64 years [3].

Clinical signs and symptoms

Clinical signs and symptoms are indistinguishable from those associated with other mass lesions within the cavernous sinus. Patients most often have cranial neuropathies, worsening vision, headaches, or retro-orbital pain. Less frequent signs or symptoms include exophthalmos, trigeminal neuralgia, and hemi- or monoparesis. Duration of symptoms has been reported to span 1 week to 10 years. Symptoms usually progress gradually but sudden onset or progression of clinical symptoms due to intratumoral hemorrhage has been reported in at least two cases [3].

Endocrine implications

Since the dura of the medial wall of the cavernous sinus separates the tumor from the pituitary gland, and the tumor only gradually encroaches on the space within the sella turcica or the hypothalamic–pituitary stalk in the suprasellar cistern, hormonal assessment is usually normal. In some cases of larger tumors, mild-moderate elevations of serum prolactin have been reported, most consistent with stalk disinhibition effect [1, 6–10]. The only reported serum prolactin level for these cases was 120 ng/mL [9]. Rarely the hyperprolactinemia associated with cavernous sinus hemangiomas can lead to clinical amenorrhea or galactorrhea [1, 6–8].

Symptoms have been reported to first appear or worsen with pregnancy in at least four patients [11, 12]. In an additional case, symptoms were reported to first appear concomitant with the administration of exogenous estrogen for Turner syndrome [13]. To our knowledge, cavernous sinus hemangiomas have yet to be assessed for the presence or absence of hormone receptors.

Neuroimaging findings

Cavernous sinus hemangiomas characteristically show no calcifications and demonstrate surrounding bony erosion or remodeling rather than hyperostotic reaction. On computerized tomography (CT) scans they tend to be either hyper- or isodense to surrounding brain on non-contrast studies. They enhance densely and homogenously with intravenous iodine-based contrast (Fig. 42.3).

Cavernous sinus hemangiomas show a subtle tumor blush in 80% of cases (Fig. 42.4) [3]. This blush occasionally requires prolonged selective arterial contrast injection to demonstrate. The blush is usually described as "flecked" in appearance with "pooling" of contrast in small collections or "lakes" [3]. Identifiable feeding vessels may or may not be present and can be multiple. When identifiable, the most common feeding vessels are the meningohypophyseal trunk, the middle meningeal artery, and the accessory middle meningeal artery, in decreasing order of frequency [3]. Arterial embolization is rarely possible due to the small size the feeding vessels and the dominance of feeders coming off the intracavernous ICA as opposed to external carotid artery dural branches.

(a)

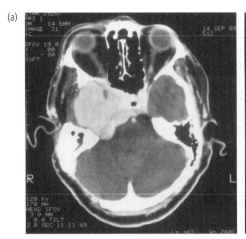

(b)

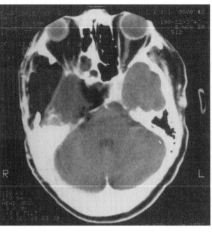

Figure 42.3 Preoperative contrast-enhanced axial CT scan of a patient with a cavernous sinus hemangioma (a) demonstrating a giant right cavernous sinus and middle cranial fossa tumor. Repeat contrast-enhanced CT scan 2 weeks after skull base microsurgical resection (b) reveals no residual tumor. (Reproduced from Linskey ME [3], with permission from Lippincott Williams & Wilkins.)

(a)

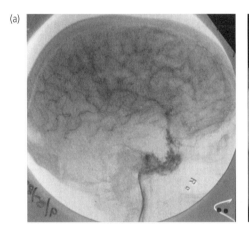

(b)

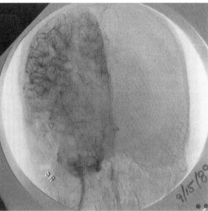

Figure 42.4 Right lateral (a) and anteroposterior (b) views of a preoperative cerebral angiogram of the same patient in Fig.42. 3. The right petrous and intracavernous ICA were displaced anteriorly and inferiorly with opening of the carotid siphon. A dense "flecked" tumor blush is apparent with pooling of contrast material in small "lakes" well into the venous phase. (Reproduced from Linskey ME [3], with permission from Lippincott Williams & Wilkins.)

(a)

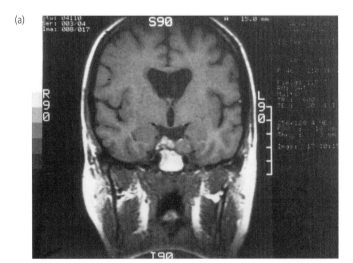

(b)

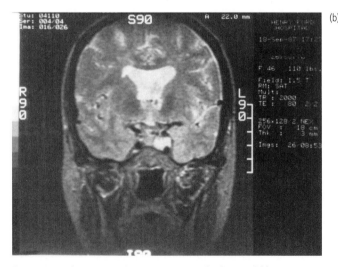

Figure 42.5 Preoperative coronal MR images of a patient with a small left cavernous sinus hemangioma. The tumor was isointense on T1-weighted images (a) (TR, 600; TE, 20) and hyperintense on T2-weighted images (b) (TR, 2000; TE, 80). (Reproduced from Linskey ME [3], with permission from Lippincott Williams & Wilkins.)

(a)

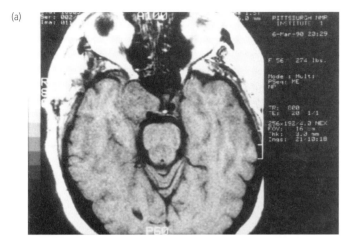

(b)

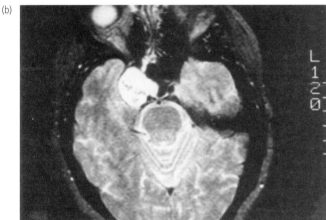

Figure 42.6 Preoperative axial MR images of a patient with a moderate-size left cavernous sinus hemangioma. The tumor was isointense on T1-weighted images (a) (TR, 800; TE, 20) and hyperintense on T2-weighted images (b) (TR, 2000; TE, 80). The tumor extended into the sella turcica. (Reproduced from Linskey ME [3], with permission from Lippincott Williams & Wilkins.)

On magnetic resonance imaging (MRI), cavernous sinus hemangiomas are usually hyperintense on T1-weighted noncontrast images, and characteristically brightly hyperintense on T2-weighted non-contrast images. They brightly enhance with gadolinium-based intravenous contrast administration (Figs 42.5 and 42.6).

Differential diagnosis

From a histopathological and epistemological standpoint, cavernous sinus hemangiomas need to be distinguished from brain parenchymal cavernous malformations (cavernomas), intraneural hemangiomas, and osseous hemangiomas, all of which can appear quite similar on microscopic histology (Fig. 42.7). Cavernous sinus hemangiomas are true benign neoplasms that grow and enlarge over time due to cellular proliferation, and arise within a dural vascular sinus. Cavernous malformations are vascular hamartomas within the larger set of cerebral vascular

malformations, which can only enlarge as a result of hemorrhage or engorgement of pre-existing vascular channels [14]. Intraneural hemangiomas are usually small lesions that arise within the substance of cranial nerves, and it remains controversial whether or not they represent intraneural hamartomas or true neoplasms. Osseous hemangiomas are true neoplasms arising in bone that can involve the skull base and orbit. They arise in a different age and sex spectrum than dural sinus hemangiomas, are routinely calcified, and tend to destroy bone. They may, on rare occasions, involve a dural sinus secondarily [15].

From a practical, pragmatic, and clinical decision-making standpoint, cavernous sinus hemangiomas need to be distinguished from two other more common benign cavernous sinus tumors: meningioma and cranial nerve schwannoma. The presence of tumor calcium or hyperostosis on CT scan favors the diagnosis of meningioma over hemangioma, but in the absence of these findings, hemangiomas cannot be distinguished from meningiomas or schwannomas on CT scan. The characteristic "flecked" tumor blush of hemangiomas on angiography is very useful for confirming the diagnosis when present. Unfortunately, it is absent in 20% of cases of hemangioma and, more and more, clinicians are moving away from invasive diagnostic angiography in favor of CT angiography or MR angiography, which are insensitive to this finding.

MRI is the major development likely explaining the acceleration in recognition and reporting of cavernous sinus hemangiomas. Prior to the late 1980s it is likely that a subset of presumed cavernous sinus meningiomas diagnosed solely on CT scan characteristics were in fact cavernous sinus hemangiomas. MR is the imaging modality that can distinguish meningioma from hemangioma in 67–80% cases. Most meningiomas are either isointense or hypointense on T1-weighted images. More importantly, 67–80% of are isointense or only mildly hyperintense on T2-weighted images (hyperintense relative to gray matter but hypointense compared with cerebrospinal fluid) [16, 17]. The only exceptions to this observation are angioblastic meningiomas and 50% of syncytial meningiomas which are also brightly hyperintense on T2-weighted images [17]. Thus MRI can distinguish between cavernous sinus hemangioma and somewhere between two of three and four of five meningiomas.

Cranial nerve schwannomas tend to be hypointense on T1-weighted images and hyperintense on T2-weighted images [18]. Thus MRI cannot distinguish between cavernous sinus hemangioma and cavernous sinus schwannoma unless the characteristic tumor blush is present on angiography (hemangioma) or there is enlargement of foramen ovale or rotundum (schwannoma). Fortunately schwannomas arising from cranial nerves III, IV, or VI are much rarer than meningioma.

Treatment

Microsurgery

Complete resection of cavernous sinus hemangiomas is curative (Fig. 42.3). However, cavernous sinus hemangiomas are

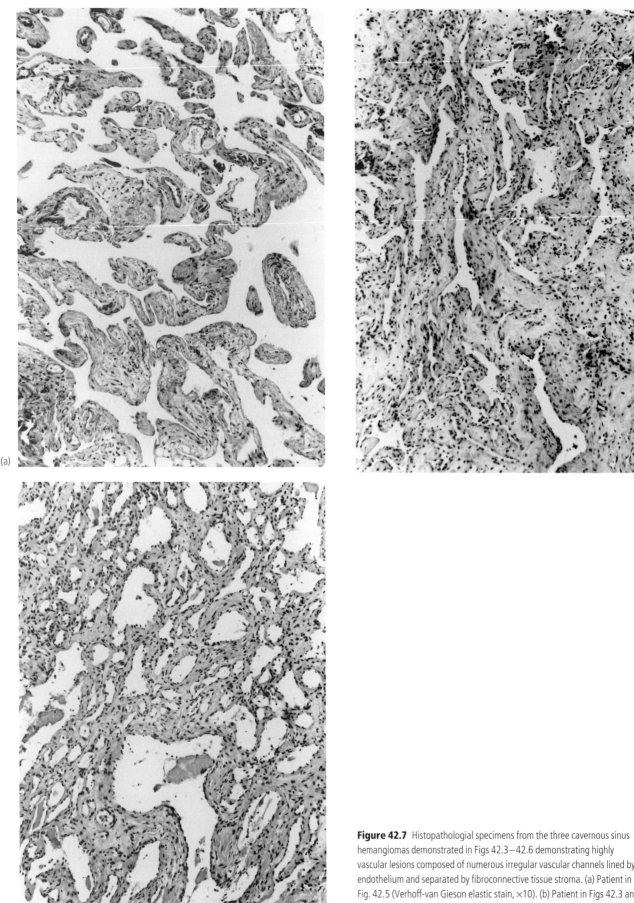

Figure 42.7 Histopathologial specimens from the three cavernous sinus hemangiomas demonstrated in Figs 42.3–42.6 demonstrating highly vascular lesions composed of numerous irregular vascular channels lined by endothelium and separated by fibroconnective tissue stroma. (a) Patient in Fig. 42.5 (Verhoff-van Gieson elastic stain, ×10). (b) Patient in Figs 42.3 and 42.4 (Masson Trichrome stain, ×10). (c) Patient in Fig. 42.6 (hematoxylin and eosin stain, ×10). (Reproduced from Linskey ME [3], with permission from Lippincott Williams & Wilkins.)

formidable surgical challenges. Prior to 1983, the surgical mortality rate for these lesions was 36% with the major etiology being excessive blood loss [3]. Specialized skull base microsurgical approaches and increasing experience with recognizing these lesions preoperatively to allow special preparation have significantly reduced the mortality rate, but significant blood loss can still be a problem. Specific vascular pedicle blood supply is rarely robust enough for therapeutic preoperative embolization. Special intraoperative techniques include avoidance of piecemeal dissection [3], temporary occlusion of the ICA, use of controlled hypotension [19], and direct intratumoral injections of fibrin glue [20] or plastic fixation material [21].

Approximately 44% of patients experience permanent worsening of their preoperative cranial nerve function after surgery (abducens palsy most common) [3]. The intracavernous ICA can usually be spared but intraoperative temporary occlusion, ICA dissection from manipulation, or permanent sacrifice in the desperate setting of uncontrollable blood loss can lead to major cerebral stroke. As a result, for these lesions, we still perform a clinical preoperative ICA balloon test occlusion (BTO) together with a BTO–cerebral blood flow (CBF) study to assess subclinical CBF reserve [3].

Stereotactic radiosurgery and fractionated radiotherapy

Fractionated radiation therapy has been used in a limited number of cases with some reported success [1, 22–27]. Fractionated radiotherapy has the advantage of being able to handle very large tumor volumes as well as treat tumors that closely abut the optic nerve near the superior orbital fissure–optic canal approximation, and/or the chiasm via suprasellar tumor extension. There are occasions where fractionated radiotherapy is the only therapeutic alternative for patients with cavernous sinus hemangiomas.

Unfortunately, fractionated radiotherapy leads to exposure of the temporal lobes as well as the hypothalamo–pituitary axis to radiation in patients who would be anticipated to have a normal expected lifespan once their benign tumor is controlled. These exposures will lead to a risk of hypopituitarism as well as cognitive decline over 10–20 years. The multiple repeated exposures (often up to 30) of a larger volume of tissue to a supra-mutagenic threshold of radiation (1–3 Gy threshold in the Israeli tinea capitis studies) also lead to a finite risk of secondary malignancy over the course of the patient's residual lifespan (3% risk at 10 years for pituitary tumor patients treated with fractionated radiotherapy).

Fortunately, stereotactic radiosurgery (SR) has emerged as a promising alternative to both microsurgery and fractionated radiotherapy for patients with cavernous sinus hemangiomas. Given in one single dose, the number of potential supra-threshold mutagenic exposures is reduced 25–30-fold. Precisely targeted with strict three-dimensional tumor conformality, the pituitary gland can usually be partially, and the pituitary stalk and hypothalamus completely, excluded from significant radiation exposure, thereby theoretically reducing the risk of hypopituitarism. The same theoretically holds true for bilateral medial temporal lobe exposure and subsequent cognitive deficits.

More than 20 cases of cavernous sinus hemangioma treated with SR have now been reported [28–35], almost all having been treated with Gamma Knife technique. Excellent neuroimaging and clinical results have been uniformly reported, albeit with limited length of imaging follow-up for slowly growing benign tumors. Should this experience hold up for a minimum of 10 years of neuroimaging follow-up, then SR is likely to become the preferred method of treatment for patients with cavernous sinus hemangiomas.

References

1. Meyer FB, Lombardi D, Scheithauer, Nichols DA. Extra-axial cavernous hemangiomas involving the dural sinuses. *J. Neurosurg.* 1990;73:187–192.
2. Boockvar JA, Stiefel M, Malhotra N, et al. Dural cavernous angioma of the posterior sagittal sinus: case report. *Surg. Neurol.* 2005;63: 178–181.
3. Linskey ME, Sekhar LN. Cavernous sinus hemangiomas: a series, a review, and a hypothesis. *Neurosurgery* 1992;30:101–107.
4. Zhang R, Zhou LF, Mao Y. Microsurgical treatment of nonmeningeal tumors of the cavernous sinus. *Zhonghua Yi Xue Za Zhi* 2005;85: 1373–1378.
5. Goel A, Muzumdar D, Sharma P. Extradural approach for cavernous hemangioma of the cavernous sinus: experience with 13 cases. *Neurol. Med. Chir. (Tokyo)* 2003;43:112–118.
6. Ishijima Y, Matsumura H, Kagayma N. Intracranial cavernous hemangioma: Report of two cases. *Arch. Jpn. Chir.* 1966;35:748–754.
7. Matias-Guiu X, Alejo M, Sole T, et al. Cavernous angiomas of the cranial nerves: Report of two cases. *J. Neurosurg.* 1990;73:620–622.
8. Namba S. Extracerebral cavernous hemangioma of the middle cranial fossa. *Surg. Neurol.* 1983;19:379–388.
9. Odake G, Tanaka K. Cavernous hemangiomas of the middle fossa: case report and review of the literature. *Neurol. Med. Chir. (Tokyo)* 1986;26:58–67.
10. Tsuiki K, Abe S, Chiba M, et al. A case of cavernous angioma of the middle cranial fossa originating in the cavernous sinus with hyperprolactinemia. *Neurol. Surg. (Tokyo)* 1987;15:301–305.
11. Finkmeyer VH, Kautzky R. Das Kavernom des sinus cavernosus. *Zentralbl. Neurochir.* 1968;29:23–30.
12. Kawai K, Fului M, Tanaka A, et al. Extracerebral cavernous hemangioma of the middle fossa. *Surg. Neurol.* 1978;8:19–25.
13. Rosenblum B, Rothman AS, Lanzieri C, Song S. A cavernous sinus hemangioma. *J. Neurosurg.* 1986;65:716–718.
14. McCormick WF. Pathology of vascular malformations of the brain. In Wilson CB, Stein BN (eds). *Intracranial Arteriovenous Malformations.* Baltimore: Williams & Wilkins, 1984:44–63.
15. Pasztor E, Szabo G, Slowik F, Zoltan J. Cavernous hemangioma of the base of the skull: report of a case treated surgically. *J. Neurosurg.* 1964;21:582–585.
16. Bradac GB, Riva A, Schorner W, Sutra G. Cavernous sinus meningiomas: an MRI study. *Neuroradiology* 1987;29:578–581.
17. Elster AD, Challa VR, Gilbert TH, et al. Meningiomas: MR and histopathologic features. *Radiology* 1989;170:857–862.
18. Watabe T, Azuma T. T1 and T2 measurements of meningiomas and neuromas before and after Gd-DTPA. *AJNR* 1989;10:463–470.

19. Ohata K, El–Naggar A, Takami T, et al. Efficacy of induced hypotension in the surgical treatment of large cavernous sinus cavernomas. *J. Neurosurg.* 1999;90:702–708.

20. Kim IM, Yim MB, Lee CY, et al. Merits of intralesional fibrin glue injection in surgery for cavernous sinus cavernous hemangiomas. Technical note. *J. Neurosurg.* 2002;97:718–21.

21. Hashimoto M, Yokota A, Ohta H, Urasaki E. Intratumoral injection of plastic adhesive material for removal of cavernous sinus hemangioma. Technical note. *J. Neurosurg.* 2000;93:1078–1081.

22. Harada T, Aoyama N, Terada H, et al. A case of extracerebral hemangioma of the middle fossa. *Prog. Comput. Tomogr. (Tokyo)* 1982;4:460–465.

23. Jamjoom AB. Response of cavernous sinus hemangioma to radiotherapy: a case report. *Neurosurg. Rev.* 1996;19:261–264.

24. Maruishi M, Shima T, Okada Y, et al. Cavernous sinus cavernoma treated with radiation therapy – case report. *Neurol. Med. Chir. (Tokyo)* 1994;34:773–777.

25. Mori K, Handa H, Gi H, Mori K. Cavernomas in the middle cranial fossa. *Surg. Neurol.* 1980;14:21–31.

26. Miserocchi G, Vaiani S, Migliore MM, Villani RM. Cavernous hemangioma of the cavernous sinus. Complete disappearance of the neoplasma after subtotal excision and radiation therapy. Case report. *J. Neurosurg. Sci.* 1997;41:203–207.

27. Tsao MN Schwartz ML, Bernstein M, et al. Capillary hemangioma of the cavernous sinus. Report of two cases. *J. Neurosurg.* 2003;98:169–174.

28. Iwai Y, Yamanaka K, Nakajima H, Yasui T. Stereotactic radiosurgery for cavernous sinus cavernous hemangioma – case report. *Neurol. Med. Chir. (Tokyo)* 1999;39:288–290.

29. Seo Y, Fukuoka S, Sasaki T, et al. Cavernous sinus hemangioma treated with gamma knife radiosurgery: usefulness of SPECT for diagnosis – case report. *Neurol. Med. Chir. (Tokyo)* 2000;40:575–580.

30. Thompson TP, Lunsford LD, Flickinger JC. Radiosurgery for hemangiomas of the cavernous sinus and orbit: technical case report. *Neurosurgery* 2000;47:778–783.

31. Kida Y, Kobayashi T, Mori Y. Radiosurgery of cavernous hemangiomas in the cavernous sinus. *Surg. Neurol.* 2001;56:117–122.

32. Nakamura N, Shin M, Tago M, et al. Gamma knife radiosurgery for cavernous hemangiomas in the cavernous sinus. Report of three cases. *J. Neurosurg.* 2002;97(5 Suppl):477–480.

33. Kuo JS, Chen JC, Yu C, et al. Gamma knife radiosurgery for benign cavernous sinus tumors: quantitative analysis of treatment outcomes. *Neurosurgery* 2004;54:1385–1393.

34. Peker S, Kilic T, Sengoz M, Pamir MN. Radiosurgical treatment of cavernous sinus cavernous haemangiomas. *Acta Neurochir. (Wien)* 2004;146:337–341.

35. Liu AL, Wang C, Sun S, et al. Gamma knife radiosurgery for tumors involving the cavernous sinus. *Stereotact. Funct. Neurosurg.* 2005;83:45–51.

43   Langerhans' Cell Histiocytosis

Matthew F. Gorman, Michelle Hermiston, and Katherine K. Matthay

Key points
- Langerhans' cell histiocytosis is a monoclonal proliferative disorder of dendritic cells.
- Langerhans' cell histiocytosis can involve a single organ system, most commonly bone, or multiple systems.
- A high index of suspicion is required to make the diagnosis of Langerhans' cell histiocytosis and pathological confirmation is needed for a definitive diagnosis.
- Treatment ranges from local control to systemic chemotherapy.
- The course of Langerhans' cell histiocytosis can range from spontaneous remission to multiply relapsing to rapidly fatal.
- Endocrinopathies, due to hypothalamic and pituitary infiltration, especially diabetes insipidus and growth hormone deficiency, are the most commonly seen long-term sequelae of Langerhans' cell histiocytosis.

Introduction

Langerhans' cell histiocytosis (LCH) includes several disorders previously known as histiocytosis X, eosinophilic granuloma, Letterer–Siwe disease, Hand–Schuller–Christian disease and diffuse reticuloendotheliosis. It can be a single-system or multi-system (more than two organ systems) disease and its pathogenesis is not fully understood. Endocrinological effects of the disease due to infiltration of the hypothalamo–pituitary axis produce some of the most striking sequelae of LCH. The natural history of the disease is variable with patients experiencing spontaneous remission, a chronic course of remission and relapse, or mortality.

Epidemiology

LCH can present at any age from neonates to adults, though it most commonly affects children aged 1–4 years [1]. Adults comprise approximately 30% of LCH cases [2]. The estimated incidence is reported in a range of 3–9 cases per million children per year with a small male predominance of 1.2–2:1 [3, 4]. As a high clinical suspicion is often required to make the diagnosis of LCH, it is likely underdiagnosed.

Etiology

The pathological cell in LCH is the Langerhans' cell, a bone marrow-derived dendritic cell [5]. These cells are normally

Clinical Endocrine Oncology, 2nd edition. Edited by Ian D. Hay and John A.H. Wass. © 2008 Blackwell Publishing. ISBN 978-1-4051-4584-8.

antigen-presenting cells; however in LCH, this ability has been lost [5]. Importantly, unlike other histiocytes, LCH cells express CD1a [5]. The etiology of the disease phenotype is not fully known but is thought to be linked to increased inflammatory activity such as a "cytokine storm" [6]. Increased levels of cytokines including granulocyte–macrophage colony-stimulating factor, interferon-γ, interleukin (IL)-1 and IL-10 have been found in LCH lesions relative to surrounding tissue [6]. The Langerhans' cell appears to be involved in a cytokine production loop with macrophages and T-lymphocytes [1].

LCH is a consistently monoclonal proliferative disease, although the factors involved in its initiation and progression are unknown. As no cytogenetic abnormality has been identified, however, theories of LCH being a reactive process also exist. Attempts to link LCH to viral diseases like HHV-6 and Epstein–Barr virus have been inconclusive [4]. Pulmonary disease seen in adults may represent a distinct entity from LCH seen in children as it is not a clonal disease [7]. Increased numbers of Langerhans' cells are seen in bronchial epithelium in association with smoking [7]. When compared to pediatric LCH, more mature cells are seen in adult pulmonary disease, further distinguishing these different disease states [7].

Symptoms and disease involvement

As noted previously, LCH can be a single-system or multi-system disease. The most common sites for single-system disease are bone, skin, and lymph nodes. The skeletal system is the most often involved in LCH and the disease extent can be monostotic or polyostotic. Patient symptoms include painless lesions to fractures and bony deformities. The lesions are usually osteolytic with a sclerotic margin on imaging studies and can involve the skull, mandible, axial skeleton, and extremities (Fig. 43.1). Skin findings include a scaly and seborrheic rash often on the scalp, behind the ears, or in the diaper region. These rashes are frequently mistaken for eczema or seborrheic dermatitis. Also seen are purplish brown papules over the trunk. Cervical lymphadenopathy is a classic finding in LCH [4].

Multi-system disease

In multi-system disease, aural discharge can represent ear involvement. In the gastrointestinal tract, LCH can result in diarrhea or malabsorption with poor growth. Rare cases of thyroid disease from direct involvement of the thyroid gland have been reported. "High-risk organs" include the liver and spleen, lungs, and bone

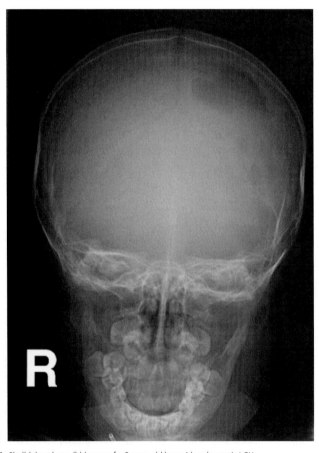

(a)

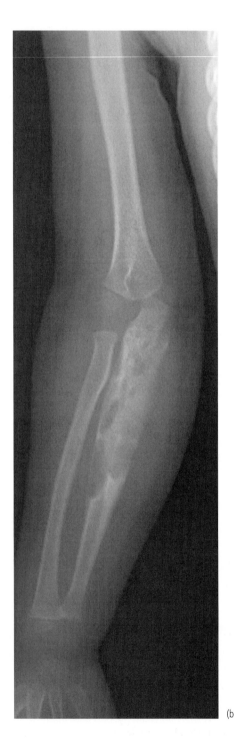

(b)

Figure 43.1 Skull (a) and arm (b) bones of a 2-year-old boy with polyostotic LCH.

marrow and are associated with a worse prognosis. Liver and spleen involvement can present with hepatosplenomegaly with hypoalbuminemia, ascites, hyperbilirubinemia, coagulopathy, and hypersplenism. While less common in children than adults, lung involvement in LCH can present with tachypnea or pneumothoraces. Cystic and nodular involvement of the lung parenchyma can eventually result in diffuse lung fibrosis. Varying degrees of cytopenias are seen with LCH involvement of the bone marrow [4].

Endocrine and central nervous system disease

Central nervous system (CNS) involvement may occur at presentation or many years after initial diagnosis. Symptoms are variable and may include ataxia, hyperreflexia, dysarthria, and dysphagia [4]. Pituitary disease results in the most significant endocrinological dysfunction associated with LCH. The mechanism of dysfunction is thought to be the infiltration of the pituitary and/or hypothalamus by Langerhans' cells which cause local tissue damage with glandular function being affected by excessive production of IL-1 and prostaglandins [8]. The posterior pituitary is more commonly involved and diabetes insipidus (DI) is the most common endocrinopathy observed in LCH. DI may develop during various times in the disease course and may occur prior to the presence of any evidence of LCH. Less frequently, other pituitary dysfunction including growth hormone deficiency, sex hormone deficiencies, and panhypopituitarism may develop over the clinical course.

Diagnosis

The diagnosis of LCH is based entirely on pathology. Unfortunately, because it is often difficult to make the diagnosis on the first pathological specimen, a strong clinical suspicion is required to facilitate repeat biopsy and the suspected diagnosis of LCH must be relayed to the pathologist to ensure adequate processing and testing of the samples. The Histiocyte Society has outlined recommended diagnostic requirements [9]. For a "presumptive diagnosis," morphology on light microscopy with H&E stain must be consistent with LCH with granulomatous lesions and the presence of "LCH cells" (homogenously stained pink cytoplasm with lobulated nuclei). For a "definitive diagnosis," light microscopy must be consistent with LCH *and* Birbeck granules (infoldings of the cell membrane possibly due to processing of antigens) must be detected in cells in the lesion on electron microscopy *and/or* the presence of positive staining for CD1a on lesional cells must be observed. Other immunohistochemical stains which can help support the diagnosis of LCH include ATPase, α-D-mannosidase, S-100 protein (seen in 50–60% of LCH cells), and the binding of peanut lectin agglutinin [4].

Staging

The goals of staging in LCH are to categorize the disease burden as single system or multi-system, to separate bony disease into

Table 43.1 Diagnostic testing

Laboratory tests
Complete blood count
Liver function tests
Coagulation studies
Urine and serum osmolality after water deprivation test
Radiological evaluation
Chest radiograph
Skeletal survey
Case-specific evaluations (depending on symptoms)
Pulmonary function tests
CT scan of chest
Bronchoalveolar lavage and lung biopsy
GI endoscopy with biopsies
Liver biopsy
Bone marrow aspirates and biopsies
Hormonal evaluations
MRI of brain and pituitary

Based on [1].

monostotic and polyostotic, and to determine the extent of organ dysfunction (seen in less than 15% of children) [4]. Recommended evaluations include complete blood counts with white blood cell differential, liver function tests including an evaluation of coagulation, DI screening with urine osmolality and a water deprivation test, and a chest X-ray with skeletal survey (Table 43.1) [1]. Further evaluation depends on the patient's clinical picture. For patients with evidence of pulmonary disease, computerized tomography (CT) scans of the chest and pulmonary function tests are indicated [1]. LCH involving the gastrointestinal system may require CT imaging of the abdomen and/or endoscopy with biopsies [1]. Patients with CNS symptoms including pituitary dysfunction should undergo a magnetic resonance imaging (MRI) scan of the brain. Hypothalamic–pituitary lesions are the most frequently seen on brain MRI [8]. Imaging findings on MRI when DI is present is a thickening with enhancement of the pituitary stalk and the loss of the pituitary "bright spot" (though not specific for LCH alone) (Fig. 43.2) [8]. Ultimately, biopsies of potentially involved organs are recommended to determine the extent of disease [1].

Treatment

Local

Therapy for LCH relies on local control measures and systemic chemotherapy depending on the extent of the disease. In monostotic disease, therapeutic options include observation, curettage, intralesional steroids, indomethacin, and rarely radiation therapy (6–10 Gy) except in vertebral or femoral neck lesions at risk of collapse [4]. For polyostotic disease, similar approaches may be used or systemic chemotherapy may be initiated with 6–12 months of a two-drug regimen of prednisone and vinblastine. In patients with skin involvement alone, observation or interventions with topical

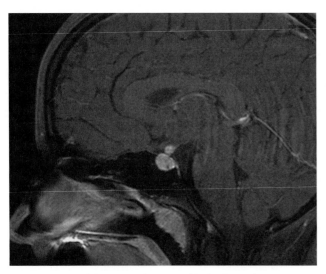

Figure 43.2 MRI of the pituitary of a 17-year-old girl with LCH who presented with DI. Note the enlarged enhancing pituitary infundibulum in this T1 postgadolinium image.

therapy of steroids, nitrogen mustard, or immune-modulating agents (such as tacrolimus) may be used. No treatment is often recommended for patients with only lymph node disease, as most spontaneously resolve.

Systemic

In patients with multi-system disease, systemic chemotherapy remains the mainstay of treatment. In current Histiocytosis Society group protocols [10], patients are divided into "risk" and "low-risk" groups mostly based on the presence or lack of "risk" organs (Table 43.2). "Risk" patients receive corticosteroids, vinblastine, and 6-mercaptopurine with or without methotrexate for 12 months. "Low-risk" patients are randomized to receive corticosteroids and vinblastine for either 6 or 12 months. Other non-standard treatment approaches include cyclosporine and anticytokine therapy. Salvage therapy for progressive or multiply relapsing disease has included myeloablative chemotherapy with allogeneic stem cell transplant, solid organ transplants, and a newer agent 2-chlorodeoxyadenosine, a purine analog, with promising results.

Hypothalamo–pituitary axis

Besides early recognition of DI and hormonal replacement, the role of radiation therapy or chemotherapy to improve the

Table 43.2 Poor prognostic factors

Involvement of high-risk organs:
   Liver
   Lungs
   Spleen
   Bone marrow
Poor response to therapy at 6 weeks

symptoms of DI and to reduce the degree of hormone replacement is controversial. Many groups have not found efficacy in radiation therapy or chemotherapy for the treatment of DI. Complete or partial responses to radiation therapy at low doses (800–1600 cGy) given to the sellar region and hypothalamus have been reported in up to 38% of patients [11]. This required a prompt institution of therapy within 7–10 days of diagnosis of DI. Damage to the hypothalamo–pituitary axis and induction of a secondary malignancy are small risks associated with this low dose of radiation given to this region. Rosenwieg's group reviewed the literature and their 20 years of experience with radiation therapy in LCH-associated DI [12]. They found only a rare response to radiation, and only in patients with partial DI. They recommend close monitoring for development of DI with the implementation of radiation therapy being justified only if done early (7–10 days).

The influence of chemotherapy on the development and prevention of DI remains unclear. In retrospective studies, a possible preventative role of chemotherapy has been postulated since a lower incidence of DI was seen in the results of more recent treatment groups that called for prompt initiation of chemotherapy [13]. This reduced incidence was not appreciated in the LCH-II groupwide protocol which used a more aggressive approach [14]. Similarly, when observation alone was compared to early chemotherapy intervention by Donadieu, no difference in DI development existed [15]. Further studies are needed to clarify this issue.

Prognosis

The outcome of LCH is dramatically variable with some patients achieving spontaneous remission, others experiencing a relapsing course with disease recurrence decades later, and still others dying from their LCH. Attempts have been made to identify factors that could aid in the prediction of outcomes. Patients with disease involving the "high-risk organs" (liver, lungs, spleen, bone marrow) have a poorer prognosis (Table 43.2). An early response to therapy is predictive of better long-term outcome. In the most recent international LCH-II study, there were 143 patients with multi-system disease receiving systemic chemotherapy [16]. All children ≥2 years of age without risk organ involvement survived [16]. A slow response to therapy, defined as ≥6 weeks, in the face of high-risk organ involvement indicated poor prognosis and a mortality rate of 66% [16]. In patients with bone lesions, recurrent disease occurs more frequently in patients with multiple bone lesions or multi-system disease [14]. Long-term survival in low-risk patients overall is estimated at 90% [14, 16].

Disease sequelae

General

Unlike many other oncological diseases, the majority of late sequelae from LCH are due to the disease itself rather than the implemented treatments. LCH involvement of organs can result

Table 43.3 Incidence of endocrine deficiencies in LCH

Group	Total patients	DI	Growth deficiencies	Other
Haupt et al. [2]	n = 182 (SS and MS)	24%	GR: 9%	
Donadieu et al. [15]	n = 589 (SS and MS)	24%	GHD: 10%	Any endocrinopathy: 24% Central hypothyroidism: 4% Gonadotropin deficiency: 3% Panhypopituitarism: 1.5%
Willis et al. [17]	n = 51 (SS and MS)	25%	GHD: 20%	Sex hormone deficiency: 16% Hypothyroidism: 14%
Bernstrand et al. [3]	n = 49 (SS and MS)	15%	GHD: 10%	Any endocrinopathy: 23% Any endocrine CNS disease: 18%
Nanduri et al. [19]	n = 144 (MS only)	35%	GHI: 14%	Any hypothalamic endocrinopathy: 35%
Grois et al. [13]	n = 1741 (SS and MS)	12%	N/A	

SS, single-system disease; MS, multi-system disease; GR, growth retardation; GHD, growth hormone deficiency; GHI, growth hormone insufficiency; N/A, not addressed.

in direct tissue destruction with eventual fibrosis or CNS gliosis [4]. The reported incidence of long-term complications varies, but is quite frequent and ranges from 45% to 75% of all-comers with LCH [2, 3, 4, 17]. As expected, patients who suffered from multi-system disease are more likely to have permanent consequences.

In patients with bony disease, skeletal complications are common and include fractures, vertebral collapse, and scoliosis. Neurological disease is often the most debilitating and may be progressive. Symptoms are neurodegenerative and may manifest years after diagnosis, even without evidence of CNS involvement at diagnosis or at reactivation [2]. The most common symptoms include ataxia, tremor, and dysarthria with some patients having compromise of higher functioning. This neurodegenerative syndrome has been associated more frequently with patients who have pituitary involvement of LCH [15]. No proven therapies exist for this condition [4].

Endocrine

The incidences of the various endocrine sequelae are shown in Table 43.3. Diabetes insipidus has been reported as the most common long-term sequela of LCH. The incidence of DI ranges from 10% to 25% of all LCH patients either during their disease course or during follow-up [2, 3, 13, 15, 17–19]. Grois et al. studied 1741 patients with LCH. At diagnosis, 6% had DI. The risk of developing DI at 5 years was 16% and at 15 years was 20% [15]. The greatest risk factor for developing DI is the presence of multi-system involvement [13]. Osseous lesions in the craniofacial bones, disease involving the eyes, ears, and oral cavity, and involvement of the CNS also appear to increase the risk of developing DI (Table 43.4) [15].

Late effects of LCH resulting from involvement of the anterior pituitary are much less common and usually do not present for years after posterior pituitary disease is seen [20]. Growth hormone (GH) deficiency, sex hormone deficiencies, central hypothyroidism, and panhypopituitarism have been reported in

long-term follow-up studies of LCH survivors. The overall incidence of GH deficiency in LCH patients is approximately 10% [3, 19]. The risk factors are similar to DI and include multi-system disease, presence of DI, and craniofacial involvement. Five- and 10-year risks for the development of GH deficiency were found to be 35% and 55% respectively in LCH patients with DI [20]. Treatment with GH supplementation has been shown to improve growth in proven GH insufficient patients with LCH, with growth velocities and final heights similar to treatment effects seen in non-LCH associated GH insufficiency [19]. The best outcomes are seen if patients are treated prior to significant growth retardation is identified [19]. Final heights are similar to non-GH insufficient LCH patients [19]. The overall cumulative risk of growth retardation at 14 years follow-up for all LCH patients was 17.6% [2]. No evidence of increased disease recurrence has been found in patients treated with GH [3, 19].

Screening recommendations for the detection of endocrinopathies in patients with a history of LCH include frequent symptom screening for polydipsia and polyuria, growth measurements, Tanner staging, and anterior pituitary hormone screening in patients with DI with or without hypothalamic-pituitary lesions on MRI [19].

The incidence of secondary malignancies has been reported at up to 5% in various long-term follow-up studies of patients with LCH [1, 2, 3, 17]. Secondary leukemias, often acute non-lymphoblastic

Table 43.4 Risk factors for the development of diabetes insipidus in LCH

Multi-system involvement
Craniofacial osseous lesions
Eye involvement
Ear involvement
Oral cavity involvement
CNS disease

leukemia, and solid tumors have been reported. Risk factors for the development of secondary cancers include therapy with etoposide and radiation therapy.

Conclusion

Langerhans' cell histiocytosis is a rare disease with a remarkably variable clinical presentation and course. While the cell of origin is known, the exact pathogenesis of LCH is not understood. The treatment ranges from observation to local control to systemic chemotherapy. Endocrinopathies, particularly DI and GH insufficiency, are the most common complications of the disease. Besides hormone replacement, no other treatment or preventive strategies have been proven efficacious for these disease sequelae.

References

1. Egeler RM, D'Angio GJ. Langerhans cell histiocytosis. *J. Pediatr.* 1995;127:1–11.

2. Haupt R, Nanduri V, Calevo MG, Bernstrand C, et al. Permanent consequences in Langerhans cell Histiocytosis patients: a pilot study from the Histiocyte Society-late effects study group. *Pediatr. Blood Cancer.* 2004;42:438–444.

3. Bernstrand C, Sandstedt B, Ahstrom L, Henter J. Long-term follow-up of Langerhans cell histiocytosis: 39 years' experience at a single centre. *Acta Paediatr.* 2005;94:1073–1084.

4. Henter JI, Tondini C, Pritchard J. Histiocyte disorders. *Clin. Rev. Oncol./Hematol.* 2004;50:157–174.

5. Favara BE. Langerhans' cell histiocytosis pathobiology and pathogenesis. *Semin. Oncol.* 1991;18:3.

6. Egeler RM, Favara BE, van Meurs M, et al. Differential *in situ* cytokine profiles of Langerhans-like cells and T cells in Langerhans cell histiocytosis: abundant expression of cytokines relevant to disease and treatment. *Blood* 1999;94:4195.

7. Bernstrand C, Cederlund K, Sandsstedt B, et al. Pulmonary abnormalities at long-term follow-up of patients with Langerhans cell histiocytosis. *Med. Pediatr. Oncol.* 2001;36:459–468.

8. Prayer D, Grois N, Prosch H, et al. MR imaging presentation of intracranial disease associated with Langerhans cell histiocytosis. *Am. J. Neuroradiol.* 2004;25:880.

9. Favara BE, Feller AC, Pauli M, et al. Contemporary classification of histiocytic disorders. The WHO committee on histioctyic/reticulum cell proliferations. Reclassification Working Group of the Histiocyte Society. *Med. Pediatr. Oncol.* 1997;29:157–166.

10. Histiocyte Society. Treatment Protocol of the Third International Study for Langerhans Cell Histiocytosis. April 2001.

11. Minehan KJ, Chen MG, Zimmerman D, et al. Radiation therapy for diabetes insipidus caused by Langerhans cell histiocytosis. *Int. J. Radiat. Oncol. Biol. Phys.* 1992;23:519–524.

12. Rosenzweig KE, Arceci RJ, Tarbell NJ. Diabetes insipidus secondary to Langerhans' cell histiocytosis: is radiation therapy indicated? *Med. Pediatr. Oncol.* 1997;29:36–40.

13. Grois N, Potschger U, Prosch H, et al. Risk factors for diabetes insipidus in Langerhans cell Histiocytosis. *Pediatr. Blood Cancer.* 2006;46:228–233.

14. Gadner H, Heitger A, Grois N, et al. Treatment strategy for disseminated Langerhans cell histiocytosis. DAL HX-83 Study Group. *Med. Pediatr. Oncol.* 1994;23:72–80.

15. Donadieu J, Rolon MA, Thomas C, et al. Endocrine involvement in pediatric-onset Langerhans' cell histiocytosis: a population-based study. *J. Pediatr.* 2004;144:344–350.

16. Gadner H, Grois N, Arico M, et al. A randomized trial of treatment for multi-system Langerhans' cell histiocytosis. *J. Pediatr.* 2001;138:728.

17. Willis B, Ablin A, Weinberg V, Zoger S, Wara WM, Matthay KK. Disease course and late sequelae of Langerhans cell histiocytosis: 25-year experience at the University of California, San Francisco. *J. Clin. Oncol.* 1996;14:2073–2082.

18. Dunger DB, Broadbent V, Yeoman E, et al. The frequency and natural history of diabetes insipidus in children with Langerhans-cell histiocytosis. *N. Engl. J. Med.* 1989;321:1157–1162.

19. Nanduri VR, Bareille P, Pritchard J, Stanhope R. Growth and endocrine disorders in multi-system Langerhans' cell histiocytosis. *Clin. Endocrinol.* 2000;53:509–515.

20. Donadieu J, Rolon MA, Pion I, et al. Incidence of growth hormone deficiency in pediatric-onset Langerhans cell histiocytosis: efficacy and safety of growth hormone treatment. *J. Clin. Endocrinol. Metab.* 2004;89:604–609.

44 Pituitary and Hypothalamic Sarcoidosis

Damian G. Morris and Shern L. Chew

Key points

- Endocrine dysfunction caused by granulomatous infiltration of the hypothalamo–pituitary region occurs in approximately 25% of patients with neurosarcoidosis.
- Disorders of water balance and reproductive dysfunction are the most common manifestations.
- The diagnosis of isolated hypothalamo–pituitary sarcoidosis can be challenging and usually requires histopathological confirmation.
- Corticosteroids are the mainstay of treatment. Immunosuppressive and immunomodulatory agents and/or radiotherapy may be used as adjunctive treatment.
- Endocrinopathies rarely improve with immunosuppression; as a result, chronic hormonal replacement therapy is usually necessary.

Introduction

Sarcoidosis is an inflammatory non-necrotizing granulomatous disease of unknown etiology. Neurological involvement occurs in approximately 5% of patients with sarcoidosis. There is a female preponderance. Neurosarcoidosis may be suspected in patients with systemic sarcoidosis who develop neurological symptoms and signs. In addition, neurosarcoidosis may be in the differential diagnosis of patients who are not known to have systemic sarcoidosis but manifest with neurological disease. Neurological signs are the presenting manifestation in approximately 50% of patients with neurosarcoidosis [1]. However, it is rare to have isolated neurosarcoidosis.

Endocrine manifestations of neurosarcoidosis

Any area of the central or peripheral nervous system can be affected by sarcoidosis. Cranial nerve abnormalities are the most frequent, with facial nerve involvement in 50%. Other neurological presentations include aseptic meningitis, hydrocephalus, and central nervous system (CNS) parenchymal mass lesions. Hypothalamo–pituitary dysfunction is the most common manifestation of the latter (occurring in 15–25% of patients), presumably due to the predilection of lesions for the basal brain areas, and any of the neuroendocrinological systems may be disturbed. Hypothalamic infiltration is the usual mode of pathology, although thickening of the pituitary stalk or direct pituitary

involvement can occur, and in these cases it must be differentiated from other causes of pituitary mass lesions.

Patients can present with a wide range of clinical signs and symptoms (see Table 44.1), as highlighted in a useful review of 91 cases of hypothalamic–pituitary neurosarcoidosis by Murialdo and Tamagno [2].

Table 44.1 The frequency of clinical signs and symptoms in hypothalamo–pituitary manifestations of neurosarcoidosis

Manifestation	Frequency
Hypogonadotropic hypogonadism	38.5%
Diabetes insipidus	37.3%
Polydipsia	31.9%
Amenorrhea	58.7% of females
Changes in pubic, axillary, body hair	25.3%
Panhypopituitarism	23.1%
Loss of libido	22.0%
Visual defects	22.0%
Impotence	33.3% of males
Malaise	9.9%
Galactorrhea	8.8% (17.4% of females)
Psycho-affective change	7.7%
Cold intolerance	7.7%
Headache	7.7%
Changes in smell, taste, hearing	5.50%
Obesity or weight gain	5.50%
Loss of body weight	5.50%

Other with frequency of <5%: Hypothermia; hypotension; anorexia; growth impairment; changes in consciousness; isolated TSH deficiency; hypodipsia; vertigo; hyperphagia; isolated ACTH deficiency; xerodermia; nausea

Adapted from Murialdo and Tamagno [2], with permission from Editrice Kurtis.

Clinical Endocrine Oncology, 2nd edition. Edited by Ian D. Hay and John A.H. Wass. © 2008 Blackwell Publishing. ISBN 978-1-4051-4584-8.

Diabetes insipidus is a common endocrine feature of neurosarcoidosis. However, other alterations to water metabolism can be manifest, including inappropriate antidiuretic hormone (ADH) secretion. In a series of seven patients with neurosarcoidosis and abnormal water balance, careful clinical evaluation revealed three patients to have evidence of ADH deficiency, and one of these also had deficient thirst [3]. One patient had excessive thirst and evidence of an inappropriately low threshold for ADH release. One other had thirst deficiency only, and two patients had excessive thirst only. One explanation for these changes is resetting of the thirst "osmostat" up in patients with deficient thirst, or down in excessive thirst, although a central effect of increased angiotensin II (mediated through elevated serum/cerebrospinal fluid [CSF] angiotensin-converting enzyme [ACE]) on drinking behavior has been purported [4].

Reproductive dysfunction is the other most common presentation of hypothalamo–pituitary neurosarcoidosis. Classically this is due to hypogonadotropic hypogonadism presumably from lesions affecting gonadotropin-releasing hormone (GnRH) neurons, although it may be secondary to hyperprolactinemia related to disinhibition of dopaminergic tone to the lactotroph cells.

Associated multiple anterior pituitary hormone failure is also relatively common, and although other isolated anterior pituitary hormone dysfunction (thyroid-stimulating hormone [TSH], adrenocorticotropic hormone [ACTH], growth hormone) has been reported this is less common.

Diagnosis and investigations

Patients can be classified as having possible, probable or definite neurosarcoidosis based on criteria devised by Zajicek in 1999 (Table 44.2) [5]. The diagnosis of definite neurosarcoidosis can only be made by histological confirmation of non-caseating granulomas, and therefore a brain biopsy is usually required. Tissue for microbiological culture including tuberculosis should also be obtained at the same time. If this is not possible then isolated neurosarcoidosis in particular can cause diagnostic difficulties and can hinder making a prompt diagnosis.

Magnetic resonance imaging (MRI) is the most sensitive and specific imaging modality for neurosarcoidosis, although this may

Table 44.2 Criteria for the diagnosis of neurosarcoidosis

Definite	Clinical presentation suggestive of neurosarcoidosis
	Exclusion of other possible diagnoses
	Presence of positive nervous system histology
Probable	Clinical presentation suggestive of neurosarcoidosis
	MRI evidence compatible with neurosarcoidosis
	Laboratory support for CNS inflammation
	Elevated levels of CSF proteins and/or cells
	Presence of oligoclonal bands
	Exclusion of alternative diagnoses together with evidence for systemic sarcoidosis (either through positive histology, including Kveim test, and/or at least two indirect indicators from gallium scan, chest imaging and serum ACE)
Possible	Clinical presentation suggestive of neurosarcoidosis with exclusion of alternative diagnoses where the above criteria are not met

Adapted from Zajicek et al. [5], with permission from Oxford University Press.

be normal in approximately 10% of patients [5]. The most common findings are multiple white-matter lesions, single or multiple parenchymal lesions, and meningeal enhancement. These are best appreciated on fluid-attenuated inversion recovery (FLAIR) sequences, T2-weighted, and gadolinium-enhanced T1-weighted images (Fig. 44.1). Many such changes are not specific to neurosarcoidosis [6]. Surrounding edema is also commonly seen.

Computerized tomography (CT) is inferior and does not always show even quite marked parenchymal change which is evident on MRI (Fig. 44.1).

CSF examination is important and is abnormal in approximately 80% of cases. Typically, CSF findings are an elevated CSF pressure, elevated protein, and increased cell counts, either raised lymphocytes or a pleocytosis including neutrophils and monocytes. Analysis of CSF T-lymphocyte populations has revealed that an elevated T CD4$^+$/T CD8$^+$ ratio appears to be a sensitive marker of neurosarcoidosis [2]. In addition, CSF glucose levels may be low, immunoglobulins elevated, and oligoclonal bands detectable. CSF ACE level may be elevated in neurosarcoidosis but is not as sensitive or specific a marker of neurosarcoidosis as may be thought (elevations also occurring in CNS infection and malignancy), and serial measurement does not appear to be a useful indicator of disease activity [7].

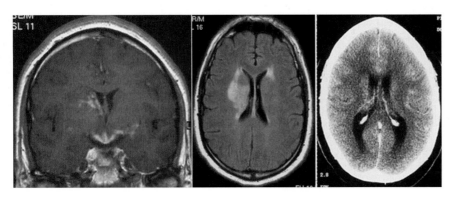

Figure 44.1 FLAIR MRI imaging (left and middle) in parenchymal neurosarcoidosis showing characteristic high signal in the hypothalamic and periventricular regions. This compares with the apparently normal CT (right) taken at the same time.

Table 44.3 Other diseases to be considered in the differential diagnosis of neurosarcoidosis

Tuberculosis/other mycobacterial infection
Fungal infection
Langerhans' cell histiocytosis
Eosinophilic granuloma
Plasma cell granuloma
Lymphocytic hypophysitis
Lymphoma
Multiple sclerosis
Vasculitis (giant cell arteritis/Wegener's granulomatosis)
Primary CNS neoplasia
Germ cell tumors

Other investigations may be useful to demonstrate extracranial sites of sarcoidosis that may be amenable to biopsy as corroborative evidence. These include plain chest radiography, thoracic CT, ^{67}Ga uptake, ^{111}In-pentetreotide imaging, and fluorodeoxyglucose positron emission tomography (PET). None of these latter isotope methods is sensitive or specific in identifying intracranial disease.

In the differential diagnosis of a patient presenting with possible neurosarcoidosis, infectious and other infiltrative diseases affecting the brain must be considered (Table 44.3). Full endocrinological assessment is necessary to detect even subtle deficits in pituitary hormone secretion, and to identify abnormalities in water balance.

Treatment

That treatment changes the natural history of neurosarcoidosis is not proven. Therefore the goals of treatment are to alleviate symptoms, and reduce tissue ischemia from perivascular inflammation, thereby aiming to reduce the likelihood of irreversible fibrosis. By using such a strategy it is hoped that with time the inflammatory process may become quiescent, allowing treatment to be discontinued or reduced.

Given the nature of the condition there have not been any randomized controlled trials to determine the optimal treatment for neurosarcoidosis, and therefore recommendations come from case reports or series [5, 8, 9], and from experience gained in treating systemic sarcoidosis.

Corticosteroids

In general, high-dose corticosteroids are the first treatment of choice unless contraindicated. For parenchymal disease including hypothalamo–pituitary involvement prednisolone is usually started at a dose of 1 mg/kg/day. If the diagnosis of neurosarcoidosis is correct then most patients exhibit a clinical response. In view of the immunosuppressive nature of prolonged corticosteroid therapy, if an infective cause for the dysfunction cannot be reliably excluded (e.g. tuberculosis) it may be appropriate to give concurrent antimicrobial therapy. Depending on the clinical response the dose of prednisolone may be gradually tapered after 2 to 4 weeks. Most patients require a maintenance dose to prevent relapse of symptoms. This is usually in the 10–15 mg/day range, but is variable from patient to patient. If patients do note a relapse then the corticosteroid dose should be doubled to at least 20 mg/day. Patients may require multiple cycles of increasing and tapering dosage regimes as the disease relapses and remits. Concomitant use of anti-seizure medication which induces liver enzyme pathways may necessitate higher oral doses of corticosteroids.

In patients with acute severe neurological signs and symptoms parenteral corticosteroids may be warranted in the form of methylprednisolone 20 mg/kg/day intravenously for 3 days followed by high-dose prednisolone.

Unfortunately, with such long-term corticosteroid regimes patients often develop the associated deleterious side effects including Cushing syndrome, diabetes mellitus and osteoporosis. Thus a wide range of other immunosuppressive agents have been tried either as steroid-sparing therapy in refractory disease or in patients with progressive disease despite aggressive corticosteroid treatment.

Immunosuppressive agents

Ciclosporin A is one of the most frequently used alternative immunosuppressive drugs in systemic sarcoidosis, and therefore its use in neurosarcoidosis is well described. Its mode of action is through suppression of helper T lymphocytes and reduction in release of interleukin-2. Ciclosporin A is given at a dose of 4–6 mg/kg/day, and blood levels should be monitored and maintained in the therapeutic range. Whilst our particular experience of this agent has not been encouraging [10], others have found it to offer some benefit in terms of reduction of corticosteroid dose, although a significant proportion of patients do relapse or progress despite combination therapy [11].

Methotrexate has also been advocated as a first-line adjuvant treatment in neurosarcoidosis, and is usually given in a dose of 10 mg weekly [5, 12]. Its mode of action as an anti-inflammatory is probably through inhibition of T lymphocyte activation and suppression of intercellular adhesion molecule expression by T lymphocytes.

Other agents that have been tried include: azathioprine, cyclophosphamide [13], chlorambucil [14], mycophenolate mofetil and cladribine [15].

Overall response rates to these various agents are variable and at best seem to offer modest adjunctive benefit. It is rarely possible to withdraw corticosteroid treatment entirely. No one agent seems to be more potent than another and choice of immunosuppressive therapy should be determined, in part, by its potential adverse effects.

Immunomodulatory agents

In addition to corticosteroids and other immunosuppressive agents, drugs used in other inflammatory conditions to modulate the immune response have also been tried in the treatment of systemic sarcoidosis and neurosarcoidosis.

Hydroxychloroquine and chloroquine have been utilized to good effect in selected patients and Sharma reports a response rate of 83% in terms of stabilization or control of symptoms in a series of 12 patients [16]. It is proposed that the effects of these drugs result from their interference with "antigen processing" in macrophages and other antigen-presenting cells. Doses of hydroxychloroquine are 200 mg twice daily and chloroquine 250 mg twice daily respectively. The ocular toxic effects of these agents were not observed at these doses in the study.

Other immunomodulatory agents that have been tried in systemic sarcoidosis are pentoxifylline and thalidomide. Both of these agents modulate the effects of tumor necrosis factor α (TNF-α), and as TNF-α has been shown to have a pivotal role in the initiation and maintenance of granulomatous inflammation and progression to fibrosis, there is good theoretical reason for their use. Their role in neurosarcoidosis is unclear.

More recently there have been increasing data on the use of anti-TNF-α antibodies in cases of systemic sarcoidosis and neurosarcoidosis refractory to corticosteroids and conventional immunosuppressants. These agents are currently licensed for use in rheumatological and inflammatory bowel disease, but have been shown to provide clinical benefit in a range of other inflammatory conditions.

The best studied of these in sarcoidosis is infliximab, a chimeric monoclonal human–murine antibody against TNF-α. There are currently five published reports on the use of infliximab in neurosarcoidosis, all with good results. These include a case of direct pituitary involvement by biopsy-proven non-caseating granuloma, presenting with hypogonadotropic hypogonadism and hyperprolactinemia. Control of this patient's disease was dependent on high-maintenance doses of prednisolone (20 mg/day), and therefore methotrexate and then cyclophosphamide were utilized. Despite these adjunctive treatments the neurosarcoidosis progressed, and treatment with infliximab was commenced, resulting in clinical and radiological improvement after 5 months [17].

We have also used infliximab in a young man with severe and refractory parenchymal neurosarcoidosis with hypothalamic involvement. However, despite an initial dramatic clinical response and concomitant radiological improvement (Fig. 44.2) to the initial course of infliximab, his disease relapsed and he unfortunately eventually died from the neurosarcoidosis.

The usual dose of infliximab is 5 mg/kg given as an intravenous infusion at 0, 2 and 6 weeks. Further maintenance doses can be given every 4 to 8 weeks. Hypersensitivity reactions can develop within 1 to 2 hours of the infusion and patients should be closely monitored during treatment. Antibodies to infliximab may develop, resulting in loss of efficacy, and development of other autoantibodies such as antiphospholipid has been reported. As with other immunosuppressive therapy reactivation of tuberculosis is a risk and prophylactic antimicrobials may need to be considered.

Other agents in this class which have also been tried with some success in sarcoidosis are etanercept and adalimumab.

Other treatments

External beam radiotherapy has been utilized in resistant cases of neurosarcoidosis with variable success [18]. It should be reserved for cases unresponsive to corticosteroid and adjunctive drug treatment, and may be more useful for localized disease including pituitary lesions [13]. It appears to be most effective at preventing the progression of local symptoms rather than reversing established neurological deficits. Total doses of 20–25 Gy are usually administered.

Neurosurgical resection of hypothalamic–pituitary lesions is not recommended unless expanding masses are causing raised intracranial pressure. Ventriculoperitoneal shunting may be necessary if hydrocephalus occurs, but is not recommended prophylactically as shunt obstruction is common due to the inflammatory process, and the presence of foreign body in the context of immunosuppression predisposes to CNS infection.

Endocrinological hormone replacement should be instituted if necessary, and dopamine agonist therapy is useful in cases of hyperprolactinemia.

Patients on long-term corticosteroids are at risk of osteoporosis, and should be on bisphosphonate therapy in addition to ensuring adequate gonadal steroid reserve.

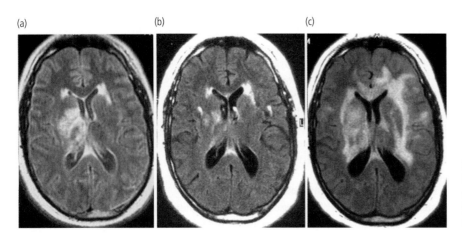

(a) (b) (c)

Figure 44.2 FLAIR MRI in a patient with hypothalamo–pituitary neurosarcoidosis treated with infliximab. Pretreatment (a), 6 weeks post first dose (b), and 5 months later (c) following a clinical relapse despite further doses of infliximab.

Prognosis

The clinical outcome of neurosarcoidosis is difficult to predict due to its heterogeneous nature, and the course of hypothalamo–pituitary disease is not clearly defined. Patients with parenchymal neurosarcoidosis tend to run a remitting/relapsing or chronically progressive course as compared to the often monophasic course of cranial neuropathy or aseptic meningitis. The vegetative hypothalamic symptoms and signs do generally respond to treatment. However, endocrinopathies rarely improve with immunosuppression; as a result, chronic hormonal replacement therapy is usually necessary.

References

1. Stern BJ. Neurological complications of sarcoidosis. *Curr. Opin. Neurol.* 2004;17:311–316.
2. Murialdo G, Tamagno G. Endocrine aspects of neurosarcoidosis. *J. Endocrinol. Invest.* 2002;25:650–662.
3. Stuart CA, Neelon FA, Lebovitz HE. Disordered control of thirst in hypothalamic–pituitary sarcoidosis. *N. Engl. J. Med.* 1980;303:1078–1082.
4. Reichlin S. Neuroendocrinology. In Wilson JD, Foster DW, Kronenberg HM, Larsen PR (eds). *Williams' Textbook of Endocrinology.* Philadelphia: W.B. Saunders, 1998:177.
5. Zajicek JP, Scolding NJ, Foster O, et al. Central nervous system sarcoidosis – diagnosis and management. *QJM* 1999; 92:103–117.
6. Pickuth D, Heywang-Kobrunner SH. Neurosarcoidosis: evaluation with MRI. *J. Neuroradiol.* 2000; 27:185–188.
7. Dale JC, O'Brien JF. Determination of angiotensin-converting enzyme levels in cerebrospinal fluid is not a useful test for the diagnosis of neurosarcoidosis. *Mayo Clin. Proc.* 1999;74:535.
8. Sharma OP. Neurosarcoidosis: a personal perspective based on the study of 37 patients. *Chest* 1997;112:220–228.
9. Chapelon C, Ziza JM, Piette JC, et al. Neurosarcoidosis: signs, course and treatment in 35 confirmed cases. *Medicine (Baltimore)* 1990;69:261–276.
10. Cunnah D, Chew S, Wass J. Cyclosporin for central nervous system sarcoidosis. *Am. J. Med.* 1988;85:580–581.
11. Stern BJ, Schonfeld SA, Sewell C, et al. The treatment of neurosarcoidosis with cyclosporine. *Arch. Neurol.* 1992;49:1065–1072.
12. Soriano FG, Caramelli P, Nitrini R, et al. Neurosarcoidosis: therapeutic success with methotrexate. *Postgrad. Med. J.* 1990;66:142–143.
13. Agbogu BN, Stern BJ, Sewell C, et al. Therapeutic considerations in patients with refractory neurosarcoidosis. *Arch. Neurol.* 1995;52:875–879.
14. Kataria YP. Chlorambucil in sarcoidosis. *Chest* 1980;78:36–43.
15. Tikoo RK, Kupersmith MJ, Finlay JL. Treatment of refractory neurosarcoidosis with cladribine. *N. Engl. J. Med.* 2004;350:1798–1799.
16. Sharma OP. Effectiveness of chloroquine and hydroxychloroquine in treating selected patients with sarcoidosis with neurological involvement. *Arch. Neurol.* 1998;55:1248–1254.
17. Carter JD, Valeriano J, Vasey FB, et al. Refractory neurosarcoidosis: a dramatic response to infliximab. *Am. J. Med.* 2004;117:277–279.
18. Menninger MD, Amdur RJ, Marcus RB Jr. Role of radiotherapy in the treatment of neurosarcoidosis. *Am. J. Clin. Oncol.* 2003;26:e115–e118.

4   Adrenal and Gonadal Tumors

45 Imaging of the Adrenal Glands

Anju Sahdev and Rodney H. Reznek

Key points

- Modern cross-sectional imaging has greatly improved the detection of functioning adrenal pathology.
- A detailed understanding of the advantages and limitations of the technology is necessary to optimally correlate and correctly interpret the appearances on adrenal pathology with clinical and biochemical findings.
- The nature of incidentally detected adrenal masses can be determined with a high degree of accuracy using computerized tomography (CT) and magnetic resonance imaging.
- New developments in imaging including positron emission tomography are likely to have an increasing role in the future in evaluating adrenal pathology.
- The development of multidetector CT has several advantages in the detection and characterization of adrenal disease. MRI with newer gradient sequences and better abdominal coils is usually used to solve problems or where ionizing radiation or administration of iodine-based contrast medium cannot be used.

Introduction

Imaging is an essential adjunct to clinical and biochemical findings in adrenal disorders. Close collaboration between the endocrinologists and radiologists is important in the selection of the appropriate imaging modality. In recent years there have been many technological advances in cross-sectional and radionucleotide imaging, many of which can be applied to investigation of adrenal pathology. The use of conventional X-rays of the abdomen is limited in adrenal investigations. Ultrasound (US) is reserved for large adrenal masses and in pediatrics.

Computerized tomography (CT)

CT is the most widely used modality in detection and investigation of adrenal disease, with good spatial resolution and ability to characterize adrenal pathology using tissue attenuation and enhancement characteristics. CT images are computer-generated grayscale representations of body parts scanned on CT. The computer allocates electronic CT values to all structures within the scanned area and arranges them as a spatial image. These CT numbers, called attenuation values, are measured in Hounsfield units (HU)

Clinical Endocrine Oncology, 2nd edition. Edited by Ian D. Hay and John A.H. Wass. © 2008 Blackwell Publishing. ISBN 978-1-4051-4584-8.

and calculated based on the linear X-ray absorption coefficient of tissues compared to water. For the purpose of grayscale, water has a standardized Hounsfield number of 0 HU, air is −1000 HU and bone is +1000 HU. Attenuation values allow body tissues to be converted and displayed as grayscale CT images. In clinical practice, the attenuation value of each tissue can be acquired by placing an electronic CT cursor over the region of interest. This ability to measure tissue attenuation values before and after administration of intravenous iodine-based contrast agents has been extensively utilized to characterize adrenal masses based on enhancement characteristics. CT of adrenal glands should be performed with narrow collimation (scan thickness <3 mm) before and after administration of intravenous contrast. Narrow collimation improves spatial resolution and administration of contrast improves contrast resolution. Together this allows detection of small adrenal lesions and more accurate attenuation value measurements. With the advent of multidetector CT (MDCT), images can be reconstructed down to 0.5 mm sections. This will improve visualization of adrenal pathology and provide multiplanar imaging comparable to MRI.

Contrast-enhanced CT is acquired after administration of iodine-based contrast media (70–100 ml) into a peripheral vein injected at a rate between 3–5 ml/s. The images are acquired 60 s and 10–15 min after completion of contrast injection. Solid adrenal lesions with attenuation values below 10 HU prior to administration of contrast agents are lipid-rich adenomas. However, 30% of adenomas are lipid poor and have attenuation values greater than 10 HU [1]. To distinguish these lipid-poor adenomas from malignant adrenal lesions, absolute and relative CT contrast washout characteristics can be used [2] (see below).

Magnetic resonance imaging (MRI)

MRI has advantages of no radiation burden to patients and better contrast resolution than CT. It has an increasing role in investigation of difficult adrenal lesions. Most adrenal imaging protocols include conventional spin-echo axial T1- and T2-weighted scans. To elucidate the nature of adrenal masses these are supplemented by chemical shift imaging (CSI) and occasionally with fat-suppressed T1-weighted images before and after administration of intravenous gadolinium. CSI is a technique that relies on detecting intracellular lipid within tissues. Typically, images are acquired in-phase, where water and fat combine to give a stronger signal in voxels where they co-exist. Images are also obtained out-of-phase where water and fat oppose and cancel each other, giving a weaker signal. Hence tissues with high intracellular lipid, such as lipid-rich adenomas, lose signal on out-of-phase images. There are several ways of assessing the degree of loss of signal intensity. Quantitative analysis can be made using a variety of ratios, essentially comparing the loss of signal in the adrenal mass with that of liver, paraspinal muscle or spleen on in-phase and out-of-phase images. Fatty infiltration of the liver (particularly in oncology patients receiving chemotherapy) and iron overload make the liver an unreliable internal standard. Fatty infiltration may also affect skeletal muscle to a lesser extent. The spleen has been shown to be the most reliable internal standard, although this may also be affected by iron overload, and provides the adrenal lesion–spleen ratio [3].

To calculate the adrenal lesion–spleen ratio (ASR), regions of interest (ROIs) are used to acquire the signal intensity (SI) within the adrenal mass and the spleen from in-phase and out-of-phase images. The ASR reflects the percentage signal drop-off within the adrenal lesion compared with the spleen and it can be calculated as follows:

$$ ASR = \left[\frac{SI\ lesion\ (out\text{-}of\text{-}phase)/SI\ spleen\ (out\text{-}of\text{-}phase)}{SI\ lesion\ (in\text{-}phase)/SI\ spleen\ (in\text{-}phase)} \right] \times 100 $$

An ASR ratio of 70 or less has been shown to be 100% specific for adenomas but only 78% sensitive [4]. Simple visual assessment of relative signal intensity loss is just as accurate but quantitative methods may be useful in equivocal cases. A signal intensity loss within an adrenal mass on out-of-phase images of greater than 20% is diagnostic of adenomas [4].

The second, better accepted, quantitative method assesses the signal loss in adrenal masses as a ratio of signal intensities on the in-phase and out-of-phase images (signal intensity index). The signal intensity index (SII) is obtained as follows:

$$ SII = [(SI\ in\text{-}phase - SI\ out\text{-}of\text{-}phase)/SI\ in\text{-}phase] \times 100 $$

Using a 5% signal loss as the minimal threshold, the technique characterizes adrenal adenomas with a reported accuracy of 100% [7].

Gadolinium-enhanced MRI improves the accuracy of MRI in differentiating adenomas from malignant lesions. As with CT, adenomas show enhancement after administration of intravenous gadolinium, with rapid washout, whereas malignant tumors and pheochromocytomas show strong enhancement but a slower washout. Gadolinium enhancement, T1 and T2 signal characteristics demonstrate considerable overlap in properties of benign and malignant lesions.

[18F]-fluorodeoxyglucose positron emission tomography (18-FDG PET)

18-FDG PET alone and in combination with CT (PET-CT) allows recognition of malignant adrenal lesions. In the presence of CT- or MRI-detected indeterminate adrenal mass, 18-FDG PET-CT has a sensitivity and specificity of 98.5% and 92% respectively for separating malignant lesions from adenomas [5]. Recent studies have reported false-positive cases of pheochromocytomas and adenomas. For the diagnosis of a malignant adrenal tumor, the positive predictive value (PPV) of 18-FDG PET was 100%, and negative predictive value (NPV) to rule out malignancy was also 100%. It is possible that 18-FDG PET may be able to detect metastatic lesions in non-enlarged adrenal glands, but the accuracy of this has not been fully evaluated. 18-FDG PET also has the advantage of simultaneously detecting metastases at other sites. The disadvantages of PET relate to its limited availability.

Scintigraphy

Radionucleotide imaging is complementary to biochemical tests and anatomical cross-sectional imaging since specific tracers exist to provide functional information. It provides metabolic information so that adrenal disease can be localized but little anatomical information is obtained. Radiopharmaceuticals can be divided into two main categories: adrenocortical (cholesterol analogs) used to depict masses resulting in adrenal cortical dysfunction and adrenomedullary (guanethidine analogs, particularly meta-iodobenzylguanidine, MIBG) agents used to image adrenomedullary disorders.

Venous sampling

Venous sampling may provide additional information especially when imaging results are equivocal. Adrenal vein cortisol levels above that of background, with undetectable levels in the contralateral adrenal vein, help lateralize an adenoma. Petrosal sinus sampling is employed to try and confirm and lateralize pituitary adrenocorticotropic hormone (ACTH) source.

Normal radiological anatomy of adrenal glands

The adrenal glands are usually well visualized as an inverted Y or V shape enclosed within the perinephric fascia with surrounding retroperitoneal fat on CT and MRI. Both adrenal medulla and cortex have similar lipid content and therefore even with sophisticated CT and MR imaging techniques these cannot be differentiated.

Normal adrenal glands are not seen on US except in young children when the adrenal glands are large. To date, normal dimensions of the adrenal glands have been described only on CT. The maximum width of the left and right adrenal bodies is 0.79 cm (SD 0.21) and 0.6 cm (SD 0.2) respectively. The right adrenal limbs are 0.14–0.49 cm and left adrenal limbs are 0.13–0.52 cm in thickness. In practice normal adrenal limb thickness should not exceed 5 mm [6].

Functional adrenal cortical disorders

Cushing syndrome

The diagnosis of Cushing syndrome depends on clinical and biochemical manifestations of hypercortisolism. Imaging helps to confirm the cause of the Cushing syndrome. In order to plan appropriate therapy it is important to distinguish between ACTH-dependent and ACTH-independent disease.

ACTH-independent Cushing syndrome
Adrenal adenomas

Hyperfunctioning ACTH-secreting adenomas, which account for most of the cases, have imaging features similar to other benign non-hyperfunctioning adrenal adenomas. They are best demonstrated on CT, are between 2 and 7 cm in size and have low or soft tissue attenuation usually enhancing after contrast administration. As 95% of these hyperfunctioning adenomas are lipid rich, they have non-contrast CT attenuation of 10 HU or lower [4]. Only 5% of these adenomas are lipid poor. MRI also readily demonstrates adrenal adenomas which have a low homogeneous signal on T1-weighted images and a signal intensity equivalent or higher than the liver on T2-weighted scans. CSI will readily identify the lipid-rich adenomas with signal loss on the out-of-phase images. After intravenous gadolinium over 90% of adenomas demonstrate a thin, hyperintense rim enhancement. The contralateral adrenal gland is either normal or atrophic due to low circulating ACTH levels [7].

Adrenal carcinoma

In our series, carcinomas accounted for 27% of ACTH-independent Cushing syndrome ranging in size between 6 and 10 cm [4]. Large adenomas may be indistinguishable from a carcinoma [8]. CT typically shows a unilateral mass, usually over 7 cm in size with necrosis, hemorrhage, fibrosis and calcification (Fig. 45.1). Direct invasion into adjacent structures (liver, kidney, IVC), nodal involvement or distant metastases favor the diagnosis of carcinoma.

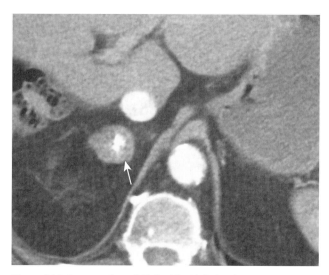

Figure 45.1 Contrast-enhanced CT of a right-sided adrenal carcinoma (arrow) causing Cushing syndrome with amorphous dense calcification and heterogeneous enhancement.

Multiplanar imaging using MRI or multidetector CT allows better assessment of invasion into adjacent structures, important for surgical planning. A large mass, high suspicion of malignancy and surrounding invasion preclude laparoscopic adrenalectomy which may be suitable for small unilateral benign adenomas.

Primary pigmented nodular adrenocortical disease (PPNAD)
On imaging, adrenal glands in PPNAD may be normal or minimally hyperplastic with multiple, benign cortical nodules (Fig. 45.2). Secondary to pigmentation, the nodules demonstrate lower T1 and T2 signal intensity on MRI compared to surrounding

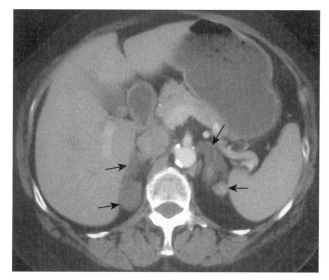

Figure 45.2 Contrast-enhanced CT showing marked nodular hyperplasia of both adrenal glands. The circulating ACTH was undetectable. The patient underwent bilateral adrenalectomy and histopathology confirmed macronodular hyperplasia in both glands.

atrophic cortical tissue. The nodules do not normally exceed 5 mm but in older patients may be 1–2 cm [9]. Histologically there are multiple pigmented nodules in both adrenal glands and atrophy of the cortex due to low circulating ACTH levels. In the absence of gradients on petrosal venous sampling and normal cross-sectional imaging, a presumptive diagnosis of PPNAD may be confirmed by bilateral uptake of ^{131}I-alsosterol scintigraphy [10]. Occasionally in older patients where nodules are 1–2 cm in size, atrophy of intervening cortex helps distinguish this from ACTH-dependent hyperplasia.

ACTH-independent macronodular adrenal hyperplasia (AIMAH)

AIMAH on imaging shows massive bilateral adrenal enlargement, nodularity and distortion of adrenal contour. Nodules vary in size from 1 mm to 5.5 cm and on CT have low attenuation in keeping with lipid-rich adenomas. Glands may extend down below the renal hila. On MRI nodules are isointense to muscle on T1 images and hyperintense to liver on T2 images. In ACTH-dependent Cushing syndrome nodules are isointense to liver on T2 images while in PPNAD nodules are hypointense on both T1- and T2-weighted images. On CSI, nodules lose signal intensity on out-of-phase images. In AIMAH intervening cortex is not hyperplastic on imaging or histology.

ACTH-dependent Cushing syndrome

ACTH-dependent Cushing's is secondary to increased ACTH production either by a pituitary adenoma or an ectopic source. Having confirmed a biochemical diagnosis it is imperative to locate the source of ACTH production. Clinically and biochemically it may be difficult to distinguish between a pituitary or occult ectopic ACTH-secreting tumor. Chronic hyperstimulation of adrenal glands results in bilateral enlargement. The largest glands, usually lobular and nodular, occur from an ectopic rather than pituitary source. Two types of hyperplasia are seen pathologically: smooth (diffuse) or nodular [11, 12]. Smooth hyperplasia is more common but may be obvious or not seen on CT (Fig. 45.3). A normal CT therefore does not exclude the diagnosis. Nodular hyperplasia can be micro- or macronodular. In the latter there is bilateral enlargement of adrenal glands with one or more nodules. The presence of a dominant unilateral nodule, reaching up to 4 cm, may be misinterpreted as hyperfunctioning adenoma, conflicting with biochemical evidence of ACTH dependence. The remainder of the glands are enlarged and nodular, aiding the imaging diagnosis of bilateral hyperplasia (Fig. 45.4).

Pituitary-dependent Cushing disease (Cushing disease)

Cushing disease is secondary to secretory pituitary adenoma. Imaging of the pituitary gland is discussed in Chapter 25.

Ectopic ACTH source

Investigation of patients with "occult" ectopic ACTH production represents a major challenge since clinical, biochemical and

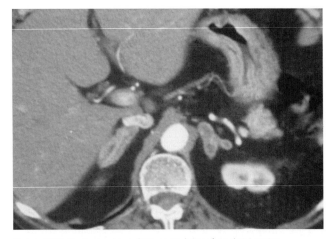

Figure 45.3 Contrast-enhanced CT acquired 60 s after administration of intravenous contrast medium. Both adrenal glands show smooth diffuse enlargement without nodularity in a patient with ACTH-dependent Cushing syndrome.

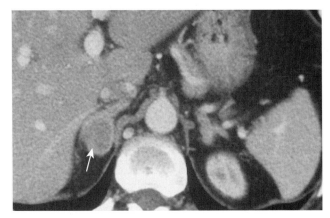

Figure 45.4 Contrast-enhanced CT acquired 60 s after administration of intravenous contrast medium. The right adrenal gland has a dominant 2 cm adrenal nodule (arrow). The diffuse nodular appearance of the left adrenal gland is important to note in this patient with bilateral adrenal hyperplasia causing Cushing syndrome, to avoid erroneously diagnosing a right adrenal adenoma.

radiological features are often indistinguishable from Cushing disease [13]. Tumors producing ectopic ACTH are usually small. The most common sites of "occult" tumors include small bronchial carcinoids (79%), thymic carcinoids, thyroid medullary carcinoma, pancreatic islet cell tumors, pheochromocytomas, mesenteric and small bowel carcinoids. CT of chest, abdomen and pelvis aids identification of the source and also detects liver and nodal metastases (Fig. 45.5). Systemic venous sampling is performed in difficult cases. In the presence of a small indeterminate pulmonary nodule, negative systemic venous sampling lends support to the pulmonary nodule being the source of ACTH. It should be noted that elevated ACTH levels in thymic veins may be due to bronchial carcinoids, mediastinal metastases, thymic carcinoid or diffuse thymic hyperplasia.

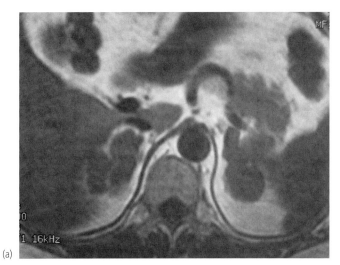

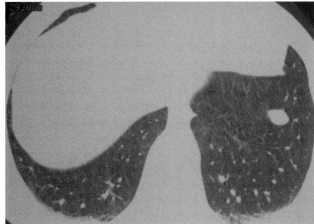

Figure 45.5 (a) Axial T1-weighted image showing massive bilateral adrenal enlargement in a patient with Cushing syndrome and elevated ACTH. The pituitary gland was normal on MRI. (b) CT of the chest on lung window setting shows a small ovoid mass in the left costophrenic angle, which was resected and was a bronchial carcinoid on histopathology.

Primary hyperaldosteronism (Conn syndrome)

Conn syndrome is a disorder characterized by aldosterone excess with suppressed renin activity that results in hypertension and usually hypokalemia. The two principal causes are aldosterone-producing adenoma (APA) and bilateral adrenal hyperplasia (BAH). Differentiating these two causes is important because solitary adenomas are surgically resected whilst BAH is managed medically. Adenomas account for 80% and BAH accounts for 20% of Conn syndrome. CT and MRI are used to differentiate between the two causes after clinical and biochemical diagnosis is established. APAs are lower attenuation on CT, less than 0 HU, than other adenomas. They demonstrate no significant contrast enhancement, rarely calcify and are small, mean size of 1.6–2.2 cm, median size of 2 cm and range between 1 and 4.75 cm. Several studies have examined performance of thin section CT (3–5 mm) in detection of APA, with sensitivities and specificities varying between 88% and 100% and 33% and 100%, respectively [30–32].

On CT if the adrenal limb width is 3 mm or greater, sensitivity for diagnosing BAH is 100% but specificity is 54% [14]. Specificity of 100% is achieved if the limb width is 5 mm or greater.

In detection of APA, MRI has a sensitivity, specificity and accuracy of 70%, 100% and 85% respectively. Eighty-six percent of adenomas and 89% of BAH glands have intracellular lipid demonstrating loss of signal intensity on CSI [15]. CT and MRI have a comparative performance in detection of APAs with sensitivity and specificity of 87–93% and 82–85% for CT and 83% and 92% for MRI, respectively [16]. There are several reasons for lack of specificity in detection of APAs, including concomitant non-functioning nodule, presence of dominant nodules in BAH and increased nodularity with age and hypertension [7, 16]. The lack of sensitivity has been attributed to the small size of the adenomas. A high specificity for detection of adenomas is desirable to avoid unsuccessful surgery in patients with BAH (Fig. 45.6).

Adrenal venous sampling for aldosterone levels is very accurate in preoperative assessment of Conn syndrome. However, even with experienced operators the procedure has high complication rates and cumulative failure rates for catheterization of the right adrenal vein of 26% [17]. A sensitivity of between 70% and 100% is achieved if the operator can catheterize both veins with a positive predictive value of 90% [18]. The complications include adrenal infarction, adrenal vein thrombosis, perforation, adrenal hemorrhage, hypotensive crisis and adrenal insufficiency. Venous sampling is therefore reserved for patients where:

- no definite adenoma is seen and the adrenal glands appear normal;
- there are bilateral nodules, which may be either macronodules of adrenal hyperplasia or multiple adenomas;
- there is disagreement between CT and MR imaging or between imaging and biochemical findings.

^{75}Se 6β-selenomethyl-19-norcholesterol imaging can be used to lateralize a Conn's adenoma in difficult cases. Dexamethasone suppression prior to scintigraphy helps to increase tracer uptake. However, bilateral tracer uptake may occur in BAH and normal

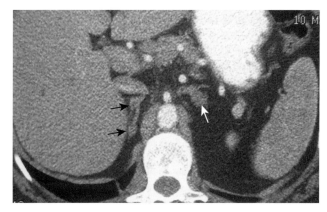

Figure 45.6 Contrast-enhanced CT acquired 60 s after administration of intravenous contrast medium. Both adrenal glands demonstrate nodular hyperplasia in this patient with Conn syndrome.

adrenal glands. With dexamethasone suppression the sensitivity and specificity of scintigraphy are 87% and 89% respectively.

Virilization

Virilization may be due to congenital adrenal hyperplasia (CAH), adrenal androgen-producing adenomas, adrenocortical carcinomas or extra-adrenal pathologies (polycystic ovaries and gonadal tumors). The role of imaging is detection or exclusion of surgically resectable sources of androgen excess in the adrenals, ovaries or testes (Fig. 45.7). In these young patients MRI or ultrasound

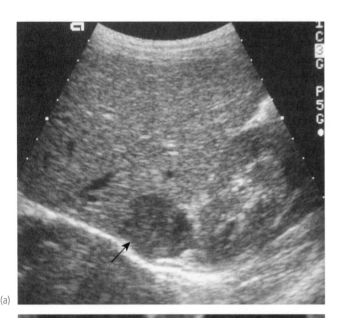

(a)

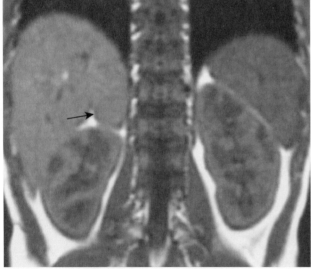

(b)

Figure 45.7 (a) A longitudinal ultrasound image through the upper abdomen of a young boy showing a hypoechoic mass in the suprarenal space (arrow). Clinically the patient had precocious puberty. (b) Coronal T1-weighted image. The mass is seen to be an adrenal mass (arrow), which was resected showing a virilizing adenoma on histopathology.

is the modality of choice to avoid ionizing radiation from CT. Venous catheterization should be reserved for patients in whom uncertainty remains as the presence of small ovarian tumors cannot be excluded biochemically or on US.

Congenital adrenal hyperplasia (CAH)
CAH is a group of autosomal recessive disorders resulting from deficiency of one of the five enzymes necessary for synthesis of cortisol. As a result there is an increase in circulating ACTH with chronic adrenal hyperstimulation. The raised ACTH results in gross enlargement of adrenal glands seen on CT and MRI. In children, enlarged, lobulated, adrenal glands with stippled echogenicity may be seen on ultrasound [19]. On CT and MRI the adrenal glands often enhance inhomogeneously and can be mass-like, indistinguishable from carcinomas. Rarely, long-term ACTH stimulation may lead to transformation of CAH into an autonomous adenoma or carcinoma. This complication occurs in patients who have had untreated CAH for many years and represents a different group from primary adrenal virilizing tumors [20].

Adrenal virilizing tumors
These are most commonly carcinomas and rarely adenomas. They usually exceed 2 cm in diameter and have the same imaging characteristics for adenomas and carcinomas.

Functioning adrenal medullary disorders

Pheochromocytomas and paragangliomas
These are neuroendocrine tumors of chromaffin cell origin. The majority (85–90%) arise in the adrenal medulla and are termed pheochromocytomas. Extra-adrenal tumors (15%) are termed paragangliomas, occur in second to third decades, afflicting men and women equally and are less hormonally active than adrenal tumors [21]. Once a clinical diagnosis of pheochromocytoma has been made, imaging studies are performed to localize the tumor and for surgical planning. Sporadic adrenal pheochromocytomas are usually large at time of diagnosis (90% larger than 2 cm) and thereby readily detected by US, CT and MRI. Pheochromocytomas in association with neuroectodermal syndromes (multiple endocrine neoplasia, von Hippel–Lindau disease, neurofibromatosis) are smaller at detection as they are often actively sought.

On ultrasound pheochromocytomas are well-defined, ovoid or round suprarenal masses. They frequently have an inhomogeneous internal architecture due to hemorrhage and necrosis. Ultrasound has a lower sensitivity for the detection of pheochromocytomas than CT or MRI as smaller lesions, particularly on the left, may be obscured by bowel gas.

Contrast-enhanced CT is highly accurate in detection of adrenal pheochromocytomas with sensitivities, specificities and positive predictive value between 93–100%, 87–94% and 90%, respectively. Prior to contrast medium administration they are of soft tissue attenuation, similar to liver, and may contain small amounts of calcification or low attenuation necrosis. Contrast medium enhancement using non-ionic contrast media has been used safely without α-adrenergic blockade [22]. After administration of contrast media, they enhance avidly and have a prolonged contrast washout phase. The amount of necrosis is variable and may present as a predominantly cystic mass. The rim of cystic lesions still retain avidly enhancing solid tissue.

On MRI, pheochromocytomas have iso- or hypointense signal intensity to liver on T1-weighted images and high signal intensity compared to liver on T2-weighted images. This typical appearance is not seen in up to 35% of patients [23]. Small areas of high T1 signal intensity corresponding to hemorrhage may present up to 20% of tumors. Larger tumors have heterogeneous signal intensity on T2-weighted images due to necrosis, hemorrhage and calcification. On CSI, pheochromocytomas do not lose signal intensity on out-of-phase images (Fig. 45.8). The typical features described above have a significant overlap with appearances of

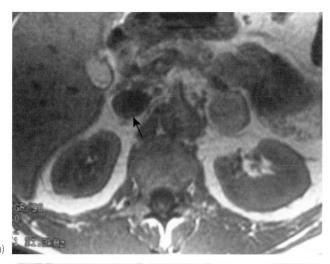

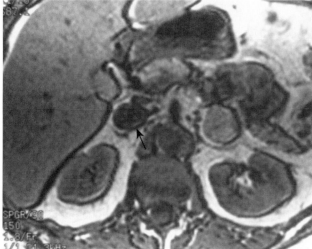

Figure 45.8 (a) Axial in-phase MRI image showing the adrenal mass with a signal intensity equivalent to the liver. (b) Axial out-of-phase MRI image showing no visual loss of signal intensity within the mass and an ASR and SII of 134% and 4% respectively confirming a non-adenoma, in this case a clinical pheochromocytoma.

necrotic adrenal metastases. Intravenous gadolinium does not assist in further differentiation as both have similar enhancement characteristics.

MRI has been shown to be equivalent to or better than CT in demonstration of extra-adrenal paragangliomas [21]. It is superior to CT in demonstration of cardiac, spinal and bladder paragangliomas [24]. Multiplanar MRI or reconstructed multidetector CT is important in neck, bladder and retroperitoneal tumors during planning of surgical resection by providing precise anatomical information. MRI is advantageous in patients with an increased risk of developing paragangliomas (predisposing syndromes or previous paragangliomas) as they require screening. In these patients combined use of MRI and ^{123}I-MIBG avoids high radiation burden associated with repeated CT.

MIBG resembles norepinephrine (noradrenaline) and concentrates in sympatho-adrenal tissue. MIBG is therefore used for imaging tumors of neural crest origin, particularly pheochromocytomas and paragangliomas. As ^{123}I-MIBG (or ^{131}I-MIBG) provides whole-body imaging, it is extremely useful in detection of extra-adrenal tumors. Metastatic lesions are detected, most commonly in the skeleton, liver, lymph nodes, peritoneum and lung. In postoperative patients, the functional nature of MIBG helps differentiate recurrent disease from scar tissue in the operative bed. ^{123}I-MIBG is more often used at diagnosis as it has better imaging characteristics, utilizes smaller doses of tracer and demonstrates small and metastatic lesions better than ^{131}I-MIBG[21]. ^{131}I-MIBG is used mainly for therapy. The sensitivity of MIBG is reported as 87–90%, lower than both CT and MRI as its performance depends on the ability of tumor to take up radionucleotide. The specificity of MIBG exceeds 90%.

Neuroblastomas and ganglioneuroblastomas

Neuroblastomas and ganglioneuroblastomas are primitive tumors derived from neuroblastic and mature ganglion cells distributed along the sympathetic nervous system. Adrenal glands are the commonest primary site of involvement. Neuroblastoma and ganglioneuroblastoma occur most frequently in infants and children. They are two of the most common malignant tumors of childhood, with 40 % arising in adrenal glands.

On gross examination ganglioneuroblastomas have variable amounts of calcification and their appearance depends upon degree of differentiation and primitive elements. Reported CT findings reflect this diversity and vary from predominantly solid to predominantly cystic masses with strands of solid tissue [25]. Neuroblastomas are aggressive tumors; the majority are irregularly shaped, lobulated, and unencapsulated. They invade adjacent organs or encase adjacent vessels and tend to be inhomogeneous owing to tumor necrosis and hemorrhage. They contain coarse, amorphous, mottled peripheral calcification in approximately 85% of cases at CT and in up to 55% of cases at conventional radiography.

CT features of neuroblastoma are a large mass, often extending across the midline to engulf and displace the aorta anteriorly (Fig. 45.9). Inhomogeneous contrast enhancement is usual. CT

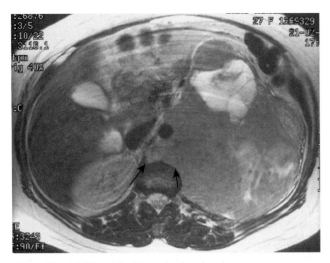

Figure 45.9 Axial T2-weighted image showing a large heterogeneous mass arising from the left adrenal gland. The mass creeps posterior to the aorta, extends across the midline and displaces the aorta anteriorly (arrows), a feature typical in neuroblastomas.

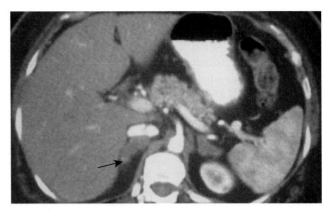

Figure 45.10 Contrast-enhanced CT of the abdomen demonstrating bilateral adrenal enlargement and fine calcification in the right adrenal gland (arrow). The patient had acute TB.

and MRI are useful for defining morphological features and precisely assessing tumor extent for planning biopsies and surgical resection. Imaging also helps determine tumor extension to retroperitoneal lymph nodes and liver, around central vessels, and into the vertebral canal. Liver metastases may take two forms: diffuse infiltration, sometimes missed at CT because it may uniformly increase parenchymal attenuation, or focal hypoenhancing masses. MRI has become the modality of choice for staging due to its multiplanar capabilities, lack of ionizing radiation and good contrast between the very high signal tumor and surrounding tissues on T2-weighted images [25]. MRI is the preferred modality for investigating intraspinal extension of primary tumor (the so-called dumbbell tumors, seen in 10% of abdominal, 28% of thoracic, and occasionally in cervical neuroblastomas) and for detection of diffuse hepatic metastases; these metastases manifest as areas of high signal intensity on T2-weighted images [25].

MIBG plays a complementary role to MRI and CT. Its advantage is being able to detect distant metastases and improving staging accuracy [26]. The reported cumulative sensitivity and specificity of ^{123}I-MIBG for detection of neuroblastoma are 69% and 85% respectively [27]. As approximately 30% of tumors are MIBG negative, normal results do not exclude the diagnosis. Routine use of MIBG is controversial; recent studies show MRI has the highest sensitivity (86%), MIBG the highest specificity (85%) and combined integrated imaging improves both sensitivity (99%) and specificity (95%) [27, 28].

Hypoadrenalism

Primary adrenal insufficiency (Addison disease), usually the result of autoimmune disease, results in small atrophic, non-calcified adrenal glands which are difficult to detect. Calcification in atrophic adrenal glands excludes primary atrophy. This is seen in granulomatous diseases [tuberculosis (TB), histoplasmosis and sarco-

idosis] (Fig. 45.10). Enlarged glands are most commonly due to TB but occasionally may be due to other causes such as amyloid, metastatic disease, hemochromatosis, fungal infections, acquired immune deficiency syndrome and adrenal hemorrhage. In acute adrenal TB, bilateral adrenal enlargement is seen in 91% of cases. This can be mass like and calcification is seen in up to 59%. Low attenuation centers with peripheral rim enhancement are seen in 47% of patients. After treatment 88% of enlarged glands decreased or returned to normal size and configuration [29].

Incidentally discovered adrenal masses

Introduction

Incidentally detected adrenal masses occur in up to 9% of all abdominal CT scans, the vast majority of these being benign adenomas. Cross-sectional imaging readily characterizes benign adrenal masses, such as lipid-rich adenomas, myelolipomas, adrenal cysts, granulomas and adrenal hemorrhage as they have characteristic diagnostic imaging findings such as intralesional fat, water or blood (Figs 45.11 and 45.12). Nevertheless, some masses elude characterization and remain indeterminate. These include lipid-poor adenomas, which are the commonest lesions, adrenal metastases, adrenal carcinomas and pheochromocytomas. The nature of any biochemical abnormality dictates further management but non-functioning masses pose the greatest difficulty. CT and MRI techniques are optimized to maximize specificity for adenomas whilst still maintaining an acceptable sensitivity.

Non-functioning adenomas versus malignant masses

Computerized tomography
Size criteria
On CT, certain imaging findings occur more frequently in malignant masses. Lesions greater than 5 cm in diameter tend to be either metastases or primary adrenal carcinomas [30]. However,

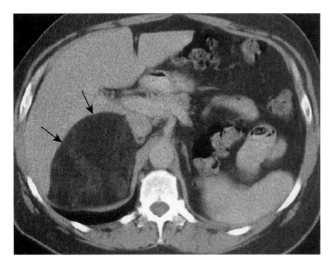

Figure 45.11 Non-contrast CT of the abdomen showing a large adrenal myelolipoma of fatty density with enhancing foci. The CT attenuation of the mass is 5 HU, characteristically higher than fat but lower than water.

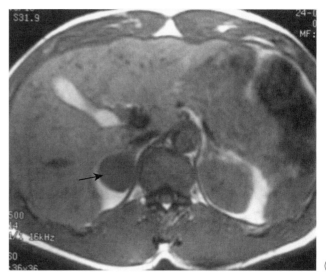

(a)

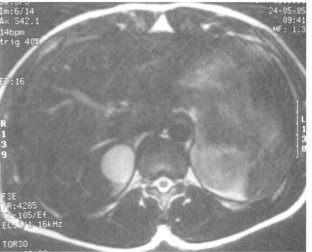

(b)

Figure 45.12 (a) Axial T1-weighted MR image showing a low fluid signal intensity right adrenal mass (arrow). (b) Axial T2-weighted MR image showing the mass has a uniform high fluid signal intensity with smooth walls and no internal architecture in keeping with an adrenal cyst.

size alone is poor at discriminating between benign and malignant lesions. In a study by Lee et al., using 3.0 cm as the size cut-off, the specificity was only 79% and the sensitivity 84% [30]. Rapid change in size also suggests malignancy as benign adenomas are slow-growing lesions. Although it has been suggested that adenomas have a smooth contour, whilst malignant lesions have an irregular shape, there is a very large overlap between the two groups and shape is therefore not a helpful differentiating feature.

Attenuation values

Adenomas have a high intracellular lipid content which lowers their attenuation value. If the attenuation value of an adrenal mass measures 0 HU or less on an *unenhanced* scan, the specificity of the mass being an adenoma is 100% but sensitivity is only an unacceptable 47%. Boland et al. [31] performed a meta-analysis of 10 studies demonstrating that if a threshold attenuation value of 10 HU was adopted on *unenhanced* scans, the specificity dropped to 98% but sensitivity increased to 71%. In clinical practice, therefore, 10 HU is the most widely used threshold attenuation value for diagnosis of an adrenal adenoma.

Contrast-enhanced CT

In routine clinical practice, many, if not the majority of adrenal masses are detected following intravenous administration of contrast which precludes measurement of their attenuation value on unenhanced scans. Also, up to 30% of benign adenomas have attenuation values greater than 10 HU on unenhanced scans and are considered to be lipid poor [1]. Malignant lesions are also lipid poor. Characterization of adrenal masses using contrast-enhanced CT utilizes differing perfusion patterns of adenomas and metastases. Adenomas enhance rapidly after contrast administration and also demonstrate rapid loss of contrast medium – a

phenomenon termed contrast washout. Metastases enhance rapidly but demonstrate a slower washout of contrast medium. In standard abdominal CT, images are acquired 60 s after contrast administration. Attenuation values of adrenal masses obtained 60 s after contrast medium injection show too much overlap between adenomas and malignant lesions to be of clinical value [32]. Adrenal masses with attenuation values less than 30 HU, on images obtained 10–15 min after contrast enhancement, are almost always adenomas. However, the percentage of contrast washout between initial enhancement (at 60 s) and delayed enhancement (at 15 min) can be used to differentiate adenomas from malignant lesions [33]. These absolute contrast medium enhancement washout values are only applicable to relatively homogeneous masses without large areas of necrosis or hemorrhage. Both lipid-rich and lipid-poor adenomas behave similarly,

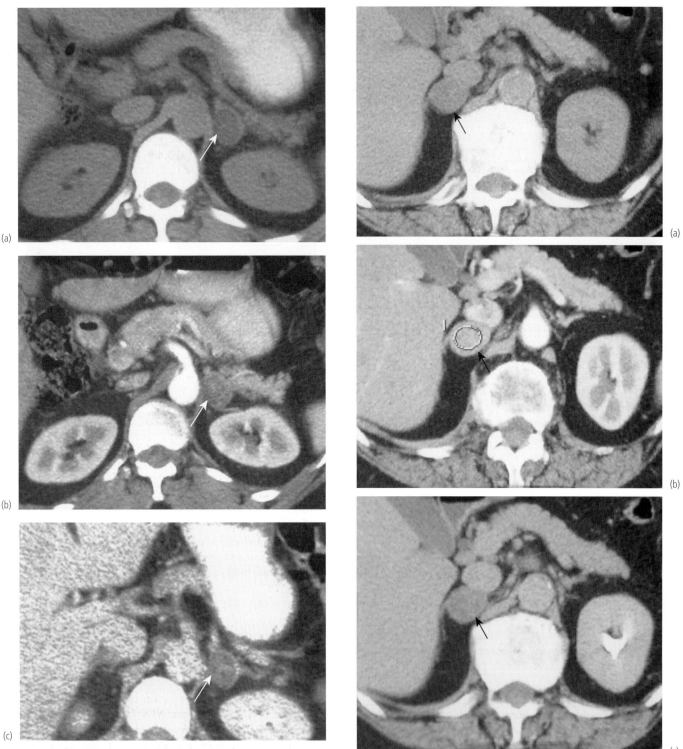

Figure 45.13 (a) Non-contrast enhanced CT showing a left adrenal mass (arrow). The attenuation of the adrenal mass prior to contrast administration is −10 HU. This would be in keeping with a lipid-rich adenoma. (b) Contrast-enhanced CT acquired 60 s after contrast administration. The attenuation value is 98 HU. (c) Contrast-enhanced CT acquired 15 min after contrast administration. The attenuation value is 30 HU. From these attenuation values the calculated absolute and relative enhancement washout figures are 73% and 69% respectively, confirming a lipid-rich adenoma.

Figure 45.14 (a) Non-contrast enhanced CT showing a right adrenal mass (arrow). The attenuation of the adrenal mass prior to contrast administration is 20 HU making this an indeterminate mass. (b) Contrast-enhanced CT acquired 60 s after contrast administration. The attenuation value is 100 HU. (c) Contrast-enhanced CT acquired 15 min after contrast administration. The attenuation value is 32 HU. From these attenuation values the calculated absolute and relative enhancement washout figures are 85% and 68%, confirming a lipid-poor adenoma.

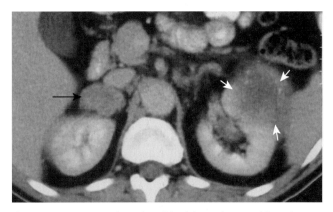

Figure 45.15 Contrast-enhanced CT of the abdomen showing a left renal cell carcinoma (white arrows) and a contralateral right adrenal metastasis (black arrow). The contralateral adrenal metastasis renders the patient stage IV disease.

as this property of adenomas is independent of their lipid content (Figs 45.13–45.15).

The percentage of absolute enhancement washout (AEW) can be calculated thus:

$$\frac{\text{Enhanced attenuation value} - \text{delayed attenuation value}}{\text{Enhanced attenuation value} - \text{non-enhanced attenuation value}} \times 100$$

Enhanced attenuation value is attenuation value of the mass, in Hounsfield units, 60 s after contrast administration.

Delayed attenuation value is the attenuation value of the mass in Hounsfield units 10–15 min after contrast administration.

If AEW is 60% or higher, this has a sensitivity of 88% and a specificity of 96% for diagnosis of an adenoma [2]. However, measurement of AEW requires an unenhanced image. Frequently, in clinical practice only post-contrast images are available. In these patients the "relative" enhancement washout (REW) can be calculated thus:

$$\frac{\text{Enhanced attenuation value} - \text{delayed attenuation value}}{\text{Enhanced attenuation value}} \times 100$$

At 15 min, if REW of 40% or higher is achieved, this has a sensitivity of 96–100% and a specificity of 100% for diagnosis of an adenoma.

More recently, AEW and REW values at 10 min have been evaluated [2]. Blake et al. [2] characterized all adrenal lesions between 0 and 43 HU. They assumed all lesions below 0 HU were benign and all lesions above 43 HU were malignant on unenhanced images. They applied minimal threshold values of AEW greater than 52% and REW of 38%. The combined protocol had a sensitivity and specificity of 100% and 98% respectively for the diagnosis of an adenoma. Therefore, combination of non-enhanced CT and enhancement washout characteristics correctly separates nearly all adrenal masses as adenomas or non-adenomas.

Histogram analysis method
This technique is applied to non-contrast CT scans [34]. A region of interest (ROI) cursor is drawn covering at least two-thirds of the adrenal mass. The individual attenuation values of all the pixels in the ROI are plotted against their frequency. This provides the range, mean and number of pixels within the ROI. The amount of lipid in the mass is proportional to the number of negative pixels (less than 0 HU) within it; 97% of adenomas contain negative pixels. 85% have more than 5% negative pixels and 83% have more than 10% negative pixels. No metastases have negative pixels. The performance and reproducibility of this method require further studies.

Magnetic resonance imaging
Early reports were enthusiastic that MRI would allow differentiation of benign from malignant adrenal masses on the basis of signal intensity differences on T2-weighted spin-echo images. Metastases and carcinomas in general have higher fluid contents than adenomas and therefore are of higher signal intensity on T2-weighted images than surrounding normal adrenal gland. Adenomas are homogeneously iso- or hypointense compared with the normal adrenal gland. However, considerable overlap exists between the signal intensities of adenomas and other lesions and up to 31% of lesions remain indeterminate. Gadolinium-enhanced MRI also demonstrates considerable overlap in characteristics of adenomas and non-adenomas, limiting its clinical applicability. The combination of spin-echo signal characteristics, gadolinium enhancement and CSI is currently 85–90% accurate in distinguishing between adenomas and non-adenomas [35] (Fig. 45.16). There are few direct comparisons between CT and MRI. Evidence from one histological study showed that because both non-contrast CT alone and CSI rely upon the same property of adenomas, namely their lipid content, the techniques correlate [36]. Our own work suggests that CSI may be more sensitive in the detection of intracellular lipid than CT.

Percutaneous adrenal biopsy
With improved imaging techniques only a small percentage of adrenal masses cannot be accurately characterized and require percutaneous biopsy for diagnosis. However, prior to percutaneous biopsy the likelihood of a pheochromocytoma must be excluded due to the risk of a biopsy-induced adrenal crisis. The NPV of adrenal biopsies has been shown to be between 98% and 100%. Percutaneous CT-guided adrenal biopsy is a relatively safe procedure in patients with a known extra-adrenal malignancy. Minor complications of adrenal biopsy include abdominal pain, hematuria, nausea and small pneumothoraces. Major complications, generally regarded as those requiring treatment, occur in 2.8–3.6% of cases and include pneumothoraces requiring intervention, and hemorrhage, with isolated reports of adrenal abscesses, pancreatitis and seeding of metastases along the needle track [37, 38].

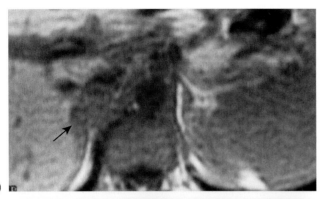

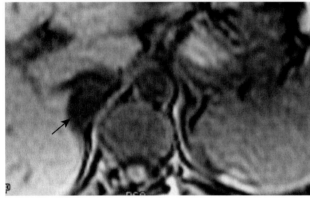

Figure 45.16 (a) Axial in-phase MR image showing a right-sided adrenal mass with intermediate signal intensity (SI = 93) lower than adjacent liver but equivalent to spleen (SI = 97). (b) Axial out-of-phase MR image showing the adrenal mass has visually lost signal intensity, suggesting an adrenal adenoma. The measured SI values of the mass and spleen are 54 and 95, respectively. These SI values produce ASR and SII values of 59% and 42% respectively, confirming an adrenal adenoma.

Other adrenal masses

Adrenal myelolipomas

Adrenal myelolipomas are rare, benign neoplasms composed of adipose and hematopoietic tissue. The imaging features are usually characteristic, allowing radiologists to make a confident diagnosis. Although frequently detected as incidental masses, they may present with pain due to hemorrhage or necrosis within the tumor [39]. Large, greater than 4 cm, lesions may be detected on US as highly echogenic masses. Myelolipomas are best assessed by CT, where fat density and hemorrhage, if present, can be demonstrated. Other fat-containing lesions of the retroperitoneum such as lipomas, liposarcomas and renal angiomyelolipomas may mimic these appearances. If the fat content of myelolipomas is small, it may be indistinguishable from other adrenal masses (Fig. 45.11).

Adrenal cyst

Adrenal cysts are uncommon. There are several types of cysts, the most frequent being endothelial (45%). These may be lymphatic or angiomatous, the former probably arising as a result of blocked lymphatics. Remaining cysts are parasitic (echinococcus) and

pseudocysts (39% of all cysts), which are presumed to result from hemorrhage. US demonstrates their cystic nature and pseudocysts may have internal septae which, unlike renal cysts, have thick walls. CT cannot reliably differentiate between cysts and adenomas as both can have identical low attenuation values [40]. US and MRI are used to differentiate (Fig. 45.12). Malignancy in cysts is difficult to exclude and requires follow-up or cyst fluid aspiration for cytology.

References

1. Caoili EM, Korobkin M, Francis IR, Cohan RH, Dunnick NR. Delayed enhanced CT of lipid-poor adrenal adenomas. *AJR Am. J. Roentgenol.* 2000;175:1411–1415.
2. Blake MA, Kalra MK, Sweeney AT, et al. Distinguishing benign from malignant adrenal masses: multi-detector row CT protocol with 10-minute delay. *Radiology* 2006;238:578–585.
3. Mayo-Smith WW, Lee MJ, McNicholas MM, Hahn PF, Boland GW, Saini S. Characterization of adrenal masses (<5 cm) by use of chemical shift MR imaging: observer performance versus quantitative measures. *AJR Am. J. Roentgenol.* 1995;165:91–95.
4. Rockall AG, Babar SA, Sohaib SA, et al. CT and MRI of the adrenal glands in ACTH-independent cushing syndrome. *Radiographics* 2004;24:435–452.
5. Metser U, Miller E, Lerman H, Lievshitz G, Avital S, Even-Sapir E. 18F-FDG PET/CT in the evaluation of adrenal masses. *J. Nucl. Med.* 2006;47:32–37.
6. Vincent JM, Morrison ID, Armstrong P, Reznek RH. The size of normal adrenal glands on computed tomography. *Clin. Radiol.* 1994;49:453–455. Erratum in: *Clin. Radiol.* 1995;50:202.
7. Reznek RH, Armstrong PA. Imaging in endocrinology: the adrenal gland. *Clin. Endocrinol.* 1994;40:561–576.
8. Newhouse JH, Heffess CS, Wagner BJ, Imray TJ, Adair CF, Davidson AJ. Large degenerated adrenal adenomas: radiologic–pathologic correlation. *Radiology* 1999;210:385–391.
9. Ohara N, Komiya I, Yamauchi K, et al. Carney's complex with primary pigmented nodular adrenocortical disease and spotty pigmentations. *Intern. Med.* 1993;32:60–62.
10. Doppman JL, Travis WD, Nieman L, et al. Cushing syndrome due to primary pigmented nodular adrenocortical disease: findings at CT and MR imaging. *Radiology.* 1989;172:415–420.
11. Sohaib SA, Hanson JA, Newell-Price JD, et al. CT appearance of the adrenal glands in adrenocorticotrophic hormone-dependent Cushing's syndrome. *AJR Am. J. Roentgenol.* 1999;172:997–1002.
12. Francis IR, Gross MD, Shapiro B, Korobkin M, Quint LE. Integrated imaging of adrenal disease. *Radiology* 1992;184:1–13. Erratum in: *Radiology* 1992;185:286.
13. Vincent JM, Trainer PJ, Reznek RH, et al. The radiological investigation of occult ectopic ACTH-dependent Cushing's syndrome. *Clin. Radiol.* 1993;48:11–17.
14. Lingam RK, Sohaib SA, Vlahos I, et al. CT of primary hyperaldosteronism (Conn's syndrome): the value of measuring the adrenal gland. *AJR Am. J. Roentgenol.* 2003;181:843–849.
15. Sohaib SA, Peppercorn PD, Allan C, et al. Primary hyperaldosteronism (Conn syndrome): MR imaging findings. *Radiology* 2000;214:527–531.
16. Lingam RK, Sohaib SA, Rockall AG, et al. Diagnostic performance of CT versus MR in detecting aldosterone-producing adenoma in

primary hyperaldosteronism (Conn's syndrome). *Eur. Radiol.* 2004; 14:1787–1792.

17. Young WF, Stanson AW, Thompson GB, Grant CS, Farley DR, van Heerden JA. Role for adrenal venous sampling in primary aldosteronism. *Surgery* 2004;136:1227–1235.

18. Sheaves R, Goldin J, Reznek RH, et al. Relative value of computed tomography scanning and venous sampling in establishing the cause of primary hyperaldosteronism. *Eur. J. Endocrinol.* 1996;134:308–313.

19. Gross MD, Falke THM, Shapiro B, Sandler MP. Adrenal glands. In Sandler MP, Patton JA, Gross MD, Shapiro B, Falke THM (eds). *Endocrine Imaging.* Norwalk, CT: Appleton and Lange, 1992:271–349.

20. Falke TH, van Seters AP, Schaberg A, Moolenaar AJ. Computed tomography in untreated adults with virilizing congenital adrenal cortical hyperplasia. *Clin. Radiol.* 1986;37:155–160.

21. Quint LE, Glazer GM, Francis IR, Shapiro B, Chenevert TL. Pheochromocytoma and paraganglioma: comparison of MR imaging with CT and I-131 MIBG scintigraphy. *Radiology* 1987;165:89–93.

22. Mukherjee JJ, Peppercorn PD, Reznek RH, et al. Pheochromocytoma: effect of nonionic contrast medium in CT on circulating catecholamine levels. *Radiology* 1997;202:227–231.

23. Varghese JC, Hahn PF, Papanicolaou N, Mayo-Smith WW, Gaa JA, Lee MJ. MR differentiation of phaeochromocytoma from other adrenal lesions based on qualitative analysis of T2 relaxation times. *Clin. Radiol.* 1997;52:603–606.

24. Sahdev A, Sohaib A, Monson JP, Grossman AB, Chew SL, Reznek RH. CT and MR imaging of unusual locations of extra-adrenal paragangliomas (pheochromocytomas). *Eur. Radiol.* 2005;15:85–92.

25. Mehta N, Tripathi RP, Popli MB, Nijhawan VS. Bilateral intraabdominal ganglioneuroblastoma in an adult. *BJR* 1997;70:96–98.

26. Kushner BH. Neuroblastoma: a disease requiring a multitude of imaging studies. *J. Nucl. Med.* 2004;45:1172–1188.

27. Pfluger T, Schmied C, Porn U, et al. Integrated imaging using MRI and 123I metaiodobenzylguanidine scintigraphy to improve sensitivity and specificity in the diagnosis of pediatric neuroblastoma. *AJR Am. J. Roentgenol.* 2003;181:1115–1124.

28. Mitjavila M. Meta-iodobenzylguanidine in neuroblastoma: from diagnosis to therapy. *Nucl. Med. Commun.* 2002;23:3–4.

29. Yang ZG, Guo YK, Li Y, et al. Differentiation between tuberculosis and primary tumors in the adrenal gland: evaluation with contrast-enhanced CT. *Eur. Radiol.* 2006;16:2031–2036. Epub 2006: 25 January.

30. Lee MJ, Hahn PF, Papanicolaou N, et al. Benign and malignant adrenal masses: CT distinction with attenuation coefficients, size, and observer analysis. *Radiology* 1991;179:415–418.

31. Boland GW, Lee MJ, Gazelle GS, Halpern EF, McNicholas MM, Mueller PR. Characterization of adrenal masses using enhanced CT: an analysis of the CT literature. *AJR Am. J. Roentgenol.* 1998;171:201–204.

32. Korobkin M, Brodeur FJ, Yutzy GG, et al. Differentiation of adrenal adenomas from nonadenomas using CT attenuation values. *AJR Am. J. Roentgenol.* 1996;166:531–536.

33. Szolar DH, Kammerhuber FH. Adrenal adenomas and nonadenomas: assessment of washout at delayed contrast-enhanced CT. *Radiology* 1998;207:369–375.

34. Bae KT, Fuangtharnthip P, Prasad SR, Joe BN, Heiken JP. Adrenal masses: CT characterization with histogram analysis method. *Radiology* 2003;228:735–742.

35. McNicholas MM, Lee MJ, Mayo-Smith WW, et al. An imaging algorithm for the differential diagnosis of adrenal adenomas and metastases. *AJR Am. J. Roentgenol.* 1995;165:1453–1459.

36. Korobkin M, Giordano TJ, Brodeur FJ, et al. Adrenal adenomas: relationship between histologic lipid and CT and MR findings. *Radiology* 1996;200:743–747.

37. Harisinghani MG, Maher MM, Hahn PF, et al. Predictive value of benign percutaneous adrenal biopsies in oncology patients. *Clin. Radiol.* 2002;57:898–901.

38. Silverman SG, Mueller PR, Pinkney LP, Koenker RM, Seltzer SE. Predictive value of image–guided adrenal biopsy: analysis of results of 101 biopsies. *Radiology* 1993;187:715–718.

39. Meyer A, Behrend M. Presentation and therapy of myelolipoma. *Int. J. Urol.* 2005;12:239–243.

40. Park BK, Kim B, Ko K, Jeong SY, Kwon GY. Adrenal masses falsely diagnosed as adenomas on unenhanced and delayed contrast–enhanced computed tomography: pathological correlation. *Eur. Radiol.* 2006;16:642–647.

46 Pheochromocytoma

Andrew Solomon and Pierre Bouloux

> **Key points**
> - Pheochromocytoma is an important secondary cause of hypertension and has a variety of clinical presentations.
> - Genetic screening is essential in familial cases and may be extended in future.
> - Investigation ideally requires biochemical confirmation of catecholamine excess followed by localization.
> - Radiological investigation may involve a variety of modalities with recent promising data arising from positron emission tomography scans.
> - Management of pheochromocytoma is medical followed by surgical; lifelong follow-up is essential.

Introduction

Pheochromocytomas and paragangliomas are chromaffin cell tumors of the sympathetic nervous system characterized by hypersecretion of catecholamines and their metabolites. Pheochromocytomas were termed as such (*phaios* = dusky color) by Pick in 1912 and are adrenomedullary tumors; paragangliomas are extra-adrenal tumors arising from the medullary neural crest.

They are uncommon, "often sought but rarely found," and occur at a rate of 1–8 per million per annum with maximum incidence between 20 and 50 years. However, the condition may occur at any age, including in children and during pregnancy (see below). Ante-mortem diagnosis is more likely in younger patients, in whom extra-adrenal and multifocal tumors are more common. Overall approximately 10% of tumors are bilateral, malignant, or extra-adrenal. Bilateral tumors are more likely to be associated with a familial syndrome. In those over 60, in whom an incidence nearer 1 in 2500 is found at autopsy, it is thought that altered baroreceptor reflexes and symptoms attributed to cardiac or cerebrovascular disease make it more likely to remain undiagnosed. Pheochromocytomas carry a mortality of 70–80% in the case of an untreated hypertensive crisis; however, successful surgery effects a cure rate of around 75% with approximately <2% perioperative mortality in expert centers. Treatment of pheochromocytoma aims to counteract excessive catecholamine secretion whilst ensuring optimal end-organ function. Following definitive therapy, follow-up is life-long; 5-year survival rates for benign and malignant tumors are around 96% and 44% respectively. Paragangliomas are more likely to be malignant and to recur. Pheochromocytomas are the underlying cause in 0.1–0.5% of those with hypertension and around 4% of those with adrenal incidentalomas – this figure is higher in those genetic conditions with a raised baseline risk such as multiple endocrine neoplasia 2 (MEN 2) and neurofibromatosis 1 (NF1).

Pheochromocytoma in pregnancy

Pheochromocytoma occurring in pregnancy is rare with only around 250 cases reported, with a key diagnostic challenge being to differentiate it from pre-eclampsia. Early resection of the tumor and careful medical follow-up are advised for successful *in utero* development and later delivery. The second trimester is thought to be the optimal time for surgery – a diagnosis made in the third trimester may be managed medically with resection at the time of cesarean section or soon after vaginal delivery. At least four cases of successful laparoscopic surgery for pheochromocytoma in pregnancy have been reported. All involved preoperative alpha blockade, and delivery of a healthy infant at term [1]. It has been noted that a cautious approach should be taken when creating the CO_2 pneumoperitoneum during such procedures.

Molecular genetics

A significantly increased understanding of the genetics of this condition has occurred in recent years, with a higher hereditary basis for pheochromocytoma uncovered than previously thought [2]. There have been five major susceptibility genes identified (*RET/VHL/SDHB/SDHD/SDHC*), the latter being associated with subunits of the succinate dehydrogenase gene – SHD (see Table 46.1). The three genes *SDHB* (Chr1p36), *SDHC* (Chr1q21) and *SDHD* (Chr1q23) encode three of the four subunits of mitochondrial complex II – succinate dehydrogenase. There is now an accessible SDH genetic database available on the internet

Clinical Endocrine Oncology, 2nd edition. Edited by Ian D. Hay and John A.H. Wass. © 2008 Blackwell Publishing. ISBN 978-1-4051-4584-8.

Table 46.1 Familial conditions at increased risk of pheochromocytoma

Familial condition	Estimated risk of pheochromocytoma	Genetic basis
MEN 2A	50%	*RET* proto-oncogene
MEN 2B	50%	*RET* proto-oncogene
Familial paraganglioma syndrome	Est. 20%	*SDHD, SDHB*
Neurofibromatosis 1	1%	*NF1*
von Hippel–Lindau	10–20%	*VHL*

including both mutations and non-pathogenic polymorphisms [3]. Mutations of these genes are specifically associated with hereditary paraganglioma syndrome (HPS). SDHD mutations confer a risk associated with the gender of the transmitting parent; age-dependent autosomal dominant paternal transmission occurs with maternal imprinting, i.e., the maternally derived gene being inactivated [4]. The risk of tumor development appears to be increased at higher altitudes in SDHD.

Recently, careful genotype–phenotype correlation in patients with the SDHB or SDHD mutations has been performed, with a preponderance of extra-adrenal and/or malignant disease found in SDHB carriers and SDHD carriers having a higher likelihood of head and neck paragangliomas plus multifocality [5].

A recent large series describing genetic screening of unselected cases has been published [6]. Over 300 patients with pheochromocytoma or functional paraganglioma were investigated, over 250 of which were apparently sporadic. The apparently sporadic group were found to harbor an 11.6% germline mutation rate.

The reasons for these findings include *de novo* mutations, an incomplete family history, or maternal genomic imprinting in SDHD carriers.

Inherited cases are often younger, with a more likely multifocal or extra-adrenal tumor.

These data have led some commentators to suggest that genetic screening is performed in all patients and that investigations are performed to seek any unsuspected findings associated with MEN 2, NF1 or von Hippel–Lindau disease (VHL). A practical approach may be to offer genetic testing to patients aged under 50 at presentation, including children. However, the sensitivity of genetic information requires explicit consent and the availability of appropriate genetic counseling.

Pathology

Biosynthesis of catecholamines occurs in central nervous system nuclei, sympathetic neurons and chromaffin cells. Chromaffin granules in pheochromocytomas are similar to those in the normal adrenal medulla. Chromaffin cells, including those found in the brain and adrenal medulla, express the phenylethanolamine-*N*-methyltransferase (PNMT) enzyme. PNMT is necessary for the methylation of norepinephrine (noradrenaline) to epinephrine (adrenaline) and is cortisol dependent. The metabolism of catecholamines occurs via two enzymatic pathways: catechol-*o*-methyltransferase (COMT) and monoamine oxidase (MAO). COMT converts epinephrine to metanephrine and norepinephrine to normetanephrine. Metanephrine and normetanephrine are oxidized MAO to vanillylmandelic acid (VMA) by oxidative deamination. MAO has an important role in regulating norepinephrine and dopamine metabolism; intravesical stores of norepinephrine are increased by MAO inhibitors. Small tumors (<50 g) have a rapid metabolic turnover, often releasing unmetabolized contents into the plasma and thus explaining how smaller tumors may cause disproportionately severe symptoms. The PNMT enzyme will not be activated as avidly in larger tumors which may outstrip corticomedullary blood supply, therefore they tend to secrete less epinephrine relative to norepinephrine; paragangliomas usually lack PNMT and therefore predominantly secrete norepinephrine.

Because of increased activation of the sympathetic nervous system (SNS), any stimulus affecting the SNS may increase norepinephrine release and precipitate a hypertensive crisis. Crises can occur without marked changes in circulating catecholamines and conversely, blood pressure may remain normal in the face of markedly raised plasma catecholamine concentrations.

Additional products secreted from these tumors include opioids and a range of peptides such as calcitonin, calcitonin gene-related peptide (CGRP), gastrin, serotonin, vasoactive intestinal peptide (VIP), neuropeptide Y (NPY), adrenocorticotropic hormone (ACTH), parathyroid hormone (PTH) and its related peptide, PTHrp – each potentially causing their attendant syndromes. Co-secretion of NPY has been claimed as a co-factor for catecholamine mediated vasoconstriction. It is thought to be involved in the mechanism of hypertensive crisis precipitated by tumor manipulation, despite adequate preoperative alpha blockade [7].

Presentation

In terms of clinical presentation, the triad of headache, palpitations and sweating is the syndrome [8] with highest specificity for the diagnosis; in addition paroxysms sometimes known as "spells" occur in only 10–17% of patients – characteristically similar in any individual patient. Pheochromocytoma is a great mimic and a wide variety of presentations have been reported. Common clinical features include palpitations, sweating, pallor, anxiety, pulmonary edema, paralytic ileus, angina and myocardial infarct or stroke. More unusual symptoms include paresthesia, pulsatile scotomas and hemianopia. Certain symptoms may assist with localization of paragangliomas; for example, if occurring in association with micturition this may suggest the presence of a bladder paraganglioma. Weight loss, pallor, orthostatic hypotension and vomiting are commonly overlooked features. In addition, objective measures of labile blood pressure, tachyarrhythmias, cardiomyopathy and "unexplained" lactic acidosis should all alert the physician to the diagnosis.

The differential diagnosis includes thyrotoxicosis, anxiety states, menopausal vasomotor symptoms, illicit drug use, alcohol and caffeine intake/withdrawal, monoamine oxidase inhibitors (MAOI) and tyramine-containing foods, autonomic dysfunction (e.g., in spinal injury, Guillain–Barré syndrome, acute intermittent porphyria, lead poisoning and abrupt withdrawal of drugs including clonidine, methyldopa and beta blockers).

Diagnosis of pheochromocytoma

There are a large number of modalities for the biochemical investigation of suspected pheochromocytoma (Table 46.2). In cases of high clinical suspicion, biochemical tests alone can provide diagnostic specificity of 95% [9]. Urinary VMA estimations

Table 46.2 Indications for screening

Young hypertensive patient
Unexplained shock
Abnormal blood pressure response to anesthesia or surgery
Hypertension refractory to several antihypertensives
Family history of pheochromocytoma, medullary carcinoma of thyroid or MEN
Neurofibromatosis or café-au-lait spots
von Hippel–Lindau syndrome
Sturge–Weber syndrome
Tuberous sclerosis
Ataxia–telangiectasia
Acromegaly
Cushing disease
Radiological evidence of adrenal mass, i.e., incidentaloma

Table 46.3 Drugs interfering with urine catecholamine measurements*

Antihypertensives and vasodilators
    ACE inhibitors
    Alpha$_1$-adrenergic blockers
    Alpha$_2$-agonists
    Beta blockers
    Calcium channel blockers
    Hydralazine
    Labetalol
Analgesics, e.g., acetaminophen, aspirin
Antibiotics, e.g., tetracycline, oxytetracycline
Antipsychotics
Bromocriptine
Drug withdrawal, e.g., alcohol, clonidine
Sympathomimetics, e.g., amphetamines, ephedrine
Stimulants, e.g., caffeine
Tricyclic antidepressants

*Depending on the assay.
ACE, angiotensin-converting enzyme.

are not found in modern protocols. The more recent forms of investigation employ measurement of catecholamines in the plasma/urine, and/or assessment of plasma/urinary metanephrines. Adjustments need to be made in cases of impaired renal function. Laboratories generally use HPLC (high performance liquid chromatography) with electrochemical detection for assays of catecholamines. In terms of urine testing, 24-h urine collection in 6 M HCl is standard – the acid stabilizes the sample; a higher pH may lower values. Random (or timed) urine samples for catecholamine/creatinine ratio can also be performed, such as during a crisis or in pediatric patients.

Plasma catecholamines may be a useful investigation in specific patients and should ideally be taken in symptomatic patients, especially when hypertensive, from an indwelling cannula after lying supine for at least 20 min. In a hypertensive individual, if the plasma norepinephrine concentration is found to be normal, the diagnosis of pheochromocytoma is very unlikely. The sensitivity and specificity of various biochemical testing methods have achieved an excellent level of understanding as a result of large well-characterized series [2] (Fig. 46.1).

Diagnostic techniques

24-h urine for unmetabolized or free catecholamines

Nearly all pheochromocytomas excrete elevated quantities of catecholamine metabolites (VMA and metanephrines) or free catecholamines. The larger tumors tend to secrete more metabolites due to intrinsic metabolic activity. A 24-h urine collection for urinary metanephrines or catecholamines is usually undertaken, but an overnight sample may be of similar accuracy and more convenient [10]. When collecting urine catecholamines, patients do not need to be on a vanilla-free diet, but must ensure collection is in an acid-containing bottle and that care is taken in terms of avoiding drugs that may cause assay interference (Table 46.3). Often a larger tumor will produce catecholamine metabolites (pre-metabolized within the tumor); smaller tumors may secrete more free catecholamines.

Plasma catecholamines

Plasma catecholamines are most useful during symptomatic episodes or during dynamic testing. Plasma norepinephrine levels exceeding 10 nmol/L or epinephrine levels exceeding 1.5 nmol/L give a high specificity*. Elevated plasma epinephrine levels suggest the tumor is of adrenal origin. Plasma catecholamines are elevated by caffeine, nicotine, exercise and certain medications. (*To convert epinephrine or normetanephrine from nmol/L to pg/mL, multiply by 183; for norepinephrine multiply by 169; and for metanephrine multiply by 197.)

Plasma free and urinary metanephrines

The measurement of plasma free metanephrines is generating significant interest, suggesting that this may become a diagnostic modality of choice in the future and is regarded as the most

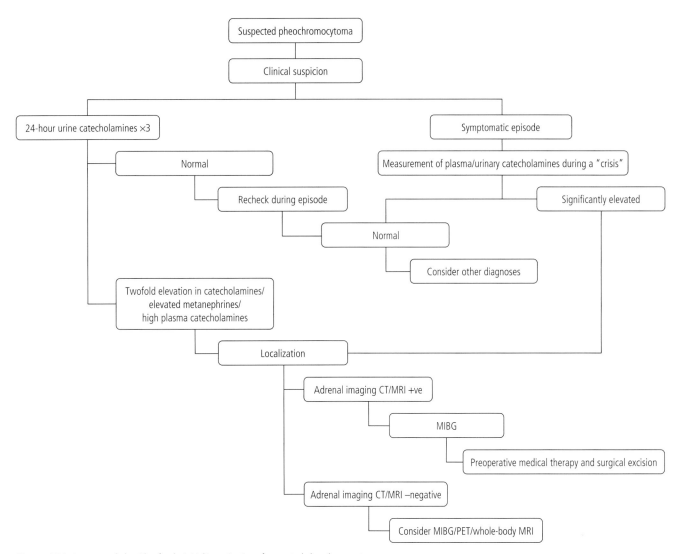

Figure 46.1 A suggested algorithm for the initial investigation of suspected pheochromocytoma.

sensitive biochemical test. If the values obtained are 3.5- to four fold above the reference range, a high level of specificity is also obtained. Recent data suggest that plasma metanephrines may provide information about the size and location of the tumor. These results were obtained from a retrospective analysis of 275 pheochromocytoma patients, followed by a prospective study of 16 additional patients [11]. Eisenhofer et al. then went on to create a sophisticated linear regression analysis incorporating a "relative tumor epinephrine content" and differentiation of a "noradrenergic" phenotype of extra-adrenal tumors to predict size and location in the prospective cohort to a correlation of $r = 0.87$ ($p < 0.001$). However, despite these data several large centers disagree on the optimal plasma investigation, partly due to up to a 15% false-positive rate of plasma metanephrines. A systematic review assessing this technique has recently been published [12]. The authors concluded that this test had a sensitivity of 96–100% and specificity of 85–100%, i.e., that a negative test could rule out pheochromocytoma. In addition urinary-fractionated metanephrines (normetanephrine

and metanephrine separately) have become increasingly available. The basis of these tests' higher sensitivity is the production of O-methylated metabolites independent of the variability of catecholamine release. In order to avoid false-positive diagnoses using these techniques, relative diagnostic likelihood can be proposed using a variety of cut-off reference ranges (Table 46.4).

In addition, it has been noted that false positive results have been associated with pharmacological effects, notably phenoxybenzamine and tricyclic antidepressants.

Plasma chromogranin A

This test is widely used in the field of neuroendocrine tumors. For pheochromocytoma, it has a sensitivity of 86% but a low specificity [7].

Venous sampling

Venous sampling is occasionally performed but is of some risk; alpha and beta blockade should be administered prior to the

Table 46.4 Biochemical test cut-off points – based on a reference group of 644 patients

	Presence of pheochromocytoma unlikely	Presence of pheochromocytoma likely
Urine		
Urinary norepinephrine (nmol/24 h)	<500	>1180
Urinary epinephrine (nmol/24 h)	<100	>170
Blood		
Norepinephrine (nmol/L)	<3.00	>7.70
Epinephrine (nmol/L)	<0.45	>1.20
Free normetanephrine (nmol/L)	<0.6	>1.4
Free metanephrine (nmol/L)	<0.3	>0.42

To convert epinephrine or normetanephrine from nmol/L to pg/mL, multiply by 183; for norepinephrine multiply by 169; and for metanephrine multiply by 197.

procedure. Reversal of the norepinephrine:epinephrine ratio ($N < 1$) in the adrenal vein is suggestive of the diagnosis.

In general, the urgency with which diagnostic information is required combined with local laboratory protocol will have significant influence on the tests actually employed. Optimal sensitivity, to avoid missing false-negative results, is more important in emergency situations. In some centers, the results of 24-h urine collections can be obtained within hours of delivery to the laboratory; in some random urine samples may be most rapidly analyzed; few centers have rapid analysis of plasma free metanephrines. In terms of imaging, CT is the modality that is most readily accessible in a state of urgency.

Radiological localization

Imaging of pheochromocytoma provides information about the site, size and nature of the mass as well as the possible identification of metastases. In addition, pheochromocytoma may be suspected following imaging for alternative indications such in the case of the adrenal "incidentaloma" [13].

• *Computerized tomography (CT) and/or magnetic resonance imaging (MRI) with or without contrast enhancement* are utilized in the vast majority of patients and are the first-line imaging modalities offering high sensitivity and – with most tumors being >3 cm – they are often visualized; however, specificity of these modalities is only around 70%. Contrast-enhanced CT is thought to be relatively safe using non-ionic media without the use of alpha blockade, although it is still advisable. Around 12% of tumors demonstrate speckled calcification and pheochromocytomas intensely enhance with contrast. Pheochromocytomas usually provide high intensity signal on T2 MRI; chemical-shift imaging is used to differentiate from lipid-containing adrenal adenomas; MRI is the preferred modality for extra-adrenal tumors or those in pregnant women or children (Fig. 46.2). CT is the usual modality for the detection of adrenal "incidentalomas,"

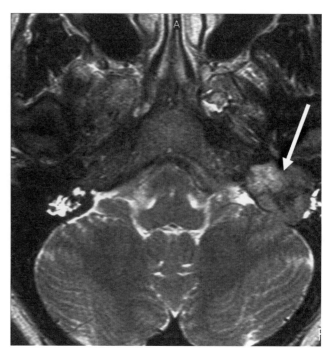

Figure 46.2 MRI scan showing left-sided norepinephrine-secreting glomus jugulare paraganglioma as part of the familial paraganglioma syndrome.

which are then screened for evidence of excessive catecholamine secretory activity. They typically enhance avidly. It should be remembered that the use of traditional iodinated contrast when imaging pheochromocytomas is regarded as risky, possibly improved by the use of non-ionic media [14].

• *Metaiodobenzylguanidine (MIBG)* is a compound similar to norepinephrine that is taken up by adrenergic tissue. This type of scan, after administration of [131]I- or ^{123}I-labeled MIBG, is especially useful in cases of extra-adrenal, residual or metastatic disease. It has around 90–96% sensitivity and 98–99% specificity. Following intravenous injection of MIBG, the patient is scanned at both 24 and 48–72 h. Potentially interfering drugs should be discontinued several weeks before the scan (Table 46.5). Radionuclide ^{123}I-MIBG scanning may be used intraoperatively.

Table 46.5 Drugs interfering with MIBG uptake*

Antihypertensives and vasodilators
    ACE inhibitors
    Alpha$_1$-adrenergic blockers
    Calcium channel blockers
    Labetalol
    Reserpine
Antipsychotics
Cocaine
Opioids
Sympathomimetics
Tricyclic antidepressants

*Depending on the assay.

Table 46.6 Comparison of sensitivity and specificity of diagnostic methods

Test	Sensitivity (%)	Specificity (%)
24-h urine catecholamines ×2	86	88
Plasma free metanephrines	99	85
Urinary-fractionated metanephrines	97	69
Urinary VMA	65	86
MRI	98	70
CT	93	70
MIBG	80	95

• *Octreotide scanning* relies on the presence of somatostatin receptors on the surface of these tumors. When used, the spleen may affect the quality of adrenal imaging.

• *Positron emission tomography (PET)* has become widely used in clinical oncology. Tumor-specific agents have been developed to image pheochromocytomas in addition to the commonly used [18F]-fluorodeoxyglucose. They include [11C]-hydroxyephedrine, [11C]-epinephrine and 6-18F-fluorodopamine. 6-18F-fluorodopamine has been shown to identify some confirmed pheochromocytomas not seen on ^{131}I-MIBG scanning. It is likely that in endocrine oncology in general and pheochromocytoma in particular, PET scanning will become an increasingly available, highly informative imaging modality [15].

Table 46.6 compares the sensitivity and specificity of the different methods.

Treatment of pheochromocytoma

Definitive therapy for pheochromocytomas is surgical, with medical therapy used perioperatively and in metastatic disease. Surgery, or at least debulking of the tumor, is the primary management strategy. The regime of alpha blockade, followed after 48 h by beta blockade is now standard. Ideally, complete excision of pheochromocytomas leads to normotension, usually in around 75% of cases. Essential hypertension may be still present after therapy.

Perioperative management

Preoperative

Phenoxybenzamine is initiated at a dose of 10 mg once daily, increasing to twice, then three times daily, later 10–20 mg four times daily. Usually a total dose of around 1 mg/kg will be sufficient. Initiation of alpha blockade can cause severe hypotension and volume filling is recommended. Further adverse effects of phenoxybenzamine include tachycardia, miosis, nasal congestion, diarrhea and fatigue. Intravenous phenoxybenzamine may be infused for 2–3 h each day for 3 days prior to surgery (0.5 mg/kg intravenously in 500 ml normal saline). The beta$_1$/beta$_2$ agonist propranolol is then added at a dose of 40–80 mg three times

daily; other beta blockers also used include nadolol, atenolol (e.g., starting at 25 mg once daily) or metoprolol (approx. 50 mg three times daily). Side effects of beta blockers include cool peripheries, bradycardia and postural hypotension. Labetalol is usually avoided as it may precipitate a hypertensive crisis.

Selective alpha-1 antagonists such as terazosin, prazosin and doxazosin are also used in some centers – they tend to reduce reflex tachycardia. An alternative approach is to use a calcium channel blocker (e.g., nicardipine) or metyrosine in the preoperative regimen. In cases of proven or suspected bilateral tumors, perioperative hydrocortisone is advised to prevent the risk of adrenal insufficiency. There is increasing interest in newer calcium channel blockers such as urapidil, used safely in a recently reported series of 18 patients [16].

The alpha-blockade pretreatment may be performed as an outpatient and adequate preoperative preparation has been suggested as a blood pressure well below 160/90 mmHg for over 24 h and minimal occurrence of ventricular ectopics on electrocardiogram (ECG).

Intraoperative management

The surgical approach to pheochromocytoma is now usually laparoscopic with conversion rates to an open procedure of 5–10%. Adrenal cortex-sparing partial adrenalectomies have been attempted in certain familial cases to preserve functional glucocorticoid-secreting tissue. A recent analysis of 165 operations at a single center suggested a 2.4% perioperative mortality rate including a 7.8% rate of splenectomy [17]. If splenectomy is envisaged – for left-sided tumors – it is prudent to provide pneumococcal and influenza vaccination preoperatively and thereafter.

In terms of the anesthetic approach, careful attention is given to continuous ECG and blood pressure monitoring, with bolus doses of phentolamine and sodium nitroprusside being useful for hypertensive episodes. Minimization of tumor palpation by the surgeon will be helpful in this respect. Intravenous propranolol or lidocaine may be used for arrhythmias; peri-arrest arrhythmias may require management according to standard protocols. Magnesium has been increasingly advocated as a useful agent in perioperative management, first described in 1985. Magnesium ions inhibit the release of catecholamines from the normal adrenal medulla and adrenergic terminals. It acts as an alpha-antagonist and antiarrhythmic. Suggested dosage is 40–60 mg/kg, often supplemented at the time of tumor manipulation. In documented cases, boluses of 1–4 g have been given followed as indicated by infusion at 1–2g/h [18]. However, the evidence for the use of magnesium is not prospective or outcome based and carefully designed trials may be organized in the future.

Postoperative management

This requires optimization of volume status, assisted by blood transfusion in cases of reduced hematocrit. Hypoglycemia, due to reduced catecholamine suppression of insulin secretion, may require dextrose infusion. There have been several published series of perioperative complications [19]. Adverse events are associated with larger tumor size, duration of anesthesia and higher preoperative levels of urinary catecholamines.

In terms of longer-term oral treatment the use of alpha and beta blockade is the therapeutic combination of choice, with a suggestion of a synergistic effect in combination with metyrosine. However, there is increasing use of metyrosine, alpha blockade and calcium channel blockers.

Pheochromocytoma crisis – treatment of a hypertensive crisis

During a pheochromocytoma crisis, the supply–demand mismatch caused by catecholamine-driven tachycardia, increased afterload, and increased myocardial oxygen demand can precipitate serious complications (Table 46.7). Clinically, two or more symptoms may occur simultaneously, with abrupt onset, with most "crises" lasting 15–60 minutes. Subjects often described a sense of impending doom, "that they are about to die," and a severe sense of anxiety. Initial management (Table 46.8) of a hypertensive crisis may involve intravenous boluses of phentolamine. Phentolamine is a short-acting non-selective competitive alpha-adrenergic blocker; its short half-life allows for repeated dosing, every few minutes if necessary. An initial dose of 1 mg can be given, and then extended towards 5 mg boluses or as a continuous infusion of 5–10 µg/kg/min made up as 100 mg phentolamine in 500 ml of 5% dextrose. Phenoxybenzamine may be used as described above, both initially orally or intravenously 0.5 mg/kg intravenously over 2–4 h; side effects include severe hypotension and watershed cerebral infarction. Commencing beta blockade within 24 h is advised. Beta blockade during a hypertensive crisis

Table 46.7 Precipitating factors for hypertensive crisis

Tumor hemorrhage
Raised intrathoracic pressure, e.g., coughing
Exercise
Parturition
Pressure on abdomen
Tumor palpation
Pneumoperitoneum
Drugs – unopposed beta blockade, glucagon, ACTH, anesthetic agents, metoclopramide, tricyclic antidepressants, opiates, intravenous contrast agents, phenothiazines, naloxone, cytotoxic agents, glucagon

Table 46.8 Complications of hypertensive crisis

Myocardial infarction
Cardiac arrhythmias
Cardiogenic shock
Pulmonary edema
Cardiomyopathy
Visual disturbances
Cerebrovascular accident
Hypertensive encephalopathy

may be achieved using esmolol (50–200 mg/kg/min intravenously).

Sodium nitroprusside may be given as a continuous infusion from a light-sensitive bag though it appears to be somewhat less potent. It is used at doses of 0.5 µg/kg/min up to 10 µg/kg/min.

Metyrosine, a competitive inhibitor of tyrosine hydroxylase, may also be used. The starting dose is usually 250 mg twice to four times per day – it may be used alone or in combination with an alpha blocker.

Malignant pheochromocytomas

Malignancy in pheochromocytoma is extremely difficult to predict but is best indicated by the aggressiveness of disease, i.e., size (often 6–8 cm), local invasion or distant metastases. The most common sites of metastasis are bone, lungs, liver and lymph nodes [8]. Although highly variable, 5-year survival rates in the setting of malignant disease average 50%. Histology may be similar to benign disease, although chromosomal ploidy has been suggested as a marker, aneuploidy and tetraploidy suggesting more aggressive disease. Management for malignant disease includes surgical excision or debulking, and long-term antihypertensive therapy. Further therapeutic options include high-dose ^{131}I-MIBG therapy, chemotherapy or radiotherapy. There is a lack of controlled studies in this field, although brief remission is the rule in these tumors which are not generally chemo- or radiosensitive. In addition, radiofrequency ablation or transarterial embolization of hepatic metastases has been performed with some response.

Conclusion

Pheochromocytoma is a heterogeneous neuroendocrine tumor associated with numerous clinical features, a variety of diagnostic modalities and the potential for surgical cure. It requires a high index of suspicion with use of focused biochemical and radiological investigations. In the future, predictive biology associated with disease susceptibility genes and targeted therapies may further improve the outlook for patients with this condition.

References

1. Kim PT, Kreisman SH, Vaughn R, Panton ON. Laparoscopic adrenalectomy for pheochromocytoma in pregnancy. *Can. J. Surg.* 2006;49:62–63.
2. Lenders JW, Eisenhofer G, Mannelli M, Pacak K. Phaeochromocytoma. *Lancet* 2005;366:665–675.
3. Bayley JP, Devilee P, Taschner PE. The SDH mutation database: an online resource for succinate dehydrogenase sequence variants involved in pheochromocytoma, paraganglioma and mitochondrial complex II deficiency. *BMC Med. Genet.* 2005;6:39.
4. Baysal BE. On the association of succinate dehydrogenase mutations with hereditary paraganglioma. *Trends Endocrinol. Metab.* 2003;14: 453–459.

5. Benn DE, Gimenez-Roqueplo AP, Reilly JR, et al. Clinical presentation and penetrance of pheochromocytoma/paraganglioma syndromes. *J. Clin. Endocrinol. Metab.* 2006;91:827–836.

6. Amar L, Bertherat J, Baudin E, et al. Genetic testing in pheochromocytoma or functional paraganglioma. *J. Clin. Oncol.* 2005;23:8812–8818.

7. Bravo EL, Tagle R. Pheochromocytoma: state-of-the-art and future prospects. *Endocr. Rev.* 2003;24:539–553.

8. Kaltsas GA, Papadogias D, Grossman AB. The clinical presentation (symptoms and signs) of sporadic and familial chromaffin cell tumours (phaeochromocytomas and paragangliomas). *Front. Horm. Res.* 2004;31:61–75.

9. Peaston RT, Weinkove C. Measurement of catecholamines and their metabolites. *Ann. Clin. Biochem.* 2004;41(Pt 1):17–38.

10. Peaston RT, Lennard TW, Lai LC. Overnight excretion of urinary catecholamines and metabolites in the detection of pheochromocytoma. *J. Clin. Endocrinol. Metab.* 1996;81:1378–1384.

11. Eisenhofer G, Lenders JW, Goldstein DS, et al. Pheochromocytoma catecholamine phenotypes and prediction of tumor size and location by use of plasma free metanephrines. *Clin. Chem.* 2005;51:735–744.

12. Sawka AM, Prebtani AP, Thabane L, Gafni A, Levine M, Young WF, Jr. A systematic review of the literature examining the diagnostic efficacy of measurement of fractionated plasma free metanephrines in the biochemical diagnosis of pheochromocytoma. *BMC Endocr. Disord.* 2004;4:2.

13. Maurea S, Caraco C, Klain M, Mainolfi C, Salvatore M. Imaging characterization of non-hypersecreting adrenal masses. Comparison between MR and radionuclide techniques. *Q. J. Nucl. Med. Mol. Imaging* 2004;48:188–197.

14. Blake MA, Kalra MK, Maher MM, et al. Pheochromocytoma: an imaging chameleon. *Radiographics* 2004;24 (Suppl 1):S87–S99.

15. Pacak K, Eisenhofer G, Goldstein DS. Functional imaging of endocrine tumors: role of positron emission tomography. *Endocr. Rev.* 2004;25:568–580.

16. Tauzin-Fin P, Sesay M, Gosse P, Ballanger P. Effects of perioperative alpha1 block on haemodynamic control during laparoscopic surgery for phaeochromocytoma. *Br. J. Anaesth.* 2004;92:512–517.

17. Plouin PF, Duclos JM, Soppelsa F, Boublil G, Chatellier G. Factors associated with perioperative morbidity and mortality in patients with pheochromocytoma: analysis of 165 operations at a single center. *J. Clin. Endocrinol. Metab.* 2001;86:1480–1486.

18. James MF, Cronje L. Pheochromocytoma crisis: the use of magnesium sulfate. *Anesth. Analg.* 2004;99:680–686, table.

19. Kinney MA, Warner ME, van Heerden JA, et al. Perianesthetic risks and outcomes of pheochromocytoma and paraganglioma resection. *Anesth. Analg.* 2000;91:1118.

47 Peripheral Neuroblastic Tumors

Bruno De Bernardi, Vito Pistoia, Claudio Gambini, and Claudio Granata

---

Key points

- Peripheral neuroblastic tumors originate from primitive cells of the neural crest and occur prevalently in the early childhood (approximately 10% of pediatric malignancies).
- NT comprise three histotypes: neuroblastoma, ganglioneuroblastoma and ganglioneuroma, characterized by different degrees of differentiation and clinical aggressiveness.
- A number of biological abnormalities have been discovered in NT with *MYCN* oncogene playing a crucial role in patients' outcome.
- Clinical presentation, histological features and biochemical–biological characteristics differ remarkably from one case to another accounting for the great variety of clinical situations ranging from extreme aggressiveness to spontaneous regression.
- Results of treatment are largely unsatisfactory for patients older than 1 year at diagnosis (more than half of cases) presenting with localized invasive and disseminated disease.

Introduction

The term "*peripheral neuroblastic tumors*" (PNT) refers to a group of tumors derived from the primitive cells of the neural crest. The main constituents of PNT are neuroblastoma, ganglioneuroblastoma and ganglioneuroma, which are histologically characterized by a different degree of differentiation and biological features [1].

From the clinical viewpoint, PNT present the greatest degree of behavioral variations among all pediatric neoplasias [2]. Most children older than 1 year at diagnosis (representing two-thirds of all cases) have extensive or metastatic disease at diagnosis and consequently a low probability of being cured with the currently available therapy. On the other hand, a minority of children have a localized resectable tumor that can be cured by surgery alone. Few other children present with localized but unresectable tumors requiring chemotherapy before resection. Lastly, in about 10% of cases (mostly infants, 0–11 months), the tumor tends to regress spontaneously, despite disseminated disease.

In the last few decades there has been a remarkable improvement in both knowledge of the biological characteristics of these tumors and the development of diagnostic techniques [3]. This has led to the delineation of subsets of patients based on clinical and biological features, and to the consequent identification of risk-related therapies [3].

Clinical Endocrine Oncology, 2nd edition. Edited by Ian D. Hay and John A.H. Wass. © 2008 Blackwell Publishing. ISBN 978-1-4051-4584-8.

Etiology and epidemiology

Etiology

The causes of PNT remain unknown. A number of reports have pointed to the possible influence of the intrauterine exposure to various substances including alcohol (fetal alcohol syndrome), anti-epileptic drugs, diuretics, tranquilizers, pain medications, fertility drugs and hair dyes. Other reports have associated a greater incidence of PNT with a variety of parental employment categories including farmers, gardeners, painters and electricians. Some authors have recently observed an increased number of PNT together with BK virus infection. None of these associations have been seen consistently nor have they been confirmed by large studies. However, the role the environment may play in the pathogenesis of PNT cannot yet be ruled out [4].

PNT have been reported with increased frequency in patients with neurofibromatosis type 1 and with Hirschsprung disease, suggesting that they may be part of a spectrum of disorders (neurocristopathies) involving the development of the neural crest.

Epidemiology

PNT represent the most frequent extracranial solid neoplasias in children up to 15 years of age. Boys are more commonly affected than girls, with a male:female ratio of 1.2:1. The overall prevalence is between 8 and 10 new cases per million children per year. PNT prevail in young children and are in fact the most common tumors arising in preschool age children (0–5 years), with median age at diagnosis of approximately 20 months. In addition, PNT represent the majority of the rare tumors diagnosed in the first month of life

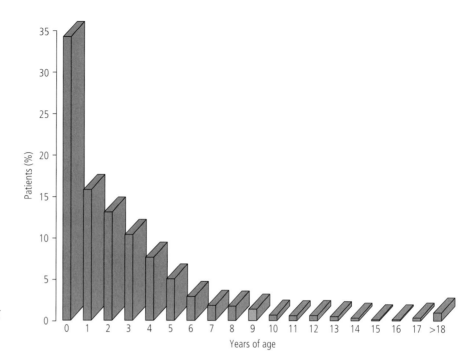

Figure 47.1 Age distribution in 2346 cases of PNT (from the Italian Neuroblastoma Registry, unpublished).

(congenital tumors). In the Italian Neuroblastoma Registry, spanning a 27-year period (1979–2005), 34% of all patients are 1 year old or younger at diagnosis, almost 80% are less than 5 years old, and 95% are less than 10 years old (Fig. 47.1). However, PNT do occur in adolescents (4%) and, albeit rarely, even in adults (1%).

Based on the much better outcome of PNT when diagnosed within the first year of life, in the early 1970s Japanese investigators activated a nation-wide screening program to detect PNT in infancy by measuring the catecholamine metabolite vanillylmandelic acid (VMA) in the urine of 6-month-old infants. This led to a striking increase in the number of identified cases of PNT. However, the overall mortality was not affected since it was later discovered that aggressive PNT appear in children above 1 year of age [5]. Based on these results, this type of screening was recently halted [6]. It is noteworthy that screening to detect urinary tract malformations and hip dislocation in infants also picks up cases of PNT that otherwise would not be identified.

Pathology and genetics

Pathology

PNT are composed of two predominant cell types: neuroblasts and Schwannian cells. Historically, PNT were categorized into three histotypes (neuroblastoma, ganglioneuroblastoma and ganglioneuroma) based on maturation, differentiation and clinical outcome.

Neuroblastoma is composed of small and uniformly sized cells with a dense, hyperchromatic nucleus and scant cytoplasm. The presence of neuritic processes, or neuropil, is a pathognomonic feature of all but the most primitive neuroblastomas. The Homer–Wright pseudorosette, another diagnostic feature of neuroblastoma

which is seen in 15–50% of cases, is composed of neuroblasts surrounding an area of eosinophilic neuropil (Plate 47.1a). Ganglioneuroma is the fully differentiated, benign counterpart of neuroblastoma. It is predominantly composed of Schwannian cells and scattered ganglion cells (Plate 47.1b). The third histotype, ganglioneuroblastoma, defines a heterogeneous group of tumors. Its histopathological features span the two extremes of maturation. Histopathological criteria for classifying these tumors and predicting clinical behavior have varied considerably. The most widely used system, developed by Shimada et al. two decades ago, was age-linked and classified PNT according to the amount of Schwannian cell stroma (poor or rich) and the degree of differentiation of neuroblasts [7]. The more recent International Neuroblastoma Pathology Classification (INPC) adds further features to the Shimada system, thus allowing greater concordance among pathologists [8]. In particular, ganglioneuroblastoma is defined as any tumor bearing both ganglioneuromatous and neuroblastic components. The latter may be observed either as multiple microscopic foci (ganglioneuroblastoma intermixed) (Plate 47.1c), or as distinct macroscopic nodule/s (ganglioneuroblastoma nodular) (Plate 47.1d). Thus, the INPC is now able to identify two prognostically favorable histotypes (ganglioneuroma and ganglioneuroblastoma intermixed). With regards to the remaining two histotypes, ganglioneuroblastoma nodular and neuroblastoma Schwannian stroma-poor, prognosis is defined on the basis of age at diagnosis, degree of differentiation of the neuroblastic component and evaluation of the mitosis–karyorrhexis index (MKI) [8].

Genetics

Several genetic defects have been identified in PNT, such as amplification of chromosomal material, chromosomal gains and losses and aneuploidy that correlate with distinct clinical entities.

In addition, epigenetic mechanisms have been found to contribute to the silencing of some putative tumor suppressor genes.

MYCN gene amplification

This is the most important of the genetic abnormalities detected in PNT, so far. The *MYCN* gene maps on chromosome 2p24 and its overexpression has oncogenic consequences, as unambiguously proven by the neoplastic transformation of normal cells upon *MYCN* transfection, and the generation of transgenic mice overexpressing *MYCN* in neuroectodermal cells that develop neuroblastoma spontaneously [9].

The amplified status of a proto-oncogene is often inferred from the cytogenetic detection of either type of chromosomal abnormality, i.e., homogeneously staining regions (HSR) or double minutes (DM). Although initial observations of neuroblastoma cell lines pointed to HSR as the hallmark of *MYCN* amplification (Plate 47.2a), subsequent studies have demonstrated that DM are the predominant configuration of amplified *MYCN* in primary PNT (Plate 47.2b). DM formation takes place in a chromosomal region other than where the amplified gene maps. Thus, in PNT the normal copies of *MYCN* at 2p24 are retained and the *MYCN* locus may be copied and multiplied extrachromosomally in DM.

MYCN gene copies in PNT cells range from 10 to 500. Analyses of large series of patients have shown that the prevalence of *MYCN* amplification is approximately 20% [1,9]. Localized and stage 4s tumors with amplified *MYCN* have a poor prognosis, whereas the outcome of the majority of stage 4 metastatic tumors is unfavorable, regardless of *MYCN* amplification [9].

1p deletion

The most frequent allelic deletions are loss of heterozygosity (LOH) of various 1p regions, where one or more tumor suppressor genes may map. 1p36 is the primary site of 1p deletion, which is often associated with *MYCN* amplification. In a small percentage of cases 1p deletion is found in the absence of *MYCN* amplification and seems to predict disease progression, but not overall survival [10]. Attempts at identifying the tumor suppressor gene(s) that have been deleted in the 1p regions of allelic deletions have been unsuccessful so far. Allelic losses of other chromosomal regions, such as 1p, 11q, 2q, 3p, 4p, 9p and 14q, have been detected in PNT.

17q gain

Another karyotypic abnormality that is consistently detected in more than half of PNT is trisomy for the long arm of chromosome 17 (17q), which often occurs as part of an unbalanced translocation between chromosomes 1 and 17. 17q gain is associated with an aggressive course of the disease [11]. The underlying mechanism may be the fusion of a gene flanking the 17q breakpoint or a dosage effect of gene mapping in the extra 17q region, such as nm23-H1, nm23-H2 and survivin, a member of the inhibitor of apoptosis proteins that is upregulated in many types of cancer. Other segmental gains have been detected on 1q, 5q, and 18q, but their characterizations are still lacking.

Aneuploidy

Aneuploidy means gain or loss of one or more chromosomes of a diploid genome and is a marker of genetic instability. Near-diploid and near-tetraploid PNT are typically found in patients older than 1 year of age in association with 1p deletion and *MYCN* amplification. These features are commonly associated with unfavorable prognosis [12]. In contrast, hyperdiploidy or near triploidy is detected in the tumors of patients below 1 year of age or in low-risk tumors (stage 1, 2 and 4s), that collectively carry a favorable prognosis and do not show structural chromosomal rearrangements [12].

Epigenetic silencing of caspase 8

Silencing of the caspase 8 gene through methylation of a 5′-flanking sequence is a common event in high-risk PNT. Caspase 8 is activated by most members of the TNF superfamily and triggers cell apoptosis. It acts as a tumor suppressor gene in many tumors, and its silencing in PNT, commonly associated with *MYCN* amplification, is prognostically unfavorable [13].

Clinical presentation, diagnosis and staging

Clinical presentation

The fact that NT may arise from any site along the chain of the sympathetic nervous system or in adrenal medulla accounts for the remarkable variety of locations of the primary tumor [1]. Table 47.1 lists the sites of the primary tumor and the relative

Table 47.1 Features of PNT in relation to primary tumor sites

Tumor site	Main symptoms and signs	Incidence (%)	Mets (%)	Outcome
Neck	Mass mimicking an adenopathy Horner syndrome	4	2	Good
Thorax				
Upper	Respiratory symptoms	6	5	Good
Lower	Accidental X-ray detection	6	2	Good
Abdomen	Central or lateral mass; symptoms related to metastatic disease (fever, pallor, anorexia, bone pain, change of mood)	70	75	Poor
Pelvis	Hypogastric mass, dysuria, stipsis	5	5	Good
Not identified	Fever, pallor, anorexia, bone pain, change of mood	1	100	Very poor
Multicentric (stage 4s)	Hepatomegaly, skin nodules	8	100	Good

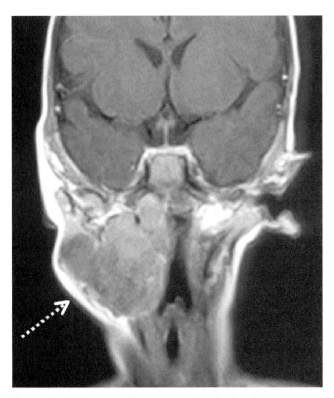

Figure 47.2 MRI T1-weighted image, coronal view, showing a large, irregular right cervical mass in close contact with the upper airway.

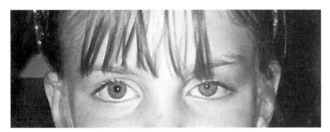

Figure 47.3 Claude Bernard Horner syndrome (anisocoria, proptosis, enophthalmos) as only clinical evidence of cervical NT.

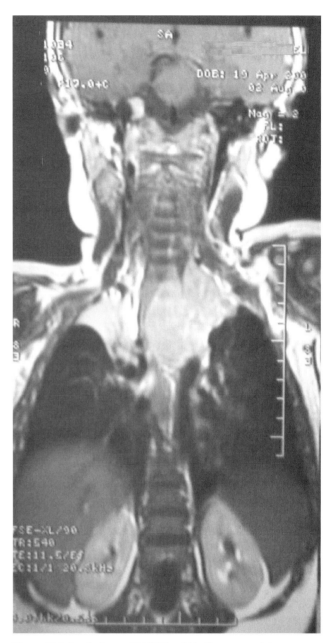

Figure 47.4 Female, 5 years old. MRI T1-weighted image, coronal view. Left cervicomediastinal mass crossing the midline. Trachea, esophagus, superior vena cava and aorta are encased by the mass.

symptoms, incidence, percentage of metastatic spread and outcome. Cervical tumors (4% of cases) mimic aspecific adenopathies and may reach a large size (Fig. 47.2). Horner syndrome is often present (Fig. 47.3). The thoracic locations of PNT represent 15% of the cases. While tumors in the upper mediastinum cause respiratory distress (Fig. 47.4), those arising in the middle and lower mediastinum are usually asymptomatic and are discovered by routine chest X-ray (Fig. 47.5). The abdomen is by far the most frequent location of PNT. The tumor may arise either in the adrenal gland (Fig. 47.6a), and be palpable as a lateral mass, or in the paravertebral or celiac ganglia (Fig. 47.6b), where it is commonly found as a central, hard, fixed, non-tender mass. Pelvic tumors are uncommon and present as suprapubic masses causing stipsis and urinary disturbances (Fig. 47.7).

Approximately half the patients have disseminated disease at the time of diagnosis, with bone marrow (Fig. 47.8) and skeleton

(Fig. 47.9) being the most commonly involved organs [1–3]. Disseminated disease is usually associated with aspecific symptoms, such as fever, pallor, anorexia, bone pain with consequent refusal to walk, and change of mood. Retro-orbital and orbital metastases are rather frequent and produce a typical appearance of proptosis and periorbital ecchymoses. Occasionally, metastatic spread is the only way the disease appears and it is associated with an especially poor prognosis. In infants, massive liver involvement, with or without the presence of bluish nodules in the subcutaneous tissue and infiltration of the bone marrow identifies stage 4s

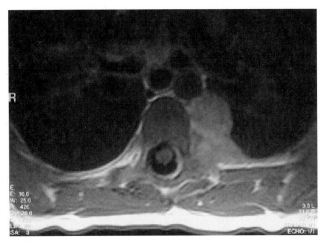

Figure 47.5 Male, 12 years old. MRI T1-weighted image, axial view, shows a left paravertebral thoracic mass. The adjacent vertebral foramina are involved without invasion of spinal canal.

(s meaning special), a peculiar clinical pattern commonly evolving toward spontaneous regression. In adolescents and adults PNT have a slow, indolent clinical course compared to children, although the distribution of primary site and pattern of metastases are similar. PNT in older patients have poor sensitivity to chemotherapy [14].

The anatomical connection between the sympathetic nervous system and spinal cord accounts for the propensity of PNT to infiltrate the intervertebral foramina, as documented by magnetic resonance imaging (MRI) in approximately one-third of patients [15]. However, only 5–8% of patients have clinical evidence of epidural compression (Fig. 47.10). Early detection of this phenomenon is crucial because symptoms may rapidly worsen, leading the child to irreversible paraplegia.

In 1–2% of cases NT present with opsoclonus–myoclonus syndrome, which includes ataxia, myoclonic movements, and erratic nystagmus ("dancing eyes" and "dancing feet" syndrome). These symptoms may precede the detection of a tumor mass and

(a)   (b)

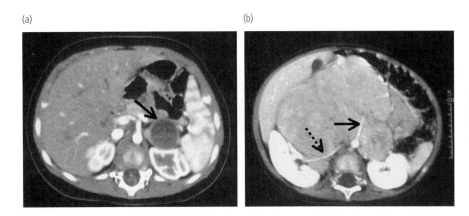

Figure 47.6 (a) Male, 5 months old. Contrast enhanced CT. Left suprarenal mass (black arrow). The mass does not encase any vital organ or large vessel. (b) Male, 3 years old. Contrast enhanced CT. Huge abdominal retroperitoneal mass displacing bowel loops and both kidneys. Aorta, celiac axis (black arrow) and renal vessels (black dotted arrow) are encased.

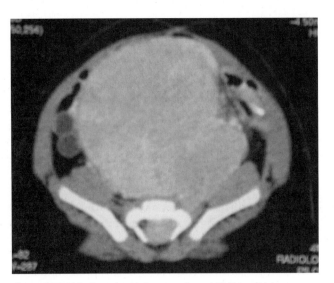

Figure 47.7 Male, 6 months old. Contrast-enhanced CT. Huge, slightly dishomogeneous pelvic mass displacing bowel loops.

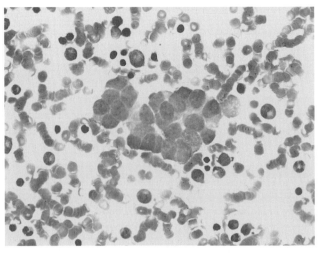

Figure 47.8 Bone marrow aspirate showing an aggregate of tumor cells (pseudorosette).

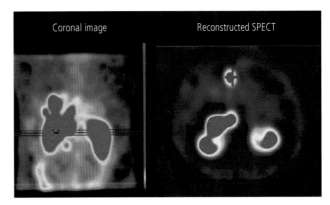

Plate 7.1 Image of ⁹⁰yttrium-octreotide obtained at 24 h in a patient with a malignant insulinoma with a liver metastasis. The primary site and liver metastasis are well shown, particularly in the SPECT image.

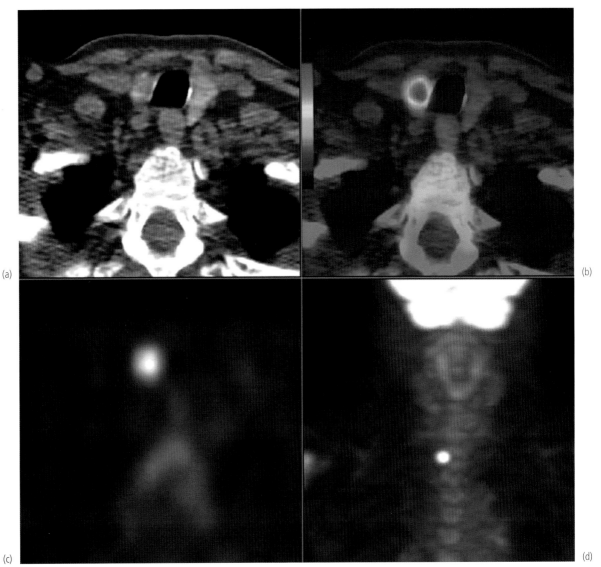

(a)

(b)

(c)

(d)

Plate 14.1 CT (a) and FDG PET with (b) and without (c and d) fused CT of a patient with a incidentally discovered solitary papillary thyroid carcinoma.

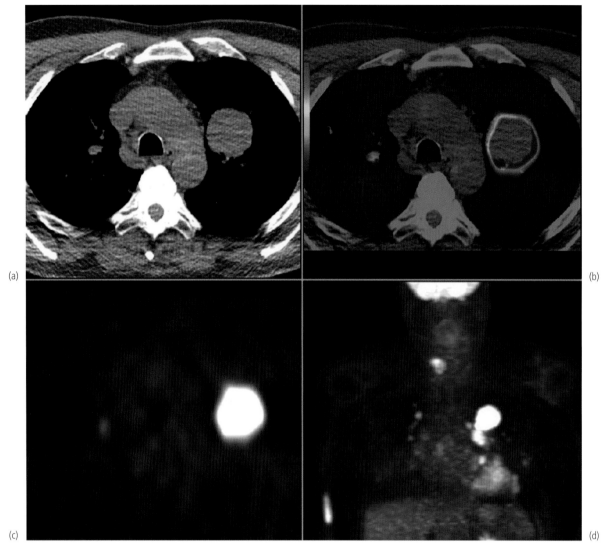

(a)

(b)

(c)

(d)

Plate 14.2 CT (a) and FDG PET with (b) and without (c and d) fused CT of a patient with left lung mass and multiple small lung tumors of metastatic papillary thyroid carcinoma. There is also a right neck recurrence.

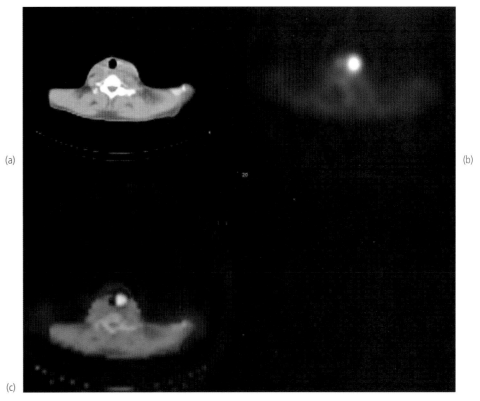

Plate 14.3 Recurrent thyroid carcinoma in the left neck is seen on CT (a), SPECT (tomographic) Octreoscan®
imaging (b), and SPECT Octreoscan® image fused with CT (c).

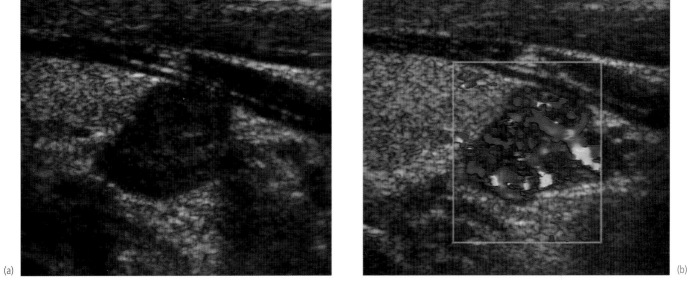

Plate 14.4 Hypervascular parathyroid adenoma at ultrasound both without (a) and with (b) color Doppler.

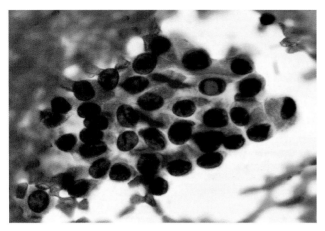

Plate 16.1 Photomicrograph (×400 magnification) of smear from fine needle aspiration biopsy of papillary thyroid carcinoma, illustrating characteristic nuclear changes including nuclear enlargement, crispness of nuclear contours, longitudinal grooves, and cytoplasmic intranuclear inclusion. (Courtesy of Prof. Thomas J. Sebo, Mayo Clinic.)

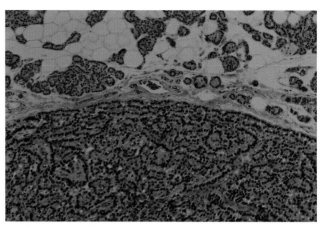

Plate 21.2 Parathyroid adenoma with mostly chief cells with follicle formation and no fat present. Note the rim of normal parathyroid gland with fat present. Hematoxylin and eosin, ×200. (Courtesy of Ricardo V. Lloyd, MD, Mayo Clinic, Rochester, MN.)

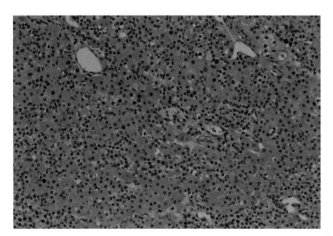

Plate 21.1 Parathyroid adenoma composed of a mix of chief and oxyphil cells with no fat present. Hematoxylin and eosin, ×200. (Courtesy of Ricardo V. Lloyd, MD, Mayo Clinic, Rochester, MN).

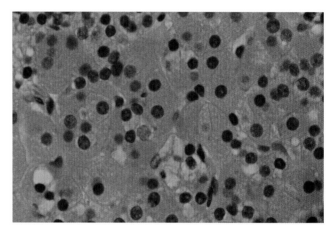

Plate 21.3 Parathyroid adenoma with mostly oxyphil cells and no fat present. Hematoxylin and eosin, ×400. (Courtesy of Ricardo V. Lloyd, MD, Mayo Clinic, Rochester, MN.)

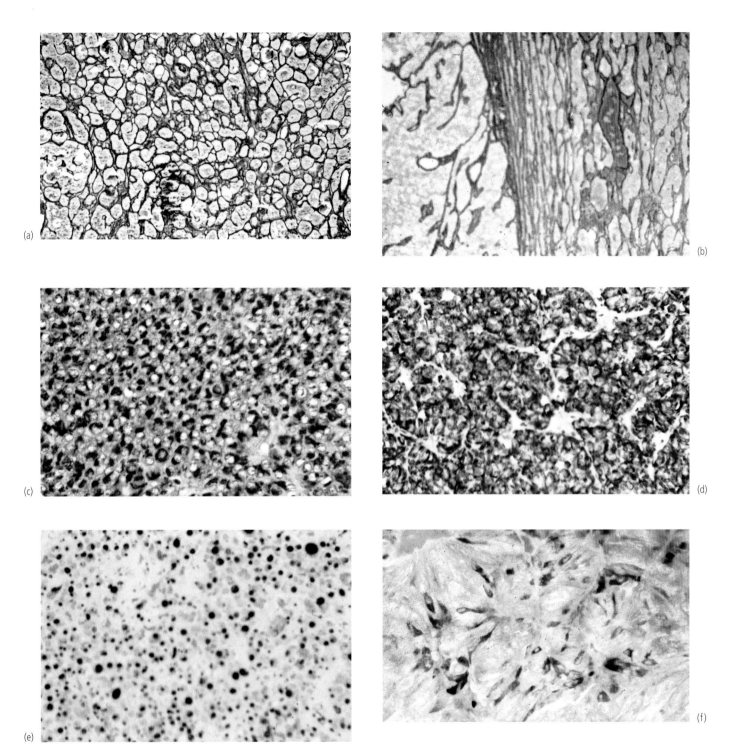

Plate 26.1 (a) Normal acinar architecture of human adenohypophysis as shown by the Gordon–Sweet silver technique for reticulin. Original magnification ×10.
(b) Within adenomas, the normal reticulin fiber network is broken down (left), whereas the reticulin fiber network of the surrounding non-tumorous gland (right) is stretched and condensed into a so-called pseudocapsule. Gordon–Sweet reticulin technique. Original magnification ×10. (c) The characteristic pattern of PRL immunoreactivity, outlining the Golgi apparatus, is shown in a PRL cell adenoma. Original magnification ×40. (d) Densely granulated GH cell adenoma displaying generalized immunoreactivity for GH. Original magnification ×25. (e) Immunostaining for cytokeratin demonstrates strong immunopositivity in the intracytoplasmic spherical fibrous bodies in a sparsely granulated GH cell adenoma. Original magnification ×25. (f) Immunostaining for FSH demonstrates immunoreactivity as well as the characteristic pseudorosette arrangement of the polar adenoma cells of a gonadotroph cell adenoma. Original magnification ×25.

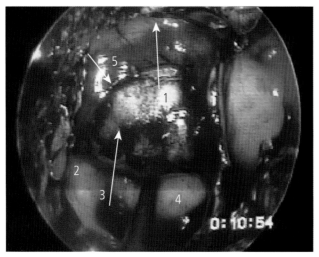

Plate 27.1 View of internal structures of sphenoid and pituitary fossa during endoscopic pituitary surgery. The bone of the pituitary fossa has been partly removed exposing the underlying dura. 1. Bone of anterior cranial fossa. 2. Bone over right carotid artery (carotid eminence). 3. Exposed dura overlying pituitary tumor. 4. Clivus. 5. Bone edge of partly resected bone of floor of pituitary fossa.

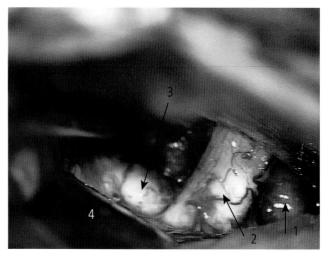

Plate 27.2 Intraoperative view of pituitary tumor during craniotomy. 1. Right carotid artery. 2. Right optic nerve. 3. Pituitary macroadenoma visible between optic nerves pushing optic chiasm superiorly. 4. Brain retractor on right frontal lobe of brain.

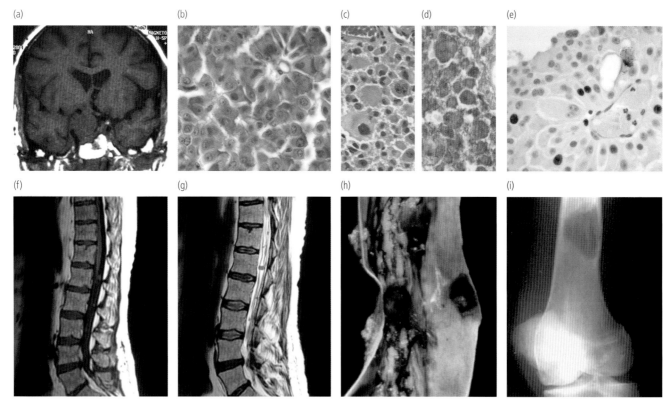

Plate 34.1 Pituitary carcinoma. (a–g) Corticotroph carcinoma following multiple sellar recurrences of an invasive macroadenoma. (a) T1 magnetic resonance imaging (MRI) of the sellar lesion several years before manifestation of metastatic disease. Note extensive extrasellar component and displacement of internal carotid arteries. (b and c) Increased cellular pleomorphism in successive biopsies; (b) early sellar recurrence, (c) spinal cord metastasis with (d) strong ACTH expression. Although p53 was not overexpressed, the metastasis showed an increased proliferation fraction (e) (MIB-1 antibody). Corresponding T1 (f) and T2 (g) MRIs of multiple spinal cord metastases. (h) Macroscopic appearances of intrathecal metastases. (i) X-ray of an osteolytic bone metastasis. (Images (h) and (i) reproduced with permission from Scheithauer BW [4], with permission from Lippincott Williams & Wilkins.)

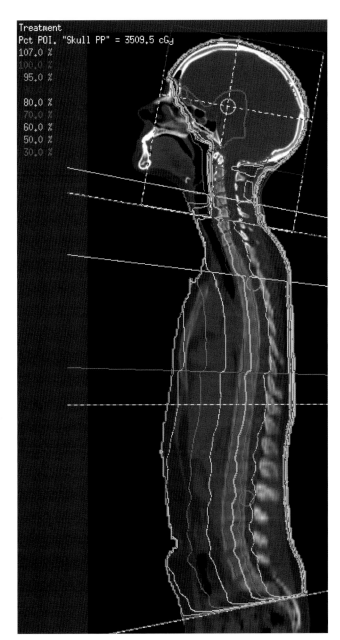

Plate 41.1 Example of a patient receiving craniospinal irradiation in a supine position using a three-dimensional computer-assisted planning process. To avoid overdoses in the field junction between the opposed lateral brain fields and the posterior spinal the junction is "feathered" on a daily basis (moving gap technique). The colored lines represent the isodose distribution with the 100% isodose (red line, prescription dose) being planned to match the posterior edge of the vertebral body.

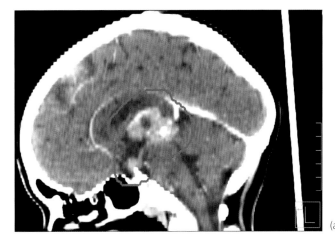

(a)

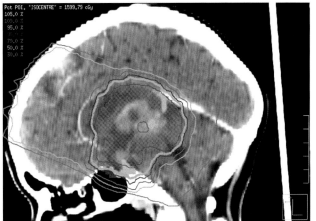

(b)

Plate 41.2 (a) Contrast-enhanced planning CT scan of head. This demonstrates a homogeneously contrast-enhancing mass lesion in the pineal and suprasellar area histopathologically verified to be a bifocal germinoma. The purple line represents the gross tumor volume plus an appropriate margin creating the planning target volume (PTV). (b) Demonstrates a 3D-generated conformal radiotherapy treatment plan to the primary tumor area for the patient seen in (a). The purple area represents the planning target volume (PTV). The enhanced green line represents the 95% isodose level encompassing the PTV. The other lines represent different levels of radiation exposure of surrounding normal tissues (e.g. purple line 70% and green line 50% isodose).

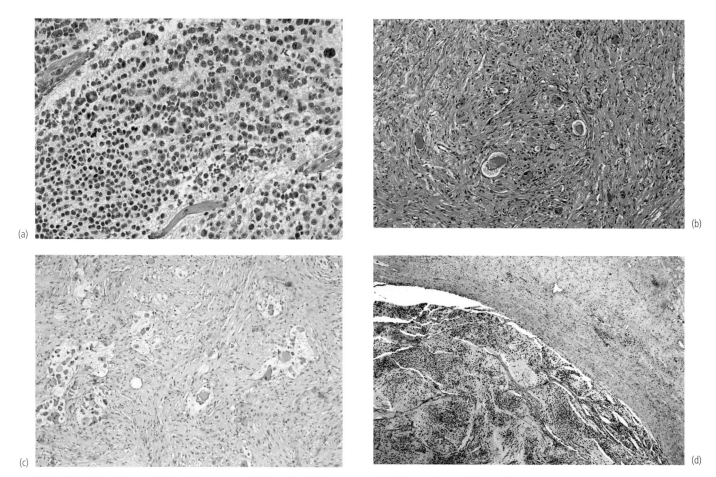

Plate 47.1 (a) Neuroblastoma (Schwannian stroma-poor), differentiated subtype, composed of differentiating neuroblastic cells, sometimes showing synchronous nuclear and cytoplasmic differentiation. Moderate amount of neuropil. H & E, ×10. (b) Ganglioneuroma (Schwannian stroma-dominant), maturing subtype. Few neuroblastic cells are identifiable that have not reached full maturation to ganglion cells. Neuroblastic and ganglion cells are individually scattered and do not form nests. H & E, ×10. (c) Ganglioneuroblastoma intermixed (Schwannian stroma-rich). Well-defined nests of neuroblastic cells in various stages of differentiation and maturing ganglion cells in a background of neuropil randomly distributed in the ganglioneuromatous tissue. H & E, ×10. (d) Ganglioneuroblastoma nodular. Thickened fibrovascular septa separate the poorly differentiated stroma-poor neuroblastoma (bottom left) from the stroma-rich ganglioneuromatous component (top right) H & E, ×2.5.

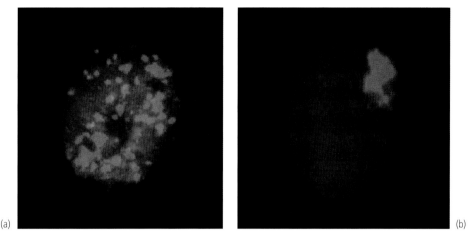

(a)   (b)

Plate 47.2 Fluorescence *in situ* hybridization (FISH) analysis using a MYCN specific probe. (a) Tumor cell from a human stage 4 primary neuroblastoma showing MYCN amplification in form of multiple red hybridization signals (white spots) indicative of DM chromosomes. (b) Cell derived from the HTLA 230 neuroblastoma cell line displaying clustering of *MYCN* hybridization signals (single spot) in a single large spot representing the HSR region. (Courtesy of Dr Annalisa Pezzolo, Laboratory of Oncology, Giannina Gaslini Children's Hospital, Genova, Italy.)

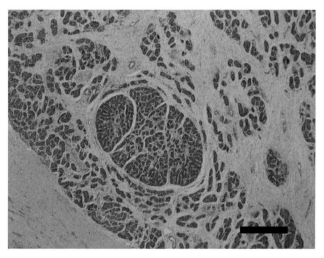

Plate 55.1 Sertoli cell nodule found in a patient with CAIS. Scale bar, 500 μm.

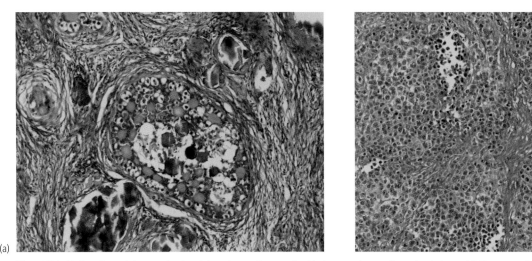

Plate 55.2 (a) Gonad containing round and oval shaped nests of germ cells with clear cytoplasm and round vesicular nuclei. The germ cells surround eosinophilic Call–Exner-like bodies, which show progressive hyalinization and calcification in many areas. Appearances are consistent with a gonadoblastoma (×10). (b) Malignant dysgerminoma has replaced the gonad which invades the serosal surface (×10). (Courtesy of Dr Dallimore and Dr Boyde, Department of Histopathology, University Hospital of Wales, Cardiff, UK.)

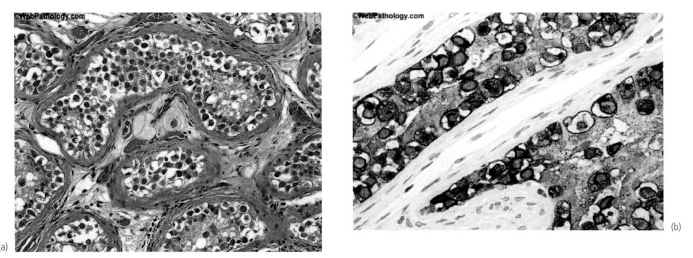

Plate 55.3 Intratubular germ cell neoplasia or carcinoma *in situ* showing large numbers of germ cells (a) staining positive for placental-like alkaline phosphatase, PLAP (b).

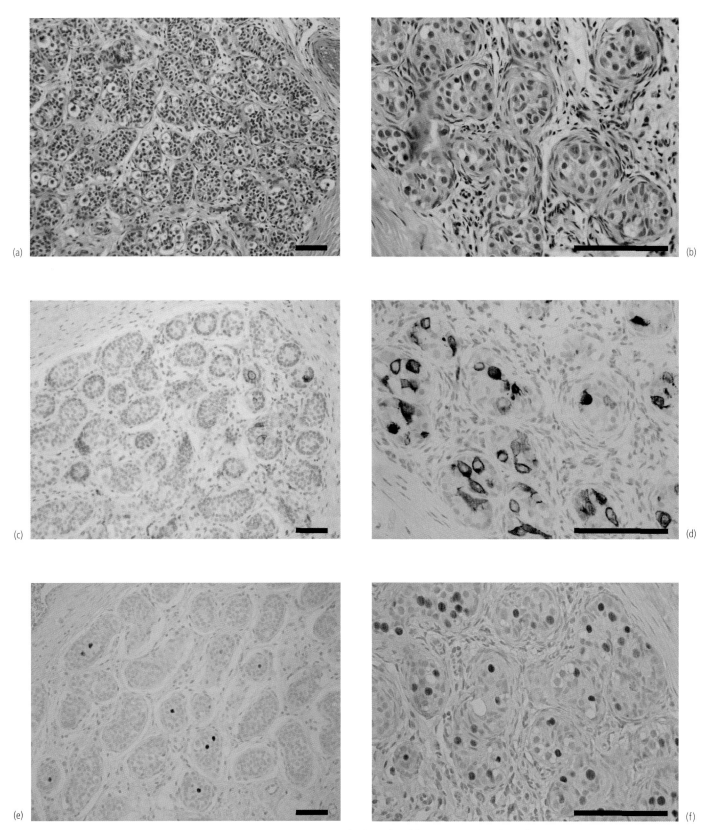

Plate 55.4 Delayed germ cell development versus carcinoma *in situ*. Sections stained with H&E (a and b), anti-PLAP antibody (c and d), or anti-AP2gamma antibody (e and f). (a, c and e) PLAP and AP2gamma positive germ cells are scattered throughout the testis, mostly located centrally in the seminiferous tubules and most germ cells are morphologically normal. This indicates delayed germ cell development rather than CIS. (b, d and f). There are foci of hyalinized seminiferous tubules containing numerous PLAP and AP2gamma positive cells, some located on the basal lamina of the seminiferous tubule, which morphologically show characteristics of CIS. Scale bars, 100 μm.

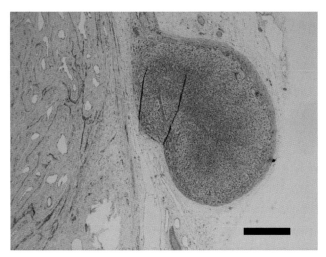

Plate 55.5 Adrenal rest. Adrenal rest attached to the testis of a patient with CAIS. Scale bar, 500 μm.

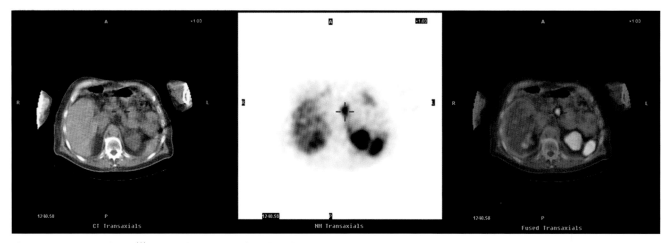

Plate 58.1 Axial images from a ^{111}In-octreotide SPECT/CT performed on a hybrid gamma camera/CT showing increased tracer uptake within a pancreatic islet cell tumor which localizes to the body of the pancreas (red cross-hairs).

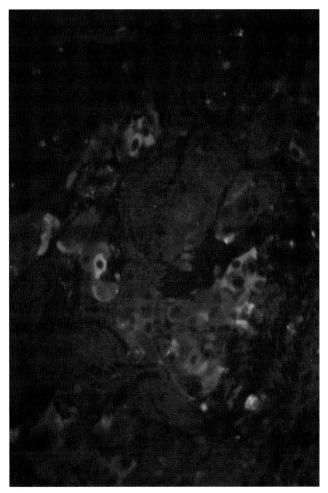

Plate 61.1 Fluorescent immunohistochemical staining of pancreatic VIPoma.

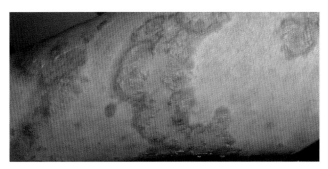

Plate 62.1 Characteristic appearances of NME on the lower limb of a patient with glucagonoma syndrome.

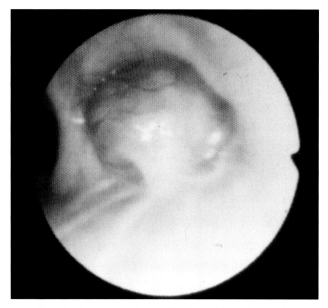

Plate 64.1 Bronchoscopic visualization of intrabronchial typical carcinoid tumor.

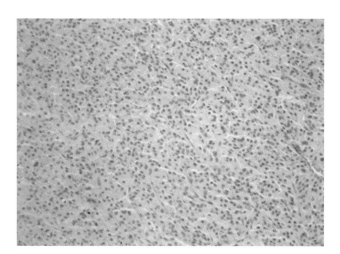

Plate 64.2 Histopathological picture of typical carcinoid.

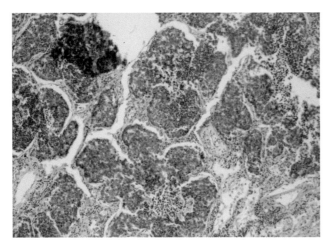

Plate 64.3 Histopathological picture of atypical carcinoid.

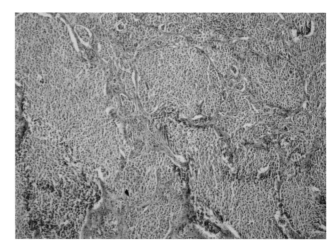

Plate 64.5 Histopathological picture of thymic neuroendocrine tumor.

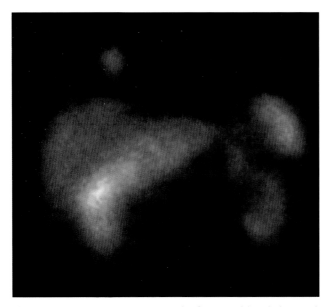

Plate 64.4 Somatostatin receptor scintigraphy of patient with bronchial carcinoid using ^{111}In-labeled octreotide.

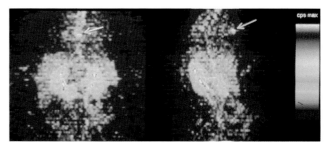

Plate 64.6 Positron emission tomography of thymic neuroendocrine tumor using C11-5-HTP PET.

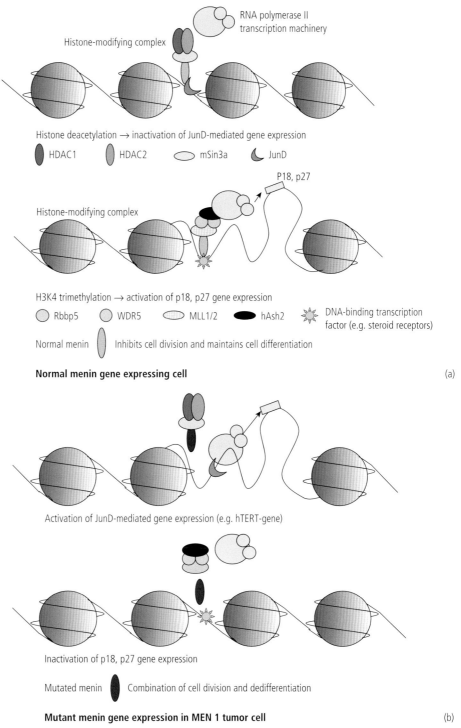

RNA polymerase II transcription machinery

Histone-modifying complex

Histone deacetylation → inactivation of JunD-mediated gene expression

HDAC1   HDAC2   mSin3a   JunD

P18, p27

Histone-modifying complex

H3K4 trimethylation → activation of p18, p27 gene expression

Rbbp5   WDR5   MLL1/2   hAsh2   DNA-binding transcription factor (e.g. steroid receptors)

Normal menin   Inhibits cell division and maintains cell differentiation

Normal menin gene expressing cell   (a)

Activation of JunD-mediated gene expression (e.g. hTERT-gene)

Inactivation of p18, p27 gene expression

Mutated menin   Combination of cell division and dedifferentiation

Mutant menin gene expression in MEN 1 tumor cell   (b)

Plate 68.1 (a) Menin as a dual regulator of gene expression. Two interconnected mechanisms of action: (1) stabilization or modification of histone proteins; (2) regulation of transcription. Menin maintains stability of cells by inhibition of cell division (co-repressor) and preserving the differentiated state (co-activator). (b) In MEN-1 tumors the inactivating mutation in *MEN1* gene results in: co-repressor function on JunD/c-Jun being defective; co-activator function on P18 and P27 being defective.

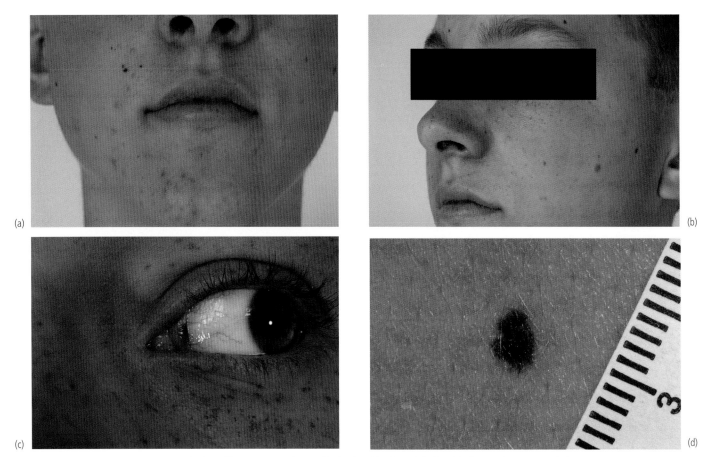

Plate 72.1 Pigmentation in Carney complex (a and b). Lentigines on the vermilion border of the lips and the face. (c) Characteristic inner-canthal pigmentation in a patient with the complex; this is considered pathognomonic of the condition but is only present in a third of the patients. (d) Blue nevus; other unusual pigmented lesions in patients with Carney complex may occur everywhere and are not unusual even in newborns with the disease.

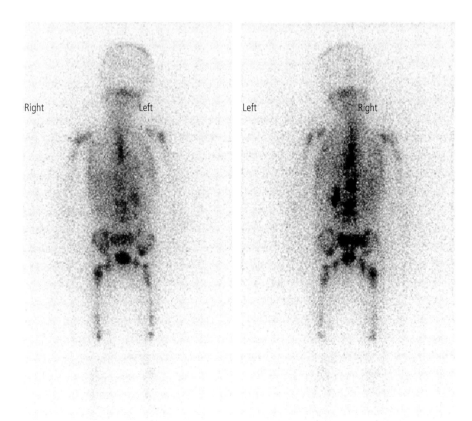

Figure 47.9 Male, 5 years old. ^{123}I-MIBG scintigraphy. Intense positivity involving almost the entire skeleton.

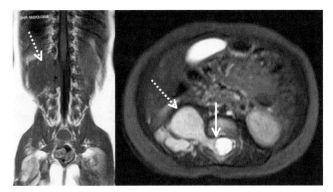

Figure 47.10 Male, 12 years old. Coronal T1-weighted MRI image (left) and axial T2-weighted image (right) show a right paravertebral mass (white dotted arrow) extending into the spinal canal and compressing the dural sac (white arrow).

Table 47.2 Diagnosis of PNT

By

unequivocal histology made from tumor tissue using light microscopy

Or

identification of unequivocal tumor cells (e.g. syncytia or immunocytologically positive clumps of cells) in the bone marrow aspirates or trephine biopsies, associated with increased catecholamine metabolites in the urine or serum

Adapted from Brodeur et al. [17], with permission from the American Society of Clinical Oncology.

may be attributable to an autoimmune mechanism involving the cerebellum and reticular system [16]. An even rarer presentation of PNT is with watery diarrhea secondary to the hyperproduction by the tumor of a vasoactive intestinal polypeptide (VIP). Diarrhea usually regresses after surgical resection of the tumor.

Diagnosis

The main co-operative groups involved with PNT adopt common criteria to diagnose the disease, evaluate its extension and measure response to therapy [17]. Accordingly, the diagnosis of PNT requires the histological confirmation or, in alternative, evidence of unequivocal bone marrow infiltration plus elevated urinary excretion of catecholamine metabolites (Table 47.2).

Thorough work-up at diagnosis in an effort to accurately define disease extension is mandatory in order to plan proper therapy (guidelines in Table 47.3). The study of the primary tumor requires modern imaging techniques including MRI or computerized tomography (CT) to better evaluate its relationship with the surrounding stuctures and to detect intraspinal extension (Fig. 47.11). Ultrasonography is useful especially to document tumor changes during therapy. Special attention must be paid to the search for bone marrow infiltration and skeletal involvement. Appropriate marrow evaluation should include morphological, histological and immunocytological studies of marrow aspirates, as well as trephine biopsies from both posterior iliac crests. Bone involvement is best

Table 47.3 INSS guidelines to evaluate disease extension

Tumor site	Recommended tests
Primary tumor	CT and/or MRI, ^{123}I-MIBG scintigraphy
Metastatic sites	
Bone marrow	Bilateral posterior iliac crest marrow aspirates and trephine biopsies are required to rule out marrow involvement. Trephine biopsies must contain at least 1 cm of marrow, excluding cartilage
Bone	^{123}I-MIBG scintigraphy: [99m]Tc scintigraphy in case of negative MIBG; plain radiographs of MIBG-positive bone segments
Lymph nodes	Clinical examination (palpable nodes), histologically confirmed; CT scan for non-palpable nodes
Abdomen/liver	CT and/or MRI
Chest	Anteroposterior and lateral chest radiographs. CT/MRI necessary if chest radiograph is positive, or if abdominal mass/nodes extend into the chest

Adapted from Brodeur et al [17], with permission from the American Society of Clinical Oncology.

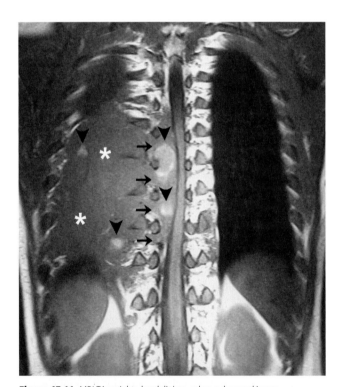

Figure 47.11 MRI T1-weighted gadolinium-enhanced coronal image. Huge thoracic mass (white asterisks) extends an intraspinal component through four, markedly enlarged neural foramina (black arrows). This component compresses and displaces the spinal cord. The mass has numerous hemorrhagic components areas (black arrowheads).

documented by ^{123}I-meta-iodobenzylguanidine (MIBG) scintigraphy, based on the preferential uptake of this radioelement by tumor cells [18]. A [99m]technetium scan may detect bone lesions in the rare cases with negative MIBG scan.

The serum assay of some tumor molecules, such as lactate dehydrogenase (LDH), ferritin, and neuron-specific enolase (NSE), is helpful since their levels correlate with tumor extension and response to therapy.

Staging

On the basis of both the quality of initial surgery and the results of the diagnostic work-up, the patient is assigned a stage number from 1 to 4s according to INSS criteria (Table 47.4). In brief, stage 1–2 defines a localized resectable tumor, stage 3 defines a tumor that infiltrates across the midline and/or invades the contralateral nodes, stage 4 means that the disease has spread to distant sites, while stage 4s defines a quite peculiar entity that affects infants and tends to regress spontaneously, despite dis-

Table 47.4 International Neuroblastoma Staging System (INSS) for PNT*

Stage	Definition
1	Localized tumor with complete gross excision, with or without microscopic residual disease; representative ipsilateral lymph nodes negative for tumor microscopically (nodes attached to and removed with primary tumor may be positive)
2A	Localized tumor with incomplete gross excision; representative ipsilateral and non-adherent lymph nodes negative for tumor microscopically
2B	Localized tumor with complete or incomplete gross excision with ipsilateral non-adherent lymph nodes positive for tumor; enlarged contralateral lymph nodes may be negative microscopically
3	Unresectable unilateral tumor infiltrating across the midline†, with or without regional lymph node involvement, or localized unilateral tumor with contralateral regional lymph node involvement, or midline tumor with bilateral extension by infiltration (unresectable) or by lymph node involvement
4	Any primary tumor with dissemination to distant lymph nodes, bone, bone marrow, liver, skin and/or other organs (except as defined in stage 4s)
4s	Localized primary tumor (as defined for stage 1, 2A or 2B) with dissemination limited to skin, liver and/or bone marrow‡ (limited to infants <1 year)

*Multifocal primary tumors (e.g., bilateral adrenal primary tumors) should be staged according to the greatest extent of the disease, as defined above, followed by a subscript M (e.g., 3_M).

†The midline is defined as the vertebral column. Tumors originating on one side and "crossing the midline" must infiltrate to or beyond the opposite side of the vertebral column.

‡Bone marrow involvement in stage 4s should be minimal, that is, less than 10% of total nucleated cells identified as malignant on bone marrow biopsy or marrow aspirate. More extensive marrow involvement will be considered to be stage IV. The MIBG scan should be negative in the marrow.

Reproduced from Brodeur et al [17], with permission from the American Society of Clinical Oncology.

Table 47.5 Distribution by stage and age of 2347 NT in the Italian Neuroblastoma Registry (unpublished)

| Stage | No. | % | Age (years) | |
			<1%	≥1%
1	469	20.0	27	13
2	247	10.5	14	7
3	435	18.5	17	20
4	997	42.5	24	60
4s	199	8.5	17	0

semination to the liver, skin or bone marrow. Table 47.5 shows the patients' distribution based on disease extension (INSS stage) and age at diagnosis (above or below 1 year) in an Italian series (unpublished).

Therapy

Treatment of children with PNT depends mainly on patient's age, disease extension and *MYCN* oncogene status. The currently employed treatment modalities include surgery, chemotherapy and radiotherapy. Differentiation therapy is given to high-risk patients in complete remission in an attempt to destroy minimal residual disease. Given the largely unsatisfactory results, there is a great need to look into novel therapies.

Surgery

Surgery is used for both diagnosis and treatment [19]. The goals of primary surgery are to establish the diagnosis by providing tumor tissue for histology and biological studies, to define tumor extension and to attempt tumor resection in the absence of risk factors documented by imaging studies. In delayed primary or second-look surgery, the surgeon evaluates the response to therapy and removes the residual tumor, whenever possible. Surgery is usually the only treatment that is needed to cure the majority of patients with localized disease, even if some micro- or macroscopic remnants of the tumor are left behind. Recently, it has been hypothesized that infants may not require surgery, but rather, only observation.

Radiation therapy

Although PNT are considered radiosensitive tumors, the role of radiation therapy in the overall therapeutic approach is still poorly defined [20]. Irradiating the primary site in the presence of *MYCN* gene amplification is a common procedure. Whether irradiation in stage 4 cases actually reduces the local relapse rate is under study. Other clinical situations that could benefit from radiation therapy include progressive liver enlargement in stage 4s and spinal cord compression, even though chemotherapy remains the treatment of choice for both cases. Lastly, external beam radiotherapy is commonly used for the palliative treatment of painful bone metastases. Experimental targeted radiotherapy uses

^{131}I-MIBG in an effort to eradicate both local residual disease and bone tumor foci [21].

Chemotherapy

Chemotherapy is the main modality for the treatment of PNT in patients with intermediate- or high-risk disease. A number of effective drugs have been identified over the last three decades through phase 1–2 studies carried out on children with refractory and recurrent PNT. These studies have identified numerous active compounds, such as alkylating agents, platinum analogs, podophilotoxins and doxorubicin, and the different ways they work. Combining these compounds has led investigators to design protocols that remarkably improved the response rate, although the cure rate remains unsatisfactory [22].

Topotecan, a topoisomerase I inhibitor, has recently shown significant antitumor activity in relapsing patients [23]. Other promising drugs under study include irinotecan and the combination of melphalan and buthionine sulfoximine. Oral etoposide is effectively used as a palliative agent and is well tolerated.

Risk-guided therapy

Treatment of PNT is determined by the predicted risk of disease recurrence, which is based on age at diagnosis, disease extension and selected biological features. Several groups pooled their data and designed a stratification model which provides the basis for co-operative studies on low-, intermediate- and high-risk patient subsets (Table 47.6).

Low risk

Predicted survival for these patients is greater than 95%. All children with stage 1, and those with stage 2A/2B and 4s without *MYCN* amplification, are included. Stage 1, 2A and 2B are managed by surgery alone. Chemotherapy is only indicated in case of recurrence. Patients with asymptomatic stage 4s follow a "wait and see" policy while those with symptoms (prevalently of a respiratory nature secondary to enlarged liver) require chemotherapy until symptoms regress. The SIOP Europe Neuroblastoma Group (SIOPEN) believes that the definition of low risk should be extended to infants with stage 4 disease as long as bone, pleura/lung and central nervous system are not involved. It must be pointed out that SIOPEN defines bone involvement as positive MIBG spots confirmed by abnormal X-ray.

Intermediate risk

This group, whose predicted survival is greater than 80%, includes patients with inoperable tumor and infants with stage IV metastatic to bone, pleura/lung and central nervous system. Both subsets are given chemotherapy in order to reduce the tumor mass and (in the latter cases) to eradicate metastatic disease.

High risk

Predicted survival is below 30%. This group includes all stage 4 patients above 1 year of age and stage 2, 3 and 4s with *MYCN* amplification. The poor prognosis of these patients has prompted

Table 47.6 Risk categories based on clinical, histological and biological features

INSS stage	Low risk	Intermediate risk	High risk
1	All	None	None
2A, 2B	Age <1 year, or Age 1–21 years with *MYCN*–,* or Age 1–21 years with *MYCN*– and FH	None	Age 1–21 years with *MYCN*+ and UH†
3	None	Age <1 year with *MYCN*–, or Age 1–21 years with *MYCN*– and FH	Age 0–21 years with *MYCN*+, or Age 1–21 years with *MYCN*– and UH
4	None	Age <1 year with *MYCN*–	Age <1 year with *MYCN*+, or age 1–21 years with *MYCN*+
4s	*MYCN*–; FH; DI‡ >1	*MYCN*–; UH or DI = 1	*MYCN*+

*MYCN+, amplified; MYCN–, not amplified; †FH, favorable histology; UH, unfavorable histology; ‡DI, DNA index .
Reproduced from Brodeur [33], with permission from Nature Publishing Group.

the design of aggressive therapeutic protocols, which include high-dose chemotherapy followed by the infusion of autologous hematopoietic stem cells. These patients also receive radiation therapy to the primary tumor site following surgical resection. Oral retinoic acid is subsequently given based on proofs of effective differentiating properties on tumor cell lines. A randomized study by the Children's Cancer Group has provided evidence that this effect also occurs *in vivo* [24].

Novel therapies

Identifying new active compounds and strategies is needed and should be actively pursued to improve the outcome of high-risk patients.

Retinoids

Retinoids are vitamin A derivatives that include all-*trans*-retinoic acid (ATRA), 9-*cis*-retinoic acid (RA), 13-*cis*-RA, and *N*-(4-hydroxyphenyl)retinamide (HPR), also known as fenretinide. 13-*cis*-RA is presently included in the protocols for high-risk patients. It likely acts by promoting maturation of residual malignant cells that are present in the patient's bone marrow after high-dose chemotherapy. HPR is a potent inducer of neuroblastoma cell apoptosis *in vitro*. In a phase I study, HPR was administered orally for as long as 28 days with good tolerability and low toxicity. Moreover, the drug plasma levels were comparable to those inducing apoptosis of neuroblastoma cell lines *in vitro* [25]. These findings were confirmed in a subsequent phase I study in which oral fenretinide was administered to 54 children with high-risk solid tumors, 39 of whom had neuroblastoma [26].

Tumor antigen-specific monoclonal antibodies (mAbs)

Both murine and chimeric mAbs directed to the G_{D2} ganglioside have been tested in phase I–II clinical trials. The mechanisms whereby anti-G_{D2} mAbs kill tumor cells are likely related to complement activation and antibody-mediated cell cytotoxicity [27].

Fusion proteins

A fusion protein in which an interleukin (IL)-2 moiety has been fused to an anti-G_{D2} moiety (EMD 273063) has shown excellent anti-neuroblastoma activity in preclinical models based upon recruitment of activated T and natural killer cells to the tumor site. In a recent phase I study the fusion protein has proven to be safe and able to activate the patient's immune system [28].

Gene therapy

All studies performed to date on PNT have enrolled patients with advanced or refractory disease, who had been vaccinated with autologous or allogeneic tumor cells transfected with cytokine genes (IL-2, IL-2 plus lymphotactin) using different protocols. Altogether, 42 patients were treated in four published studies using different schedules and vaccines [29]. Clear immunological changes, such as IL-2-related eosinophilia and the generation of tumor specific cytotoxic T lymphocytes and antibodies, were detected in the peripheral blood of vaccinated children. Several objective tumor responses were observed. [30].

Anti-angiogenesis

The degree of vascularity is associated with poor prognosis in PNT, and the high expression of several angiogenic factors, especially vascular endothelial growth factor (VEGF), has been detected in advanced stages. Bevacizumab (Avastin) is a humanized anti-VEGF mAb with anti-angiogenic and antitumor activity in preclinical models that is now being widely tested in the clinical setting. No trials have been carried out so far.

Imatinib mesylate (STI-571 or Gleevec) is a selective inhibitor of the Abl tyrosine kinase activity in chronic myelogenous leukemia (CML) cells, that also targets the tyrosine kinase activities of c-Kit (the receptor for stem cell factor) and of platelet-derived growth factor receptor (PDGFR). Imatinib inhibits the growth of human neuroblastoma cells (both *in vitro* and *in vivo*), which express both c-Kit and PDGFR-a and b. This inhibition is related to suppression of PDGFR or c-Kit phosphorylation and to the inhibition of VEGF expression, leading to impaired neoangiogenesis. Thus, Gleevec may be a promising candidate for PNT treatment [31].

Liposomal tumor and vascular targeting

Liposomes coated with anti-G_{D2} mAbs or with peptides targeted to the tumor vasculature can be used in preclinical models as carriers of various molecules endowed with anti-neuroblastoma activity, such as retinoids [32], cytotoxic drugs and antisense oligonucleotides. This strategy spares normal tissues from drug toxicity since it selectively targets the tumor cells.

Acknowledgments

The authors are indebted to Dr Riccardo Haupt for providing the INBR data, Ms Sara Calmanti for editing the manuscript and Ms Valerie Perricone for reviewing the text.

References

1. Castleberry RP. Neuroblastoma. *Eur. J. Cancer* 1997;33:1430–1437.

2. De Bernardi B, Milanaccio C, Occhi M. Neuroblastoma. In Sheaves R, Jenkins PJ, Wass JAH (eds). *Clinical Endocrine Oncology*. Oxford: Blackwell Science, 1997:306–311.

3. Caron HN, Pearson ADJ. Neuroblastoma. In Voute PA, Barrett A, Stevens MCG, Caron HN (eds). *Cancer in Children*, 5th edn. Oxford: Oxford University Press, 2005:337–352.

4. Brodeur GM, Maris JM. Neuroblastoma. In Pizzo PA, Poplack DG (eds). *Principles and Practice of Pediatric Oncology*, 4th edn. Philadelphia: Lippincott Williams & Wilkins, 2002:895–938.

5. Kaneko Y, Kanda N, Maseki N, et al. Current urinary mass screening for catecholamine metabolites at 6 months of age may be detecting only a small portion of high-risk neuroblastomas: a chromosome and N-myc amplification study. *J. Clin. Oncol.* 1990;8:2005–2013.

6. Tsubono Y, Hisamichi S. A halt to neuroblastoma screening in Japan. *N. Engl. J. Med.* 2004;350:2010–2011.

7. Shimada H, Chatten J, Newton WA Jr, et al. Histopathologic prognostic factors in neuroblastic tumors: definition of subtypes of ganglioneuroblastoma and an age-linked classification of neuroblastomas. *J. Natl Cancer Inst.* 1984;73: 405–416.

8. Shimada H, Ambros IM, Dehner LP, et al. The International Neuroblastoma Pathology Classification (the Shimada System). *Cancer* 1999;86: 364–372.

9. Tonini GP, Boni L, Pession A, et al. *MYCN* oncogene amplification in neuroblastoma is associated with worse prognosis, except in stage 4s: the Italian experience with 295 children. *J. Clin. Oncol.* 1997;15:85–93.

10. Caron H, van Sluis P, Buschman R, et al. Alleic loss of chromosome 1p as a predictor of unfavorable outcome in patients with neuroblastoma. *N. Engl. J. Med.* 1996;334:225–230.

11. Bown N, Cotterill S, Lastowska M, et al. Gain of chromosome arm 17q and adverse outcome in patients with neuroblastoma. *N. Engl. J. Med.* 1999;340:1954–1961.

12. Look AT, Hayes FA, Shuster JJ, et al. Clinical relevance of tumor cell ploidy and N-myc gene amplification in childhood neuroblastoma. A Pediatric Oncology Group study. *J. Clin. Oncol.* 1991;9:581–591.

13. Teitz T, Wei T, Valentine MB, et al. Caspase 8 is deleted or silenced preferentially in childhood neuroblastomas with amplification of MYCN. *Nat. Med.* 2000;6:529–535.

14. Conte M, Parodi S, De Bernardi B, et al. Neuroblastoma in adolescents: the Italian experience. *Cancer* 2006;106:1409–1417.

15. De Bernardi B, Pianca C, Pistamiglio P, et al. Neuroblastoma with symptomatic spinal cord compression at diagnosis: treatment and results with 76 cases. *J. Clin. Oncol.* 2001;19:183–190.

16. Gambini C, Conte M, Bernini G, et al. Neuroblastic tumors associated with opsoclonus–myoclonus syndrome: histological, immunohistochemical and molecular features of 15 Italian cases. *Virchows Arch.* 2003;442:555–562.

17. Brodeur GM, Pritchard J, Berthold F, et al. Revisions of the international criteria for neuroblastoma diagnosis, staging, and response to treatment. *J. Clin. Oncol.* 1993;11:1466–1477.

18. Claudiani F, Stimamiglio P, Bertolazzi L, et al. Radioiodinated meta-iodobenzylguanidine in the diagnosis of childhood neuroblastoma. *Q. J. Nucl. Med.* 1995;39:21–24.

19. La Quaglia MP. Surgical management of neuroblastoma. *Semin. Pediatr. Surg.* 2001;10:132–139.

20. Halperin EC, Cox EB. Radiation therapy in the management of neuroblastoma: the Duke University Medical Center experience 1967–1984. *Int. J. Radiat. Oncol. Biol. Phys.* 1986;12:1829–1837.

21. Garaventa A, Bellagamba O, Lo Piccolo MS, et al. ^{131}I-metaiodobenzylguanidine (^{131}I-MIBG) therapy for residual neuroblastoma: a mono–institutional experience with 43 patients. *Br. J. Cancer* 1999;81:1378–1384.

22. De Bernardi B, Nicolas B, Boni L, et al. Disseminated neuroblastoma in children older than one year at diagnosis: comparable results with three consecutive high-dose protocols adopted by the Italian Co-Operative Group for Neuroblastoma. *J. Clin. Oncol.* 2003;21:1592–1601.

23. Garaventa A, Luksch R, Biasotti S et al. A phase II study of topotecan with vincristine and doxorubicin in children with recurrent/refractory neuroblastoma. *Cancer* 2003;98:2488–2494

24. Matthay KK, Villablanca JG, Seeger RC, et al. Treatment of high–risk neuroblastoma with intensive chemotherapy, radiotherapy, autologous bone marrow transplantation, and 13-*cis*-retinoic acid. Children's Cancer Group. *N. Engl. J. Med.* 1999;341:1165–1173.

25. Garaventa A, Luksch R, Lo Piccolo MS, et al. Phase I trial and pharmacokinetics of fenretinide in children with neuroblastoma. *Clin. Cancer Res.* 2003;9:2032–2039.

26. Villablanca JG, Krailo MD, Ames MM, et al. Phase I trial of oral fenretinide in children with high–risk solid tumors: a report from the Children's Oncology Group (CCG 09709). *J. Clin. Oncol.* 2006;24:3423–3430.

27. Yu AL, Uttenreuther-Fischer MM, Huang CS, et al. Phase I trial of a human–mouse chimeric anti-disialoganglioside monoclonal antibody ch14.18 in patients with refractory neuroblastoma and osteosarcoma. *J. Clin. Oncol.* 1998;16:2169–2180.

28. Neal ZC, Yang JC, Rakhmilevich AL, et al. Enhanced activity of hu14.18-IL2 immunocytokine against murine NXS2 neuroblastoma when combined with interleukin 2 therapy. *Clin. Cancer Res.* 2004;10:4839–4847.

29. Tonini GP, Pistoia V. Molecularly guided therapy of neuroblastoma: a review of different approaches. *Curr. Pharm. Dev.* 2006;12:2303–2317.

30. Bowman LC, Grossmann M, Rill D, et al. Interleukin-2 gene-modified allogeneic tumor cells for treatment of relapsed neuroblastoma. *Hum. Gene Ther.* 1998;9:1303–1311.

31. Beppu K, Jaboine J, Merchant MS, et al. Effect of imatinib mesylate on neuroblastoma tumorigenesis and vascular endothelial growth factor expression. *J. Natl Cancer Inst.* 2004;96:46–55.

32. Raffaghello L, Pagnan G, Pastorino F, et al. Immunoliposomal fenretinide: a novel antitumoral drug for human neuroblastoma. *Cancer Lett.* 2003;197:151–155.

33. Brodeur GM. Neuroblastoma: biological insights into a clinical enigma. *Nat. Rev. Cancer* 2003;3:203–216.

Primary Hyperaldosteronism

Mark Sherlock and Paul M. Stewart

Key points

- Primary hyperaldosteronism is increasing in prevalence with the commonest cause now being bilateral adrenal hyperplasia rather than adrenal adenoma.
- The majority of patients with primary hyperaldosteronism are normokalemic, therefore physicians need to have a high index of suspicion for this condition in hypertensive patients.
- In recent years aldosterone has been implicated in premature cardiovascular disease and as a result the diagnosis and appropriate treatment of primary hyperaldosteronism are increasingly important.
- A knowledge is needed of the strengths and weaknesses of each investigation for diagnosing primary hyperaldosteronism and subtype differentiation, including awareness of complicating factors in the interpretation of results.
- The optimum treatment of aldosterone-producing adenomas is surgical resection, and of bilateral adrenal hyperplasia is with mineralocorticoid receptor antagonists.

Introduction

Primary hyperaldosteronism (PA) was first characterized as a syndrome of hypertension, hypokalemia, suppressed plasma renin activity (PRA) and increased aldosterone secretion by Jerome Conn in 1955 [1]. In recent years a number of studies have indicated that PA is the commonest form of secondary hypertension; indeed, PA has been found to occur in up to 10% of all individuals attending hypertension clinics [2]. The diagnosis of PA is particularly important as it can lead to targeted medical or surgical therapy, which can either cure or permit easier pharmacological control of hypertension in these patients. Normalization of plasma aldosterone levels has become increasingly important in light of studies linking aldosterone excess to cardiac fibrosis and vascular inflammation [3] in what is now described as an aldosterone-induced vasculopathy [4].

There are a number of recognized causes of PA: bilateral adrenal hyperplasia (BAH) and aldosterone-producing adenomas (APA) (the two most common forms) and less commonly glucocorticoid-remediable hypertension, adrenal carcinomas, primary adrenal hyperplasia and renin-responsive APA. Screening for PA in the past 10 years has seen a dramatic change in the relative prevalences of the different etiologies of PA with BAH now being the commonest form of PA.

Clinical Endocrine Oncology, 2nd edition. Edited by Ian D. Hay and John A.H. Wass. © 2008 Blackwell Publishing. ISBN 978-1-4051-4584-8.

Regulation of aldosterone secretion

In normal physiology, aldosterone secretion is regulated by three well-established stimulators, namely the renin–angiotensin system, adrenocorticotropic hormone (ACTH) and serum potassium. The most potent physiological stimulator of aldosterone secretion is angiotensin-II (ATII), followed by serum potassium and ACTH, which has a minor role in the normal control of aldosterone secretion. In the normal adrenal gland aldosterone is secreted from the zona glomerulosa, cortisol from the zona fasciculata and sex steroids from the zona reticularis. The synthesis of aldosterone in the zona glomerulosa requires the action of two distinct but related CYP_{450} enzymes: 11β-hydroxylase and aldosterone synthase (Fig. 48.1). The genes encoding these enzymes have been cloned (*CYP11B1* and *CYP11B2*, respectively), they have 95% sequence homology and lie adjacent to each other on chromosome 8q22.

Classification of primary hyperaldosteronism

PA can be classified into the following four groups.

Aldosterone-producing adenoma

These benign tumors are usually small (0.5–2.5 cm), unilateral and solitary (Fig. 48.2). Aldosterone secretion is partly autonomous; it was previously believed that APAs were responsive to ACTH but not ATII; however, recent reports have shown that 50% of APAs are responsive to ATII [5]. Adenoma occur more frequently in females with a male–female ratio of 1:2 and the

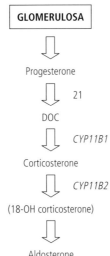

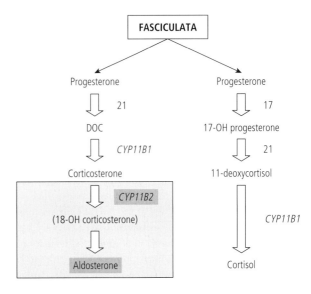

Figure 48.1 In the normal adrenal gland, only the zona glomerulosa synthesizes aldosterone because it expresses aldosterone synthase (a product of the *CYP11B2* gene). Both the zona glomerulosa and zona fasciculata express 11β-hydroxylase (a product of *CYP11B1* gene) but cortisol can be synthesized in the zona fasciculata because it expresses 17α-hydroxylase. The gray area indicates the mechanism of aldosterone synthesis in patients with GRA.

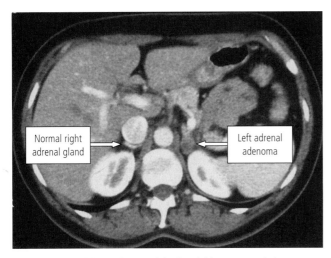

Figure 48.2 CT abdomen showing a left adrenal aldosterone-producing adenoma (APA).

Figure 48.3 CT abdomen showing bilateral adrenal hyperplasia (BAH) (arrows indicate hyperplastic adrenal glands).

average age group of affected patients is between 30 and 50 years. A familial form of PA which is associated with APAs and BAH exists and is called familial hyperaldosteronism type II (FH-II). Linkage has been found with a locus in chromosome 7p22, but the implicated gene is unknown [6].

Unilateral APAs were previously thought to be the most common cause of PA; however, with an increase in screening of hypertensive patients with the plasma aldosterone concentration/plasma renin activity (PAC/PRA) ratio BAH is now the most prevalent cause of PA.

Bilateral adrenal hyperplasia

In contrast to APA this condition is more common in men with a male:female ratio of 4:1 and peak incidence occurs in the sixth decade. In this condition aldosterone secretion is exquisitely sensitive to circulating ATII (but not ACTH) and thus it can be considered to be an exaggeration of the normal physiological aldosterone response to ATII. ATII infusion studies indicate enhanced

aldosterone secretion in BAH when compared to hypertensive subjects. Less marked changes are seen in patients with essential hypertension when categorized on the basis of PRA levels, with patients with low-renin hypertension demonstrating a more marked ATII-stimulated aldosterone response than those with high renin levels. Because of this many authors have suggested that BAH merely represents one end of the spectrum of low-renin essential hypertension. Microscopically, hyperplasia of the zona glomerulosa is found bilaterally (occasionally it may be unilateral), and may be associated with microscopic or macroscopic nodules (Fig. 48.3).

Glucocorticoid-remediable aldosteronism (GRA)

Also referred to as glucocorticoid- or dexamethasone-suppressible hyperaldosteronism, GRA was first described in 1967 by Sutherland and colleagues [7] in a father and son with a hypokalemic hypertensive syndrome. It is an autosomal dominantly inherited condition and is now recognized as the commonest monogenic form of human hypertension.

In the normal adrenal gland the zona fasciculata does not contain aldosterone synthase and therefore aldosterone is not synthesized; instead both corticosterone and cortisol are synthesized under the control of ACTH which regulates 11β-hydroxylase. In the zona glomerulosa cortisol cannot be synthesized in the absence of 17α-hydroxylase. Corticosterone (B), however, can be metabolized further to 18-OHB and aldosterone by aldosterone synthase which is regulated primarily by ATII [8].

Subjects with GRA have two normal copies of genes encoding aldosterone synthase and 11β-hydroxylase, but they also have an abnormal gene duplication. This chimeric gene duplication combines the 5′ ACTH-responsive promoter sequence of *CYP11B1* (encoding 11β-hydroxylase) fused to the 3′ *CYP11B2* (encoding aldosterone synthase). As a result aldosterone synthase is expressed ectopically in the zona fasciculata but is under the regulation of ACTH, not ATII. Provided this break point occurs 5′ to exon 4 of the *CYP11B2* gene then the chimeric gene will convert corticosterone to aldosterone. This chimerism also results in the synthesis of the hybrid steroids 18-oxocortisol and 18-hydroxycortisol (Figs 48.1 and 48.4).

Surprisingly these patients are usually normokalemic unless they have been treated with non-potassium-sparing diuretics. As a result clinicians must be aware of the need to screen for this condition in certain circumstances even in the setting of normokalemia.

As a result the recommendations to screen for this condition include [8]:

1 Patients diagnosed with primary hyperaldosteronism without a demonstrable tumor (like BAH, microscopically the adrenal glands show micronodular and macronodular hyperplasia in GRA).
2 Young patients (<30 years of age) with suppressed plasma renin activity.
3 Family history of hypertension or cerebral hemorrhage before the age of 30.
4 Refractory hypertension.
5 Members of known GRA kindreds.

The dexamethasone suppression test (DST) is an easily performed screening test for this condition with 0.5 mg of dexamethasone administered orally every 6 h for 48 h. Patients with GRA will suppress plasma aldosterone to <4 ng/dl (<111 pmol/L) at 8:00 h on day 3. The DST is a sensitive screening test but its specificity is low, leading to a high false-positive rate. The measurement of 24 h urinary 18-hydroxycortisol and 18-oxocortisol levels is less practical than the DST as a screening test as these assays are only available in specialized centers; that being said, a urinary level of 18-hydroxycortisol >378.5 ng/dL (10 nmol/L) is highly suggestive of GRA. Initial genetic screen includes a long-PCR, which if positive should be confirmed by Southern blot. Genetic testing can be arranged through the international GRA registry (http://www.brighamandwomens.org/gra).

The treatment of GRA should be with dexamethasone (0.125–0.25 mg) or prednisolone (2.5–5 mg), titrated to achieve normotension. Mineralocorticoid receptor antagonists are also effective in the management of associated hypertension, as are epithelial sodium channel antagonists [8].

Miscellaneous

Aldosterone-producing adrenocortical carcinoma, primary adrenal hyperplasia and aldosterone-producing renin-responsive adenoma are all rare causes of primary hyperaldosteronism. Carcinomas may secrete aldosterone in isolation, or concomitantly with glucocorticoids and sex steroids. In patients presenting with these tumors the hypertension and hypokalemia are severe, and the aldosterone levels, which are unresponsive to ACTH, are very high. The best diagnostic criterion is the size of the tumor: the majority are in excess of 3 cm and often associated with metastases. Primary adrenal hyperplasia is characterized by bilateral hyperplastic adrenal glands that resemble BAH morphologically, but in terms of hormonal studies and treatment resemble APA. Finally aldosterone-producing renin-responsive adenoma mimics APA morphologically but biochemically behaves more like BAH.

Clinical features

Few symptoms and no specific physical findings accompany the syndrome of PA. The symptoms are non-specific, and are due to hypertension and potassium depletion. They include:

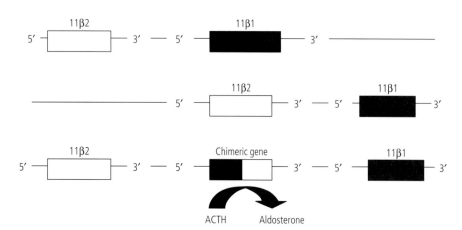

Figure 48.4 GRA results from a chimeric gene which occurs because of an unequal crossover between CYP11B1 and CYP11B2 genes at meiosis. The chimeric gene results in the expression of an enzyme in the zona fasciculata which can synthesize aldosterone from corticosterone but which is regulated by ACTH and not ATII.

• headaches, usually bitemporal but unrelated to the height of the arterial pressure

• thirst, polyuria and nocturia secondary to hypokalemic nephropathy

• paresthesia, tetany, weakness of proximal muscle groups and intermittent paralysis; a positive Trousseau's or Chvostek's sign may be seen due to potassium depletion and alkalosis

• tachycardia with or without palpitations

• edema is surprisingly rare as there is concomitant renal loss of sodium (the "escape" phenomenon).

Hypertension is initially volume mediated as a result of the mineralocorticoid-excess state, though this is soon followed by an increase in peripheral vascular resistance. Aldosterone increases vascular tone by a number of mechanisms including the potentiation of catecholamine and ATII-induced vasoconstriction and by inhibiting endothelial relaxation [9]. Blood pressure levels vary greatly from near normal to severely elevated, but malignant hypertension is rare. Postural hypotension in the absence of a reflex tachycardia may occur, due to a blunted baroreceptor response secondary to potassium depletion. Vascular changes in the fundi are usually minimal, but occasionally Keith–Wagner group III or IV changes can be observed.

Diagnosis and differential diagnosis

Every patient with hypertension should have serum electrolytes measured. Spontaneous hypokalemia (serum potassium concentration <3.5 mmol/L) is uncommon in patients with uncomplicated and untreated hypertension and when present strongly suggests associated mineralocorticoid excess. However, up to 70% of patients with surgically confirmed primary hyperaldosteronism will have normal serum potassium concentrations and therefore the clinician must have a high index of suspicion for PA in all hypertensive patients [10, 11]. Patients presenting with hypokalemia on diuretic therapy should be screened by discontinuing the diuretic therapy, replacing potassium stores and testing using the PAC/PRA ratio in 4 weeks provided serum potassium is >3.6 mmol/L.

In addition to the presence of hypertension and hypokalemia, abnormal results of routine clinical laboratory tests should raise suspicion that primary hyperaldosteronism is present; for example, mild metabolic alkalosis (serum bicarbonate >30 mmol/L) and relative hypernatremia (serum sodium >142 mmol/L) are frequent findings. The effect of chronic potassium depletion on insulin secretion and action produces an elevated fasting plasma glucose level in approximately 25% of patients. Table 48.1 includes a guide as to which patients should be screened for primary hyperaldosteronism.

Screening tests

The commonest screening test for PA is the plasma aldosterone concentration/plasma renin activity (PAC/PRA) ratio. The

Table 48.1 Which patients should be screened for primary hyperaldosteronism?

1 All patients with hypokalemia whether spontaneous or diuretic induced (as when present hypokalemia is a strong indicator of PA; however <30% of patients with PA will have biochemical hypokalemia)

2 Patients who remain hypertensive despite triple antihypertensive therapy (including a diuretic)

3 Patients with a history of hypertension or stroke in immediate family members less than 50 years of age

4 Patients with an adrenal incidentaloma

PAC/PRA has simplified the screening of patients for PA as it can be performed in the outpatient clinic with the patient in the seated position. However, this simplicity of testing does come at the expense of a high false positive rate. Ideally, the use of this ratio should be center based, with normal ranges established for prevailing population salt intakes [10].

Interpreting the PAC is crucial in the assessment of PA as all patients with a suppressed PRA will have an increased PAC/PRA ratio. Therefore the PAC value should be greater than 15 ng/dl (416 pmol/L) in a patient with a fully suppressed PRA and a PAC/PRA ratio >30 (ng/dl)/(ng/ml/h) to indicate PA. It has been shown previously that all patients with aldosterone levels <9 ng/dl (250 pmol/L) demonstrated normal suppression during a fludrocortisone suppression test regardless of the initial PAC/PRA.

Importantly, the serum potassium must be above 3.6 mmol/L to allow interpretation of aldosterone levels as hypokalemia can suppress aldosterone secretion. If the serum potassium is <3.6 mmol/L then the patient should be given supplemental potassium and tested once the serum potassium is >3.6 mmol/L. The interpretation of the PAC/PRA is further confounded by the fact that the patients being screened are frequently already on a number of antihypertensive agents at the time of presentation [12]. In particular, beta blockers can raise the PAC/PRA by decreasing to a greater extent the PRA compared to the PAC [12, 13], leading to an increase in false-positive results. Conversely, diuretics (including spironolactone), angiotensin-converting enzyme inhibitors, calcium channel blockers and angiotensin II receptor blockers tend to reduce PAC/PRA, which in turn will lead to an increase in false-negative results. Patients should have, if possible, a period of washout from the above medications for 4 weeks prior to testing. As these patients often have severe hypertension this may not be feasible without the addition of other classes of antihypertensive agents. The most neutral class of antihypertensive agent on the renin–angiotensin–aldosterone system are the alpha receptor blockers (doxazosin/prazosin) and these therefore may be the best choice of agent if one has to discontinue other antihypertensive agents before screening for PA with the PAC/PRA [12, 14].

If the patient's blood pressure is not controlled with alpha receptor blockade then a calcium channel blocker would be the next drug of choice (although as mentioned above, these have been associated with a slight reduction in the PAC/PRA). The angiotensin-converting enzyme (ACE) inhibitor fosinopril has also been shown not to interfere with the diagnosis of PA but this should be kept as a third-line agent for patients who have severe hypertension despite full-dose alpha blocker and calcium channel blocker [12]. Of note, non-steroidal anti-inflammatory agents should also be discontinued if possible as they cause increased renal sodium retention, leading to a suppression of renin and retention of potassium leading to aldosterone secretion and therefore a falsely elevated PAC/PRA ratio [6] resulting in a false-positive screening test.

Confirming the diagnosis of primary aldosteronism

An increased PAC/PRA is a screening test and is not by itself diagnostic of primary hyperaldosteronism as between 30% and 50% of patients with a positive PAC/PRA will show normal suppression of plasma aldosterone on further confirmatory tests. Therefore a suppression test should be performed to demonstrate that the aldosterone secretion is inappropriately elevated for a high salt diet and not normally suppressible [12, 15]. The most widely used tests are the saline load test (either oral or intravenous) and the fludrocortisone suppression test (FST).

Saline load test

The intravenous saline load consists of the infusion of 2 L of 0.9% NaCl solution over 4 h and the subsequent measurement of plasma aldosterone. If aldosterone is >5 ng/dl (139 pmol/L) after the saline infusion, PA is diagnosed. If aldosterone is <5 ng/dl (139 pmol/L), then PA can be excluded [16]. Post-saline load plasma aldosterone values between 5 and 10 ng/dL (139–277 pmol/L) represent a gray zone but most clinicians consider these patients to be affected by PA (more often caused by adrenal hyperplasia than by adrenal adenoma).

The oral saline load is performed with the patient subjected to a high sodium diet (300 mmol sodium per day for 3 days). Of note, a high sodium diet can increase kaliuresis and hypokalemia, therefore daily monitoring of serum potassium is essential and vigorous replacement of potassium is often required. On the last day of the high salt diet, a 24-h urine collection is obtained to measure urinary sodium excretion. PA is diagnosed if a post-saline load 24-h urinary aldosterone excretion is >12 μg/day (33.3 nmol/day), with a concomitant urinary sodium excretion >200 mEq/24 h (to document adequate sodium repletion).

Fludrocortisone suppression test

The fludrocortisone suppression test (FST) is the most reliable test to confirm the diagnosis of PA. Fludrocortisone acetate (0.1 mg) is administered every 6 h along with slow-release sodium chloride (30 mmol) every 8 h for 4 days. PA is diagnosed if the upright plasma aldosterone levels measured at 10:00 h at the conclusion of 4 days' administration of fludrocortisone are >5 ng/dl (139 pmol/L) [6, 10].

Distinction between the subtypes and localization

Because the treatment of APA, BAH and GRA varies, it is essential to distinguish between them correctly (see Fig. 48.5). The distinction between the subtypes of PA involves the use of adrenal imaging techniques, genetic analysis, pharmacological testing and catheter sampling studies. Previously, posture studies were used to differentiate between BAH and APA: APA aldosterone secretion is sensitive to changes in ACTH (but not ATII), BAH aldosterone secretion is sensitive to changes in angiotensin II levels (but not ACTH) but these are not a reliable test with up to 50% of APAs responding to ATII [5]. For the same reason the captopril suppression test may also be less useful than previously reported.

Radiological investigations

Before undertaking radiological investigations it is essential to have confirmed the diagnosis of PA as there is a high incidence of non-functioning adrenal "incidentalomas" in the normal population.

Adrenal computerized tomography (CT) scanning

Adrenal CT scanning is the initial radiological investigation of patients with confirmed PA with a sensitivity of >85% for adenomas larger than 1 cm; however, most APAS are <1 cm in diameter. CT scans of the adrenal glands should be high resolution with fine cuts (2.5–3 mm) as this gives the best sensitivity in identifying adrenal nodules (Figs 48.2 and 48.3) [5]. Adrenal CT scan has an estimated overall sensitivity of 50%, which is higher than magnetic resonance (MR), therefore MR should only be used in patients with contraindications for CT scanning [10]. Adrenal imaging alone is inadequate for the differential diagnosis between APA and BAH. An adrenal nodule in a patient with confirmed PA can be an APA, an incidentaloma or a macronodule in a hyperplastic gland in a patient with BAH.

Patients with PA who have adrenal adenomas >3 cm in diameter should be suspected of having an aldosterone-producing carcinoma. Patients with BAH have either normal-appearing glands or changes consistent with bilateral nodular hyperplasia.

Adrenal scintigraphy with radiolabeled iodocholesterol

Adrenal imaging with iodocholesterol (^{131}I-6-iodomethyl-19-norcholesterol, NP-59) provides a non-invasive means of differentiating patients with APA from those with BAH and identifies the site of the adenoma when present. NP-59 accumulates in the adrenals, and scintigraphy is carried out 5 days after administration. Theoretically, patients with APA concentrate radioactivity at the site of the tumor, whereas patients with IHA usually show diffuse uptake (aldosterone-producing carcinomas show little or no uptake). In practice, however, adrenal scintigraphy is less reliable due to a high rate of equivocal or misleading results independent of whether pretreatment with dexamethasone is used or

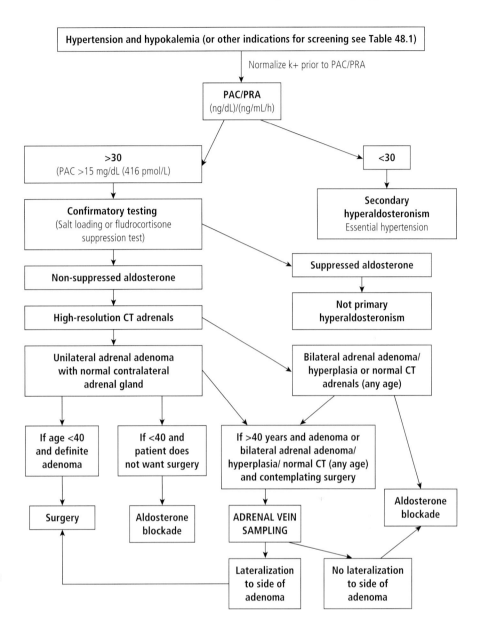

Figure 48.5 Flowsheet for the assessment of patients with suspected primary hyperaldosteronism (k+ = potassium, PAC/PRA = plasma aldosterone concentration/plasma renin activity).

not. However, in some centers it is still used successfully and therefore it may be helpful in selected patients [17].

Adrenal vein sampling (AVS)

Bilateral adrenal vein sampling is the most accurate test for differentiating between APAs and IHA [18]. However, AVS is invasive, technically demanding and requires skill and experience. AVS must be performed by an experienced radiologist as there is an appreciable incidence of complications, including venous thrombosis and extravasation of dye into the adrenal gland which if bilateral may lead to adrenal insufficiency. Considering these factors AVS should only be performed if surgery is an option in management of the patient, otherwise PA should be managed with medical therapy.

The adrenal veins are very small and therefore it may be difficult to place the catheter tip within the vein (catheterization of the right adrenal vein is particularly difficult) and the sample may be obtained from near the orifice of the vein. To ensure that the catheter is in the correct position, serum cortisol is measured simultaneously with aldosterone (which also allows for correction of any dilutional effect). Unfortunately, there is no universally accepted cut-off level of cortisol that determines the success of catheter positioning; ratios reported vary between >2 and >3 between cortisol levels in the adrenal vein and in the peripheral vein to indicate that the catheter is in the adrenal vein [6, 10]. ACTH infusion is performed by some groups in order to avoid fluctuation of aldosterone and cortisol secretion which may result in misleading results of the aldosterone to cortisol ratio (ACR).

AVS is considered to show lateralization when the adrenal venous aldosterone/cortisol ratio is at least two times the peripheral concentration on one side (this figure ranges from >2 to >5 depending on center) [10] and no higher than peripheral on the contralateral side [6]; however a complete contralateral suppression does not appear to always be necessary.

Treatment

Surgery

When a functional unilateral adrenal adenoma is confirmed, the treatment of choice is unilateral total adrenalectomy. Laparoscopic adrenalectomy is the procedure of choice as it associated with shorter hospital stays and lower morbidity than open adrenalectomy [19]. Patients should be adequately prepared preoperatively (ideally for 6 weeks) with spironolactone or amiloride (see below) and the blood pressure response to these agents preoperatively has been used as a predictor of response to adrenalectomy. If the patient is not adequately blocked there is anesthetic risk of hypokalemia and hypertension, but perhaps more importantly of a mineralocorticoid-deficient state postoperatively. If preoperative medical therapy has been inadequate and the renin–angiotensin drive to aldosterone secretion from the "normal" contralateral adrenal remains suppressed, there is a real risk of hyperkalemia postoperatively. Patients should be encouraged to have a generous sodium intake for a few weeks postoperatively to help ameliorate this effect. This risk of postoperative hyperkalemia may be exacerbated by spironolactone which has a long half-life and may still be effective for several days after discontinuation of the drug, therefore spironolactone should be discontinued immediately following surgery, if not before. Rarely these adenomas may secrete aldosterone and cortisol and for the same reason glucocorticoid deficiency should be anticipated postoperatively.

Cure rates following unilateral adrenalectomy for APA range from 30% to 60% [6, 19]. In the case of cure potassium levels are normalized rapidly after surgery and blood pressure typically returns to normal within 1–3 months, but may take considerably longer. Surgery is effective in less than 20% of cases of BAH and should therefore be avoided.

Pharmacological therapy

Pharmacological therapy is indicated in all patients preoperatively and long term for patients who are unsuitable surgical candidates or who have BAH or GRA. Spironolactone, a mineralocorticoid receptor antagonist, is the most commonly used agent in the treatment of PA. Doses are given initially as 25–50 mg twice daily, increasing as required to a maximum daily dose of 400 mg. This is usually extremely effective in correcting hypokalemia although it may take some time to return blood pressure to normal. Spironolactone, particularly in high doses, inhibits testosterone biosynthesis and antagonizes peripheral androgen action resulting in gynecomastia (often painful), reduced libido and erectile impotence in males and menstrual irregularity in females (due to progesterone receptor agonist action). Other side effects include nausea and abdominal pain. Importantly, serum

potassium and creatinine levels must be monitored carefully during therapy with spironolactone.

Amiloride can be used as a first-line agent or in patients intolerant of spironolactone. Dose starts at 10 mg/day often needing to be increased to 30–40 mg/day. Side effects are rare but include headache, fatigue and nausea. In the occasional patient who is intolerant to both spironolactone and amiloride, triamterene can be used in doses of 100–300 mg/day.

In 2002 the selective aldosterone receptor antagonist eplerenone was approved by the United States Food and Drug Administration for the treatment of hypertension. There have been no published trials evaluating eplerenone in the treatment of PA, but a number of trials looking at its efficacy in the treatment of "essential hypertension" and post-myocardial infarct heart failure have been encouraging [20]. The doses of eplerenone recommended for the treatment of congestive cardiac failure post myocardial infarction are 25 mg once per day initially with an increase following 4 weeks to 50 mg once per day if tolerated. In patients receiving eplerenone for the treatment of hypertension this dose can be increased further; however, doses of greater than 100 mg per day are not recommended as they have no greater effect on blood pressure than 100 mg per day or are associated with increased risk of hyperkalemia. Eplerenone has the advantage of having 0.1% of the binding affinity to the androgen receptor and <1% of the binding affinity to the progesterone receptor compared with spironolactone and as such an incidence of adverse events similar to placebo [19]. Spironolactone has been shown in the RALES study to decrease the progression of congestive cardiac failure and mortality (particularly sudden cardiac death) in a cohort of patients with congestive cardiac failure (NYHA Class III or IV) [21]. The effectiveness of aldosterone blockade was confirmed in the EPHESUS study which showed a decreased mortality in patients with systolic left ventricular dysfunction following myocardial infarct treated with eplerenone [22]. It should be noted that in both these studies all patients also had optimum medical treatment with diuretics, ACE inhibitors and beta blockers.

Antihypertensive treatment is frequently required in addition to the above medications. Because intracellular calcium is an important second messenger in the synthesis and action of aldosterone, calcium antagonists have been used with good success. Aldosterone secretion in patients with BAH is extremely sensitive to circulating ATII and perhaps the most effective antihypertensive in such patients are the ACE inhibitors. Hypervolemia in patients with PA may also lead to antihypertensive agent resistance and low doses of thiazide diuretic can be useful in combination with potassium-sparing diuretics.

Conclusion

Primary hyperaldosteronism is increasing in prevalence with the commonest cause now being BAH rather than the classic adrenal adenoma first described by Conn in 1955, and should be considered in the context of a spectrum of low renin hypertension. The knowledge that the majority of patients with PA are normokalemic has led to an increase in screening for PA in hypertensive patients. In recent years aldosterone has been implicated in premature cardiovascular disease and as a result the diagnosis and appropriate treatment of PA may be even more important than previously thought. In the screening and diagnosis of PA, the clinician must be aware of the strengths and weaknesses of the investigations used and factors which may complicate the interpretation of the results obtained.

References

1. Conn JW. Presidential address. I. Painting background. II. Primary aldosteronism, a new clinical syndrome. *J. Lab. Clin. Med.* 1955;45:3–17.

2. Young WF, Jr. Minireview: primary aldosteronism–changing concepts in diagnosis and treatment. *Endocrinology* 2003;144:2208–2213.

3. Rossi G, Boscaro M, Ronconi V, et al. Aldosterone as a cardiovascular risk factor. *Trends Endocrinol. Metab.* 2005;16:104–107.

4. Struthers AD. Aldosterone-induced vasculopathy. *Mol. Cell. Endocrinol.* 2004;217:239–241.

5. Mulatero P, Veglio F, Pilon C, et al. Increased diagnosis of primary aldosteronism, including surgically correctable forms, in centers from five continents. *J. Clin. Endocrinol. Metab.* 2004;89:1045–1050.

6. Stowasser M, Gordon RD. Primary aldosteronism. *Best Pract. Res. Clin. Endocrinol. Metab.* 2003;17:591–605.

7. Sutherland DJ, Ruse JL, Laidlaw JC. Hypertension, increased aldosterone secretion and low plasma renin activity relieved by dexamethasone. *Can. Med. Assoc. J.* 1966;95:1109–1119.

8. McMahon GT, Dluhy RG. Glucocorticoid-remediable aldosteronism. *Arq. Bras. Endocrinol. Metabol.* 2004;48:682–686.

9. Stewart PM., Mineralocorticoid hypertension. *Lancet* 1999;353:1341–1347.

10. Mulatero P, Dluhy RG, Giachetti G, et al. Diagnosis of primary aldosteronism: from screening to subtype differentiation. *Trends Endocrinol. Metab.* 2005;16:114–119.

11. Young WF Jr, et al. Primary aldosteronism: diagnosis and treatment. *Mayo Clin. Proc.* 1990;65:96–110.

12. Mulatero P, Rabbia F, Milan A, et al. Drug effects on aldosterone/plasma renin activity ratio in primary aldosteronism. *Hypertension* 2002;40:897–902.

13. Seiler L, Rump LC, Schulte-Monting J. et al. Diagnosis of primary aldosteronism: value of different screening parameters and influence of antihypertensive medication. *Eur. J. Endocrinol.* 2004;150:329–337.

14. Stowasser M, Gordon RD, Rutherford JC, et al. Diagnosis and management of primary aldosteronism. *J. Renin Angiotensin Aldosterone Syst.* 2001;2:156–169.

15. Lim PO, Dow E, Brennan G, et al. High prevalence of primary aldosteronism in the Tayside hypertension clinic population. *J. Hum. Hypertens.* 2000;14:311–315.

16. Holland OB, Brown H, Kuhnert L, et al. Further evaluation of saline infusion for the diagnosis of primary aldosteronism. *Hypertension* 1984;6:717–723.

17. Lumachi F, Marzola MC, Zucchetta P, et al. Non-invasive adrenal imaging in primary aldosteronism. Sensitivity and positive predictive value of radiocholesterol scintigraphy, CT scan and MRI. *Nucl. Med. Commun.* 2003;24:683–688.

18. Magill SB, Raff H, Shaker JL, et al. Comparison of adrenal vein sampling and computed tomography in the differentiation of primary aldosteronism. *J. Clin. Endocrinol. Metab.* 2001;86:1066–1071.

19. Young WF Jr. Primary aldosteronism – treatment options. *Growth Horm. IGF Res.* 2003;13 (Suppl A):S102–108.

20. Moore TD, Nawarskas JJ, Anderson JR. Eplerenone: a selective aldosterone receptor antagonist for hypertension and heart failure. *Heart Dis.* 2003;5:354–363.

21. Pitt B, Zannad F, Remme WJ, et al. The effect of spironolactone on morbidity and mortality in patients with severe heart failure. Randomized Aldactone Evaluation Study Investigators. *N. Engl. J. Med.* 1999;341:709–717.

22. Pitt B, Remme W, Zannad F, et al. Eplerenone, a selective aldosterone blocker, in patients with left ventricular dysfunction after myocardial infarction. *N. Engl. J. Med.* 2003;348:1309–1321.

49 Adrenal Causes of Cushing's Syndrome

John R. Lindsay and A. Brew Atkinson

> **Key points**
> - Adrenal adenomas/carcinomas account for around 10–20% of cases of Cushing's syndrome.
> - Computerized tomography/magnentic resonance imaging provides excellent delineation of adrenal gland morphology and should be employed once the diagnosis of adrenocorticotropic hormone-independent Cushing's syndrome has been secured biochemically.
> - Laparoscopic adrenal surgery has replaced open adrenalectomy as the treatment of choice for most small or medium-sized adrenal tumors.
> - The recognition of bilateral adrenal hyperplasia caused by aberrant receptors offers the potential for targeted pharmacological therapies.
> - Adrenal cancer is associated with low 5-year survival rates; extensive surgery, mitotane and tumor bed irradiation should be considered until more effective chemotherapeutic regimens become available. If possible patients should be enrolled in clinical trials.

Introduction

Cushing's syndrome is a constellation of clinical and biochemical abnormalities resulting from chronic excess of cortisol of any etiology. There are two major classifications of the syndrome: adrenocorticotropic hormone (ACTH)-dependent and ACTH-independent Cushing's syndrome. The presentation, investigation and treatment of ACTH-dependent Cushing's syndrome are discussed elsewhere (see Chapter 31). This chapter will consider the adrenal causes of Cushing's syndrome.

ACTH-independent Cushing's syndrome

There are a number of ACTH-independent causes of the syndrome (Table 49.1). Adrenal adenomas and carcinomas account for around 10–20% of all cases of Cushing's syndrome, with equal frequencies of adenoma and carcinoma in adults. These tumors are less common in men than in women. The majority of tumors arise spontaneously and are not associated with chronic ACTH stimulation. With small tumors the clinical picture is usually that

Table 49.1 Etiologies of adrenal Cushing's syndrome

Adrenocortical adenoma
Adrenocortical carcinoma
Adrenocortical macronodular hyperplasia (partially ACTH-dependent)
Primary pigmented nodular adrenocortical disease

Clinical Endocrine Oncology, 2nd edition. Edited by Ian D. Hay and John A.H. Wass. © 2008 Blackwell Publishing. ISBN 978-1-4051-4584-8.

of glucocorticoid excess, although purely virilizing or mixed adrenocortical adenomas may occur. Large tumors are more likely to be malignant and often show clinical evidence of both glucocorticoid excess and excess androgen production. Occasionally, adrenal carcinomas may also secrete aldosterone, deoxycorticosterone or estrogens. While many cases with adrenal Cushing's syndrome due to adrenal adenoma present with clinically apparent disease, there is increasing recognition of incidental adrenal adenoma in around 3–4% of the population with the advent of routine imaging techniques. Adrenal incidentaloma may be accompanied by subclinical Cushing's syndrome in between 5–20% of cases [1]. Diagnosis and management of subclinical Cushing's syndrome are clinically important due to its association with complications of the metabolic syndrome, which include hypertension, obesity, and diabetes and also the potential of precipitating adrenal insufficiency during surgery for patients in whom the subclinical Cushing's syndrome has led to suppression of the contralateral gland. A previous NIH consensus conference provided a detailed framework for the evaluation of these cases [2].

Presentation

The symptoms and signs of Cushing's syndrome are well known to clinicians. It is difficult to rival the excellent description of the disease provided by Harvey Cushing himself [3]. Cushing described a patient with cessation of menses, increasing obesity, headache, nausea, vomiting and palpitations, purpuric outbreaks, a definite growth of hair on the face with thinning of the hair on the scalp, muscular weakness and backache. On physical examination the patient was undersized, kyphotic and of most extraordinary appearance. Her round face was dusky and cyanosed with an abnormal growth of hair, particularly noticeable on the sides of the forehead, upper lip and chin. Her abdomen had the appearance of a full-term pregnancy. The breasts were hypertrophied and pendulous, and there were pads of fat over the supraclavicular and posterior cervical regions. The cyanotic appearance of the skin was particularly apparent over the body and lower extremities which were spotted by subcutaneous ecchymoses. Numerous purple striae were present over the stretched skin and a fine hirsuties was present over the back, hips and around the umbilicus. The skin, which everywhere was rough and dry, showed considerable pigmentation. The peculiar tense and painful adiposity affecting face, neck and trunk was in marked contrast to her comparatively spare extremities.

As well as the classic features described above, other abnormalities have been reported in Cushing's syndrome. Hypertension, type 2 diabetes mellitus and osteoporosis are prevalent. An increased incidence of opportunistic infections such as cryptococcosis, aspergillosis, nocardiosis and *Pneumocystis jiroveci* pneumonia have been reported, with the signs and symptoms of infection often masked by the hypercortisolism. The prevalence of the various signs and symptoms has been well reviewed.

It is not often possible to differentiate between the various causes of Cushing's syndrome on the basis of symptoms and signs alone but certain features may suggest a specific etiology. Adrenal adenomas usually present with a clinical picture of mild hypercortisolism of a gradual onset. Androgenic manifestations such as hirsutism are usually absent. With adrenal carcinomas, clinical features of glucocorticoid and androgen hypersecretion have a much more rapid onset and are rapidly progressive. Hypercortisolism is usually marked. Hypokalemia is common. Abdominal pain, abdominal masses and evidence of hepatic or pulmonary metastases are common at diagnosis.

Diagnosis of Cushing's syndrome

The diagnosis of Cushing's syndrome is the first essential step in investigation prior to proceeding to differential diagnosis.

Differential diagnosis

Having established the diagnosis of Cushing's syndrome, one proceeds to differential diagnosis [4]. Proper treatment of Cushing's syndrome depends crucially on establishing the precise etiology. The mainstays of the differential diagnostic tests have been the high-dose dexamethasone suppression test, the metyrapone test, and measurement of plasma ACTH, potassium and dehydro-epiandrosterone sulfate (DHEA-S) [4]. For ACTH-dependent cases bilateral inferior petrosal sampling for ACTH levels, the serum cortisol response to exogenous corticotropin-releasing hormone (CRH) and specialist magnetic resonance imaging (MRI) are helpful.

Whereas it is often difficult to establish precisely the site of abnormality in ACTH-dependent Cushing's syndrome, there is usually no great difficulty in establishing the differential diagnosis

of ACTH-independent Cushing's syndrome. Primary adrenal lesions can be readily identified using the combination of computerized tomography (CT) scanning of the adrenals and the demonstration of undetectable or very low plasma ACTH levels. To avoid falsely low values, samples for ACTH determination should be collected in pre-chilled ethylenediaminetetra-acetic acid tubes, with transport in an ice bath and with prompt refrigerated centrifugation and plasma separation [4]. In addition, there is generally no suppression of cortisol with high-dose dexamethasone, no rise in plasma 11-deoxycortisol or urinary steroids following metyrapone, and no response of cortisol to CRH. Both adrenal adenomas and carcinomas causing Cushing's syndrome are readily apparent on CT scan.

CT scanning produces excellent delineation of the adrenal gland morphology because of the characteristically abundant perinephric and adrenal fat in Cushing's syndrome. Adrenocortical adenomas producing Cushing's syndrome are usually larger than 2 cm and are of low tissue density on CT. The contralateral gland usually appears normal but can appear atrophic secondary to the feedback reduction in ACTH levels. The differential diagnosis for an adrenal mass in a patient with Cushing's syndrome includes a pheochromocytoma producing ACTH, a metastasis from an ectopic ACTH carcinoma, an incidental mass such as a non-functioning adenoma or a metastasis from a known or unknown primary tumor. Adrenal adenomas display low attenuation values in pre-contrast scans that may help differentiate adenomas from non-adenomatous lesions, including malignancies. If the attenuation value is greater than 10 Hounsfield units (HU) at non-contrast imaging then contrast-enhanced scanning should be performed. Over 50% washout of contrast material on 10-minute delayed CT is diagnostic of an adenoma.

Adrenal scintigraphy with cholesterol-based radiopharmaceuticals such as 75Se-selenocholesterol or NP-59 can also be used to image unilateral functional adenomas with absence of radiopharmaceutical in the contralateral gland. However, this is not usually necessary.

Adrenal carcinomas are rare with an estimated incidence of 0.5–2 per million population. The majority measure at least 6 cm at diagnosis and are often heterogeneous with areas of necrosis and calcification. Some carcinomas may be smaller and resemble adenomas. Carcinomas invade adjacent organs such as the liver (Fig. 49.1). Such invasion can be assessed using ultrasonography, CT and MRI scanning. Direct invasion into the inferior vena cava, involvement of regional lymph nodes and metastases to the liver, lung and bone can all occur. Adrenocortical carcinomas show no uptake of cholesterol-based radiopharmaceuticals unless they are well differentiated, which is rare.

MRI will readily identify functioning adrenal adenomas and carcinomas but may not adequately differentiate adenoma from carcinoma on the basis of relative signal intensities. For indeterminate lesions chemical shift MRI or adrenal biopsy may be performed [5]. With chemical shift MRI, the sensitivity and specificity for differentiating adenomas from metastases range from 81% to 100% and 94% to 100%, respectively [5]. Furthermore,

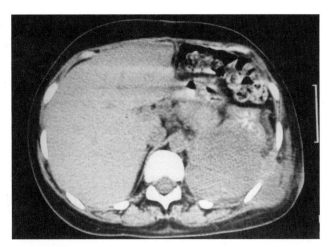

Figure 49.1 CT scan of adrenals, which shows a large left-sided adrenal carcinoma with invasion of surrounding structures.

MRI is superior to CT for assessment of tumor thrombosis in blood vessels, particularly the inferior vena cava and adrenal and renal veins.

Positron emission tomography (PET) performed with fluorine-18 fluorodeoxyglucose (FDG) is a promising novel modality that in several earlier trials had 100% sensitivity but lower specificity (80–100%) for differentiating malignant from benign adrenal masses [5]. More recently combined PET/CT was shown to have increased sensitivity for detection of metastatic lesions [6]. PET has particular utility in cases in which CT or MRI features are indeterminate but none of the existing isotopes are specific for malignancy. In one recent study PET altered management in 5 of 28 cases with adrenocortical carcinoma at the expense of one false positive. PET may prove to have a useful complementary role to standard imaging modalities but further studies are required to determine its overall efficacy.

Fine needle aspiration biopsy (FNAB) is not routinely employed for evaluation of adrenal masses but is most useful for cases in which the adrenal lesion cannot be characterized by standard or nuclear medicine imaging modalities discussed earlier. Adrenal biopsies are safe, accurate and are associated with complication rates less than 3%. While several series have demonstrated the utility and safety of FNAB in the absence of needle track extension, this complication remains a theoretical possibility. Advances in fine needle aspiration technology may also allow improvements in diagnostic accuracy. Needless to say, it is important to carefully exclude pheochromocytoma before embarking on such a strategy.

Rare causes of ACTH-independent hypercortisolism

While adrenal Cushing's syndrome is usually due to a benign (adenoma) or malignant (carcinoma) unilateral adrenocortical tumor, approximately 10% of cases occur due to bilateral ACTH-independent adrenocortical macronodular hyperplasia (AIMAH) or primary pigmented nodular adrenocortical disease (PPNAD). In both cases the clinical presentation may lead to clinically overt or subclinical Cushing's syndrome.

The earliest example of AIMAH is food-dependent Cushing's syndrome[7/8], which was described by Lacroix et al. [8], who later demonstrated that gastric inhibitory polypeptide (GIP) exerted an abnormal adrenocortical response in two patients with AIMAH, both with low fasting cortisol levels that increased with food. Since then a wide range of ectopic or eutopic hormone receptors have been implicated in AIMAH, including receptors for V-1 vasopressin, beta-adrenergic receptors, luteinizing hormone (LH)/human chorionic gonadotropin (HCG) receptors and serotonin 4 (5-HT4) receptors [8]. Patients typically have bilateral large adrenal nodules of varying size which are often up to several centimeters in diameter. These nodules often co-exist with a hyperplastic adrenal cortex. ACTH levels tend to be low or undetectable and cortisol levels fail to show 50% suppression during a high-dose dexamethasone suppression test. A range of testing protocols has been developed in order to identify stimuli to aberrant receptors and potential therapeutic targets. These include dynamic tests of steroidogenesis to stimuli including posture, standard mixed meal, ACTH, gonadotropin-releasing hormone, thyrotropin-releasing hormone, glucagon and metoclopramide. A change in plasma cortisol of 50% or greater is characterized as a positive response, 25–49% increase as partial and less than 25% as no response [8].

PPNAD is a rare cause of Cushing's syndrome, which is characterized by small to normal adrenal glands containing multiple, small, deeply pigmented adrenal nodules. This condition is described in more detail in Chapter 72. PPNAD may occur sporadically, or can be inherited in an autosomal dominant pattern as part of Carney complex (pigmented skin lesions, spotty facial pigmentation, myxomas, testicular and pituitary tumors). Most commonly, PPNAD is characterized by a paradoxical, more than 50% rise in urine free cortisol excretion on the second day of the high-dose dexamethasone suppression test [9].

It is important to be aware of these rare conditions, as they can be associated with unusual biochemistry while in addition nodular hyperplasia of the adrenals with a solitary or dominant nodule may be misdiagnosed as a hyperfunctioning adrenal adenoma.

Pathophysiology and molecular biology of adrenal causes of Cushing's syndrome

Adrenocortical tumors are associated with a variety of genetic syndromes, whose clinical features and molecular defects are summarized in Table 49.2. Two loci, 2p16 and 17q22–24 that are associated with the development of Carney complex have provided useful insights into adrenal pathophysiology and development of adrenocortical tumors. In particular, heterozygous mutations at the 17q22–24 locus, which acts as the regulatory subunit R1A of protein kinase A (PRKAR1A), have been identified in around 45% of index cases of Carney complex and 80% of families of those presenting with Cushing's syndrome. Effects on PRKAR1A interactions on the cyclic AMP signaling pathway may contribute to tumorigenesis and have been implicated as a potential tumor suppressor gene.

Table 49.2 Genetic syndromes predisposing to adrenocortical tumors

Syndrome	Clinical features	Molecular defects
Beckwith–Wiedemann	Macrosomia, macroglossia, omphalocele, visceromegaly, hemihypertrophy, neonatal hypoglycemia, and various tumors (nephroblastoma, adrenocortical carcinoma, neuroblastoma, and hepatoblastoma)	Allelic loss or imprinting error of the 11p15 chromosomal region (genes for H19, p57^{KIP2}, and IGF-II)
Li–Fraumeni	Familial susceptibility to various cancers (e.g., breast, adrenal cortex, brain, leukemia)	Germline mutation in the gene for p53
McCune–Albright	Polyostotic fibrous dysplasia, cafe au lait spots, precocious puberty, endocrine tumors	Mosaicism for activating mutation in the *GNAS1* gene
Carney	Primary pigmented nodular adrenocortical disease, schwannomas, myxomas, lentigines	Defect mapped to the 2p16 locus
Multiple endocrine neoplasia type 1	Hyperparathyroidism, pancreatic–duodenal tumors, and pituitary tumors	Germline mutation in the *menin* gene

IGF, insulin-like growth factor.
(Reproduced from Gicquel C et al. *Endocrinol. Metab. Clin. North Am.* 2000;29:1–13, with permission from Elsevier Ltd.)

Increasingly, the role of ectopic expression of abnormal hormone receptors in adrenal Cushing's syndrome has been explored [8]. Ectopic receptors are more common in AIMAH, and rare in adrenal adenoma [10]. While the clinical and biochemical responses to aberrant stimuli have been well characterized, the molecular mechanisms remain unknown and no mutations in the coding regions or these receptors have been identified [11]. The majority of cases are sporadic, occurring in the fifth to sixth decade, with an equal prevalence among the genders [8]. The identification of illicit membrane hormone receptors offers the potential for targeted pharmacological strategies for treatment of adrenal Cushing's syndrome. Therapy with octreotide in GIP-dependent Cushing's syndrome was an effective treatment in several cases with food-dependent Cushing's syndrome but only in the short term, with adrenalectomy eventually being required for control of hypercortisolism. Similarly, beta blockade with propranolol was partially effective, as primary and then adjunctive therapy following unilateral adrenalectomy, in one case with catecholamine-dependent Cushing's syndrome [8]. More recently, leuprolide acetate was used to control hypercortisolism in one case with LH/hCG-dependent AIMAH [8].

Adrenal carcinomas appear to be monoclonal in origin [12] although their pathogenesis may involve multiple genetic changes. The molecular and genetic bases of adrenal adenoma and carcinoma have been intensively studied [13]. Germline mutations of the tumor suppressor gene p53 are responsible for features of the Li–Fraumeni syndrome that result, in affected individuals, in the development of a variety of carcinomas including adrenocortical carcinoma [14]. Similarly, Beckwith–Wiedemann syndrome is associated with chromosomal derangements at 11p15 and multifocal neoplasia, including adrenocortical carcinoma. Gicquel

demonstrated the potential predictive value of structural changes at chromosome 17p and 11p15 and the malignant clinical phenotypes, which were correlated [15].

Activating mutations of the ACTH receptor have previously been excluded as a common factor in the pathogenesis of adrenal tumors. There is some evidence that cAMP-dependent mitogenic pathways may be important, as activating mutations in the cyclase inhibitory Giα subunit have been detected in both adenomas and occasional carcinoma. However, our knowledge of the molecular biology of these tumors remains incomplete and much work remains to be done to show any proof of similarity to other cancers that may allow more rational selection of chemotherapeutic regimens in the future.

Treatment of adrenal causes of Cushing's syndrome

Adrenal adenomas can be successfully treated by unilateral adrenalectomy, which can be achieved by either laparoscopic or open procedure. Despite a lack of controlled trials laparoscopic adrenal surgery has largely replaced the open procedure and has proved to be as effective for small or medium-sized tumors but with less associated morbidity [16]. Laparoscopic adrenalectomy was described in 1992 and has since been employed in around 500 cases of cortisol-secreting adrenal adenoma. While the procedure is advantageous in terms of a shorter recovery time and reduced surgical morbidity, it may not be suitable for larger tumors (greater than 8 cm) or when adrenocortical carcinoma is evident during perioperative assessment [16]. In view of the efficacy of existing surgical techniques for management of functioning adrenocortical adenomas it is unclear as to the potential future role of less invasive procedures including CT-guided percutaneous acetic acid injection therapy. While this treatment may result in resolution of adrenocortical hyperfunction, limitations including the inability to determine histopathology may curtail its future use.

The prognosis for cortisol-producing adenomas following treatment with adrenalectomy is excellent. Postoperatively, all patients have adrenal insufficiency because of suppression of ACTH secretion and hence of the contralateral adrenal gland. Adequate glucocorticoid replacement therapy is therefore mandatory but mineralocorticoid therapy is not usually required. Glucocorticoid therapy must be continued until complete recovery of the hypothalamo–pituitary–adrenal axis has occurred. This can take up to or even longer than 24 months [17].

In this context the identification of cases with bilateral macronodular disease, caused by stimulation of aberrant receptors, might be of value. Ideally, as discussed earlier, targeted medical therapy might be offered for control of hypercortisolism, thereby obviating the need for a surgical procedure and long-term post-surgical hypoadrenalism. Unfortunately the majority of these strategies have proven ineffective for longer-term treatment [8]. It is in this setting that definitive treatment with bilateral adrenalectomy, which in the modern era is safe and effective in experienced hands, should be considered [18].

Treatment of adrenocortical carcinoma is much less satisfactory and the mortality rate is high. Many patients have widespread metastases at the time of diagnosis. Five-year survival rates are in the range 15–47%, with a mean survival time after therapy of around 18 months [19]. The clinical staging at diagnosis was the most important prognostic factor in the recent series reported by Ng, whereas the effect of age, gender, or tumor functional status was not significant [19].

Extensive surgery, if possible, is the first step in therapy, serving to reduce the tumor mass and the degree of hypercortisolism. Curative surgery should result in absent steroid secretion since the pituitary output of ACTH is suppressed. Adjuvant tumor bed irradiation should be considered in cases with no macroscopic evidence of residual tumor after initial surgery, as it may reduce the risk of local recurrence; however, at present there is no evidence of improved survival using this modality in the longer term.

Persisting non-suppressible plasma cortisol following surgery indicates residual metastatic tumor. After operation, mitotane is usually employed, which is associated with around a 30% response rate, although its impact on survival is uncertain. It is generally effective in controlling hormonal hypersecretion but does not have a significant effect on survival. It is given in doses of between 6 and 12 g daily, but severe side effects (nausea, vomiting and diarrhea) limit its use in high doses in many patients. Because mitotane affects the metabolism of cortisol, plasma cortisol or urinary free cortisol should be monitored in these patients and, if necessary, dexamethasone given as replacement steroid therapy. The utility of a high-dose mitotane therapeutic schedule was recently tested and may reduce the interval between starting treatment and achieving the therapeutic range [20]. A free plasma mitotane testing service has recently become available in Europe (www.lysodren-europe.com), which may aid prompt dose titration and reduce associated side effects. Higher response rates, of the order of 58%, were previously observed using a dosing strategy to achieve plasma mitotane levels within 14–20 mg/L. Metyrapone and aminoglutethimide can also be given in attempts to control steroid hypersecretion, and ketoconazole should also be considered.

A range of alternative chemotherapeutic regimens have been attempted including cisplatin, etoposide, doxorubicin, 5-fluorouracil, vincristine, suramin and gossypol but with variable results. Etoposide, doxorubicin and cisplatin may be added to mitotane, but were previously associated with similar overall response rates to mitotane used alone (48.6%) in a recent prospective phase II trial. Kirschner recently reviewed the emerging range of potential therapies for adrenocortical carcinoma [13]. Current and future trials are underway to examine effects of competitive inhibitors of multi-drug resistance protein (MDR1) such as Tariquidar used in combination with mitotane. Vascular targeted therapies include the use of anti-vascular endothelial growth factor antibodies using bevacizumab and attempts to disrupt established tumor vasculature [13]. In order to determine the clinical utility of these novel treatment strategies a series of international clinical trials are underway. Due to the low prevalence of adrenocortical cancer all patients should be referred for assessment at a specialist center and be considered for inclusion in a controlled trial such as the FIRM ACT study (First International Randomized Trial for Locally Advanced and Metastatic Adrenocortical Tumors; www.firm-act.org) [13].

Conclusion

Cushing's syndrome is an unusual and unpleasant condition, which carries a high mortality if undetected or untreated. Following careful assessment and confirmation of hypercortisolism by biochemical means, it is imperative to accurately define the underlying cause. ACTH-independent Cushing's syndrome accounts for 10–20% of cases and can usually be readily distinguished from ACTH-dependent causes. Radiological and other imaging techniques help further define the underlying etiology, which is most often an adrenal adenoma or carcinoma, although aberrant receptors should be borne in mind in those with bilateral adrenal enlargement. Surgical treatment of adrenal adenomas is highly successful. Novel drug treatments or bilateral adrenalectomy can be used in cases with bilateral adrenocortical macronodular hyperplasia. In contrast, adrenal carcinomas have a very poor prognosis but combined surgical and chemotherapeutic treatment may help improve survival. Better agents are required urgently.

References

1. Terzolo M, Bovio S, Reimondo G, et al. Subclinical Cushing's syndrome in adrenal incidentalomas. *Endocrinol. Metab. Clin. North Am.* 2005;34:423–439.

2. NIH state-of-the-science statement on management of the clinically inapparent adrenal mass ("incidentaloma"). *NIH Consens. State Sci. Statements* 2002;19:1–25.

3. Cushing H. The basophil adenomas of the pituitary body and their clinical manifestations (pituitary basophilism). *Bull. Johns Hopkins* 1932;50:137–195.

4. Lindsay JR, Nieman LK. Differential diagnosis and imaging in Cushing's syndrome. *Endocrinol. Metab. Clin. North Am.* 2005;34:403–421.

5. Mayo-Smith WW, Boland GW, Noto RB, Lee MJ. State-of-the-art adrenal imaging. *Radiographics* 2001;21:995–1012.

6. Leboulleux S, Dromain C, Bonniaud G, et al. Diagnostic and prognostic value of 18-fluorodeoxyglucose positron emission tomography in adrenocortical carcinoma: a prospective comparison with computed tomography. *J. Clin. Endocrinol. Metab.* 2005;91:920–925.

7. Hamet P, Larochelle P, Franks DJ, Cartier P, Bolte E. Cushing syndrome with food-dependent periodic hormonogenesis. *Clin. Invest. Med.* 1987;10:530–533.

8. Lacroix A, Ndiaye N, Tremblay J, Hamet P. Ectopic and abnormal hormone receptors in adrenal Cushing's syndrome. *Endocr. Rev.* 2001;22:75–110.

9. Stratakis CA, Sarlis N, Kirschner LS, et al. Paradoxical response to dexamethasone in the diagnosis of primary pigmented nodular adrenocortical disease. *Ann. Intern. Med.* 1999;131:585–591.

10. Groussin L, Perlemoine K, Contesse V, et al. The ectopic expression of the gastric inhibitory polypeptide receptor is frequent in adrenocorticotropin-independent bilateral macronodular adrenal hyperplasia, but rare in unilateral tumors. *J. Clin. Endocrinol. Metab.* 2002;87:1980–1985.

11. Antonini SR, Baldacchino V, Tremblay J, Hamet P, Lacroix A. Expression of ACTH receptor pathway genes in glucose-dependent insulinotrophic peptide (GIP)-dependent Cushing's syndrome. *Clin. Endocrinol. (Oxf.)* 2006;64:29–36.

12. Gicquel C, Leblond-Francillard M, Bertagna X, et al. Clonal analysis of human adrenocortical carcinomas and secreting adenomas. *Clin. Endocrinol. (Oxf.)* 1994;40:465–477.

13. Kirschner LS. Emerging treatment strategies for adrenocortical carcinoma: a new hope. *J. Clin. Endocrinol. Metab.* 2006;91:14–21.

14. Reincke M, Karl M, Travis WH, et al. p53 mutations in human adrenocortical neoplasms: immunohistochemical and molecular studies. *J. Clin. Endocrinol. Metab.* 1994;78:790–794.

15. Gicquel C, Bertagna X, Gaston V, et al. Molecular markers and long-term recurrences in a large cohort of patients with sporadic adrenocortical tumors. *Cancer Res.* 2001;61:6762–6767.

16. Young WF, Jr., Thompson GB. Laparoscopic adrenalectomy for patients who have Cushing's syndrome. *Endocrinol. Metab. Clin. North Am.* 2005;34:489–499, xi.

17. Graber AL NR, Nicholson WE, Island DP, Liddle GW. Natural history of pituitary-adrenal recovery following long-term suppression with corticosteroids. *J. Clin. Endocrinol. Metab.* 1965:11–16.

18. McCance DR, Russell CF, Kennedy TL, Hadden DR, Kennedy L, Atkinson AB. Bilateral adrenalectomy: low mortality and morbidity in Cushing's disease. *Clin. Endocrinol. (Oxf.)* 1993;39:315–321.

19. Ng L, Libertino JM. Adrenocortical carcinoma: diagnosis, evaluation and treatment. *J. Urol.* 2003;169:5–11.

20. Faggiano A, Leboulleux S, Young J, Schlumberger M, Baudin E. Rapidly progressing high o,p'DDD doses shorten the time required to reach the therapeutic threshold with an acceptable tolerance: preliminary results. *Clin. Endocrinol. (Oxf.)* 2006;64:110–113.

50 Adrenal Incidentalomas

Maria Verena Cicala, Pierantonio Conton, Anna Patalano, and Franco Mantero

> **Key points**
> - The estimated prevalence of adrenal incidentalomas in the general population is around 4%.
> - The main diagnostic purpose is the identification of hypersecreting tumors and malignant neoplasia.
> - Around 70% of incidentalomas are benign non-hypersecreting cortical adenomas.
> - Subclinical cortisol-secreting tumors are the most frequently found among the hypersecreting tumors. Adrenal carcinoma accounts for approximately 5%.
> - Minimal endocrine work-up includes overnight 1 mg dexamethasone suppression test for cortisol, aldosterone/PRA ratio in hypertensives and urinary metanephrines.
> - Imaging techniques (computerized tomography, magnetic resonance imaging, isotope scan, positron emission tomography) are fundamental in defining the nature of the mass.
> - Surgery is indicated in most hypersecreting tumors and in the suspicion of malignancy.
> - A 2- to 3-year follow-up may be adequate for other cases.

Introduction

The term "adrenal incidentaloma" indicates an adrenal mass discovered unexpectedly by an imaging procedure performed for reasons other than suspected adrenal pathology.

The differential diagnosis of an adrenal mass is extensive, with common causes including benign or malignant, hormonally active or inactive primary adrenal tumors, tumors metastasizing to the adrenal gland, infections, hemorrhage and compensatory hypertrophy.

Abdominal imaging procedures that may reveal an adrenal incidentaloma are performed for non-specific symptoms (36%), abdominal pain (36%) – including ill-defined discomfort or biliary and renal colic, postoperative follow-up (8%), acute abdomen (1.5%), abdominal trauma (1.5%) and various other reasons (17%). A retrospective multicenter study in Italy analyzed 1004 incidentalomas. At diagnosis, hypertension was seen in 41% of patients, obesity in 28% and diabetes in 10%. In patients with pheochromocytoma 45% were normotensive [1].

Causes and prevalence

In normal subjects, the prevalence of adrenal incidentalomas may depend on the type of imaging performed. The current prevalence of unsuspected adrenal masses is approximately 0.7–4.3% without

Clinical Endocrine Oncology, 2nd edition. Edited by Ian D. Hay and John A.H. Wass. © 2008 Blackwell Publishing. ISBN 978-1-4051-4584-8.

difference between the left and right side (10% are bilateral masses). This is probably an underestimation and the prevalence of this "new" clinical entity will probably continue to increase as a result of technological advances [2]. In autopsy series, the prevalence of previously undiagnosed adrenal masses ranges between 1.4% and 8.7% [3].

In addition to the source of data (autopsies versus clinical series) and the reasons for imaging (cancer work-up, non-endocrinological symptoms and general health screening), age also influences the prevalence of clinically apparent masses. The prevalence of incidentalomas detected at autopsy is less than 1% for patients under 30 years of age and increases to 7% in patients aged 70 years or more. The frequency peaks between the fifth and seventh decades of life [4], suggesting a compensatory growth in response to local ischemic damage due to atherosclerotic disease, although it may merely reflect the larger number of diagnostic procedures performed in older patients.

The differential diagnosis of this clinical problem must consider Cushing syndrome, pheochromocytoma, primary aldosteronism, primary and metastatic malignancy, myelolipoma, and non-hypersecretory cortical adenoma. Table 50.1 summarizes the prevalence of adrenal incidentalomas (reported by the AI-SIE) and the histological diagnoses are illustrated in Fig. 50.1 [4].

The majority of adrenal incidentalomas are non-hypersecretory adenomas, with a reported prevalence ranging from 36% to 94% (74% in our series) in patients with no family history of cancer; but many patients with adrenal incidentalomas have revealed isolated or multiple mild hypothalamo–pituitary–adrenal abnormalities.

A situation of cortisol excess without the classic clinical signs is a common finding in patients with incidental adrenal adenomas

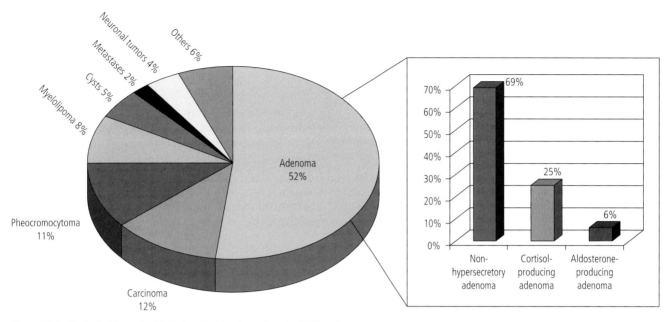

Figure 50.1 Histological diagnosis of 376 adrenal incidentalomas from the AI-SIE study.

Table 50.1 Prevalence (%) of causes of adrenal incidentaloma in AI-SIE series (on 1004 incidentalomas)

Type of tumor	AI-SIE (n 1004 incidentalomas)
Non-hypersecretory adrenal adenomas	74.0
Hypersecretory tumors	
Cortisol-secreting adenomas	9.2
Pheochromocytomas	4.2
Aldosteronomas	1.4
Adrenal carcinomas	4.0
Other adrenal masses	
Myelolipomas	3.0
Cysts	1.9
Ganglioneuromas	1.5
Metastases	
Unselected patients	0.7

and it is called subclinical Cushing syndrome. The term subclinical autonomous glucocorticoid hypersecretion (SAGH) has recently been proposed to define this condition [5]. The prevalence of hypercortisolism in patients with clinically inapparent adrenal masses ranges from 5% to 47% in various studies using different protocols and diagnostic criteria [6–8].

Approximately 0.01–0.1% of hypertensive patients have a pheochromocytoma. This rare catecholamine-producing tumor can carry a significant morbidity and mortality if it is not diagnosed early. Its clinical manifestations vary but most patients with adrenal incidentaloma subsequently found to harbor a pheochromocytoma lack these features, and the diagnosis is easily missed or delayed. These "silent" pheochromocytomas may still be lethal, however. Clinically silent pheochromocytoma is not so rare and its prevalence in patients with adrenal incidentalomas has been estimated at 1.5–13% [9].

Primary aldosteronism is more common nowadays than was previously reported. The prevalence of mineralocorticoid-secreting masses in hypertensive patients with adrenal incidentalomas is estimated at 1.6–5% [10].

The most feared diagnostic possibility in cases of incidentally discovered adrenal masses is adrenal cancer (ACC), because of its poor prognosis, with a mean survival of approximately 18 months and a 5-year survival of around 16% [11]. Adrenocortical carcinoma is rare, with an incidence ranging from 0.6 to 2 cases per million population. The prevalence of primary adrenal carcinoma in clinically inapparent adrenal masses correlates with the size of the mass. ACC accounts for 2% of tumors up to 4 cm in size, 6% of tumors from 4.1 to 6 cm, and 25% of tumors larger than 6 cm. The larger the diameter of the mass, the higher the risk of it being malignant. Most publications report a predominance of female cases (up to 90% in some series). These tumors may be functional or non-functional, the former reportedly accounting for 26–94% of cases; the steroids synthesized often have a low biological activity.

The adrenal glands are common sites of metastases from extra-adrenal malignancies because of their high vascularity. Though adrenal metastases are typically bilateral and larger than 3 cm, they may also be unilateral and small. In patients with a history of malignant disease, metastases are the most common cause of incidental adrenal masses of any size, accounting for 50–75% of all incidentalomas in such patients [12]. Carcinomas of the lung, breast, kidney and gastrointestinal tract, and melanoma or lymphoma are the most common sources of adrenal metastases.

Some incidental adrenal masses are cases of infiltrative disease, fungi and tuberculosis, hemorrhage and lesions masquerading as adrenal but arising from adjacent organs (kidney, pancreas, gallbladder, spleen, lymph nodes).

Pathogenesis of adrenocortical tumors

The pathogenesis of adrenal tumors is not well understood. However, the molecular mechanisms that lead to adrenocortical tumor formation are increasingly being studied, both in genetic syndromes associated with adrenocortical neoplasms and in sporadic tumors. Several genetic syndromes facilitate the onset of adrenocortical tumors. Some of the molecular targets responsible have been identified in the Beckwith–Wiedemann, Li–Fraumeni, multiple endocrine neoplasia type 1 (MEN 1) and McCune–Albright syndromes. Cushing syndrome secondary to primary pigmented nodular adrenocortical disease may also be found in Carney syndrome, which is an autosomal dominant disease due to *PRKAR1A* mutations.

As mentioned earlier, the sporadic type of pheochromocytoma is the most frequent, but up to 30% of cases may be part of a hereditary syndrome including MEN 2, von Hippel–Lindau disease (VHL), neurofibromatosis type 1 (NF-1) and paraganglioma syndrome which are associated with an autosomal dominant inheritance pattern and variable penetrance.

A few molecular alterations are known that could give rise to adrenal tumors, which include overexpression of the insulin-like growth factor II (IGF-II) gene, somatic mutations of β-catenin gene, K-ras mutation; also germline mutations in the p53 tumor suppressor gene contribute to the high cancer risk.

Clinical aspects

Patients with a clinically inapparent adrenal mass require a complete history and physical examination, biochemical evaluation for hormone excess and possibly additional radiological studies [1]. Hormone screening may retrospectively reveal a significant number of cases of clinically unsuspected hormone-secreting adrenal tumors.

Central obesity, hypertension, glucose intolerance or osteoporosis may point to glucocorticoid hypersecretion (SAGH), or subclinical Cushing syndrome.

The clinical manifestations of pheochromocytoma vary from symptomatic (headache, palpitations, diaphoresis, anxiety and sustained or paroxysmal hypertension, orthostatic hypotension and hyperglycemia) to asymptomatic.

Patients with adrenal incidentalomas who have normal kalemic values should also be screened to rule out primary hyperaldosteronism, particularly if they have arterial hypertension. In its classic form, primary aldosteronism presents with aldosterone (ALD) excess, low plasma renin activity (PRA) and hypokalemia, but several reports indicate that normokalemic primary aldosteronism is the most common presenting sign of the disease, while the hypokalemic variant probably only occurs in the more severe cases.

Androgen hypersecretion, sometimes associated with glucocorticoid excess, is seldom encountered in adrenal incidentalomas (mainly in ACC). It may become particularly evident in females and in puberty, with an increase in secondary sexual characteristics and hirsutism; androgen excess in males leads instead to infertility, gynecomastia and decreased libido.

Non-hypersecretory adrenal incidentalomas also produce "mass effects" in the case of sizable lesions compressing adjacent organs, in which case a differential diagnosis with adrenal cancer is warranted.

Hormonal assessment (functional status evaluation)

Essential hormone screening involves measuring plasma cortisol, urinary free cortisol and adrenocorticotropic hormone (ACTH). The rationale for the 1-mg dexamethasone suppression test is to detect subclinical hypercortisolism. After taking 1 mg dexamethasone the previous evening, a serum cortisol below 5 µg/dl (<138 nmol/L) at 08:00 used to be considered negative, but this cut-off level has recently been reduced to 1.8 µg/dl (50 nmol/L) [5].

It is also important to measure midnight cortisol levels in hypertensive patients with adrenal incidentalomas. The biological justification for this is that a high midnight cortisol level appears to be the earliest and most sensitive marker of Cushing syndrome. Patients with midnight serum cortisol levels higher than 5.4 g/dl more often have hypertension, hyperglycemia and a history of cardiovascular or cerebrovascular events than those with lower midnight cortisol levels, suggesting that a high midnight cortisol concentration is a valuable clue for earmarking a subgroup of patients with clinically inapparent adrenal adenoma at greater risk of cardiovascular and metabolic disease [13]. Midnight salivary cortisol may be a more convenient tool than serum cortisol.

The most reliable biochemical tests used for diagnosing pheochromocytoma are plasma or urinary metanephrines (normetanephrine and metanephrine). Dynamic testing with clonidine suppression should be reserved for dubious cases. Glucagon testing can trigger a hypertensive crisis and is not to be recommended. Because of its inadequate sensitivity and specificity, chromogranin A offers no additional benefit over the use of catecholamines or their metabolites for the initial diagnosis of pheochromocytoma [14].

A higher than normal ratio of plasma aldosterone concentration to plasma renin activity (PAC/PRA ratio) in the upright posture is widely accepted as a screening test for hyperaldosteronism, because it has proved highly sensitive [15]. Depending on the assay used to detect PAC, the PRA lower detection level, and the normal reference ranges for PAC and PRA at a given center, the ratio is considered above normal when it is greater than 20–50, where the PAC and PRA are expressed in ng/dl and ng/ml/h, respectively. Normokalemia does not rule out aldosteronism because a significant number of patients (7–38%) with aldosteronism are normokalemic (sodium restriction leads to potassium retention, minimizing hypokalemia). Patients undergoing this test should be off all antihypertensive treatment for at least 2–3 weeks and off anti-aldosterone drugs for at least 6 weeks to rule out any interference [16]. Other confirmatory tests include the captopril test and the saline or fludrocortisone suppression test.

The routine assessment of dehydroepiandrosterone sulfate (DHEAS), a marker of adrenal androgen excess, has been recommended, but there is still some controversy over its real value. Low DHEAS levels are frequently observed in patients with SCS (subclinical Cushing syndrome) and adrenocortical adenomas, but the sensitivity and specificity of this parameter are both low (51% and 65%, respectively), and so is its diagnostic power (positive predictive value of 10%). High DHEAS levels are frequently seen in patients with adrenocortical carcinoma, but other studies have found no convincing data to show that DHEAS helps distinguish malignant from benign masses.

Another endocrine alteration, commonly observed in patients with adrenal masses, is an exaggerated 17-OH-progesterone (17-OHP) response to the ACTH test, but its significance is still not clear. It has been suggested that an unrecognized 21-hydroxylase defect could result in ACTH secretion and predispose to adenoma formation, but genetic studies very rarely confirmed this hypothesis.

An enhanced 17-OHP response was also seen in the majority of patients with subclinical Cushing syndrome (68%), and this endocrine alteration returned to normal in most of the patients who underwent unilateral adrenalectomy. The mechanism of enhanced 17-OHP response in adrenocortical tumors consequently remains to be elucidated; it might merely be a sign of a disrupted intratumoral steroidogenesis [17].

Imaging studies

The imaging studies that are most commonly and most effectively used to identify and discriminate between different types of adrenal masses are computerized tomography (CT), magnetic resonance imaging (MRI), and adrenal scintigraphy.

The CT scan is the most often used to assess adrenal masses. Adrenocortical adenomas usually appear on scans as small, homogeneous, round masses with smooth margins and a large intracytoplasmic lipid content, which enables a quantitative evaluation by measuring the attenuation value of the lesions (expressed in Hounsfield units, HU). Adenomas usually have attenuation values below 18 HU on unenhanced CT, and most lesions smaller than 4 cm appear to be benign [18].

In the case of a mass with a high attenuation value (>20 HU), when a metastasis is suspected and pheochromocytoma excluded, ultrasound or CT-guided fine needle aspiration biopsy may be useful for evaluating adrenal lesions, with a sensitivity of 81–100%, a specificity of 83–100%, and an accuracy of 91% (4).

On CT, pheochromocytomas usually appear as rounded or oval masses with a similar density to the liver. Large medullary tumors may reveal a cystic component due to central necrosis

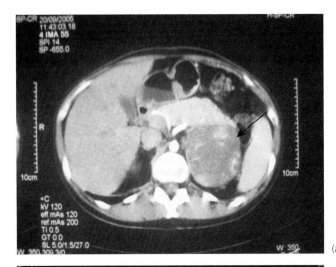
(a)

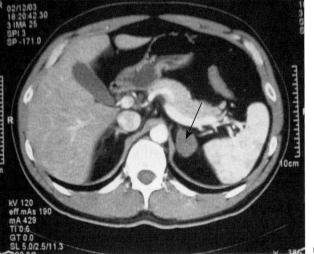
(b)

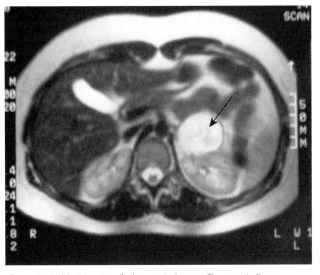
(c)

Figure 50.2 (a) CT imaging of adrenocortical cancer. The arrow indicates a large ACC. (b) CT imaging of adrenal adenoma. They appear as a small, homogeneous, round masses with smooth margins and attenuation values below 18 HU. (c) MRI T2-weighted imaging of pheochromocytoma. It is typically hyperintense on T2-weighted images.

or hemorrhage. (Fig. 50.2 shows the imaging characteristics of adrenal lesions on CT.)

MRI is an accurate method for defining adrenal masses. Both T1 and T2 relaxation times have been studied to distinguish between adenomas, metastases and pheochromocytomas. Malignancies usually show high signal intensity on T2-weighted images, whereas most benign tumors have isointense or low signal intensity on both T1- and T2-weighted images. The sensitivity of CT and MRI proved similar in the differential diagnosis of adrenal tumors, but MRI was more specific in confirming a clinical suspicion of pheochromocytoma. Pheochromocytoma is typically isointense with respect to the liver on T1-weighted images and hyperintense on T2-weighted images; adrenal carcinomas and metastases may have a similar T2-weighted hyperintensity.

Adrenocortical scintigraphy using ^{131}I-6β-iodomethyl-19-norcholesterol (NP-59) or Se-methyl norcholesterol facilitates its *in vivo* functional characterization, and can be particularly useful in association with CT or MRI in cases of ACC, which normally show no uptake.

Most malignant tumors show an enhanced glycolytic metabolism with an increased uptake of deoxyglucose that can be visualized by PET using ^{18}F-2-fluoro-D-deoxyglucose (FDG).

Treatment and follow-up

Adrenalectomy should be considered for patients with a functioning adrenal mass having significant clinical repercussions that might be improved by its resection, or in the event of any biochemical evidence of pheochromocytoma.

When surgery is recommended on the basis of the dimensions of the mass, the cut-off is 6 cm. Lesions that are less than 4 cm and are defined as low risk by imaging criteria are unlikely to have malignant potential and are generally not resected. The need and strategy for routine follow-up in this group are unclear. For

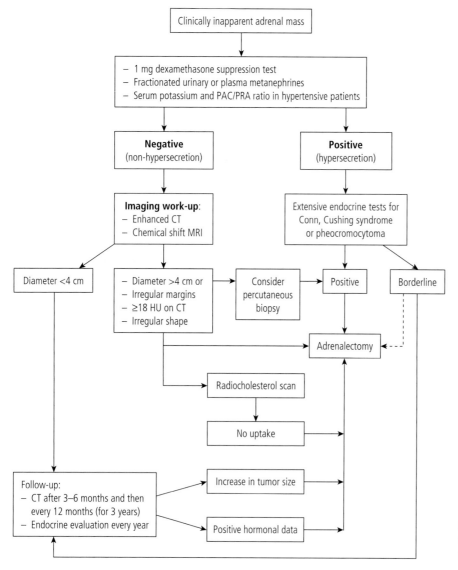

Figure 50.3 Approach to the management of adrenal incidentaloma. PAC, plasma aldosterone concentration; PRA, plasma renin activity.

lesions between 4 and 6 cm, either close follow-up or adrenalectomy is considered a reasonable approach [19].

The treatment of choice is via a laparoscopic access, while open surgery is preferable in the case of malignancy.

As for pheochromocytomas, preoperative treatment with adrenergic alpha$_1$-antagonists (prazosin, doxazosin) is important. There is no standardized therapeutic approach for cases with no clinical or laboratory signs, or for cases in which imaging shows the features of a benign lesion. Although the natural history of subclinical Cushing syndrome is still not entirely clear, adrenalectomy is considered for cases with associated hypertension, obesity, diabetes mellitus and osteoporosis. Adrenalectomy is also indicated in cases of primary hyperaldosteronism. For malignant adrenocortical lesions, surgery is the first and most important treatment option and its radicality decides the prognosis.

Long-term follow-up indicates that the majority of incidentalomas remain stable with time; only 5–10% increase in size or in function. In patients whose lesions have not been excised, CT repeated 6 to 12 months after the initial study is reasonable. Fig. 50.3 shows a flow-chart of adrenal incidentaloma management [17].

This observation is based on longitudinal studies of up to 10 years reporting that the risk for developing adrenal cortical carcinoma is extremely low. The risk for tumor hyperfunction seems to plateau after 3 to 4 years.

References

1. Mantero F, Terzolo M, Arnaldi G, et al. A survey on adrenal incidentaloma in Italy. *J. Clin. Endocrinol. Metab.* 2000;85:637–644.
2. Glazer HZ, Weyman PJ, Sagel SS, Levitt RG, McClennan BL. Nonfunctioning adrenal masses: incidental discovery on computed tomography. *Am. J. Roentgenol.* 1982;139:81–85.
3. Masumori N, Adachi H, Hokfelt B. Detection of adrenal and retroperitoneal masses in a general health examination. *Urology* 1968;52:572–576.
4. Mantero F, Albiger N. A comprehensive approach to adrenal incidentalomas. *Arq. Bras. Endocrinol. Metab.* 2004;48:583–591.
5. Mansmann G, Lau J, Balk E, Rothberg M, Miyachi Y, Bornstein SR. The clinically inapparent adrenal mass: update in diagnosis and management. *Endocr. Rev.* 2004;25:309–340.
6. Rossi R, Tauchmanova L, Luciano A, et al. Subclinical Cushing's syndrome in patients with adrenal incidentaloma: clinical and biochemical features. *J. Clin. Endocrinol. Metab.* 2000;85:1440–1448.
7. Terzolo M, Osella G, Ali A, et al. Subclinical Cushing's syndrome in adrenal incidentaloma. *Clin. Endocrinol. (Oxf.)* 1998;48:89–97.
8. Emral R, Uysal AR, Asik M, et al. Prevalence of subclinical Cushing's syndrome in 70 patients with adrenal incidentaloma: clinical, biochemical and surgical outcomes. *Endocr. J.* 2003;50:399–408.
9. Mannelli M, Ianni L, Cilotti A, Conti A. Pheochromocytoma in Italy: a multicentric retrospective study. *Eur. J. Endocrinol.* 1999;141:619–624.
10. Vierhapper H. Determination of aldosterone/renin ratio in 269 patients with adrenal incidentaloma. *Exp. Clin. Endocrinol. Diabetes* 2007;115:518–521.
11. Nawar R, Aron D. Adrenal incidentalomas – a continuing management dilemma. *Endocrine-Related Cancer* 2005;12:585–598.
12. Liu AM, Maeda S, Hosone M, et al. Use of electron microscopic evaluation for the diagnosis of adrenal cortical carcinoma in fine needle aspiration cytology: a case report and review of the literature. *Med. Electr. Microsc.* 2001;34:190–197.
13. Terzolo M, Bovio S, Pia A, et al. Midnight serum cortisol as a amarker of increased cardiovascular risk in patients with a clinically inapparent adrenal adenoma. *Eur. J. Endocrinol.* 2005;153:307–315.
14. Lenders JW, Eisenhofer G, Mannelli M, Pacak K. Phaeochromocytoma. *Lancet* 2005;366:665–675.
15. Young WF, Jr. Minireview: primary aldosteronism – changing concepts in diagnosis and treatment. *Endocrinology* 2003;144:2208–2013.
16. Mantero F, Bedendo O, Opocher G. Does dynamic testing have a place in the modern assessment of endocrine hypertension? *J. Endocrinol. Invest.* 2003;26:92–98.
17. Mantero F, Arnaldi G. Management approaches to adrenal incidentalomas. *Endocrinol. Metab. Clin. North Am.* 2000;29:107–125.
18. Szolar DH, Kammerhuber FH. Adrenal adenomas and non adenomas: assessment of washout at delayed contrast-enhanced CT. *Radiology* 1998;207:369–375.
19. Grumbach M, Biller BMK, Braunstein GD, et al. Management of the clinically inapparent adrenal mass. *Ann. Intern. Med.* 2003;138:424–429.

51 Androgen-secreting Tumors

Quirinius Barnor, Tom R. Kurzawinski, and Gerard S. Conway

Key points

- Androgen-secreting tumors usually present with virilization in women and can be of either adrenal or ovarian origin.
- Adrenal tumors may be malignant and ovarian tumors are usually benign.
- A short history of hyperandrogenism and a serum testosterone concentration above 144 ng/dL (5.0 nmol/L) are suggestive of a tumorous cause for androgen excess.
- Ultrasound of the ovary and computerized tomography of the adrenal glands usually localize the source.
- Surgical removal is the mainstay of treatment.

Epidemiology and pathology

Androgen-secreting tumors are rare. In a retrospective clinical observation of 950 women presenting with hyperandrogenic syndromes only 0.2% presented with androgen-secreting tumors [1]. The age range of presentation is variable with approximately 50% of adrenal androgen-secreting tumors affecting women under 50 years of age [2] and a similar proportion of ovarian androgen-secreting tumors affecting women under 30 years of age [3].

Ovarian tumors

Virilizing ovarian tumors account for less than 1% of all ovarian tumors [3]. The majority of the androgen-secreting ovarian tumors are sex cord–stromal tumors. Androgen excess has also been reported in epithelial tumors (mostly mucinous cystadenocarcinoma), germ cell tumors, Brenner tumors, stromal carcinoids, metastatic signet-ring cell (Krukenberg) and colonic adenocarcinomas [4]. The occurrence of virilization in these tumors is probably due to stromal luteinization as a reactive phenomenon to the presence of the expansile ovarian lesion. Rare cases of ovarian hemangiomas have also presented with hyperandrogenic syndromes [5].

Sex cord–stromal tumors (SCST)

Ovarian sex cord–stromal tumors constitute 5–8% of all ovarian malignancies [3,6], about 90% of functioning ovarian tumors and over 60% of the case reports of androgen-secreting ovarian tumors

(Table 51.1). They are derived from sex cords and the ovarian stroma or mesenchyme of the embryonic gonad that constitute the intraovarian matrix supporting the germ cells. Granulosa cells and Sertoli cells are derived from sex cord cells while the theca

Table 51.1 Summary of 70 case reports ascertained from Medline between 1995 and 2005 using search terms "ovarian neoplasm" and "androgen excess"

Histological class of ovarian tumor	Median (range) age of onset (years)	Prevalence %
Adult granulosa cell	17(13–30)	2.9
Thecomas	34(19–49)	2.9
Sclerosing stromal	–	1.4
Sertoli–Leydig cell		13.0
Sertoli–Leydig cell	33(11–69)	8.7
Stromal–Leydig cell	24(22–58)	4.3
Steroid cell		33.3
Pure Leydig cell (hilar and non-hilar types)	43(35–80)	15.9
Steroid cells not otherwise specified	12(6–93)	17.4
Others		
Luteoma of pregnancy	25(22–28)	5.8
Cystadenoma	–	1.4
Cystadenocarcinomas	–	2.9
Gyandroblastoma	–	2.9
Brenner	–	1.4
Hyperthecosis	–	1.4
Stromal luteoma	–	1.4
Endometroid adenocarcinoma	–	2.9
Germ cell tumors	–	5.8
*Miscellaneous	52(15–70)	22.1

*Miscellaneous includes leiomyoma, transitional cell, endometrial, metastases and tumors with no histological information.

Clinical Endocrine Oncology, 2nd edition. Edited by Ian D. Hay and John A.H. Wass. © 2008 Blackwell Publishing. ISBN 978-1-4051-4584-8.

cells, Leydig cells and fibroblasts are from mesenchymal cells. The majority of these tumors are of low malignant potential, affect a young age group and have good long-term prognosis. Granulosa, theca and Sertoli cells are usually estrogen secreting but can also secrete androgens or have mixed sex steroid output. They present with variety of symptoms across different age groups from pre-cocious puberty, menometrorrhagia to postmenopausal bleeding as well as with endometrial carcinoma and hyperandrogenism. Sertoli–Leydig cells and steroid cells, on the other hand, produce predominantly androgens.

Granulosa cell tumors

Granulosa cell tumors (GCT) are the most common SCST, account for about 70% of malignant sex cord-stromal tumors and are mostly estrogen secreting although some secrete androgen. Two main pathological subtypes exist: adult granulosa cell tumor (AGCT) and juvenile granulosa cell tumor (JGCT). These subtypes are classified according to histopathological findings. AGCTs account for 95% of all GCTs, have an average size of about 12 cm in diameter and present in the peri- or postmenopausal age group with endome-trial hyperplasia [3, 7]. AGCTs are predominantly cystic tumors with compartments filled with blood or fluid which are separated by solid tissue. On microscopic examination they grow in a wide variety of patterns including microfollicular, macrofollicular, insular, trabecullar, solid tubular and hollow-tubular patterns. JGCTs, which affect mainly prepubertal children causing pseudo-precocity, are solidcystic neoplasms containing hemorrhagic fluid. The microscopic appearance is of a solid cellular tumor with focal areas of follicle formation that are less well differentiated than the adult type. The prognosis of JGCTs is excellent because most present as stage IA disease (tumors limited to one ovary with intact capsule and no presence of malignant cells in ascitic fluid). Conversely, AGCTs of all patterns have malignant potential and a high late recurrence rate even three or more decades after surgery.

Thecoma

Theca cell tumors account for approximately 1% of ovarian neoplasms [3, 7]. Thecomas are the most hormonally active sex cord-stromal tumors and can be divided into typical and luteinized subtypes. More than 80% of affected women are aged over 60 at presentation with postmenopausal uterine bleeding which, in over 20% of instances, is the result of endometrial carcinoma. Theca cell tumors appear as solid masses of varying sizes, occasionally with cystic change. The typical thecoma is composed of swollen lipid-laden stromal cells that resemble theca cells with varying numbers of fibroblasts. Luteinized thecomas contain steroid-type cells resembling luteinized theca and luteinized stromal cells. Half of luteinized thecomas are estrogenic, 40% are non-functioning, and 10% are androgenic. The luteinized thecoma subgroup occurs in a younger age group compared to the typical thecoma.

Sclerosing stromal cell tumors

Sclerosing stromal cell tumors are amongst the benign sex cord–stromal tumors accounting for less than 5% of the total SCSTs [3, 7]. These tumors are usually unilateral and the majority present in women under 30 with menstrual irregularity, although a few cases have androgenic features. At microscopic examination, these tumors are hypervascular with prominent areas of sclerosis. They are characterized by the presence of pseudolobular pattern, in which cellular areas are separated by edematous and collagen-ous hypocellular tissue.

Sertoli–Leydig cell tumors (SLCT)

SLCTs contain a combination of Sertoli cells, Leydig cells and fibroblasts. Sertoli cell tumors account for only 4% of SLCT and are usually non-functioning [3]. Pure Leydig cell tumors are also classified as steroid cell tumors. Sertoli–Leydig cell tumors are divided into four subtypes: well differentiated, intermediately dif-ferentiated, poorly differentiated, and retiform. Seventy-five per-cent of people with Sertoli–Leydig tumors are younger than 30 years of age and virilization occurs in only about 30% of women. Tumors with retiform or heterologous components are usually cystic while the other subtypes are rarely so. Most of the tumors are unilateral and 80% are diagnosed as stage I disease. Sertoli–Leydig cell tumors in patients with virilization are often small and dif-ficult to detect, even with transvaginal ultrasonography.

Steroid cell tumors (SCT)

Steroid cell tumors, which constitute only 0.1% [3, 7] of all ovarian tumors, are composed entirely of cells resembling typical steroid hormone-secreting cells, such as lutein cells, Leydig cells and adrenocortical cells and are the most common group in a review of androgen-secreting tumor case reports (see Table 51.1). This tumor group includes stromal luteoma, Leydig cell tumor and steroid cell tumor not otherwise specified. Some tumors in the last category are malignant, whereas those in the first two categories are benign. At gross examination, stromal luteomas are well-circumscribed solid tumors within the ovary. They are difficult to identify because they are almost always smaller than 3 cm in diameter.

Sex cord tumors with annular tubules

The sex cord tumors with annular tubules account for 6% of sex cord-stromal tumors and 30% are associated with Peutz–Jeghers syndrome (PJS) of which 15% are in turn associated with adenoma malignum of the cervix [3, 8]. They are characterized by the presence of simple and complex solid ringlike tubules. PJS-associated sex cord tumors with annular tubules are usually small, multifocal, calcified, bilateral and benign while PJS-independent tumors are typically large, rarely multifocal or calcified unilateral and one-fifth are malignant.

Ovarian tumors with functioning stroma

Various ovarian tumors with both estrogenic and androgenic manifestations have been reported. Epithelial tumors such as especially mucinous cystadenomas or carcinomas most commonly have estrogenic stroma. Among the ovarian tumors with an androgenic stroma, one-third are metastatic ovarian tumors mostly of gastric origin, 20% are primary mucinous cystic tumors and the remainder comprise Brenner tumors, teratomas, and carcinoid tumors [3].

Adrenocortical tumors

Virilizing adrenal tumors are relatively rare and are usually adrenocortical carcinomas. Adrenocortical carcinoma is a rare malignancy (0.02% of all cancers) with an incidence of 1 per million and is more common in women than men [9]. There is a bimodal age distribution with a peak of incidence in children less than 5 years of age and in adults in their fourth or fifth decades of life. Adrenocortical cancers occur sporadically or as part of a familial cancer syndrome such as Li–Fraumeni syndrome arising from germline mutations of the TP63 gene located at 17p13; Beckwith–Wiedemann syndrome characterized by overgrowth disorders and increased risk of Wilms tumors, neuroblastoma and hepatoblastoma (gene locus 11p15.5) and multiple endocrine neoplasia (MEN) type 1 caused by mutation of the *menin* gene at 11q13. Fifty to 80% of adrenocortical tumors are functional of which 40% secrete cortisol, causing Cushing syndrome, and 25% secrete both cortisol and androgen, causing a virilizing form of Cushing syndrome. Malignant adrenal tumors have a greater propensity to virilize compared to adrenal adenomas because they tend to secrete higher levels of dihydroepiandrosterone (DHEA). The majority of children with adrenal carcinoma present with virilizing syndromes and therefore present relatively early and have a relatively good prognosis [2, 10, 11].

Clinical presentation of androgen-secreting tumors

Androgen-secreting ovarian and adrenal tumors can present with features of mild hyperandrogenism or severe virilization which may be accompanied by the effects of excess estrogen or cortisol or with mass effects and metastases.

Features of hyperandrogenism
The natural history of hyperandrogenism from tumors is frequently short and more severe compared to that from nonneoplastic androgen excess such as polycystic ovarian syndrome

and congenital adrenal hyperplasia. Presentations vary according to age and degree of androgen excess which is related to the size and type of tumor. Adult women may present with muscular male body habitus, deepening of voice, clitorimegaly, increased libido, breast atrophy, menstrual irregularities and infertility. Cutaneous manifestations include hirsutism (involving the face, chin, chest and perineum – male pattern pubic hair), alopecia (usually male pattern, vertex and crown hair loss), oily skin, acne vulgaris and male sweat changes (malodorous perspiration). There may be associated metabolic effects including hyperlipidemia, impaired glucose tolerance and hypertension. Pregnant women with virilizing tumors can rarely give birth to virilized girls; even though the fetus is usually protected from androgen excess by the action of placental aromatase, this mechanism can be overwhelmed.

Androgen excess before puberty is responsible for clinical manifestations that vary with sex. Prebubertal boys present with pseudoprecocious puberty comprising penile enlargement, hair development in androgen-dependent areas of the skin and other secondary sexual characteristics. Girls present with signs of virilization including acne, hirsutism and clitorimegaly. In both sexes there is an increase in height velocity and somatic development as well as accelerated skeletal maturation. Premature epiphyseal fusion leads to short stature.

Features due to mass effect and malignancy
Other clinical features associated with the mass effect and malignancy of the ovarian tumors include weight loss, abdominal mass/swelling, abdominal pain, ascites, hydrothorax (including Meig syndrome). Thrombophlebitis migrans and fever from tumor necrosis may also be present. Malignant adrenal tumors may result in abdominal swelling and pain as well as peripheral edema and varicoceles.

Features due to individual tumor characteristics
Sex cord tumors with annular tubules and associated Peutz–Jeghers syndrome can present with intestinal polyposis and intussusception. Granulosa cell and theca cell tumors may produce estrogen resulting in endometrial hyperplasia or carcinoma causing menometrorrhagia or postmenopausal bleeding. Cushing syndrome, with or without virilization, is the most frequent presentation in functioning adrenocortical carcinoma often with a rapid development of clinical features. Muscle weakness may be relatively spared because of the anabolic effect of androgens. Hypertension and hypokalemia are more common in adrenal carcinomas compared with benign adenomas.

Screening and diagnosis

Screening for an androgen-secreting tumor should be considered for women in the upper 5% of serum testosterone concentrations. For instance, a 144 ng/dL (5.0 nmol/L) cut off is frequently used as a guide and one report of a small series found that a testosterone level of 210.4 ng/dL (7.3 nmol/L) or above fully discriminated tumorous from non-tumorous hyperandrogenism but that a cut-off of 86.5 ng/dL (3.0 nmol/L) for serum testosterone had a specificity of 53% below the age of 40 and 95% above 40 years [12]. The differential diagnosis in young girls is congenital adrenal hyperplasia, in adult women is polycystic ovarian syndrome and the postmenopausal age group is stromal hyperplasia.

The evaluation of hyperandrogenism includes history, physical examination, biochemical investigations and localization with imaging. The main objectives of investigation are to confirm biochemical evidence of androgen excess and to localize the source and cause of androgen excess using a combination of adrenal and ovarian suppression tests and imaging.

Endocrine evaluation

The endocrine work-up of a subject with a suspected androgen-secreting tumor includes a full androgen profile comprising total serum testosterone, androstenedione, dehydroepiandrosterone sulfate (DHEAS) and a screen of related hormones: serum luteinizing hormone (LH), follicle-stimulating hormone (FSH), estradiol, 17-hydroxyprogesterone (17-OHP) and 24-h urinary collection for cortisol.

High DHEAS levels are at best suggestive of adrenal androgen excess, particularly adrenocortical carcinoma [12]. Patients with 17-OHP value, greater than 1.57 ng/dL (5.0 nmol/L) may require adrenocorticotropic hormone (ACTH) stimulation or urinary steroid profile using mass spectrometry to exclude late-onset congenital adrenal hyperplasia. Adrenal suppression can be performed using the low-dose dexamethasone suppression test (LDDST) and ovarian suppression can be achieved using a combined oral contraceptive pill or analogs of gonadotropin-releasing hormone (GnRH). Amongst the components of an androgen profile total serum testosterone is generally the most informative with little additional information coming from androstenedione and DHEAS measurements.

Adrenal suppression (LDDST)

The LDDST involves collection of blood samples for plasma testosterone and cortisol at 09:00 h before and after eight doses of dexamethasone given as 0.5 mg every 6 h for 48 h. The second blood sample is obtained 6 h after the last dose of dexamethasone. In a small series of 11 women with androgen-secreting tumors all 11 failed to suppress serum testosterone by 40% compared to 1% of women with non-tumorous hyperandrogenism [12]. In this series, a combination of clear history, serum testosterone and imaging was effective in identifying the tumorous group so the efficacy of the LDDST in routine practice is unclear, particularly as rare cases of androgen suppression by glucocorticoid have also been reported. Whether this test in useful in discriminating adrenal from ovarian tumors has not been established.

Ovarian suppression and stimulation

Blood samples for LH, FSH, and testosterone can be taken before and after administration of an oral contraceptive pill (ovarian suppression test). With GnRH analogs, samples can be taken in the stimulatory phase or suppressive phase after administration of super-active analogs [13, 14] or after suppression with a GnRH antagonist [15]. In one series of five women, suppression of androgen excess with a GnRH analog was achieved in all cases irrespective of ovarian histology [16]. It seems therefore that false negatives for this test are rare and that most ovarian androgen-secreting tumors are gonadotropin dependent.

Imaging

Ovary
Pelvic ultrasonography is the most useful imaging modality for ovarian tumors and the wider use of power Doppler may add to the utility of this tool [17]. Ultrasound will also provide additional information on estrogen status from uterine size and endometrial thickness which will vary according to age and exposure to estrogen. Magnetic resonance imaging (MRI) of pelvic organs can be used to demonstrate gross pathological features of the various sex cord–stromal ovarian tumors.

Adrenal
Abdominal computerized tomography (CT) is the most useful imaging modality in adrenal tumors as surrounding fat allows for good delineation of adrenal margins. CT attenuation is usually less than 10 Hounsfield units for a benign adrenal adenoma while adrenocortical carcinomas usually have higher attenuation, features of inhomogeneity, irregular borders and invasion of surrounding tissues. Adrenal MRI can also be helpful in distinguishing between malignant potential. T1-weighted images of adrenocortical carcinomas are hypointense and T2 images are slightly hyperintense relative to liver and spleen. The sensitivity and specifity of MRI for differentiation of benign and malignant adrenocortical lesions range between 81–89% and 92–99%, respectively [18].

As non-functioning adrenal nodules or incidentalomas are so common, functional imaging may be required before committing to surgery. Positron emission tomography (PET scanning) using ^{18}F-fluorodeoxyglucose (FDG) has been thought to distinguish between malignant and benign adrenal tumors. In one report of adrenal tumors only malignant adrenal tumors had FDG uptake compared to benign adrenal tumors [19]. FDG-PET has been used in tumor localization as well as follow-up of a rare case of ectopic Cushing's presenting with androgen excess [20].

Radiocholesterol scintigraphy using ^{131}I-6-beta-iodo-methyl-norcholesterol (NP-59) has been used to identify benign cortical tumors. High NP-59 uptake tumors are likely to be benign while little or no uptake is more likely to be adrenocortical carcinoma although this distinction is less reliable than with FDG-PET [21].

Selective adrenal and ovarian venous sampling
Ovarian and adrenal venous catheterization and sampling contribute little further diagnostic information in differential diagnosis of hyperandrogenism beyond that derived from history, standard biochemical testing and imaging [22]. The main indications for

this procedure are when the suspicion of an androgen-secreting tumor is high but imaging is negative or when there is uncertainty over whether an identified mass is functional.

Management

Surgery is the mainstay of treatment for both adrenal and ovarian androgen-secreting tumors. Medical treatment is an option for women with benign ovarian tumors in whom surgery is not straightforward such as in the case of extensive adhesions [15]. Malignant ovarian tumors and adrenocortical carcinomas secreting androgens are relatively insensitive to either chemotherapy or radiotherapy.

Laparoscopic oophorectomy is the favored procedure for benign ovarian tumors. Open surgery may be indicated if hysterectomy is also being considered because of accompanying endometrial hyperplasia due to co-secretion of estrogen. In malignancies, *en bloc* resection of invaded organs and, if necessary, peri-aortic/retroperitoneal lymphadenectomy will be required. In some cases surgical debulking is the only option possible. Some sex cord–stromal tumors require definitive surgical staging. This will include multiple biopsies from high yield sites, omentectomy, pelvic and para-aortic sampling. When surgery fails to offer a cure then adjuvant therapy with vincristine, actinomycin D, cyclophosphamide (VAC) and cisplatinum combination therapy may be of benefit in some ovarian tumors.

With respect to adrenal lesions, preoperative imaging assessing the size, homogeneity, margins of the tumor and presence of potential metastases is important in choosing between laparoscopic or open adrenalectomy. It remains uncertain whether the frequency of local recurrence and peritoneal seeding is different between open and laparoscopic approaches. Lesions up to 6 cm in diameter which appear benign are ideal candidates for laparoscopic adrenalectomy, which can be performed trans- or retroperitoneally. Larger tumors up to 10 cm, inhomogeneous and with areas of necrosis but with clear margins and preserved capsule can be considered for laparoscopic approach but with low threshold for conversion to an open procedure. Tumors larger than 10 cm with irregular borders and infiltrative features should always be removed by an open procedure, which should consist of *en bloc* resection of invaded organs and retroperitoneal lymphadenectomy. Liver metastases can be treated simultaneously with segmental liver resection or radiofrequency ablation. All tumors should be removed aiming at clear resection margins (R0 resection) and intact capsule. Tumor spillage results in increased rates of loco-regional recurrence and poor prognosis. In univariate analysis, tumor size, clear resection margins, Ki67 (>5%), capsular invasion, invasion of blood vessels, and age were associated with reduced overall survival [23, 24].

Adjuvant therapy is available for those individuals with adrenal lesions who are not cured by surgery. Mitotane alone or in combination with cytotoxic drugs such as etoposide, doxorubicin, cisplatin and streptozotocin remains the treatment of choice.

Mitotane has been shown to have a modest effect in unresectable, metastatic or residual disease with overall response between 14–36% but no proven survival benefit Monitoring of drug levels is important for optimum results [10, 24]. Postoperative radiotherapy to the adrenal bed after resection for adrenal carcinoma is effective in reducing the risk of local recurrence, but has no survival benefit [24].

Prognosis

The prognosis is excellent in benign tumors. Hirsutism will improve postoperatively but clitorimegaly, male pattern alopecia and the deepening of voice are likely to persist. The prognosis of malignant tumors depends on the stage of disease at presentation and the size of the tumor. The overall prognosis in patients with adrenocortical carcinoma is still poor. Recent data from the German ACC Registry demonstrate an overall 5-year survival of 43%. Survival is clearly stage-dependent with a 5-year survival of 90% in stage I, 57% in stage II, 45% in stage III, and 20% in stage IV [24]. The age of presentation of adrenocortical carcinomas is also important. The overall 5-year survival in treated adrenocortical carcinomas is between 23% and 60% and that of pediatric adrenocortical carcinoma about 54%(9–11).

References

1. Carmina E, Rosato F, Janni A, Rizzo M, Longo RA. Extensive clinical experience: relative prevalence of different androgen excess disorders in 950 women referred because of clinical hyperandrogenism. *J. Clin. Endocrinol. Metab.* 2003;91:2–6.
2. Latrinico AC, Chruousos GP Extensive personal experience: adrenocortical tumors. *J. Clin. Endocrinol. Metab.* 1997;82:1317–1324.
3. Koonings PP, Campbell K, Mishell DR, Jr, Scully Grimes DA. Relative frequency of primary ovarian neoplasm: a 10 year review. *Obstet. Gynecol.* 1989;74:921.
4. Nezhat F, Slomovitz BM, Saiz AD, Cohen JC. Ovarian mucinous cystadenocarcinoma with virilisation. *Gynaecol. Oncol.* 2002;84:468–472.
5. Gucer F, Ozyilmaz F, Balkanli-Kaplan P, Mulayim N, Aydin O. Ovarian haemagioma presenting with hyperandrogenism and endometrial cancer: a case report. *Gynecol. Oncol.* 2004; 94:821–824.
6. Quirk JT, Natarrajan N. Ovarian cancer incidence in the United States 1992–1999. *Gynecol. Oncol.* 2005;97:519–523.
7. Tavassoli FA, Norris HJ. Sertoli tumours of the ovary. A clinicopathological study of 28 cases with ultrastructural observations. *Cancer* 1980;46:2281–2297.
8. Podczaski E, Kaminski PF, Pees RC, Singapuri K, Sorosky JI. Peutz–Jeughers syndrome with ovarian sex cord tumour with annular tubules and cervical adenoma malignum. *Gynecol. Oncol.* 1991;42:74–78.
9. Allolio B, Hahner S, Weiman D, Fassnatch M. Management of adrenocortical carcinoma. *Clin. Endocrinol.* 2004;60:273–287.
10. Roman S. Adrenocortical carcinoma. *Curr. Opin. Oncol.* 2006;18:36–42.
11. Sidhu S, Sywak M., Robinson B, Delbridge, L. Adrenocortical cancer: recent clinical and molecular advances. *Curr. Opin. Oncol.* 2004;16: 13–18.

12. Kaltsas GA, Isidori MA, Kola BP, et al. The value of the low dose dexamethasone suppression test in the differential diagnosis of hyperandrogenism. *J. Clin. Endocrinol. Metab.* 2003;88:2634–2643.

13. Ibanez L, Potau N, Zampolli M, et al. Source of localization of androgen excess in adolescent girls. *J. Clin. Endocrinol. Metab.* 1994;79:1778–1784.

14. Picon MJ, Lara JI, Sarasa JL, et al. Use of a long–acting gonadotrophin–releasing hormone analogue in a postmenopausal woman with hyperandrogenism due to a hilus cell tumour. *Eur. J. Endocrinol.* 2000;142:619.

15. Stephens JW, Katz JR, McDermott N, et al. An unusual steroid–producing ovarian tumour: case report. *Hum. Reprod.* 2002;17:1468–1471.

16. Pascale MM, Pugeat M, Roberts M, et al. Androgen suppressive effect of GnRH agonist in ovarian hyperthecosis and virilizing tumours. *Clin. Endocrinol.* 1994;41:571–576.

17. Marret H, Sauget S, Giraudeau B, Body G, Tranquart F. Power Doppler vascularity index for predicting malignancy of adnexal masses. *Ultrasound Obstet. Gynecol.* 2005;25:508–513.

18. Honigschnab S, Gallo S, Niederle B. How accurate is MR imaging in characterisation of adrenal masses update of long term studies. *Eur. J. Radiol.* 2002;41:113–122.

19. Jenebaum F, Groussin L, Foehrenbach H. F-Fluorodeoxyglucose positron emission tomography as a diagnostic tool for malignancy of adrenal tumours. Preliminary report of 13 consecutive patients. *Eur. J. Endocrinol.* 2004;150:789–792.

20. Markou A, Manning P, Kaya B, Datta SN, Bomanji JB, Conway GS. (18F) fluoro-2-deoxy-D-glucose positron emission tomograghy imaging of thymic carcinoid tumour presenting with recurrent Cushing's syndrome. *Eur. J. Endocrinol.* 2005;152:521–525.

21. Maurea S, Klain M, Mainoli C. The diagnostic role of radionuclide imaging in evaluation of patients with non hypersecreting adrenal masses. *J. Nucl. Med.* 2001;42:884–892.

22. Kaltsas GA, Mukherjee JJ, Kola B, et al. Is ovarian and adrenal venous catheterization and sampling helpful in the investigation of hyperandrogenic women? *Clin. Endocrinol.* 2003;59:34–43.

23. Walz MK, Petersenn S, Koch JA, Mann K, Neumann HP, Schmid KW. Endoscopic treatment of large primary adrenal tumours. *Br. J. Surg.* 2005;92:719–723.

24. Fassnacht M, Hahner S, Koschker A, et al. German Adrenal Network GANIMED. The German Adrenocortical Cancer Registry – Analysis of the First 285 Patients. Presented at Endo 2006, The Endocrine Society 88th Annual Meeting.

52 Functional Ovarian Tumors

Nia Jane Taylor and Niall Richard Moore

Key points

- Arise from germ cells, sex cord–stromal cells or epithelial cells.
- Most sex cord–stromal and granulosa cell tumors are confined to the ovary.
- Epithelial tumors tend to show early peritoneal and lymphatic spread.
- Tumors vary in appearance from small solid to large multicystic masses on all forms of imaging.
- Imaging appearances are rarely specific to tumor type.

Introduction

Functional tumors of the ovary are defined as those which produce estrogen or androgen and hence have a hormonal effect. Primary tumors of the ovary can be broadly classified into three main groups based on their origin: those arising from the surface epithelium, those arising from germ cells and those derived from ovarian stromal and sex cord elements. It is the sex cord–stromal tumors, which represent approximately 8% of ovarian neoplasms, that have a tendency to manifest with tumor-mediated endocrinopathy. These hormonal effects include pseudoprecocious puberty, post-menopausal bleeding and virilization. Unlike the more common epithelial neoplasms, 75% of which are stage III or IV at diagnosis, sex cord–stromal tumors are commonly stage I at presentation, are therefore primarily treated surgically and generally have a good prognosis. The frequency of sex cord–stromal tumors is similar throughout the world, they affect all ages and there is no apparent racial predisposition. This group of neoplasms has a range of radiological appearances from small solid lesions to large multicystic masses. However, there are characteristic appearances which, together with clinical clues, can aid diagnosis.

Most other ovarian tumors can also produce sexual hormones in their stroma. For example, metastatic ovarian tumors often have androgen-producing stroma whilst mucinous cystadenoma has been reported to produce estrogens.

Tables 52.1 and 52.2 list the ovarian causes of hyperandrogenism and hyperestrogenism.

Ovarian stromal and sex cord–derived cells

Ovarian sex cord–stromal tumors arise from two groups of cells in the ovary: stromal cells and sex cords. Stromal cells derive from

Clinical Endocrine Oncology, 2nd edition. Edited by Ian D. Hay and John A.H. Wass. © 2008 Blackwell Publishing. ISBN 978-1-4051-4584-8.

Table 52.1 Ovarian causes of hyperestrogenism

Sex cord-stromal tumors
  Steroid cell tumors
    Stromal luteoma
  Granulosa stromal tumor
    Granulosa cell tumor
    Thecoma
    Sclerosing stromal tumor
  Sex cord tumor with annular tubules
Surface epithelial tumors
  Serous tumors
  Mucinous tumors
  Endometroid tumors
Metastatic tumors

Table 52.2 Ovarian causes of hyperandrogenism

Sex cord–stromal tumors
  Sertoli stromal tumors
    Sertoli–Leydig cell tumor
  Steroid cell tumors
  Leydig cell tumor
  Stromal luteoma
  Steroid cell tumor not otherwise specified
  Granulosa stromal tumors
  Sclerosing stromal tumor
Gynandroblastoma
Gonadoblastoma
Ovarian carcinoid
Surface epithelial tumors
  Brenner tumor
Metastatic tumor
Tumor-like lesions
  Polycystic ovary syndrome
  Stromal hyperplasia
  Stromal hyperthecosis
  Hyperreactio luteinalis
  Pregnant luteoma

the genital ridge mesonephros mesenchyma, which forms the undifferentiated gonad. Stromal cells include fibroblasts, theca cells and Leydig cells. The primitive sex cords form from the celomic epithelium (primordial peritoneum) and grow into the mesenchyme of the genital ridge. They form the cords of the testis but regress as recognizable structures in the developing ovary. Cells arising from the primitive sex cords include granulosa cells in the normal ovary, Sertoli cells in the testis and Sertoli cells in ovarian tumors.

Sex cord–stromal tumors usually have more than one cell type within the tumor. For example, Sertoli–Leydig cell tumors have both sex cord (Sertoli cell) and stromal origins (Leydig cells and fibroblasts).

The radiological appearance of sex cord–stromal tumors varies from a small solid mass to a large multicystic lesion. Sertoli–Leydig cell tumors, fibrothecomas and sclerosing stromal tumors are usually solid masses; granulosa cell tumors are mostly large multicystic masses with solid components.

Sertoli–Leydig cell tumors

Sertoli stromal tumors include tumors with varying combinations of Sertoli cells, Leydig cells and fibroblasts. The three main subtypes are Sertoli–Leydig cell tumors, Leydig cell tumors (classified as steroid cell tumors), and Sertoli cell tumors (4% of Sertoli stromal tumors but normally non-functioning in women). Sertoli–Leydig cell tumors are by far the most common tumor in this group. They are also the most common virilizing ovarian tumors, although they represent only about 0.5% of all ovarian neoplasms [1].

Sertoli–Leydig cell tumors are broadly divided into four histological subtypes: well differentiated (predominant tubular pattern), intermediately differentiated (sheets of immature cells with some stroma), poorly differentiated (immature Sertoli cells with little or no stroma), and retiform. Three of these subtypes have variants that contain heterologous elements [2].

The heterologous tissue most often contains mucinous epithelium, sometimes with small foci of carcinoid. Less commonly, and generally in poorly differentiated neoplasms, mesenchymal components including fetal-type cartilage and, very rarely, rhabdomyosarcoma may be present. As a result, the histological characteristics of these tumors can be extremely varied and they are commonly confused with other tumors. It is particularly important to distinguish such heterologous tumors from pure sarcomas and teratomas. The retiform neoplasms may mimic serous borderline tumors or even serous carcinomas. Well-differentiated Sertoli–Leydig cell tumors, however, are characteristically composed of tubules of epithelial cells, usually steroid secreting, interspersed in a fibrous stroma. These tubules resemble the tubules of the testis.

Sertoli–Leydig cell tumors tend to present at a younger age than most sex cord–stromal tumors with 75% occurring in patients under 30 years of age [2], with a mean age of 25 years. The presenting symptoms are related to clinical signs of androgenic activity with virilization occurring in approximately 30%. This is

attributable to the Leydig cells, which produce androgens, and manifests as amenorrhea or virilized secondary sexual characteristics. Fifty percent of tumors have no hormonal manifestations. Rarely, the tumor may be estrogenic [3].

As a result of their histological variability, Sertoli–Leydig cell tumors have a varied gross appearance. Most, however, are solid or solid with cystic areas. This is reflected on imaging with the majority of tumors appearing solid. On ultrasound, a well-defined hypoechoic mass is the most common finding. Computerized tomography (CT) usually demonstrates an enhancing solid mass, occasionally with intratumoral cysts within the solid portions of the tumor. Calcifications are rare.

On magnetic resonance imaging (MRI), these tumors are generally seen as solid masses with the extent of the fibrous stroma present influencing the signal intensity on T2-weighted sequences. They do not, however, demonstrate the very low signal intensity characteristic of fibromas [4]. On T1-weighted images, they are hypointense and enhance intensely and heterogeneously.

Patients with virilizing tumors tend to present early, hence androgenically active tumors are commonly small and difficult to visualize, even with transvaginal ultrasonography [2]. Color Doppler imaging can be helpful but if the tumor cannot be localized on imaging, ovarian vein sampling may be required to lateralize and locate the lesion [4].

Tumors with retiform and heterologous components are more often cystic and occasionally show larger multicystic areas, appearing indistinguishable from granulosa cell tumors. The cystic areas are intermediate signal on T1-weighted images and high signal on T2-weighted sequences but are not commonly hemorrhagic.

Sertoli–Leydig cell tumors are usually unilateral and 80–90% are stage I or only involve the surface of the ovary at the time of diagnosis. However, 10–20% may behave in a malignant manner, with poorly differentiated tumors most commonly doing so [3]. A small subset of malignant Sertoli–Leydig cell tumors has been reported in patients with Peutz–Jeghers syndrome. Recurrence tends to occur relatively soon after initial diagnosis, in contrast to granulosa cell tumors. Relatively few recurrences have been reported after a 5-year latency.

Stage and histological differentiation are the most important predictors of clinical outcome. In the majority of cases, surgical resection alone is required, with unilateral salpingo-oophorectomy usually preferred in order to preserve fertility.

Granulosa cell tumors

Granulosa cell tumors (GCT) include tumors made up of granulosa cells, theca cells and fibroblasts in varying degrees and combinations. They account for 2–5% of all ovarian tumors and 70% of sex cord–stromal tumors [5]. The granulosa cell is a hormonally active component of the ovarian stroma and is responsible for estradiol production. Granulosa cell tumors are the commonest clinically estrogenic ovarian tumor [1].

GCT have similar gross appearances but are divided into two subtypes based on histopathological findings: juvenile (5%) and adult (95%) [5]. Both subtypes commonly produce estrogen and a clinical endocrinopathy is often the reason for early diagnosis.

Juvenile GCT tend to occur in prepubertal children and women under 30 years of age. The mean age of patients with juvenile GCT is 13 years, with just 3% occurring in patients over the age of 30 years [4]. In premenarchal girls, excess estrogen results in isosexual precocity (more accurately termed pseudoprecocity). It is manifest by the development of the breasts, followed by secondary sexual characteristics and irregular uterine bleeding. Somatic and skeletal development is also accelerated [6]. Juvenile GCT accounts for about 10% of cases of pseudoprecocity [4].

In postmenarchal patients, juvenile GCT may also present with symptoms of excess estrogen, causing irregular and excessive uterine bleeding. This may be preceded by months or even years of amenorrhea.

Adult GCT can occur at any age but is most commonly found in peri- and postmenopausal women. Median age at diagnosis is 50–54 years [5]. In women of reproductive age, prolonged exposure of the endometrium to tumor-derived estradiol can cause atypical or excessive uterine bleeding or even secondary amenorrhea. In older women, postmenopausal bleeding is the most common presentation with endometrial polyps and carcinoma reported in 3–25% of cases [1]. Endometrial carcinoma occurs twice as often as in the premenopausal group [7].

Very occasionally, infertility can be the presentation – possibly as a result of unregulated inhibin secretion by the GCT with consequent negative feedback on follicle-stimulating hormone (FSH) secretion by the anterior pituitary [5].

Rarely, GCT may be androgen secreting with hirsutism or virilizing features. However, Sertoli–Leydig cell tumors should first be considered.

In both adult and juvenile GCT, persistent abdominal or pelvic pain is a common presentation due to a large pelvic mass which can be hemorrhagic. The mass can also cause ovarian torsion with acute onset of pelvic pain.

On imaging, juvenile GCT is usually a solid and cystic neoplasm with no evidence of fat or calcification. The solid component is usually high signal on T2-weighted MR images and demonstrates contrast enhancement on T1-weighted sequences. The cysts may contain hemorrhagic fluid. Uterine manifestations of excess estrogens may be identified on ultrasound or MRI with enlarged uterus and thickened endometrium. Ascites is an occasional finding. Extra-ovarian GCT have been reported – these are thought to be related to the derivation of sex cord–stromal tumors from epithelium of the celom and mesonephric duct.

Juvenile GCT has an association with Ollier disease (multiple enchondromatosis) and Maffuci syndrome (enchondromatosis with multiple soft tissue cavernous hemangiomas) and should be considered as the primary differential diagnosis for an ovarian mass in patients with these conditions.

The imaging features of adult GCT range from entirely cystic to entirely solid masses [8]. This is reflected on ultrasound (Fig. 52.1)

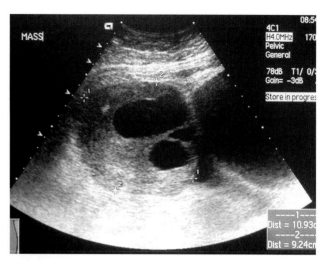

Figure 52.1 Transabdominal ultrasound demonstrating a mixed solid and cystic granulosa cell tumor arising in the right ovary.

and CT (Fig. 52.2) where the tumors are most commonly seen as multilocular cystic masses with thick septations and solid components but a predominantly solid small mass arising from the ovary (Fig. 52.3) is also well recognized. Calcification is rare. Metastases, although uncommon, appear on CT as peritoneal-bases nodules, similar to epithelial neoplasms, or as cystic liver lesions.

On MRI, the histological variability results in a spectrum of findings: solid with mild enhancement; solid with heterogeneity due to intratumoral hemorrhage (Fig. 52.4), infarct, fibrous degeneration and irregularly arranged tumor cells [1]; multilocular cystic and completely cystic. However, unlike serous and mucinous epithelial tumors, GCT do not have intracystic

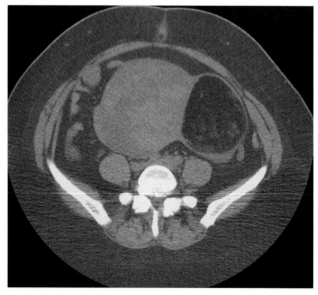

Figure 52.2 CT image demonstrating a well-defined complex left ovarian mass with a multicystic/solid component medially representing a granulosa cell tumor together with a typical mature cystic teratoma laterally.

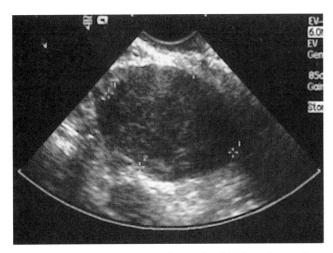

Figure 52.3 Transabdominal ultrasound image of a solid right ovarian granulosa cell tumor.

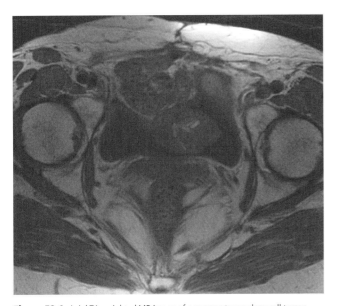

Figure 52.4 Axial T1-weighted MR image of a recurrent granulosa cell tumor involving the bladder dome. The high signal intensity within the metastases represents hemorrhage.

papillary projections. The most distinctive MRI finding is that of the large encapsulated multilocular cystic lesion filled with watery fluid or hemorrhage. The septa are low signal on T2-weighted sequences. The septa and solid portions enhance strongly giving a sponge-like appearance.

As with juvenile GCT, the uterus must also be assessed and is often found to be larger with thicker and brighter endometrium on T2 sequences when compared with healthy postmenopausal women. Endometrial biopsy should be considered due to the concurrent risk of adenocarcinoma.

Juvenile GCT tend to be less well differentiated than adult GCT but prognosis is excellent because most present as stage I disease. Mortality for patients with stage IA juvenile GCT is only 1.5%.

Despite a frequently large size at presentation, recurrence is less likely than adult GCT after simple resection. If they do recur, however, they tend to do so within the first 3 years of the initial diagnosis and are then usually rapidly fatal with early intra-abdominal spread. Adult GCT have a potential for clinically malignant behavior and not uncommonly recur 10–20 years after surgery. For adult GCT, however, average survival after recurrence is 5 years.

The staging system for GCT is adapted from that used for epithelial ovarian cancer as originally defined by the International Federation of Obstetrics and Gynaecology (FIGO [9]; Table 52.3), although the prognostic significance of certain features within the FIGO classification (such as positive cytology and surface involvement) has not been well defined for patients with GCT.

Seventy-eight to 91% of adult GCT present with stage I disease [5]. The remainder have advanced disease with variable involvement of the pelvis, intra-abdominal organs and peritoneum. Rarely, patients present with metastatic disease involving liver, lungs or bone. Only 5% are bilateral. The 5-year survival for stage I disease ranges from 85% to 95%. Ten-year survival remains high at 84–95%. For stage II, 5-year survival is 55–75% and 10-year survival 50–65%. Stage III/IV, however, has a 22–50% 5-year and 17–33% 10-year survival rate due to the potential for late relapse and death in patients with advanced disease [5]. Late recurrence means that long-term follow-up of this patient group is required.

Table 52.3 Staging system for ovarian neoplasms

Stage	
0	No evidence of primary tumor
I	Tumor confined to ovaries
IA	Tumor limited to one ovary, capsule intact
	No tumor on ovarian surface
	No malignant cells in ascites or peritoneal washings
IB	Tumor limited to both ovaries, capsules intact
	No tumor on ovarian surface
	No malignant cells in ascites
IC	Tumor limited to one or both ovaries but capsule ruptured, tumor on ovarian surface or malignant cells in ascites
II	Tumor involves one or both ovaries with pelvic extension
IIA	Extension or metastases to uterus or fallopian tubes
	No malignant cells in ascites
IIB	Extension to other pelvic organs
	No malignant cells in ascites
IIC	IIA/B with malignant cells in ascites
III	Tumor involves one or both ovaries with microscopically confirmed peritoneal metastases outside the pelvis and/or regional lymph node metastases
IIIA	Microscopic peritoneal metastases beyond the pelvis
IIIB	Macroscopic peritoneal metastases beyond the pelvis 2 cm or less in greatest dimension
IIIC	Peritoneal metastases beyond the pelvis more than 2 cm in dimension and/or regional lymph node metastases
IV	Distant metastases beyond the peritoneal cavity (includes liver parenchymal metastases)

Reproduced from [9], with permission from FIGO.

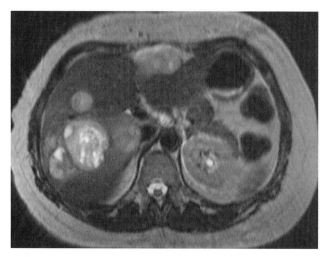

Figure 52.5 Axial T2-weighted MR image of the liver demonstrating multiple hepatic parenchymal metastases within the right lobe and a capsular metastasis involving the left lobe.

The median time to relapse is 4–6 years after initial diagnosis, with 17% of relapses reported over 10 years after diagnosis and relapses over 20 years later also occurring [4, 8, 10]. The pelvis is the most common site of relapse with local pelvic recurrence only reported in 30–45%, with 55% having some degree of extrapelvic spread [5]. Upper abdominal disease usually involves the peritoneal surface but visceral metastases (Fig. 52.5) can occur.

Stage is the most important prognostic factor for GCT; stage III/IV at presentation; stage I with large tumor size, high mitotic index or possible tumor rupture.

The management of GCT is predominantly surgical and fertility-preserving unilateral salpingo-oophorectomy may be sufficient in young patients with stage I disease. Ten percent of GCT actually occur in pregnancy and should be surgically removed at 16–18 weeks' gestation. The indolent nature of the adult form and its propensity for late relapse, however, require prolonged clinical follow-up with tumor marker studies such as inhibin and estradiol.

Fibrothecomas and thecomas

Thecomas and fibrothecomas form a spectrum of benign tumors extending from lipid-rich thecomas, composed of cells that resemble theca interna cells with little fibrosis, to pure fibromas with no theca cells. Differentiation is frequently difficult and the many tumors with populations of both theca cells and fibroblasts are labelled fibrothecomas. Together, this tumor group constitutes about half of all gonadal stromal tumors and approximately 46% of ovarian neoplasms [4]. These tumors are almost always benign but rare cases of tumors with low malignant potential have been reported [11]. Estrogenic activity depends on their histological origin with those of a predominantly fibrous origin having no estrogenic activity and those of predominantly thecal derivation being hormonally active.

Fibrothecomas and thecomas with estrogenic activity are less common than GCT and occur in older women with a mean age at presentation of 59 years. Approximately 60% of patients are postmenopausal. The theca cells of thecomas and fibrothecomas have abundant lipid in the cytoplasm giving a yellowish appearance on gross examination. These cells are responsible for the estrogenic effect of these tumors. Like adult GCT, these tumors commonly manifest with uterine bleeding and associated endometrial hyperplasia. Endometrial adenocarcinoma has been reported in 20% of cases [2].

A rare subtype of fibrothecomas, the luteinized thecoma, contains steroid-type cells resembling luteinized theca and luteinized stromal cells. They occur in a younger age group than typical fibrothecomas; 39% are non-functioning, 50% are estrogenic and 11% are androgenic, producing virilization [2].

On ultrasound, fibrothecomas appear most commonly as solid hypoechoic masses with marked sound wave attenuation at the posterior wall. On CT, they have been described primarily as well-defined solid, homogeneous or slightly heterogeneous masses (Fig. 52.6) [11]. Differentiation of these tumors from other solid ovarian masses is often not possible. Nonetheless, accurate diffentiation has important clinical and therapeutic implications.

On MRI, the imaging characteristics of these tumors depend on the amount of fibrocollagenous stroma present. In general, small tumors are well defined with homogeneous low signal on T1- and T2-weighted images (Fig. 52.7), similar to the appearance of fibromas. Thecomas with little or no fibrosis show high signal intensity similar to the appearance of malignant tumors. The prominent lipid component of these lesions can be demonstrated by chemical shift MRI, similar to the evaluation of adrenal adenomas.

Larger lesions tend to be lobulated and homogeneously low signal on T1- but heterogeneous on T2-weighted sequences owing to edema and cystic degeneration. Calcification and hemorrhage are rare. Free intraperitoneal fluid may be seen [1, 11]. The degree

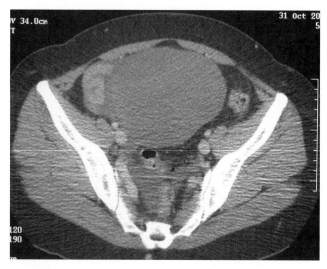

Figure 52.6 Axial CT image demonstrating a large homogeneous solid density mass in a woman who presented with pelvic pain. Histology revealed a thecoma.

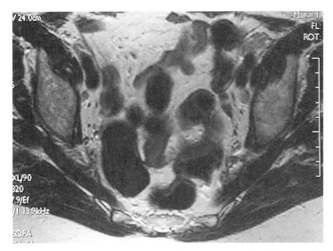

Figure 52.7 Axial T2-weighted MR image demonstrating a uniformly low signal right ovarian thecoma. Ultrasound had suspected a pedunculated uterine fibroid. Thecoma was confirmed at oophorectomy.

of contrast enhancement also varies with the amount of fibrous stroma present.

Benign Brenner tumors can mimic fibrothecoma with dense fibrous stroma demonstrating low signal intensity on T2 sequences but intratumoral edema is rare and they often demonstrate extensive amorphous calcification in the solid component on CT.

Fibrothecomas with extensive cystic degeneration occasionally have a multilocular "stained-glass appearance" in which the loculi show variable signal intensities on both T1 and T2 sequences [12]. This is most commonly seen in mucinous cystadenoma and cystadenocarcinoma of the ovary but also in endometrioma, mature cystic teratoma, struma ovarii, uterine leiomyoma with extensive cystic degeneration, as well as fibrothecomas. Thus, large ovarian fibrothecomas with extensive cystic degeneration can readily be mistaken for malignant tumors.

Estrogenic activity produces the secondary uterine changes seen with GCT: uterine enlargement and endometrial thickening on ultrasound and MRI. If the tumor is androgenic, the uterus may be atrophic.

Occasionally, it can be difficult to distinguish a fibrothecoma with a significant fibrous component from intraligamentous or pedunculated leiomyoma, which frequently appear as adnexal masses with typically very low signal on T2-weighted MRI. The presence of two normal ovaries, a pedicle to the uterus, or multiple vessels/flow voids along the interface between uterus and juxtauterine mass imply uterine origin – the latter is known as the "bridging vascular sign" [13].

Steroid cell tumors

Steroid cell tumors are ovarian neoplasms composed entirely of cells resembling typical hormone-secreting cells: lutein cells, Leydig cells and adrenocortical cells. They include stromal luteomas and Leydig cell tumors, both benign, and steroid cell tumors not otherwise specified, one-third of which may behave in a malignant fashion. All three tumor types can be virilizing and stromal luteomas can produce estrogen. Rarely, steroid cell tumors are associated with Cushing syndrome.

Steroid cell tumors account for 0.1–0.2% of all ovarian tumors. They affect a wide age range but are most commonly found in the fifth and sixth decades [4].

Stromal luteomas are very similar to, and frequently associated with, stromal hyperthecosis, a non-neoplastic lesion characterized by proliferation of ovarian stromal cells. Leydig cell tumors are characterized histologically by the presence of intracytoplasmic crystals of Reinke. Most steroid cell tumors, however, are not classifiable as either of these cell types and are thus called steroid cell tumor not otherwise specified.

Hormonally active steroid cell tumors are frequently difficult to identify due to their small size at presentation, commonly nodules under 3 cm. They are almost always unilateral solid tumors. Occasionally small areas of cystic change or necrosis may be seen but this is rare compared to GCT and Sertoli–Leydig cell tumors. On transabdominal ultrasound and CT, they are frequently not detected. Transvaginal ultrasound with color Doppler or MRI may be more sensitive. On T1-weighted images, small lesions have a high signal intensity probably related to their lipid content [4]. However, pure Leydig cell tumors, whilst having a low attenuation on CT, do not have a high signal on T1-weighted MRI despite the abundance of lipid in the cytoplasm. On T2-weighted images, signal intensity is usually intermediate. Steroid cell tumors do enhance intensely, reflecting a rich vascularity.

Sclerosing stromal tumor

Sclerosing stromal tumors are rare benign sex cord–stromal tumors that belong to the granulosa stromal subset. They are predominantly fibrotic masses that occur generally in young women, 80% in the second and third decade. The commonest clinical symptom is menstrual irregularity but tumors can have either estrogenic or androgenic manifestations.

On ultrasound, sclerosing stromal tumors are solid and cystic adnexal masses that may have centrally located round or cleft-like cysts. Color Doppler imaging reveals prominent vascularity in the peripheral portion and intercystic spaces. This can produce a "spoke-wheel" appearance [14].

On MRI, they are usually solid masses with homogeneous signal intensity, slightly higher than that of muscle on T1 sequences. The pseudolobulation results in a heterogeneous appearance with low signal intensity nodules and high signal oedematous stroma on T2-weighted images [2]. Hyperintense cystic areas and focal edema may be present in large masses. A thick peripheral hypointense rim represents compressed ovarian cortex and capsule due to a slow-growing tumor. Ascites may be seen but is rare.

On dynamic contrast-enhanced MRI, the hypervascularity of sclerosing stromal tumors seen on ultrasound results in striking early peripheral enhancement with centripetal progression, the highly vascular nodules enhancing more than the collagenous stroma [1]. This pattern differentiates these tumors from fibro-thecomas with cystic degeneration that show only slight early enhancement and delayed accumulation of contrast. Centripetal progression also differentiates these tumors from ovarian meta-stases and malignant epithelial tumors, which tend to occur in older patients.

Surgical removal of the tumor is curative. There is no local or distant recurrence [1]. Malignant sclerosing stromal tumor has not been reported to date.

Sex cord tumor with annular tubules

Sex cord tumor with annular tubules is an estrogen-producing sex cord–stromal tumor that is histologically intermediate between GCT and Sertoli cell tumor [4]. It is characterized by sex cord cells in the form of a ring with nuclei orientated around a central hyalinized body. Thirty percent of these tumors occur in patients with Peutz–Jeghers syndrome and they occur in almost 100% of females with Peutz–Jeghers syndrome where they are associated with low-grade mucinous tumors of the cervix. This patient group is also susceptible to GCT and malignant Sertoli–Leydig cell tumors.

When associated with Peutz–Jeghers syndrome, sex cord tumors with annular tubules are small, benign and, in two-thirds, bilateral. The ovaries frequently show multifocal histological involvement. In the absence of this syndrome, these tumors are usually large, unilateral and are malignant in 20% of cases [4]. They are usually solid masses.

Gynandroblastomas

Gynandroblastomas are extremely rare sex cord–stromal tumors that can be a cause of hyperandrogenism. They are made up of both well-differentiated ovarian cell types (granulosa stromal cells) and testicular cell types (Sertoli stromal cells) [4]. They are 100% malignant. Imaging features have not been reported.

Ovarian tumors with functioning stroma

It is not uncommon for ovarian tumors to contain stromal cells and have estrogenic or androgenic manifestations. Surface epithelial tumors, especially mucinous cystadenomas, are the most common type to have an androgenic stroma [2]. They are multilocular cystic masses with varying signal intensities in each locule – the "stained-glass appearance" [12]. The appearance can be similar to GCT. Serous and endometroid tumors can also have an estrogenic stroma.

More than 60 ovarian tumors have been reported with an androgenic stroma [2]. Of these, one-third are metastatic ovarian tumors (mostly gastric in origin), and one-fifth are primary muci-nous cystic tumors. Brenner tumors, carcinoids and teratomas can also have androgen-producing stroma [15].

Metastatic ovarian tumors may be mainly solid or multilocular cysts and tend to be well-demarcated lesions with varying amounts of low signal components on T2-weighted MRI [2]. Metastatic tumors arising from the gastrointestinal tract are frequently bilateral. They distinctively have hypointense solid components with internal hyperintensity on T1 and T2 images respectively.

Ovarian carcinoids with androgen-producing stroma may produce the "stained-glass appearance" in a multilocular cystic mass. They frequently also have an enhancing low signal mural nodule.

Functional ovarian tumors in pregnancy

Virilization during pregnancy caused by ovarian tumors with functioning stroma is a rare but well-recognized phenomenon and has been reported in many tumor types. Hormonally active sex cord–stromal tumors also occur in pregnancy. However, such tumors often cannot be readily classified and are designated as sex cord–stromal tumors unclassified [16].

Differential diagnosis on imaging

Functional ovarian tumors range in radiological appearance from small solid masses to large multicystic lesions. However, there are important radiological features that aid diagnosis.

The vast majority of sex cord–stromal tumors are either benign (fibrothecomas, sclerosing stromal tumors) or confined to the ovary at diagnosis (Sertoli–Leydig cell tumors, GCT). In contrast, epithelial neoplasms have a propensity for early peritoneal and lymphatic spread resulting in radiological findings such as peri-toneal and perihepatic diaphragmatic nodules and omental cake. Furthermore, sex cord–stromal tumors do not demonstrate papil-lary projections, a distinctive feature of epithelial neoplasms. Calcification is rare, unlike germ cell neoplasm. However, it must be remembered that a number of the more common ovarian neoplasms can have functioning stroma, particularly ovarian metastases.

References

1. Jung SE, Rha SE, Lee JM, et al. CT and MRI findings of sex cord–stroma tumor of the ovary. *Am. J. Roentgenol.* 2005;185:207–215.
2. Tanaka YO, Tsunoda H, Kitagawa Y, at al. Functioning ovarian tumors: direct and indirect findings at MR imaging. *Radiographics* 2004;34;5147–5166.
3. Young RH, Scully RE. Ovarian Sertoli–Leydig cell tumors a clinico-pathological analysis of 200 cases. *Am. J. Surg. Pathol.* 1985;9:543–569.
4. Outwater EK, Wagner BJ, Mannion C, et al. Sex cord–stromal and steroid cell tumours of the ovary. *Radiographics* 1998;18:1523–1546.
5. Schumer ST, Cannistra SA. Granulosa cell tumor of the ovary. *J. Clin. Oncol.* 2003;21:1180–1189.

6. Young RH, Dickersin GR, Scully RE. Juvenile granulosa cell tumor of the ovary: a clinicopathological analysis of 125 cases. *Am. J. Surg. Pathol.* 1984;8:575–596.

7. Gusberg SB, Kardon P. Proliferative endometrial response to theca-granulosa cell tumors. *Am. J. Obstet. Gynecol.* 1971;111:633–643.

8. Ko SF, Wan YL, Ng SH, et al. Adult ovarian granulosa cell tumors: spectrum of sonographic and CT findings with pathologic correlation. *Am. J. Roentgenol.* 1999;172:1227–1233.

9. FIGO staging of ovarian cancer. www.figo.org.

10. Jung SE, Lee JM, Rha SE, et al. CT and MR imaging of ovarian tumors with emphasis on differential diagnosis. *Radiographics* 2002;22:1305–1325.

11. Troiano RN, Lazzarini KM, Scoutt LM, et al. Fibroma and fibrothecomas of the ovary: MR imaging findings. *Radiology* 1997;204:795–798.

12. Tanaka YO, Nishida M, Yurosaki Y, et al. Differential diagnosis of gynaecological "stained glass" tumors on MRI. *Br. J. Radiol.* 1999;72:414–420.

13. Kim JC, Kim SS, Park JY. "Bridging vascular sign" in the MR diagnosis of exophytic uterine leiomyoma. *J. Comput. Assist. Tomogr.* 2000;24:57–60.

14. Lee MS, Cho HC, Lee YH, et al. Ovarian sclerosing stromal tumors: gray scale and color Doppler sonographic findings. *J. Ultrasound Med.* 2001;20:413–417.

15. Tanaka YO, Ide Y, Nishiada M, et al. Ovarian tumor with functioning stroma. *Comput. Med. Imaging Graph.* 2002;26:193–197.

16. Young RH. Sex cord–stromal tumors of the ovary and testis: their similarities and differences with consideration of selected problems. *Mod. Pathol.* 2005;18:581–598.

53 Endocrine Aspects of Ovarian Tumors

John H. Shepherd and Lisa Wong

Key points
- Ovarian tumors can have estrogenic or androgenic endocrine manifestations.
- Majority of hormone-producing ovarian tumors arise from sex cord–stromal tumors and germ cell tumors of the ovary.
- Other types of benign or malignant primary or metastatic tumor of the ovary can also have endocrine effects.
- Conservative surgery can be an option in these tumors in young patients desirous of preserving their fertility.
- Modern chemotherapy has improved the survival and fertility options for these women.

Introduction

Most hormonally active ovarian tumors arise from sex cord–stromal and germ cell tumors of the ovary. They account for approximately 5% of all malignant neoplasms. However, almost every type of benign, malignant, primary and metastatic ovarian neoplasm has been reported to have estrogenic and androgenic manifestations [1]. The endocrinologic syndromes manifested in ovarian neoplasia reflect an over-production of sex steroids, estrogenic or androgenic hormones which has specific effects on the hormone-sensitive target organs. The clinical manifestations depend on both the amount of hormone secreted and the age of the patient.

Sex cord–stromal tumors

Ovarian sex cord–stromal tumors (OSCST) are derived from the sex cords and ovarian stroma of the ovary. They are uncommon malignancies and account for 5% of all ovarian tumors [1, 2]. They are composed of the "female" cells such as the granulosa cells, theca cells and their luteinized derivatives and the "male" cells such as the Leydig and Sertoli cells. Sex cord–stromal tumors tend to present at an early stage and run a slow indolent course and are generally associated with a good prognosis. Some women may present with endocrinologic manifestations secondary to steroid production. A classification of sex cord–stromal tumors of the ovaries is shown in Table 53.1.

Granulosa cell tumors

Granulosa cell tumors account for 70% of all feminizing ovarian tumors. They are, however, considered to be rare cancers and

Table 53.1 Classification of sex cord–stromal tumors

Granulosa-stromal tumors
  Granulosa cell tumor
    Adult type
    Juvenile type
  Thecoma-fibroma tumors
    Thecoma
      Typical
      Luteinized
    Fibroma-fibrosarcoma
      Fibroma
      Cellular fibroma
      Fibrosarcoma
  Sclerosing stromal tumor
  Unclassified
Sertoli–Leydig cell tumors (androblastomas/arrhenoblastoma)
  Well differentiated
  Intermediate differentiation
  Poorly differentiated
  With heterologous elements
Gynandroblastoma
Sex cord tumor with annular tubules
Unclassified

account for only 2–5% of all ovarian malignancies. Between 32% and 39% occur in women younger than 40 years and about 5% occur in the prepubertal period. They are classified into the adult type or juvenile type.

The unique features of these tumors lie in their capacity to secrete estrogens and a propensity for late recurrence, sometimes 10 to 20 years after the initial surgical excision. About two-thirds of patients have endocrine manifestations due to hormone secretion by the tumor, leading to an early diagnosis. The natural history is characterized by slow growth, local spread and late recurrence. The long-term prognosis is very favorable and the

Clinical Endocrine Oncology, 2nd edition. Edited by Ian D. Hay and John A.H. Wass. © 2008 Blackwell Publishing. ISBN 978-1-4051-4584-8.

majority (85–90%) of patients present with stage I disease which is associated with an excellent 5-year survival of greater than 90% [3].

The clinical and pathologic characteristics of tumors which present at the menopause are different from those that occur in children and younger patients. Scully [1] described a form of granulosa cell tumors that was different in appearance and nearly always occurred in the first 20 years of life. Thus granulosa cell tumors are usually classified into the adult or juvenile form.

Adult type granulosa cell tumors

Adult type granulosa cell tumors are more common than the juvenile form and account for 95% of all granulosa cell tumors. They usually occur in the late reproductive and early menopausal age groups, between 45 and 55 years of age. The signs and symptoms relate mainly to menstrual dysfunction in the form of metrorrhagia, menorrhagia, oligomenorrhea or amenorrhea. In the postmenopausal woman, it can cause postmenopausal bleeding. These symptoms are related to the estrogen secretion by the tumor. Due to the hyperestrogenic state, 50–60% of patients develop endometrial hyperplasia and 5–10% are at risk of endometrial cancer [3]. These patients are also at risk of breast cancer. Like all ovarian tumors, they can also present with non-specific symptoms related to tumor size such as abdominal distension, bloating and abdominal or pelvic pain. Occasionally, these tumors are androgenic and virilization has been reported in up to 7% of patients [4]. Androgenic manifestations include hirsutism, clitorimegaly, deepening of the voice, amenorrhea and breast atrophy.

Histological characteristics include three typical gross appearances of solid and cystic with hemorrhage within the cysts, solid and yellow or cystic, either multiloculated or uniloculated. Bilateral tumors are uncommon and account for 2–8% of cases. Microscopic examination follows a variety of distinctive patterns, with the cells growing diffusely or in islands, intersecting bands, thin columns, or tubules separated by fibrothecomatous stroma. Call–Exner bodies may be present. The key feature is the appearance of the tumor cell nuclei, which is usually pale and grooved.

On imaging with computerized tomography (CT) and magnetic resonance imaging (MRI) scans, these tumors can have the appearance of solid masses, tumors with hemorrhagic or fibrotic changes, multilocular cystic lesions or completely cystic tumors.

Juvenile type of granulosa cell tumor

The juvenile type occurs in younger women and has a natural history and histological characteristics which are very different from the adult type. It accounts for 85% of granulosa cell tumors that occur before puberty. The majority of cases are associated with the rapid development of isosexual precocious pseudoprecocity such as breast enlargement, development of pubic and axillary hair, irregular menstrual bleeding, advanced somatic and skeletal development and other secondary sexual characteristics. Five percent of tumors are bilateral. Reported series of juvenile type of granulosa cell tumors have shown that 44% to 80% occur during the first decade of life and the majority, between 73.6% and 100%, are stage I at diagnosis [5]. The prognosis was excellent with reports of 5-year survival between 94.4% and 100%.

Histologically, these tumors show immature follicles which contain more mucin, the number of Call–Exner bodies are minimal and the cell nuclei are dark and rarely grooved whereas pale and grooved nuclei are common in the adult form. The solid and follicular pattern, luteinization of the cells and immaturity of the nuclei with a brisk mitotic rate distinguish it from the adult form.

The stage of the disease is the most important prognostic factor for all granulosa cell tumors. Poor prognostic features include tumor rupture, high mitotic index, lymphatic invasion and tumor size. More recently, DNA ploidy and S-phase fraction determined by cytometry have also been shown to be of prognostic significance.

The management of granulosa cell tumors is mainly surgical. There are currently no data to support any form of adjuvant therapy for completely staged stage I granulosa cell tumors. Evans and colleagues reported a 9% risk of recurrence for stage IA disease [2].

Inhibin has been shown to be a useful tumor marker for granulosa cell tumors. Studies have shown that both inhibin A and B are produced by sex cord stromal tumors and some studies have suggested that inhibin B is the major form produced by malignant granulosa cells but does not discriminate as well as the alpha subunit [6]. Jobling and colleagues, in a prospective study [7], demonstrated a sevenfold elevation of inhibin levels before surgery and rising inhibin levels several months before clinical recurrence. The long natural history of granulosa cell tumors with its tendency for late recurrences marks the importance of extended follow-up.

Thecoma-fibromas

Thecomas are defined as theca cells with a small fibroblastic component. They occur mainly in the perimenopausal and postmenopausal age groups. They can secrete estrogen and present with similar symptoms of abnormal vaginal bleeding or with a pelvic mass. Occasionally, these tumors are masculinizing in nature and cause virilization. Most reported series of thecomas have shown that these tumors are almost entirely unilateral and associated with an excellent 5-year survival rate of 100% [4]. Thecomas are almost always benign tumors and are about one-third as common as granulosa cell tumors. Thecomas can be associated with endometrial hyperplasia and give rise to malignant endometrial lesions and this association emphasizes the need for dilatation and curettage where a more conservative surgical approach is undertaken. Thecomas have also been associated with pregnancy and can cause cyst rupture.

Gross examination reveals a solid tumor that ranges in color from uniformly yellow to white mottled with yellow. Microscopic examination shows a diffuse proliferation of stromal cells laden with clear lipid vacuoles separated by fibromatous tissue.

Surgery remains the mainstay of treatment. For younger women, ovarian cystectomy or unilateral salpingo-oophorectomy together with dilatation and curettage is recommended. Total hysterectomy with bilateral salpingo-oophorectomy is advised for patients where fertility is not a concern. There is no role for adjuvant radiation therapy or chemotherapy.

Sclerosing stromal tumors

These are rare tumors that occur mainly in young women. They are generally benign in nature and present with menstrual abnormalities. Surgical resection is advocated and there is usually no local or distant recurrence.

Sertoli–Leydig cell tumors

Sertoli–Leydig cell tumors are rare tumors and comprise about 0.5% of all ovarian tumors. The terms arrhenoblastoma, androblastoma and gonadal stromal tumor of android type have been used as synonyms for this tumor.

These tumors commonly occur at an average age of 25 years, with 70–75% occurring during the second and third decade of life. Pure Leydig cell tumors may be virilizing and are virtually always benign. Sertoli–Leydig cell tumors cause virilization in a third of cases. The characteristic clinical features are that of defeminization and virilization which can present as oligomenorrhea, atrophy of the breasts and genitals. Signs of virilization include clitorimegaly, hirsutism, acne, deepening of the voice and increased libido. Occasionally, the body mass increases and temporal balding occurs. Biochemical markers include an elevation of plasma testosterone and occasionally, elevated levels of plasma androstenedione, 17-ketosteroids and corticosteroids have been reported. Occasionally, Sertoli–Leydig cell tumors can present with hyperestrogenism. Symptoms relating to estrogen excess include menstrual irregularities, isosexual precocious puberty and postmenopausal bleeding. Endometrial stimulation can occur and cause endometrial hyperplasia and well-differentiated adenocarcinoma. Serum alpha fetoprotein (AFP) can also be elevated. However, less than 50% of patients with Sertoli–Leydig cells tumors have no endocrine manifestation and present with abdominal swelling and bloatedness.

Gross examination shows a predominantly mixed solid–cystic lobulated tumor with the solid areas being yellow–orange, reflecting a high lipid content. Microscopically, these tumors are classified into four categories: well differentiated, intermediately differentiated, poorly differentiated tumors and heterologous tumors. Heterologous tumors contain cell types which are foreign to the gonad and include cells from the cartilage, skeletal muscle and gastrointestinal epithelium.

Sertoli–Leydig cell tumors are usually unilateral and if well differentiated, have an excellent prognosis and rarely spread beyond the ovary of origin. These tumors are bilateral in less than 5% of cases and 97% of these tumors are stage I at diagnosis. The prognosis is related to the stage and grade of disease. Tumor recurrence classically occurs early (66–70% within 1 year) and locally.

The treatment of these tumors is mainly surgical. Young and Scully reported no recurrence in patients who had well-differentiated stage I tumors and a recurrence rate of 7% in patients with stage I tumors of intermediate or poor differentiation [8]. The overall 5-year survival rate has been reported to be 70–90% [9].

Gynandroblastoma

Gynandroblastomas are rare tumors and account for less than 1% of all ovarian stromal tumors. These tumors are derived from undifferentiated gonadal mesenchyme which has a bisexual potential and differentiation could occur along both female as well as male directed cell lines. Thus signs and symptoms of both estrogen and androgen excess are present.

The majority of these tumors occur in the third to fifth decade and 60% of cases have symptoms of virilization. Endometrial hyperplasia is also common and pelvic masses are often palpable. These tumors commonly present with primary amenorrhea, virilization or developmental abnormalities of the genitalia. The majority of cases (80%) are phenotypic women and the remainder are phenotypic men with cryptorchidism, hypospadias and internal female genital secondary sex organs. Biochemical changes could include elevated serum testosterone, urinary 17-ketosteroids or elevated serum estradiol. Lesser elevations of androstenedione, dihydroepiandrosterone and dihydrotestosterone have also been observed.

Gross examination shows that these tumors are commonly 7 to 10 cm in size and appear solid yellow–white with cystic areas. Microscopic examination classically includes the presence of both granulosa–theca cell elements as well as Sertoli–Leydig cell elements mixed together.

The management for gynandroblastomas is similar to that of the other sex cord–stromal cell tumors of the ovary. Surgery is the mainstay of treatment. The prognosis is generally excellent for early-stage disease. Serum androgen or estrogen levels if elevated could be used as markers of disease recurrence during follow-up.

Sex cord tumors with annular tubules

Sex cord tumors with annular tubules are now classified separately from the unclassified group of sex cord–stromal tumors. It is thought that these tumors arose from granulosa cells and then developed in a pattern more closely associated with Sertoli cells. Some regard these tumors as variants of Sertoli cell tumors. A peculiar feature of this tumor is that 30–36% of cases are associated with Peutz–Jeghers syndrome and these cases tend to have bilateral tumors.

These tumors can present in a variety of ways due to the overproduction of estrogen. They can cause menstrual disturbances and in young children, they can cause sexual precocity.

Surgery is the main treatment modality. However, in patients with Peutz–Jeghers syndrome, careful evaluation of the contralateral ovary is necessary.

Management of sex cord–stromal tumors

Surgery

Surgery remains the mainstay of treatment for OSCST. As the majority, 95%, of OSCST are unilateral and at least 95% are confined to the ovary, a strong argument could be made for conservative surgery with unilateral salpingo-oophorectomy for young women with stage IA disease. Careful surgical staging should be performed and this would entail random biopsies of the omentum, peritoneum and retroperitoneal lymph nodes if appropriate. Dilatation and curettage should also be performed to exclude a concomitant endometrial pathology. Radical surgery with total hysterectomy bilateral salpingo-oophorectomy is recommended if fertility is not an issue and for patients with higher than stage IA disease.

Prognostic factors

Stage is the most important prognostic factor for granulosa cell tumors. Chan et al. showed that age less than 50 years, smaller tumor size and absence of residual disease were independent prognostic factors for improved survival [10]. Other prognostic factors include tumor rupture, mitotic index, capsular and lymphatic invasion and DNA ploidy. For Sertoli–Leydig cell tumors, histologic differentiation and the presence of heterologous elements are also prognostic factors.

Postoperative adjuvant therapy should be considered for patients with advanced-stage disease or stage I disease with poor prognostic factors such as large tumor size, high mitotic index or tumor rupture.

Chemotherapy

Chemotherapy has been recommended for patients with extensive residual disease, inoperable recurrences and metastases [11]. Various combination chemotherapeutic agents have been used for treatment of OSCST of the ovary. For OSCST, experience with actinomycin, 5-fluorouracil and cyclophosphamide regimen and vincristine, actinomycin and cyclophosphamide regimen (VAC) has been well documented. The combination of cisplatin, vinblastine and bleomycin (PVB) was also popular and response rates ranged from 57% to 92% [12]. Subsequently, the substitution of etoposide for vinblastine resulted in the bleomycin, etoposide and cisplatin (BEP) regimen which proved to be equally active but less toxic. Recently, the efficacy of taxanes has been compared with BEP regimen for OSCST [13]. Brown et al. [13] reported that for primary OSCST, there was no significance difference in response rate, progression-free survival and overall survival for patients treated with BEP versus taxanes. For recurrent disease, the response rate was higher for BEP-treated (71%) than for taxane-treated patients (37%) although this was not shown to be statistically significant. Taxanes were shown to be less toxic than BEP and the combination of taxane with platinum chemotherapy warrants further investigations.

Radiotherapy

The value of radiotherapy for OSCST is unclear. Definite activity has been demonstrated and studies have shown that prolonged survival was observed for granulosa and Sertoli–Leydig cell tumors. It is generally agreed that there was no benefit of radiotherapy for stage I disease although radiotherapy may have a role in prolonging disease-free survival in advanced or recurrent disease [3].

Hormonal therapy

Hormonal treatment may play a role for metastatic granulosa cell tumors. Progesterone, tamoxifen and gonadotropin-releasing hormone agonist analog have shown stabilization or partial response of the tumor.

Germ cell tumors

Ovarian germ cell tumors (OGCT) comprise about 20% of all ovarian tumors and the malignant forms account for less than 5% of all ovarian tumors. They can present with endocrine manifestations. Most of these tumors occur in young women and extirpation of disease revolves around decisions concerning child bearing and the probabilities of tumor recurrence. Recent developments in chemotherapy have dramatically changed the prognosis for many patients with malignant germ cell tumors of the ovary. A classification of germ cell tumors of the ovary is shown in Table 53.2.

Table 53.2 Classification of germ cell tumors

Germ cell tumors
  Dysgerminoma
  Endodermal sinus tumor (yolk sac tumor)
  Embryonal carcinoma
  Polyembryoma
  Choriocarcinoma
  Teratoma
    Immature
    Mature
  Monodermal or highly specialized
    Struma ovarii
    Carcinoid
    Struma ovarii and carcinoid
    Mixed forms
Tumors composed of germ cells and sex cord stroma derivative
  Gonadoblastoma
  Mixed germ cell–sex cord stroma tumor

Dysgerminoma

Dysgerminoma is an uncommon tumor, accounting for 1–2% of primary ovarian tumors and 3–5% of ovarian malignancies. They commonly occur in adolescence and early adulthood. This is the ovarian counterpart of the testicular seminoma. Dysgerminoma is the only germ cell tumor in which the contralateral ovary may be involved in 10–15% of cases [14]. An elevated human chorionic gonadotropin (HCG) and lactate dehydrogenase (LDH) level may be present in these patients.

The clinical presentation is that of abdominal distension and the presence of a pelvi-abdominal mass on examination. Occasionally menstrual and endocrine abnormalities may be the presenting symptoms.

Gross examination shows a firm or fleshy cream-colored tumor, which is often lobulated. Microscopically, the parenchymal cells are large, uniform, round or polygonal. The nuclei are round, vesicular, containing one or more nucleoli with abundant glycogen. A lymphocytic infiltrate is characteristic.

Dysgerminomas have a predilection for lymphatic spread and are known for their acute sensitivity to irradiation. Historically, surgery followed by radiation has resulted in an excellent cure rate. More recently, combination chemotherapy has resulted in good cure rates in young women desirous of future child bearing. As 70% of patients are stage I at diagnosis and the majority are younger than 30 years, conservative surgery and preservation of fertility are major considerations.

Conservative surgery can be considered for stage IA lesions although the other ovary should be carefully inspected. The resected specimen should be carefully evaluated for the presence of germ cell elements other than dysgerminoma. When the dysgerminoma is not pure and contains small areas of more malignant histology, the prognosis and therapy are determined by the other germ cell elements.

Adjuvant radiotherapy or chemotherapy has not been shown to be of benefit in stage IA disease. Asadourian and Taylor reported a 10-year survival of 91% after conservative surgery with a 20% risk of recurrence [14]. Ninety percent of recurrences occur within the first 2 years and can be successfully eradicated with chemotherapy or radiotherapy. These data strongly support the initial conservative approach with preservation of fertility.

More advanced lesions should be treated with adjuvant chemotherapy. Radiotherapy may be appropriate in patients where fertility is not an issue and where there may be some contraindication to chemotherapy.

Endodermal sinus tumor

Endodermal sinus tumors are also commonly known as yolk sac tumors of the ovary. These tumors originate from the germ cells that differentiate into the extra-embryonal yolk sac. The median age at presentation is 19 years and clinical presentation is that of abdominal discomfort and a pelvi-abdominal mass. They can cause elevated alpha fetoprotein levels.

Microscopically, the tumor is arranged in tubules with loose reticular stroma. Schiller–Duval bodies are also sometimes seen. The prognosis for patients with these tumors has been unfavorable although the use of combination chemotherapy has improved the outlook. These tumors are not sensitive to radiotherapy and conservative surgery with chemotherapy has resulted in a number of successful pregnancies.

Embryonal carcinoma

Embryonal carcinomas of the ovary are highly malignant tumors that mainly occur in children and adolescents. The mean age at diagnosis is 15 years. This tumor accounts for 4% of the malignant germ cell tumors of the ovary. It usually presents with an abdominal mass associated with hormonal abnormalities such as irregular menstrual bleeding, precocious puberty or hirsutism. Tumor markers such as HCG and AFP are commonly elevated. Microscopically, the tumor consists of cells with eosinophilic cytoplasm arranged in papillary or gland-like formations. Atypical mitotic figures and multinucleated giant cells are commonly seen. Stage I tumors have been shown to have survival rates of 50% [15].

Polyembryoma

Polyembryoma is a rare ovarian germ cell tumor and is commonly associated with immature teratomas. It is a highly malignant tumor and usually presents when locoregional spread has occurred.

Choriocarcinoma

Choriocarcinoma of the ovary are tumors that undergo differentiation towards trophoblastic structures. They can be classified as gestational choriocarcinoma or non-gestational choriocarcinoma, and we will limit our discussion here to the non-gestational choriocarcinoma. The diagnosis is made when both cytotrophoblast and syncytiotrophoblast are present. In the majority of cases, the tumor is admixed with other germ cell elements and their presence is diagnostic of non-gestational choriocarcinoma.

The tumor occurs mainly in children and young adults. Non-gestational choriocarcinomas tend to be large and necrosis and hemorrhage are usual features. The HCG level is characteristically elevated in these tumors and in prepubescent children, signs of precocious puberty, breast development, growth of axillary and pubic hair and uterine bleeding are common presentations.

As these are highly malignant tumors, the prognosis for these tumors has been poor. However, the advent of modern combination chemotherapy has been effective in achieving prolonged remissions.

Teratoma

Mature cystic teratomas are benign tumors that consist of mature elements derived from all three germ cell layers. They are very common and account for 95% of all ovarian teratomas and about 25% of all ovarian neoplasms. These tumors are multicystic and contain hair, teeth, bone or cartilage intermixed with sticky keratinous and sebaceous debris. They are bilateral in 12% of cases. Malignant transformation in the mature tissues occurs in 1–2% of cases and transformation into squamous cell carcinoma occurs in 1% of dermoid cysts.

The clinical presentation is related to its size, compression symptoms, torsion or chemical peritonitis resulting from intra-peritoneal spillage of the cholesterol-laden debris.

Mature solid teratoma is a very rare ovarian neoplasm that occurs mainly in children and young adults. They are usually unilateral and benign although peritoneal implants may be present, composed entirely of mature glial tissue. The prognosis is excellent with surgical resection of the ovarian tumor.

Immature teratomas are tumors derived from the three germ layers but containing immature or embryonal structures. They are also known as malignant teratoma, solid or embryonal teratoma. They are uncommon tumors and comprise less than 1% of ovarian teratoma. They usually occur in the first two decades of life and rarely after the menopause. These tumors are graded histologically based on the amount and degree of cellular immaturity and are usually unilateral. The prognosis is related to the histological grade, stage of disease, size of tumor and both nature and quantity of immature element present.

Treatment is mainly surgical with unilateral salpingo-oophorectomy and wide sampling of peritoneal implants. If the primary tumor is grade 0 or 1 and all peritoneal implants are grade 0, no adjuvant therapy is needed. However, if the primary tumor is grade 2 or 3 or if the implants are grade 1, 2 or 3, combination chemotherapy is useful.

Struma ovarii are generally benign tumors which are composed of predominantly mature thyroid tissue. Some patients present with clinical hyperthyroidism and malignant transformation is unusual.

Carcinoid tumors usually arise in association with gastrointestinal or respiratory epithelium present in mature cystic teratoma. These patients may present with the typical carcinoid syndrome.

Gonadoblastoma

Gonadoblastomas are rare tumors composed of mixed germ cells and sex cord–stromal cells. Patients usually present with endocrine symptoms such as primary amenorrhea, virilization or developmental abnormalities of the genitalia or a pelvic mass. Eighty percent of patients are phenotypic women, the majority of which are virilized, and 20% are phenotypic men with cryptorchidism, hypospadias and internal female sex organs.

Management of germ cell tumors

Surgery

The current surgical approach to OGCT has been derived mainly from data from the Armed Forces Institute of Pathology in the 1970s [16]. These reports show that the median age of patients with OGCT occurs in the teenage years and that most of these tumors are unilateral except for dysgerminomas, in which 10–15% of tumors are bilateral. Thus, for most cases of OGCT, a unilateral salpingo-oophorectomy with careful staging and preservation of the contralateral ovary and the uterus is considered the appropriate surgical management. Routine biopsy of the contralateral ovary should be avoided as this could lead to future infertility from peritoneal adhesions or ovarian failure. Meticulous technique and avoidance of unnecessary surgery are important.

Even in patients with advanced disease, preservation of reproductive function is still possible if the contralateral ovary is normal. Evidence from several large series suggests an at least equivalent survival after conservative surgery compared with bilateral salpingo-oophorectomy with or without hysterectomy [17]. In the current age and with advances in the field of reproductive medicine, conserving the ovary could offer the option of oocyte retrieval with a surrogate uterus, while conserving the uterus could leave the option of donor eggs and *in vitro* fertilization and embryo transfer into the womb. If, however, bilateral ovarian masses were found at laparotomy, then the more suspicious ovary should be resected and the other ovary should be biopsied. If the other ovary contains tumor or is dysgenetic, then bilateral salpingo-oophorectomy is indicated.

For patients with advanced disease, the same principles of cytoreductive surgery for epithelial ovarian tumors should still apply with maximal resection to achieve minimal residual disease. However, OGCT, especially dysgerminomas, are generally more chemosensitive than epithelial ovarian tumors. Therefore the surgeon must take this into consideration and must exercise thoughtful intraoperative judgement in weighing the relative benefit of each cytoreductive maneuver for these chemosensitive tumors.

Surgery alone is sufficient for patients with stage IA, grade 1 pure immature teratoma or stage I pure dysgerminoma. Postoperative treatment is recommended for stage I, grade 2 immature teratoma.

Chemotherapy for OGCT

Ovarian germ cell tumors are highly chemosensitive malignancies. Many of the strategies evolved from experience with testicular germ cell tumors. In the 1970s, the first effective combination chemotherapy for OGCT was the vincristine, actinomycin-D and cyclophosphamide (VAC) regimen. The GOG reported a cure rate of 82% in stage I disease and less than 50% in metastatic disease[18]. The introduction of cisplatin-based chemotherapy using cisplatin, vinblastine and bleomycin (PVB) led to a significant improvement of survival [19]. PVB regimens demonstrated an improved cure rate of 95% or better for stage I and II disease, 80% for stage III disease and 60% for stage IV disease. In 1977, the Charing Cross Hospital in London developed an alternative approach using an alternating chemotherapy schedule (POMB/ACE) which includes cisplatinum, vincristine, methotrexate, bleomycin (POMB) and actinomycin-D, cyclophosphamide and etoposide (ACE). This regimen was designed to minimize the development of drug resistance as well as maximizing tumor recovery. Subsequently the substitution of etoposide for vinblastine proved to be equally active but less toxic. Combination chemotherapy with bleomycin, etoposide and cisplatin (BEP) became the most widely used regimen and has become the standard of care for OGCT [20]. Reports comparing PVB and BEP showed that BEP showed excellent activity with less toxicity [21]. Several studies have reported an impressive disease-free survival with BEP ranging from 92% to 96% [22]. The excellent outcome suggests there is no role for second-look surgery in patients with completely resected OGCT after chemotherapy [18]. Successful pregnancies have been reported after chemotherapy and this demonstrates the fact that the reproductive potential is unaffected after chemotherapy [23]. The incidence of infertility in these patients attempting conception ranged from 5% to 10% which corresponds to the background incidence rate of infertility in the general population.

Radiotherapy

Radiation therapy has been the traditional postoperative treatment for patients with metastatic dysgerminoma. However, radiation therapy usually renders these young patients infertile. Currently chemotherapy has replaced radiotherapy as the postoperative treatment of choice with dysgerminoma and radiotherapy should be reserved as a salvage option in selected patients.

Summary

In summary, although the majority of hormonally active tumors of the ovary arise form sex cord–stromal and germ cell tumors of the ovary, they form only a small proportion of all ovarian tumors. Potentially any type of benign or malignant ovarian tumor could have estrogenic or androgenic manifestations. The majority of these tumors occur in young women. These tumors are highly sensitive to chemotherapy and fertility-sparing surgery should be considered for these women.

References

1. Scully RE, Young RH, Clement PB. *Tumours with Functioning Stroma. Tumours of the Ovary, Maldeveloped Gonads, Fallopian Rube, and Broad Ligament*, 3rd edn. Washington, DC: Armed Forces Institute of Pathology, 1998:373–378.

2. Evans AT III, Gaffey TA, Malkasian GD Jr, Annegers JF. Clinico-pathologic review of 118 granulosa and 82 theca cell tumors. *Obstet. Gynecol.* 1980;55:231–238.

3. Savage P, Constenla D, Fisher C, et al. Granulosa cell tumours of the ovary: demographics, survival and the management of advanced disease. *Clin. Oncol. (R. Coll. Radiol.)* 1998;10:242–245.

4. Anikwue C, Dawood MY, Kramer E. Granulosa and theca cell tumours. *Obstet. Gynecol.* 1978;51:214–220.

5. Young RH, Dickersin GR, Scully RE. Juvenile granulose cell tumour of the ovary: a clinicopathologic analysis of 125 cases. *Am. J. Surg. Pathol.* 1984;8:575–596.

6. Robertson DM, Cahir N, Burger HG, Mamers P, Groome N. Inhibin forms in serum from postmenopausal women with ovarian cancers. *Clin. Endocrinol.* 1999;50:381–386.

7. Jobling T, Mamers P, Healy DL, et al. A prospective study of inhibin in granulosa cell tumours of the ovary. *Gynecol. Oncol.* 1994;55:285–289.

8. Young RH, Scully RE. Ovarian Sertoli–Leydig cell tumors: A clinico-pathological analysis of 207 cases. *Am. J. Surg. Pathol.* 1985;9:543–569.

9. Disaia PJ, Creasman WT. Germ cell, stromal, and other ovarian tumors. In: *Clinical Gynecologic Oncology*, 4th edn. St Louis: Mosby-Year Book Inc., 1993:426–457.

10. Chan JK, Zhang M, Kaleb V, et al. Prognostic factors responsible for survival in sex cord stromal tumours of the ovary – A multivariate analysis. *Gynecol. Oncol.* 2005;96:204–209.

11. Homesley HD, Bundy BN, Hurteau JAS, Roth LM. Bleomycin, etoposide and cisplatin combination therapy of ovarian granulosa cell tumours and other stromal malignancies: a gynecologic oncology group study. *Gynecol. Oncol.* 1999;72:131–137.

12. Zambetti M, Escobedo A, Pilotti S, De Palo G. Cisplatinum/vinblastine/bleomycin combination chemotherapy in advanced or recurrent granulosa cell tumours of the ovary. *Gynecol. Oncol.* 1990;36:317–320.

13. Brown J, Shvartsman HS, Deavers MT, et al. The activity of taxanes compared with bleomycin, etoposide, and cisplatin in the treatment of sex cord–stromal ovarian tumours. *Gynecol. Oncol.* 2005;97:489–496.

14. Asadourian LA, Taylor HB. Dysgerminoma: an analysis of 105 cases. *Obstet. Gynecol.* 1969;33:370–375.

15. Kurman RJ, Norris HJ. Embryonal carcinoma of the ovary – a clinicopathologic entity distinct from endodermal sinus tumour resembling embryonal carcinoma of the adult testis. *Cancer* 1976;38:2420–2433.

16. Kurman RJ, Norris HJ. Malignant mixed germ cell tumours of the ovary. A clinical and pathologic analysis of 30 cases. *Obstet. Gynecol.* 1976;48:578–589.

17. Slayton RE, Park RC, Silverberg SG, Shingleton H, Creasman WT, Blessing JA. Vincristine, dactinomycin, and cyclophosphamide in the treatment of malignant germ cell tumours of the ovary. A Gynecologic Oncologic Group Study. *Cancer* 1985;56:243–248.

18. Gershenson DM. Management of early ovarian cancer: germ cell and sex cord–stromal tumours. *Gynecol. Oncol.* 1994;55:S62–72.

19. De Palo G, Zambetti M, Pilotti S, et al. Nondysgerminomatous tumours of the ovary treated with cisplatin, vinblastine and bleomycin: longterm results. *Gynecol. Oncol.* 1992;47:239–246.

20. Williams S, Blessing JA, Liao SY, et al. Adjuvant therapy of ovarian germ cell tumours with cisplatin, etoposide and bleomycin: a trial of Gynecologic Oncologic Group. *J. Clin. Oncol.* 1994;12:701–706.

21. Williams SD, Birch R, Einhorn LH, Irwin L, Greco FA, Loehrer P. Treatment of disseminated germ cell tumours with cisplatin, bleomycin, and either vincristine or etoposide. *N. Engl. J. Med.* 1987;316:1435–1440.

22. Dimopoulos MA, Papadopoulos M, Andreopoulou E, et al. Favorable outcome of ovarian germ cell malignancies treated with cisplatin or carboplatin-based chemotherapy: a Hellenic Cooperative Oncology Group study. *Gynecol. Oncol.* 1998;70:70–74.

23. Low JJH, Perrin LC, Crandon AJ, Hacker NF. Conservative surgery to preserve ovarian function in patients with malignant ovarian germ cell tumours. *Cancer* 2000;89:391–398.

54 Testicular Germ Cell Cancers

R. Timothy D. Oliver

> **Key points**
> - Testicular germ cell cancer is a tumor of increasing interest to endocrinologists, given the emerging evidence for a role of intrauterine exposure to endocrine factors in its causation. It is also of interest because of the insights it gives to the possible causes of metabolic syndrome which is an increasing problem in long-term follow-up studies.
> - Study of biology of carcinoma *in situ* provides clear evidence that seminoma and non-seminoma are derived from the same stem cell.
> - While new and improved salvage therapy is available for the minority failing treatment, most recent progress has come from development of ways of safely minimizing treatment through combined chemotherapy and surgical approaches.

Introduction

There is little dispute that the stem cells, which are the source of more than 90% of testicular cancer in young adults, the spermatogonia, are hormone dependent. Equally the occurrence of ectopic endocrinopathy from inappropriate hormone production by this group of tumors now collectively known as germ cell cancers (GCCs) was discovered long before those from other tumor sites. This was because the Aschheim Zondek test for ovulation in frogs enabled the demonstration of what subsequently become known as human chorionic gonadotropin (hCG) in males with testis cancer and gynecomastia [1].

Despite this, apart from the demonstration of carcinoma *in situ*, changes in a small minority of biopsies from men with infertility [2] and more than 90% of GCCs [3], in recent years there has been very little input from endocrinologists into either the pathogenesis of testis cancer or its treatment. Despite an overall cure rate today in excess of 95% [4], there is increasing evidence, as this chapter aims to summarize, of a need for more input in both understanding the cause and managing the late effects of treatment. This is particularly so as late follow-up of cured patients demonstrates that 20% develop second non-testicular cancers within 20 years of radiation [5] when their average age would be only 55, while after excessive dosage of etoposide in excess of 1% develop leukemias [6]. In addition, there is increasing evidence that testicular atrophy is one of the most significant risk factors for this tumor and metabolic syndrome of androgen deficiency with hypertension, vascular and hearing problems are well-documented late effects of cure of these

Clinical Endocrine Oncology, 2nd edition. Edited by Ian D. Hay and John A.H. Wass. © 2008 Blackwell Publishing. ISBN 978-1-4051-4584-8.

patients, even those cured by surgery alone [7]. This is leading to considerable pressure to do trials risking less treatment in the more curable good-risk patients, which is not without risk, as the 10% worse survival in trials of carboplatin [8] and similar worse results in trials to justify stopping the use of bleomycin [8] illustrate.

It is the aim of this chapter to focus on the relevance of modern endocrinology to pathogenesis and treatment of testicular GCC and attempt to identify areas for the future where there may be a case for involvement of endocrinologists in development of new strategies for this disease.

Epidemiology [9]

Geographical epidemiology

Testis germ cell tumors are the most frequent malignancy in males in caucasian populations between the age of 20 and 34, when the lifetime risk is 1 in 500. In non-caucasian, particularly African, populations they are very rare, with the exception of the New Zealand Maori. Germ cell tumors are exceptionally rare prior to puberty, although there is a small peak in the first year of life, presumably reflecting the influence of intrauterine hormone milieus. It is this observation which may explain why the clinical behavior of these tumors is more like a delayed pediatric tumor than an early-onset adult tumor in terms of response to chemotherapy and radiotherapy.

The peak age incidence in adults (20–45 years) precisely coincides with the period of maximum sexual activity in the male and recently, coincident with evidence of earlier onset of puberty and evidence of earlier onset of sexual activity, the incidence has begun to peak earlier providing compelling evidence to suggest that the tumor, at least initially, must have some dependence on hormone factors.

Table 54.1 Danish testis cancer incidence and overview of literature reports on sperm counts during the last 50 years

	Danish incidence of testis cancer (per 100 000)	No. of studies (no. of cases)	Median of reported mean sperm count	Proportion with sperm count >100 × 10⁶/mL
<1960	4.7	10 (1612)	107	46%
1960–81	6.3	20 (2265)	84	25%
1982–90	8.6	31 (10 679)	72	17%

Modified from [10].

Table 54.2 Semen analysis on normal males and germ cell cancer patients

	Median sperm count	<20 (×100/mL)	≥20 (×100/mL)
Normal male fertile (n = 104)	84	11.5%	89%
Infertile (n = 53)	10	68%	36%
Testis tumor stage I survivor (n = 16)	7.5	75%	25%
Metastatic pre-chemo (n = 24)	10	71%	29%
Metastatic post-chemo (n = 27)	7.0	70%	29%
Testis conservation chemo (n = 10)	2.65	90%	10%

Atrophy-induced gonadotropin drive as the final common pathway of testis tumor development

As Table 54.1 demonstrates there has been a worldwide decline in sperm count [10] coincident with the rising incidence of GCC [11]. This is leading to increasing acceptance that gonadal atrophy with loss of feedback inhibition of the hypothalamus and increased gonadotropin drive, thus allowing less time for repair of DNA damage, may be the final common pathway in tumor development [11, 12]. Support for this comes from the demonstration that more than 70% of patients have evidence of reduced spermatogenesis from their contralateral "normal" testis (Table 54.2).

Exogenous atrophogens acting post puberty

That chemical-induced atrophy could be a factor comes from the discovery that military dogs returning from Vietnam after exposure to the defoliant, Agent Orange, had an increased incidence of seminoma. Furthermore, returning members of the US armed forces from Vietnam, in addition to reduced sperm counts [13], were also found to have an increased risk of GCC [14]. Attention has also focused on other agricultural organochlorine chemicals as possible contributing factors. They are well known to cause damage to the germinal epithelium [13] and also chronic immune suppression [15], which, in the setting of massive accidental overdose such as occurred in Bhopal, India, and in Minnesota, can be associated with the development of a human immunodeficiency virus (HIV)-negative type of acquired immune deficiency syndrome (AIDS). The observation from Israel that substantial reduction (greater than 90%) in the levels of this group of fat-soluble

chemicals in milk following a ban on their use between 1976 and 1986 was associated with a 28% reduction in breast cancer in women under the age of 45 and 19% in women between 45 and 64 [16], may provide an explanation as to why one study has observed a significant association between consumption of milk and risk of GCC [17], while a report from Denmark has claimed that organic food farmers have higher than average sperm counts.

That agricultural organochlorine compounds are not the only gonadal atrophogens involved is supported from a case–control epidemiological risk factor study involving 794 patients and controls [18, 19]. It confirmed the well-known association with undescended testis, and supported the idea that early operation reduced the incidence. It demonstrated a significant association with testicular trauma, always held in suspicion because of recall bias, and orchitis (possibly supporting the long discussed association with mumps [20]), venereal disease and infertility, suggesting that there may be multiple interacting atrophogens involved. This study also demonstrated that early puberty and a sedentary lifestyle increase risk possibly due to increased apoptosis of germ cells produced by heat [21], while late onset of puberty and more than average exercise (known from studies in women to reduce gonadotropin production and reduce breast cancer risk) is protective, providing added evidence that gonadotropin drive is important in development of these tumors.

There have been two reports suggesting that serum follicle-stimulating hormone (FSH) levels may be of prognostic significance in the clinical behavior of GCC. The first from Norway demonstrated, confirmed by a recent clinical trial [22], that patients with an elevated FSH had a higher than average risk for the development of tumors in the contralateral testis (Table 54.3). This suggests that early stages of GCC, which as the next section indicates could include seminoma, may be hormone dependent.

The only factor that does not fit with this hypothesis is the observation that germ cell tumor incidence decreases after its peak at 30–35 years when FSH levels are rising in association with a declining sperm count. A possible explanation could be that the vulnerable stem cells or the Sertoli cells become menopausal and are switched off or exhausted at this stage or there is an organ resistance to FSH. Recent evidence that inhibin has a wide pleiotropic tumor-suppressive effect provides one avenue in need of further investigation to explain this paradox.

There are two therapeutic options that might emerge from these observations on the prognostic significance of elevated FSH

Table 54.3 FSH level and risk of contralateral tumor after unilateral orchidectomy

Hoff Wanderas et al. [23]	Number of cases	Elevated FSH level
Patients with second GCC	13	77%
Control patients	26	15%
Oliver et al. [22]	Number of cases	Median FSH (iu/L)
Patients with second GCC	12	19.9
Control patients	985	9.3

on development of metastases and tumors in the contralateral testis. The first is that such patients at diagnosis might benefit from endocrine replacement, to suppress the hypothalamus and reduce gonadotropin drive. The second therapeutic option that could be explored arising out of these observations is the possibility of using short-term luteinizing hormone releasing hormone analogs to treat carcinoma *in situ*. Old experimental animal data now supported from some recent clinical observations [24, 25] emerging from study of the effects of hormone treatment on the immune system (i.e., its ability to induce lymphocytosis and thymic regeneration), suggests that endocrine therapy might have an immunoadjuvant effect, which could enable short-term endocrine therapy completely to reject premalignant cells. It has been speculated that this may explain why some patients with prostate cancer can have durable remissions after stopping hormone therapy [26].

Modern views on GCC pathology

It is increasingly accepted that most tissue cell growth is regulated in an endocrine manner by positive growth factors (cellular oncogenes) stimulating growth and negative inhibitors of growth (suppressor genes) inhibiting replication and enhancing cellular differentiation. Understanding this endocrinology is increasingly important in cancer as mutation in the set of genes called cellular oncogenes (so called because mutated forms of these genes were found in oncogenic viruses), leads to increased growth of cancers as do deletions of DNA material controlling suppressor genes [27].

It is more than 15 years since the early cytogenetic data of Atkin first led to the suggestion that non-seminomas with modal DNA content of 2.8 N may, at least in part, arise by clonal evolution from seminoma with a modal DNA content of 3.6 N in association with chromosomal loss [12]. The subsequent discovery of premalignant carcinoma *in situ* lesions in testis biopsies from men with infertility, and the association of this pathological feature with all types of GCC (Table 54.4) [2] has been particularly important for understanding the cytogenetics. This was because these cells had higher chromosome numbers than both seminoma

and non-seminoma and a minority of tumors containing both seminoma and non-seminoma elements had a gradient in DNA content between carcinoma *in situ*, seminoma and non-seminoma components. This led to the conclusion that in the majority of patients the chromosomal loss occurred before the development of the solid tumor element. Support for this concept has come from immunochemical studies on carcinoma *in situ* elements in the residual rim of normal testis [29].

It is clear from reviewing the data presented in Table 54.5 that for all parameters examined patients with combined seminoma/non-seminoma display characteristics that are intermediate between those of pure seminoma and pure non-seminoma. It is this gradient, taken with the morphological similarity between seminoma cells and spermatogonia, that justifies applying the principles used in grading other solid cancers to seminoma and considering it as grade 1 or well-differentiated GCC (G1 GCC) with respect to its cell of origin [12]. On this basis, combined tumors with both cell types would be considered as grade 2 or intermediate differentiated GCC (G2 GCC) and pure non-seminoma (so-called malignant teratoma in the British Testicular Tumour Panel classification) without any cells resembling the differentiated stem cell would be considered as undifferentiated or grade 3 (G3 GCC).

Although this scheme explains very clearly the relationship between seminoma and the embryonal carcinoma elements it does not explain the occurrence of extra-embryonic tissues such as trophoblast and yolk sac or fetal tissues such as cartilage, glandular or neural elements. The increasing frequency with which immunocytochemistry is identifying these elements in other solid tumors such as bladder cancer [30] and classifying them as metaplastic components provides a possible solution

Table 54.4 Risk factors for carcinoma in situ (CIS)

Subpopulation	Prevalence of CIS
General Danish male population	<0.8%
Cryptorchidism	2.0–3.0%
Infertility	0.4–1.1%
Unilateral GCC*	5.0–6.0%
Unilateral GCC†	94.0%
Extragonadal GCC	35.0%
Androgen insensitivity	25.0% (4/12)
Gonadal dysgenesis	100% (4/4)

*Contralateral testis.
†Ipsilateral testis.
GCC, germ-cell cancer.
Data from [28].

Table 54.5 Combined tumors as an intermediate prognosis subgroup of testicular germ cell tumors

Group	Seminoma (n = 248) (%)	Combined seminoma/non-seminoma (n = 116) (%)	Non-seminoma (n = 241) (%)
Proportion presenting in stage I	79	51	41
Relapse stage I after adjuvant chemotherapy	1	6	0
Relapse stage I after surveillance only	23	31	38
Primary cure of all metastatic patients	91	93	86
Proportion of metastatic cases with high markers	0	16	21
Cure rate low markers	91	94	92
Cure rate high markers	–	89	65

The median age for stage I patients with: seminoma is 36 years; non-seminoma, 29 years; combined seminoma/non-seminoma, 31 years. The median age for metastatic patients with: seminoma is 42 years; non-seminoma, 29 years; combined seminoma/non-seminoma, 37 years.
Data from [12].

for improving the precision of classification in combination with a grading classification. The report from Murty and colleagues that GCC with somatic elements have a higher level of loss of heterozygosity than other GCC [31] provides a justification for considering the clonal grading evolution and fetal/somatic tissue differentiation as two separate dimensions of GCC development.

Contribution of immune response to prognostication of metastatic seminoma

Although considerable skepticism persists about the practical relevance of the concept of immune surveillance in cancer, the 60% durable complete remission of patients with superficial bladder cancer treated by intravesical bacille Calmette–Guérin (BCG) and its durability correlating with degree of interleukin-2 induction, the high response rate of wart virus-induced tumors to α-interferon and the occurrence of up to 5% durable (more than 5 years) complete remission of terminal renal cancer and melanoma patients after interleukin-2 regimens, are the most convincing evidence that even today there are limited areas of gain from immunotherapy. The evidence that the survival of cancer patients might be improved if it were possible to reduce the immunosuppression occurring after prolonged anesthesia for surgical procedures, blood transfusion, pregnancy or in heavy smokers provideadditional reasons for clinical awareness of the relevance of immune suppression. Although immunosuppression, whether in HIV-positive individuals or transplant recipients, increases instances of some malignancies, HIV status, though originally effecting survival of GCC, in the era of highly active retroviral therapy does not effect cure rate [32].

As discussed earlier, seminoma is the germ cell tumor of which the morphology most closely resembles the original starting stem cell, the spermatogonium, and can therefore be functionally considered as well differentiated. This tumor's excessive levels of lymphocyte infiltrate and high frequency of spontaneous regression have long been well established. The idea discussed earlier that GCC develop in a clonal way in association with chromosomal loss from near tetraploid carcinoma *in situ* via seminoma (DNA content 3.6 N) and combined tumors (mixed content populations) to embryonal carcinoma (DNA content 2.6 N) fits closely to the accepted clonal evolution with increasing escape from immune surveillance from grade 1 to grade 3 tumors in other adult cancers and explains why seminoma, like other grade 1 tumors such as bladder cancer, demonstrates more evidence for the importance of antitumor immune response.

Intrauterine exposure to "xeno-estrogens" and GCC development

While the data discussed in the preceding sections clearly establish that events after puberty do accelerate the development of GCC, more recently it has become clear that events occurring

in utero play possibly an even more important role in terms of the initial initiation of the primary step in causing malignant transformation. The observation was that the risk of familial GCC of siblings was double that of father sons; the observation that dizygotic twins had a higher risk than monozygotic twins supports the view that intrauterine environmental factors make an important contribution to later post-pubertal development of GCC.

Because it is known that mothers bearing dizygous twins have higher levels of estrogen than those of monozygous twins, one environmental factor long suspected is estrogen [33], though other factors such as radiation and smoking may also be involved. Endocrine studies in normal twins show higher inhibin in dizygous twins [34], suggesting the need for more information on the role of this hormone in testis cancer.

More recently there has been more direct evidence of how intrauterine environmental factors might act through mutation of c-KIT. Three points have emerged from these studies: first, the c-KIT mutation is not in the germ line; second, it is the same mutation in both testes, suggesting that it is developing before 16 weeks when the germ cell arrives in the developing testis; the final point demonstrating the importance of c-KIT mutation for initiation but not maintenance of GCC growth is the observation that it is occasionally found to be lost when the tumor is fully developed, though it is present in the intratubular germ cell neoplasia cells. This suggests that, though necessary for initiation of the cancer, it plays a hit and run role and is not necessary for the later stages and can be lost with the other genetic material lost during clonal development.

Clinical management [8, 35]

Clinical use of oncofetal markers

Although known about for a long time since the advent of the Aschheim Zondek test [1], the real era of tumor markers began with the advent of radioimmunoassays and today use of such assays is an integral part of patient management. Marker decline rate at the appropriate half-life (36 h for β-hCG and 6 days for alpha fetoprotein) after orchidectomy in patients without obvious metastases is a routine way to establish the absence of metastasis and in some centers also for the response of metastases to chemotherapy, although this is more disputed because many patients with metastases develop post-treatment surges due to tumor lysis. This third main area is on detection of relapse, although it cannot be relied on totally as one-third of relapses are marker negative and are picked up by scans [36].

Although alpha fetoprotein and β-hCG are the most frequently used tumor markers for clinical monitoring of patients, other markers have been used to a lesser extent. The most valuable is lactic dehydrogenase (LDH), particularly the isoform LDH-1 which in clinical practice can be measured by the assay for hydroxybutyric dehydrogenase (HBD) performed at a high temperature of 37 °C (98.6 °F). This, as well as predicting patients with a high risk of metastases resistant to chemotherapy, is also paradoxically positive in seminoma patients, who, by definition have a low hCG and are alpha fetoprotein negative. Placental alkaline phosphatase is another marker that is specific for seminoma although false positives in smokers have limited the reliability of the assay.

Currently, as far as prognostication is concerned, tumor marker levels are proving more important than actual anatomical volume of metastases in defining a prognostic index to identify patients with high, intermediate and low chance of cure by modern chemotherapy.

Clinical behavior and response to treatment

The last 80 years have seen the overall cure rate of testicular GCC rise from 15% to 95%. Although a major part of this has occurred in the last 30 years since the introduction of cisplatin-based chemotherapy (Table 54.6), there has been a continuous improvement since the end of the 19th century. Table 54.7 lists current standard and experimental approaches.

Metastatic disease

During the last 15 years of development of curative chemotherapy for GCC as summarized in Table 54.8, there have been four

Table 54.6 Improved outcome from chemotherapy for metastatic germ cell cancer

	1978–	1986–
Number of cases	128	128
Undergoing RPLND	32%	30%
Actuarial survival at 10 years	75%	93%
Late relapse	4%	0.8%
Dead from GCC	23%	6%
Other causes	2%	0%

RPLND, retroperitoneal lymph node dissection.
Data from [4].

Table 54.7 Current practice and new trials for different stages of germ cell cancer

	Seminoma		Non-seminoma	
	Accepted	Trial	Accepted	Trial
Stage I	Radiation Carboplatin (×1)	PET/CT v MRI lymphogram	Surveillance RPLND	BEP v BEC (×1 course)
Stage II	Radiation	Carboplatin AUC 10	RPLND + BEP (×2) or BEP ×3	Laparoscopic lymph node biopsy
Stage III/IV	BEP (×3)	As non-seminoma	*Good risk*: BEP ×3 *Poor risk*: BEP ×4	BEP ×4 vs. cBOP/BEP

Table 54.8 Primary cisplatin-based chemotherapy regimen for metastatic grade 2/3 germ cell cancer

	Initial no. of cases			Subsequent series		
	Year	No. of cases	Progression free	Year	No. of cases	Progression free
BVP	1977	50	64%	1981	171	73%
VAB	1981	45	49%	1986	147	72%
POMB	1980	43	66%	1983	69	83%
BOP	1978	34	35%	1984	29	83%

Data from [8].

principal regimens used for metastatic patients, primarily in non-seminoma (for review see [8]). Though each has shown a learning curve (Table 54.8) large-scale clinical trials have now established a consensus that the combination of bleomycin, etoposide and cisplatin (BEP), developed by the substitution of etoposide instead of vinblastine in Einhorn's original bleomycin, vinblastine, and platinum (BVP) regimen [8, 37, 38], is the most effective and this is now the standard for all stages and histological subgroups. This is a 3–5 day treatment normally given as an inpatient for three or four courses every 21 days depending on the extent of the disease. Although total alopecia is universal and cumulative lethargy and anemia result in the patient being unable to work during the 3 months of treatment, there are only rarely serious infectious episodes and recovery is rapid. Return to work by 4–5 months and return of fertility by 18–24 months is the norm. Complete remission is not achieved after four courses in about 30–35% of patients and these proceed to surgical staging with excision of as much disease as possible. These operations can be quite extensive and in a small minority necessitate grafting of the aorta and nephrectomy. This may seem excessive when 75% of the operations fail to demonstrate viable malignancy. However, two-thirds of the negative specimens contain mature teratoma and this can, after 5–10 years, revert to non-germ cell malignancy, which fails to respond to germ cell-type treatment.

Salvage therapy and dose intensification for poor-risk patients

GCC, as well as having the highest primary cure of metastatic disease, has a wide range of options for second and-third-line therapy. As well as two second-line regimens, which cure 30–40% of relapses (one based on incorporating ifosfamide with cisplatin and etoposide and the other giving bleomycin, vincristine and cisplatin weekly to counteract the fast-growing clones), a further 15–20% are cured by high-dose chemotherapy given with a stem cell transplant as third-line treatment (for review see [39]). Currently, debate continues as to whether the high-dose procedure, which in all initial series has been associated with a treatment-related mortality, is now safe enough to be used at an early stage in patients with a high prediction of poor response. Considerable effort has been invested to establish criteria for dividing patients into good-, intermediate- and poor-risk patients although with more than 45% cured in the poor-risk groups, employment of treatments that have a treatment-related mortality, high risk of loss of fertility and other systematic effects it is as yet not seen to offer a major advantage over early intervention in poor-risk patients if they do not show clearcut evidence of early response. This is particularly so given the encouraging results seen with new drugs and schedules developed for salvage regimens.

Risking less treatment for good-risk patients

Today more than 60% of patients have good-risk characteristics with in excess of 90% cure. This includes metastatic seminoma and patients with stage II/III disease as well as small to moderate volume of lung metastases but not liver, brain or bone. Risking less treatment in such patients is even more difficult than dose intensifying. There have been three attempts, which are summarized in Table 54.9, the first trying to eliminate the need for bleomycin, which in the early days caused a rare (1%) but lethal lung toxicity. These trials gave conflicting results (for review see [8]) although with significantly worse relapse-free survival in three of the four trials, dosage reduction rather than elimination has become the approach today.

Carboplatin, an analog of cisplatin with less nephro- and neurotoxicity, first licensed in 1984 for ovarian cancer, can be given on an outpatient basis. It is still not known if there is a safe dose for GCC. Two large trials and one smaller one have all observed just under 10% less cure (for review see Table 54.8). However, there is evidence that much higher doses can safely be used in older ladies with ovarian cancer [40] and even higher doses can be used in combination with stem cell support as curative third-line therapy. Given that the initial carboplatin dose–response phase I/II study showed a very steep dose–response curve (Table 54.10), it is possible that the previous studies have underdosed and it is likely that there may be a safer dose that can be given. The critical issue is

Table 54.9 Overview of trials in good-risk patients

	No. of trials	No. of cases	Progression free
Platinum combination			
+ Bleomycin	4	434	86%
– Bleomycin	4	425	77%
Combination +			
Cisplatin	3	256	91%
Carboplatin	3	240	79%
No. of courses:			
BEP × 4	2	96 + 395	92% + 89%
BEP × 3	2	88 + 397	92% + 91%

Data from [8].

Table 54.10 Relapse and area under curve (AUC) optimization of carboplatin dose for germ cell cancer

AUC	No. of cases	Relapse rate (%)
<4	8	50
4–4.5	20	10
4.6–5.0	73	4
>5.0	20	0

Data from [41].

whether the small but real gains in terms of less hospitalization, deafness, hypertension and peripheral neuropathy will provide enough stimulus to encourage investment in the large-scale trials necessary now that the drug is nearly out of patent and the drug companies are no longer interested in sponsoring new trials even with new cisplatin analogs.

The third study to reduce treatment in good-risk patients compared three with four courses of chemotherapy, and this seems to demonstrate that three courses can be safely used.

Early-stage tumors

Stage I seminoma

For more than 50 years radiation has been favored as the standard of care for stage I seminoma because of the high radiocurability and technical problems of surgical node dissection. The emergence in the last 10 year of reports that 20% of these young patients may develop second tumors by 20 years [46] (Table 54.11) has led to a re-examination of this issue initially by reducing radiation volume and dose though the occurrence of late relapse and atypical sites of metastasis [42] has raised doubts about this strategy. The success of chemotherapy compared to radiation in bulky metastatic seminoma, which has proven chemocurable even with single agent cisplatin [43], has led to trials using first two, then a single course of carboplatin as an adjuvant. In a randomized trial involving 1477 patients comparing one course of carboplatin and radiation, a similar relapse rate of 3% was achieved [22]. In addition, in the short term carboplatin produced less acute toxicity. However, more unexpectedly there was a 72% reduction of 5-year risk of

Table 54.11 Mortality of seminoma patients after radiotherapy

	No. of cases	15-year survey O/E	30-year survey O/E
London Hospital (1951–1990) [45]	136	82%/92%	48%/70%
MD Anderson (1951–1999) [46]	453	87%/95%	39%/57%
SMR all cases	<15 vs. >15	1.3	1.85
SMR cardiac	<15 vs. >15	1.2	1.85
SMR cancer	<15 vs. >15	1.75	2.02

O/E, observed–estimated ratio; SMR, standardized mortality ratio.

second tumors in the contralateral testis. Clearly, 5 years is inadequate follow-up to be sure that there are no late toxicities, though with 415 followed for 5 and 82 followed for 10 years and no relapse after 30 months [44], these results are better than are available for the newer radiation schedules.

Stage I non-seminoma (for review see [35])

The toxicity of BVP cisplatin-based combination treatment was initially so bad that it was not thought safe to use it as adjuvant treatment for early-stage disease and it very early on became evident that relapse following radiation increased risk of toxic death from this BVP treatment. As a result, centers using radiation rather than surgery for early-stage non-seminoma rapidly learnt to use tumor marker and computerized tomography (CT) radiological surveillance for these patients [36] and detected most of the 35% of patients who relapsed at a very early stage so that overall survival was identical to those who had retroperitoneal lymph node surgery and suffered a long known but little discussed complication of surgery, i.e., loss of ejaculation. However, the surgeons did provide important information of the inaccuracy rate of the first-generation CT scans with 40% of negative scans proving to have histologically positive nodes and, more significantly, 25% of early radiological stage II cases found to have false-positive scans. They also demonstrated that two courses of adjuvant treatment would eliminate a 50% risk of relapse of those patients found to be pathological stage II and so ushered in the era of adjuvant chemotherapy without surgery for stage I patients with a high risk of relapse which produced similar over-all survival.

The surgeons meanwhile went on to improve their technique and identify the nerves responsible for ejaculation and performed nerve-sparing operations that enabled preservation of ejaculation in most but not all patients. Some also began to use laparoscopy and Da Vinci robot to diminish morbidity of surgery, and continued to prove the inaccuracy (Table 54.12) of even second- and third-generation CT scans. Medical oncologists, increasingly aware of this inaccuracy, learnt to defer treatment in such stage II patients as they had done for stage I patients until it was clear from either rising tumor markers or enlarging nodes on follow-up scans that the patient had active disease. In addition they demonstrated in pilot studies that adjuvant studies in high-risk patients with

Table 54.12 Open versus laparoscopic RPLND for clinical stage I and II non-seminoma

	Pathological stage I (%)	Pathological stage II (%)
Open RPLND		
Clinical stage I (n = 308)	71	29
Clinical stage II	37	67
Laparoscopic RPLND		
Clinical stage I	77.8	22.2
Clinical stage II	36	64

Data from [45, 46].

one course of BEP produced as good survival as two courses and in a randomized trial showed that one course of BEP as adjuvant produced a lower relapse rate than retroperitoneal lymph node dissection (RPLND).

Future trials

Today, with the increasing safety net of new drugs and new schedules for salvaging patients who fail first-line chemotherapy, confidence is growing for risking less treatment in this group of highly curable cancers. In addition, patients, because of increasing awareness of the curability, are being diagnosed earlier with smaller tumors and less advanced metastases. As a result increasing numbers are being treated with surveillance, encouraged by newer modalities for staging early-stage cases such as PET scan and ferromagnetic MRI lymphoscintigraphy. With laparoscopic RPLND and sentinel lymph node sampling [47] offering lower morbidity techniques for validating the accuracy of the newer staging techniques, it is possible that even for early-stage II seminomas, surgical lymph node staging may become more common.

The demonstration in patients who had such extensive disease that they were unfit for orchidectomy that chemotherapy can cure primary tumors as well as metastases has led to increasing interest in using chemotherapy as treatment for primary tumors. Taken with the results from a pilot study of using chemotherapy to preserve the primary testis in 28 patients with tumors in a solitary testis [48] which achieved 75% successful testis preservation and recovery of fertility using chemotherapy ± lumpectomy and the recent finding of a 72% reduction of second tumors after one course of carboplatin [22], this has raised the possibility that in the long term testis preservation could be as safe as breast preservation.

Conclusion

The exquisite chemosensitivity of GCC is demonstrated by the fact that even in the third-line setting there are drugs that can cure one in five patients, while in the earliest stage of the disease, that is stage I seminoma, most of a 25% risk of relapse has been eliminated by a single dose of carboplatin. Today overall more than 95% of patients presenting with a testicular GCC can expect to be cured by orchidectomy, combined with BEP for patients with metastases. It is clear that the last 25 years have seen a revolution in treatment of this tumor, although with the demonstration that testis-conserving chemotherapy is possible and the development of less toxic drugs for use as an outpatient, there will remain important clinical studies that will stimulate interest in this tumor for a long time to come.

The advances of the last decade in molecular biology have also transformed our understanding of the genetics of development of testicular GCC, with increasing support for the view that clonal evolution from carcinoma *in situ* through seminoma and combined seminoma/non-seminoma to pure non-seminoma is a realistic possibility to explain the myriad cell types found in this group of tumors.

It is, however, the epidemiology and specifically understanding the role in tumor development of gonadotropin and sex hormone-driven proliferation of germ cells under the circumstances of chemical, viral and traumatic atrophic damage that is of increasing interest to the endocrinologist. In addition to the need for finding approaches to deal with the increased incidence of metabolic syndrome problems found in these patients, even those treated by orchidectomy alone, at the therapeutic level the possibility of using short-term endocrine treatment for the premalignant changes is another area with potential for interesting collaboration between oncologists and endocrinologists in the next decade.

References

1. Ferguson R. Quantitative behaviour of prolan A in teratoma testis. *Am. J. Cancer* 1933;18:269–295.

2. Shakkbaek N. Possible carcinoma-in-situ of the testis. *Lancet* 1972;2: 516–517.

3. Jacobsen GK, Henriksen OB, von der Maase H. Carcinoma in-situ of testicular tissue adjacent to malignant germ cell tumours. A study of 105 cases. *Cancer (Philadelphia)* 1981;47:2260–2262.

4. Ravi R, Oliver RT, Ong J, et al. A single-centre observational study of surgery and late malignant events after chemotherapy for germ cell cancer. *Br. J. Urol* 1997;80:647–652.

5. van Leeuwen FE, Stiggelbout AM, Vandenbeltdusebout AW, et al. Second tumours after radiation treatment of testicular germ cell tumors. *J. Clin. Oncol.* 1993;11:2286–2287.

6. Boshoff CB, Begent RHJ, Oliver RTD, et al. Secondary tumours following etoposide containing therapy for germ cell cancer. *Ann. Oncol.* 1995;6:35–40.

7. Nuver J, Smit AJ, Wolffenbuttel BH et al. The metabolic syndrome and disturbances in hormone levels in long-term survivors of disseminated testicular cancer. *J. Clin. Oncol.* 2005;23:3718–3725.

8. Shelley M, Oliver RTD, Mason M. Testicular germ cell cancer. *Evidence-based Oncology* 2003;34:365–373.

9. Oliver R. Epidemiology of testis cancer. In Vogelzang N, Shipley W, Scardino P, Debruyne F (eds). *Comprehensive Textbook of Genitourinary Oncology*, 3rd edn. Philadephia: Lippincott Williams & Wilkins, 2005: 547–558.

10. Carlsen E, Giwercman A, Keiding N, Skakkebaek NE. Evidence for decreasing quality of semen during the past 50 years. *Br. Med. J.* 1992;305:609–612.

11. Oliver RTD. Atrophy, hormones, genes and viruses in aetiology of germ cell tumours. *Cancer Surveys* 1990;9:263–268.

12. Oliver RTD, Leahy M, Ong J. Combined seminoma/non-seminoma should be considered as intermediate grade germ cell cancer (GCC). *Eur. J. Cancer* 1995;31A:1392–1394.

13. Destefano F, Annest JL, Kresnow M. Semen characteristics of Vietnam veterans. *Reprod. Toxicol.* 1989;3:165–173.

14. Tarone RE, Hayes HM, Hoover RN, Rosenthal JF. Service in Vietnam and risk of testicular cancer. *J. Natl Cancer Inst.* 1990;83:1497–1499.

15. Bekesi J, Roboz J, Solomon S, Fischbein A, Selikoff I. Altered immune function in Michigan residents exposed to polybrominated biphenyls. *Immunotoxicology* 1983;1:181–191.

16. Westin JB, Richter E. The Israeli Breast Cancer anomaly. *Ann. N. Y. Acad. Sci.* 1990;609:269–279.

17. Davies TW, Palmer CR, Ruja E, Lipscombe JM. Adolescent milk, dairy product and fruit consumption and testicular cancer. *Br. J. Cancer* 1996;74:657–660.

18. Chilvers CEO, Forman D, Oliver RTD, et al. Social, behavioural and medical factors in the aetiology of testicular cancer – results from the UK study. *Br. J. Cancer* 1994;70:513–520.

19. Forman D, Chilvers C, Oliver R, Pike M. The aetiology of testicular cancer: association with congenital abnormalities, age at puberty, infertility and exercise. *Br. Med. J.* 1994;308:1393–1399.

20. Beard CM, Benson RC, Kelalis PP. The incidence and outcome of mumps orchitis in Rochester, Minnesota 1935–1974. *Mayo Clin. Proc.* 1977;52:3–7.

21. Mieusset R, Bujan L. The potential of mild testicular heating as a safe, effective and reversible contraceptive method for men. *Int. J. Androl.* 1994;17:186–191.

22. Oliver RTD, Mason MD, Mead GM, et al. Radiotherapy versus singe-dose carboplatin in adjuvant treatment of stage 1 seminoma: a randomised trial. *Lancet* 2005;366:293–300.

23. Hoff Wanderas E, Fossa SD, Heilo A, Stenwig AE, Norman N. Serum follicle stimulating hormone – predictor of cancer in the remaining testis in patients with unilateral testicular cancer. *Br. J. Urol.* 1990;66:315–317.

24. Oliver RTD, Joseph JV, Gallagher CJ. Castration-induced lymphocytosis in prostate cancer: possible evidence for gonad/thymus endocrine interaction in man. *Urol. Int.* 1995;54:226–229.

25. Sperandio P, Tomio P, Oliver RTD, Fiorentino MV, Pagano F. Gonadal atrophy as a cause of thymic hyperplasia after chemotherapy. *Br. J. Cancer* 1996;74:991–992.

26. Shaw G, Wilson P, Cuzick J, Prowse D, Oliver RTD. International study into the use of intermittent therapy in the treatment of carcinoma of the prostate (ISICAP), a meta-analysis of 1446 patients. *BJU Int.* 2006;99:1056–1065.

27. Vogelstein B, Fearon ER, Hamilton SR, et al. Genetic alterations during colorectal-tumor development. *N. Engl. J. Med.* 1988;319: 527–532.

28. Giwercman A, von der Maase H, Skakkebaek NE. Epidemiological and clinical aspects of carcinoma in situ of the testis. *Eur. Urol.* 1993;23:104–114.

29. Berney D, Lee A, Randle SJ, Jordan S, Shamash J, Oliver RTD. The frequency of intratubular embryonal carcinoma: implications for the pathogenesis of germ cell tumours. *Histopathology* 2004;45:155–161.

30. Oliver RTD, Nouri AME, Crosby D, et al. Biological significance of Beta hCG, HLA and other membrane antigen expression on bladder tumours and their relationship to tumour infiltrating lymphocytes (TIL). *J. Immunogenetics* 1989;16:381–390.

31. Murty V, Bosi G, Houldsworth J, et al. Allelic loss and somatic differentiation in human male germ cell tumours. *Oncogene* 1994;9:2245–2251.

32. Powles T, Bower M, Daugaard G, et al. Multicenter study of human immunodeficiency virus-related germ cell tumors. *J. Clin. Oncol.* 2003;21:1922–1927.

33. Sharpe R. Reproductive biology – another ddt connection. *Nature* 1995;375:538–539.

34. Sutcliffe A, Spoudeas H, Devaki N, et al. Comparison of serum FSH and Inhibin B levels berween adult male dizygotic and monozygotic twins. *Hum. Reprod.* 2006;21:447–450.

35. Oliver RTD. Emerging controversies in the management of stage 1 germ cell cancers. *Br. J. Urol. Int.* 2003;92:1–5.

36. Freedman LS, Parkinson MC, Jones WG, et al. Histopathology in the prediction of relapse of patients with stage 1 testicular teratoma treated by orchidectomy alone. On behalf of MRC Testicular Tumour Subgroup (Urological Working Party). *Lancet* 1987;ii:294–298.

37. Einhorn LH, Donohue JP. Cis-diaminodichloroplatinum, vinblastine, and bleomycin combination chemotherapy in disseminated testicular cancer. *Ann. Intern. Med.* 1977;87:293–298.

38. Peckham MJ, Barrett A, Liew KH, et al. The treatment of metastatic germ-cell testicular tumours with bleomycin, etoposide and cisplatin (BEP). *Br. J. Cancer* 1983;47:613–619.

39. Oliver R. High-dose chemotherapy in germ cell cancer salvage regimens: where next? *Nature Clin. Pract. Urol.* 2005;2:590–591.

40. Jodrell DI, Egorin MJ, Canetta RM. Relationships between carboplatin exposure and tumour response and toxicity in patients with ovarian cancer. *J. Clin. Oncol.* 1992;10:520–528.

41. Childs WJ, Nicholls EJ, Horwich A. The optimisation of carboplatin dose in carboplatin, etoposide and bleomycin combination chemotherapy for good prognosis metastatic non-seminomatous germ cell tumours of the testis. *Ann. Oncol.* 1992;3:291–296.

42. Oliver RTD. One-dose carboplatin in seminoma. *Lancet* 2005;366:1526.

43. Oliver RTD, Lore S, Ong J, et al. Alternatives to radiotherapy in management of seminoma. *Br. J. Urol.* 1990;65:61–67.

44. Oliver T, Mead G, Mason M, et al. The sword of Damocles and the treatment of stage I seminoma. *J. Clin. Oncol.* 2006;24:2599–600.

45. Steiner H, Peschel R, Janetschek G, et al. Long-term results of laparoscopic retroperitoneal lymph node dissection: a single-center 10-year experience. *Urology* 2004;63:550–555.

46. Stephenson AJ, Bosl GJ, Motzer RJ, et al. Retroperitoneal lymph node dissection for nonseminomatous germ cell testicular cancer: impact of patient selection factors on outcome. *J. Clin. Oncol.* 2005;23:2781–2788.

47. Satoh M, Ito A, Kaiho Y, et al. Introperative, radio-guided sentinel lymph node mapping in laparoscopic lymph node dissection for stage I testicular carcinoma. *Cancer* 2005;103:2067–2072.

48. Oliver RTD, Ong J, Berney D, Nargund V, Badenoch D, Shamash J. Testis conserving chemotherapy in germ cell cancer: its potential to increase understanding of the biology and treatment of carcinoma-in-situ. *APMIS* 2003;111:86–92.

55 Neoplasia and Intersex States

Sabine E. Hannema and Ieuan A. Hughes

> **Key points**
> - "Intersex" has now been renamed as "disorders of sex development".
> - Germ cell tumors are the most common tumors in disorders of sex development.
> - Tumor risk is higher in gonadal dysgenesis and low in complete androgen insensitivity syndrome.
> - Useful tumor markers include OCT 3/4 and AP2γ.
> - Gonads left *in situ* require long-term monitoring.

Introduction

Disorders of sex development have been known to exist for hundreds of years, but only recently have the underlying molecular genetic causes been identified. The terms that were originally used to describe these disorders, such as hermaphrodite and sex reversal, are now deemed confusing and patient unfriendly. Therefore, new terminology has been proposed; "disorders of sex development" (DSD) is now used to describe congenital conditions in which development of chromosomal, gonadal, or anatomical sex is atypical (Table 55.1). This can be subdivided into sex chromosome DSD, such as Turner and Klinefelter syndrome; 46,XY DSD, comprising disorders of testicular development, disorders of androgen synthesis and disorders of action; 46,XX DSD, including disorders of ovarian development and androgen excess [1].

The risk of gonadal tumors is increased, but not to the same extent, in all types of DSD. One of the challenges for clinicians who work with individuals with DSD is to estimate this risk and advise on appropriate management. Should gonadectomy be performed, and at what age? If not, how should patients be followed up to identify (pre)malignant lesions as early as possible? Research into the pathogenesis of germ cells tumors, their occurrence in DSD, and methods to detect premalignant changes through gonadal biopsy has provided evidence that can guide clinical practice.

Normal sex determination

The gonads are formed during the fifth week of gestation in humans, and between E10 and E11.5 in mice, in a region of the

Table 55.1 Classification of disorders of sex development (DSD)

1. Sex chromosome DSD	a. 45,X (Turner syndrome and variants)
	b. 47,XXY (Klinefelter syndrome and variants)
	c. 45,XO/46,XY (Mixed gonadal dysgenesis)
	d. 46,XX/46,XY (Ovotesticular DSD)
2. 46, XY DSD	a. Disorders of gonadal development
	i. Complete gonadal dysgenesis (Swyer syndrome)
	ii. Partial gonadal dysgenesis
	iii. Gonadal regression
	iv. Ovotesticular DSD
	b. Disorders in androgen synthesis or action
	i. LH receptor defects (e.g., Leydig cell hypoplasia, aplasia)
	ii. Androgen biosynthesis defect (e.g., 17βHSD deficiency)
	iii. Defect in androgen action (e.g., CAIS and PAIS)
	c. Other
	i. Disorders of AMH and AMH receptor (persistent Mullerian duct syndrome)
	ii. e.g., Severe hypospadias, cloacal exstrophy
3. 46, XX DSD	a. Disorders of gonadal development
	i. Gonadal dysgenesis
	ii. Ovotesticular DSD
	iii. Testicular DSD (e.g., SRY+, duplication SOX9)
	b. Androgen excess
	i. Fetal (e.g., 21-hydroxylase deficiency)
	ii. Fetoplacental (aromatase deficiency, POR)
	iii. Maternal (e.g., luteoma, exogenous)
	c. Other
	i. e.g., cloacal exstrophy, vaginal atresia, MURCS

LH, luteinizing hormone; 17βHSD, 17β-hydroxysteroid dehydrogenase; AMH, anti-Mullerian hormone; POR, cytochrome P450 oxidoreductase; MURCS, Mullerian, renal, cervicothoracic somite abnormalities.

Clinical Endocrine Oncology, 2nd edition. Edited by Ian D. Hay and John A.H. Wass. © 2008 Blackwell Publishing. ISBN 978-1-4051-4584-8.

intermediate mesoderm known as the urogenital ridge. This region consists of the pronephros, which includes the adrenal primordium, the mesonephros, from which the gonad arises, and the metanephros, from which the definitive kidney forms. Proliferation of the celomic epithelium and the underlying mesenchyme results in formation of the gonad primordium. The epithelium grows into the mesenchyme to form the primary sex cords (Fig. 55.1). Primordial germ cells migrate from the yolk sac through the gut mesentery and colonize the gonad between E10 and E11.5 in mice [2]. There are three different founding cell populations that have the capacity to differentiate into either testicular or ovarian cell types. The supporting cell precursors can develop into Sertoli cells in the testis, or granulosa cells in the ovary, whereas a common steroidogenic precursor cell lineage may give rise to Leydig cells in the testis and theca cells in the ovary. The connective cell lineage differentiates into peritubular myoid cells in the XY gonad and stromal cells in the XX gonad.

In the female fetus, germ cells form nests and enter meiosis but arrest at diplotene of the first meiotic division. The primary or medullary sex cords degenerate and secondary or cortical sex cords develop. They surround the germ cell nests forming primordial follicles (Fig. 55.1).

In the male fetus, germ cells are sequestered inside the primary sex cords forming testis cords. They enter mitotic arrest in mice for approximately 1 week and resume mitosis after birth. When germ cells are located outside the testis, they enter meiotic arrest, similar to germ cells in the ovary, suggesting a testicular factor is needed to prevent a programmed arrest in meiosis [3]. Germ cells

are not required for testis formation but are essential for formation of ovarian follicles [3].

The seminiferous cords develop into the seminiferous tubules, tubuli recti and rete testis. Once the tunica albuginea forms as the fibrous capsule of the testis, they lose their connection with the surface epithelium. Leydig cells differentiate from the mesenchyme in between the seminiferous tubules at around 8–9 weeks' gestation in humans and start producing testosterone. Sertoli cells produce anti-Mullerian hormone (AMH) slightly earlier.

Early development of the indifferent gonad is regulated by a number of genes (Figs 55.2 and 55.3). Wilms' tumor 1 (*WT1*) encodes a variety of protein products with different functions. Homozygous deletion of the *WT1* gene in mice results in failure of kidney and gonad development, and the mice die *in utero* [4]. In addition, heterozygous deletions cause genitourinary

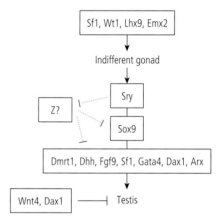

Figure 55.2 Genes involved in regulation of gonadal development. Diagram showing some of the genes thought to be important for early development of the indifferent gonad, and for subsequent differentiation into a testis. Wnt4 and Dax1 may act as antitestis factors.

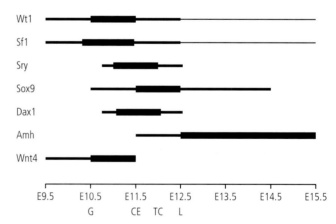

Figure 55.3 Temporal pattern of gene expression in the mouse gonad. Shown are expression patterns of several genes involved in testis development. The thickness of the line corresponds to expression levels. Underneath the time scale is indicated when the indifferent gonad is first distinguishable (G), when proliferation of the celomic epithelium increases in the XY gonad (CE), when Sertoli cells differentiate and testicular cords form (TC) and when Leydig cells differentiate (L). (Adapted from figures by Swain and Lovell-Badge [5] and Veitia et al. [6].)

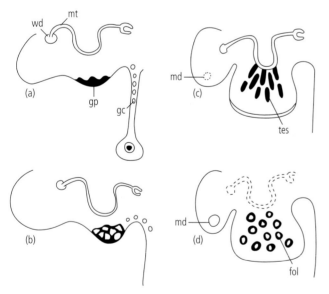

Figure 55.1 Gonadal development. (a) Schematic drawing of the gonad at 4 weeks' gestation. The celomic epithelium and underlying mesenchyme proliferate and form the gonad primordium (gp). (b) Indifferent gonad at 5 weeks' gestation. Primary sex cords form and germ cells (gc) colonize the gonad. (c) Testis. Testis cords (tes) have developed; the Mullerian duct (md) regresses. (d) Ovary. Primordial follicles (fol) have developed; the Wolffian duct (wd) regresses. mt, mesonephric tubule.

abnormalities and an increased risk of kidney tumors in humans [5]. Heterozygous missense mutations result in Denys–Drash syndrome and a donor splice mutation causes Frasier syndrome, both associated with 46,XY DSD [5]. Lhx9 and Emx2 are two transcription factors required for the formation of indifferent gonads in mice [3, 6–8]. Both WT1 and Lhx9 are thought to regulate expression of steroidogenic factor 1 (*SF1*), an orphan nuclear receptor [9]. *Sf1* is expressed in several endocrine organs, such as the adrenals, pituitary and hypothalamus [5]. In embryos lacking *Sf1*, the adrenals do not form and between E10.5–12 the gonads cease to develop and start to degenerate [10]. In humans, *SF1* mutations have been associated with 46,XY DSD, with or without primary adrenal failure [11–14]. *Sf1* may also have a later role, in male specific gonadal development [3]. After *Sry* (sex determining region of the Y) expression starts (see below), *Sf1* levels are higher in the testis than in the ovary [5].

Once the bipotential gonad has formed, the process of sex determination begins. The genetic sex of the embryo is established at fertilization with the inheritance of an X or Y chromosome from the father. Only one gene on the Y chromosome, *SRY*, is required to initiate differentiation of the gonad into a testis. Expression of *Sry* is sufficient to induce male development of XX mice [15] and mutations of the *Sry* gene can result in female development in XY mice and humans [5]. SRY acts within the supporting cell lineage to direct their fate to that of Sertoli cells [16]. These cells probably induce differentiation of the rest of the testis through cell–cell interaction and/or secreted products [2, 5]. Wnt4 is also required for early testis development and Sertoli cell differentiation; it is believed to act downstream of *Sry* but upstream of Sertoli cell markers *Sox9* (SRY-related HMG box9) and *Dhh* (Desert hedgehog) [17].

SRY contains a high mobility group (HMG) box type of DNA-binding domain (DBD), which is essential to its function. Such domains bind and bend DNA, so it is likely that SRY functions by changing chromatin configuration. Another gene involved in controlling chromatin organization and associated with gonadal development is *ATRX* [2]. *ATRX* mutations cause testicular dysgenesis in humans [2]. *DAX1* (dose sensitive sex reversal-congenital adrenal hypoplasia critical region on the X 1) encodes a nuclear receptor. Despite its initial characterization as an anti-testis gene, it is now thought to be an early mediator of testicular development, downstream of *SRY* [2]. Disruption of *Dax1* causes 46,XY DSD on certain genetic backgrounds. How *Dax1* is involved in both protestis and antitestis pathways is not clear. Its role may differ according to cell types and stages in gonadal development or alternatively, its specific effect may be dosage dependent [2].

The *SRY*-related gene *SOX9* also acts downstream of SRY. Heterozygous *SOX9* mutations can cause 46,XY DSD, as well as bone pathology (campomelic dysplasia) in humans. Haploinsufficiency probably causes this phenotype and protein levels need to exceed a threshold to be effective [5]. Duplication of a genomic region containing *SOX9* was reported in a case of 46,XX testicular DSD, suggesting that *SOX9* expression is sufficient to induce testis differentiation [18]. Similarly, disruption and constitutive expression of *Sox9* in mice lead to 46,XY gonadal dysgenesis and 46, XX testicular DSD, respectively [19, 20]. *Sox9* expression patterns are more conserved across vertebrates than *Sry* expression, indicating that it may be a common gene downstream of different sex-determining mechanisms [5, 6].

Dmrt1 encodes a zinc finger-like DNA-binding protein. It is initially expressed in gonads of both sexes, but becomes male-specific by E13.5–E14.5 in mice [3]. *DMRT1* is also expressed in the XY gonad at the time of testis determination in humans [6]. Disruption of this gene results in hypoplastic testes with disorganized seminiferous tubules that lack germ cells in mice [7]. In humans, partial deletion of 9p, the chromosomal region where *DMRT1* is located, causes dysmorphic features and 46,XY DSD [6].

Differentiation and proliferation of Leydig cells seem to require *Dhh*, as well as the gene aristaless-related homeobox *ARX* [2]. *Dhh* is expressed in a male-specific manner by Sertoli cells, whereas one of the hedgehog receptors, patched 1, is expressed by interstitial cells [2]. Mice lacking *Dhh* have small testes with depressed spermatogenesis, resulting in infertility [7]. They show abnormalities of the peritubular tissue, arrested Leydig cell maturation and, as a consequence, cryptorchidism and undermasculinized external genitalia [21]. Mutations in *DHH* are associated with 46,XY complete gonadal dysgenesis in humans [22]. ARX is expressed in interstitial cells other than Leydig cells and may act as a paracrine factor [2]. Mutations of this gene cause X-linked lissencephaly with abnormal genitalia in humans [23].

Wnt4 appears to antagonize the testis pathway. It is initially expressed in the genital ridge and mesonephros, but is subsequently downregulated in the testis (after E11.5), whereas expression is maintained in the ovary [24]. Studies of *Wnt* knockout mice indicate that *Wnt4* may be important for suppression of steroid synthesis in the ovary, as well as for post-meiotic maintenance of oocytes [24]. Duplication of a part of 1p that contains *WNT4* has been found in a case of 46,XY DSD [25]. Wnt4 induces *Dax1* expression *in vitro*, and *Wnt4* knockout mice show reduced *Dax1* expression in gonads, suggesting increased *DAX1* expression may be the cause of 46,XY DSD in this patient [25]. The expression pattern of *Dax1* in the gonad is similar to that of *Wnt4*. After initial expression in both the male and female gonad from E11.5, it is downregulated in the testis but not in the ovary by E12.5 [5, 6]. This timing is consistent with the notion that Sry could either downregulate *Wnt4* or interfere with the Wnt signaling cascade to prevent *Dax1* expression [25]. *Dax1* may also be able to act as an antitestis factor; overexpression causes 46,XY gonadal dysgenesis in mice with weak alleles of *Sry* [26], and duplication of the part of the X-chromosome that contains *DAX1* has the same effect in humans [27]. It has been proposed that *Dax1* may compete with *Sry* to control target gene activation [26]. However, XX mice with *Dax1* deletions develop ovaries, suggesting *Dax1* is not the only repressor of testis-specific genes [28].

Once a testis has formed, masculinization of the fetus is dependent on normal androgen synthesis. Absence of normal luteinizing hormone (LH)/LH receptor interaction, or a mutation in one of the genes encoding enzymes necessary for the production of testosterone and dihydrotestosterone, such as 17β-hydroxysteroid dehydrogenase or 5α-reductase, can lead to abnormal phenotypic sex. Normal tissue responsiveness to androgens is another prerequisite for masculinization, and mutations in the X-linked androgen receptor gene can lead to genital ambiguity or a female phenotype.

Classification of gonadal tumors

Individuals with DSD are at increased risk of gonadal tumors. Germ cell tumors are the most common and most serious type of tumor. Of the five categories of germ cell tumors, type II is the most relevant to DSD [29]. Type II tumors originate from primordial germ cells or gonocytes. Initially, a premalignant lesion develops, known as intratubular germ cell neoplasia unclassified or carcinoma *in situ* (CIS). In the dysgenetic gonad a different premalignant lesion is more commonly found, known as a gonadoblastoma. This is a tumor composed of germ cells and immature Sertoli or granulosa-like cells, and sometimes Leydig or lutein-like cells. These premalignant lesions can progress to an invasive tumor: a seminoma or non-seminoma (in testes) or a dysgerminoma or non-seminoma (in ovaries and dysgenetic gonads).

Type I tumors, teratomas and yolk sac tumors, have also been described in individuals with DSD [30]. In addition to germ cell tumors a number of other, mostly benign tumors have been observed in DSD, such as granulosa cell tumors, Sertoli cell tumors and Leydig cell tumors [29, 31]. Sertoli cell nodules, which are regions of tightly packed hypoplastic seminiferous tubules lacking germ cells, are commonly found in gonads from individuals with 46,XY DSD and in cryptorchidism (Plate 55.1). It is unclear how they form, but it has been suggested they are the result of a malformative process of congenitally hypoplastic seminiferous tubules rather than a benign, neoplastic proliferation of Sertoli cells [32].

Clinical disorders in which gonadal tumors occur

An increased risk of germ cell tumors exists in many but not all types of DSD. The presence of Y chromosomal material seems to determine which groups are at risk. The existence of a locus on the Y chromosome that predisposes dysgenetic gonads to develop gonadoblastoma (gonadoblastoma locus on the Y chromosome or GBY) was postulated some time ago [33]. Subsequently this locus was mapped to a small region on the Y chromosome, containing seven known genes. One of these, testis-specific protein Y-encoded or *TSPY*, seems most likely to act as an oncogene in germ cells [34].

The precise risk of germ cell tumors in the different forms of DSD is not clear. In many studies, results are difficult to interpret because of imprecise diagnoses. Only reliance on a clinical diagnosis was possible until recently, with several disorders that result in a similar phenotype being grouped together. Further confusion was caused by using terms and synonyms to describe DSD variants

that lacked clarity in definitions. The diagnosis of CIS is difficult to establish in children with DSD. Gonadectomy in DSD is often performed before or just after puberty so that accurate incidence figures for germ cell tumors in all disorders are difficult to obtain. A recent review estimated the risk highest in Frasier syndrome (60%) and Denys–Drash syndrome with 46,XY karyotype (40%), although limited data were available and positive cases may be overrepresented due to selection bias [29] (Table 55.2). No data are available for patients with gonadal dysgenesis due to specific gene mutations, other than for *WT1*. Gonadal dysgenesis in general was associated with a risk of 12%, but this figure is based on a heterogeneous group which includes abnormalities of sex chromosomes as well as mutations in genes involved in early development of the indifferent gonad. In 46,XY gonadal dysgenesis the risk was estimated to be 30%, whereas mixed gonadal dysgenesis/asymmetrical gonadal differentiation had a lower risk of 15%. This figure may be an underestimation because of early gonadectomies. The risk for individuals with a 45,X/46,XY karyotype was 15–40%. Gonadoblastoma is the most frequently encountered lesion in this group, followed by dysgerminoma [29]. CIS is much less common and non-seminoma very rare. Interestingly, the risk of germ cell tumors is much lower in ovotesticular DSD (2.6%), a condition characterized by the presence of both testicular and ovarian tissue [29].

Germ cell tumors are less common in androgen insensitivity syndrome (approximately 5.5%) than in gonadal dysgenesis, but this figure is affected by the practice of early gonadectomies [29]. The risk is very low in children [35], but increases after puberty, reaching as high as 33% at 50 years [36]. Partial androgen insensitivity syndrome (PAIS) characterized by varying degrees of masculinization is associated with a higher risk of 15%; this compares with 0.8% in complete androgen insensitivity syndrome (CAIS). The difference may be explained by the decline in germ cell numbers being more rapid in CAIS [37]. It was hypothesized that the risk may be lower still in CAIS patients with AR gene mutations that completely abolish androgen action as compared to mutations associated with some residual androgen function. However, we did not observe such an association where CIS was found in a 17-year-old CAIS girl with a frameshift mutation in the AR gene [35]. No large studies of DSD due to androgen biosynthetic and LH receptor defects are available, so it is not possible to comment on the risk of malignancy in these specific disorders. One case of CIS was found in a series of six patients with 17β-hydroxysteroid dehydrogenase deficiency [37].

Individuals with 46,XX DSD caused by androgen excess (from an adrenal or exogenous origin) are not at increased risk of germ cell tumors. However, they may have testicular tumors due to adrenal rests (see "Other conditions").

Origin of tumors

It is thought that CIS might be the result of a developmental arrest of fetal germ cells. These may subsequently undergo malignant

Table 55.2 Risk of germ cell malignancies in forms of DSD and recommended action [28]

Risk (category)	Disorder	Risk (%)	Recommended action	No. studies	No. patients
High	GD[1] (+Y[2]) intra-ab	15–35	Gonadectomy[3]	12	>350
	PAIS non-scrotal	15	Gonadectomy[3]	3	80
	Frasier	60	Gonadectomy[3]	1	15
	Denys–Drash (+Y)	40	Gonadectomy[3]	1	5
Intermediate	Turner (+Y)	12	Gonadectomy[3]	11	43
	17β-HSD	28	Monitoring Possibly biopsy	2	7
Low	CAIS	0.8	Biopsy[4] Possibly irrad/ gonadectomy	3	120
	Ovotesticular DSD	3	Removal of testicular tissue if raised female	3	426
	Turner (−Y[5])	1	None	11	557
Unknown	5α-reductase def.	0	Unresolved	1	3
	Leydig cell hypoplasia	0	Unresolved	1	2
	GD (+Y[2]) scrotal	?	Biopsy[4], irrad?	0	0
	PAIS scrotal gonad	?	Biopsy[4], irrad?	0	0

Recommended actions are indicated, as well as the number of studies and patients included in the review [28]. In PAIS, 17β-HSD deficiency and ovotesticular DSD, the decision regarding gonadectomy is largely determined by sex of rearing. In low-risk groups such as CAIS, patients may opt for gonadectomy for psychological or cosmetic (inguinal testes) reasons.

GD, gonadal dysgenesis; intra-ab, intra-abdominal testes; PAIS, partial androgen insensitivity syndrome; non-scrotal, non-scrotal testes; 17β-HSD, 17β-hydroxysteroid dehydrogenase deficiency; CAIS, complete androgen insensitivity syndrome; 5α-reductase def., 5α-reductase deficiency; irrad, local irradiation with 18 Gy.

[1]Gonadal dysgenesis, including not further specified, 46XY, 46X/46XY, mixed, partial, complete.

[2]GBY positive, including the TSPY gene.

[3]At time of diagnosis.

[4]At puberty, allowing investigation of at least 30 seminiferous tubules.

[5]PCR detection of Y-chromosomal sequences (in particular the GBY region) is implicated if a marker is identified by karyotyping.

transformation. This hypothesis is based on the similarity of gonocytes and CIS cells with respect to morphology and expression of certain proteins [38, 39]. DSD, as well as cryptorchidism and Down syndrome, are associated with delayed differentiation of germ cells which may explain the increased risk of germ cells tumors in all these disorders.

Patients with insufficient androgen production or action almost exclusively have CIS as a precursor lesion, similar to normal males. However, in patients with gonadal dysgenesis, precursor lesions are mainly gonadoblastomas (92% versus 8% CIS) [29]. It has been suggested that gonadoblastomas arise in undifferentiated gonadal tissue or primitive sex cords, normally found in the early gonad before SRY expression. The undifferentiated cells persist, however, in the dysgenetic gonad. It is possible that gonadoblastomas are more common than CIS in dysgenetic gonads, because the development of gonadoblastomas takes place more rapidly than the formation of CIS [40]. Alternatively, immature germ cells may survive in undifferentiated gonadal tissue, more suited to their environment in the embryo than in normally differentiated seminiferous cords. Others hypothesize that germ cells in the dysgenetic gonad start to develop along the female pathway but are arrested at the stage of oocytic clusters when germ cells enter meiotic prophase. These clusters closely resemble an early form of gonadoblastoma (microfollicular pattern). Expansion of

proliferating germ cells within these nests leads to the formation of a more advanced form of gonadoblastoma (coronary pattern), which may progress to an invasive dysgerminoma [41]. Examples of the histology are shown in Plate 55.2.

Invasive germ cell tumors rarely occur before puberty in CAIS [31, 35]. Stimulation of germ cells to proliferate may occur as a result of the increase in hormone levels at puberty. FSH may play a role, as levels are normal or elevated in postpubertal patients with CAIS [31]. FSH can indirectly stimulate germ cell proliferation in mice, independent of the LH–testosterone axis [42]. Another possible source of stimulation is estrogens which are increased in CAIS compared with normal males [31]. Estrogens induce somatic cells of the mouse fetal gonadal ridge *in vitro* to produce c-Kit ligand, stimulating primordial germ cell growth [43]. If the somatic cells of the testis in CAIS are capable of a similar response to estrogens, then c-Kit ligand could activate the Kit receptor. This is expressed by germ cells that fail to differentiate normally and also by CIS cells [39]. Estrogens also directly increase proliferation of gonocytes purified from 3-day-old rats, although not in gonocytes from 2-day-old rats [44]. Another study using cultures of testes from day E14.5 rat fetuses showed negative effects of estrogens on gonocyte numbers [45]. Alternatively, the developmentally delayed germ cell may spontaneously acquire premalignant characteristics over time as a result of progressive genetic instability [39]. The latter explanation appears to be the case in gonadal dysgenesis, where germ cell tumors occur at a much earlier age [29, 46].

As noted already, the relation between abnormal germ cell development and germ cell tumors is not only present in DSD, but also thought to exist in normal males. In fact, testicular cancer is postulated to be part of a testicular dysgenesis syndrome which also includes abnormal spermatogenesis, cryptorchidism and hypospadias [47]. The incidence of each component appears to be increasing. It has been suggested that the testicular dysgenesis syndrome is the result of an adverse effect on the development of the fetal testis due to a combination of genetic factors and an imbalance in fetal androgen/estrogen dynamics caused by environmental endocrine disruptors [48].

Tumor markers

In addition to morphology, immunohistochemical analysis of several tumor markers is used to identify (pre)malignant germ cells such as placental-like alkaline phosphatase (PLAP) (Plate 55.3). Another commonly used marker is proto-oncogene c-*kit* product KIT, which is a membrane tyrosine kinase receptor for stem cell factor [48–51]. Two more tumor markers recently described are transcription factors activator protein-2gamma (AP2gamma) and OCT3/4 [52–55]. These markers are normally expressed by fetal germ cells, and small numbers of positive cells may be found in the first year of life [36, 50–52, 56–59] (Table 55.3). Thereafter, expression is limited to (pre)malignant germ cells. Testis-specific protein y-encoded (TSPY) is abundantly expressed in both immature and (pre)malignant germ cells, but is also present in spermatogonia in the normal adult testis [60].

Expression of tumor markers may be prolonged in DSD because of delayed development [34, 36, 39, 52, 59, 61]. It is therefore difficult to determine whether cells expressing these markers are developmentally delayed germ cells or (pre)malignant cells. In such cases it is useful to examine the distribution of positive cells throughout the testis, and the position of these cells in the seminiferous tubule [34, 36]. When testis development is delayed, positive cells are distributed evenly throughout the gonad and mostly located in the middle of the seminiferous tubules, whereas in CIS positive cells are found in clusters confined to a specific region of the gonad and mostly located on the basal membrane (Plate 55.4). Most developmentally delayed germ cells appear to differentiate or undergo apoptosis, but some may make contact with the basal lamina and then progress to (pre)malignancies [28, 34].

Some tumor markers may be essential for malignant potency of germ cells. OCT3/4 plays a role in maintaining pluripotency of embryonic stem cells [62]. It is expressed in primordial germ cells but is downregulated when oocytes enter the first meiotic prophase in female embryos and when gonocytes differentiate to infantile spermatogonia in male embryos [28, 59]. There is a strong correlation between high levels of OCT3/4 and the aggressive nature of malignancy in embryonic stem cell-derived tumors [63]. This may also hold true for other tumors. TSPY is believed to be involved in mitotic proliferation of spermatogonia and may therefore also be important for proliferation of (pre)malignant germ cells [33, 60].

The tumor markers can only be used to identify (pre)malignant changes in gonadal tissue obtained at biopsy or gonadectomy. Seminal fluid analysis for the presence of CIS cells would be a more convenient way of monitoring patients but this technique is currently not sufficiently sensitive [64]. Circulating serum tumor markers have yet to be identified.

Management

The options for management include leaving the gonads *in situ*, which has the advantage of no need for hormone replacement and potential fertility, versus gonadectomy, which avoids a risk of germ cell tumors and virilization at puberty in those raised as females. Appropriate monitoring is essential if gonads are left in place long term.

The following recommendations were proposed following an international consensus meeting on DSD [1] (Table 55.2). Gonadectomy at the time of diagnosis is recommended in high-risk groups, which include GBY-positive gonadal dysgenesis with intra-abdominal gonads, PAIS with non-scrotal testes, Frasier syndrome and Denys–Drash syndrome. In GBY-positive gonadal

Table 55.3 Expression of tumor markers during germ cell development, in (pre)malignancies of the testis and in the adult ovary

Protein	ES	PGC	Gono	Spgon	Spcyt	Sptid	CIS	GB	Sem	Nonsem	Ovary
PLAP	−	+	+	−	−	−	+	+	+	EC	−
AP2γ	?	?	+	−	−	−	+	+	+	EC	−
OCT3/4	+	+	+	−	−	−	+	+	+	EC	−
KIT	?	+	+/−	−	−	−	+	+	+/−	−	+
TSPY	?	?	+	+	−	−	+	+	+	−	−
VASA	?	+/−	+/−	+	+	+	+/−	+/−	+/−	−	+

ES, embryonic stem cells; PGC, primordial germ cells; Gono, gonocyte; Spgon, spermatogonia; Spcyt, spermatocytes; Sptid, spermatids; CIS, carcinoma *in situ*; GB, gonadoblastoma; Sem, seminoma; Nonsem, non-seminoma; EC, embryonal carcinoma.
(Based on [28,38].)

dysgenesis with scrotal testes and PAIS with scrotal testes, the tumor risk is thought to be intermediate; testicular biopsy is recommended at puberty. The sensitivity of a biopsy in detecting CIS is estimated to be 95% [65]. If CIS is found, irradiation may have a place in preventing progression to invasive tumors, as shown in normal adult males [65]. However, this management strategy needs to be evaluated in cases of DSD. Perhaps gonadal biopsy should also be recommended in 17β-HSD deficiency where the tumor risk is intermediate.

The risk of germ cell tumors seems low in CAIS, but these patients should be monitored by serial ultrasound and, if necessary, testicular biopsies. Ovotesticular DSD is another category of low tumor risk, but testicular tissue should be removed if patients are raised female. In Turner syndrome, the presence of a marker chromosome in the karyotype is associated with the presence of Y chromosomal material (including GBY), which in turn increases the risk of gonadoblastoma [28]. This is an indication to perform further molecular genetic analysis. Gonadectomy is recommended if GBY-positive, but no action is needed in its absence. Biopsy and gonadectomy specimens should be fixed appropriately to allow morphological and immunohistochemical analyses [34, 66].

The precise tumor risk is not known for all DSD categories, so that management strategy for some groups is not possible. Future studies should include associations between gonad histology and detailed molecular markers to assess gonadal dysgenesis sub-types and other conditions such as in LH and LH-receptor mutations and disorders of androgen biosynthesis.

Other conditions

Failure of complete testicular descent into the scrotum, cryptorchidism, is one of the most frequent congenital abnormalities and affects approximately 3% of male births [7]. The condition is associated with a 4–10-fold increased risk of germ cell tumors [67–70]. Similarities in tumor risk between cryptorchid testes and testes from patients with DSD suggests a commonality of ectopic gonad position causing abnormal testis development and increased tumor risk. However, there is evidence that androgen signaling is also abnormal in cryptorchidism [71]. Sertoli cells in nodules of hypoplastic or dysgenetic seminiferous tubules from cryptorchid testes show reduced or absent AR expression, whereas germ cell development and maintenance of spermatogenesis are found in areas with AR positive Sertoli cells. Consequently, it is not possible to distinguish between the effects of insufficient androgen action and abnormal testis location. The similarities between the dysgenetic, cryptorchid and androgen-insensitive gonad also suggest a possible common developmental defect [34]. Development of germ cells is slightly delayed in Down syndrome, with a moderate (0.5%) risk of germ cell tumors [28].

Patients with congenital adrenal hyperplasia do not have an increased risk of germ cell tumors. However, they may have adrenal rests that can present in males as testicular tumors (Plate 55.5).

Adrenal rests arise from aberrant adrenal cortical cells that have adhered to, and migrated with, the gonad during embryogenesis. Autopsy studies indicate their presence in association with 7.5% of testes in normal male infants less than 1 year old [72]. In congenital adrenal hyperplasia, the adrenal rests can become hyperplastic under the influence of adrenocorticotropic hormone and have been reported in 50–95% of affected males and are associated with a higher risk of infertility [73, 74]. The most common presenting feature is testicular enlargement, often bilaterally. The adrenal rest "tumors" appear hypoechogenic on ultrasound, are peripherally located and tend to be minimally disruptive to the surrounding testis tissue [75]. They generally occur when treatment is inadequate and they may atrophy when restoration of glucocorticoid treatment suppresses elevated ACTH levels. Alternatively, testis-sparing surgery can be performed to remove the adrenal rest; this resolves any pain and discomfort, but seldom improves testicular function [76]. It is recommended that ultrasound examination of the testes be undertaken from puberty onwards, together with regular self-examination of the scrotal contents.

References

1. Hughes IA, Houk C, Ahmed SF, Lee PA, LWPES/ESPE Consensus Group. Consensus statement on management of intersex disorders. *Arch. Dis. Child.* 2006;91:554–563.
2. Brennan J, Capel B. One tissue, two fates: molecular genetic events that underlie testis versus ovary development. *Nat. Rev. Genet.* 2004;5:509–21.
3. Capel B. The battle of the sexes. *Mech. Dev.* 2000;92:89–103.
4. Kreidberg JA, Sariola H, Loring JM, et al. WT-1 is required for early kidney development. *Cell* 1993;74:679–691.
5. Swain A, Lovell-Badge R. Mammalian sex determination: a molecular drama. *Genes Dev.* 1999;13:755–767.
6. Veitia RA, Salas-Cortés L, Ottolenghi C, Pailhoux E, Cotinot C, Fellous M. Testis determination in mammals: more questions than answers. *Mol. Cell. Endocrinol.* 2001;179:3–3016.
7. Nef S, Parada LF. Hormones in male sexual development. *Genes Dev.* 2000; 14:3075–86.
8. Miyamoto N, Yoshida M, Kuratani S, Matsuo I, Aizawa S. Defects of urogenital development in mice lacking *Emx2. Development* 1997;124:1653–1664.
9. Wilhelm D, Englert C. The Wilms tumor suppressor WT1 regulates early gonad development by activation of *Sf1. Genes Dev.* 2002;16: 1839–1851.
10. Luo X, Ikeda Y, Parker KL. A cell-specific nuclear receptor is essential for adrenal and gonadal development and sexual differentiation. *Cell* 1994;77:481–490.
11. Achermann JC, Ito M, Ito M, Hindmarsh PC, Jameson JL. A mutation in the gene encoding steroidogenic factor-1 causes XY sex reversal and adrenal failure in humans. *Nat. Genet.* 1999;22:125–126.
12. Achermann JC, Ozisik G, Ito M, et al. Gonadal determination and adrenal development are regulated by the orphan nuclear receptor steroidogenic factor-1, in a dose-dependent manner. *J. Clin. Endocrinol. Metab.* 2002;87:1829–1833.

13. Correa RV, Domenice S, Bingham NC, et al. A microdeletion in the ligand binding domain of human steroidogenic factor 1 causes XY sex reversal without adrenal insufficiency. *J. Clin. Endocrinol. Metab.* 2004;89:1767–1772.

14. Lin L, Philibert P, Ferraz-de-Souza B, et al. Heterozygous missense mutations in steroidogenic factor 1 (SF1/Ad4BP, NR5A1) are associated with 46,XY disorders of sex development with normal adrenal function. *J. Clin. Endocrinol. Metab.* 2007;92:991–999.

15. Koopman P, Gubbay J, Vivian N, Goodfellow P, Lovell-Badge R. Male development of chromosomally female mice transgenic for *Sry*. *Nature* 1991;351:117–121.

16. Sekido R, Bar I, Narv'aez V, Penny G, Lovell-Badge R. SOX9 is up-regulated by the transient expression of SRY specifically in Sertoli cell precursors. *Dev. Biol.* 2004;274:271–279.

17. Jeays-Ward K, Dandonneau M, Swain A. *Wnt4* is required for proper male as well as female sexual development. *Dev. Biol.* 2004;276:431–440.

18. Huang B, Wang S, Ning Y, Lamb AN, Bartley J. Autosomal XX sex reversal caused by duplication of *SOX9*. *Am. J. Med. Genet.* 1999;87:349–353.

19. Chaboissier M, Kobayashi A, Vidal VIP, et al. Functional analysis of *Sox8* and *Sox9* during sex determination in the mouse. *Development* 2004;131:1891–1901.

20. Bishop CE, Whitworth DJ, Qin Y, et al. A transgenic insertion upstream of *Sox9* is associated with dominant XX sex reversal in the mouse. *Nat. Genet.* 2000;26:490–494.

21. Clark AM, Garland KK, Russell LD. *Desert hedgehog (Dhh)* gene is required in the mouse testis for formation of adult-type Leydig cells and normal development of peritubular cells and seminiferous tubules. *Biol. Reprod.* 2000;63:1825–1838.

22. Canto P, Söderlund D, Reyes E, Méndez JP. Mutations in the *Desert hedgehog (DHH)* gene in patients with 46,XY complete pure gonadal dysgenesis. *J. Clin. Endocrinol. Metab.* 2004;89:4480–4483.

23. Kitamura K, Yanazawa M, Sugiyama N, et al. Mutation of *ARX* causes abnormal development of forebrain and testes in mice and X-linked lissencephaly with abnormal genitalia in humans. *Nat. Genet.* 2002;32:359–369.

24. Vainio S, Heikkilä M, Kispert A, Chin N, McMahon AP. Female development in mammals is regulated by Wnt-4 signalling. *Nature* 1999;397:405–409.

25. Jordan BK, Mohammed M, Ching ST, et al. Up-regulation of WNT-4 signaling and dosage sensitive sex reversal in humans. *Am. J. Hum. Genet.* 2001;68:1102–1109.

26. Swain A, Narvaez V, Burgoyne P, Camerino G, Lovell-Badge R. *Dax1* antagonizes *Sry* action in mammalian sex determination. *Nature* 1998;391:761–767.

27. Bardoni B, Zanaria E, Guioli S, et al. A dosage sensitive locus at chromosome Xp21 is involved in male to female sex reversal. *Nat. Genet.* 1994;7:497–501.

28. Yu RN, Ito M, Saunders TL, Camper SA, Jameson JL. Role of *Ahch* in gonadal development and gametogenesis. *Nat. Genet.* 1998;20:353–357.

29. Cools M, Drop SLS, Wolffenbuttel KP, Oosterhuis JW, Looijenga LHJ. Germ cell tumours in the intersex gonad: old paths, new directions, moving frontiers. *Endocr. Rev.* 2006;27:468–484.

30. Morris JM. The syndrome of testicular feminization in male pseudohermaphrodites. *Am. J. Obstet. Gynecol.* 1953;65:1192–1211.

31. Quigley CA, De Bellis A, Marschke KB, El-Awady MK, Wilson EM, French FS. Androgen receptor defects: historical, clinical, and molecular perspectives. *Endocr. Rev.* 1995;16:271–321.

32. Regadera J, Martínez-García F, Paniagua R, Nistal M. Androgen insensitivity syndrome: an immunohistochemical, ultrastructural, and morphometric study. *Arch. Pathol. Lab. Med.* 1999;123:225–234.

33. Page DC. Hypothesis: a Y-chromosomal gene causes gonadoblastoma in dysgenetic gonads. *Development* 1987;101(Suppl):151–155.

34. Lau YC. Gonadoblastoma, testicular and prostate cancers, and the TSPY gene. *Am. J. Hum. Genet.* 1999;64:921–927.

35. Hannema SE, Scott IS, de Meyts ER, Skakkebaek NE, Coleman N, Hughes IA. Testicular development in the complete androgen insensitivity syndrome. *J. Pathol.* 2006;208:518–527.

36. Manuel M, Katayama KP, Jones Jr HW. The age of occurrence of gonadal tumors in intersex patients with a Y chromosome. *Am. J. Obstet. Gynecol.* 1976;124:293–300.

37. Cools M, van Aerde K, Kersemaekers A, et al. Morphological and immunohistochemical differences between gonadal maturation delay and early germ cell neoplasia in patients with undervirilization syndromes. *J. Clin. Endocrinol. Metab.* 2005;90:5295–5303.

38. Skakkebaek NE, Berthelsen JG, Giwercman A, Muller J. Carcinoma-in-situ of the testis: possible origin from gonocytes and precursor of all types of germ cell tumours except spermatocytoma. *Int. J. Androl.* 1987;10:19–28.

39. Rajpert-De Meyts E, Bartkova J, Samson M, et al. The emerging phenotype of the testicular carcinoma in situ germ cell. *APMIS* 2003;111:267–278.

40. Cools M, Stoop H, Kersemaekers AF, et al. Gonadoblastoma arising in undifferentiated gonadal tissue within dysgenetic gonads. *J. Clin. Endocrinol. Metab.* 2006;91:2404–2413.

41. Pauls K, Franke FE, Büttner R, Zhou H. Gonadoblastoma: evidence for a stepwise progression to dysgerminoma in a dysgenetic ovary. *Virchows Arch.* 2005;447:603–609.

42. Allan CM, Garcia A, Spaliviero J, et al. Complete Sertoli cell proliferation induced by follicle-stimulating hormone (FSH) independently of luteinizing hormone activity: evidence from genetic models of isolated FSH action. *Endocrinology* 2004;145:1587–1593.

43. Moe-Behrens GHG, Klinger FG, Eskild W, Grotmol T, Haugen TB, De Felici M. Akt/PTEN signaling mediates estrogen-dependent proliferation of primordial germ cells *in vitro*. *Mol. Endocrinol.* 2003;17:2630–2638.

44. Li H, Papadopoulos V, Vidic B, Dym M, Culty M. Regulation of rat testis gonocyte proliferation by platelet-derived growth factor and estradiol: identification of signaling mechanisms involved. *Endocrinology* 1997;138:1289–1298.

45. Lassurguère J, Livera G, Habert R, Jégou B. Time- and dose-related effects of estradiol and diethylstilbestrol on the morphology and function of the fetal rat testis in culture. *Toxicol. Sci.* 2003;73:160–169.

46. Pena-Alonso R, Nieto K, Alvarez R, et al. Distribution of Y-chromosome-bearing cells in gonadoblastoma and dysgenetic testis in 45,X/46,XY infants. *Mod. Pathol.* 2005;18:439–445.

47. Skakkebaek NE, Rajpert-De Meyts E, Main KM. Testicular dysgenesis syndrome: an increasingly common developmental disorder with environmental aspects. *Hum. Reprod.* 2001;16:972–978.

48. Bay K, Asklund C, Skakkebaek NE, Andersson A. Testicular dysgenesis syndrome: possible role of endocrine disrupters. *Best Pract. Res. Clin. Endocrinol. Metab.* 2006;20:77–90.

49. Manivel JC, Jessurun J, Wick MR, Dehner LP. Placental alkaline phosphatase immunoreactivity in testicular germ-cell neoplasms. *Am. J. Surg. Pathol.* 1987;11:21–29.

50. Koide O, Iwai S, Baba K, Iri H. Identification of testicular atypical germ cells by an immunohistochemical technique for placental alkaline phosphatase. *Cancer* 1987;60:1325–1330.

51. Giwercman A, Andrews PW, Jørgensen N, Müller J, Græm N, Skakkebæk NE. Immunohistochemical expression of embryonal marker TRA-1-60 in carcinoma in situ and germ cell tumors of the testis. *Cancer* 1993;72:1308–1314.

52. Hamilton-Dutoit SJ, Lou H, Pallesen G. The expression of placental alkaline phosphatase (PLAP) and PLAP-like enzymes in normal and neoplastic human tissues. An immunohistological survey using monoclonal antibodies. *APMIS* 1990; 98:797–811.

53. Hoei-Hansen CE, Nielsen JE, Almstrup K, et al. Transcription factor AP-2gamma is a developmentally regulated marker of testicular carcinoma *in situ* and germ cell tumors. *Clin. Cancer Res.* 2004;10: 8521–8530.

54. Cheng L. Establishing a germ cell origin for metastatic tumors using OCT4 immunohistochemistry. *Cancer* 2004;101:2006–2010.

55. Jones TD, Ulbright TM, Eble JN, Cheng L. OCT4:a sensitive and specific biomarker for intratubular germ cell neoplasia of the testis. *Clin. Cancer Res.* 2004;10:8544–8547.

56. Cheng L, Thomas A, Roth LM, Zheng W, Michael H, Abdul Karim FW. OCT4: A novel biomarker for dysgerminoma of the ovary. *Am. J. Surg. Pathol.* 2004;28:1341–1346.

57. Jørgensen N, Giwercman A, Müller J, Skakkebæk NE. Immunohistochemical cells. *Histopathology* 1993;22:373–378.

58. Jørgensen N, Rajpert-De Meyts E, Græm N, Müller J, Giwercman A, Skakkebæk NE. Expression of immunohistochemical markers for testicular carcinoma *in situ* by normal human fetal germ cells. *Lab. Invest.* 1995;72:223–231.

59. Armstrong GR, Buckley CH, Kelsey AM. Germ cell expression of placental alkaline phosphatase in male pseudohermaphroditism. *Histopathology* 1991;18:541–547.

60. Rajpert-de Meyts E, Hanstein R, Jorgensen N, Graem N, Vogt PH, Skakkebaek NE. Developmental expression of *POU5F1* (OCT-3/4) in normal and dysgenetic human gonads. *Hum. Reprod.* 2004;19: 1338–1344.

61. Schnieders F, Dörk D, Arnemann J, Vogel T, Werner M, Schmidtke J. Testis-specific protein, y-encoded (TSPY) expression in testicular tissues. *Hum. Mol. Genet.* 1996;5:1801–1807.

62. Rajpert-De Meyts E, Jørgensen N, Müller J, Skakkebæk NE. Prolonged expression of the *c-kit* receptor in germ cells of intersex fetal testes. *J. Pathol.* 1996;178:166–169.

63. Niwa H, Miyazaki J, Smith AG. Quantitative expression of Oct-3/4 defines differentiation, dedifferentiation or self-renewal of ES cells. *Nat. Genet.* 2000;24:372–376.

64. Hoei-Hansen CE, Carlsen E, Jorgensen N, Leffers H, Skakkebaek NE, Rajpert-De Meyts E. Towards a non-invasive method for early detection of testicular neoplasia in semen samples by identification of fetal germ cell-specific markers. *Hum. Reprod.* 2007;22: 167–173.

65. McLachlan RI, Rajpert-De Meyts E, Hoei-Hansen CE, de Kretser DM, Skakkebaek NE. Histological evaluation of the human testis – approaches to optimising the clinical value of the assessment: Mini review. *Hum. Reprod.* 2007; 22:2–16.

66. Gidekel S, Pizov G, Bergman Y, Pikarsky E. Oct-3/4 is a dose-dependent oncogenic fate determinant. *Cancer Cell.* 2003;4:361–370.

67. Dieckmann KP, Skakkebaek NE. Carcinoma in situ of the testis: review of biological and clinical features. *Int. J. Cancer* 1999;83: 815–822.

68. Verp MS, Simpson JL. Abnormal sexual differentiation and neoplasia. *Cancer Genet. Cytogenet.* 1987;25:191–218.

69. Cortes D. Cryptorchidism – aspects of pathogenesis, histology and treatment. *Scand. J. Urol. Nephrol. Suppl.* 1998;196:1–54.

70. Pinczowski D, McLaughlin JK, Lackgren G, Adami HO, Persson I. Occurrence of testicular cancer in patients operated on for crptorchidism and inguinal hernia. *J. Urol.* 1991;146:1291–1294.

71. Regadera J, Martínez-García F, González-Peramato P, Serrano A, Nistal M, Suárez-Quian C. Androgen receptor expression in Sertoli cells as a function of seminiferous tubule maturation in the human cryptorchid testis. *J. Clin. Endocrinol. Metab.* 2001;86:413–421.

72. Dahl EV, Bahn RC. Aberrant adrenal cortical tissue near the testis in human infants. *Am. J. Pathol.* 1962;40:587–598.

73. Cabrera MS, Vogiatzi MG, New MI. Long term outcome in adult males with classic congenital adrenal hyperplasia. *J. Clin. Endocrinol. Metab.* 2001;86:3070–3078.

74. Stikkelbroeck NMML, Otten BJ, Pasic A, et al. High prevalence of testicular adrenal rest tumors, impaired spermatogenesis, and Leydig cell failure in adolescent and adult males with congenital adrenal hyperplasia. *J. Clin. Endocrinol. Metab.* 2001;86:5721–5728.

75. Avila NA, Premkumar A, Shawker TH, Jones JV, Laue L, Cutler JGB. Testicular adrenal rest tissue in congenital adrenal hyperplasia: findings at Gray-scale and color Doppler US. *Radiology* 1996;198: 99–104.

76. Claahsen-van der Grinten HL, Otten BJ, Takahashi S, et al. Testicular adrenal rest tumours in adult males with congenital adrenal hyperplasia: evaluation of pituitary-gonadal function before and after successful testis-sparing surgery in 8 patients. *J. Clin. Endocrinol. Metab.* 2006;Epub:1.

56 Gestational Trophoblastic Neoplasia

Tim Crook and Michael J. Seckl

> **Key points**
> - Gestational trophoblastic neoplasia is a group of uncommon disorders involving abnormal proliferation of trophoblast.
> - The etiology involves loss of normal imprinting of specific genes, together with acquired epigenetic changes.
> - Measurement of serum human chorionic gonadotropin has a key role in the diagnosis, management and follow-up of patients.
> - Gestational trophoblastic neoplasia is an intrinsically chemosensitive disease and the great majority of patients with these disorders are cured by chemotherapy, usually without impairment of fertility.
> - Understanding invasiveness in gestational trophoblastic neoplasia may provide clues to the mechanisms of metastasis in solid tumors.

Introduction

Normal gestational trophoblast arises from the peripheral cells of the blastocyst in the first few days immediately following conception. Trophoblast tissue forms two layers: (1) an inner cytotrophoblast of mononucleated cells which migrate out and fuse to form (2) an outer syncytiotrophoblast of large multinucleated cells. The syncytiotrophoblast invades the endometrium producing the placenta. When the mechanisms that normally regulate proliferation and invasiveness are lost, the trophoblast tissue may grow abnormally and cause disease. The term gestational trophoblastic disease (GTD) encompasses a spectrum of disorders of progressively greater malignant potential, the underlying pathobiology of which is abnormal proliferation of trophoblastic tissue. Trophoblasts are specialized epithelial cells derived from the outermost layer of the blastocyst. When GTD arises, the normal regulatory mechanisms controlling growth of trophoblastic tissue are lost and the excessively proliferating trophoblast may invade through the myometrium. The World Health Organization has classified GTD into two premalignant diseases, termed complete and partial hydatidiform mole (CM and PM), and three malignant disorders – invasive mole, gestational choriocarcinoma and placentalsite trophoblastic tumor [1]. The latter are also collectively known as gestational trophoblastic tumors (GTT) or gestational trophoblastic neoplasia (GTN). Each form of GTD has distinct properties as discussed below. Although relatively uncommon, these tumors are important to recognize because they are almost always curable with, in most cases, preservation of fertility.

Clinical Endocrine Oncology, 2nd edition. Edited by Ian D. Hay and John A.H. Wass. © 2008 Blackwell Publishing. ISBN 978-1-4051-4584-8.

Table 56.1 Features of partial moles (PM) and complete moles (CM)

	PM	CM
Karyotype	Triploid	Diploid
	Maternal & paternal	Paternal
	69,XXY (58%)	46,XX (90%)
	69,XXX (40%)	46,XY (10%)
	69,XYY (2%)	
Malignant sequelae	<1:200	1:16
Uterus enlarged for age	Often no	Yes

Some data are from Andrea et al. [30].

Moles

PM and CM are distinct pathobiological entities with characteristic genetic, histological and clinical features, some of which are summarized in Table 56.1. Despite these differences, management of CM and PM is similar (see below). Diagnosis of moles is usually during the first trimester, the most common presenting symptom being vaginal bleeding. Other features include uterine size being larger than expected for age (complete mole), hyperemesis gravida and abnormally elevated serum human chorionic gonadotropin (hCG) levels.

Gestational trophoblastic tumors

Invasive mole is a CM or PM that penetrates and invades the myometrium. It is usually diagnosed because serial urine or serum hCG measurements reveal a plateaued or rising hCG level in the weeks after evacuation of the mole. Patients may complain of persistent vaginal bleeding or lower abdominal pains and/or swelling as a result of hemorrhage from leaking tumor-induced vasculature as the trophoblast invades through the myometrium, or because of vulval, vaginal or intra-abdominal metastases. The tumor may also involve other pelvic structures, including the bladder or rectum, producing hematuria or rectal bleeding, respectively.

Choriocarcinoma is the most aggressive form of GTD, often growing and metastasizing rapidly throughout the body. It may arise from any type of pregnancy, including a normal term pregnancy, miscarriage, routine termination of pregnancy [2–4], a CM [3] or a PM [5]. CM is probably the most common antecedent to choriocarcinoma, being 29–83% in various studies across the world [1], whereas the incidence of choriocarcinoma following term delivery without a history of CM is approximately 1:50 000. Choriocarcinoma appears as a soft, largely hemorrhagic mass. This mass fails to stimulate the connective tissue support normally associated with tumors and induces hypervascularity of the surrounding maternal tissues. This may account for its highly metastatic and hemorrhagic behavior. Indeed, although presenting symptoms may include vaginal bleeding, abdominal pain and pelvic mass, one third of patients with choriocarcinoma present with symptoms of distant metastasis rather than gynecological features. Common sites of metastasis include lungs, liver and brain, but any site may be involved. As such, choriocarcinoma should always be included in the differential diagnosis of metastatic cancer in female patients of child-bearing age.

Placental-site trophoblastic tumor (PSTT) is likely to constitute about 1% of all malignant trophoblastic tumors. It is a rare, slow-growing form of GTD arising from intermediate trophoblasts at the implantation site and so produces little hCG [6]. PSTT can follow term delivery, non-molar abortion and CM. Recently, a case of PSTT following a PM was described [7]. Like choriocarcinoma, the causative pregnancy may not be the immediate antecedent pregnancy. Unlike choriocarcinoma, metastasis occurs later in the natural history of the disease and patients frequently present with gynecological symptoms alone.

Genetics

PMs are all triploid or, rarely, tetraploid with at least two paternal chromosome sets but also some maternal contribution. Triploidy occurs in 1–3% of all recognized conceptions, and in about 20% of spontaneous abortions with abnormal karyotypes. However, triploids due to two sets of maternal chromosomes do not become PMs [8, 9]. CMs are cytogenetically diploid, with a 46,XX karyotype, of which both X chromosomes are of paternal origin. CMs most frequently occur following fertilization of an anuclear ovum by a 23X spermatozoon followed by duplication to form a 46,XX homozygote [10]. However, in up to 25% of CM, the anuclear ovum is fertilized by two spermatozoa, resulting in heterozygous 46,XY or 46,XX heterozygotes [11]. A 46,YY genotype has never been observed and is presumed to be non-viable. Interestingly, in additional to the paternally derived nuclear DNA, there are some maternal genes in CM, including the mitochondrial

genome [12]. Rarely, CM develops from a fertilized ovum which retains maternal nuclear DNA, giving rise to a biparental mole [13].

Three closely related imprinted genes on chromosome 11p15 may be involved in GTT development and in other overgrowth syndromes [14]. These are: H19, a putative tumor suppresser gene, the cyclin-dependent kinase inhibitor p57kip2 (both normally maternally expressed) by the maternal allele; and the paternally expressed insulin-like growth factor-II (IGF-II). While p57kip2 showed the expected pattern of expression in CM and choriocarcinoma and some post-term tumors showed biallelic expression of both H19 and IGF-II, there is increasing evidence that loss of the normal imprinting patterns of these genes may be an important factor in the development of GTT.

In the search for genes predisposing to GTD, linkage and homozygosity analysis of biparental CM suggested the involvement of a gene mapping at chromosome 19q13.3–13.4 [15]. In two families with biparental CM, mutations were detected in the gene *NALP7* which maps in this region [16]. However, genetics analysis of two families from China has revealed no homozygosity in members of either family in this region, implying the existence of other susceptibility genes in distinct locations of the genome, consistent with genetic heterogeneity of this condition [17].

Epigenetics

Transformation of hydatidiform moles into GTT almost certainly involves multiple additional molecular genetic events. Accordingly, there is considerable interest in identification of genes in which changes in expression are associated with malignant progression. Evidence is now emerging that acquired epigenetic changes, principally transcriptional silencing, may have an important role in this process. Several recent studies have sought evidence of methylation-dependent transcriptional silencing in specific genes in moles and choriocarcinoma. From these studies it is becoming clear that such epigenetic changes are common in both moles and GTT. In one study, it was shown that transcriptional silencing of the tumor suppressor PTEN, mediated by aberrant hypermethylation, occurs at a higher frequency in PM and CM than in normal placentas [18].

In another study, six candidate genes from diverse functional groups that are known targets for transcriptional silencing in common solid tumors were analyzed in a series of moles and choriocarcinomas (Table 56.2; [19]). Three of the genes (E-cadherin, HIC-1, p16INK4a) were aberrantly hypermethylated in moles and four of the six (E-cadherin, HIC-1, p16INK4a and TIMP3) hypermethylated in choriocarcinoma. Fifteen of the 54 moles ultimately required chemotherapy (see Table 56.3 for indications for chemotherapy) and p16INK4a hypermethylation was correlated with this. These studies suggest that epigenetic analysis of molar tissue might have utility in assessing risk of malignant progression and/or prediction of clinical outcome, although additional work is clearly required. The mismatch repair genes *hMLH1* and *hMSH2* are abundantly expressed in cytotrophoblasts from normal placentas,

Table 56.2 Genes epigenetically inactivated in gestational trophoblastic disease

Gene	Methylation in moles	Methylation in chorio.	Ref.
p16 INK4a	Yes	Yes	[19]
E-cadherin	Yes	Yes	[19]
HIC-1	Yes	Yes	[19]
GSTP1	No	No	[19]
TIMP3	No	Yes	[19]
DAPK	No	No	[19]
PTEN	Yes	Yes	[18]
hMLH1	Yes	Not done	[18]
hMSH2	Yes	Not done	[18]

Table 56.3 Indications for chemotherapy

1 Histological evidence of choriocarcinoma
2 Evidence of metastases in brain, liver or gastrointestinal tract, or radiological opacities >2 cm on chest X-ray
3 Pulmonary, vulval or vaginal metastases unless hCG falling
4 Heavy vaginal bleeding or evidence of gastrointestinal or intraperitoneal hemorrhage
5 Rising or plateaued hCG after evacuation
6 Serum hCG >20 000 iu/L more than 4 weeks after evacuation, because of the risk of uterine perforation
7 Raised hCG 6 months after evacuation even if still falling

Any of the above are indications to treat following the diagnosis of GTD.

but expression is transcriptionally downregulated by aberrant hypermethylation in hydatidiform moles. These results imply that the loss of genome stability usually maintained by expression of hMLH1 and hMSH2 contributes to the pathogenesis of GTT [18]. It remains to be established whether down-regulation of mismatch repair genes contributes to the chemosensitivity of GTT. The use of microarray technology has revolutionized studies of gene expression in human cancer. Using this methodology, differential gene expression has been studied in a cell line derived from normal trophoblasts of a first-term placenta and two choriocarcinoma cell lines [20]. Twenty-three genes were reported to be differentially expressed in the choriocarcinoma lines compared to the normal trophoblasts. Among these genes, methylation-dependent transcriptional silencing of tissue inhibitor of metalloproteinase 3 (TIMP3) was confirmed (see also Xue at al. [19]). Insulin growth factor binding protein 3 (IGFBP3) was a second gene of obvious interest reported to be down-regulated in choriocarcinoma in this study [20]. Undoubtedly, numerous further differentially expressed genes await description in normal trophoblasts, hydatidiform mole and choriocarcinoma which will shed new light on the pathogenesis of these conditions. Furthermore, it is not possible at present to predict which patients with a CM or PM will develop GTT. As such, all these patients must be rigorously followed up with hCG monitoring. Gene expression profiling and/or epigenetic analysis may in future afford a novel means to identify individual patients

at risk of these sequelae and ultimately obviate the need for such long-term hCG follow-up.

hCG

In the UK all women with GTD are registered for centralized hCG follow-up. Serial measurements of this hormone are central to the safe and effective management of GTD and so the methods used to determine hCG levels are vitally important. HCG is a glycoprotein hormone comprising an alpha and beta subunit but only the latter is specific to hCG. An elevated hCG is found in pregnancy and all forms of GTD, but can also arise from non-gestational tumors such as germ cell and even epithelial tumors, may be normal for an individual or the result of a false-positive interaction in the hCG assay. The beta subunit of hCG in pregnancy is usually intact and may be hyperglycosylated but in disease multiple isoforms of hCG can be produced. Consequently, assays used to monitor hCG in GTD and other cancers should detect all beta hCG isoforms, something that most commercial assays fail to do. We are fortunate at Charing Cross Hospital to have an hCG assay suitable for monitoring hCG in GTD and cancer. Measurement of hCG has a vital role in diagnosis, monitoring and assessment of response to chemotherapy in GTD. The amount of hCG produced correlates with tumor volume, a serum hCG of 5 iu/L corresponding to approximately 104–105 viable tumor cells. Consequently, these assays are several orders of magnitude more sensitive than the best imaging modalities available today. In addition, hCG levels can be used to determine prognosis and response to treatment [21].

Investigations and treatment

Most women presenting with molar disease have an ultrasound that shows no evidence of a normal pregnancy and instead the uterus may contain a variable amount of mixed echogenic material. This combined with a positive pregnancy test is highly suggestive of either CM or PM. Suction evacuation of the uterine cavity is the standard initial gynecological management of PM and CM. All patients are then registered for centralized hCG follow-up in the UK. In the majority of patients the hCG returns to normal and no more treatment is required but 16% of patients with CM and <0.5% with PM develop persistent GTD. This can be invasive mole, choriocarcinoma or, very rarely, PSTT and is diagnosed by a plateaued or rising hCG post evacuation. Other reasons to consider chemotherapy are listed in Table 56.3. Re-evacuation or biopsy at this point to confirm malignant change is rarely performed because of the risk of life-threatening bleeding and/or uterine perforation from these highly vascularized and invasive tumors. Staging investigations include a pelvic Doppler ultrasound (US) to determine uterine size/local tumor extent and vascularity and a chest X-ray. If lung metastases are present then an MRI brain is essential to exclude CNS spread. A lumbar puncture to determine the CSF–serum hCG ratio, which should be less than

1:60, is required if the magnetic resonance imaging (MRI) is normal. For women presenting with a GTT following another type of pregnancy or where more extensive disease is suspected then computerized tomography (CT) body, MRI brain and pelvis are required and sometimes fluorodeoxyglucose-positron emission tomography scans can help to complete staging. This information combined with the history and hCG level is plugged into a scoring system (Tables 56.4 and 56.5) that enables us to determine the risk of the patient's tumor becoming resistant to single-agent chemotherapy. Those patients with a low risk (Charing Cross score 0–8, FIGO score 0–6) receive single drug therapy whilst those scoring >8 or >6 receive combination agent treatment.

At Charing Cross Hospital low-risk patients receive single-agent methotrexate with folinic acid rescue which cures approximately two thirds of women, the remaining third needing to change treatment to achieve cure. Patients with a high risk receive an intensive regimen consisting of etoposide, methotrexate and actinomycin D (EMA), alternating weekly with cyclophosphamide and vincristine, otherwise known as Oncovin® (CO). The cumulative 5-year survival of patients treated with this schedule is 86%, with no deaths from GTT beyond 2 years after the initiation of chemotherapy [22]. Frequent measurement of the serum hCG is a simple way to detect drug resistance at an early stage as the hormone levels will stop falling and may start to rise long before there are other clinical changes. In patients receiving methotrexate for low-risk disease, if the hCG is <100 iu/L when drug resistance occurs, the disease can often be cured simply by substituting actinomycin D, although this drug is rather more toxic than

Table 56.4 Scoring system for gestational trophoblastic tumors (Charing Cross Scoring System)

Score prognostic factor	0	1	2	6
Age (years)	<39	>39	–	–
Antecedent pregnancy (AP)	Mole	Abortion or unknown	Term	–
Interval (end of AP to chemotherapy in months)	<4	4–7	7–12	>12
hCG (iu/L)	103–104	<103	104–105	>105
Number of metastases	0	1–3	4–8	>8
Site of metastases	None, lung, vagina	Spleen, kidney	GI tract	Brain, liver
Largest tumor mass	–	3–5 cm	>5 cm	–
Prior chemotherapy	–	–	Single drug	>2 drugs

The total score for a patient is obtained by adding the individual scores for each prognostic factor. Low risk, 0–8; high risk, ≥9. Patients scoring 0–8 currently receive single-agent therapy with methotrexate and folinic acid, while patients scoring ≥9 receive combination drug therapy with EMA/CO. hCG, human chorionic gonadotropin; GI, gastrointestinal.

Table 56.5 Scoring system for gestational trophoblastic tumors (modified FIGO scoring system)

Score prognostic factor	0	1	2	4
Age (years)	<40	≥40	–	–
Antecedent pregnancy (AP)	Mole	Abortion	Term	–
Interval (end of AP to chemotherapy in months)	<4	4–6	7–13	>13
hCG (iu/L)	<103	103–104	104–105	>105
Number of metastases	0	1–4	5–8	>8
Site of metastases	Lung	Spleen, kidney	GI tract	Brain, liver
Largest tumor mass	–	3–5 cm	>5 cm	
Prior chemotherapy	–	–	Single drug	>2 drugs

The total score for a patient is obtained by adding the individual scores for each prognostic factor. Low risk, 0–6; high risk, ≥7.

methotrexate. Low-risk risk patients failing methotrexate whose serum hCG is >100 iu/L are treated with the EMA–CO regimen outlined above. This treatment protocol saves virtually all low-risk patients [23], but some high-risk patients develop drug-resistant disease. Fortunately, most of these can still be salvaged with platinum and/or taxane-based regimens [24, 25] but unlike some other highly chemosensitive malignancies, the value of high-dose chemotherapy is less clear [26].

On completion of therapy, the pelvic US should be repeated to confirm that the masses have disappeared, or at least reduced in size. This ensures that the masses did not originate from some other pathology. Chest X-rays and other scans are repeated if they previously showed abnormalities to serve as a baseline for future comparisons. Any residual masses are not removed provided the hCG is normal as there is no evidence that this decreases the risk of subsequent relapse [27].

Long-term outlook and summary

The overall risk of relapse is 3% and most are cured because hCG surveillance detects recurrence at an early stage. Fertility does not appear to be impaired by either methotrexate or EMA–CO treatment although the latter does bring forwards the menopause date by 3 years [28]. Importantly, methotrexate alone does not induce second tumor, but EMA-CO does have a slight but significant effect in this context. Indeed, there is a slight excess of leukemias, melanoma, breast and bowel cancer in women who have received EMA-CO with an overall increased risk of 1.5-fold compared to the general age-matched population [29].

Thus the long-term outlook for women with GTT is excellent and treatment failures are fortunately rare.

References

1. WHO. Gestational trophoblastic diseases. Technical Report series 692. Geneva: World Health Organization, 1983:7–81.

2. Wake N, Tanaka K-I, Chapman V, Matsui S, Sandberg AA. Chromosomes and cellular origin of choriocarcinoma. *Cancer Res.* 1981;41:3137–3143.

3. Fisher RA, Newlands ES, Jeffreys AJ, et al. Gestational and non-gestational trophoblastic tumours distinguished by DNA analysis. *Cancer* 1992;69:839–845.

4. Seckl MJ, Gillmore R, Foskett M, Sebire NJ, Rees H, Newlands ES. Routine terminations of pregnancy–should we screen for gestational trophoblastic neoplasia? *Lancet* 2004;364:645–646.

5. Seckl MJ, Fisher RA, Salerno G, et al. Choriocarcinoma and partial hydatidiform moles. *Lancet* 2000;356:366–339.

6. Shih IM, Kurman RJ. The pathology of intermediate trophoblastic tumors and tumor-like lesions. *Int. J. Gynecol. Pathol.* 2001;20:31–47.

7. Palmieri C, Fisher RA, Sebire NJ, et al. Placental site trophoblastic tumor arising from a partial hydatidiform mole. *Lancet* 2005;366:688.

8. Jacobs PA, Hunt PA, Matsuuro JS, Wilson CC. Complete and partial hydatidiform mole in Hawaii: cytogenetics, morphology and epidemiology. *Br. J. Obstet. Gynaecol.* 1982;89:258–266.

9. Lawler SD, Fisher RA, Pickthall VG, Povey S, Wyn Evans M. Genetic studies on hydatidiform moles I: the origin of partial moles. *Cancer Genet. Cytogenet.* 1982;4:309–320.

10. Kajii T, Ohama K. Androgenetic origin of hydatidiform mole. *Nature* 1977;268:633–634.

11. Ohama K, Kajii T, Okamoto E, et al. Dispermic origin of XY hydatidiform mole. *Nature* 1981;292:551–552.

12. Edwards YH, Jeremiah SJ, McMillan SL, Povey S, Fisher RA, Lawler SD. Complete hydiatidiform moles combine maternal mitochondria with paternal nuclear genome. *Ann. Hum. Genet.* 1984;48:119–127.

13. Fisher RA, Newlands ES. Gestational trophoblastic disease: molecular and genetic studies. *J. Reprod. Med.* 1998;43:81–97.

14. Li M, Squire JA, Weksberg R. Overgrowth syndromes and genomic imprinting: from mouse to man. *Clin. Genet.* 1998;53:165–170.

15. Hodges MD, Rees HC, Seckl MJ, Newlands ES, Fisher RA. Genetic refinement and physical mapping of a biparental complete hydatidiform mole locus on chromosome 19q13.4. *J. Med. Genet.* 2003;40:e95.

16. Murdoch S, Djuric U, Mazhar B, et al. Mutations in NALP7 cause recurrent hydatidiform moles and reproductive wastage in humans. *Nat. Genet.* 2006;38:300–302.

17. Zhao J, Moss J, Sebire NJ, et al. Analysis of the chromosomal region 19q13.4 in two Chinese families with recurrent hydatidiform mole. *Hum. Reprod.* 2006;21:536–541.

18. Chen H, Ye D, Xie X, Lu W, Zhu C, Chen X. Mismatch repair gene promoter methylation and expression in hydatidiform moles. *Arch. Gynecol. Obstet.* 2005;272:35–39.

19. Xue WC, Chan KY, Feng HC, et al. Promoter hypermethylation of multiple genes in hydatidiform mole and choriocarcinoma. *J. Mol. Diagn.* 2004;6:326–324.

20. Feng H, Cheung AN, Xue WC, et al. Down-regulation and promoter methylation of tissue inhibitor of metalloproteinase 3 in choriocarcinoma. *Gynecol. Oncol.* 2004;94:375–382.

21. Bagshawe KD. Risk and prognostic factors in trophoblastic neoplasia. *Cancer* 1976;38:1373–1385.

22. Bower M, Newlands ES, Holden L, et al. EMA/CO for high-risk gestational trophoblastic tumours: results from a cohort of 272 patients. *J. Clin. Oncol.* 1997;15:2636–2643.

23. McNeish IA, Strickland S, Holden L, et al. Low-risk persistent gestational trophoblastic disease: outcome after initial treatment with low-dose methotrexate and folinic acid from 1992 to 2000. *J. Clin. Oncol.* 2002;20:1838–1844.

24. Jones WB, Schneider J, Shapiro F, Lewis JLJ. Treatment of resistant gestational choriocarcinoma with taxol: a report of two cases. *Gynaecol. Oncol.* 1996;61:126–130.

25. Newlands ES, Mulholland PJ, Holden L, Seckl MJ, Rustin GJ. Etoposide and cisplatin/etoposide, methotrexate, and actinomycin D (EMA) chemotherapy for patients with high-risk gestational tropho-blastic tumors refractory to EMA/cyclophosphamide and vincristine chemotherapy and patients presenting with metastatic placental site trophoblastic tumors. *J. Clin. Oncol.* 2000;18:854–859.

26. El-Helw LM, Seckl MJ, Haynes R, et al. High-dose chemotherapy and peripheral blood stem cell support in refractory gestational trophoblastic neoplasia. *Br. J. Cancer* 2005;93:620–621.

27. Powles T, Savage P, Short D, Young A, Pappin C, Seckl MJ. Residual lung lesions after completion of chemotherapy for gestational trophoblastic neoplasia: should we operate? *Br. J. Cancer* 2006;94:51–54.

28. Woolas RP, Bower M, Newlands ES, Seckl MJ, Short D, Holden L. Influence of chemotherapy for gestational trophoblastic disease on subsequent pregnancy outcome. *Br. J. Obstet. Gynaecol.* 1998;105:1032–1035.

29. Rustin GJS, Newlands ES, Lutz J-M, et al. Combination but not single agent methotrexate chemotherapy for gestational trophoblastic tumours (GTT) increases the incidence of second tumours. *J. Clin. Oncol.* 1996;14:2769–2773.

30. Andrea A, Franceschi S, Ferlay J, Smith J, La Vecchia C. Epidemiology and aetiology of gestational trophoblastic disease. *Lancet Oncol.* 2003;4:670–678.

5 Neuroendocrine Tumors and the Clinical Syndromes

57 Classification of Neuroendocrine Tumors

Adeel Ansari, Karim Meeran, and Stephen R. Bloom

Key points
- Neuroendocrine tumors are slow growing and have an indeterminate prognosis.
- Current classification serves as a guide to prognosis and treatment, but this is less precise than classification of other tumors.
- The anatomical site of origin may affect prognosis.
- Appendiceal carcinoids when found incidentally almost never metastasize.

Introduction

Neuroendocrine cells were first described by Paul Langerhans in 1869. The definition of neuroendocrine cells has since changed over and over again. In 1969 these cells were described as APUD "amine precursor uptake and decarboxylation" cells, as they accumulate amine precursors and decarboxylate them to produce peptide hormones and biogenic amines identical to those found in neurones. With immunocytochemistry an increasing number of similar cells producing and secreting peptides have been identified in the gut, pancreas and nervous system – leading to the term "neuroendocrine." Neuroendocrine cells are now described on the following criteria: the production of a neurotransmitter, neuromodulator or neuropeptide hormone; the presence of dense-core secretory granules from which the hormones are released by exocytosis in response to an external stimulus; and the absence of axons and synapses [1].

Neuroendocrine tumors are a heterogeneous group of tumors arising from these neuroendocrine cells. They include gastrointestinal carcinoids, islet cell pancreatic tumors, chromophobe pituitary tumors, medullary carcinoma of the thyroid and pheochromocytomas.

Epidemiology

The apparent incidence of neuroendocrine tumors is rising with improvements in the diagnosis and classification of these tumors. Neuroendocrine tumors currently account for 0.5% of all malignancies. Recent studies have reported rates of 2–3 per 100 000 per year, with a female preponderance under the age of 50 years.

Clinical Endocrine Oncology, 2nd edition. Edited by Ian D. Hay and John A.H. Wass. © 2008 Blackwell Publishing. ISBN 978-1-4051-4584-8.

Gastrointestinal neuroendocrine tumors account for a majority of the neuroendocrine tumors. Most of these are sporadic, but association with genetic syndromes and familial clustering are reported. About 20% of patients with neuroendocrine tumors develop secondary cancers. There is now an increase in the survival of these patients and hence, prevalence is also relatively high [2, 3].

Classification of neuroendocrine tumors

Neuroendocrine tumors have long been a source of clinical and pathological interest. In 1907 the term "karzinoid" was used to classify all neuroendocrine tumors. Subsequently neuroendocrine tumors from the gastrointestinal tract as well as those from other sites of origin were classified as carcinoids.

In 1963 it was suggested that the carcinoid tumors should be classified according to their embryonic site of origin into foregut carcinoids (respiratory tract, stomach, proximal duodenum, biliary system, pancreas), midgut carcinoids (distal duodenum, lower jejunum, ileum, appendix, proximal colon) and hindgut carcinoids (distal colon and rectum) [4]. However, this classification was unreliable as it classified tumors, for example lung and gastrointestinal tract endocrine tumors, with distinctive morphological, functional and clinical patterns into the same group.

In 1980 the World Health Organization (WHO) classification of neuroendocrine tumors separated the gastrointestinal tumors from those with other origin. The gastrointestinal neuroendocrine tumors, which make up about 90% of the neuroendocrine tumors, were classified as carcinoids. The remaining, which include endocrine tumors of the pancreas and thyroid, paragangliomas, small cell lung carcinomas and Merkel cell tumors of the skin, were the exception. On the basis of various staining techniques, the carcinoids were then sub-classified into enterochromaffin cell carcinoids, gastrin cell carcinoids and other carcinoids. However, this classification caused confusion and misinterpretation.

The general use of the term "carcinoid" to classify neuroendocrine tumors is not accurate and fails to incorporate the wide spectrum of neoplasms that originate from different neuroendocrine cell types and produce a wide variety of biologically active agents. The definition and prognosis of neuroendocrine tumors vary from site to site. In 1994 Capella et al. suggested replacing the term "carcinoid" with the term "neuroendocrine tumor" so that all neoplasms with neuroendocrine features would be included. They proposed a new classification based on clinical and pathological features. The tumors are initially distinguished according to the site of origin and then subdivided into tumors with benign behavior, tumors with uncertain behavior, low-grade malignant and high malignant neoplasms. The separations are made on the basis of the histological differentiation, size, extension into surrounding tissues and angioinvasion [5]. This was supported by Rindi et al. similarly classifying the tumors based on their characteristics into benign, uncertain and malignant tumors [6]. The hormonal function and clinical associations of the neuroendocrine tumors are related to their clinical behavior and hence, are also of importance in classifying these tumors. Tumors are termed functioning neuroendocrine tumors if there is elevated serum hormone concentration and clinical syndrome with hyperfunction symptoms, whereas those without significant plasma hormone rise and lacking the symptoms are termed non-functioning neuroendocrine tumors.

The most recent 2000 WHO classification follows the same principle [7]. This classification is based on histopathological and biological characteristics, including tumor size and location/origin, cellular grading, cell proliferation markers, local or vascular invasion and the production of biologically active substances. They have also introduced the term "neuroendocrine carcinoma". The tumors are classified on the basis of the histopathological and biological characteristics as: (1) well-differentiated neuroendocrine tumors that show a benign or uncertain malignancy; (2) well-differentiated neuroendocrine carcinomas that are more aggressive due to the presence of metastasis; (3) poorly differentiated neuroendocrine carcinomas that have a high grade of malignancy and a poor prognosis; and (4) mixed exocrine–endocrine tumors.

Histopathology and biology of neuroendocrine tumors

The histopathology of neuroendocrine tumors helps to classify these tumors according to their origin, biochemical behavior and prognosis. Traditionally the differentiation of endocrine tumors was made using light microscopy, silver staining and electron microscopy. Now the differentiation is aided by immunohistochemistry of general neuroendocrine markers and cell-specific markers [7, 8]. Neuroendocrine cells secrete specific peptides and biogenic amines that are tumor specific (such as insulin in insulinoma) and have diagnostic and prognostic implications. The general neuroendocrine markers include the granular markers (chromogranin A (CgA) and synaptophysin) and the cytosol-based markers (neuron-specific enolase (NSE) and the protein gene product 9.5) [8]. Non-functioning neuroendocrine tumors stain positive for these markers but are not associated with a particular clinical syndrome.

DNA analysis is of little benefit in classifying these tumors, but the nuclear antigen Ki-67 is useful in indicating the proliferative capacity of the tumors [7, 9]. Survival is negatively correlated with a high Ki-67 protein expression.

Neuroendocrine tumors are mostly well-differentiated tumors. "Well-differentiated neuroendocrine tumors" show characteristic features of a solid, trabecular or glandular arrangement (histologically), tumor cell monomorphism with absent or low cytological atypia, and a low mitotic (<2 mitoses/mm^2) and proliferative status (<2% Ki-67 positive cells). These tumors are slow growing but can have a higher mitotic (>2 mitoses/mm^2) and proliferative index (>2% Ki-67 positive cells) – "well-differentiated neuroendocrine tumor with uncertain malignancy."

"Well-differentiated neuroendocrine carcinomas" are characterized by the presence of metastasis and/or invasiveness of the tumor. Well-differentiated neuroendocrine cells stain diffusely and intensely positive for the granular and cytosol-based markers. These well-differentiated tumors are composed of one or more endocrine cell types, which reflect the normal endocrine cell population of the organ of origin.

Poorly differentiated neuroendocrine carcinomas are tumors that grow in the form of large, ill-defined solid aggregates with central abundant necrosis. These poorly differentiated tumors have a characteristic cellular atypia with a high mitotic index (>10 mitoses/mm^2) and proliferative status (>15% Ki-67 positive cells). They have a diffuse reactivity for neurone-specific enolase, protein gene product 9.5 and synaptophysin but only a scant reactivity for chromogranin A or cell-specific secretory products on immunohistochemistry.

The mixed exocrine–endocrine carcinomas are tumors in which the exocrine and endocrine cell populations are intimately mixed. The endocrine cell comprises about one-half of the tumor tissue, but the biological behavior is dependent on the exocrine component [7, 9, 10].

Neuroendocrine tumors of the pancreas

The endocrine pancreas is made up of the islets of Langerhans with four types of cells, namely glucagon, insulin, somatostatin, and pancreatic polypeptide causing the islet cell tumors. Few serotonin-producing enterochromaffin cells are also scattered in the exocrine tissue. Pancreatic endocrine tumors can stain for these cell types and their hormones, individually or in combination. Pancreatic endocrine tumors may contain ectopic cells not typically found in the endocrine pancreas: gastrin-producing cells, vasoactive intestinal peptide-producing cells, growth hormone-releasing factor, and adrenocorticotropin-producing cells [7].

Pancreatic neuroendocrine tumors are generally well-differentiated tumors that synthesize and secrete particular

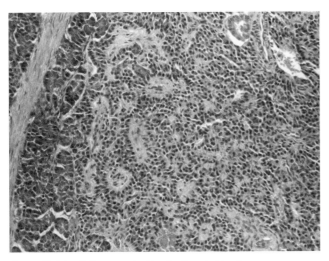

Figure 57.1 Insulin immunostained in cells of a typical insulinoma.

hormones. The symptoms of functional pancreatic neuroendocrine tumors depend on the hormones secreted, whereas symptoms of the non-functional tumors depend on the gross tumor mass. About 50% of the pancreatic neuroendocrine tumors are functioning tumors. Insulinomas make up the majority (75%) of pancreatic neuroendocrine tumors. Insulinomas are associated with hypersecretion of insulin and the subsequent development of related symptoms. (see Fig. 57.1). These tumors are small solitary benign tumors (1–2 cm), but a small proportion (approx. 10%) are multiple and malignant. Insulinomas that are <2 cm in size and non-invasive are classified as well-differentiated endocrine tumors with benign behavior. They have malignant behavior when >3 cm in size or with the presence of angioinvasion [7, 8]. Patients with benign tumors have a normal life expectancy after successful surgery, but malignant insulinomas have a 10-year survival of 29% [11].

About 60% of functioning tumors of the glucagon-producing cell-, gastrin-producing cells, vasoactive intestinal peptideproducing cells and adrenocorticotropin-producing cells, causing glucagonoma, gastrinoma, VIPoma, and Cushing syndrome,

respectively, are malignant. They are grossly invasive, metastatic to regional lymph nodes and the liver and on diagnosis are mostly >2 cm in size. These tumors are classified as low-grade malignant when >2 cm in size or in the presence of angioinvasion [7, 8]. Angioinvasion is of significant relevance in the classification of the pancreatic neuroendocrine tumors such that a tumor is considered malignant if angioinvasion is present, even if no other features suggestive of malignancy are present [12].

Glucagonomas are associated with a clinical syndrome of excess glucagon. About 60–70% of these are malignant and are typically large at 3–5 cm. These tumors stain positive for glucagon-producing cells, but often also stain positive for pancreatic polypeptide-, insulin- and somatostatin- producing cells. Atypical glucagon cell granules are found in functional glucagonomas, but typical cell granules are seen in the non-functioning tumor.

Pancreatic gastrinomas give rise to the Zollinger–Ellison syndrome and have a malignancy rate of 50–60%. Most of the pancreatic gastrinomas stain positive for gastrin and about half also stain for pancreatic polypeptide, insulin and/or somatostatin cells.

Pancreatic VIPomas are sporadic tumors. They are usually large (>2 cm) and similarly about 60% have already developed metastases to the lymph nodes and liver at the time of diagnosis.

Serotonin-producing tumors of the pancreas are rare. Again, these are relatively large with a high rate of metastasis on diagnosis. These tumors are commonly associated with the carcinoid syndrome. They have a poor prognosis due to delayed diagnosis and treatment. Pancreatic somatostatinomas are rare, usually large and present with symptoms of somatostatin excess [5, 7, 8].

The clinical features (Table 57.1) of functioning neuroendocrine tumors help distinguish them from the adenocarcinomas, but as many as 50% of pancreatic neuroendocrine tumors may be non-functional and hence clinically indistinguishable from adenocarcinoma of the pancreas. The distinction is important because treatment of neuroendocrine tumors is different from that of adenocarcinomas. Non-functioning tumors account for 20% of all pancreatic endocrine tumors. They do not have an associated syndrome caused by hormonal hypersecretion and their symptoms relate to the gross tumor bulk. They are usually large

Table 57.1 Pancreatic neuroendocrine tumors and their syndromes

Tumor	Frequency of pancreatic neuroendocrine tumors (%)	Malignancy (%)	Clinical syndrome
Insulinoma	70–75	<10	Hypoglycemia, weight gain
Gastrinoma	20–25	>50	Abdominal pain, diarrhea, peptic ulcers
VIPoma	3–5	>50	Secretory diarrhea, hypokalemia, achlorhydria, metabolic acidosis, flushing
Glucagonoma	1–2	>70	Necrolytic migratory erythema, diabetes, cachexia, thromboembolic disease
PPoma	<1	>60	Pain, weight loss, diarrhea
Somatostatinoma	<1	>50	Steatorrhea, diabetes, gallstones, weight loss
Serotoninoma/ carcinoid	<1	90	Classic carcinoid syndrome, flushing, diarrhea, wheeze, cardiac fibrosis, pellagra dermatosis

PPoma, pancreatic polypeptide-secreting tumor.
Adapted from [15].

and have metastasized at time of diagnosis. Histologically these tumors may stain positive for insulin, glucagon and polypeptide on immunohistochemistry. Survival rates of 65% and 49% at 5 and 10 years respectively have been reported for non-functioning pancreatic tumors [13]. Poorly differentiated neuroendocrine carcinomas of the pancreas are highly malignant tumors, diagnosed as small cell carcinomas, and have a poor prognosis with a life expectancy of 1 year.

Neuroendocrine tumors of the gastrointestinal tract

The gastrointestinal mucosa has a number of endocrine cell types. The histamine-producing enterochromaffin-like cells, gastrin-producing G cells and secretin, cholecystokinin, motilin or gastric inhibitory polypeptide cells are found in the upper small intestine. Serotonin-producing enterochromaffin cells or somatostatin D cells are scattered throughout the gastrointestinal tract, and enteroglucagon L cells and neurotensin cells are present in the lower small intestine, appendix, colon, and rectum. The enterochromaffin-like cells are the main component of the gastric endocrine tumors. Gastrin and somatostatin cells are the main component of the duodenal endocrine tumors, enterochromaffin cells for tumors of the jejunum, ileum, appendix, and proximal colon, and enteroglucagon cells for tumors of the distal colon and rectum. More so, neuroendocrine tumors arising in different parts of the gastrointestinal tract show different pathogenetic, histological and clinical patterns (see Table 57.2). The term "carcinoid" used in classification previously is applied to the well-differentiated endocrine tumors of the gastrointestinal tract, while the well-differentiated endocrine carcinomas are termed "malignant carcinoid." [7].

Gastric neuroendocrine tumors

Gastric neuroendocrine tumors are mainly well-differentiated, non-functioning enterochromaffin-like cell tumors arising in the corpus or fundus mucosa. Occasionally gastrinomas and a few histamine and 5-hydroxytryptophan-producing enterochromaffin cell tumors with metastases and functional carcinoid syndrome have been reported. The gastrin-producing enterochromaffin-like tumors are usually benign [7]. They have been found to be associated with diffuse type A chronic atrophic gastritis, achlorhydria, and marked hypergastrinemia causing enterochromaffin cell hyperplasia. Chronic atrophic gastritis-associated tumors are typically slow growing with low rates of local and distant metastases and low mortality rates. About 10% of the enterochromaffin-like cell gastric neuroendocrine tumors have also been found to be associated with hypertrophic gastropathy and hypergastrinemia due to Zollinger–Ellison syndrome in multiple endocrine neoplasia type 1 (MEN 1). They are generally <1.5 cm, limited to the mucosa and submucosa, and have a good prognosis. Malignant enterochromaffin-like cell tumors also arise in the corpus or fundus mucosa and are sporadic tumors. They are usually solitary, >1 cm in diameter, highly

aggressive and have often metastasized on diagnosis with a high mortality rate. The poorly differentiated carcinomas arise in any part of the stomach and have a poor survival. True mixed exocrine-endocrine carcinomas are rare [7, 10].

Neuroendocrine tumors of duodenum and upper jejunum

Duodenal tumors are generally uncommon and mostly arise in the first or second part of the duodenum. Gastrinomas account for two-thirds of the duodenal neuroendocrine tumors. Non-functioning small gastrin tumors are confined to the mucosa–submucosa of the proximal duodenum and have a benign behavior. Functioning gastrinomas can occur at any part of the duodenum and are also found in the upper jejunum. They are often multiple, associated with Zollinger–Ellison syndrome in MEN 1, usually small and are metastatic to regional lymph nodes. They may also be metastatic to the liver, but this is usually late compared with metastasis to regional lymph node, which are often larger than the primary tumor. Most functional gastrin cell tumors fall into the classification of low-grade malignant behavior, as sporadic or MEN-associated gastrinomas, whereas the non-functioning gastrin tumors have benign behavior. Somatostatin cell tumors, gangliocytic paragangliomas, serotonin-producing enterochromaffin cell tumors and small cell carcinomas occur in the second part of the duodenum with preponderance for the ampulla and papilla. Somatostatin-producing tumors account for 15% of all duodenal neuroendocrine tumors, are usually large, deeply invasive, and metastatic to regional lymph nodes. They often cause obstruction of bile flow and may be associated with neurofibromatosis, but are rarely functional. Somatostatinomas fall into the classification of non-functioning well-differentiated duodenal neuroendocrine tumors with low-grade malignant potential. The serotonin-producing enterochromaffin cell tumors are rare, typically non-functioning, confined to the mucosa–submucosa, and are benign with a better prognosis than duodenal gastrinomas or somatostatinomas. These tumors are also classified as non-functioning well-differentiated tumors with low malignant potential. The gangliocytic paragangliomas are deep in the duodenal wall invading the muscularis propria and have a pseudoinfiltrative pattern of growth, but are benign. These are classified as neuroendocrine tumor with benign behavior. A few malignant cases have been reported. However, the small cell carcinomas are poorly differentiated, invasive and highly malignant. More often, at the time of diagnosis they have metastasized into the regional lymph nodes and liver [5, 7, 8, 14].

Neuroendocrine tumors of the ileum, cecum, colon and rectum

Neuroendocrine tumors of the ileum and cecum are mostly well-differentiated serotonin and substance-P producing enterochromaffin cell tumors. They are deeply invasive, causing local obstructive symptoms, and are associated with reactive fibrosis. The tumors are frequently multiple and have a distinct histological structure made up of well-demarcated solid nests with peripheral palisading of highly granular, serotonin-rich tumor cells

Table 57.2 Summary of the WHO classification of gastroenteropancreatic neuroendocrine tumors

Classification	Well-differentiated endocrine tumor	Well-differentiated endocrine tumor	Well-differentiated endocrine carcinoma	Poorly differentiated endocrine carcinoma
Site	**Benign behavior**	**Low-grade malignant**	**Low-grade malignant**	**High-grade malignant**
Pancreas	Confined to pancreas <2 cm, <2 mitoses per 10 HPF <2% Ki-67 positive cells No vascular invasion	Confined to pancreas ≥2 cm >2 mitoses per 10 HPF >2% Ki-67 positive cells or vascular invasion	Well to moderately differentiated Mitotic rate often higher (2–10 per 10 HPF) Ki-67 index >5% Gross local invasion and/or metastases	Necrosis common >10 mitoses per 10 HPF >15% Ki-67 positive cells Prominent vascular and/or perineural invasion
	– functioning: insulinoma – non-functioning	– functioning: gastrinoma, insulinoma, VIPoma, glucagonoma, or somatostatinoma – non-functioning	– functioning: gastrinoma, insulinoma, VIPoma, glucagonoma, or somatostatinoma – non-functioning	Small cell carcinoma
Stomach	Confined to mucosa–submucosa, ≤1 cm No vascular invasion	Confined to mucosa–submucosa, >1 cm or vascular invasion	Well- to moderately differentiated Invasion to muscularis propria or beyond or metastases	Small cell carcinoma
	Non-functioning: – ECL tumor associated with chronic atrophic gastritis (CAG) or MEN 1 – serotonin-producing tumor – gastrin-producing tumor	Non-functioning: – ECL tumor associated with CAG or MEN 1 or sporadic – serotonin-producing tumor – gastrin-producing tumor	Functioning or non-functioning: – ECL tumor usually sporadic – serotonin-producing tumor – gastrin-producing tumor	Usually non-functioning Occasionally with Cushing syndrome
Duodenum, upper jejunum	Confined to mucosa–submucosa, ≤1 cm No vascular invasion	Confined to mucosa–submucosa, >1 cm or vascular invasion	Well- to moderately differentiated Extending beyond submucosa or beyond or metastases	Small cell carcinoma
	Non-functioning: – gastrin-producing tumor – serotonin-producing tumor – gangliocytic paraganglioma	– gastrin-producing tumor, functioning or non-functioning, sporadic or MEN 1 associated – somatostatin-producing tumor with or without Recklinghausen – serotonin-producing tumor, non-functioning	– gastrin-producing tumor, functioning or non-functioning, sporadic or MEN 1 associated – somatostatin-producing tumor with or without Recklinghausen – serotonin-producing tumor, non-functioning or functioning (any size or extension) – malignant gangliocytic paraganglioma	
Ileum, colon, rectum	Confined to mucosa–submucosa, ≤1 cm (small intestine) ≤2 cm (large intestine) No vascular invasion	Confined to mucosa–submucosa, >1 cm (small intestine) >2 cm (large intestine) or vascular invasion	Well to moderately differentiated Invasion to muscularis propria or beyond or metastases	Small cell carcinoma
	Non-functioning: – serotonin-producing tumor – enteroglucagon-producing tumor	Non-functioning: – serotonin-producing tumor – enteroglucagon-producing tumor	– serotonin-producing tumor with or without carcinoid syndrome – enteroglucagon-producing carcinoma	
Appendix	Non-functioning Confined to appendiceal wall ≤2 cm No vascular invasion	Enteroglucagon-producing Confined to subserosa >2 cm or vascular invasion	Well to moderately differentiated Invasion to mesoappendix or beyond or metastases	Small cell carcinoma
	Non-functioning: – serotonin-producing tumor	Non-functioning: – enteroglucagon-producing tumor	– serotonin-producing tumor with or without carcinoid syndrome	

Adapted from [7] and [16].

surrounding an inner part of smaller, less granulated, polyhedral cells. Small proportions of these tumors are functional, causing the carcinoid syndrome, and are metastatic to the liver.

Neuroendocrine tumors of the colon are rare. They are poorly differentiated neuroendocrine carcinomas that have usually metastasized by the time they are diagnosed and hence, have a poor prognosis. They are mostly synaptophysin cell tumors, and rarely serotonin- and somatostatin- producing cell tumors. Neuroendocrine tumors of the rectum have a better prognosis and include enteroglucagon- and polypeptide-producing cell tumors. They are mostly small tumors expanding in the submucosa and have a distinctive trabecular structure. They usually only metastasize if >2 cm in size [5, 7, 8, 14].

Neuroendocrine tumors of the appendix

Neuroendocrine tumors of the appendix account for about 20% of the gastrointestinal neuroendocrine tumors. They are usually found incidentally in the appendicectomy specimens from patients with appendicitis. The tumors mostly stain positive for enterochromaffin cells producing serotonin and substance P and are seen in the mucosa and deep mucosa of the tip of the appendix. Most tumors are confined to the appendix and are benign, despite often infiltrating the muscularis propria. A tiny proportion of these tumors have metastasis to regional lymph nodes when the size is >2.5 cm. The serotonin-producing cell tumors never metastasize to the liver and development of carcinoid syndrome is rare. Rare enteroglucagon-producing neuroendocrine tumors are also found in the appendix. Goblet cell tumors have also been identified in the appendix and these represent the mixed exocrine–endocrine neuroendocrine tumors that are low grade malignant with a poorer prognosis [5, 7, 8, 14].

Conclusion

Neuroendocrine tumors are generally slow growing but prognosis depends on the tumor site, histological type, degree of differentiation, mitotic rate, Ki-67 index, tumor size, depth, location and presence of lymph node or liver metastases. The definition and classification of neuroendocrine cells and tumors have been revised repeatedly over decades in an attempt to improve prediction of prognosis. The recent 2000 WHO classification defines these tumors based on the above factors into well-differentiated neuroendocrine tumors (benign or uncertain malignancy), well-differentiated neuroendocrine carcinomas (low-grade malignancy), poorly differentiated neuroendocrine carcinomas (high-grade malignancy) and mixed tumors. Recent studies [17] have suggested that this WHO classification is feasible for evaluating the characteristics of neuroendocrine tumors and the prognosis and considering them jointly with the clinical and biological features of the tumor to prescribe appropriate treatment.

References

1. Langley K. The neuroendocrine concept today. *Ann. N. Y. Acad. Sci.* 1994;15:1–17.
2. Modlin IM, Lye KD, Kidd M. A 5-decade analysis of 13,715 carcinoid tumors. *Cancer* 2003;97:934–959.
3. Taal BG, Visser O. Epidemiology of neuroendocrine tumours. *Neuroendocrinology* 2004;80(Suppl 1):3–7.
4. William ED, Sandler M. The classification of carcinoid tumours. *Lancet* 1963;1:238–239.
5. Capella C, Heitz PU, Höfler H, et al. Revised classification of neuroendocrine tumors of the lung, pancreas and gut. *Digestion* 1994;55(Suppl 3):11–23.
6. Rindi G, Capella C, Solcia E. Cell biology, clinicopathological profile and classification of gastroenteropancreatic endocrine tumours. *J. Mol. Med.* 1998;76:413–420.
7. Solcia E, Klöppel G, Sobin LH, in collaboration with 9 pathologists from 4 countries. *Histological Typing of Endocrine Tumours*, 2nd edition. World Health Organization International histological classification of tumours. Berlin: Springer Verlag, 2000.
8. Rindi G, Villanacci V, Ubiali A. Biological and molecular aspects of gastroenteropancreatic neuroendocrine tumors. *Digestion* 2000; 62(Suppl 1):19–26.
9. Klöppel G, Heitz PU, Capella C, et al. Pathology and nomenclature of human gastrointestinal neuroendocrine (carcinoid) tumors and related lesions. *World J. Surg.* 1996;20:132–141.
10. Rindi G, Luinetti O, Cornaggia M, et al. Three subtypes of gastric argyrophil carcinoid and the gastric neuroendocrine carcinoma: a clinicopathologic study. *Gastroenterology* 1993;104:994–1006.
11. Service FJ, McMahon MM, O'Brien PC, et al. Functioning insulinoma – incidence, recurrence, and long-term survival of patients: a 60-year study. *Mayo Clin. Proc.* 1991;66:711–719.
12. La Rosa S, Sessa F, Capella C, et al. Prognostic criteria in nonfunctioning pancreatic endocrine tumours. *Virchows Arch.* 1996;429:323–333.
13. Bartsch DK, Schilling T, Ramaswamy A, et al. Management of nonfunctioning islet cell carcinomas. *World J. Surg.* 2000;24:1418–1424.
14. Klöppel G, Anlauf M. Epidemiology, tumour biology and histopathological classification of neuroendocrine tumours of the gastrointestinal tract. *Best Pract. Res. Clin. Gastroenterol.* 2005;19:507–517.
15. Barakat MT, Meeran K, Bloom SR. Neuroendocrine tumours. *Endocr. Relat. Cancer* 2004;11:1–18.
16. Ramage JK, Davies AH, Ardill J, et al. Guidelines for the management of gastroenteropancreatic neuroendocrine (including carcinoid) tumours. *Gut* 2005;54(Suppl 4)iv:1–16.
17. Bajetta E, Catena L, Procopio G, et al. Is the new WHO classification of neuroendocrine tumours useful for selecting an appropriate treatment? *Ann. Oncol.* 2005;16:1374–1380.

58 Imaging of Gastrointestinal Neuroendocrine Tumors

Andrew F. Scarsbrook and Rachel R. Phillips

Key points

- Gastrointestinal neuroendocrine tumors are rare neoplasms with varying malignant potential depending on tumor location and type.
- Tumors present with symptoms related to mass effect, with a constellation of symptoms related to hormonal hypersecretion or with metastatic disease.
- Tumors may arise sporadically or be associated with syndromes, particularly multiple endocrine neoplasia type 1 (MEN 1) and neurofibromatosis type 1. Following diagnosis of a pancreaticoduodenal neuroendocrine tumor, the possibility of multiple endocrine neoplasia type 1 or neurofibromatosis type 1 should always be excluded.
- Accurate preoperative localization and staging are essential to guide surgical resection, the only curative option. A combined approach using both anatomical (ultrasound, computerized tomography, magnetic resonance imaging) and functional imaging (somatostatin receptor scintigraphy) is usually required.
- Co-registration of structural and functional imaging is often of incremental value in localizing the site of the primary tumor and any metastatic disease. Debulking of metastatic disease, whether within the mesentery, lymph nodes or the liver, may offer symptomatic relief.

Introduction

The gastrointestinal (GI) tract contains mucosal neuroendocrine cells throughout its length. Consequently, GI neuroendocrine tumors (NET) can arise from any component of the alimentary tract including organs which develop from the GI tract embryologically such as the lung, biliary tract, pancreas and liver. NET have a variable malignant potential depending on their site of origin and may spread via the lymphatics or hematogenously to regional lymph nodes, the liver, bone or the brain. GI tract NET have a reported incidence of 1/100 000, but this is likely to be an underestimate, the incidence at autopsy being higher, 8/100 000 [1].

NET arising from the GI tract can be divided into two distinct groups.

1 Carcinoid tumors that arise from: the foregut (lung, thymus, esophagus, stomach, duodenum, liver, biliary tract, and pancreas): the midgut (small bowel, appendix, right-sided colon, and ovary or testis): and hindgut (left-sided colon and rectum). The vast majority of tumors arise within the small bowel, appendix and proximal right colon.

2 Islet cell or pancreaticoduodenal NET including gastrinomas, insulinomas, glucagonomas, VIPomas, pancreatic polypeptidomas, and somatostatinomas.

Carcinoid and islet cell tumors usually arise sporadically but may be associated with rarer endocrine syndromes. Multiple endocrine neoplasia type 1 (MEN 1) is associated with pancreaticoduodenal neuroendocrine (often multiple) and foregut carcinoid tumors (lung, thymus and gastric). Von Hippel-Lindau syndrome (VHL) is associated with pancreatic NET and neurofibromatosis type 1 (NF1) is associated with duodenal carcinoid tumors.

There has been a recent shift in NET classification to a histologically based system with subtyping based on cellular differentiation [2]. For the purposes of this chapter on imaging, however, the traditional classification of NET by site of embryological origin will be used.

Imaging techniques in gastrointestinal neuroendocrine tumors

Imaging of neuroendocrine tumors is often challenging and requires meticulous attention to detail. A combination of anatomical and functional techniques is usually required but varies according to tumor type and location. Imaging techniques include ultrasonography (transabdominal, endoscopic and intraoperative),

Clinical Endocrine Oncology, 2nd edition. Edited by Ian D. Hay and John A.H. Wass. © 2008 Blackwell Publishing. ISBN 978-1-4051-4584-8.

computerized tomography (CT), magnetic resonance imaging (MRI), angiography, arterial stimulation and venous sampling (ASVS) and a variety of functional imaging techniques including somatostatin receptor scintigraphy (SRS), meta-iodobenzyl-guanidine (MIBG) scintigraphy and positron emission tomography (PET). Co-registration of structural and functional imaging is often of incremental value to accurately localize the primary tumor and any metastatic disease [3]. The key roles of imaging are to accurately localize and stage suspected tumors, monitor response to treatment and detect new manifestations of established disease.

Imaging of GI carcinoid tumors

Over 90% of all carcinoid tumors arise within the GI tract. Clinical presentation is often non-specific and tumors can remain undiagnosed for many years. Recent advances in CT, MRI, ultrasonography and scintigraphy have improved detection, which may partially explain why disease incidence has increased by 50% in the last 25 years. Patients with midgut NET have an increased risk of synchronous gastrointestinal or genitourinary tract carcinomas possibly due to tumorigenic peptide secretion by the carcinoid tumor [4].

Imaging of foregut tumors

Gastric carcinoid

Nine percent of GI tract carcinoid tumors arise within the stomach [5]. There are three subtypes: Type I (70–80%) is associated with hypergastrinemia and chronic atrophic gastritis and is usually diagnosed coincidentally. The typical appearance is multiple, small (<2 cm) nodules within the gastric fundus/body and metastatic disease is rare. Type II (5–6%) occurs almost exclusively in MEN 1 patients with gastrinoma-associated hypergastrinemia. Appearances consist of multiple, small, antral/fundal nodules, usually detected at surveillance endoscopy and metastatic disease is uncommon. Type III (14–25%) occurs in the absence of underlying gastric pathology. Typically there is a large solitary mass in the gastric body/fundus, indistinguishable from a gastric carcinoma. This subtype is more aggressive and may be metastatic at diagnosis. Preoperative staging with cross-sectional imaging (CT or MRI) and SRS is indicated.

Barium studies are often negative but may demonstrate a polyp(s), which may ulcerate. Gastroscopy and biopsy are required for subtyping. Endoscopic ultrasound (EUS) demonstrates depth of invasion and typically shows a hypoechoic, submucosal mass extending into the muscularis propria/serosa. At CT, enhancing submucosal nodule(s) (Fig. 58.1) or a mass may be seen. Visualization is improved by using water as oral contrast. At MRI, tumors are mildly hyperintense on T2-weighted and isointense on T1-weighted imaging and may enhance following intravenous gadolinium.

Biliary carcinoid

Extrahepatic biliary carcinoid is very rare, most cases arising within the gallbladder. Patients present with jaundice and pain.

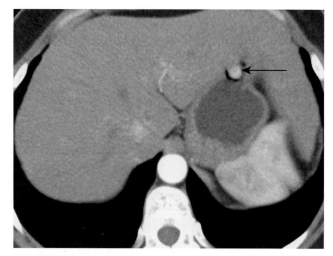

Figure 58.1 Image from a contrast-enhanced CT showing a small enhancing gastric nodule (arrow) in a patient with Type I gastric carcinoid.

Local invasion and metastases are less common than with cholangiocarcinoma, which is indistinguishable on imaging.

Duodenal carcinoid

Two to 3% of GI carcinoid tumors arise within the duodenum [6]. Most occur in the first or second part, except in NF1 patients where the tumor is characteristically periampullary and may present with biliary obstruction. Approximately one-third of patients have lymph node or hepatic metastases at presentation.

Most duodenal carcinoid tumors are detected coincidentally at endoscopy and biopsy is essential for diagnosis. Barium studies may demonstrate either a focal intraluminal polyp(s) within the proximal duodenum, occasionally with ulceration, or a focal mural mass. CT, using a multi-phasic acquisition, demonstrates a focal duodenal mass with arterial enhancement in most cases. The primary tumor is not detected in 10%. MRI may demonstrate a low T1-weighted, heterogeneously enhancing, polypoid or submucosal mass with ulceration. EUS and SRS are useful to evaluate the extent of local and distant disease.

Imaging of midgut tumors

Appendiceal carcinoid

Up to 50% of GI carcinoid tumors arise from the appendix and these are usually discovered incidentally following appendicectomy. Ninety percent are smaller than 1.5 cm and 25-year follow-up suggests that they almost never recur [7]. Patients with larger tumors have an increased risk of metastatic disease. Imaging is not necessary in most patients with small coincidental tumors. In patients with larger tumors (>1.5 cm), CT and SRS should be used to assess local and distant disease.

Small bowel carcinoid

About 33% of GI carcinoid tumors arise from the small intestine, most commonly within the distal ileum/ileocecal region. Tumors rarely obstruct the bowel lumen, but invasion through the muscularis mucosa is common and results in desmoplasia and associated mesenteric, omental and peritoneal fibrosis. This can cause intermittent small bowel obstruction and/or bowel wall ischemia. The primary tumor(s) is usually small (1–2 cm), sub-mucosal/intramural and may be very difficult to detect. There are multiple primaries in 29–40% and a synchronous malignancy (usually GI) is present in 29–53% of patients. Even if the primary is less than 1 cm, nodal and liver metastases are present in about 70% of patients at presentation.

Barium studies rarely detect the primary tumor(s) but may demonstrate a smooth, intraluminal filling defect(s) in the dis-tal ileum. More commonly, retraction, fixation and tethering of small bowel loops in association with an exocentric, partially calcified, mesenteric mass are seen.

Cross-sectional imaging using CT or MR requires a meticulous technique for detection of small primary tumors, which are not localized in 40% of scans. At CT, small, enhancing, submucosal lesions can be obscured by oral, iodinated, contrast media and water should be used instead. A triphasic technique using thin, contiguous slices acquired prior to intravenous contrast and during arterial and venous phase enhancement is essential. This technique enables detection of sub-centimeter bowel wall abnor-malities. On CT or MR, the primary tumor may also appear as focal asymmetric bowel wall thickening, with MR signal intensity isointense to muscle on T1-weighted and isointense or mildly hyperintense to muscle on T2-weighted imaging (Fig. 58.2a).

Extraluminal mesenteric extension is frequently present and is well demonstrated on CT. Mesenteric involvement has a char-acteristic spiculated/stellate configuration (Fig. 58.2b) and there is calcification in up to 70%. At MR, mesenteric lymph node exten-sion and desmoplastic reaction appears hypo- or isointense on T1-weighted and isointense on T2-weighted imaging; the stranding enhances following gadolinium. Calcification is not usually appre-ciated on MR. The radiating strands are not due to tumor infiltration but represent fibrotic proliferation/desmoplasia due to vasoactive hormone release by the primary tumor(s). Thickened small bowel loops representing tumor infiltration and/or ischaemia due to vessel sclerosis/angulation are also well demonstrated (Fig. 58.2c). Sub-sequent 3D image reconstruction allows multiplanar evaluation and is of incremental value in small lesion detection. In addition, arterial phase images (CT angiogram) can be processed to accurately determine the extent of any vascular encasement due to mesenteric involvement, a vital aid prior to surgical debulking (Fig. 58.2d).

Conventional angiography is infrequently used due to the improved detection of small bowel tumors using CT, MRI and scintigraphy. On rare occasions, angiography is still performed and may demonstrate a vascular blush at site of the primary tumor.

Imaging of hindgut tumors

Colonic carcinoid

Carcinoid tumors arising from the colon are generally aggressive and have a poor prognosis. Colonic tumors may be sessile, bulky (>5 cm), fungating, intraluminal lesions or annular, constricting lesions and are occasionally polypoid or submucosal. The differ-ential diagnosis is adenocarcinoma. Fifty to 60% of patients have metastases to the liver, lymph nodes, mesentery or peritoneum at diagnosis.

Rectal carcinoid

Rectal carcinoid tumors are usually small, less than 2 cm, poly-poidal, submucosal lesions above the dentate line, on the anterior or lateral rectal wall. Most are incidental, asymptomatic and have low malignant potential; however, if large, there is a greater incidence of metastatic disease.

Barium studies do not have high detection rates in the rectosig-moid; however, they are more accurate in the cecum and ascend-ing colon. EUS is used to determine the depth of involvement in rectal carcinoid tumors which appear as a hypoechoic submucosal mass which may extend into the muscularis propria or serosa.

Imaging of metastatic carcinoid tumors

Midgut carcinoid is often metastatic at presentation. Hepatic meta-stases are well depicted on CT or MR and more distant disease involving the lungs, bones and peritoneum can also be assessed. Liver metastases are common and are characteristically hypervas-cular being most easily detected on arterial phase CT images (Fig. 58.3a). At MR, liver metastases are often complex cystic lesions with low T1-weighted and high T2-weighted signal (Fig. 58.3b) and moderately intense arterial phase enhancement following gado-linium. Larger metastases may show heterogeneous enhancement and central necrosis. Functional imaging frequently demonstrates tracer uptake within hepatic metastases unless they are predomin-antly cystic. Guided biopsy can be performed under CT or (more frequently) ultrasound guidance. Less common sites of metastatic disease include the pancreas, ovaries, lungs and mediastinum.

Somatostatin receptor scintigraphy

Midgut carcinoid tumors express somatostatin receptors and scintigraphy using radiolabeled somatostatin analogs (SRS) is widely used as a first-line sensitive method of diagnosing, staging and monitoring patients with GI carcinoid tumors. SRS is a useful staging tool because it is a whole-body technique that can detect lesions as small as 6 mm and may identify unsuspected sites of metastatic disease. SRS is also important for assessing patients suitable for palliative radiolabeled octreotide therapy and for monitoring therapeutic response in these patients.

Single photon emission computed tomography (SPECT) sig-nificantly increases the sensitivity and accuracy of SRS compared to planar scintigraphy alone (Fig. 58.4a, b). Correlation with contem-porary cross-sectional imaging is required to improve anatomical localization.

Use of image fusion software facilitates co-registration of ana-tomical (CT or MRI) and scintigraphic (SPECT) data and aids localization. Recently hybrid CT–gamma camera systems have been introduced and these are a highly accurate method of tumor and metastatic disease localization [8].

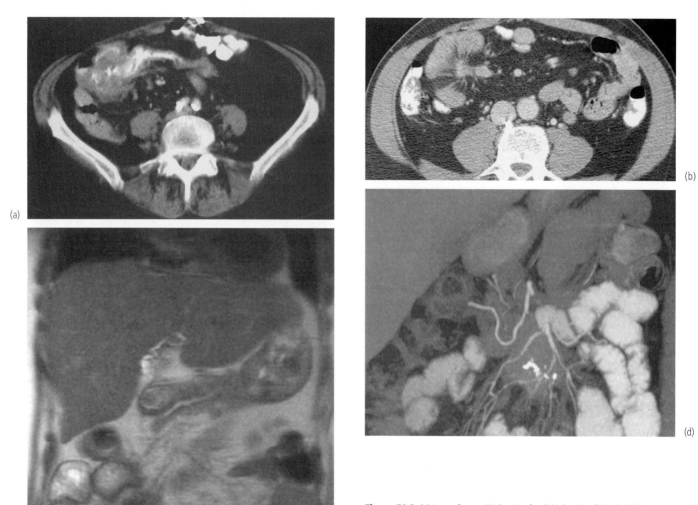

Figure 58.2 (a) Image from a CT showing focal thickening of the distal ileum and ileocecal junction in a patient with midgut carcinoid. (b) Image from a CT showing the characteristic desmoplastic reaction within the small bowel mesentery of a patient with ileal carcinoid. (c) Coronal image from a T2-weighted MR image showing multiple loops of thickened distal ileum, mesenteric fibrosis and a mesenteric mass (arrow) in a patient with midgut carcinoid. (d) Coronal reconstructed image from the arterial phase acquisition of a CT showing a mesenteric mass that encases several of the ileal branches of the superior mesenteric artery in a patient with ileal carcinoid.

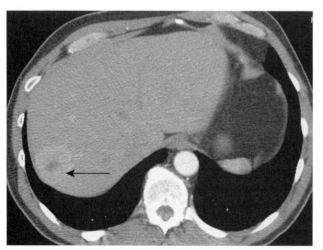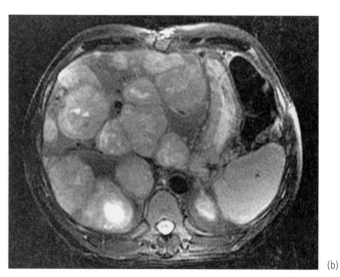

Figure 58.3 (a) CT image from the hepatic arterial phase acquisition showing an avidly enhancing carcinoid liver metastasis (arrow) in the right lobe of the liver with central necrosis. The patient had a primary midgut tumor in the ileum. (b) Axial T2-weighted MR image showing multiple carcinoid liver metastases. The patient had a primary pancreatic carcinoid tumor which is a very rare primary site.

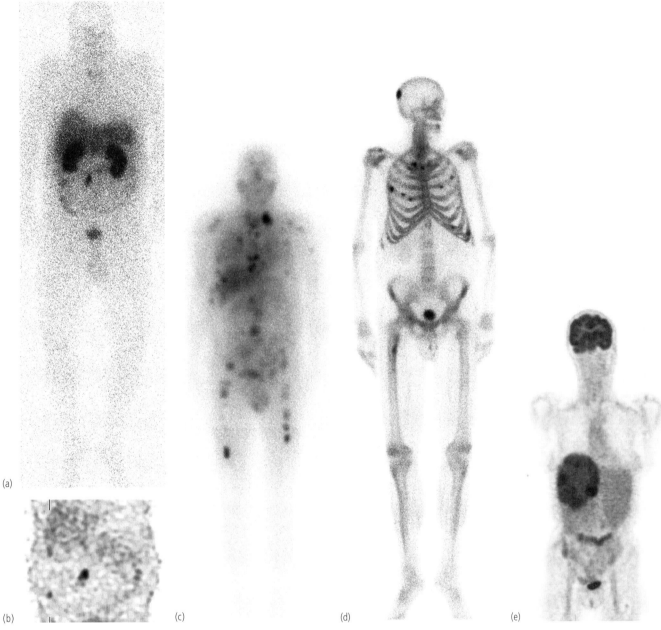

Figure 58.4 (a) 24 h planar and (b) 24 h coronal SPECT images (anterior) from a [111]Indium-octreotide scintigram showing tracer uptake within the mid abdomen due to a mesenteric carcinoid nodal mass and more subtle uptake within the right iliac fossa which corresponded to the primary ileal carcinoid tumor within the distal small bowel. (c) Anterior 24 h planar image from a ^{131}I-MIBG scintigram in a patient with metastatic ileal carcinoid showing multiple abnormal areas of tracer uptake throughout the marrow-containing bones and the liver. (d) Anterior planar image from a [99m]technetium-MDP bone scintigram showing multiple areas of abnormal tracer uptake within the bones due to metastases from a midgut carcinoid tumor. (e) Coronal image from an ^{18}F-FDG PET scan showing abnormal tracer uptake within the liver due to a poorly differentiated primary hepatic carcinoid tumor.

MIBG scintigraphy

Iodinated MIBG (^{123}I or ^{131}I) should be used as a complementary functional imaging technique, particularly in patients with midgut carcinoid tumors. MIBG scintigraphy has a lower overall sensitivity than SRS and is positive in ~50% [9]. The technique is most useful if other imaging methods have failed to localize disease or when therapeutic ^{131}I-MIBG is being considered (Fig. 58.4c).

Bone scintigraphy

Bone metastases are relatively uncommon in carcinoid disease, arising more often from hindgut tumors, and are usually osteoblastic. Radiographic signs may be subtle and easily missed; however, sclerotic bony deposits are more readily demonstrated on cross-sectional imaging. MRI provides the most sensitive detection of marrow metastases (sensitivity ~100%) and appearances are identical to bony metastases from other primary tumors. Bone scintigraphy is also a reliable method of identifying bony metastases with a sensitivity of 90% (Fig. 58.4d). MIBG and octreotide scintigraphy may underestimate bony deposits in 50–80% of carcinoid patients and bone scintigraphy is often complementary in patients with advanced gastrointestinal NET and bone pain. Carcinoid tumors and any metastatic disease may have similar or variable affinity for different radiotracers; as a result no single functional test is perfect and a combination of different techniques frequently helps provide a comprehensive map of disease.

PET-CT

PET-CT shows the potential to be a definitive localization and staging method in patients with NET. However, the ubiquitous oncological PET tracer, fluorine-18-fluoro-deoxyglucose (FDG) often fails to localize well-differentiated NET because of their low metabolic rate [10]. Conversely, poorly differentiated NET have a high glucose turnover and can be FDG avid (Fig. 58.4e).

The amine precursor uptake and transport characteristics of NET offer highly specific PET tracer targets. Various radiolabeled serotonin precursors have been utilized for GEP-NET localization. Of these, perhaps carbon-11-5-hydroxytryptophan (5-HTP) and gallium-68-DOTA-octreotide (DOTATATE) show the greatest promise, with reported sensitivities for detection of NET as small as 2 mm exceeding all other techniques [10]. At present, these tracers are restricted to a few highly specialized centers.

With the recent advances in functional and anatomical imaging and the increased survival time of patients due to new treatment modalities, more unusual sites of metastatic disease can occasionally be demonstrated including soft tissue, breast, cardiac, scalp and orbital deposits.

Imaging of islet cell tumors

Neuroendocrine tumors of the pancreas are collectively referred to as islet cell tumors (Table 58.1). Islet cell tumors are rare with an incidence of approximately 1 in 100 000 [11]. Usually they are functionally active and present with a recognizable clinical syndrome due to hormonal hypersecretion. Twenty-five percent of islet cell tumors are non-functioning and present at a late stage with mass effect. Tumors have varying malignant potential and are usually sporadic but are occasionally associated with inherited syndromes. Diagnosis is often made from the combination of clinical presentation, biochemical and imaging findings. Of the more commonly occurring tumors the majority of insulinomas are benign, whilst most gastrinomas and non-functioning tumors are malignant.

Table 58.1 Islet cell tumor subtypes

	Insulinoma	Non-functioning	Gastrinoma	VIPoma	Glucagonoma	Somatostatinoma
Presentation	Episodic hypoglycemia	Abdominal pain, weight loss, jaundice	Abdominal pain, diarrhea, ZE syndrome	Diarrhea, hypokalemia, achlorhydria	Diabetes, weight loss, glossitis, erythema	Diabetes
Relative frequency	60% of cases	25% of cases	20% of cases	3% of cases	1% of cases	Rare <1% of cases
Age in years at presentation	30–60	50–60	30–50	40–50	50 (sporadic) 30 (if in MEN 1)	50–60
Tumor location	Most intrapancreatic (any location) Rarely extrapancreatic in duodenum, lung, cervix	Usually within pancreatic head	90% within gastrinoma triangle ~50% in duodenum, small bowel or stomach	80% intrapancreatic, usually within tail 10–20% extrapancreatic in retroperitoneal sympathetic chain or adrenal medulla	Pancreatic body and tail	50% pancreas 50% duodenum
Multiplicity	Usually solitary 10% multiple	Usually solitary	Often multiple	Rarely multiple	Usually solitary	Usually solitary
Size	Small 90% <2 cm	Large	Small	Large >2 cm	2–4 cm	2 cm or larger
Malignancy	10%	90%	60%	50–70%	70%	50%
Associations	5% MEN 1 IF so, then multiple and malignant in 25%		25% MEN 1 IF so, multiple and malignant in 25%	Rarely associated with MEN 1	Rarely associated with MEN 1	50% of duodenal tumors associated with NF1

ZE, Zollinger–Ellison syndrome.

The key roles of imaging are accurate tumor localization and staging, detection of new manifestations of disease and distinction from adenocarcinoma of the pancreas, which generally has a poorer prognosis. No single imaging technique is uniformly successful and a combination of different modalities is often complementary [12].

Islet cell tumors can usually be distinguished from pancreatic carcinoma by a variety of imaging features including presence of calcification (in 20% of islet cell tumors (Fig. 58.5a), but only 2% of carcinomas), central necrosis/cystic degeneration (Fig. 58.5b), lack of vascular encasement and/or ductal dilatation, or rarely due to the presence of tumor thrombus extending into the portal vein.

There is considerable debate regarding the ideal imaging strategy for patients with suspected pancreaticoduodenal NET. The best approach will vary according to local expertise and availability but generally consists of a combination of SRS with ultrasonography (especially EUS) and thin-slice CT or MRI. Invasive angiographic techniques and other functional imaging methods are much less frequently used.

Ultrasound

Transabdominal ultrasound is readily available but is operator dependent and only has a sensitivity of 50–60% in most centers. Detection is greatest for larger tumors (>3 cm) but is poor in those less than 1 cm. Tumors are generally well circumscribed and hypoechoic compared to normal pancreatic parenchyma; 10% are isoechoic and may only be detected due to glandular distortion. Larger tumors may be more heterogeneous with central necrosis and unclear margins, features implying malignancy. Liver metastases are usually hyperechoic, especially if due to a gastrinoma; transabdominal ultrasound has a sensitivity of 63% for their detection. Ultrasonic contrast may improve the detection rate.

Endoscopic ultrasound is much more sensitive with an overall sensitivity of 93% [13], but is less widely available, highly operator dependent and invasive. EUS is particularly useful for detection of

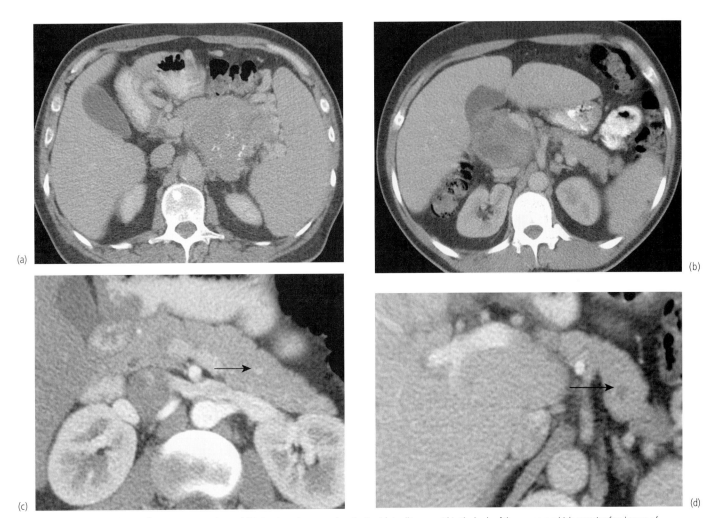

(a)

(b)

(c)

(d)

Figure 58.5 (a) Axial image from a contrast-enhanced CT showing a large non-functioning islet cell tumor within the body of the pancreas which contains focal areas of calcification. (b) Axial contrast-enhanced CT image showing a large heterogeneous mass within the head of the pancreas with central necrosis. Biopsy confirmed a malignant non-functioning pancreatic neuroendocrine tumor. (c) Axial CT image during arterial phase enhancement showing a tiny hypervascular insulinoma within the body of the pancreas (arrow). (d) Axial image from a contrast-enhanced CT showing a small cystic insulinoma within the pancreatic tail (arrow).

small tumors (<2 cm) (see Fig. 58.7b) and is more accurate than other modalities in evaluating peripancreatic lymph nodes and determining the relationship of the tumor(s) to vessels and ducts. There is reduced accuracy in tumors arising from the pancreatic tail, stomach or duodenal wall where the sensitivity falls to ~50%.

Intraoperative ultrasound has a very high sensitivity of up to 97% when combined with surgical palpation. This technique is particularly useful for localization of multiple lesions and can also be used to assess liver metastases and their exact relationship to other hepatic structures at the time of surgery.

CT

CT is the most common modality used for tumor localization due to its wide availability. It has an overall sensitivity for detection of insulinoma of 30–80%. Detection rates for other types of islet cell tumor are higher because these are generally larger at presentation. Biphasic, thin-section CT combined with EUS has a reported sensitivity of 100% [14]. CT has a reduced sensitivity in detection of multiple, extrapancreatic or pancreatic tail tumors.

The primary tumor(s) and metastases are often small (50% <1.3 cm) and isodense on unenhanced CT and many are non-contour deforming. Typically, islet cell tumors are hypervascular and avidly enhance following contrast (Fig. 58.5c). Occasionally

insulinomas are hypovascular, cystic (Fig. 58.5d), necrotic or calcified. Increased size, inhomogeneity, central necrosis and invasion of retroperitoneal structures suggest malignancy.

Careful attention to CT technique is critical. Following acquisition of unenhanced images using water as oral contrast, we perform a thin-section (1.5–3 mm) triple-phase, dynamic study after injecting 150 ml of intravenous contrast at 3–5 ml per second. Images are acquired during the arterial phase at 20–30 s, the pancreatic parenchymal phase at 40–70 s and during the portal venous phase at 60–70 s after the start of the injection. Precise timing depends on cardiac output and can be tailored to the individual patient by using a pump injector with triggering of the arterial phase image acquisition when contrast arrives within the proximal aorta. The field of view should cover the entire upper abdomen allowing detection of an extrapancreatic primary tumor and assessment of any metastatic disease.

MRI

MRI is the most sensitive technique for evaluating extrapancreatic extension and monitoring response to treatment. Islet cell tumors have decreased protein and hydrogen protons compared to the normal pancreas and are therefore of low signal on T1-weighted and high on T2-weighted sequences (Fig. 58.6a). If the tumor is

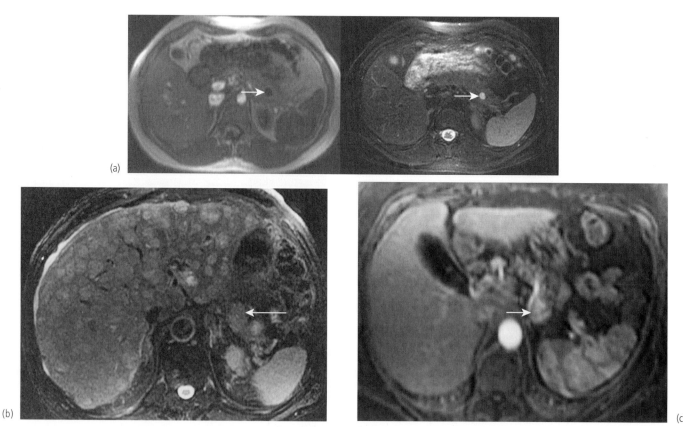

Figure 58.6 (a) T1- and T2-weighted axial MR images showing a small insulinoma (arrows) within the tail of the pancreas which has low T1 and high T2 signal. (b) Axial T2-weighted MR image in a patient with a metastatic pancreatic neuroendocrine tumor (somatostatinoma). There are innumerable liver metastases which have the same signal characteristics as the primary tumor within the tail of the pancreas (arrow). (c) Reformatted axial T1-weighted, gadolinium-enhanced MR image showing an insulinoma within the tail of the pancreas (arrow).

desmoplastic, it may be of decreased signal on T2-weighted sequences and demonstrate little enhancement. Functioning tumors are usually solid, small and homogeneous. There may be multiple small tumors especially if there is underlying MEN 1. Cystic/necrotic change may be demonstrated, particularly if the tumor is non-functioning.

Liver and nodal metastases have similar signal characteristics to the primary tumor (Fig. 58.6b). MRI is more accurate than CT for detection of small tumors and liver metastases [15]. There may be associated findings such as gastric wall hypertrophy or small bowel wall thickening due to elevated gastrin levels in patients with a gastrinoma.

The MRI technique should be optimized to allow the greatest chance of tumor localization. Important aspects include use of a phased array body coil (which improves signal to noise ratio), image acquisition using rapid breath hold sequences (to avoid respiratory motion artefacts) and contiguous thin slices. A combination of in and out of phase T1-weighted, fat-suppressed T2-weighted and fat-suppressed T1-weighted volume acquisitions prior to and sequentially following intravenous gadolinium injection are the critical sequences. Most tumors are hypervascular and optimally demonstrated on arterial phase images. The precise arterial phase for image acquisition is determined using a timing run following a small bolus of intravenous contrast. Subsequent CT or MR image manipulation and the use of multiplanar reformatting can allow distinction of an occult tumor from adjacent vessels (Fig. 58.6c).

Functional imaging

Many islet cell tumors express somatostatin receptors, particularly subtype 2 (SSRT-2) [16]. Consequently, SRS is widely employed as a highly sensitive method of localizing and staging patients with islet cell tumors (Fig. 58.7). The sensitivity of the technique varies according to the NET type (Table 58.2) and is proportional to the number of SSRT-2 receptors expressed on the cell surface. Insulinomas and poorly differentiated pancreatic NET typically have reduced numbers of receptors and SRS is less sensitive in these tumor types [16].

As with SRS in patients with GI carcinoid tumors, SPECT image acquisition and use of hybrid SPECT/CT significantly increase the sensitivity and accuracy of the technique (Plate 58.1). MIBG scintigraphy has a much lower sensitivity than SRS with only 9% of pancreatic NET showing uptake [9]. At present PET has a very limited role in imaging of patients with islet cell tumors and is limited to a few highly specialized centers.

Imaging of metastatic islet cell tumors

The detection and appropriate management of metastases improve prognostic and therapeutic consequences for patients with islet cell tumors. Most commonly, malignant islet cell tumors metastasize to local lymph nodes (50%), the liver (30%) and bone (7%) and less commonly to the lungs, mediastinum, peritoneum, spleen, brain and meninges [17]. SRS allows assessment of the biological activity of residual tumor. Hepatic metastases are usually hypervascular with the same imaging characteristics as

the primary tumor but vary in shape and size. Approximately 80–90% of liver metastases larger than 1–2 cm are visualized. CT or US-guided biopsy allows histological confirmation of presumed islet cell tumor metastases.

Islet cell bone metastases are usually osteosclerotic; however, 10% may be purely osteolytic, become sclerotic when healed or mixed osteolytic/osteosclerotic. There may be hyperintense epidural involvement. As with metastatic GI carcinoid tumors, bone scintigraphy, SRS and MR are useful for evaluation of suspected bony deposits.

CT or MR occasionally demonstrates peritoneal metastases, which manifest with ascites and omental soft tissue nodules.

Suggested imaging algorithms

The detection rate of GI neuroendocrine tumors varies depending on local expertise and the availability of different imaging techniques. A wide variety of different cross-sectional and functional imaging modalities can be employed with the optimal imaging strategy depending upon the clinical scenario. Suggested imaging algorithms for localization and staging of a suspected GI-NET (Fig. 58.8) or for disease monitoring and detection of new manifestations (Fig. 58.9) as used in our radiology department are provided.

Conclusion

The imaging of GI neuroendocrine tumors is often challenging and requires meticulous technique. In general, the combination of contrast-enhanced, thin-section, CT or MRI with functional imaging enables accurate tumor localization in most cases. SRS is widely available and a highly sensitive method of staging most tumors, perhaps with the exception of insulinomas, and should be employed as the first-line functional imaging technique [18]. Accuracy is improved with SPECT and anatomical–functional image fusion. EUS is often complementary in patients with islet cell, gastric, duodenal, and rectal NET. In a small number of cases,

Table 58.2 Sensitivity of somatostatin receptor scintigraphy in gastrointestinal NET

Tumor type	SSTR-2 expression	SRS sensitivity
Glucagonoma	80–100%	100%
Carcinoid	80–100%	85–95%
VIPoma	80–100%	88%
Non-functioning islet cell	80–100%	82%
Somatostatinoma	80–100%	80%
Gastrinoma	80–100%	73%
Insulinoma	50–70%	50–60%

Adapted from information in [16].

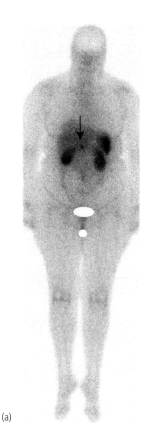

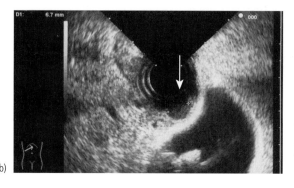

Figure 58.7 (a) 24 h anterior planar image from an ^{111}In-octreotide scintigram showing focal abnormal tracer uptake within the upper abdomen which was subsequently shown to be a duodenal gastrinoma following (b) endoscopic ultrasound-guided biopsy (arrow).

(a)

(b)

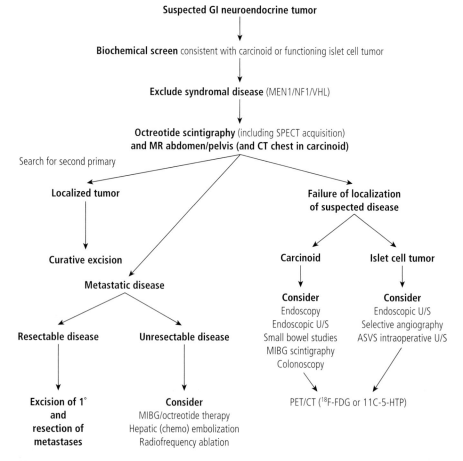

Suspected GI neuroendocrine tumor

↓

Biochemical screen consistent with carcinoid or functioning islet cell tumor

↓

Exclude syndromal disease (MEN1/NF1/VHL)

↓

Octreotide scintigraphy (including SPECT acquisition) **and MR abdomen/pelvis (and CT chest in carcinoid)**

Search for second primary

Localized tumor

↓

Curative excision

Metastatic disease

Resectable disease   **Unresectable disease**

Excision of 1° **and** **resection of** **metastases**

Consider MIBG/octreotide therapy Hepatic (chemo) embolization Radiofrequency ablation

Failure of localization of suspected disease

Carcinoid   **Islet cell tumor**

Consider Endoscopy Endoscopic U/S Small bowel studies MIBG scintigraphy Colonoscopy

Consider Endoscopic U/S Selective angiography ASVS intraoperative U/S

PET/CT (^{18}F-FDG or 11C-5-HTP)

Key
MEN1, multiple endocrine neoplasia type 1; NF1, neurofibromatosis type 1; VHL, von Hippel–Lindau disease; SPECT, single photon emission computed tomography; U/S, ultrasound; MIBG, ^{123}I–metaiodobenzylguanidine; ASVS, arterial stimulation and venous sampling; ^{18}F-FDG, fluorine-18-fluorodeoxyglucose; ^{11}C-5-HTP, carbon-11-5-hydroxytryptophan; PET/CT, positron emission tomography/computed tomography

Figure 58.8 Algorithm for investigation of suspected GI tract neuroendocrine tumors. (Adapted from information in [19, 20]).

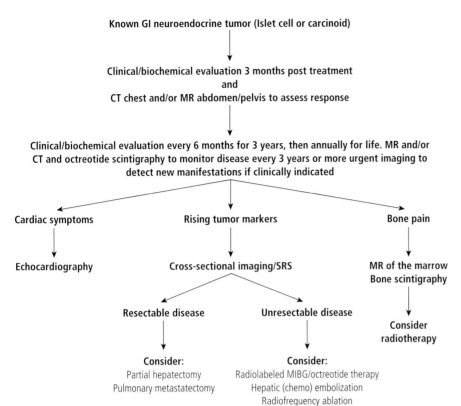

Figure 58.9 Algorithm for assessment of treatment response, disease monitoring and detection of new manifestations of GI-NET. (Adapted from information in [19, 20]).

intraoperative ultrasound, angiography or more specialized functional imaging methods may be required. MIBG scintigraphy is best used as second line in patients with metastatic carcinoid tumors and negative SRS or in patients being considered for palliative MIBG therapy. Bone scintigraphy can be complementary in patients with bone pain and suspected metastatic NET. Hybrid PET/CT using a variety of novel tracers shows great promise as the imaging modality par excellence once it becomes more widely available.

Screening for associated syndromes including NF1 and MEN 1 in patients with gastropancreaticoduodenal NET is advisable. In addition, the possibility of a synchronous gastrointestinal or genitourinary tumor should always be considered in patients with midgut carcinoid tumors.

References

1. Oberg K, Astrup L, Eriksson B, et al. Guidelines for the management of gastroenteropancreatic neurondocrine tumours. *Acta Oncol.* 2004; 43:617–625.
2. Solcia E, Kloppel G, Sobin LH. Histological typing of endocrine tumours, second edition. In *International Histological Classification of Tumours.* Berlin: World Health Organization, Springer, 2000.
3. Plockinger U, Rindi G, Arnold R, et al. Guidelines for the diagnosis and treatment of neuroendocrine gastrointestinal tumours. A consensus statement on behalf of the European Neuroendocrine Tumour Society. *Neuroendocrinology* 2004;80:394–424.
4. Gore RM, Berlin JW, Mehta UK, et al. GI carcinoid tumours: appearance of the primary and detecting metastases. *Best Pract. Res. Clin. Endocrinol. Metab.* 2005;19:245–263.
5. Delle Fare G, Capurso G, Annibale B, et al. Gastric neuroendocrine tumors. *Neuroendocrinology* 2004;80(Suppl 1):16–19.
6. Levy AD, Taylor LD, Abbott RM, et al. Duodenal carcinoids: imaging features with clinical-pathologic comparison. *Radiology* 2005;237: 967–972.
7. Kvols L. Carcinoids of the appendix. *Neuroendocrinology* 2004; 80(Suppl 1):33–34.
8. Pfennenberg AC, Eschmann SM, Hozer M, et al. Benefit of anatomical-functional image fusion in the diagnostic work-up of neuroendocrine neoplasms. *Eur. J. Nucl. Med. Molec. Imaging* 2003; 30:835–843.
9. Kaltsas G, Korbonits M, Heintz E, et al. Comparison of somatostatin analogue and meta-iodobenzylguanidine radionuclides in the diagnosis and localization of advanced neuroendocrine tumours. *J. Clin. Endocrinol. Metab.* 2001;86:895–902.
10. Pacak K, Eisnehofer G, Goldstein DS. Functional imaging of endocrine tumors: role of positron emission tomography. *Endocr. Rev.* 2004;25:568–580.
11. Power N, Reznek RH. Imaging islet cell tumours. *Imaging* 2002;14: 147–159.
12. Ricke J, Klose K-J, Mignon M, et al. Standardisation of imaging in neuroendocrine tumours; results of a European Delphi process. *Eur. J. Radiol.* 2001;37:8–17.
13. Anderson MA, Carpenter S, Thompson NW, et al. Endoscopic ultrasound is highly accurate and directs management in patients with neuroendocrine tumours of the pancreas. *Am. J. Gastroenterol.* 2000;95:2271–2277.

14. Noone TC, Hosey J, Firat Z, et al. Imaging and localization of islet cell tumours of the pancreas on CT and MR. *Best Pract. Res. Clin. Endocrinol. Metab.* 2005;19:195–211.

15. Owen NJ, Sohaib SAA, Peppercorn PD, et al. MRI of pancreatic neuroendocrine tumours. *Br. J. Radiol.* 2001;74:968–973 .

16. Reubi JC. Somatostatin and other peptide receptors as tools for tumour diagnosis and treatment. *Neuroendocrinology* 2004;80:51–56.

17. Debray MP, Geoffroy O, Laissy JP, et al. Imaging appearances of metastases from neuroendocrine tumours of the pancreas. *Br. J. Radiol.* 2001;74:1065–1070.

18. Ramage JK, Davies AHG, Ardill J, et al. Guidelines for the management of gastroenteropancreatic neuroendocrine including carcinoid tumours. *Gut* 2005;54(Suppl IV):iv1–iv16.

19. Kaltsas GA, Besser GM, Grossman A. The diagnosis and medical management of advanced neuroendocrine tumours. *Endocr. Rev.* 2004;25:458–511.

20. Guidelines from Neuroendocrine Tumors, National Comprehensive Cancer Network. Clinical Practice Guidelines in Oncology, v.1.2003.

59 Insulinomas and Hypoglycemia

Adrian Vella and F. John Service

> **Key points**
> - In the absence of self-induced hypoglycemia, insulinoma is the commonest cause of hyperinsulinemic hypoglycemia.
> - Diagnosis depends on the demonstration that a patient's symptoms occur during hypoglycemia and resolve with correction of plasma glucose.
> - Non-insulinoma pancreatogenous hypoglycemia syndrome is a recently recognized clinical entity where patients experience neuroglycopenia after meals and not in the fasting state.
> - Localization procedures should only be used after hyperinsulinemic hypoglycemia has been confirmed.
> - Insulinomas associated with multiple endocrine neoplasia syndrome type 1 tend to occur at a younger age, are frequently multiple and are more likely to recur.

Introduction

The observation that symptoms similar to those arising from overtreatment of diabetes mellitus with insulin could occur in non-diabetic patients led to the speculation of hyperinsulinemia as a cause of hypoglycemia in such patients. Support for the existence of hyperinsulinism was provided in 1926 by the identification, at the Mayo Clinic, of a malignant pancreatic islet cell tumor in a surgeon who presented with episodes of severe hypoglycemia and who was found to have a metastatic islet cell tumor [1]. Following his death, postmortem extracts of tissue metastatic to the liver were noted to cause marked hypoglycemia in laboratory animals. In the two decades after the identification of insulinoma as the source of excessive insulin secretion, it was recognized that food deprivation provoked hypoglycemia. Consequently, the prolonged fast evolved as the chief diagnostic test when the measurement of blood glucose during a spontaneous episode of hypoglycemia was not feasible.

Whipple's triad

In clinical practice, patients attribute many symptoms to hypoglycemia. Many of these are common and non-specific. Therefore, to correctly attribute these symptoms to a hypoglycemic disorder, a low plasma glucose level must be documented at the time that spontaneous symptoms occur and subsequently, one must

demonstrate that symptoms are relieved through the correction of the low glucose level (<50 mg/dl – 2.7 mmol/L). This is Whipple's triad: symptoms occur at the time of hypoglycemia, and resolve with the administration of glucose [2]. A normal plasma glucose level reliably obtained during the occurrence of spontaneous symptoms eliminates the possibility of a hypoglycemic disorder and no further evaluation is required. Normoglycemia during symptoms cannot be ascribed to spontaneous recovery of glycemia from prior hypoglycemia. Indeed, the opposite may occur where symptoms resolve despite persistence of low blood glucose [3]. Reflectance meter measurements are not reliable in these situations and can provide misleading information. Often, the measurement of plasma glucose level is not feasible when spontaneous symptoms occur during activities of ordinary life. Under such circumstances, the decision by a physician to proceed with further evaluation depends on a detailed history. A history of neuroglycopenic symptoms or a confirmed low plasma glucose level (<50 mg/dl – 2.7 mmol/L) warrants further testing.

Occasional individuals have plasma glucose levels in the 40–50 mg/dl range while fasting, without overt neuroglycopenic symptoms. Assuming that there is no evidence of β-cell hypersecretion and β-hydroxybutyrate concentrations (see below) are elevated it is unlikely that this represents a hypoglycemic disorder. It is important to emphasize that when a hypoglycemic disorder is suspected, the presence or absence of neuroglycopenia must be sought through simple tests of cognition such as recall, subtraction of serial sevens, etc.

Biochemical criteria for the diagnosis of a hyperinsulinemic hypoglycemic disorder in the presence of documented blood glucose levels near or below 45 mg/dl (2.5 mmol/L) include concomitant insulin levels equal to or greater than 3 µU/ml (18 pmol/L; measured by an immunochemiluminometric assay – ICMA) and

Clinical Endocrine Oncology, 2nd edition. Edited by Ian D. Hay and John A.H. Wass. © 2008 Blackwell Publishing. ISBN 978-1-4051-4584-8.

elevated C-peptide levels (≥200 pmol/L measured by ICMA) with a negative sulfonylurea screen. Although insulin and C-peptide levels are secreted in equimolar amounts, the different half-lives (4–6 min for insulin, 11–14 min for C-peptide) explain the discrepancy between values. The insulin/C-peptide ratio is the same for people with insulinoma as it is for normal subjects.

Hypoglycemic disorders – classification

Prior classifications of hypoglycemic disorders have attempted to differentiate between disorders that cause fasting versus postprandial hypoglycemia. However, it is sometimes difficult to differentiate between the two and some causes of hypoglycemia cause both fasting and postprandial symptoms [3]. A classification we prefer recognizes that persons who appear healthy have hypoglycemic disorders that differ from those persons who are ill.

The adult patient who appears healthy and who has a history of episodes of neuroglycopenia usually has a hyperinsulinemic hypoglycemic disorder. In such situations, the causes of hyperinsulinemic hypoglycemia may encompass the following conditions: factitial hypoglycemia from insulin or sulfonylurea, insulinoma, non-insulinoma pancreatogenous hypoglycemia syndrome (NIPHS), and insulin autoimmune hypoglycemia.

In persons with co-existing disease, it may be sufficient to recognize the underlying disease and its association with hypoglycemia and to take action to minimize recurrences of hypoglycemia. Confirmation of the suspected mechanism of the hypoglycemia may be sought, such as elevated insulin-like growth factor II levels in non-β-cell tumor hypoglycemia [4] and low levels of cortisol in adrenal insufficiency [5]. Hospitalized patients are often severely ill with multisystem disease. They are at risk for iatrogenic hypoglycemia (insulin added to total parenteral nutrition), as well as for any hypoglycemia that may be produced by the underlying disease. In determining the cause of hypoglycemia in a hospitalized seriously ill patient, a diligent examination of the medical record may be more profitable than examination of the patient [6].

Causes of hyperinsulinemic hypoglycemia

Insulinoma
Insulinomas are the commonest functioning islet cell tumors. More than 80% are solitary benign tumors with an indolent course. Indeed, patients may tolerate symptoms of hypoglycemia for many years prior to seeking medical attention [7]. Surgical enucleation is the treatment of choice. The experience at our institution between July 1982 and October 2004 showed that the mean time from symptom onset to diagnosis was over 4 years (50 months), and one patient had experienced symptoms for 52 years. Cure should be expected in patients without the multiple endocrine neoplasia type 1 (MEN 1) syndrome. In such patients there is only a 7% recurrence rate [8].

Non-insulinoma pancreatogenous hypoglycemia syndrome (NIPHS)
NIPHS is a recently recognized clinical entity where patients experience neuroglycopenic symptoms 2 to 4 h postprandially and not in the fasting state [9]. These patients exhibit positive responses to the selective arterial calcium stimulation test indicative of beta cells hyperfunction. Following gradient-guided partial pancreatectomy, there was amelioration of symptoms. Pancreatic tissue from these patients showed evidence of islet hyperplasia and nesidioblastosis. No disease-causing mutation was detected in the Kir6.2 and SUR1 genes, which have been associated with familial persistent hyperinsulinemic hypoglycemia of infancy. This syndrome is being increasingly recognized in patients who have undergone bariatric surgery [10].

Insulin autoantibody hypoglycemia
This is a rare disorder where hyperinsulinemic hypoglycemia is associated with high titers of antibodies to human insulin that occur in the absence of prior exposure to exogenous insulin [11]. Hypoglycemia occurs in the presence of normal pancreatic islets because the insulin autoantibodies initially bind secreted insulin and then release this bound insulin independently of prevailing glucose concentrations. The hypoglycemia is not associated with any change in sequentially measured titers of insulin antibodies. Measurement of insulin antibodies during the evaluation of a patient with hypoglycemia is required to make the diagnosis although very high serum insulin concentrations are unique to this disorder [12].

Diagnostic tests used in the evaluation of suspected hypoglycemia

The 72-h fast
The 72-h fast is the classic diagnostic test for hypoglycemia. Ideally, it should be conducted in a setting where the care-givers have experience in conducting such a study. Standardized procedures should be followed and access to a method for rapid and accurate measurement of plasma glucose should be available. The fast may be conducted to establish that hypoglycemia is truly the basis for the patient's symptoms or to establish that hypoglycemia is due to fasting hyperinsulinemia because Whipple's triad has already been demonstrated.

In a fast performed for the first purpose, Whipple's triad must be demonstrated. Measurement of β-cell polypeptide products and screening for the presence of sulfonylureas (or other hypoglycemic agents) in the serum provide other important adjunctive data. In patients who do not exhibit symptoms or signs of hypoglycemia and in those without severely depressed plasma glucose concentrations (below 45 mg/dl – 2.5 mmol/L), the fast should be terminated at 72 h. The fast should be terminated earlier if a patient has both symptoms of hypoglycemia and a plasma glucose level in the hypoglycemic range.

The decision to end the fast may not be easy to make when documentation of Whipple's triad is the goal. Because of possible delays in the availability of the results of plasma glucose testing, the bedside reflectance meter may have to serve as a guide to glucose levels. Some patients have slightly depressed glycemic levels without symptoms or signs of hypoglycemia. Other patients may reproduce during fasting the symptoms they experience in ordinary life but may have plasma glucose levels that are sometimes in, and sometimes above, the hypoglycemic range. In such instances, the attribution of symptoms to hypoglycemia is difficult, especially if all additional measurements made during fasting are normal. To complicate matters, young lean healthy women and, to a lesser degree, some men may have plasma glucose levels in the range of 40 mg/dl (2.2 mmol/L) or even lower. Careful examination and testing for subtle signs or symptoms of hypoglycemia should be conducted repeatedly when the patient's plasma glucose level is near or in the hypoglycemic range. To end fasting solely on the basis of a low plasma glucose level in the absence of symptoms or signs of hypoglycemia jeopardizes the possibility of discriminating between normal persons and those with hypoglycemia not mediated by insulin.

On the other hand, concluding that a fast is negative on the basis of no symptoms or signs is also a source of error. It is essential to monitor patients closely during the fast and to be vigilant for subtle signs of neuroglycopenia. In our experience, the prolonged (72-h) fast has been terminated within 12 h in 35% of patients with insulinoma, within 24 h in 75%, and within 48 h in 92% [13]. Extending the fast to 96 h did not alter results in patients with a negative 72-h fast. The interpretation of insulin, C-peptide, and proinsulin concentrations during the prolonged supervised fast depends on the concomitant plasma glucose concentration. The normal overnight fasting ranges for these polypeptides do not apply when the plasma glucose is 50 mg/dl or lower and probably 60 mg/dl or lower.

When an ICMA for insulin with a sensitivity of 0.1 μU/ml (0.6 pmol/L) is used, insulin-mediated hypoglycemic disorders are characterized by plasma insulin concentrations of 3 μU/ml (18 pmol/L) or higher [14] (Fig. 59.1). Persons with non-insulin-mediated hypoglycemic disorders and healthy persons with

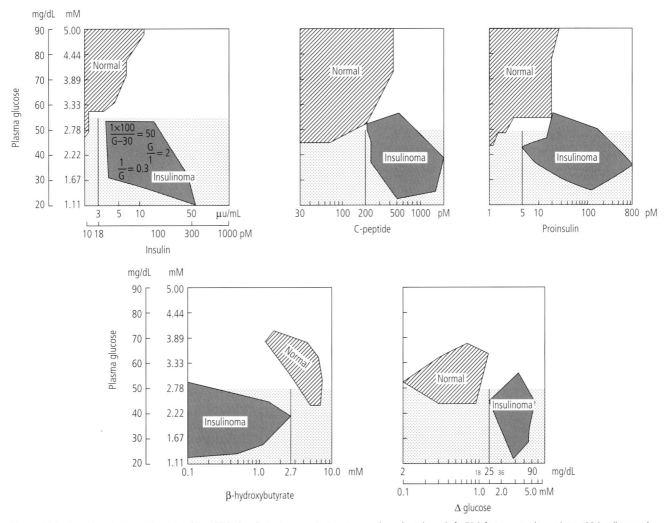

Figure 59.1 Plasma insulin, C-peptide, proinsulin and β-hydroxybutyrate concentrations in normal people at the end of a 72-h fast compared to patients with insulinoma who developed Whipple's triad during the fast. Also shown is the response in glucose (Δglucose) to intravenous glucagon. Shaded areas represent plasma glucose levels ≤50 mg/dl. (Reproduced from Service FJ. Hypoglycemic disorders. *N. Engl. J. Med.* 1995; 332:1144–1152, with permission from the Massachusetts Medical Society.)

plasma glucose of 50 mg/dl (2.7 mmol/L) or less have lower insulin concentrations. Persons with insulinomas have insulin concentrations that rarely exceed 100 µU/ml (600 pmol/L). Values of 1000 µU/ml (6000 pmol/L) or greater suggest recent insulin administration or the presence of insulin antibodies. Criteria for hyperinsulinemia using C-peptide and proinsulin (each measured by ICMA) are levels of 200 pmol/L or greater and 5 pmol/L or greater, respectively.

Measurement of plasma β-hydroxybutyrate at the end of a fast is used as an insulin surrogate as ketone production is extremely sensitive to insulin and is suppressed by hyperinsulinemia. Another insulin surrogate is the response of plasma glucose to intravenous glucagon at the end of the fast. Insulin suppresses glycogenolysis and stimulates glycogen synthesis. A plasma glucose increment of 25 mg/dl (1.38 mmol/L) or greater above the terminal fasting plasma glucose suggests the presence of hyperinsulinemia to a degree that prevented glycogenolysis during the fast [15]. Both insulin surrogates (β-hydroxybutyrate and glucose response to intravenous glucagon) are applicable when the plasma glucose is 60 mg/dl (3.3 pmol/L) or lower at the end of the fast. A rising concentration of β-hydroxybutyrate may indicate a negative fast [16].

Screening for the presence of oral hypoglycemic agents (during the fast and at the time of hypoglycemia) is an essential component of the prolonged supervised fast. The pattern of plasma glucose and β-cell polypeptides produced by secretagogues that stimulate endogenous insulin secretion is identical to that observed in persons with insulinoma.

Mixed meal test

For persons with a history of neuroglycopenic symptoms within 5 h of food ingestion, a mixed meal test may be conducted. Unfortunately, there are no standards for the interpretation of this procedure. At our center, patients eat a meal similar to the meal that led to symptoms during ordinary life activities. The test is considered positive if the patient experiences neuroglycopenic symptoms when concomitant plasma glucose is low (≤50 mg/dl – 2.7 mmol/L). There are no standards for the interpretation of levels of β-cell polypeptides measured during this test. A positive mixed meal test does not provide a diagnosis, only biochemical confirmation of the history. Because patients with insulinoma may have neuroglycopenic symptoms after meals and, in some instances, only after meals, patients with a positive mixed meal test may require a prolonged (72-h) fast. In patients with a positive mixed meal test (a history of neuroglycopenia postprandially confirmed biochemically) and a negative prolonged (72-h) fast, the possibility of NIPHS should be considered [9]. These patients should undergo a selective arterial calcium stimulation test [17]. The 5-h oral glucose tolerance test has no role as a diagnostic test for hypoglycemia because a substantial percentage of healthy persons may have a plasma glucose nadir of 50 mg/dl (2.7 mmol/L or lower) [18].

Insulin antibodies

Insulin antibodies may be present in patients using (or abusing) animal insulin. Patients who use human insulin usually have no detectable insulin antibodies since this is less antigenic than the form derived from animals. On occasion insulin antibodies are pathogenic, causing insulin autoimmune hypoglycemia.

Selective arterial calcium injection

The diagnosis of a hypoglycemic disorder should be made biochemically prior to attempts at localization. However, since the description of NIPHS as a clinical entity, this test has been increasingly used as a diagnostic test. Previously, the knowledge that calcium infusion can stimulate insulin secretion from an insulinoma together with selective arterial injection and venous sampling had been used to regionalize insulinomas [19]. Given the difficulties in interpreting insulin and C-peptide concentrations in patients with chronic renal failure it has been considered to be the test of choice for the evaluation of a possible insulinoma in such patients [20].

A catheter is sequentially inserted into the gastroduodenal, superior mesenteric and splenic arteries. This is used to inject calcium. The second catheter is placed in the right hepatic vein via the inferior vena cava. With the intra-arterial injection of calcium, a two- to three-fold step-up of insulin when measured 20, 40 and 60 s after calcium injection in the venous effluent will regionalize the hyperinsulinism to the head of the pancreas (gastroduodenal artery), the uncinate (superior mesenteric artery), and the body or tail (splenic artery).

Patients with NIPHS also exhibit a similar response. In our experience although we assume NIPHS to be a diffuse process, such a response is not invariably seen in all three regions of the pancreas. An arteriogram obtained at the same time allows assessment of the pancreatic circulation, thereby detecting aberrancies of the vasculature that may falsely regionalize the site of hypersecretion.

Localization procedures

As with most endocrine disorders documentation of abnormal function, i.e., hyperinsulinemic hypoglycemia, is essential prior to embarking on anatomic localization. The choice of imaging modalities has been the subject of much debate. We believe that the choice is dependent on the expertise and technology available at a particular center as well as the patient characteristics (previous abdominal surgery, obesity, etc.).

Transabdominal ultrasonography

This method is non-invasive, relatively inexpensive, and anatomically precise. However, it is very dependent on the expertise of the operator. Its ability to reliably visualize the pancreas in obese individuals is limited. Most insulinomas are hypoechoic with a distinct interface between the normal pancreas and the tumor. They are most likely to be visualized when embedded within the pancreas. If situated on the pancreatic surface, the tumor is often indistinguishable from surrounding fat. Ultrasound examination should also include visualization of the uncinate process behind the superior mesenteric vein.

Endoscopic ultrasonography

Endoscopic ultrasonography overcomes some of the limitations imposed by body habitus or gastrointestinal tract air on transabdominal ultrasonography [21]. It is most likely to localize tumors in the head of the pancreas and is less likely to visualize tumors in the body and tail. Again the technique is highly dependent on operator expertise. It is of little use in patients who have undergone Roux-en-Y gastric bypass surgery.

Intraoperative ultrasonography

Intraoperative ultrasonography completely overcomes the limitations of body habitus or overlying air. When coupled with the experience and knowledge of a highly qualified ultrasonographer, it is invaluable to localization of tumors. It is especially useful in the detection of multiple islet cell tumors as encountered in MEN. Furthermore, the relationship of the tumor to the ducts and adjacent blood vessels can be determined [22].

Computed tomography (CT)

CT is safe, simple to perform and operator independent. However, previously reported sensitivities for this test ranged from 20% to 40%. The advent of spiral CT together with dynamic imaging of intravenous bolus infusion of contrast has produced a remarkable increase in the sensitivity of CT for the detection of insulinoma with reported sensitivities ranging between 60–90% [23]. CT imaging is also helpful in the detection of metastatic disease.

Arteriography

Previously considered to be the gold standard for the localization of insulinomas, the use of arteriography has declined due to improvements in alternative imaging modalities. It is invasive, expensive, and requires considerable technical expertise to perform and interpret. Currently we tend to employ arteriography solely as part of the selective intra-arterial calcium stimulation procedure described above.

MEN 1

MEN 1 is a Mendelian disorder that was first described by Wermer in 1963 and is characterized by the origin of tumors in two or more endocrine glands within a single patient [24]. The glands affected in MEN 1 are the pituitary, pancreas and parathyroids. MEN 1 is also associated with adrenocortical tumors that may be functional. Skin lesions such as angiofibromas and lipomas may also occur in some patients. MEN 1 is inherited in an autosomal dominant fashion. Mutations in the *MEN1* gene (located in chromosome 11q13) cause the disease [25, 26]. More than 10% of mutations arise *de novo* [27]. The gene is thought to act as a tumor suppressor and most of the disease-associated mutations inactivate the gene product [28]. Tumors in MEN 1 exhibit somatic loss of heterozygosity at chromosome 11q13.

Insulinomas that accompany this syndrome tend to occur at an earlier age [29]. Although they comprise about one third of

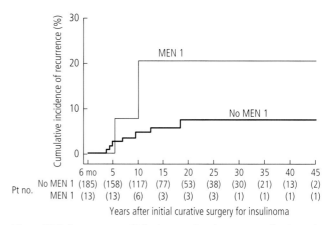

Figure 59.2 Recurrence rates (defined as occurring after a symptom-free interval of 6 months after removal of insulinoma). The recurrence rate is higher in patients with MEN 1 and the disease-free interval is shorter than in patients with sporadic insulinoma. (Reproduced from Service et al. [8], with permission.)

pancreatic islet cell tumors seen in MEN 1, they occur more often before 40 years of age and are the commonest tumor seen before age 20. Insulinomas may be the first manifestation of MEN 1 but usually occur after a diagnosis of primary hyperparathyroidism. They may be associated with gastrinomas although the tumors may arise at different times.

In contrast to the single adenoma found in the overwhelming majority of patients with sporadic insulinoma, many patients with MEN 1 have multicentric benign disease as well as a higher incidence of recurrence (21%) [30] (Fig. 59.2). Conservative pancreatic resection in this setting is likely to lead to recurrent disease. Distal subtotal pancreatic resection to the level of the portal vein combined with enucleation of tumors in the head of the pancreas (guided by intraoperative ultrasonography for safe removal) whenever possible is thought to be the optimal treatment. Preservation of endocrine and exocrine pancreatic function may not be possible in these situations. In contrast to the gastrinomas accompanying MEN 1, which are typically found in the duodenal wall [31], this has not been our experience with insulinoma.

Malignant insulinomas

Malignant insulinomas represent approximately 5% to 10% of all insulinomas [13]. Histological appearance, the number of mitotic figures and other conventional markers of cell dedifferentiation are not sufficient to classify these tumors as malignant. The presence of local invasion or liver or lymph node metastases is required.

The clinical presentation of patients with malignant insulinomas is usually indistinguishable from the symptoms of patients with benign disease. Metastases can also secrete insulin and therefore complete resection will be required to alleviate symptoms completely. Aggressive attempts at resection are recommended because of the relatively indolent nature of these tumors especially when compared to pancreatic adenocarcinoma. A 10-year

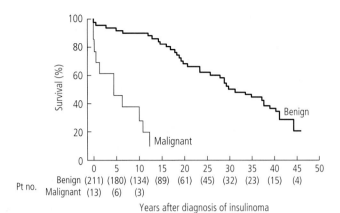

Figure 59.3 Patients with malignant insulinoma have a decreased survival compared to patients with benign insulinoma. (Reproduced from Service et al. [8], with permission.)

survival rate of 29% has been reported in patients with malignant insulinomas [13] (Fig. 59.3).

Resection of hepatic metastases has been performed. Based on a report combining islet cell tumors and carcinoids in 74 patients operated on at the Mayo Clinic, hepatic resection was performed with less than a 3% mortality rate, provided effective palliation, and probably prolonged survival [32]. Palliative resection should be considered only when at least 90% of the tumor bulk can be excised.

Conclusion

Insulinoma is the most common but not the only cause of endogenous hyperinsulinemic hypoglycemia. Diagnosis depends on confirming that hypoglycemia is indeed the cause of the patient's symptoms. Subsequently once the mechanism of hypoglycemia has been determined, efforts can be undertaken to localize the insulinoma. The localization techniques used may depend on the expertise available. Insulinomas are typically single, benign tumors that can safely be enucleated by an experienced surgeon. More extensive resection is usually indicated in MEN 1 syndrome.

References

1. Wilder RMA, Power MH. Carcinoma of the islands of the pancreas: Hyperinsulinism and hypoglycemia. *JAMA* 1927;89:348–355.
2. Whipple AO. Islet cell tumors of the pancreas. *Can. Med. Assoc. J.* 1952;66:334–342.
3. Service FJ. Diagnostic approach to adults with hypoglycemic disorders. *Endocrinol. Metab. Clin. North Am.* 1999;28:519–532, vi.
4. Daughaday WH. Hypoglycemia in patients with non-islet cell tumors. *Endocrinol. Metab. Clin. North Am.* 1989;18:91–101.
5. Samaan NA. Hypoglycemia secondary to endocrine deficiencies. *Endocrinol. Metab. Clin. North Am.* 1989;18:145–154.
6. Limburg PJ, Katz H, Grant CS, Service FJ. Quinine-induced hypoglycemia. *Ann. Intern. Med.* 1993;119:218–219.
7. Nelson RL, Rizza RA, Service FJ. Documented hypoglycemia for 23 years in a patient with insulinoma. *JAMA* 1978;240:1891.
8. Service FJ, McMahon MM, O'Brien PC, Ballard DJ. Functioning insulinoma – incidence, recurrence, and long-term survival of patients: a 60-year study. *Mayo Clin. Proc.* 1991;66:711–719.
9. Service FJ, Natt N, Thompson GB, et al. Noninsulinoma pancreatogenous hypoglycemia: a novel syndrome of hyperinsulinemic hypoglycemia in adults independent of mutations in Kir6.2 and SUR1 genes. *J. Clin. Endocrinol. Metab.* 1999;84:1582–1589.
10. Service GJ, Thompson GB, Service FJ, Andrews JC, Collazo-Clavell ML, Lloyd RV. Hyperinsulinemic hypoglycemia with nesidioblastosis after gastric-bypass surgery. *N. Engl. J. Med.* 2005;353:249–254.
11. Service FJ, Palumbo PJ. Factitial hypoglycemia. Three cases diagnosed on the basis of insulin antibodies. *Arch. Intern. Med.* 1974;134:336–340.
12. Basu A, Service FJ, Yu L, Heser D, Ferries LM, Eisenbarth G. Insulin autoimmunity and hypoglycemia in seven white patients. *Endocr. Pract.* 2005;11:97–103.
13. Service FJ, Dale AJ, Elveback LR, Jiang NS. Insulinoma: clinical and diagnostic features of 60 consecutive cases. *Mayo Clin. Proc.* 1976;51:417–429.
14. Kao PC, Taylor RL, Service FJ. Proinsulin by immunochemiluminometric assay for the diagnosis of insulinoma. *J. Clin. Endocrinol. Metab.* 1994;78:1048–1051.
15. O'Brien T, O'Brien PC, Service FJ. Insulin surrogates in insulinoma. *J. Clin. Endocrinol. Metab.* 1993;77:448–451.
16. Service FJ, O'Brien PC. Increasing serum betahydroxybutyrate concentrations during the 72–hour fast: evidence against hyperinsulinemic hypoglycemia. *J. Clin. Endocrinol. Metab.* 2005;90:4555–4558.
17. Brown CK, Bartlett DL, Doppman JL, et al. Intraarterial calcium stimulation and intraoperative ultrasonography in the localization and resection of insulinomas. *Surgery* 1997;122:1189–1193; discussion 1193–1194.
18. Lev-Ran A, Anderson RW. The diagnosis of postprandial hypoglycemia. *Diabetes* 1981;30:996–999.

Table 59.1 Causes of hypoglycemia

Islet disorders	Insulinoma
	NIPHS/post gastric bypass hypoglycemia
	Persistent hyperinsulinemic hypoglycemia of infancy
Immune disorders	Insulin autoimmune syndrome
	Insulin receptor antibody hypoglycemia
Neoplastic disorders	Tumor-mediated hypoglycemia
Medication	Prescribing error or factitial use of sulfonylureas or insulin
	Quinine
	Propoxyphene
	Salicylates
	Haloperidol
	Ethanol
Systemic illness	Panhypopituitarism or isolated ACTH deficiency
	Fulminant hepatic failure
	Renal failure
	Cyanotic congenital heart disease
	Starvation or anorexia nervosa

ACTH, adrenocorticotropic hormone.

19. Doppman JL, Miller DL, Chang R, Shawker TH, Gorden P, Norton JA. Insulinomas: localization with selective intraarterial injection of calcium. *Radiology* 1991;178:237–241.

20. Basu A, Sheehan MT, Thompson GB, Service FJ. Insulinoma in chronic renal failure: a case report. *J. Clin. Endocrinol. Metab.* 2002;87:4889–4891.

21. Rosch T, Lightdale CJ, Botet JF, et al. Localization of pancreatic endocrine tumors by endoscopic ultrasonography. *N. Engl. J. Med.* 1992;326:1721–1726.

22. Grant CS. Surgical aspects of hyperinsulinemic hypoglycemia. *Endocrinol. Metab. Clin. North Am.* 1999;28:533–554.

23. McAuley G, Delaney H, Colville J, et al. Multimodality preoperative imaging of pancreatic insulinomas. *Clin. Radiol.* 2005;60:1039–1050.

24. Wermer P. Endocrine adenomatosis and peptic ulcer in a large kindred. inherited multiple tumors and mosaic pleiotropism in man. *Am. J. Med.* 1963;35:205–212.

25. Larsson C, Skogseid B, Oberg K, Nakamura Y, Nordenskjold M. Multiple endocrine neoplasia type 1 gene maps to chromosome 11 and is lost in insulinoma. *Nature* 1988;332:85–87.

26. Chandrasekharappa SC, Guru SC, Manickam P, et al. Positional cloning of the gene for multiple endocrine neoplasia-type 1. *Science* 1997;276:404–407.

27. Bassett JH, Forbes SA, Pannett AA, et al. Characterization of mutations in patients with multiple endocrine neoplasia type 1. *Am. J. Hum. Genet.* 1998;62:232–244.

28. Agarwal SK, Guru SC, Heppner C, et al. Menin interacts with the AP1 transcription factor JunD and represses JunD-activated transcription. *Cell* 1999;96:143–152.

29. Trump D, Farren B, Wooding C, et al. Clinical studies of multiple endocrine neoplasia type 1 (MEN 1). *Q. J. Med.* 1996;89:653–669.

30. O'Riordain DS, O'Brien T, van Heerden JA, Service FJ, Grant CS. Surgical management of insulinoma associated with multiple endocrine neoplasia type I. *World J. Surg.* 1994;18:488–493; discussion 493–4.

31. Thompson NW, Vinik AI, Eckhauser FE. Microgastrinomas of the duodenum. A cause of failed operations for the Zollinger–Ellison syndrome. *Ann. Surg.* 1989;209:396–404.

32. Que FG, Nagorney DM, Batts KP, Linz LJ, Kvols LK. Hepatic resection for metastatic neuroendocrine carcinomas. *Am. J. Surg.* 1995;169:36–42; discussion 42–43.

60 Gastrinomas (Zollinger–Ellison Syndrome)

Matthew L. White and Gerard M. Doherty

Key points
- Approximately 75% of gastrinomas occur sporadically, and 25% occur in association with the multiple endocrine neoplasia type 1 syndrome. All gastrinomas should be treated as potentially malignant tumors.
- A gastrin level greater than 1000 pg/ml in the setting of increased gastric acid secretion is virtually pathognomic for Zollinger–Ellison syndrome.
- The initial imaging study to localize a gastrinoma is a high-quality spiral computerized tomography scan.
- Patients with sporadic Zollinger–Ellison syndrome in the absence of unresectable metastases should be offered surgical exploration with curative intent, even if no tumor can be localized. Long-term survival is determined by primary tumor size, liver metastases, and complete tumor resection.
- The multiple endocrine neoplasia type 1 syndrome can be managed, but not cured, and requires continued attention for parathyroid, pituitary, and pancreatic disease.

Gastrin

Gastrin is the primary hormone responsible for gastric acid production and is produced by G cells largely in the gastric antrum. Gastrin is derived from a sequential cleavage process. Preprogastrin is translated from mRNA and subsequently cleaved in the rough endoplasmic reticulum to progastrin. Progastrin undergoes further processing in the Golgi network and secretory granules to form a peptide of 34 amino acids, known as gastrin 34 (G_{34}). Removal of 17 amino acids at the amino terminus of G_{34} yields gastrin 17 (G_{17}). G_{34} is found mostly in the duodenum, whereas G_{17} is found mostly in the gastric antrum [1].

Gastrin release is largely stimulated by a protein-rich meal; ingestion of glucose and fat do not cause gastrin release. Postprandial gastric distension activates cholinergic neurons to also stimulate gastrin release. As distension diminishes, vasoactive intestinal peptide (VIP) is released which stimulates somatostatin secretion, inhibiting further gastrin release [2]. Luminal pH has a strong effect on gastrin. As postprandial luminal pH falls below 3.0, gastrin release is inhibited. Gastrin-releasing peptide (GRP) has also been found to stimulate antral G cells.

Gastrin has physiologic effects in addition to stimulating acid secretion. It acts as a trophic hormone for gastrointestinal mucosa and may influence gastric motility. Gastrin may also play a role in carcinogenesis, as patients with pernicious anemia and hypergastrinemia have an increased incidence of gastric carcinoid

tumors from enterochromaffin-like (ECL) cells. In addition, glycine-extended gastrin has demonstrated growth-promoting effects on human colon cancer cell lines *in vitro* [3], and increased serum gastrin levels have been found in those with colon cancer [4]. Chronic gastric infection with *Helicobacter pylori* is associated with increased gastrin levels that decrease after eradication of the infection. Evidence suggests that the increased acid production seen with *H. pylori* is not simply due to increased parietal cell sensitivity to gastrin.

Inflammatory cytokines produced in the gastric mucosa, including tumor necrosis factor-α (TNF-α), interleukin (IL)-1β, and interferon-γ (IFN-γ), increase gastrin release, stimulating parietal and enterochromaffin cells to increase acid secretion. TNF-α also decreases antral D cells, leading to decreased somatostatin production [5]. Eradication of *H. pylori* infection has been shown to significantly increase the density of antral D cells.

Gastrin release and resultant acid production are regulated by complex interactions of endocrine, paracrine, neural, and chemical pathways, illustrated in Fig. 60.1.

Gastrinoma (Zollinger–Ellison syndrome)

The gastrinoma was originally described by Zollinger and Ellison in 1955 after seeing two patients with hypersecretion of gastric acid, severe jejunal ulcer disease, and islet cell tumors of the pancreas. They suggested that the pancreatic tumors were secreting an ulcerogenic factor causing the syndrome. Several years of investigation led to the discovery of gastrin as the responsible hormone. The Zollinger–Ellison syndrome (ZES) is due to excessively high levels of circulating gastrin produced by neuroendocrine tumors

Clinical Endocrine Oncology, 2nd edition. Edited by Ian D. Hay and John A.H. Wass. © 2008 Blackwell Publishing. ISBN 978-1-4051-4584-8.

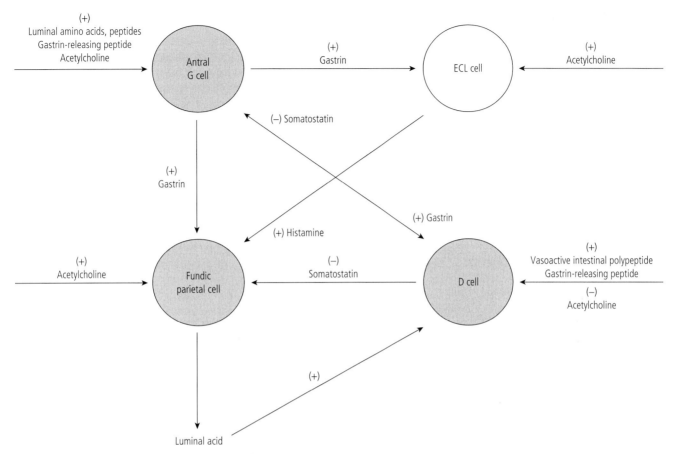

Figure 60.1 Control of gastrin release and resultant acid production.

of the gastrointestinal tract. A majority of patients present with a tumor in the gastrinoma triangle; this triangle has vertices at the junction of the cystic and common bile ducts, the junction of the second and third parts of the duodenum, and the junction of the neck and body of the pancreas [6]. Gastrinomas are not common, occurring in approximately 0.5 to 4 per million per year [7]. However, they are the second most diagnosed pancreatic islet cell tumors after insulinoma, and they are found in about 0.1% of patients with primary duodenal ulcers. Seventy-five percent of gastrinomas occur sporadically, and 25% occur in association with the multiple endocrine neoplasia type 1 (MEN 1) syndrome. Malignancy is an important concern, as historically about 60% of gastrinomas were found to have metastasized at the time of diagnosis. All gastrinomas should be treated as potentially malignant tumors, as benign-appearing tumors have been associated with metastases to the liver or lymph nodes.

ZES may resemble routine peptic ulcer disease, especially with the widespread use of proton pump inhibitors. However, certain conditions with ulcer disease should raise concern and prompt workup for ZES (Table 60.1). These conditions include: (1) ulcers that are multiple or atypical in site, such as distal to the duodenal bulb, (2) ulcers refractory to medical or surgical treatment, (3) ulcers that recur after standard treatment, (4) peptic ulcer disease associated with diarrhea, (5) prominent gastric rugal folds on

Table 60.1 Conditions in peptic ulcer disease associated with gastrinoma

Ulcers that are multiple or atypical in site, such as distal to the duodenal bulb
Ulcers refractory to medical or surgical treatment
Ulcers that recur after standard treatment
Peptic ulcer disease associated with diarrhea
Prominent gastric rugal folds on endoscopy or UGI series
Extensive family history of peptic ulcer disease
Ulcers associated with hyperparathyroidism

endoscopy or upper gastrointestinal (UGI) series, (6) extensive family history of peptic ulcer disease, and (7) ulcers associated with hyperparathyroidism. A finding of hyperparathyroidism with peptic ulcer disease should raise suspicion for the MEN 1 syndrome.

Diagnosis

Measuring fasting serum gastrin levels is the first step in the biochemical diagnosis of ZES. Ideally antisecretory therapy should be stopped 1 week prior to measurement, although this may not be possible due to the severity of disease. Patients with gastrinoma will typically have fasting serum gastrin levels above 200 pg/ml. A gastrin level greater than 1000 pg/ml in the setting of increased

Table 60.2 Differential diagnosis of hypergastrinemia

Normal to low gastric acid secretion
  Vagotomy
  Pernicious anemia
  Antisecretory treatment
  Short gut syndrome
  Chronic atrophic gastritis
  Renal failure
High gastric acid secretion
  Antral G-cell hyperplasia or hyperfunction
  Retained excluded gastric antrum
  Gastric outlet obstruction
  H. pylori gastritis (acid can be low)
  Zollinger–Ellison syndrome

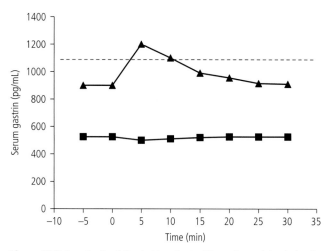

Figure 60.2 Secretin stimulation test in patients with gastrinoma (triangles) and antral G-cell hyperplasia (squares).

gastric acid secretion is virtually pathognomic for ZES. Fasting hypergastrinemia is not sufficient to diagnose ZES, as elevated gastrin levels can also occur in other conditions. Hypergastrinemia includes a differential diagnosis that is separated into two divisions: high and normal to low acid secretion (Table 60.2). Conditions associated with normal to low acid secretion include vagotomy, pernicious anemia, treatment with proton pump inhibitors, short gut syndrome, chronic atrophic gastritis, and renal failure. Conditions associated with high acid secretion include antral G-cell hyperplasia or hyperfunction, retained excluded gastric antrum, gastric outlet obstruction, *H. pylori* gastritis (acid can be low), and ZES.

The diagnosis of ZES is supported by acid hypersecretion on gastric acid analysis: basal acid output (BAO) greater than 15 mEq/h, BAO greater than 5 mEq/h in patients with previous vagotomy or ulcer operations, or a BAO greater than 60% of maximal acid concentration (MAO). The BAO/MAO ratio is usually greater than 0.6 in ZES due to hypergastrinemia causing almost maximal stimulation of the parietal cells. About 50% of ZES patients will have a BAO greater than 30 mEq/h. Finding low normal or decreased acid production without a history of gastric surgery or recent antisecretory therapy excludes the diagnosis of ZES.

Circulating levels of chromogranin A, a non-specific neuroendocrine tumor product, may provide additional evidence for a gastrinoma. Serum chromogranin A is a generic marker for neuroendocrine tumors that is elevated in most patients with ZES. Levels do appear to correlate with tumor burden, yet chromogranin A can be markedly elevated in ZES without the presence of liver metastasis [8].

Provocative tests

Once hypergastrinemic hyperacidity has been established, provocative testing can help to differentiate between ZES and the other causes of hypergastrinemic hyperacidity (Table 60.2). Several provocative tests have been used historically to clarify the diagnosis of gastrinoma, including a standardized meal, calcium infusion, and pentagastrin infusion. However, injection with

secretin is currently the provocative test of choice for ZES due to its simplicity, lack of side effects, and better discrimination [9]. The secretin test begins with drawing a gastrin level. Secretin is then given as an intravenous bolus dose of 2 μ/kg with gastrin samples drawn every 5 min for 30 min. A paradoxical rise in the gastrin level by at least 200 pg/ml is unique to the patient with ZES (Fig. 60.2). Patients with other causes of hypergastrinemic hyperacidity do not demonstrate this characteristic rise in gastrin after infusion with secretin.

Tumor localization

After a biochemical diagnosis has been made, localizing a gastrinoma can be challenging. Figure 60.3 shows a recommended approach to localization. The initial study to localize a gastrinoma is a high-quality spiral computerized tomography (CT) scan. The sensitivity of CT in detecting gastrinomas varies widely from 30% to 85%, but has greatly improved with newer techniques. CT has the advantage of identifying the anatomic extent of the primary tumor while also assessing for metastases. CT has the disadvantage of identifying lesions without regard to histology or function.

Somatostatin receptor scintigraphy (SRS) is a technique that takes advantage of the increased concentration of somatostatin receptors expressed by gastrinomas. Octreotide, a somatostatin analog, is labeled with ^{111}In and injected intravenously. The tracer binds to large numbers of somatostatin receptors on gastrinomas, making the tumors detectable scintigraphically. The sensitivity of SRS ranges from 20% to 80%, depending on the particular population under investigation. Significant false-negative rates have been reported; a negative SRS examination in a patient with biochemical disease should be viewed with skepticism. SRS does have the advantages of assessing the whole body for disease and identifying tumors functionally. However, SRS lacks anatomic specificity, so it must be combined with anatomic imaging techniques, such as CT, to define the extent of tumor.

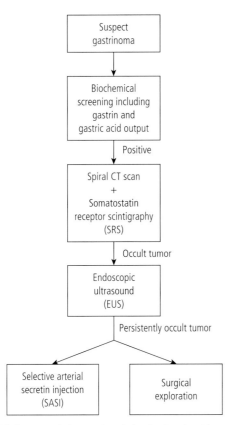

Figure 60.3 Recommended approach to the localization of gastrinomas.

Endoscopic ultrasound (EUS) is the best imaging technique to detect small pancreatic tumors, with sensitivity exceeding 75% for pancreatic tumors. It can image the parenchyma of the pancreas and peripancreatic lymph nodes with great precision. The disadvantage of EUS is its limited anatomic scope. It is less useful in detecting duodenal wall gastrinomas, and it cannot image other possible sites of disease, such as the liver or chest. Endoscopic ultrasound is also highly dependent on the experience of the person(s) performing the examination. This modality may be most helpful in patients with a positive biochemical screen but no imageable disease on SRS or CT scan [10].

Selective arterial secretin injection (SASI) was described in 1987 as a method for localizing gastrinomas not seen by conventional techniques [11]. Secretin is injected into one of three arteries feeding the pancreas: gastroduodenal, superior mesenteric, or splenic artery. Blood is collected from a hepatic vein, and gastrin levels reveal the location of the tumor because each injected artery supplies a different portion of the pancreas and/or duodenum. Gastrin levels peak earlier and higher when injecting secretin into the artery supplying the gastrinoma. The sensitivity of SASI is greater than 90%, and it has essentially replaced portal venous sampling for localizing a primary gastrinoma.

Selective visceral angiography has been used to demonstrate the vascular supply of gastrinomas in the pancreatic region. The sensitivity of angiography is better for insulinoma than gastrinoma, and it is less useful for localizing duodenal wall tumors or lymph node metastases. The introduction of newer modalities, like SRS and EUS, has decreased the need for an invasive test like angiography.

Treatment

Treatment of ZES has two principal aims: to control the secretion of acid and to completely excise gastrinoma tissue. Incomplete excision also appears to favorably alter the natural history of the disease, and palliative treatment options are available for unresectable disease.

Medical treatment

Medical management of gastrinoma has undergone tremendous changes since the original description of the syndrome in 1955. Total gastrectomy was initially the treatment to achieve long-term survival. With the introduction of the H2 blocker cimetidine in 1977, a new non-operative strategy existed. However, this new medicine was not a panacea and had undesirable antiandrogen effects at high doses, such as gynecomastia, breast tenderness, and impotence. Medical therapy again advanced with the introduction of two new H2 blockers, famotidine and ranitidine. These two new drugs more effectively inhibited gastric acid secretion without the bothersome side effects.

A recent advance in treatment has come with proton pump inhibitors (PPIs), a class of drugs that bind to the H^+/K^+ ATPase enzyme and strongly inhibit parietal cell acid secretion. PPIs are tolerated very well and can control acid hypersecretion in most ZES patients with once- or twice-daily dosing. Compared to H2 blockers, PPIs have a longer duration of action and are more effective at suppressing acid secretion. Concern has arisen that the achlorhydria produced by PPIs might increase the incidence of gastric carcinoids, as this has been demonstrated in rats. While an increase in gastric carcinoids has not been seen with PPI treatment, evidence does suggest that a hypergastrinemic state causes advanced changes in gastric ECL cells [12]. Therefore, non-operated ZES patients should undergo long-term endoscopic surveillance, to monitor both ECL changes and the effectiveness of antisecretory therapy.

The somatostatin analog octreotide has been shown to decrease both gastric acid and gastrin levels in ZES. Octreotide is not currently considered first-line therapy for ZES, but there is evidence to suggest that it may be a useful adjunct. One small series reported that about 50% of tumors demonstrated some antigrowth effects with octreotide therapy [13]. Further study may demonstrate more long-term benefits of controlling hypergastrinemia.

Surgical treatment

The role of surgical treatment for ZES has changed dramatically. Initially, total gastrectomy was performed to remove the affected organ from its hypergastrinemic environment. The introduction of H2 blockers and PPIs has made effective long-term acid control possible, virtually eliminating hyperacidity as an indication to operate. Long-term survival for ZES patients is now determined only by the natural history of the disease; this can be altered by surgical intervention.

Surgical resection of primary gastrinomas likely decreases the chance for liver metastases, the most important negative predictor of survival [14]. Patients with sporadic ZES in the absence of unresectable metastases should be offered surgical exploration with curative intent, even if no tumor can be localized. Currently greater than 90% of non-imageable tumors are still found and removed [15]. During exploration, it is essential that the entire abdomen be assessed for extrapancreatic and extraduodenal gastrinomas. Primary lymph node tumors have been described, and cure has been achieved solely by lymph node removal.

It was originally thought that duodenal gastrinomas comprised less than 15% of all gastrinomas. However, recognition of duodenal microgastrinomas, which are often not palpable through the duodenal wall and missed on preoperative imaging studies, has led some surgeons to routinely perform duodenotomy (opening the duodenum) [16]. In one recent series duodenotomy was directly attributed to an increased cure rate, from 34% to above 50% [17]. Gastrinomas in the duodenum and head of the pancreas are often enucleated or excised. Pancreaticoduodenectomy (Whipple procedure) is usually reserved for large, locally advanced tumors in the duodenum or pancreatic head. Tumors in the body and tail of the pancreas may either be excised or resected, depending on their proximity to the pancreatic duct. Finding a solitary liver lesion warrants resection; cures have been reported even in the absence of an extrahepatic primary tumor. Liver transplantation for multiple metastases is controversial, but is potentially curative and has shown benefit in highly selected patients [18].

Lifelong surveillance is required after surgical treatment. Patients should be followed with serial gastrin measurements at regular intervals during their first postoperative year. An elevated gastrin level signals residual gastrinoma tissue. A secretin provocation test may detect residual gastrinoma tissue, even with a normal gastrin level. It is reasonable to perform a secretin test 3 months postoperatively and then annually for all eugastrinemic patients who have undergone "curative" resection [9]. A combination of CT scan and SRS is useful for evaluating patients with recurrent hypergastrinemia. Endoscopic ultrasound may demonstrate small pancreatic tumors not imageable by SRS or CT scan. Imaging may reveal a new lesion amenable to resection.

The surgical management of ZES with MEN 1 is controversial. These patients usually present with primary hyperparathyroidism before symptoms of a gastrinoma are present. Parathyroidectomy should be performed before laparotomy for gastrinoma; normalizing serum calcium often reduces gastrin levels and gastric acid secretion. Most patients have multiple tumors in both the pancreas and duodenum, many of which are microscopic and undetectable. The traditional approach in most centers has been to maintain patients on antisecretory therapy with surveillance until tumor localization is possible. One surgical series with the longest follow-up found that surgical intervention was not curative in MEN 1, but likely delays malignant progression [19].

Palliative treatment

Antitumor efforts for unresectable metastatic gastrinomas include long-acting somatostatin analogs alone or combined with α-interferon. These agents demonstrate the ability to decrease the size of gastrinomas in 20% of patients and cause cessation of growth in roughly half of patients; it is unknown whether they affect survival. Chemotherapy with doxorubicin, streptozocin, ±5-fluorouracil shrinks tumors in 5–50% of patients. However, it has not been shown to prolong survival and can have considerable toxicity [20]. Cytoreductive surgery for liver metastases has shown benefit. In one series, debulking of neuroendocrine hepatic metastases extended 5- and 10-year survival if at least 90% of metastatic disease was resected [21]. If surgical treatment is not feasible or is refused, hepatic artery embolization (HAE) can be used to treat pain and hormone output by liver metastases.

Multiple endocrine neoplasia type 1

MEN 1 is an autosomal dominant syndrome, caused by inactivating mutations of the *MEN1* gene locus that codes for the tumor suppressor protein, menin. The clinical presentation of MEN 1 classically includes hyperparathyroidism due to multiple parathyroid adenomas, pituitary adenomas, and pancreatic neuroendocrine tumors. Carriers of MEN 1 may also display multiple lipomas, cutaneous angiofibromas, adrenal or thyroid adenomas, and bronchial or thymic carcinoid tumors [10].

The most common MEN 1-related cause of death is malignant pancreatic endocrine tumors. Microscopic examination of the duodenum and pancreas in this population demonstrates multiple neuroendocrine tumors, often grossly undetectable. It is common for MEN 1 kindreds to develop functional endocrine tumors of the pancreas, most of which are gastrinomas, about 20% insulinomas, 3% glucagonomas, and 1% VIPomas.

Patients with MEN 1 usually present with primary hyperparathyroidism before symptoms of a gastrinoma are present. Parathyroidectomy should be performed before laparotomy for gastrinoma; normalizing serum calcium often reduces gastrin levels and gastric acid secretion. Surgical resection of primary gastrinomas in patients with and without MEN 1 likely decreases the chance of developing liver metastases [14]. Thus, patients with imaging studies demonstrating resectable tumor should have surgical exploration with intraoperative ultrasound. Resection of liver metastases in patients with MEN 1 may prolong survival, although this has not been demonstrated conclusively [22].

MEN 1 is not currently a curable syndrome, making surveillance for all patients with MEN 1 essential. Patients should be evaluated at least annually, with more frequent assessments necessitated by the course of their disease. Surveillance follows the same pattern and employs the same modalities as screening in unoperated patients. Biochemical hormone levels are the most sensitive screening test for parathyroid, pituitary, and pancreatic disease, and can provide some reassurance if levels are normal. Imaging studies should be conducted at some interval, even with normal

Table 60.3 Staging of gastrinomas

Stage	Tumor	Tumor size (cm)	Lymph nodes	Distant metastases
0	T0	None	N0	M0
I	T1	≤1.0	Any N	M0
	T2	1.1–2.0		
II	T3	2.1–2.9	Any N	M0
	T4	≥3.0		
III	Any T	Any size	Any N	M1

Adapted from Ellison et al. [23], with permission from the American College of Surgeons.

biochemistry, to evaluate for non-functional tumors. A combination of pancreatic imaging with CT scan and SRS provides the best coverage of the abdomen and thorax. Endoscopic ultrasound is useful for sensitive assessment of the pancreas and may be most helpful in patients with a positive biochemical screen but no imageable disease on SRS or CT scan [10].

Staging

A staging system was proposed by Ellison in 1995 and revised in 2006 (Table 60.3) [23]. Analysis of 106 patients with gastrinoma over a 50-year period found that survival was determined by three independent factors: primary tumor size, liver metastases, and complete tumor resection. Survival was independent of age at diagnosis, sex, presence of lymph node metastases, normal postoperative serum gastrin, and MEN status. The overall 10- and 20-year survival rates for stage I tumors (primary ≤2 cm without liver metastases) were 78% and 65%; stage II (primary >2 cm without liver metastases), 70% and 46%; and stage III (liver metastases), 33% and 26%, respectively.

Conclusion

Gastrinomas are neuroendocrine pancreatic tumors that cause hyperacidity by secreting large amounts of gastrin. A gastrinoma should be suspected in patients with: (1) ulcers that are multiple or atypical in site; (2) ulcers refractory to medical or surgical treatment; (3) ulcers that recur after standard treatment; (4) peptic ulcer disease associated with diarrhea; (5) prominent gastric rugal folds; (6) extensive family history of peptic ulcer disease; and (7) ulcers associated with hyperparathyroidism. Seventy-five percent of gastrinomas are sporadic and 25% are associated with the MEN 1 syndrome. All gastrinomas should be treated as potentially malignant tumors that can metastasize and cause death. A biochemical diagnosis of ZES is made by documenting hypergastrinemia in the setting of hyperacidity; provoking a paradoxical rise in gastrin with the secretin test clinches the biochemical diagnosis. The initial imaging study to localize a gastrinoma is a high-quality spiral CT scan. Combining newer modalities with

CT has increased the ability to localize gastrinomas. Patients with sporadic ZES in the absence of unresectable metastases should be offered surgical exploration with curative intent, even if no tumor can be localized. Parathyroidectomy should be performed before laparotomy for gastrinoma in patients with MEN 1. Patients with metastases have a number of options, including chemotherapy, debulking, hepatic artery embolization, and sometimes liver transplantation. Long-term survival for patients with ZES is determined by primary tumor size, liver metastases, and complete tumor resection.

References

1. Sawada M, Dickinson CJ. The G cell. *Annu. Rev. Physiol.* 1997;59: 273–298.
2. Mulholland MW. Gastric anatomy and physiology. In Mulholland MW, Lillemoe K, Doherty G, et al. (eds). *Greenfield's Surgery: Scientific Principles and Practice*, 4th edition. Philadelphia, PA: Lippincott Williams & Wilkins, 2006:709–721.
3. Stepan VM, Sawada M, Todisco A, et al. Glycine-extended gastrin exerts growth-promoting effects on human colon cancer cells. *Mol. Med.* 1999;5:147–159.
4. Thorburn CM, Friedman GD, Dickinson CJ, et al. Gastrin and colorectal cancer: a prospective study. *Gastroenterology* 1998;115:275–280.
5. Suerbaum S, Michetti P. *Helicobacter pylori* infection. *N. Engl. J. Med.* 2002;347:1175–1186.
6. Stabile BE, Morrow DJ, Passaro E, Jr. The gastrinoma triangle: operative implications. *Am. J. Surg.* 1984;147:25–31.
7. Oberg K, Eriksson B. Endocrine tumours of the pancreas. *Best Pract. Res. Clin. Gastroenterol.* 2005;19:753–781.
8. Tomassetti P, Migliori M, Simoni P, et al. Diagnostic value of plasma chromogranin A in neuroendocrine tumours. *Eur. J. Gastroenterol. Hepatol.* 2001;13:55–58.
9. Wilson SD. Gastrinoma. In Clark OH, Duh Q-Y, Kebebew E (eds). *Textbook of Endocrine Surgery*, 2nd edition. Philadelphia: WB Saunders, 2005:745–756.
10. Doherty GM. Multiple endocrine neoplasia type 1. *J. Surg. Oncol.* 2005;89:143–150.
11. Imamura M, Takahashi K, Adachi H, et al. Usefulness of selective arterial secretin injection test for localization of gastrinoma in the Zollinger–Ellison syndrome. *Ann. Surg.* 1987;205:230–239.
12. Peghini PL, Annibale B, Azzoni C, et al. Effect of chronic hypergastrinemia on human enterochromaffin-like cells: insights from patients with sporadic gastrinomas. *Gastroenterology* 2002;123:68–85.
13. Shojamanesh H, Gibril F, Louie A, et al. Prospective study of the antitumor efficacy of long-term octreotide treatment in patients with progressive metastatic gastrinoma. *Cancer* 2002;94:331–343.
14. Fraker DL, Norton JA, Alexander HR, et al. Surgery in Zollinger–Ellison syndrome alters the natural history of gastrinoma. *Ann. Surg.* 1994;220:320–330.
15. Norton JA, Fraker DL, Alexander HR, et al. Surgery to cure the Zollinger–Ellison syndrome. *N. Engl. J. Med.* 1999;341:635–644.
16. Thompson NW, Vinik AI, Eckhauser FE. Microgastrinomas of the duodenum: a cause for failed operations of the Zollinger–Ellison syndrome. *Ann. Surg.* 1989;209:396–404.
17. Norton JA, Alexander HR, Fraker DL, et al. Does the use of routine duodenotomy (DUODX) affect rate of cure, development of liver

metastases, or survival in patients with Zollinger–Ellison syndrome? *Ann. Surg.* 2004;239:617–625; discussion 626.

18. van Vilsteren FG, Baskin-Bey ES, Nagorney DM, et al. Liver transplantation for gastroenteropancreatic neuroendocrine cancers: defining selection criteria to improve survival. *Liver Transpl.* 2006;12:448–456.

19. Hausman MS, Jr, Thompson NW, Gauger PG, et al. The surgical management of MEN 1 pancreatoduodenal neuroendocrine disease. *Surgery* 2004;136:1205–1211.

20. Jensen RT. Gastrinomas: advances in diagnosis and management. *Neuroendocrinology* 2004;80 (Suppl 1):23–27.

21. Sarmiento JM, Heywood G, Rubin J, et al. Surgical treatment of neuroendocrine metastases to the liver: a plea for resection to increase survival. *J. Am. Coll. Surg.* 2003;197:29–37.

22. Norton JA, Alexander HR, Fraker DL, et al. Comparison of surgical results in patients with advanced and limited disease with multiple endocrine neoplasia type 1 and Zollinger–Ellison syndrome. *Ann. Surg.* 2001;234:495–505.

23. Ellison EC, Sparks J, Verducci JS, et al. 50-year appraisal of gastrinoma: recommendations for staging and treatment. *J. Am. Coll. Surg.* 2006;202:897–905.

61 VIPomas

Vian Amber and Stephen R. Bloom

> **Key points**
> - Verner–Morrison syndrome, WDHA (watery diarrhea, hypokalemia and achlorhydria) and VIPomas are terms for tumors that secrete high levels of vasoactive intestinal peptide.
> - The cardinal symptom is massive watery diarrhea resulting in hypokalemia, hypochlorhydria and acidosis.
> - Overall, 90% of VIPomas are pancreatic and 10% are extrapancreatic associated with tumors arising along the sympathetic chain and adrenal medulla.
> - Diagnosis is based on detection of vasoactive intestinal peptide plasma levels and radiographic tumor localization.
> - Surgery is the treatment of choice, but octreotide, glucocorticoid and chemotherapy are effective palliative treatment.

VIPoma and the WDHHA syndrome

VIPoma is a rare neuroendocrine tumor that secretes vasoactive intestinal peptide (VIP) [1]. It is more common in adults in whom the pancreas is the main site of tumor origin compared to children where the majority of reported cases are in the adrenal and extra-adrenal neurogenic sites. Women are more likely to have VIPomas with a female to male ratio of 3:1, while in children and adolescents there is an equal sex distribution. Though VIPomas are uncommon they are the third commonest functional neuroendocrine tumor of the pancreas (2%) after insulinoma (50%) and gastrinoma (30%) discussed in Chapters 59 and 60 respectively. They can occur as part of multiple endocrine neoplasia (MEN) and have a poor prognosis because of larger tumor size and a high rate of metastasis at the time of diagnosis [2].

VIPomas synthesize and excrete large amounts of VIP resulting in the classic symptoms of intractable watery diarrhea, hypochlorhydria, hypokalemia and severe hyperchloremic metabolic acidosis (WDHHA). Other synonyms for the syndrome include Verner–Morrison syndrome, named after the two physicians who first described the symptoms of watery diarrhea, hypokalemia and achlorhydria (WDHA) in patients with non-insulin secreting pancreatic tumors, in 1958 [3]. It was also known as "pancreatic cholera" [4], because of the resemblance of the secretory diarrhea to that caused by *Vibrio cholerae*. The culprit VIP was not identified until 1970 when Said and Mutt [5] extracted the peptide from animal gut which was consequently sequenced by Bodanszky in 1973 [6].

The secretory diarrhea, though profuse, is insidious in onset and present for 3–4 years prior to diagnosis. However, with the tumor and disease progression, this becomes severe with life-threatening electrolyte abnormalities and acid–base imbalance, as a consequence cardiac dysrhythmias, tetany, neuromuscular dysfunction, shock and cardiovascular collapse may frequently occur. The patient excretes large amounts (six to eight times per day) of what is described as "dilute tea" stool, accompanied by massive electrolyte loss, mainly that of sodium and potassium amounting to ~6900 mg sodium and ~11 700 mg potassium loss per 24 h (~300 mmol/24 h). Other clinical and biochemical features of VIPoma include facial/head and neck flushing, hyperglycemia, hypercalcemia, and hypomagnesemia (Tables 61.1 and 61.2). The facial flushing may occur in 8–20% of the patients, on tumor palpation and is associated with marked hypotension. It can be

Table 61.1 Clinical features of VIPoma and the WDHHA syndrome

Symptoms
Watery diarrhea (persistent)
Cardiac arrhythmias
Tetany
Neuromuscular dysfunction
Hypotension
Vascular collapse
Facial flushing
Weight loss*
Abdominal distension*
Malnutrition*
Sweating*
Hypertension*

*More pronounced in children.

Clinical Endocrine Oncology, 2nd edition. Edited by Ian D. Hay and John A.H. Wass. © 2008 Blackwell Publishing. ISBN 978-1-4051-4584-8.

Table 61.2 Biochemical abnormalities and causative factors

Biochemical abnormalities	Causative factor
Hypokalemia Hypomagnesemia Hyponatremia	VIP activation of cAMP, increased intestinal motility, fecal loss, activation of renin-angiotensin system
Metabolic acidosis (hyperchloremic)	VIP-induced fecal loss of bicarbonate Inhibition of gastric acid secretion
Hypochlorhydria (rarely achlorhydria)	VIP, inhibition of gastric acid secretion
Hypercalcemia	PTHrP, dehydration, possible PTH
Hyperglycemia	GIP-like effect, glucagon cosecretion

PTHrP, parathyroid hormone related peptide.

Table 61.3 Differential diagnosis of secretory diarrhea

Laxative
  Exogenous stimulant laxative abuse, e.g. senna, castor oil, cascara
  Endogenous laxatives (dihydroxy bile acids)
Infection
  Vibrio cholerae
  Escherichia coli
Neoplasm
  Neuroendocrine tumors of the gut, e.g., VIPoma, carcinoid, gastrinoma
  Carcinoma of the lung
  Medullary thyroid cancer
  Villous adenoma of the rectum
  PPoma
Infantile causes
  Congenital dysautonomia
  Congenital chloridorrhea
  Enteric structural anomalies
Systemic mastocytosis
Immunoglobulin A deficiency
Idiopathic secretory diarrhea

patchy, erythematous or urticarial in nature [7]. In children, weight loss, malnutrition and abdominal distension have been reported as the presenting features with persistent watery diarrhea [8]. These have also been reported in adults in advanced cases.

Etiological factors of secretory diarrhea that need to be considered in the differential diagnosis of VIPoma include stimulant laxative abuse, bacterial infection, other neuroendocrine tumors and villous adenoma of the rectum (Table 61.3). Although the main manifestation of Zollinger–Ellison syndrome is peptic ulceration, diarrhea may be the presenting feature in 10% of the patients. Similarly medullary carcinoma of the thyroid and carcinoid syndrome may present with watery diarrhea. Though very rare, there are reported cases of WDHHA occurring in association with large cell carcinoma of the lung, co-secreting calcitonin and VIP [9], and systemic mastocytosis.

Pathophysiology

VIP is a 28-amino-acid neuropeptide widely synthesized peripherally by the amine precursor uptake and decarboxylation cells (APUD) in the gastrointestinal tract, pancreas, adrenal and the extra-adrenal sympathetic chain neurons. It is also expressed in the central nervous system in the hypothalamus, hippocampus and the cortex. VIP is a product of post-translational processing of a larger molecular form (170-amino acid) known as preproVIP, which is cleaved to form VIP, histidine methionine peptide (PHM) (27-amino acid) and other peptide fragments. VIP has structural homology with gastric inhibitory peptide (GIP), glucagon, gastrin, secretin, pancreatic polypeptide, thyrocalcitonin, prostaglandin, and PHM, which may account for most of its actions. VIP has a glucagon-like effect counteracting the effects of insulin, resulting in stimulation of hepatic gluconeogenesis and glycogenolysis.

Most of the clinical symptoms correspond to the known biological actions of VIP. Activation of cAMP production by the gut resulting in increased intestinal secretion and motility accounts for the principal symptom of watery diarrhea. This in turn causes massive loss of water and electrolytes from the gut, especially that

of sodium, potassium and magnesium. Profound life-threatening hypokalemia and hypomagnesemia ensue and are further enhanced by activation of the renin–angiotensin system. Other disturbances of acid–base balance, for example metabolic acidosis, develop as a result of bicarbonate loss due to increased secretion of alkaline pancreatic juice. Acidosis is aggravated by the inhibitory action of VIP on gastric acid secretion. The latter also causes hypochlorhydria and hyperchloremia.

In addition to the structural homology with other peptides (discussed above), VIP is reported to be co-secreted in various combinations with these peptides by various pancreatic and non-pancreatic tumors. As these have similar actions to VIP on the gut they may act synergistically, enhancing the severity of the symptoms. The glucagon-like effect of VIP in stimulating hepatic gluconeogenesis and glycogenolysis is implicated in the hypeglycemia seen in adult patients. Though there is no clear explanation for the occurrence of hypercalcemia, it has been attributed to dehydration and parathyroid hormone related peptide (PTHrP) in almost all the cases. Co-existence of hyperparathyroidism in MEN 1 has been implicated in some cases (Table 61.3). Similarly it is not clear why facial flushing occurs in VIPoma, but VIP's action in causing smooth muscle relaxation, leading to vascular dilatation, prostaglandin and catecholamine secretion, might be causative factors.

Diagnosis

Although VIPomas are rare, early diagnosis is important for providing curative and/or palliative treatment aiming to improving patients' quality of life. In suspected cases with secretory diarrhea diagnosis can be based on detection of elevated levels of VIP. This is found in all cases of VIPoma. However, due to the short half-life of circulating VIP (2 min) diagnosis can be confirmed by measuring the histidine-methionine fragment, pancreatic polypeptide, and neurotensin. The former is co-secreted with VIP by VIPomas and is more stable in plasma. Pancreatic polypeptide and neurotensins are secreted by VIPomas in 75% and 10% of cases respectively. It is worth noting that false-positive high plasma levels can be found in patients with hepatic cirrhosis, severe liver and renal failure, bowel ischemia and dehydration due to other causes. In these patients high VIP concentration should be interpreted with caution. Likewise a single normal VIP level in patients with secretory diarrhea may not exclude VIPoma in a symptomatic patient.

VIP can be measured as part of a gut hormone profile using highly sensitive and specific radioimmunoassay methods. In general these depend on the competition between radioactively labeled and unlabeled hormone. Gut hormones are highly labile peptides that require careful patient preparation, sample collection and handling protocols. Whole blood samples with added protease inhibitor (Trasylol, to prevent breakdown of the peptide) should be collected following an overnight fast. This needs to be transported on ice with early separation and freezing until analysis. The normal reference interval for plasma VIP is 0–103.5 pg/mL (0–30 pmol/L).

Measurement of other gut peptides may provide useful information in the diagnosis of other underlying neuroendocrine tumors and/or detection of the tumor origin. For example, high levels of pancreatic polypeptides are detected in primary pancreatic tumors, high gastrin levels in Zollinger–Ellison syndrome and glucagon in glucagonoma (see Chapter 62). Diarrhea due to causes other than VIPoma and other neuroendocrine tumors may respond to fasting depending on the underlying etiological factor (Table 61.3); however, secretory diarrhea due to VIPoma persists beyond a 48-h fast. Measuring fecal volume, osmolality, and electrolyte may further assist in confirming the diagnosis. In addition, routine biochemical blood investigations can identify hypokalemia, hypomagnesemia and other metabolic acid–base disturbances. It is essential to investigate 24-h urinary catecholamine excretion, especially in children, to exclude adrenal tumors.

Once the diagnosis is confirmed, various imaging modes and venous sampling are the mainstay for tumor localization (Table 61.4).

Table 61.4 Detection sensitivity of various imaging techniques

Imaging	Detection sensitivity
Ultrasound	
Transabdominal	25–70%
Endoscopic	79–100%
Intraoperative	100% for pancreatic tumors
	Less effective for extrapancreatic
Spiral CT (enhanced)	44–80%
Gadolinium-enhanced MRI	64–100%
Scintigraphy	
Somatostatin	80%
VIP	100%

Histological examination is important in the final diagnosis following tumor excision (Plate 61.1).

Tumor localization

In general, localization of islet cell tumors presents a challenge to the clinician. Despite the availability of diagnostic imaging and biochemical investigations a number of cases are overlooked and undiagnosed until after metastasis to the liver (Fig. 61.1). In adults, up to 90% of primary VIPomas originate in the pancreas. In a recent review of 76 patients with neuroendocrine tumors, 63.6% of the total number of VIPomas originated in the pancreas [10]. The remainder were in the duodenum or retroperitoneum. VIPomas may also occur as part of MEN 1 though this is very rare. In a series of 580 patients with MEN 1, 50% had duodeno-pancreatic tumors but VIPoma was present in only 1% [2]. Other extrapancreatic primary VIPomas are extremely rare in adults though they have been reported in the lungs, colon, liver, kidneys

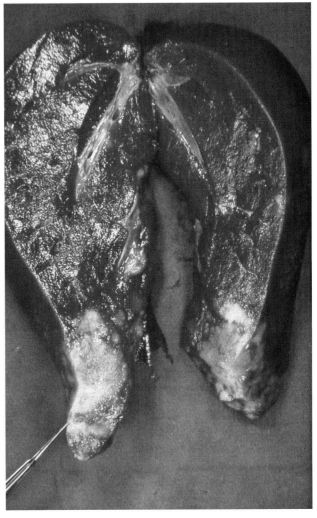

Figure 61.1 Pancreatic VIPoma, metastatic tumor in the liver.

and the skin. Pancreatic tumors are mostly malignant and may secrete VIP and/or other neuroendocrine peptide hormones [11]. As discussed earlier co-secretion of other peptides may denote tumor origin. In children VIPomas are increasingly associated with ganglioneuromas, ganglioneuroblastomas, neurofibromas and other tumors in the adrenal area and neurogenic sites along the sympathetic chain. In a series of 62 patients with raised VIP, 10 had ganglioneuroblastoma, of which 70% were children [12]. In another six reported cases of persistent diarrhea in children, all had ganglioneuroblastoma with raised VIP and urinary catecholamine, except for two in whom the VIP was not done [8]. Therefore, investigation of urinary catecholamine may provide useful information in these cases.

Most VIPomas are large (3–8 cm in diameter) or even metastasized by the time of diagnosis. First-line imaging techniques including transabdominal ultrasound, computerized tomography (CT), octreotide scanning, magnetic resonance imaging (MRI) and gadolinium-enhanced magnetic resonance are able to identify larger tumors (Table 61.4). Other methods with enhanced sensitivity are available to detect smaller sized tumors, but are costly and require specialized equipment and expertise. Spiral CT scanning is a two-phase data acquisition of the pancreas in both arterial and parenchymal phases following intravenous contrast enhancement. It has increased sensitivity (50%) for detecting tumors as small as 5 mm in size. More invasive techniques such as endoscopic or intraoperative ultrasound have an increased detection sensitivity of 80% and 90% respectively. In highly suspicious cases where no tumor can be identified using the above methods selective arteriography and venous sampling have been reported to provide higher diagnostic sensitivity. However, transhepatic portal venous sampling only allows functional localization without pinpointing the exact anatomical position of the tumor. Seemingly, it is ineffective in localizing multiple or extrapancreatic tumors. Somatostatin receptor-positive tumors <1 cm in size can successfully be detected by octreotide scintigraphy. VIPomas are 100% sensitive to ^{123}I VIP scintigraphy and 80% to somatostatin scintigraphy.

Treatment

Treatment should be divided into acute life-saving supportive measures and prolonged curative and/or palliative treatment. In acute crises, the initial treatment should be focussed on fluid and electrolyte replacement. Once the patient is stabilized curative treatment in the form of surgical removal, if practically possible, is the therapy of choice. This is feasible in patients with large localized non-metastatic tumors, for example VIP-secreting ganglioneuroblastomas in children and well-defined non-metastatic pancreatic tumors in adults. However, 50% of pancreatic tumors are diagnosed after metastasis to the liver. In these cases surgical debulking might be of palliative benefit, though not effective in all. Similarly, hepatic embolization may provide palliation in patients with extensive hepatic disease. Combined medical and surgical treatments have been reported to provide a better possible outcome in patients with metastatic disease. Somatostatin analogs such as octreotide therapy have been shown to have a dual action; in the short term they provide symptomatic relief of diarrhea and in the long term may cause tumor shrinkage [13]. Relief of symptoms and provision of a better quality of life on octreotide have also been reported in patients in whom tumor localization has failed. Octreotide relieves diarrhea by suppressing VIP secretion. This has been shown to be effective in 80% of the cases. Ironically, a proportion of patients may develop octreotide resistance after the first year of treatment. In such cases, and in advanced metastatic disease, adjuvant chemotherapy should be used. The relatively non-toxic regimen of streptozocin and 5-fluorouracil has been shown to be effective with response rates of >50%. Repeated radiofrequency ablation has also been found to resolve clinical and biochemical abnormalities in patients with metastatic VIPoma [14]. In addition, patients with severe diarrhea who have failed to respond to octreotide have been shown to benefit from high-dose steroids [15].

Prognosis depends on the time of diagnosis, tumor size and metastatic state. Generally children with VIP-secreting ganglioneuroblastomas have good prognosis. A 5-year survival rate in 241 adult patients with VIPoma was shown to be 89% in those with pancreatic and 68.5% in those with neurogenic tumors. The rate was lower at 59.6% in patients with metastatic disease [16].

Conclusion

VIPomas are neuroendocrine tumors of which 90% originate in the pancreas; the remainder are extrapancreatic. In children they are mainly benign and associated with tumors arising from the sympathetic chain and adrenal medulla. VIPomas secrete massive amounts of VIP causing the classic symptoms of watery diarrhea, hypokalemia, hypochlorhydria and metabolic acidosis with life-threatening consequences. VIPomas may arise as an individual tumor or as part of a multiple endocrine neoplasia. Co-secretion of other peptides with VIP is responsible for additional symptoms characterizing the tumor. Prompt diagnosis and differentiation from other causes of secretory diarrhea should be sought. Tumors are large and mostly metastasize by the time of diagnosis. However, early successful localization using biochemical and imaging investigations can result in effective resection and cure. In metastatic disease, medical treatment in the form of chemotherapy, somatostatin analog and high-dose glucocorticoids have been effective in palliation.

References

1. Bloom SR, Polak JM, Pearse AG. Vasoactive intestinal peptide and watery–diarrhoea syndrome. *Lancet* 1973;2:14–16.
2. Levy-Bohbot N, Merle C, Goudet P, et al. Prevalence, characteristics and prognosis of MEN 1–associated glucagonomas, VIPomas,

and somatostatinomas: study from the GTE (Groupe des Tumeurs Endocrines registry. *Gastroenterol. Clin. Biol.* 2004;28:1075–1081.

3. Verner JV, Morrison AB. Islet cell tumor and a syndrome of refractory watery diarrhea and hypokalemia. *Am. J. Med.* 1958;25:374–380.

4. Rambaud JC, Modigliani R, Matuchansky C, et al. Pancreatic cholera. Studies on tumoral secretions and pathophysiology of diarrhea. *Gastroenterology* 1975;69:110–122.

5. Said SI, Mutt V. Polypeptide with broad biological activity: isolation from small intestine. *Science* 1970;169:1217–1218.

6. Bodanszky M, Klausner YS, Said SI. Biological activities of synthetic peptides corresponding to fragments of and to the entire sequence of the vasoactive intestinal peptide. *Proc. Natl Acad. Sci. USA* 1973;70:382–384.

7. Bloom SR, Polak JM. Gut hormones. *Adv. Clin. Chem.* 1980;21:177–244.

8. Murphy MS, Sibal A, Mann JR. Persistent diarrhoea and occult VIPomas in children. *Br. Med. J.* 2000;320:1524–1526.

9. Pratz KW, Ma C, Aubry MC, et al. Large cell carcinoma with calcitonin and vasoactive intestinal polypeptide-associated Verner–Morrison syndrome. *Mayo Clin. Proc.* 2005;80:116–120.

10. Nikou GC, Toubanakis C, Nikolaou P, et al. VIPomas: an update in diagnosis and management in a series of 11 patients. *Hepatogastroenterology* 2005;52:1259–1265.

11. Long RG, Bryant MG, Yuille PM, et al. Mixed pancreatic apudoma with symptoms of excess vasoactive intestinal polypeptide and insulin: improvement of diarrhoea with metoclopramide. *Gut* 1981;22:505–511.

12. Long RG, Bryant MG, Mitchell SJ, et al. Clinicopathological study of pancreatic and ganglioneuroblastoma tumours secreting vasoactive intestinal polypeptide (VIPomas). *Br. Med. J. (Clin. Res. Ed.)* 1981;282:1767–1771.

13. Arnold R, Frank M, Kajdan U. Management of gastroenteropancreatic endocrine tumors: the place of somatostatin analogues. *Digestion* 1994;55(Suppl 3):107–113.

14. Moug SJ, Leen E, Horgan PG, M. et al. Radiofrequency ablation has a valuable therapeutic role in metastatic VIPoma. *Pancreatology* 2006;6:155–159.

15. Katapadi K, Kostandy G, Katapadi M. et al. Role of IV steroids in treatment of VIPoma. *Infect. Med.* 1998;15:410–414.

16. Soga J, Yakuwa Y. VIPoma/diarrheogenic syndrome: a statistical evaluation of 241 reported cases. *J. Exp. Clin. Cancer Res.* 1998;17:389–400.

62 Glucagonomas

Niamh M. Martin, Karim Meeran, and Stephen R. Bloom

Key points

- Glucagonomas are rare, with an estimated annual incidence of 1 per 20 000 000.
- Glucagonomas are usually greater than 2 cm in diameter at presentation. The larger they are, the greater the incidence of malignancy and in the majority of cases of sporadic glucagonomas, metastases have occurred at presentation.
- Necrolytic migratory erythema is the presenting feature of glucagonoma syndrome in approximately 70% of cases. Even if necrolytic migratory erythema is absent at diagnosis, most patients with a glucagonoma eventually develop this hallmark clinical finding.
- In glucagonoma syndrome, somatostatin analogs (e.g. octreotide) may be useful in reducing circulating bioactive glucagon and inducing remission of clinical symptoms. Octreotide is particularly useful as a prompt and effective treatment of necrolytic migratory erythema, providing improvement within 48–72 h of initiating treatment.
- Surgical resection, by enucleation or by distal pancreatectomy and splenectomy, is the only treatment that may be curative if the glucagonoma is localized.

Introduction

Glucagonomas are rare, slow-growing tumors arising from the alpha cells of the pancreas, which secrete various forms of glucagon and other peptides derived from the pre-proglucagon gene. In 1942, Becker and colleagues published the first report of glucagonoma syndrome, involving a female patient with diabetes mellitus, anemia, weight loss and an unusual erythematous migratory rash [1]. Following death from acute left iliac venous thrombosis, autopsy revealed a malignant pancreatic islet cell tumor, of unknown cell type. Twenty years after Becker's original description, McGavran et al. described a female patient with "bullous and eczematoid dermatitis of the hands, feet and legs," vulvovaginitis, diabetes mellitus, normocytic anemia and hepatomegaly, in whom a metastatic pancreatic α-cell carcinoma was discovered [2]. McGavran and colleagues were the first to associate these features with hyperglucagonemia, identifying elevated glucagon concentrations in tumor tissue and peripheral blood from this patient. Wilkinson first coined the term "necrolytic migratory erythema" (NME) in 1973, to describe the distinctive erosive cutaneous eruptions which may be associated with glucagonomas (shown in Plate 62.1) [3]. In 1974, all of these clinical features were encompassed by the term "glucagonoma syndrome" [4]. Pseudoglucagonoma syndrome is the existence of NME in the absence of a glucagon secreting-neoplasm and may be associated with cirrhosis, celiac sprue, pancreatitis, inflammatory bowel disease and generalized malabsorption syndromes.

Metabolic effects of excess glucagon

The pre-proglucagon gene is expressed in the pancreas, intestine and brain, resulting in a single pro-glucagon mRNA transcript that is identical in all tissues. The different forms of glucagon and glucagon-related peptides present in each tissue reflect tissue-specific post-translational processing of pro-glucagon. The molecular hallmark of glucagonomas appears to be the extreme variability in the post-translational processing of pro-glucagon, resulting in heterogeneity of the secreted forms of glucagon and glucagon-related peptides such as glucagon-like peptide-1 (GLP-1). The presence of various forms of glucagon and glucagon-like peptides, each having different biological activities, confuses the relationship between measured total circulating glucagon-like immunoreactivity and various manifestations of the glucagonoma syndrome [5].

Glucagon is a powerful hyperglycemic agent, stimulating hepatic glycogenolysis, hepatic gluconeogenesis and inhibiting hepatic glycogen synthesis. Glucagon also has a pronounced catabolic effect, stimulating lipolysis and enhancing amino acid catabolism.

Clinical features

Glucagonomas are rare, with an estimated annual incidence of 1 per 20 000 000, and represent 8–13% of all functional endocrine

Clinical Endocrine Oncology, 2nd edition. Edited by Ian D. Hay and John A.H. Wass. © 2008 Blackwell Publishing. ISBN 978-1-4051-4584-8.

pancreatic tumors. Patients usually present between 40 and 70 years and although initial reports described a female predominance, more recent studies suggest a more equal sex distribution [6]. Glucagonomas are most commonly sporadic, and only rarely associated with multiple endocrine neoplasia type 1 (MEN 1). The most common site for primary glucagonomas is the pancreatic tail [6, 7] and extrapancreatic glucagonomas are rare. Glucagonomas are usually greater than 2 cm in diameter at presentation. Smaller glucagonomas tend to be benign and the larger they are, the greater the incidence of malignancy; 60–80% larger than 5 cm are malignant. In the majority of cases of sporadic glucagonomas, metastases have occurred at presentation [6, 7].

The most common presenting feature of glucagonoma syndrome is weight loss. Gastrointestinal disturbances may commonly occur, with the most frequent feature being diarrhea. Anorexia and abdominal discomfort are also features, with the latter often reflecting tumor bulk from hepatomegaly.

NME is the presenting feature of glucagonoma syndrome in approximately 70% of cases [6]. Even if NME is not present at diagnosis, most patients with a glucagonoma eventually develop this hallmark clinical finding and there are only a few published cases of glucagonoma in which NME has never developed. NME is cyclical in nature, consisting of macules, central bullae formation and crusted plaques occurring mainly at friction sites [8]. Lesions extend centrifugally, resulting in a serpiginous pattern and becoming confluent. Usually after 1–2 weeks, the central part of the lesion heals, giving the lesions an annular appearance and leaving postinflammatory hyperpigmentation. Therefore, the overall picture is of lesions in various stages of the cycle. The eruption is characterized by a pattern of spontaneous remissions and exacerbations without identifiable precipitating factors. Lesions are often intensely itchy and painful, with a predilection for areas subject to greater pressure and friction such as the perineum, buttocks, groin, lower abdomen, and lower extremities. Involvement of the perineal skin predisposes to inflammation of the vaginal and urethral mucosa. This may result in recurrent urinary tract infections in women and secondary infection of cutaneous lesions with *Candida albicans* and *Staphylococcus aureus* [9].

Diabetes mellitus is present in approximately two-thirds of those with the glucagonoma syndrome [6]. As with NME, this may not be a presenting feature, but usually develops with time and often before NME in those who develop both. Although earlier reports proposed that diabetes mellitus associated with the glucagonoma syndrome was mild [5], it has been proposed more recently that this may not be the case, since these individuals often require insulin therapy [6]. Diabetic ketoacidosis is rare, although this has been reported.

Glossitis and angular cheilitis are common presentations in glucagonoma syndrome. Typically, the tongue is beefy red, smooth, shiny, and tender. Neurologic and psychiatric symptoms occur in 20% of patients and include dementia, psychosis, depression, ataxia, optic atrophy, retrobulbar neuritis, fecal and urinary incontinence. Thromboembolism has been described in up to 30% of all cases of glucagonoma syndrome [9], which is not a feature of

other pancreatic endocrine tumors. This most often occurs in the deep veins of the legs and pulmonary arteries. Thromboembolism accounts for more than half of all deaths attributable to the glucagonoma syndrome.

Secondary endocrine syndromes may develop in glucagonoma patients even many years after initial diagnosis. Zollinger–Ellison syndrome is the most commonly associated endocrine syndrome [6, 7]. Pancreatic polypeptide (PP), produced by the D_1 cells of the islets of Langerhans, is also commonly elevated in glucagonoma patients, although this rarely produces clinical manifestations [7].

Multiple endocrine neoplasia and glucagonomas

Glucagonomas may occur in association with MEN 1, although much less commonly than gastrinomas and insulinomas. Between 5% and 17% of patients with glucagonoma have been reported to have MEN 1 [6, 7]. Age at presentation is younger in those with MEN 1 (median 33 years) compared to sporadic glucagonomas. However, this may actually reflect earlier detection following regular screening for neuroendocrine tumors in MEN 1 patients.

Investigation and diagnosis

The diagnosis of glucagonoma is made on the basis of an elevated fasting plasma glucagon [174 pg/mL (>50 pmol/L)], in association with characteristic clinical features and a demonstrable neuroendocrine tumor and/or metastatic deposits.

Laboratory features

Plasma glucagon is measured by specific radioimmunoassay and other causes of an elevated glucagon such as renal failure, hepatic failure, severe stress and continued hypoglycemia should be excluded. Chromatographic analysis of plasma glucagon in the glucagonoma syndrome frequently shows unusual molecular forms [5]. Greater immunoreactivity tends to appear in the high molecular weight position on gel chromatography, presumably because tumors do not adequately process proglucagon. Interestingly, larger tumors may be less efficient in glucagon production [6]. High plasma levels of GLP-1, co-produced with pancreatic glucagon by glucagonomas, have also been described. Circulating levels of the neuroendocrine tumor marker chromogranin A may be elevated. Multiple hormone secretion has been described in glucagonoma syndrome with approximately one-fifth of glucagonoma patients having an elevated fasting plasma gastrin [6, 7]. A similar proportion of patients have elevated PP [7], although as discussed, this is not usually clinically relevant. Other hormones increased in glucagonoma syndrome include insulin, 5-hydroxyindoleacetic acid, insulin, calcitonin, and adrenocorticotropic hormone (ACTH) [6]. Plasma glucose is commonly elevated.

Hypoaminoacidemia is a common feature of glucagonoma syndrome [4]. Low levels of multiple amino acids in serum and urine have been noted, which improve after resection of the glucagonoma [6]. Hypovitaminosis B may develop due to persistent stimulation of carbohydrate metabolism as a result of hyperglucagonemia. Variable plasma zinc levels have been reported in glucagonoma syndrome. Approximately one-third of cases of glucagonoma display a normocytic and normochromic anemia [7], although macrocytosis has also been described. Despite the association of glucagonomas with thromboembolism, coagulation tests are usually normal.

Imaging

Diagnostic imaging of glucagonomas includes ultrasound, computerized tomography (CT), magnetic resonance imaging (MRI), somatostatin receptor scintigraphy (SRS) and positron emission tomography (PET) (Fig. 62.1). Ultrasound may be useful in identifying hepatic metastases, but is not usually sensitive enough to identify the primary tumor. Endoscopic ultrasound is becoming more widely used in localizing small pancreatic tumors. However, this technique is better at identifying lesions in the pancreatic head rather than the pancreatic tail, where the majority of glucagonomas are located [10]. Similarly, glucagonomas are usually of significant size at presentation to be identified by the less invasive investigations such as contrast-enhanced CT. MRI is an alternative to CT, although there are few data available on its use. Glucagonomas and their metastases are commonly hypervascular, making selective visceral angiography particularly useful in localizing the tumor and identifying small hepatic metastases [10, 11]. SRS may be helpful when planning treatment with a somatostatin analog. More recently, PET has been reported to be a useful tool in detecting both the primary tumor and its metastases. In the largest study of glucagonomas to date, there was evidence of metastatic spread at presentation in 100% of cases [6]. Therefore, it is important to identify local (e.g., peripancreatic lymph nodes) and distant (e.g., liver, lung, adrenal gland, bone) metastases prior to planning treatment.

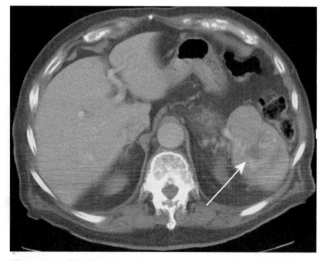

Figure 62.1 Abdominal CT scan showing glucagonoma in the pancreatic tail (identified by arrow).

Histopathology

Skin biopsy of NME often provides the first histopathological evidence for diagnosis in glucagonoma syndrome. Preferably, a biopsy of the edge of an early lesion should be taken for diagnosis. Histopathology shows necrolysis, edema, pallor of the epidermis, cleft formation, mild perivascular lymphocytic and histiocytic infiltration [8]. Cleft formation, which is highly characteristic of NME, results from necrosis of the upper layers of stratum spinosum, known as "sudden death," with separation from the minimally affected underlying epidermis [9]. Another specific feature on histological examination of the skin is necrolysis of the upper epidermis with vacuolated keratinocytes, leading to focal or confluent necrosis. However, often histological examination shows only non-specific, subacute dermatitis. Skin biopsy findings may be very similar to other dermatoses such as pellagra, zinc deficiency, acrodermatitis enteropathica, and annular chronic lupus erythematosus.

With conventional histology, glucagonomas show no more remarkable features other than general endocrine morphology [5]. General markers of neuroendocrine differentiation, including chromogranin A and neuron-specific enolase, may be present. Peptide immunocytochemistry using antibodies to pre-proglucagon may be useful in confirming the diagnosis of glucagonoma. However, it is important to use antibodies to all possible derivatives of the precursor form of glucagon, due to the wide variety of forms of glucagon often secreted by the tumor. Using electron microscopy, a variable number of secretory granules can be seen. In general, benign glucagonomas are fully granulated, whereas malignant ones are not [5]. The secretory granules may resemble the granules of pancreatic α-cells, but may be entirely atypical, particularly in malignant tumors.

Pathogenesis

The exact pathogenesis of NME remains unclear and is likely to be multifactorial. Since surgical resection of glucagonomas or treatment with somatostatin analogs may resolve NME, glucagon itself may induce NME. Amino acid deficiency may contribute to the pathogenesis of NME, since patients with glucagonomas and hypoaminoacidemia show resolution of NME following intravenous amino acid administration, even without normalization of serum amino acid levels. However, hypoaminoacidemia is unlikely to be the sole cause of NME, since normalizing amino acid levels does not always abolish NME. Zinc deficiency is another possible cause of NME, particularly as there are clinical and histological similarities between the dermatitis seen in NME and that of either acrodermatitis enteropathica (congenital zinc deficiency) or acquired zinc deficiency. Zinc supplementation has been associated with a resolution of NME. Plasma zinc levels are variable in glucagonoma syndrome and do not necessarily correlate with tissue zinc concentrations. Hypovitaminosis B may also contribute to NME and may explain the similarities between NME and other cutaneous manifestations of vitamin B deficiency such as pellagra.

Enhanced lipolysis may lead to deficiencies of essential fatty acids, which have been reported to be associated with dermatitis similar to NME. Liver dysfunction may contribute to NME by increasing serum glucagon and via hypoalbuminemia, which may potentiate the release of fatty acids and their conversion to inflammatory mediators and reduce zinc transport in the plasma.

The weight loss characteristic of glucagonoma patients is also multifactorial. Glucagon is a major catabolic hormone and this action is likely to promote this weight loss, at least in part. In addition, glucagon-related peptides, such as GLP-1, which may be present in large quantities in glucagonoma syndrome, also have inhibitory effects on appetite and body weight. PP, which is often co-secreted with glucagon in glucagonoma syndrome, can alter energy balance by stimulating weight loss, reducing food intake and increasing energy expenditure. Diarrhea associated with glucagonoma syndrome, resulting from both hyperglucagonemia and co-secretion of other peptides that alter gut motility, such as PP, vasoactive intestinal peptide (VIP) and gastrin, may further contribute to the weight loss. Extensive hepatic metastases may contribute to anorexia.

Similarly, the development of diabetes mellitus in glucagonoma syndrome may also be multifactorial, resulting from more than just a direct effect of glucagon on glucose metabolism. Glucagon and GLP-1 increase insulin secretion and therefore, the development of diabetes mellitus in glucagonoma syndrome probably depends on the relative concentrations of insulin and glucagon, which ultimately determine the net effect on hepatic glucose production. Significantly, other hormones co-secreted with glucagon in glucagonomas such as PP, VIP, ACTH and somatostatin can also promote hyperglycemia. Tumor load *per se* may play a part, particularly with large pancreatic tumors and extensive hepatic metastatic disease.

The generalized hypoaminoacidemia which is characteristic of glucagonoma syndrome may reflect increased hepatic conversion of amino acid nitrogen to urea nitrogen, resulting in decreased blood amino acid concentrations and increased clearance of circulating amino acids. A reduction in circulating glucagon using surgical debulking and somatostatin analogs can reduce amino acid catabolism.

The etiology of the normocytic normochromic anemia typical of glucagonoma syndrome has not been fully elucidated, but may reflect an inhibitory effect of glucagon on erythropoiesis. Similarly, the predisposition to thromboembolism with glucagonomas is unclear. Although no consistent abnormalities in coagulation have been described in hyperglucagonemia, glucagon increases platelet aggregation which may have a contributory effect.

Treatment

Medical

The use of somatostatin analogs in the management of glucagonomas was first described in 1986 [12]. Although octreotide does not prevent tumor growth, it may inhibit post-translational processing of proglucagon to glucagon, thereby reducing circulating bioactive glucagon and inducing remission of clinical symptoms. Octreotide is particularly useful as a prompt and effective treatment of NME, providing improvement within 48–72 h of initiating treatment [9]. Similarly, other symptoms such as diarrhea and weight loss may also improve. Somatostatin analogs have a variable effect on glucose intolerance and adjuvant glucose-lowering therapy with oral hypoglycemic agents or insulin may be required.

A number of chemotherapy agents have been used in the treatment of advanced metastatic glucagonoma, including 5-fluorouracil (5-FU), doxorubicin, streptozocin, and dacarbazine. However, their efficacy is limited. 5-FU and streptozocin in combination may be superior to streptozocin alone in the treatment of advanced islet cell carcinoma. Dacarbazine may have a role in treating glucagonomas resistant to streptozocin. Interferon-α has also been used both alone and in conjunction with somatostatin analogs in the treatment of metastatic glucagonoma, although evidence regarding its efficacy is conflicting and its use is often limited by side effects. Current opinion suggests that cytotoxic chemotherapy is withheld until symptoms become unresponsive to somatostatin or unless rapidly progressive disease intervenes [6].

Most patients with glucagonoma syndrome are treated empirically with oral zinc sulfate supplementation, regardless of plasma zinc levels. Infusions of amino acids and fatty acids have been used with variable success. Various other treatments for NME, including topical agents, oral steroids, radiation/UV light, methotrexate and dapsone, have all been used [9].

Patients with concomitant Zollinger–Ellison syndrome should be treated with proton pump inhibitors. The high incidence of thromboembolic disease associated with glucagonomas means that all patients should be treated with anticoagulants such as aspirin, warfarin or heparin.

Surgical

Surgical resection, by enucleation or by distal pancreatectomy and splenectomy, is the only treatment that may be curative if the glucagonoma is localized. Even if there is evidence of metastases at presentation, debulking surgery may lead to palliation of symptoms, particularly if there is extensive hepatic disease. There are recent reports of patients with a glucagonoma and hepatic metastases who have benefited from resection of the primary tumor and subsequent liver transplantation.

Hepatic embolization for metastatic disease

Hepatic metastases are supplied by the hepatic artery, yet the liver parenchyma has a dual blood supply from the hepatic artery and portal vein. Therefore, embolization of these metastases can occur via the hepatic arterial blood supply, resulting in devascularization and necrosis, whilst portal blood supply to the hepatic parenchyma is preserved. This may result in symptomatic improvement, even without normalizing fasting plasma glucagon. Hepatic chemoembolization combines this approach with the targeted local delivery of chemotherapy agents such as doxorubicin and cisplatin.

Prognosis

Although the majority of patients with glucagonoma syndrome present with evidence of metastases the slow-growing nature of these tumors can results in a relatively good prognosis. Five-year survival may range from 66% to 85% [7, 13] and may increase to 83% in those without hepatic metastases in whom complete resection of the primary tumor is possible [13].

References

1. Becker SW, Kahn D, Rothman S. Cutaneous manifestations of internal malignant tumours. *Arch. Dermatol. Syphilol.* 1942;45:1068–1080.
2. McGavran MH, Unger RH, Recant L, et al. A glucagon-secreting alpha-cell carcinoma of the pancreas. *N. Engl. J. Med.* 1966;274:1408–1413.
3. Wilkinson DS. Necrolytic migratory erythema with carcinoma of the pancreas. *Trans. St Johns Hosp. Dermatol. Soc.* 1973;59:244–250.
4. Mallinson CN, Bloom SR, Warin AP, et al. A glucagonoma syndrome. *Lancet* 1974;2:1–5.
5. Bloom SR, Polak JM. Glucagonoma syndrome. *Am. J. Med.* 1987;82:25–36.
6. Wermers RA, Fatourechi V, Wynne AG, et al. The glucagonoma syndrome. Clinical and pathologic features in 21 patients. *Medicine (Baltimore)* 1996;75:53–63.
7. Frankton S, Bloom SR. Gastrointestinal endocrine tumours. Glucagonomas. *Baillière's Clin. Gastroenterol.* 1996;10:697–705.
8. Kovacs RK, Korom I, Dobozy A, et al. Necrolytic migratory erythema. *J. Cutan. Pathol.* 2006;33:242–245.
9. Chastain MA. The glucagonoma syndrome: a review of its features and discussion of new perspectives. *Am. J. Med. Sci.* 2001;321:306–320.
10. Hammond PJ, Jackson JA, Bloom SR. Localization of pancreatic endocrine tumours. *Clin. Endocrinol. (Oxf.)* 1994;40:3–14.
11. Wawrukiewicz AS, Rosch J, Keller FS, et al. Glucagonoma and its angiographic diagnosis. *Cardiovasc. Intervent. Radiol.* 1982;5:318–324.
12. Boden G, Ryan IG, Eisenschmid BL, et al. Treatment of inoperable glucagonoma with the long-acting somatostatin analogue SMS 201-995. *N. Engl. J. Med.* 1986;314:1686–1689.
13. Chu QD, Al-kasspooles MF, Smith JL, et al. Is glucagonoma of the pancreas a curable disease? *Int. J. Pancreatol.* 2001;29:155–162.

63 Somatostatinomas

John A.H. Wass

Key points
- Somatostatinomas are very rare.
- There are two main types: one is pancreatic, which is almost invariably metastatic, and the other is duodenal.
- Features relate either to the effects of somatostatin or to the malignancy.

Introduction

Somatostatin was isolated in 1973 by Paul Brazeau in Roger Guillemin's laboratory. It was found to have a widespread distribution, not only in the hypothalamus and brain but also in the gastrointestinal tract. Sixty-five percent of the body's somatostatin is in the gut, mostly in the D cells of the gastric and intestinal epithelium. It is also present in the myometric and submucosal plexuses. The highest concentration is in the antrum of the stomach and there is a gradual decrease of concentrations down the gastrointestinal tract. Five percent of the body's somatostatin is in the pancreas.

Infused somatostatin, which has a short half-life of 3 min, has a large number of actions on the pituitary gland, the endocrine and exocrine pancreas, gastrointestinal tract, other hormones and on the nervous system (Table 63.1). Of importance in the gastrointestinal tract, gastrin and cholecystokinin (CCK) are inhibited. In the pancreas, insulin and glucagon are inhibited. Non-endocrine actions include inhibition of gastric acid secretion, pancreatic exocrine function, gallbladder contraction and intestinal motility. Intestinal absorption of nutrients including glucose, triglycerides and amino acids is also inhibited [1].

Somatostatin exists in two main forms: as a 14-amino-acid peptide (SMS 14) present mainly in the pancreas and the stomach, and as a 28-amino-acid peptide present mainly in the intestine. Somatostatin 14 is the peptide present in enteric neurons.

Somatostatin receptors are present on many cell types including the parietal cells of the stomach, G cells, D cells themselves and cells of the exocrine and endocrine pancreas. A large number of tumors also have somatostatin receptors and these include pituitary adenomas, endocrine pancreatic tumors, carcinoid tumors, paragangliomata, pheochromocytomas, small cell lung carcinomas, lymphomas and meningiomas. Five different somatostatin

Table 63.1 Actions of exogenously administered somatostatin on endocrine and exocrine secretion

Endocrine secretion	Exocrine secretion
Inhibits the secretion of:	Inhibition of:
Pituitary	Gastric acid secretion
Growth hormone	Gastric emptying rate
Thyroid-stimulating hormone	Pancreatic exocrine function:
	volume, electrolytes and enzyme content
Gastrointestinal tract	
Gastrin	
Cholecystokinin	Gallbladder contraction
Secretin	Intestinal motility
Vasoactive intestinal peptide	
Gastrin-inhibiting peptide	Intestinal absorption of nutrients
Motilin	Splanchnic blood flow
Enteroglucagon	
Pancreatic polypeptide	Renal water reabsorption
Insulin	Activity of some central nervous system neurons
Glucagon	
Somatostatin	Excitation of:
Other peptides	Activity of some neurons
Renin	
Growth hormone-releasing hormone	

receptors have been cloned (SSTR1 to SSTR5) and all are on different chromosomes. These have a varying affinity for somatostatin 14 and somatostatin 28 and varying tissue distribution.

Somatostatin can act either as an endocrine hormone or in a paracrine or autocrine way. It probably also has luminal effects in the gastrointestinal tract. Lastly it can act as a neurotransmitter [2].

Somatostatinoma

Somatostatinomas are rare tumors with an incidence of about 1:40 000 000. Two main types exist: pancreatic somatostatinomas, which are large tumors often associated with features of

Clinical Endocrine Oncology, 2nd edition. Edited by Ian D. Hay and John A.H. Wass. © 2008 Blackwell Publishing. ISBN 978-1-4051-4584-8.

Table 63.2 Comparison of pancreatic and duodenal somatostatin

Pancreatic	Duodenal
Large multihormonal and syndromes	Pure somatostatin
Invariably metastatic	Psammoma bodies
Somatostatinoma syndrome	40% metastatic

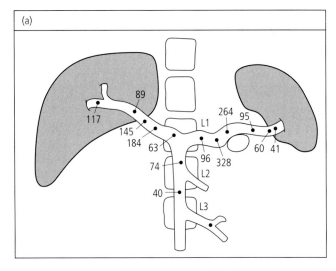

somatostatin excess, and duodenal tumors, which are usually small and more amenable to surgical resection (Table 63.2) [3]. They occur with approximately equal frequency.

Pancreatic somatostatinoma

Somatostatinoma syndrome was first described in 1977 [5]. Cases have been reported with features as in Table 63.3. The syndrome consists of cholelithiasis due to inhibition of CCK production. Almost certainly the decline in gastrointestinal motility allows increased biliary cholesterol to develop which is probably another factor. This has been demonstrated with octreotide therapy but not with somatostatinoma syndrome. Mild diabetes occurs and has often been present for many years before diagnosis. It is probably due to suppression of insulin secretion; diarrhea and steatorrhea also occur and this relates to the inhibition of pancreatic exocrine function. Hypochlorhydria relates to the inhibition of gastric acid secretion and gastrin. Anemia, abdominal pain and weight loss are also present and are non-specific. They are probably related to the size of the tumor, which is usually large, and also to the fact that it is malignant. Those tumors are often diagnosed late and distant metastases may be present in lymph nodes, liver or bone.

Plasma and tissue levels of somatostatin are elevated. These somatostatin-secreting cells often also secrete adrenocorticotropic

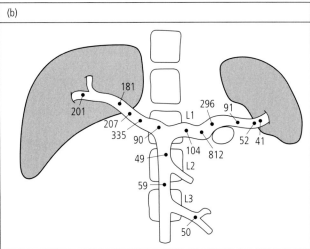

Figure 63.1 Transhepatic catheterization showing a tumor secreting both insulin and somatostatin. The tumor was located at the head of the pancreas and the patient presented with hypoglycemia. (a) Plasma insulin levels (mu/L); (b) plasma somatostatin levels (pg/ml).

hormone, calcitonin, insulin or some other peptides. This means that Cushing syndrome, flushing or hypoglycemia (if there is co-secretion of insulin; Fig. 63.1) may be present [4].

Duodenal somatostatinoma

Duodenal somatostatinomas tend to be smaller and present earlier. They may not be associated with abnormal circulating somatostatin levels. The vast majority occur near the ampulla of Vater, where they tend to cause obstructive biliary disease. They can also occur in the jejunum, cystic duct, colon and rectum. Some are associated with neurofibromatosis type 1 and multiple endocrine neoplasia type 1, and a case has been reported in association with von Hippel–Lindau syndrome. At presentation paraduodenal lymph nodes are often involved because there is a

Table 63.3 Features of pancreatic somatostatinoma

Hyperglycemia	35%
Cholelithiasis	64%
Steatorrhea	45%
Hypochlorhydria	
Weight loss	
Diarrhea	
Abdominal pain	
Anemia	
Elevated plasma and tissue somatostatin	
Tumors immunostain for chromogranin A	
Histologically malignant, may be associated with ACTH, calcitonin, gastrin and insulin secretion	

ACTH, adrenocorticotropic hormone.

high malignancy rate, although this is low grade and metastases at diagnosis, while invariable for pancreatic somatostatinoma, are not so with the duodenal variety. None of the duodenal somatostatinoma patients have developed the full-blown somatostatinoma syndrome but diabetes and gallstones have been noted in some cases.

Histologically these are psammomatous tumors. Treatment is with surgery if this is feasible, chemotherapy and if necessary hepatic embolization [6].

Survival rates

Postoperative 5-year survival rates in patients with metastatic disease are 30–60%. Patients with no metastatic involvement have a 5-year survival of around 100%.

References

1. Schultz A. Somatostatin: physiology and clinical application. *Clin. Endocrinol. Metab.* 1994;8:215–236.
2. Moayedoddin B, Booya F, Wermers RA, et al. Spectrum of malignant somatostatin-producing neuroendocrine tumors. *Endocr. Pract.* 2006;12:394–400.
3. Krejs GJ, Orci L, Conlon JN, et al. Somatostatinoma syndrome. Biochemical, morphological and clinical features. *N. Engl. J. Med.* 1979;301:285–292.
4 Wright J, Abolfathr A, Penman E, Marks V. Pancreatic somatostatinoma presenting with hypoglycaemia. *Clin. Endocrinol.* 1980;12:603–608.
5. Soga J, Yakuwa Y. Somatostatinoma/inhibitory syndrome: a statistical evaluation of 173 reported cases as compared to other pancreatic endocrinomas. *J. Exp. Clin. Cancer Res.* 1999;18:13–22.
6. Oberg K, Eriksson B. Endocrine tumours of the pancreas. *Best Pract. Res. Clin. Gastroenterol.* 2005;19:753–781.

64 Lung and Thymic Neuroendocrine Tumors

Dan Granberg and Kjell Öberg

Key points

- Neuroendocrine lung tumors (bronchial carcinoids) are rare tumors affecting all ages, harboring a malignant potential. Distant metastases may occur late. Long-term follow-up is important.
- Between 15% and 50% of the patients are asymptomatic, diagnosed on routine chest X-ray. Presenting symptoms include cough, hemoptysis, recurrent pneumonias, wheezing and dyspnea. Endocrine symptoms are uncommon.
- Radical surgery is the only treatment that may be curative, and leads to an excellent prognosis in most patients. As much lung parenchyma as possible should be spared.
- Neuroendocrine thymic tumors are rare and aggressive. About 20% are part of multiple endocrine neoplasia type 1 syndrome. One-third of sporadic tumors present with Cushing syndrome.
- Surgery is the only curative treatment. Radiotherapy is frequently indicated. Chemotherapy or targeted irradiation treatment may be tried in patients with metastatic disease.

Introduction

Lung and thymic neuroendocrine tumors belong to the group of so-called foregut neuroendocrine tumors; they have been previously described as carcinoids and this term is still used in most presentations. However, the new WHO classification of neuroendocrine tumors should be used [1].

Neuroendocrine pulmonary tumors are divided into bronchial carcinoids, large cell neuroendocrine carcinomas and small cell lung cancer. Bronchial carcinoids are further subdivided into typical and atypical carcinoids, depending on their appearance in light microscopy. According to the new definition, accepted by WHO, typical carcinoids have <2 mitoses/2 mm^2 (10 high-power fields) and no necrosis, while atypical carcinoids have 2–10 mitoses/2 mm^2 (10 high-power fields). Necrosis may be present [1]. Like other neuroendocrine tumors, bronchial carcinoids express neuroendocrine markers on immunohistochemistry and may also secrete hormones, giving rise to various endocrine symptoms.

Thymic neuroendocrine tumors (TNETS) are a rare entity. Since the first description by Rosai and Higa in 1972 [2], approximately 150 cases have been reported in the literature. These tumors are frequently associated with endocrine disorders (Cushing syndrome) or multiple endocrine neoplasia type 1 (MEN 1) and carry a poor prognosis.

Clinical Endocrine Oncology, 2nd edition. Edited by Ian D. Hay and John A.H. Wass. © 2008 Blackwell Publishing. ISBN 978-1-4051-4584-8.

Neuroendocrine lung tumors (bronchial carcinoids)

Epidemiology, etiology

Bronchial carcinoids are rare tumors, although the incidence has increased during the last decades. The reason for this is not known. The incidence is about 0.7/100 000 in caucasians and 0.5/100 000 in black people. Women are slightly more affected than men [3]. The disease is most common in middle ages, but occurs in all ages, even in children. Carcinoid is the most frequent respiratory tumor in children and adolescents. The etiology is unknown, except that patients with MEN 1 have a higher risk. Smoking is not a risk factor.

Pathology

Macroscopic findings

Bronchial carcinoids may be located centrally (60–84%) in the main or lobar bronchi, or peripherally. Central tumors are often larger (0.9–10 cm, mean 3.1 cm) than peripheral ones (0.5–6 cm, mean 2.4 cm). Central carcinoids may be seen at bronchoscopy as a polypoid, highly vascular endobronchial tumor. The color may vary from cherry-red to white-yellow or brownish-yellow (Plate 64.1). The tumor often infiltrates the surrounding lung parenchyma. Peripheral carcinoids are located in segmental bronchi or more distally. They may be multiple and surrounded by small satellite lesions, named tumorlets. Peripheral tumors are not accessible by bronchoscopy.

Histopathology and immunohistochemistry

Typical carcinoids consist of small polyhedral cells with small round or oval nuclei. The chromatin is finely granular and the cytoplasm is acidophilic. The cells are regularly arranged in nests, sheets, ribbons or spindling structures, separated by a fibrovascular stroma. Necrosis is not seen in typical carcinoids. Mitoses are few or absent (Plate 64.2). Atypical carcinoids are characterized by nuclear pleomorphism, hyperchromatism, abnormal nuclear to cytoplasmic ratio, prominent nucleoli and areas of increased cellularity with disorganized architecture. Necrosis may occur, and mitoses are more frequent (Plate 64.3). At electron microscopy, typical carcinoids display an abundance of membrane-bound secretory granules, while atypical carcinoids have fewer granules, diffusely distributed in the cytoplasm [4].

Since bronchial carcinoids are of epithelial origin, they show positive immunohistochemistry for cytokeratin. Most of the tumors stain positive for the common neuroendocrine markers chromogranin A, synaptophysin and neuron-specific enolase. In addition, many of the tumors stain positive for various hormones, such as adrenocorticotropic hormone (ACTH), serotonin, gastrin-releasing peptide (GRP)/bombesin, pancreatic polypeptide, human chorionic gonadotropin α-subunit, calcitonin, leucine, enkephalin and growth hormone-releasing hormone. Positive staining for multiple hormones is common [4, 5]. Expression of S-100 protein may be found, usually in peripheral tumors. Positive staining for the standard form of the adhesion molecule CD44, as well as for the retinoblastoma gene product, is usually found in typical carcinoids. The oncoproteins p53 and bcl-2, however, usually stain negative in typical carcinoids but more often positive in atypical carcinoids.

Genetic alterations

Deletions in the *MEN* 1 locus at 11q are common in both typical and atypical carcinoids. Homozygous somatic inactivation of the *MEN1* gene has been found in 36% of sporadic bronchial carcinoids. Atypical carcinoids may have deletions in 10q or 13q. Aneuploidy is detected in 5–32% of typical carcinoids and 17–79% of atypical carcinoid tumors.

Clinical presentation

Between 13% and 51% of patients with bronchial carcinoids are asymptomatic, and the tumor is diagnosed on routine chest X-ray. Common symptoms include cough, hemoptysis, recurrent pneumonias with or without persisting lung infiltrate on chest X-ray, wheezing, dyspnea and chest pain [5, 6]. The patient is often misdiagnosed for several years as having "asthma," frequently resulting in a delay in correct diagnosis. Endocrine symptoms are uncommon. The classic carcinoid syndrome with flush, diarrhea, wheezing, right-sided valvular heart disease and elevated urinary 5-HIAA is seen in 2–12% of the patients, usually only

when liver metastases are present. Occasionally, secretion of histamine may give rise to an atypical carcinoid syndrome (not to be confused with atypical carcinoids!) with generalized flushing, edema, lacrimation, bronchoconstriction and diarrhea. Ectopic Cushing syndrome, due to secretion of ACTH or corticotropin-releasing factor (CRF), occurs in 2–6% of the patients. These tumors are often small and may be difficult to detect on computerized tomography (CT) or magnetic resonance imaging (MRI) scan. Acromegaly, caused by production of growth hormone-releasing hormone, is rare.

Typical carcinoid tumors metastasize in 5–20% of patients, while up to 70% of patients with atypical carcinoid tumors develop metastases. Metastases most frequently occur to regional lymph nodes, but also distantly to the liver, bones, brain, subcutis, mammary glands and adrenals. Metastases may occur late, up to 20 years after surgery for the primary tumor.

Diagnosis

Chest X-ray reveals the tumor in more than 60% of the patients. In cases with central tumors, signs of bronchial obstruction may be seen, with peripheral atelectasis and pneumonic infiltrates in a lobe or a segment. CT scan, which is more sensitive, should always be performed in order to clarify the extent of the tumor and detect satellite lesions and enlarged lymph nodes. MRI may be an alternative to CT scan.

About two-thirds of bronchial carcinoids are detectable on scintigraphy with ^{111}In-labelled octreotide (octreoscan®) [7] (Plate 64.4). Octreoscan® should be done preoperatively in all patients, both for detection of distant metastases and to clarify if the tumor is somatostatin receptor positive and thus possible to follow up with octreoscan®. In cases with ectopic Cushing syndrome, octreoscan® is especially useful, since the primary tumor is often small and difficult to detect on CT or MRI scan.

Positron emission tomography (PET) with ^{11}C-5-hydroxytryptophan is a sensitive method for detection of neuroendocrine tumors [8], and is especially valuable in patients with ectopic Cushing syndrome. PET with ^{18}F-fluorodeoxyglucose is, however, usually of limited value for diagnosis of bronchial carcinoid tumors, since these tumors are slowly growing and often display lower glucose uptake than expected for malignant tumors.

Central tumors are accessible via bronchoscopy, which is performed in most patients. It is important to take biopsies, which can usually be done safely despite the risk of bleeding. Brushing or sputum cytology is frequently uninformative, since the tumor is often covered by a layer of normal mucosa. Peripheral tumors may be reached by transthoracic CT-guided needle biopsy, although the differential diagnosis to small cell lung cancer may be difficult and misdiagnosis is not uncommon.

Measurement of plasma chromogranin A should be made in all patients before surgery of the primary tumor, but is usually normal if the tumor has not metastasized. If chromogranin A is elevated, a CT or ultrasound of the abdomen is warranted to search for liver metastases. Analysis of urinary cortisol or 5'HIAA is, however, not recommended routinely, but is only indicated if the patient displays endocrine symptoms.

Differential diagnoses

Alternative diagnoses when a tumor is found on chest X-ray or CT scan include other benign or malignant lung neoplasms, hamartoma and metastasis from another primary tumor. It may sometimes be difficult on histological examination to differentiate between atypical lung carcinoid and small cell lung carcinoma. Staining for the proliferation marker Ki67 may aid in the differential diagnosis. In one study, all small cell lung cancers had a proliferative activity of >25%, while all lung carcinoids had <10% Ki67-positive cells [9].

Treatment

Radical surgery is the only possible cure for patients with bronchial carcinoids. The aim is to remove the tumor and all affected lymph nodes, sparing as much lung parenchyma as possible. Possible procedures include local excision, sleeve resection, wedge or segmental resection, lobectomy, bilobectomy and pneumonectomy. During the surgery, it is mandatory to perform a thorough lymph node dissection, aided by frozen sections. In patients with atypical carcinoids, at least a lobectomy should be performed. Endoscopic removal of the tumor by YAG-laser is usually not recommended, since the tumor often grows deeply into the surrounding tissue and radical removal thus is difficult to obtain by laser resection. This method should be reserved for palliation in those cases where surgery is not possible. In a limited number of patients, surgery may be considered after previous laser treatment to cause reduction of the tumor and allow postobstructive infiltrates to resolve.

External radiotherapy is mainly used for palliative treatment of bone or brain metastases. Radiotherapy against the primary tumor area may be used in patients with inoperable tumors and may also be considered after surgery in patients with atypical carcinoids and uncertain radicality or lymph node metastases. Targeted irradiation therapy with ^{111}In, ^{90}Y or ^{177}Lu labeled somatostatin analogs is an alternative in patients with metastatic bronchial carcinoids showing high octreotide uptake on octreoscan®.

The treatment of metastatic bronchial carcinoids (Table 64.1) is disappointing. Chemotherapy has been tried with various combinations, such as cisplatin or carboplatin + etoposide, docetaxel or paclitaxel + doxorubicin, streptozotocin + 5-fluorouracil or doxorubicin, cyclophosphamide + doxorubicin + vincristine or temozolomide as monotherapy; however, only a limited number of responses or stabilization of the disease for short periods of time has been obtained [10]. A recent study has shown that many bronchial carcinoids express the tyrosine kinase receptors c-kit, platelet-derived growth factor receptor (PDGFR)α and PDGFRβ

Table 64.1 Treatment of metastatic bronchial carcinoids

Chemotherapy
   cisplatin/carboplatin + etoposide
   docetaxel/paclitaxel + doxorubicin
   streptozotocin + 5-fluorouracil/doxorubicin
   cyclophosphamide + doxorubicin + vincristine
   temozolomide
Biotherapy
   α-interferon
   octreotide/lanreotide
Targeted radiotherapy
   ^{177}Lu-octreotate
   ^{90}Y-octreotide
   ^{111}In-octreotide
Liver embolization
Particles: gel-foam polyvinyl alcohol, tris-acryl-gelatin microspheres
Chemoembolization: doxorubicin, cisplatin, mitomycin-C, streptozotocin
SIRT: ^{90}Y-labeled resin microspheres

and endothelial growth factor receptor (EGFR) [11]. This finding makes it possible to treat patients harboring metastatic bronchial carcinoids with tyrosine kinase inhibitors.

Biotherapy with α-interferon and somatostatin analogs such as octreotide or lanreotide may in selected cases result in stabilization of the disease or even objective responses, but is mainly indicated for palliation of the classic or atypical carcinoid syndrome or Cushing syndrome. Other possibilities to relieve Cushing syndrome include ketoconazole, metyrapone or mitotane.

Hepatic arterial embolization may be used for debulking or growth stabilization of liver metastases. Embolization can be performed either with particles, such as gel-foam (Spongostan™), polyvinyl alcohol (Ivalon™) or tris-acryl-gelatin microspheres (Embospheres™), or with cytotoxic drugs (doxorubicin, cisplatin, mitomycin-C or streptozotocin) followed by particles. Another method for debulking of liver metastases is selective internal radiation therapy (SIRT), which means liver embolization with resin microspheres labelled with [90]Y. This method has shown promising results in patients with primary hepatocellular cancer and metastatic colorectal cancer and has recently been introduced for treatment of patients with neuroendocrine tumors with liver metastases. Patients with a limited number of liver metastases, not more than 3 cm in diameter, may benefit from radiofrequency ablation.

Prognosis

The prognosis for most patients with typical bronchial carcinoids is excellent. A majority is cured by radical surgery, even in the presence of lymph node metastases. Five- and 10-year survival rates are 85–100% and 90–100% respectively [12, 13]. Poor prognostic factors include lymph node metastases at diagnosis, presence of satellite lesions (tumorlets) and high proliferative rate assessed by immunohistochemistry for Ki67. On the other hand, positive immunohistochemistry for the standard form of the adhesion molecule CD44, as well as positive nuclear staining for the metastasis suppressor gene *nm23*, has been shown to correlate with decreased risk for distant metastases and death [14]. Patients with atypical bronchial carcinoids have a considerably worse prognosis. The risk of recurrence and distant metastases is high, and 5- and 10-year survival rates are only 40–76% and 18–60% respectively [15].

Since metastases may develop late, patients with bronchial carcinoids must be followed for a long time, at least 10 years. The follow-up should include CT scan of the thorax and CT or ultrasound of the abdomen and measurement of plasma chromogranin A. Octreoscan® (in patients with somatostatin receptor-positive tumors) or conventional bone scintigraphy is recommended about every third year. Special attention should be paid to patients with atypical carcinoids or high proliferative rate, Ki67 index ≥5%.

Thymic neuroendocrine tumors (carcinoids) (TNETS)

Epidemiology, etiology

The overall age-adjusted incidence of neuroendocrine tumors of the thymus (TNETS) is 0.01/100 000 individuals, with a clear male preponderance. The incidence is about three times more frequent in men than in women [3]. Tumors have been described in patients from 8 years of age up to 87 years, but occur more frequently in the middle ages. There seems to be a clear correlation with cigarette smoking. TNETS are associated with other endocrine diseases, e.g. MEN 1. Teh reported that approximately 20% of patients with thymic neuroendocrine tumors present with MEN 1 syndrome [16]. Patients with thymic neuroendocrine tumors and MEN 1 are predominantly men and smokers but usually do not present any endocrine symptoms related to the thymic tumor [17]. Cushing syndrome has been reported in about one-third of sporadic cases, but never in MEN 1 patients. In contrast approximately 10% of patients with ectopic ACTH syndrome have a sporadic neuroendocrine carcinoma of the thymus. Recently ectopic growth hormone-releasing hormone (GHRH) secretion alone and GHRH and ACTH associated secretion by a thymic carcinoid tumor have been reported in one MEN 1 patient and one patient with sporadic tumor.

Histopathology and immunohistochemistry

The gross appearance of a TNETS is similar to that of thymomas, but they are rarely encapsulated. Microscopically the tumor exhibits a ribbon-like growth pattern with rosette formation in a fibrovascular stroma. The cells are small, round or oval, with eosinophilic cytoplasm and uniformly round nuclei. Immunohistochemical studies reveal positive staining for chromogranin A, synaptophysin and neuron-specific enolase (Plate 64.5). Electron microscopy shows the presence of secretory granules. A new classification has been adopted according to specific criteria (mitotic activity, presence of necrosis and cytological atypia) [18]. A grade 1 neuroendocrine carcinoma previously called typical carcinoid has less than 10 mitoses/100 high power fields, no necrosis and minimal pleomorphism. A grade 2 neuroendocrine carcinoma previously called atypical carcinoid presents more than 10 mitoses/100 high power fields and also presents necrosis and moderate pleomorphism. A grade 3 neuroendocrine carcinoma, previously large cell neuroendocrine carcinoma and small cell carcinoma, presents more mitoses and also necrosis and pleomorphism. All subtypes of neuroendocrine thymic tumors show positive immunohistochemical staining for chromogranin A and synaptophysin.

Genetic alterations

About 20% of patients with thymic neuroendocrine tumors are associated with MEN 1 [19]. It is also quite common that the thymic tumor is diagnosed at the same time as hyperparathyroidism in MEN 1 patients. It has also been reported that parathyroid hormone (PTH) or parathyroid hormone related peptide (PTHrP) is secreted from thymic neoplasm and PTHrP is known to exhibit neuroendocrine and growth factor activities produced by epithelial cells of the mature thymus. Less frequently, thymic involvement may be the first diagnosed disorder in MEN 1 syndrome. Clusters of affected individuals have been reported in some families. Linkage of heterozygosity studies in the 11q13–*MEN1* region was negative and the absence of genotype-phenotype correlation is confirmed in most studies [19]. A role for a putative tumor suppressor gene on chromosome 1p is suggested in the pathogenesis of a subset of thymic NETS. The observation of a male preponderance for thymic neuroendocrine tumors is intriguing and the action that sex hormones exert on thymus proliferation and maturation has been discussed. Sex hormones have a strong influence in the development of thymus and estrogens act as inhibitors of thymoma growth.

Clinical presentation

About one-third to half of the patients with sporadic TNETS present with Cushing syndrome [18, 19]. Most thymic neuroendocrine tumors show an aggressive biological behavior from the time of presentation. Symptoms are related to effects of the tumor mass, with chest pain, cough and dyspnea. Superior vena cava syndrome is described in about 20% of cases. Cushing syndrome is reported in about one-third of sporadic tumors. In those patients who present with Cushing syndrome, there is no difference in sex distribution. Other non-endocrine syndromes associated with TNETS are polymyositis, polyarthritis, pericarditis and clubbing. Association with the carcinoid syndrome or myasthenia gravis has never been described, not even in metastatic disease. The majority of patients have local invasion of the tumor and metastatic spread occurs by the hematogenous and lymphatic route. Mediastinal lymph node metastases are frequently observed at presentation. Distant metastatic sites include lung, bone, adrenal glands, liver and spleen in order of frequency. Distant metastases are observed in approximately 20% of patients with thymic neuroendocrine tumors with a protracted clinical course.

Diagnosis

A thymic neuroendocrine tumor is usually diagnosed as an anterior mediastinal mass usually revealed by chest X-ray or CT scan, by accident or in the context of periodical, clinical follow-up of MEN 1 patients. The most reliable imaging technique is still a matter of debate. Routine chest X-ray may not be adequate for screening and follow-up of thymic NETS, because the profile of the great vessel and the heart does not allow diagnosis until the tumor reaches a metastatic stage. CT scan has been diagnostic in most instances, particularly in MEN 1 patients, and should for screening purposes be performed every 2–3 years. Chest X-ray should be performed yearly in MEN 1 members [18, 19]. Somatostatin receptor scintigraphy (octreoscan®) has been confirmed in several studies as an excellent pre- and postoperative diagnostic procedure and is of importance for staging of the disease [20]. However, uptake in bone metastases might be low. Other scintigraphic tracers such as ^{99m}Tc methoxyisobutylisonitrile have been reported to co-localize thymic and parathyroid involvement in MEN 1 patients. Magnetic resonance imaging (MRI) is sometimes recommended for early detection of thymic involvement. MRI may play a crucial role in detecting pericardial or large vessel invasion and thereby assessing the indication of surgical treatment and its modality. The role of positron emission tomography (PET) in the detection of thymic carcinoid remains to be established. A preliminary report has evidenced the efficacy of this diagnostic test using FDG. However, others have reported that thymic biopsies, performed on the basis of increased thymic uptake of FDG, revealed only normal thymic tissue. The use of ^{11}C-5-hydroxytryptophan is preferable for its specificity and accuracy in neuroendocrine tumors and has been effective in the diagnosis of patients with ectopic ACTH-secreting thymic NETS that were negative with octreoscan®, MRI and CT [21] (Plate. 64.6). The biochemical diagnosis of neuroendocrine thymic tumors includes urinary cortisol and plasma chromogranin A, neuron- specific enolase, plasma ACTH, GHRH, PTH and sometimes PTHrP. If there is a family history a full MEN 1 screening program should be performed. No patients have so far presented a carcinoid syndrome; therefore U-5-HIAA is not of any value.

Treatment

Surgery is the only cure for TNETS. Aggressive surgical treatment, including complete surgical excision with local lymph node resection and postoperative irradiation, offers the best chance for prolonged survival [18]. In patients with MEN 1 syndrome prophylactic thymectomy should be performed in association with parathyroidectomy, which may prevent the risk of later development of thymic malignancy. Median sternotomy is often indicated as a surgical approach, but occasionally in case of large and invasive tumors, the addition of an anterior (or posterior/lateral) thoracotomy should be considered to obtain better exposure of the involved hemithorax. Sampling lymphadenectomy is mandatory for staging and planning of future medical treatment. The role of neoadjuvant/adjuvant treatment (chemotherapy) or radiotherapy alone or in combination has not been assessed because of the low number of cases. Some authors recommend postoperative radiotherapy to prevent local recurrence of invasive tumors (45–60 Gy). There are no standard regimens of chemotherapy and only occasional experiences have been reported in the literature. Ifosfamide and etoposide have been attempted with short-lasting responses and the same for 5FU, streptozotocin, etoposide or cisplatinum. Recently five out of six patients with thymic carcinoid responded to temozolomide, with stabilization of the disease for up to 8 months [22]. Most successful has been a multi-disciplinary treatment including aggressive surgery, neoadjuvant chemotherapy and hormonal treatment including somatostatin analogs (octreotide/lanreotide). The majority of thymic neuroendocrine tumors express somatostatin receptor type 2 and therefore tumor-targeted radioactive treatment with ^{90}Y-DOTA-octreotide or ^{177}Lu-DOTA-octreotate might be of value [20]. No data have so far been presented.

Prognosis

Neuroendocrine thymic carcinomas are rare and aggressive tumors that are often characterized by local invasive growth and metastatic disease. The 5-year survival rate has been reported to be 60–100% for localized disease, 40% for regional and only 29% for patients with distant metastases.

References

1. Travis WD, Colby TV, Corrin B, Shimosato Y, Brambilla E. Countries ICwLHSaPf. *Histological Typing of Lung and Pleural Tumours*, 3rd edition. Berlin: Springer, World Health Organization, 1999.

2. Rosai J, Higa E. Mediastinal endocrine neoplasm, of probable thymic origin, related to carcinoid tumor. Clinicopathologic study of 8 cases. *Cancer* 1972;29:1061–1074.

3. Modlin IM, Lye KD, Kidd M. A 5-decade analysis of 13 715 carcinoid tumors. *Cancer* 2003;97:934–959.

4. Warren WH, Memoli VA, Gould VE. Immunohistochemical and ultrastructural analysis of bronchopulmonary neuroendocrine neoplasms. I. Carcinoids. *Ultrastruct. Pathol.* 1984;6:15–27.

5. McCaughan BC, Martini N, Bains MS. Bronchial carcinoids – review of 124 cases. *J. Thorac. Cardiovasc. Surg.* 1985;89:8–17.

6. Bertelsen S, Aasted A, Lund C, et al. Bronchial carcinoid tumors – a clinicopathologic study of 82 cases. *Scand. J. Thorac. Cardiovasc. Surg.* 1985;19:105–111.

7. Granberg D, Sundin A, Janson ET, Öberg K, Skogseid B, Westlin J-E. Octreoscan in patients with bronchial carcinoid tumours. *Clin. Endocrinol.* 2003;59:793–799.

8. Örlefors H, Sundin A, Garske U, et al. Whole-body 11C-5-hydroxytryptophan positron emission tomography as a universal imaging technique for neuroendocrine tumors – comparison with somatostatin receptor scintigraphy and computed tomography. *J. Clin. Endocrinol. Metab.* 2005;90:3392–3400.

9. Aslan DL, Gulbahce HE, Pambuccian SE, Manivel JC, Jessurun J. Ki-67 immunoreactivity in the differential diagnosis of pulmonary neuroendocrine neoplasms in specimens with extensive crush artifact. *Am. J. Clin. Pathol.* 2005;123:874–878.

10. Granberg D, Eriksson B, Wilander E, et al. Experience in treatment of metastatic pulmonary carcinoid tumors. *Ann. Oncol.* 2001;12:1383–1391.

11. Granberg D, Wilander E, Öberg K. Expression of tyrosine kinase receptors in lung carcinoids. *Tumor Biol.* 2006;27:153–157.

12. Schrevens L, Vansteenkiste J, Deneffe G, et al. Clinical-radiological presentation and outcome of surgically treated pulmonary carcinoid tumours: a long-term single institution experience. *Lung Cancer* 2004;43:39–45.

13. Chughtai TS, Morin JE, Sheiner NM, Wilson JA, Mulder DS. Bronchial carcinoid – twenty years' experience defines a selective surgical approach. *Surgery* 1997;122:801–808.

14. Granberg D, Wilander E, Öberg K, Skogseid B. Prognostic markers in patients with typical bronchial carcinoid tumors. *J. Clin. Endocrinol. Metab.* 2000;85:3425–3430.

15. Dusmet ME, McKneally MF. Pulmonary and thymic carcinoid tumors. *World J. Surg.* 1996;20:189–195.

16. Teh BT. Thymic carcinoids in multiple endocrine neoplasia type 1. *J. Intern. Med.* 1998;243:501–504.

17. Fukai I, Masaoka A, Fujii Y, et al. Thymic neuroendocrine tumor (thymic carcinoid): a clinicopathologic study in 15 patients. *Ann. Thorac. Surg.* 1999;67:208–211.

18. Filosso PL, Actis Dato GM, Ruffini E, Bretti S, Ozzello F, Mancuso M. Multidisciplinary treatment of advanced thymic neuroendocrine carcinoma (carcinoid): report of a successful case and review of the literature. *J. Thorac. Cardiovasc. Surg.* 2004;127:1215–1219.

19. Ferolla P, Falchetti A, Filosso P, et al. Thymic neuroendocrine carcinoma (carcinoid) in multiple endocrine neoplasia type 1 syndrome: the Italian series. *J. Clin. Endocrinol. Metab.* 2005;90:2603–2609.

20. Ferone D, van Hagen MP, Kwekkeboom DJ, et al. Somatostatin receptor subtypes in human thymoma and inhibition of cell proliferation by octreotide in vitro. *J. Clin. Endocrinol. Metab.* 2000;85:1719–1726.

21. Eriksson B, Bergstrom M, Sundin A, et al. The role of PET in localization of neuroendocrine and adrenocortical tumors. *Ann. N. Y. Acad. Sci.* 2002;970:159–169.

22. Ekeblad S, Sundin A, Janson ET, et al. Temozolomide as monotherapy is effective in treatment of advanced malignant neuroendocrine tumors. *Clin. Cancer Res.* 2007;13:2986–2991.

65 Carcinoid Syndrome

Thorvardur R. Halfdanarson and Timothy J. Hobday

Key points

- Carcinoid tumors are uncommon malignancies of the neuroendocrine system which commonly result in the carcinoid syndrome by overproduction of various biologically active substances.
- The key manifestations of the carcinoid syndrome are cutaneous flushing, diarrhea, bronchospasm and fibrosis of the heart valves, the mesentery and retroperitoneal tissues.
- The diagnosis is established by imaging studies, biopsy and confirming an overproduction of chromagranin A as well as biologically active amines such as serotonin.
- The treatment is primarily surgical but somatostatin analogs and hepatic artery embolization or chemoembolization can result in prolonged palliation of symptoms.
- Cytotoxic chemotherapy has limited effect but therapy with new agents such as radiolabeled somatostatin analogs and targeted agents holds promise in the management of patients with carcinoid tumors.

Introduction

Carcinoid tumors of the gastrointestinal tract are uncommon malignant tumors, most frequently located in the small bowel, and belong to the family of gastroenteropancreatic neuroendocrine tumors (GEP-NET). The cell of origin of these tumors derives from the disseminated gastrointestinal neuroendocrine cells found within the mucosa of the gut. Carcinoid tumors are generally more indolent than adenocarcinomas of the gastrointestinal tract and patients may enjoy prolonged survival despite metastatic disease. Carcinoids frequently secrete biologically active substances including amines and hormones that may result in the characteristic carcinoid syndrome. The word carcinoid was first used by Oberndorfer who used the term "*karzinoide*" to describe tumors that appeared to behave in a more benign fashion than the more commonly encountered adenocarcinomas of the gut. The most commonly used classification of carcinoid tumors rests on the presumed embryological site of origin but the accuracy of this classification has been challenged with the advent of molecular studies of these tumors. This classification still retains some value and provides a simple way of grouping these tumors according to the site of origin.

Epidemiology and prognosis

Autopsy studies have shown higher incidence of carcinoid tumors than population-based epidemiological series, suggesting that many

carcinoid tumors are asymptomatic and go undiagnosed in life. The overall annual incidence of carcinoids in the United States in 1997 was estimated to be 38.4 per 1 million individuals and had increased from 8.5 per million in 1973, with the incidence being higher in African American patients for most carcinoids, except for appendiceal and bronchopulmonary tumors. Similar but somewhat lower incidence rates have been reported by European investigators. Increasing incidence has also been noted in Europe over the last two decades. The observed increase in incidence rates may partly be explained by greater awareness and better diagnostic techniques, including specific tumor markers, improved accuracy of pathologic evaluation and newer imaging modalities.

Among all sites of carcinoid tumors, the gastrointestinal (GI) tract is the most common. Data derived from the Surveillance, Epidemiology and End Results (SEER) Program of the National Cancer Institute in addition to previously collected data from the End Results Group (ERG) and the Third National Cancer Survey (TNCS) found that GI carcinoids constituted 67.6% of all carcinoids diagnosed in the period of 1992–1999 [1]. The bronchopulmonary complex is the second most common site for carcinoids, accounting for 25.3% of the cases diagnosed. Of all 10 878 carcinoid tumors identified in the SEER registry from 1973–1999, 3105 (28.5%) were found in the small intestine. Forty-four percent of all GI carcinoids were located within the small intestine, of which more than a half were found in the ileum. The incidence of GI carcinoids increases gradually from the stomach to the ileum, possibly reflecting the increasing density of neuroendocrine cells in the distal small bowel.

Carcinoid tumors metastasize frequently but the potential for metastasis depends on the anatomic location. Overall, up to one-quarter of all carcinoid tumors are metastatic at the time of diagnosis.

Clinical Endocrine Oncology, 2nd edition. Edited by Ian D. Hay and John A.H. Wass. © 2008 Blackwell Publishing. ISBN 978-1-4051-4584-8.

Table 65.1 Five-year survival of patients with carcinoid tumors according to anatomic location and stage in the 1992–1999 SEER registry [1]

| Anatomic location | 5-year survival (%) according to stage (SEER staging system) | | | |
	Localized	Regional	Distant	All stages
Stomach	69	38*	21	63
Small bowel	60	73	50	61
Colon	76	72	30	62
Rectum	91	49	32	88
Tracheobronchial	81	77	26	74

*The 5-year survival of regional gastric carcinoids reported here derives from the SEER 1973–1991 data.
Adapted from Modlin et al. [1], with permission from John Wiley & Sons.

The SEER 1992–1999 registry of carcinoid tumors reported a metastatic rate of 13% when all sites were considered [1]. Cecal carcinoids metastasize most frequently and more than 40% have distant metastases and more than 80% are either regionally advanced with local invasion or lymph node metastases or metastatic to other organs (defined as non-localized by SEER) at the time of diagnosis. Of appendiceal and small bowel carcinoids, 39% and 58% are non-localized and 10% and 22% are metastatic respectively [1]. Non-localized appendiceal carcinoids are more common in recent series and that may be partially explained by improved sampling of regional lymph nodes at the time of resection.

The 5-year survival of patients with all types and all stages of carcinoid tumors was 67.2% according to the SEER data from 1992–1999 and had increased modestly compared to the earlier years of the SEER database [1]. Table 65.1 shows the survival according to the location and stage of the carcinoid tumors as seen in the SEER registry for the years 1992–1999 [1]. Similar survival figures have been reported by European investigators. The survival is heavily dependent upon the stage of the disease and patients with metastatic and locally advanced disease have a shorter survival. The survival also depends on the location of the primary tumor with bronchopulmonary, rectal and appendiceal carcinoids having the best overall 5-year survival. The 5-year survival rates of patients with small intestinal and appendiceal carcinoids according to the SEER 1992–1999 data were 62% for localized disease, 74% for regional disease and 48% for metastatic disease. Other adverse prognostic factors are the size of the primary tumor, atypical histology, higher Ki-67 proliferation index, carcinoid heart disease and high levels of 5-hydroxy-indoleacetic acid (5-HIAA).

Clinical presentation

The presentation of carcinoid tumors primarily depends upon the location of the tumor and its ability to produce bioactive chemicals resulting in the carcinoid syndrome. Carcinoid tumors can secrete

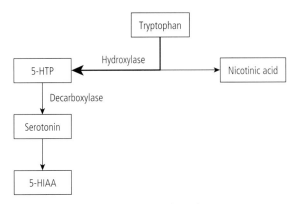

Figure 65.1 Tryptophan metabolism and synthesis of serotonin.

multiple biologically active substances, including the amines serotonin (5-hydroxytryptamine, 5-HT), 5-hydroxytryptophan (5-HTP), and catecholamines. Carcinoids may also secrete other substances such as chromogranins, and tachykinins like kallikrein and neurokinins. Under normal circumstances, dietary tryptophan is metabolized into nicotinic acid and only a very small proportion is converted to 5-HTP. Carcinoid tumors result in an overproduction of 5-HTP at the cost of nicotinic acid and patients with carcinoid syndrome may thus experience deficiency of nicotinic acid, resulting in pellagra. 5-HTP is decarboxylated to serotonin which in turn is converted to 5-hydroxyindolacetic acid (5-HIAA) that can be quantified in urine (Fig. 65.1).

Many patients are asymptomatic or minimally symptomatic and may be diagnosed after undergoing abdominal imaging studies or endoscopic examinations for unrelated reasons. Only a minority of the patients with carcinoids suffer from the carcinoid syndrome and the prevalence of the syndrome appears to be declining, likely due to earlier diagnosis. An overview of 748 worldwide reported cases of the carcinoid syndrome estimated the prevalence to be 8.4% of all patients with carcinoid tumors with significant variability depending on the location of the tumor, the extent of the disease, the time lapsed since diagnosis and ethnic origin of the patients [2]. The prevalence of carcinoid syndrome is highest in patients with tumors in the small bowel, the ileocecal region and ovary where it is present in almost one-third of patients. Other investigators have reported a higher incidence of the carcinoid syndrome in patients with carcinoid tumors but some of the earlier reports may be affected by selection bias. The carcinoid syndrome is rarely seen in patients with carcinoid tumors of the hindgut [2]. Pulmonary carcinoids rarely cause the carcinoid syndrome and when they do, the symptoms often differ from those seen in typical midgut carcinoids. The carcinoid syndrome is also infrequently seen in other foregut carcinoids, such as carcinoid tumors of the stomach.

Classic symptoms of the carcinoid syndrome include flushing, diarrhea and wheezing. The flushing is the most commonly occurring and characteristic symptom of the carcinoid syndrome. It typically involves the face, neck and the upper torso and usually begins abruptly and may last from less than a minute up to 30 min.

The flushes frequently go unnoticed by the patient but may be observed by relatives. Flushes can be associated with feeling of skin warmth, pruritus, tachycardia and a fall in the blood pressure and flushes may be provoked by certain foods, alcohol and exercise. Flushes can also be triggered pharmacologically, for example with catecholamines and pentagastrin. As the disease progresses, the flushes may become more prolonged, diffuse and take on a cyanotic hue. The differential diagnosis of cutaneous flushing includes menopausal symptoms, reactions to alcohol and drugs as well as less common causes such as systemic mastocytosis and pheochromocytoma. Flushes associated with bronchial carcinoids frequently last longer than flushes secondary to midgut carcinoids and have different characteristics. The flushes may have a more red than violaceous color and are frequently associated with other symptoms such as salivation, lacrimation, periorbital edema, hypotension, tachycardia and palpitations.

Diarrhea is commonly seen in patients with the carcinoid syndrome and may be secondary to excessive production of serotonin resulting in gastrointestinal hypermotility and does not have to be associated with the flushing. Bronchospasm and wheezing are also seen in a minority of patients and β-agonist bronchodilators may on rare occasions trigger vasodilatation in these patients. Diarrhea in patients with carcinoid tumors can also be seen secondary to ileal resection and therapy with somatostatin analogs which may cause steatorrhea.

Under certain circumstances, patients with carcinoid tumors may develop a life-threatening variant of the carcinoid syndrome called carcinoid crisis where large amounts of biologically active substances are released, resulting in flushing, tachycardia arrhythmia, bronchospasm, hypertension or hypotension that may be resistant to fluid resuscitation. The most common circumstances leading to carcinoid crisis are induction of anesthesia, surgery, and liver embolization procedures. This complication can be prevented with the use of somatostatin analogs prior to the anesthesia or the procedure. Immediate therapy with high doses of octreotide is required once carcinoid crisis is suspected.

Carcinoid heart disease is a common complication of the carcinoid syndrome and may eventually occur in up to 50% of patients and can be the presenting feature. There is a great variability in the severity of carcinoid heart disease with many patients being asymptomatic and others suffering from severe valvular disease and heart failure [3]. Deposition of fibrous tissue on the cardiac valves decreases their mobility and characteristically leads to tricuspid regurgitation. The pathogenesis of carcinoid heart disease is not fully understood but higher levels of urinary 5-HIAA are associated with increased risk. The right side of the heart is predominantly involved, probably secondary to the inactivation of the carcinoid humoral products in the lungs. The onset of symptoms of carcinoid heart disease is insidious and the symptoms are non-specific. Dyspnea on exertion is an early sign that is later followed by more florid findings of right-sided heart failure such as peripheral edema, jugular venous distension and ascites. Carcinoid heart disease is known to adversely affect the survival of patients with carcinoid tumors, with one study

showing a median survival of only 1.6 years compared to 4.6 years in carcinoid patients without cardiac involvement. Cardiac valve surgery effectively ameliorates symptoms of heart failure and may improve survival [3].

Another peculiar complication of carcinoid tumors is fibrosis of mesenteric and retroperitoneal tissues and more rarely the lungs [4]. The incidence of fibrosis among patients with carcinoids is not fully known but has been reported in up to 50% of cases. The etiology of the fibrosis is still largely unknown but may be related to production and release of serotonin and various tissue growth factors. Mesenteric fibrosis may result in impaired motility, mesenterial ischemia, abdominal pain and bowel obstruction needing surgical intervention. Retroperitoneal fibrosis can cause ureteral obstruction and renal failure. Pulmonary and cutaneous fibrosis appears to be uncommon and is usually associated with advanced carcinoid tumor.

Diagnosis

Carcinoid tumors of the GI tract are frequently symptomatic and the symptoms can be related to the primary tumor or metastatic disease. Many patients are incidentally diagnosed following imaging studies or endoscopic examinations for other reasons. Abdominal pain and intestinal obstruction are commonly seen. Patients may be diagnosed after undergoing a diagnostic or therapeutic laparotomy or laparoscopy for evaluation of recurrent abdominal pain. Other patients are diagnosed after presenting with features of the carcinoid syndrome. When approaching a patient suspected of a carcinoid tumor, it is helpful to think of the diagnostic strategy as having two main components: the biochemical confirmation of carcinoid syndrome and the topographic localization of the disease. Figure 65.2 depicts an algorithm for diagnosis and therapy of carcinoid tumors.

Biochemical diagnosis

When confronted with a patient presenting with symptoms suggestive of carcinoid syndrome, measuring the 24-h urinary excretion of 5-HIAA is a reasonable first step. This test is widely available but somewhat cumbersome and has to be interpreted with caution. The results can be spuriously high after ingestion of certain foods rich in serotonin, such as bananas, avocado, plums, tomatoes and pineapple. Elevated 5-HIAA is a very specific test for carcinoid when performed correctly with a reported specificity of 88–100% but a lower sensitivity of 73%.

Chromogranin A (CgA) is a protein and a member of the chromogranin family. It is stored in secretory granules of neuroendocrine cells and can be measured in the plasma of patients with neuroendocrine tumors. CgA is not specific for carcinoids and is also frequently elevated in the serum of patients with other neuroendocrine tumors, both functioning and non-functioning. The levels of CgA have been found to correlate with tumor volume and prognosis and CgA may serve as a valuable tool for detection of carcinoid tumor recurrence [5].

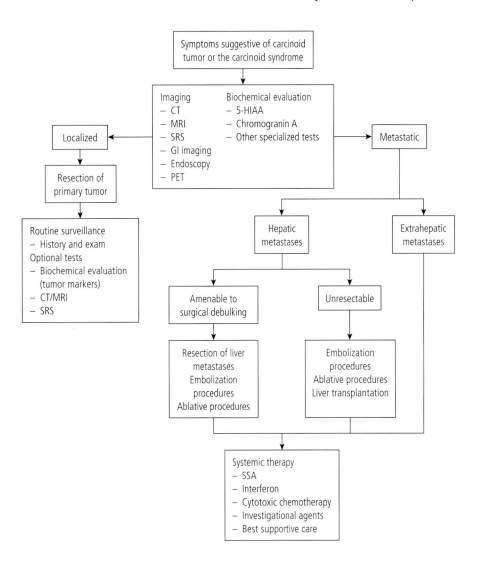

Figure 65.2 Diagnosis and management of carcinoid tumors. SSA, somatostatin analogues; SRS, somatostatin receptor scintigraphy.

Other, but less frequently utilized methods for biochemical diagnosis include serotonin levels in plasma and platelets and provocation tests using either pentagastrin or epinephrine. Platelet serotonin levels have been found to be very specific for midgut carcinoids but the test is not widely available. Provocation tests with pentagastrin are rarely used any more and may trigger life-threatening carcinoid crises.

Imaging studies

Somatostatin receptor scintigraphy has revolutionized the imaging of carcinoid tumors. Many patients are still, however, diagnosed after computerized tomography (CT) or small bowel imaging studies have been obtained to evaluate abdominal pain or other gastrointestinal symptoms.

CT, magnetic resonance imaging and barium studies

These imaging modalities are very helpful in the initial evaluation of patients suspected of having carcinoid tumor. CT or magnetic resonance imaging (MRI) characteristically shows mass lesion and mesenteric fibrosis and stranding and can also reveal meta-

static lesions in the liver and lymph nodes. MRI is more sensitive than CT for diagnosis of liver metastasis but the sensitivity of CT can be enhanced with careful sequencing of intravenous contrast administration and image acquisition. Hepatic arterial phase images are required for accurate CT diagnosis of hepatic metastases. Calcifications are frequently seen within the primary tumor or mesenteric lymph nodes. Barium studies may show mural thickening, kinking and angulation of the small bowel and changes consistent with intraluminal tumor and constriction.

Somatostatin receptor scintigraphy

Somatostatin receptor scintigraphy (SRS), frequently called octreoscan® is a valuable tool in the evaluation of patients with neuroendocrine tumors [6]. The use of SRS in patients with carcinoid tumor is based on the fact that 70–90% of carcinoid tumors express somatostatin receptors. The most commonly used SRS utilizes an indium-labeled somatostatin analog, octreotide (^{111}In-DTPA-octreotide). The radiolabeled octreotide is injected intravenously and images are obtained with single photon emission computed tomography (SPECT) 24 h later. If the uptake of the radiolabeled octreotide is slow or the background radio-activity is obscuring, the SPECT can be repeated 48 h after the injection. The reported sensitivity of SRS in detecting carcinoid tumors is between 80% and 100%. SRS frequently identifies primary carcinoid tumors and metastases in locations such as bone and lymph nodes that are not as well seen with more conventional imaging studies such as CT and MRI. SRS can be used as the first imaging study in patients suspected of carcinoid as the entire body can be evaluated and distant metastases identified, allowing more focused evaluation with other and more conventional imaging modalities. SRS can be used to predict responses to somatostatin analog therapy and it is also useful in selecting patients for therapy with radiolabeled octreotide analogs as described later.

Positron emission tomography (PET)

PET has been increasingly used for accurate staging in patients with various malignancies. Radiolabeled glucose ($[^{18}F]$ fluoro-deoxyglucose or FDG) is the most commonly used tracer. FDG-PET has not been found to be as useful for evaluating patients with carcinoids, likely because of the lower proliferative rate of carcinoid tumors. Poorly differentiated neuroendocrine tumors may, however, be detected with conventional FDG-PET. Recently, alternative radioactive tracers have been used in detecting carcinoids. Such tracers include the ^{11}C-labeled amine precursor 5-hydroxy-L-tryptophan (5-HTP) and 3,4-dihydroxy-phenylalanine (DOPA). PET scans using these tracers have shown improved sensitivity in detecting carcinoids when compared to SRS and CT [6].

Therapy

Surgical therapy of the primary tumor and locoregional metastases

Resection of the primary tumor and adjacent locoregional disease, if possible, may relieve symptoms and improve survival. Carcinoid heart disease and high output of 5-HIAA appear to be risk factors for perioperative complications. The risk of carcinoid crisis can be substantially reduced with the use of perioperative and intraoperative intravenous octreotide.

Mesenteric metastases are common in patients with carcinoid tumors and extensive mesenteric fibrosis may be challenging in the surgical management of these patients. Peritoneal metastases are also a frequent finding in patients undergoing resection for carcinoid tumors. Resection of mesenteric metastases and debulking of peritoneal metastases may alleviate or prevent symptoms in patients with carcinoid tumors.

Management of hepatic metastases

Liver metastases are frequently encountered in patients with carcinoid tumors and may markedly impair the quality of life in these patients. Patients with metastatic carcinoid tumors commonly suffer from the carcinoid syndrome and the presence of hepatic metastases is a major prognostic factor for shortened survival. Hepatic metastases can be treated by resection, tumor embolization and percutaneously with either cryoablation or radio-frequency ablation. Therapy directed against the liver metastases may markedly decrease symptoms in these patients and improve their quality of life.

Surgical therapy

Resection of hepatic metastases

No randomized studies have evaluated the usefulness of hepatic resection in the management of carcinoid tumors metastatic to the liver. Multiple retrospective series have, however, shown that hepatic resections can successfully palliate pain and alleviate the symptoms of the carcinoid syndrome and decrease the levels of 5-HIAA. Unfortunately most patients relapse in the ensuing years. Despite the high relapse rates, many patients do well for several years following debulking surgery with good control of carcinoid symptoms without needing systemic therapy. The largest reported series of patients undergoing hepatic resection comes from the Mayo Clinic and includes 120 patients with carcinoid tumors. This retrospective review showed a 5-year survival of 61% which significantly exceeds the expected survival of carcinoid patients with hepatic metastases not undergoing liver resection [7]. Other and smaller studies have supported improved survival following hepatic resection and suggested that rare patients may even be cured with an aggressive surgical approach. In general, hepatic resection is most helpful if at least 90% of tumor bulk can be resected and/or ablated with intraoperative radiofrequency ablation (RFA).

Liver transplantation

Orthotopic liver transplantation (OLT) has been used in highly selected cases of carcinoid tumors where metastases are limited to the liver. OLT is very effective in palliating the symptoms of the carcinoid syndrome and can prolong survival in highly selected patients but unfortunately, recurrences are common. Lehnert reviewed the experience with 103 patients reported in the literature [8]. The 2- and 5-year overall survival rates following OLT were 60% and 47% respectively but less than 24% were free of recurrence at 5 years. Age greater than 50 years and OLT combined with extensive upper abdominal resection such as Whipple procedure were associated with worse prognosis on multivariate analysis. Patients younger than 50 years old who underwent a limited resection had a median survival in excess of 8 years and a 5-year overall survival of 65%. Other studies have suggested that certain biomarkers, such as increased expression of Ki-67 and aberrant E-cadherin expression, predict shorter survival following OLT.

The indications for OLT are currently unclear and the limited supply of donor livers further limits the use of OLT as a therapeutic modality. Extrahepatic disease needs to be ruled out prior to embarking on OLT and patients generally need a laparoscopy to evaluate the presence of peritoneal spread. Using uniform criteria for OLT, a staging laparotomy and avoiding extensive associated surgical resections may result in prolonged disease-free survival and overall survival. A small series from the Mayo Clinic reported the experience with OLT in eight patients with carcinoid tumor metastatic to the liver. All eight patients were recurrence free after a median follow-up time of 22 months (range 4–84 months) [9].

Interventional radiology

Hepatic artery embolization and chemoembolization

Hepatic artery embolization procedures are increasingly being utilized in the management of neuroendocrine tumors metastatic to the liver. Embolization procedures are most commonly used when medical therapy with somatostatin analogs or interferons has been unsuccessful in controlling symptoms of the carcinoid syndrome or if the patient is not a candidate for more aggressive surgical therapy such as resection of liver metastases. Vascular occlusion therapy of liver metastases relies on the dual blood supply of the liver. Hypervascular tumors such as carcinoid metastases mainly receive their blood supply via the hepatic artery while the blood supply to the liver parenchyma derives from both the hepatic artery and the portal circulation. Selective hepatic artery embolization (HAE) and chemoembolization (HACE) have been utilized in the management of patients with neuroendocrine liver metastases resulting in palliation of symptoms and tumor shrinkage. HAE is performed by selectively injecting embolization materials such as gel foam powder into the branch of the hepatic artery supplying the liver metastases. This method results in objective tumor responses in up to 70% of treated patients. Hepatic artery chemoembolization relies on the same technique with the addition of cytotoxic agents to the embolization material. The most commonly used cytotoxic drugs are doxorubicin and streptozocin. Symptom improvement and biochemical responses have been reported in 60–100% of patients treated with HACE and objective responses are seen in 33–86% of patients. HAE and HACE have not been compared in a randomized clinical trial but retrospective studies suggest that these two modalities have similar efficacy in patients with carcinoid tumors [10]. Substantial palliation in the majority of patients is to be expected following a successful embolization procedure regardless of whether chemotherapy is added or not. The embolization is generally well tolerated but a minority of patients will experience a flare of their carcinoid symptoms and even a carcinoid crisis following the procedure that can be controlled with intravenous octreotide. Abdominal pain and elevated serum transaminases are commonly seen following embolization procedures. Severe and fatal adverse effects may occur but are rare.

Ablative therapy

Radiofrequency ablation (RFA) has been used successfully to treat liver metastases in patients with carcinoid tumors. This technique can be used either percutaneously or intraoperatively after the liver lesions have been localized with the aid of ultrasound [11]. Ethanol injection therapy has also been used but there are concerns regarding the inhomogeneous distribution of the ethanol within the tumor and this therapy has now largely been supplanted by RFA and cryoablation. Several studies support the use of RFA in selected patients with liver metastases. The largest study included laparoscopic ablation of 234 metastases in 34 patients and reported symptom improvement in 95% of patients with a mean duration of symptom control in excess of 10 months.

Systemic therapy

Systemic therapy with somatostatin analogs is the mainstay of treatment in patients with advanced and symptomatic carcinoid tumors. Chemotherapy has limited benefits but can be used in selected cases not responsive to other therapies.

Somatostatin analogs

Somatostatin is a naturally occurring polypeptide with a strong inhibitory effect on various exocrine and endocrine functions. Somatostatin has also been shown to have antiproliferative effects and antiapoptotic effects in various tumors. Despite the antiproliferative effects observed *in vitro*, objective tumor responses are uncommonly seen in clinical practice. There are five subtypes of somatostatin receptors (SSTR) and subtype 2 (SSTR2) is expressed in up to 100% of neuroendocrine tumors depending on studies. The synthetic somatostatin analogs octreotide and lanreotide are very useful in the management of carcinoid tumors and can be administered subcutaneously every 8 h. Somatostatin analogs (SSA) are remarkably effective in ameliorating the symptoms of carcinoid syndrome, are generally well tolerated and may exert cytostatic effects on tumor cells *in vivo*. Therapy with SSA frequently results in decreased urinary 5-HIAA and a lowering of serum chromogranin A. This likely reflects inhibition of hormone synthesis and release rather than a decrease in the tumor mass.

Multiple studies have confirmed the usefulness of SSA in clinical practice [12]. Table 65.2 lists selected studies that evaluated the effect of various SSAs in the management of gastroenteropancreatic neuroendocrine tumors including carcinoid tumors. Symptomatic responses are seen in 65–100% of patients treated with either octreotide or lanreotide and stable disease is observed in 35–80%. Biochemical response is expected in up to 80% of patients. Studies have shown that tachyphylaxis develops after a median time of 12 months of therapy but worsening symptoms can often transiently be palliated by using higher doses of SSA. Long-acting formulations of both octreotide and lanreotide have been developed and these formulations are much more convenient than the short-acting forms of the drug, allowing for a single injection every 2–4 weeks.

Octreotide LAR (Sandostatin LAR®) is a slow-release formulation of octreotide acetate that can be administered intramuscularly every 4 weeks. Octreotide LAR was compared to subcutaneous octreotide in randomized trial and the two formulations were found to be equally effective in controlling the symptoms of the carcinoid syndrome [13]. Given the increased convenience of octreotide LAR, it has largely supplanted the use of subcutaneous short-acting octreotide. Short-acting octreotide is recommended at the beginning of the therapy to ensure adequate tolerance and

Table 65.2 Somatostatin analogs in the management of gastroenteropancreatic neuroendocrine tumors

Study (first author and year published)	No. of patients	Agent	Dosage	Response (%)			
				OR	SD	BR	SR
Arnold 1996	52	OCT	200 μg three times daily	0	36.5	74	NR
Maton 1989	107	OCT	Various doses	7.5	39	79.4	67.3
Kvols 1987	22	OCT	150–500 μg three times daily	NR	NR	68.2	100
di Bartolomeo 1996	58	OCT	500–1000 μg three times daily	3	46.5	77	73
Ricci 2000	15	LAR	20 mg monthly	7	40	41	82
Tomassetti 1998	16	LAR	20 mg monthly	0	87.5	81	100
Rubin 1999	26 vs. 22/20/25	OCT vs. LAR	300–900 μg/day vs. 10/20/30 mg monthly	NR	NR	NR	58 vs. 67/71/62
Eriksson 1997	19	LAN	4 mg three times daily	5	70	58	NR
Faiss 1999	30	LAN	5 mg three times daily	6.7	37	NR	NR
Ricci 2000	25	LAN-P	30 mg every 14 days	8	40	42	65
Ruszniewski 1996	39	LAN-P	30 mg every 14 days	0	NR	18	30–39
Wymenga 1999	55	LAN-P	30 mg every 14 days	6	81	38	42

BR, biochemical response; LAN, lanreotide; LAN-P, prolonged release lanreotide; LAR, long-acting octreotide; NR, no response; OCT, octreotide; OR, objective response; SD, stable disease; SR, symptomatic response.
Adapted from Delaunoit et al. [12], with permission from *Mayo Clinic Proceedings*.

may also be needed for up to 2 weeks until the octreotide LAR has achieved a steady state. A commonly prescribed dose of subcutaneous octreotide is 150 μg three times daily followed by octreotide LAR at the dose of 20 mg intramuscularly. Higher doses of octreotide LAR may be needed to control the symptoms and occasionally patients will need subcutaneous octreotide for breakthrough symptoms. Similar results have been observed for long-acting formulations of lanreotide. There are currently two long-acting formulations of lanreotide available: lanreotide LA (Somatuline®) and lanreotide autogel (Somatuline Autogel®).

A new somatostatin analog, pasireotide (SOM230), has been evaluated in patients refractory to octreotide LAR in a phase II study and found to be safe and effective, improving the symptoms of 25% of these patients. Pasireotide has agonistic activity on somatostatin receptors 1, 2, 3 and 5 (SST1, SST2, SST3 and SST5) and compared to octreotide it has higher affinity for SST1, SST3 and SST5. The safety profiles of octreotide and pasireotide are similar.

The SSAs are generally well tolerated and the most frequently encountered side effects are usually mild. Common side effects include flatulence, diarrhea, steatorrhea and abdominal pain. Less common side effects are hyperglycemia, injection-site reactions and gastric atony. Gallstones or gallbladder sludge may be seen in up to 50% of treated patients but symptomatic gallstones or acute cholecystitis are uncommon and probably occur in less than 1% of treated patients.

Interferons

Interferons (IFNs) have been used for advanced carcinoids for decades but the antitumor mechanism of IFNs remains incompletely understood [14]. Numerous trials have evaluated IFNs in the management of carcinoid tumors and there is substantial heterogeneity in the study designs, the methods of assessing tumor response and the results reported. The two most extensively studied IFNs are recombinant IFN-α and human leukocyte interferon. Tumor responses are uncommon and usually minimal and a complete response to IFN therapy is exceedingly rare. Partial responses were reported in 0–25% of patients and stable disease in an additional 35%. Symptomatic and biochemical responses are more frequent and seen in 25–50% of patients. A median duration of response of 34 months has been reported with stability achieved in 39% of patients.

Interferons have numerous adverse effects which in addition to a rather inconvenient administration schedule limit their usefulness in the management of carcinoid tumors. The most frequently encountered adverse reactions include flu-like symptoms, weight loss, fatigue, depression, hepatotoxicity and cytopenias. Somatostatin analogs and IFNs appear to have comparable efficacy but the frequency of IFN side effects and the cumbersome administration schedule have made SSA a much more feasible option in the management of patients with carcinoid tumors. There may still be a role for IFNs in the management of carcinoid patients progressing despite therapy with SSA.

Combination therapy with somatostatin analogs and interferons

Several studies have evaluated the combination of SSA and IFN. Earlier studies had shown that the combination of these two agents was effective in a substantial proportion of patients progressing on either drug when given alone. The benefits appear to be primarily related to stability of the disease and clinical and biochemical responses. Tumor responses were uncommon when the combination was used.

Two recent, randomized clinical trials have further clarified the role of combination therapy [15, 16]. A trial of 80 patients with metastatic gastroenteropancreatic neuroendocrine tumors, including 29 with carcinoid tumors, showed no improvement in tumor responses when combination therapy was used compared with lanreotide or IFN alone. The combination therapy did, however, seem to improve the control of diarrhea and flushing to a greater degree than either drug alone at the cost of increased side effects [15]. Another trial evaluated the response of combination therapy in 68 patients with metastatic carcinoid tumors and showed that the combination therapy did not improve overall survival when compared to octreotide alone but patients receiving the combination therapy had reduced risk of progression [16]. The 5-year survival rate was 36.6% in the octreotide-only arm vs. 56.8% in the combination arm but the difference was not significant. The progression rates were significantly lower in the combination arm versus the octreotide arm or 18.1% vs. 54.3% respectively.

Radiolabeled somatostatin analogs

Carcinoid tumors are relatively resistant to external beam radiation therapy and clinical trials have found limited efficacy for this treatment modality. Radiation therapy still retains some value in treating symptomatic metastases, especially bone metastases. Somatostatin analogs labeled with radionuclides appear to be a more promising form of radiotherapy. Several studies have now confirmed the safety and efficacy of radiolabeled SSA [17]. The rationale behind this therapy is that SSA linked to radionuclides will bind to somatostatin receptors on the surface of the tumor cells and then become internalized to exert their cytotoxic effects. The most frequently utilized radionuclides used are ^{111}In, ^{90}Y and ^{177}Lu. These radionuclides differ in particles emitted, particle energy and distance of tissue penetration. The radionuclides are usually conjugated to either octreotide or octreotate. The results of a single-institution series using ^{177}Lu labeled octreotate (^{177}Lu-DOTATATE) were recently reported [18]. This study included 70 patients with carcinoid tumors. There were no complete responses in the patients with carcinoid tumors but partial responses were seen in 20% and minor response or stable disease was observed in additional 62%. The median time to progression was more than 36 months in the entire cohort of patients.

Treatment with peptide receptor radionuclides is generally well tolerated. The most commonly encountered adverse effects are nausea, vomiting and abdominal pain. Nephrotoxicity has been observed but may possibly be prevented with concurrent infusion of amino acids. Hepatotoxicity can be seen but these patients commonly have extensive liver metastases. Hematological toxicity is usually mild and manifests as transient lowering in blood counts. Myelodysplastic syndromes have been reported in a few patients receiving radiolabeled SSA and appear to be related to higher radiation doses.

Chemotherapy

Carcinoid tumors are inherently resistant to cytotoxic chemotherapy and no single drug or drug combination has emerged as a standard regimen in the setting of advanced disease. Furthermore, there is no convincing evidence that cytotoxic chemotherapy prolongs survival in these patients. Studies evaluating single-agent chemotherapy have shown response rates ranging from 0% to 20%. Doxorubicin and dacarbazine are among the most effective single agents reported with a partial response of 21% and 16% respectively. Combination chemotherapy regimens have resulted in partial responses in 10–30% of cases. These regimens typically contain streptozocin, doxorubicin, dacarbazine and 5-fluorouracil. Complete responses are rare and the survival of patients is less than 1–2 years in these trials. Commonly used cytotoxic drugs such as the taxanes and gemcitabine have minimal efficacy in carcinoid tumors. Future trials will evaluate the combination of cytotoxic chemotherapy and novel agents [19].

Novel therapies

The limited selection of effective drugs in patients with carcinoid tumor progressing on biological therapy has led to an exploration of novel agents (Table 65.3). Carcinoid tumors frequently express vascular endothelial growth factor receptors (VEGFR) and endothelial growth factor receptors (EGFR). Several small molecules including receptor tyrosine kinase inhibitors and mammalian target of rapamycin (mTOR) inhibitors have been studied in phase II trials.

Gefitinib is an inhibitor of the EGFR tyrosine kinase domain that has been studied in patients with advanced neuroendocrine tumors including carcinoids. Preliminary results indicate that disease stability can be achieved with gefitinib monotherapy. A phase II trial in 57 patients with radiographic confirmation of progressive disease at study entry resulted in a 6-month progression-free survival rate of 61% but objective tumor responses were rare [20].

Sunitinib is an inhibitor of VEGFR and platelet-derived growth factor (PDGFR) and other receptor tyrosine kinases. Sunitinib showed a minimal response rate of 2% but a high rate of stable disease (93%) in a recent phase II trial that included 43 patients

Table 65.3 Novel agents being evaluated in the management of carcinoid tumor*

Tyrosine kinase inhibitors (TKI)†
Gefitinib
Imantinib
Sunitinib
Vatalanib
Sorafenib
Antiangiogenic agents (other than TKI)
Bevacizumab
Thalidomide
mTOR inhibitors
Everolimus (RAD001)
Temsirolimus (CCI-779)

*Many of the studied agents were used concurrently with somatostatin analogs or cytotoxic chemotherapy.

†The tyrosine kinase inhibitors may have antiangiogenic properties.

with carcinoid tumors. The median time to progression was 42 weeks [21].

Bevacizumab is a humanized monoclonal antibody directed against VEGF. Inhibition of angiogenesis is thought to be one mechanism of action responsible for its effects in multiple solid tumors. Bevacizumab has been studied in patients with advanced carcinoid tumor receiving octreotide. Patients received bevacizumab, pegylated interferon-α or both and the results have been reported in abstract form. Therapy with bevacizumab resulted in improved progression-free survival and an observed decrease in tumor blood flow. A partial response was seen in 3 of the 20 patients receiving bevacizumab but stability was achieved in 16 patients [22].

The mTOR pathway is important for cell proliferation. mTOR is a downstream mediator in the PI3K/Akt signaling pathway and the mTOR kinase inhibitors temsirolimus (CCI-779) and everolimus (RAD001) are being evaluated in patients with advanced neuroendocrine tumors. Preliminary results have shown good tolerability and some antitumor activity but the studies are ongoing. A phase II study of RAD001 and depot octreotide in 32 patients with advanced neuroendocrine tumors including 18 carcinoids showed a partial response in two carcinoid patients. Stable disease was observed in 10 patients [23].

Conclusion

Carcinoid tumors are uncommon tumors of the neuroendocrine system that commonly manifest at the metastatic stage with characteristic symptoms of overproduction and secretion of various biologically active substances. The carcinoid syndrome is most frequently secondary to metastatic midgut carcinoid tumors but can be seen in carcinoids of other locations. The classic symptoms of flushing and diarrhea can be successfully controlled with somatostatin analogs in the majority of patients but many patients will eventually become refractory to such therapy. Surgical resection of the primary tumor and hepatic metastases as well as hepatic artery embolization procedures are important parts of the treatment, can effectively control symptoms and may improve survival. Liver transplantation may be an option for carefully selected patients with disease limited to the liver. Cytotoxic chemotherapy is not very effective in the treatment of these tumors but novel targeted agents as well as radiolabeled somatostatin analogs hold promise as effective therapy in patients with advanced carcinoid tumors.

References

1. Modlin IM, Lye KD, Kidd M. A 5-decade analysis of 13,715 carcinoid tumors. *Cancer* 2003;97:934–959.
2. Soga J, Yakuwa Y, Osaka M. Carcinoid syndrome: a statistical evaluation of 748 reported cases. *J. Exp. Clin. Cancer Res.* 1999;18: 133–141.
3. Connolly HM, Pellikka PA. Carcinoid heart disease. *Curr. Cardiol. Rep.* 2006;8:96–101.
4. Modlin IM, Shapiro MD, Kidd M. Carcinoid tumors and fibrosis: an association with no explanation. *Am. J. Gastroenterol.* 2004;99: 2466–2478.
5. Eriksson B, Öberg K, Stridsberg M. Tumor markers in neuroendocrine tumors. *Digestion* 2000;62(Suppl 1):33–38.
6. Öberg K, Eriksson B. Nuclear medicine in the detection, staging and treatment of gastrointestinal carcinoid tumours. *Best Pract. Res. Clin. Endocrinol. Metab.* 2005;19:265–276.
7. Sarmiento JM, Heywood G, Rubin J, Ilstrup DM, Nagorney DM, Que FG. Surgical treatment of neuroendocrine metastases to the liver: a plea for resection to increase survival. *J. Am. Coll. Surg.* 2003;197: 29–37.
8. Lehnert T. Liver transplantation for metastatic neuroendocrine carcinoma: an analysis of 103 patients. *Transplantation* 1998;66: 1307–1312.
9. van Vilsteren FG, Baskin-Bey ES, Nagorney DM, et al. Liver transplantation for gastroenteropancreatic neuroendocrine cancers: Defining selection criteria to improve survival. *Liver Transpl.* 2006;12:448–456.
10. Gupta S, Johnson MM, Murthy R, et al. Hepatic arterial embolization and chemoembolization for the treatment of patients with metastatic neuroendocrine tumors: variables affecting response rates and survival. *Cancer* 2005;104:1590–1602.
11. Atwell TD, Charboneau JW, Que FG, et al. Treatment of neuroendocrine cancer metastatic to the liver: the role of ablative techniques. *Cardiovasc. Intervent. Radiol.* 2005;28:409–421.
12. Delaunoit T, Rubin J, Neczyporenko F, Erlichman C, Hobday TJ. Somatostatin analogues in the treatment of gastroenteropancreatic neuroendocrine tumors. *Mayo Clin. Proc.* 2005;80:502–506.
13. Rubin J, Ajani J, Schirmer W, et al. Octreotide acetate long-acting formulation versus open-label subcutaneous octreotide acetate in malignant carcinoid syndrome. *J. Clin. Oncol.* 1999;17:600–606.
14. Shah T, Caplin M. Endocrine tumours of the gastrointestinal tract. Biotherapy for metastatic endocrine tumours. *Best Pract. Res. Clin. Gastroenterol.* 2005;19:617–636.
15. Faiss S, Pape UF, Böhmig M, et al. Prospective, randomized, multicenter trial on the antiproliferative effect of lanreotide, interferon alfa, and their combination for therapy of metastatic neuroendocrine gastroenteropancreatic tumors – the International Lanreotide and Interferon Alfa Study Group. *J. Clin. Oncol.* 2003;21:2689–2696.
16. Kölby L, Persson G, Franzén S, Ahrén B. Randomized clinical trial of the effect of interferon alpha on survival in patients with disseminated midgut carcinoid tumours. *Br. J. Surg.* 2003;90:687–693.
17. Kaltsas GA, Papadogias D, Makras P, Grossman AB. Treatment of advanced neuroendocrine tumours with radiolabelled somatostatin analogues. *Endocr. Relat. Cancer* 2005;12:683–699.
18. Kwekkeboom DJ, Teunissen JJ, Bakker WH, et al. Radiolabeled somatostatin analog [177Lu-DOTA0,Tyr3]octreotate in patients with endocrine gastroenteropancreatic tumors. *J. Clin. Oncol.* 2005; 23:2754–2762.
19. Schnirer, II, Yao JC, Ajani JA. Carcinoid – a comprehensive review. *Acta Oncol.* 2003;42:672–692.
20. Hobday TJ, Holen K, Donehower R, et al. A phase II trial of gefitinib in patients (pts) with progressive metastatic neuroendocrine tumors (NET): a Phase II Consortium (P2C) study. *J. Clin. Oncol.* (Meeting Abstracts) 2006;24(18 Suppl):4043.

21. Kulke M, Lenz H, Meropol N, et al. Results of a phase II study with sunitinib malate (SU11248) in patients (pts) with advanced neuroendocrine tumours (NETs). *European Journal of Cancer Supplements*. ECCO 13 Abstract Book 2005;3:204.

22. Yao JC, Ng C, Hoff PM, et al. Improved progression free survival (PFS), and rapid, sustained decrease in tumor perfusion among patients with advanced carcinoid treated with bevacizumab. *J. Clin. Oncol.* (Meeting Abstracts) 2005;23(16 Suppl):4007.

23. Yao JC, Phan AT, Chang DZ, et al. Phase II study of RAD001 (everolimus) and depot octreotide (Sandostatin LAR) in patients with advanced low grade neuroendocrine carcinoma (LGNET). *J. Clin. Oncol.* (Meeting Abstracts) 2006;24(18 Suppl):4042.

66 Appendiceal and Hindgut Carcinoids

Humphrey J.F. Hodgson

> **Key points**
> - Appendiceal and rectal carcinoid tumors are often benign, asymptomatic and incidental.
> - Colonic carcinoids are generally malignant.
> - The carcinoid syndrome is very uncommon but not unknown with carcinoids arising from these sites.
> - If required, treatment is surgical.

Introduction

Carcinoid was a term introduced to describe tumors which differed from cancers in their more differentiated appearance and more benign course. Neuroendocrine tumor is now the preferred term, and a World Health Organization classification has been produced linking different sites and histological appearances of these tumors [1]. In the mid- and hindgut, the term carcinoid remains the common usage.

The vast majority of appendiceal and hindgut carcinoids identified during life are benign, incidentally found and asymptomatic lesions: a yet greater number probably remain undetected. A routine health survey of over 20 000 Japanese teachers, involving proctosigmoidoscopy, revealed asymptomatic rectal carcinoids in 0.07% [2]. In reported series of carcinoid tumors – i.e. series biased to cases that have become symptomatic or have been resected at surgery – appendiceal carcinoids are generally similar in frequency to the rectal tumors, although again they are predominantly incidental findings at appendicectomy [3]. The appendiceal and hindgut carcinoids merit attention in this volume because of their neuroendocrine origin, and the occasional propensity of appendiceal and proximal colonic carcinoids to give rise to the carcinoid syndrome, when sufficient active products reach the systemic circulation to cause the characteristic picture of diarrhea, flushing, and associated symptoms.

Normal neuroendocrine system of the appendix, colon and rectum

The colon and rectum contain scattered neuroendocrine cells at a density nearly approaching that of the small intestine [4]. The cells

Clinical Endocrine Oncology, 2nd edition. Edited by Ian D. Hay and John A.H. Wass. © 2008 Blackwell Publishing. ISBN 978-1-4051-4584-8.

characteristically lie between the epithelial cells of the colonic crypts, rather than between the surface epithelial cells, and the endocrine cell density in the proximal colon and rectum is of the order of $2 \times 10^5/cm^2$, less in the midportion of the colon and descending colon. Neuroendocrine cells in the colon and rectum have been classified into four types on granular and staining appearances, type 1 being the enterochromaffin-like (ECL) cell. The type 1 cell granules are 150–450 nm in size, and serotonin staining is positive; this cell type is generally acknowledged as the usual cell of origin of carcinoid tumors. Types 2, 3 and 4 are neuroendocrine on morphological grounds, although only type 4 has well-characterized contents, peptide YY (PYY) and glicentin. Some hindgut carcinoid tumors stain for glicentin and PYY, but often in association with other peptides and products including serotonin. Chromogranin positivity may be found in all. Although it is unclear, on general biological grounds it seems reasonable that all these neuroendocrine cell types should be capable of giving rise to tumors.

Etiopathogenesis of appendiceal and hindgut carcinoids

Appendiceal and hindgut carcinoids are not generally associated with the genetic abnormalities characteristic of the multiple endocrine neoplasia type 1 syndrome, in contrast to a significant proportion of foregut carcinoids. A variety of chromosomal sites of loss of heterozygosity are reported however, though the genes remain to be identified [5].

Midgut and hindgut carcinoids

Contrary to expectations, the embryological hindgut commences at approximately the midportion of the transverse colon; appendiceal and proximal colonic carcinoids therefore lie in midgut territory, and distal colonic (very rare) and rectal tumors are of hindgut origin. The generally accepted rule is that midgut carcinoids tend to be active secretors of serotonin and other products, and therefore have the potential to give rise to the carcinoid syndrome if they metastasize to the liver, whilst hindgut tumors tend not to secrete not give rise to the carcinoid syndrome. In addition, there are general staining characteristics of ECL cells and their tumor derivatives, some of which tend to vary between midgut and hindgut. ECL cells stain with potassium chromate, reflecting the serotonin content. Midgut ECL cells and tumors tend to be argentaffin, taking up and reducing silver, whilst hindgut cells and tumors do this less frequently, although they may be argyrophilic, taking up silver when in the presence of a reducing agent. With the more general usage of chromogranin A staining to recognize neuroendocrine tumors, the use of silver stains has become less frequent. A variety of reports delineate expression of recently described markers [6, 7], though evidence on the hindgut tumors is generally scanty.

Relative frequency of distal carcinoid tumors and association with carcinoid syndrome

A survey combining three different tumor registers and over 13 000 patients identified the appendix as the site of 13% of neuroendocrine tumors, the rectum 14%, the colon 21% and – for comparison – the ileum also 14% [3]. Occasionally tumors may be multiple, more so when in the ileum than in the colon or rectum. These figures will understate the frequency of small asymptomatic carcinoids. As discussed elsewhere, the carcinoid syndrome requires the access of vasoactive substances to the systemic circulation, and for tumors arising in the portal system this generally requires metastasis to the liver or extensive retroperitoneal spread. In addition whilst midgut carcinoids are rich in serotonin, hindgut carcinoids in general are not; thus whilst the ileal carcinoids are well recognized as leading to the carcinoid syndrome, appendiceal, colonic and rectal carcinoids do so rarely. Overall about 9% of ileal carcinoids, and 7% of colonic carcinoids, but only one in 300 appendiceal and one in 500 rectal carcinoids lead to the carcinoid syndrome. Very rarely, lower rectal carcinoids draining directly via inferior hemorrhoidal veins into the systemic circulation may cause the syndrome; the stuff of single case reports! The carcinoid syndrome is fully covered in Chapter 65.

Macroscopic appearances

The typical gut carcinoid tumor is submucosal, usually small (<1 cm), and yellow due to a high lipid content. As carcinoid tumors grow, they tend to spread outwards, rather than into the lumen, but growth is often very slow. Unchanging clinical appearance of a rectal carcinoid over 9 years has been documented [8]. It is generally stated that all carcinoids are potentially malignant, although as already mentioned this is rare in the appendix and rectum, much more common in the colon. The carcinoid cells may spread through the muscle layers of the gut, and penetrate the serosa and invade lymphatics. Mucosal ulceration over the tumor is rare and suggests, but does not establish, malignancy. In response to locally secreted factors, carcinoid tumors may be associated with a marked desmoplastic reaction, fibrosis in surrounding connective tissue, which may make macroscopic interpretation of tumor

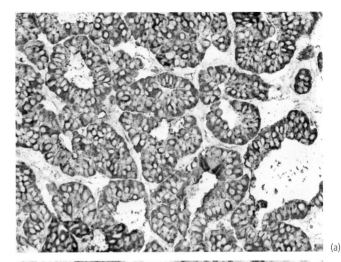

(a)

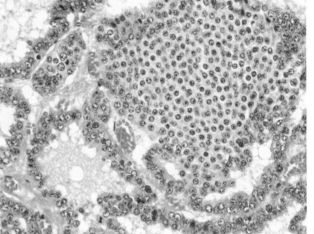

(b)

Figure 66.1 Carcinoid tumor demonstrating a nested pattern of neuroendocrine cell differentiation, with strong positive chromogranin staining (chromgranin and H&E: each 20×) (courtesy of Dr Federica Grillo).

spread and invasion difficult; some pathologists therefore require the presence of metastases before they will classify carcinoids as malignant. Metastasis is, in general, to lymph nodes and the liver, although bone and skin and nearly any organ may be involved.

Appendiceal carcinoids are generally at the tip of the appendix. Colonic carcinoids are most commonly found in the cecum. Rectal carcinoids are typically 8–10 cm from the anal verge, and characteristic clinical features of a yellow, smooth, submucosal swelling, generally less than 1 cm across, very firm or hard to palpation, may allow clinical differentiation from other rectal lesions. Carcinoids may be multicentric.

Microscopic appearances

Rather monotonous neuroendocrine cells with eosinophilic granular cytoplasm may be arranged in trabecular, glandular, insular (islets surrounded by connective tissue), mixed or undifferentiated patterns. Appendiceal tumors are, in general, insular; rectal are trabecular, insular or glandular. In the colon and rectum, confusion can occur because the cells become admixed with colonic or rectal crypts, giving a misleading appearance of malignancy, or mimicking the appearances of colitis cystica profunda. Marked desmoplasia was noted in 7% of rectal carcinoids in one series.

Of colorectal (predominantly rectal) carcinoids, a minority (but in one series 28%) are reported as argentaffin. Many more (55–75%) are argyrophilic; the majority stain positively for neuron-specific enolase (e.g. 87%) and chromogranin (58%) [9]. Many specific products are identified: for example, serotonin 4–45%, pancreatic polypeptide 45%, glucagon 10%, gastrin 3%, somatostatin 3%, adrenocorticotropic hormone (ACTH) 1%. Substance P, insulin, encephalin and β-endorphin are occasionally recognized and, in the majority of tumors, more than one product is present. Cholecystokinin (CCK), motilin, neurotensin and calcitonin have been stated to be absent. Carcinoembryonic antigen and prostatic acid phosphatase are relatively commonly identified (24% and 82%, respectively); this raises an important consideration, as carcinoids may be misdiagnosed as carcinomas by inexperienced pathologists.

The composite adenocarcinoid may also cause diagnostic confusion: a tumor predominantly of the appendix with malignant epithelial as well as neuroendocrine elements. Now it is appreciated that clonal specialization can occur in carcinomas, these are generally interpreted as primarily carcinomas rather than carcinoids, and specific genetic mutations within them are beginning to be delineated [10].

Clinical features and management

Appendiceal carcinoids

Most appendiceal carcinoids are identified histologically when appendicectomy has been performed for other reasons. As most of the tumors are at the tip, they are unlikely to induce obstructive appendicitis. Local infiltration into the mesoappendix may occur, or marked desmoplasia, and they may predispose to appendicitis by reducing motility of the organ.

What needs to be done when an appendiceal carcinoid has been detected, either at operation or subsequently by the histopathologist? Tumor size is critical. Those <1 cm virtually never metastasize [11]. For a large (>2 cm) tumor, or one with a marked desmoplastic reaction identified surgically, a right hemicolectomy should be performed as for cecal carcinomas. In the in-between group, tumors that show meso-appendiceal invasion or vascular invasion, or high proliferative indices (e.g., high Ki-67 expression) may well be appropriate for the "cancer surgery" operation. If a small tumor is found only at histopathological examination after appendicectomy, usually nothing needs to be done, but a second-look hemicolectomy has been recommended if there is tumor infiltration into the meso-appendix or lymphatic invasion. With reported 5-year survival rates of over 98%, clinicians and patients can be optimistic about appendiceal carcinoid tumors.

The previously mentioned adenocarcinoid, or goblet cell carcinoid, has a high malignant potential and needs a cancer-orientated approach.

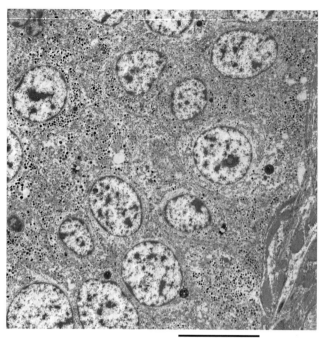

Figure 66.2 Characteristic EM staining of dense neuroendocrine granules in carcinoid tumor (2650×) (courtesy of J Lewin).

Colonic carcinoids

Colonic carcinoids, as opposed to rectal carcinoids, are rare. They are almost always poorly differentiated neuroendocrine carcinomas. Unless presenting with metastatic disease, the characteristic presentation of colonic carcinoid tumors is with pain or obstruction, or with bleeding, although surveillance colonoscopy in cancer prevention programs will also yield some. Those in the proximal colon, of midgut origin, are more likely to have an associated desmoplastic reaction. Treatment of symptomatic lesions is clearly by surgical resection with a cancer-type operation. There is little reported experience of endoscopic resection of small tumors with fulguration of the base as used for rectal carcinoids (see below); this technique is less applicable to submucosal lesions in the colon than in the rectum due to the risk of colonic perforation. Overall 5-year survivals of ~60% are reported.

Rectal carcinoids

As already mentioned, most recent series indicate that rectal carcinoids are relatively common – and constitute perhaps 15% of gastrointestinal neuroendocrine tumors and may indeed be more common than appendiceal carcinoids [3]. They are most likely to be identified as incidental findings at proctosigmoidoscopy in individuals over the age of 40. Despite their submucosal location, endoscopic biopsies are almost always diagnostic. The majority will be small, less than 1 cm, and metastasis at that stage is extremely rare. Endoscopic biopsy, with fulguration of the base, appears curative [2]. Endoscopic ultrasound or magnetic resonance can define the lack of transmural spread. Between 1 and 2 cm in size, the incidence of metastasis is again very low, perhaps 5%, but at this size a more formal operating room transanal approach may be appropriate. Over 4 cm in size, the chances of metastatic disease are very high, so formal cancer operations are indicated for all tumors over 2 cm, or if imaging suggests local spread of smaller tumors [8]. Overall survival rates of 85–90% are reported.

Management of metastatic disease

The oncological management of disseminated tumors from these sites is similar to that for metastatic midgut carcinoids described in the preceding chapter.

Tumor markers in management

The classic tumor marker of the carcinoid syndrome – urinary 5-OH indole-acetic acid – has little relevance to the majority of appendiceal and hindgut carcinoids as they are so rarely associated with the carcinoid syndrome. Elevations in blood chromogranin A may be of more relevance, as they can occur in the absence of the carcinoid syndrome or metastases, and high levels are an important sign of poor prognosis, but again most work has concentrated on foregut and midgut (ileal and jejunal) tumors and little information is available on hindgut tumors [12].

References

1. Rindi G, Capella C, Solcia E. Introduction to a revised clinicopathological classification of neuroendocrine tumors of the gastroenteropancreatic tract. *Q. J. Nucl. Med* 2000;44:13–21.

2. Matsui K, Iwase T, Kitagawa M. Small, polypoid-appearing carcinoid tumors of the rectum: clinicopathologic study of 16 cases and effectiveness of endoscopic treatment. *Am. J. Gastroenterol.* 1993;88: 1949–1953.

3. Modlin IM, Kidd M, Latich I, Zikusoka MN, Shapiro MD. Current status of gastrointestinal carcinoids. *Gastroenterology* 2005;128: 1717–1751.

4. Lluis F, Thompson JC. Neuroendocrine potential of the colon and rectum. *Gastroenterology* 1988;94:832–844.

5. Leotlela PD, Jauch A, Holtgreve-Grez H, Thakker RV. Genetics of neuroendocrine and carcinoid tumours. *Endocr. Relat. Cancer* 2003;10:437–450.

6. Kloppel G, Anlauf M. Epidemiology, tumour biology and histopathological classification of neuroendocrine tumours of the gastrointestinal tract. *Best Pract. Res. Clin. Gastroenterol.* 2005;19: 507–517.

7. La Rosa S, Rigoli E, Uccella S, Chiaravalli AM, Capella C. CDX2 as a marker of intestinal EC-cells and related well-differentiated endocrine tumors. *Virchows Arch.* 2004;445:248–254.

8. Jetmore AB, Ray JE, Gathright JB Jr, et al. Rectal carcinoids: the most frequent carcinoid tumor. *Dis. Colon Rectum* 1992;35:717–725.

9. Federspiel BH, Burke AP, Sobin LH, Shekitka KM. Rectal and colonic carcinoids. A clinicopathologic study of 84 cases. *Cancer* 1990;65:135–140.

10. Modlin IM, Kidd M, Latich I, et al. Genetic differentiation of appendiceal tumor malignancy: a guide for the perplexed. *Ann. Surg.* 2006;244:52–60.

11. Moertel CG, Weiland LH, Nagorney DM, Dockerty MB. Carcinoid tumor of the appendix: treatment and prognosis. *N. Engl. J. Med.* 1987;317:1699–1701.

12. Janson ET, Holmberg L, Stridsberg M, et al. Carcinoid tumors: analysis of prognostic factors and survival in 301 patients from a referral center. *Ann. Oncol.* 1997;8:685–690.

67 Chemotherapy for Neuroendocrine Tumors

Rebecca L. Bowen and Maurice L. Slevin

Key points

- Cytotoxic chemotherapy has been of relatively limited use in neuroendocrine tumors.
- Activity has been demonstrated with streptozocin, 5-fluorouracil and cisplatin/etoposide.
- Activity of cytotoxics appears greater in more poorly differentiated tumors.
- Novel agents, such as anti-vascular endothelial growth factor and tyrosine kinase inhibitor drugs, may yield better results.
- Promising response rates have been documented with interferon although response durations are short.

Introduction

The role of cytotoxic chemotherapy in neuroendocrine tumors remains unclear. Standard agents have limited efficacy and often significant toxicity which limits their therapeutic use. It is therefore important to consider each type of neuroendocrine tumor, therapy and patient individually. Although treatment with somatostatin analogs can usually control hormonal symptoms, they rarely induce tumor regression [1].

Cytotoxic chemotherapy

Streptozocin

Streptozocin-based regimens produce modest antitumor activity in patients with advanced neuroendocrine cancers often at the expense of quite considerable toxicity [2, 3]. In pancreatic islet cell tumors response rates for chemotherapy, including combinations of streptozocin, dacarbazine, 5-fluorouracil and adriamycin range from 40% to 70%. The combination of streptozocin and doxorubicin may confer a significant advantage in terms of both progression-free and overall survival [4–7] but not all of these studies looked at tumor differentiation.

Dacarbazine

Dacarbazine has been studied as an alternative to streptozocin and in carcinoid tumors may be at least as effective as the streptozocin-based regimens and response rates of 8–16% have been reported [7, 8]. In advanced pancreatic islet cell tumors up to one-third of patients may respond to dacarbazine [9]. However, as with streptozocin, toxicity remains a limiting factor in its use.

Clinical Endocrine Oncology, 2nd edition. Edited by Ian D. Hay and John A.H. Wass. © 2008 Blackwell Publishing. ISBN 978-1-4051-4584-8.

Fluorouracil

Fluorouracil in various combinations or alone is another reasonable alternative with a favorable response rate and less associated toxicity. Fluorouracil may be administered in a daily oral regime, which is advantageous in terms of convenience for the patient and for the cancer center [10].

Combination chemotherapy

The most impressive response rates to systemic chemotherapy have been demonstrated in poorly differentiated and anaplastic neuroendocrine tumors [11]. A small study of 45 patients treated with cisplatin and etoposide produced an objective response rate of just 7% in well-differentiated tumors and overall regression rate of 67% in those patients with anaplastic disease. Median time to progression was 8 months with a median survival of 19 months [12]. This regimen is often favored in pulmonary carcinoid as the disease represents one end of a spectrum which includes small cell carcinoma of the lung for which the treatment of choice would be cisplatin in combination with etoposide.

A recent small prospective study using an irinotecan/cisplatin combination (irinotecan, 65 mg/m^2, and cisplatin, 30 mg/m^2, administered weekly for 2 of every 3 weeks) suggested activity in aggressive neuroendocrine tumor subtypes. Toxicities were mild but again it was an ineffective regimen for patients with well-differentiated tumors [13].

Chemotherapy with arterial chemoembolization

The best responses in pancreatic islet cell carcinoma have been seen where systemic chemotherapy is used in combination with arterial chemoembolization. One study used two consecutive hepatic artery chemoembolization infusions with polyvinyl alcohol sponge (150 mg) and 150 mg cisplatin followed by an intra-arterial infusion of cisplatin. Up to 70% response rates were seen with durable remissions. However, side effects included paralytic ileus requiring nasogastric suction and moderate granulocytopenia [14].

Table 67.1 A summary of cytotoxic chemotherapy in neuroendocrine tumors

	Tumor types	Advantages	Disadvantages
Streptozocin combinations [4–7]	Pancreatic islet cell tumors	Some single agent activity Survival benefit in combination	Toxicities
Dacarbazine [7–9]	Pancreatic islet cell tumors	Some single agent activity	Toxicities
Fluorouracil [10]		Daily oral regime Less toxicity	
Cisplatin/etoposide [12]	Pulmonary carcinoid	Good responses in anaplastic NET	Marked toxicity
Cisplatin/irinotecan [13]	Aggressive NET	Minimal toxicity	
Cisplatin/arterial cisplatin chemoembolization [14]	Pancreatic islet cell tumors	Good response Durable remission	Marked toxicity Small study numbers
Interferon-α [1, 16]	Metastatic carcinoid	Symptomatic benefit in 60–70%	Marked toxicity Short response durations
Bevacizumab [18]	Metastatic carcinoid	Single agent activity Control of hormone output	Early data
SU11248 [19]	Aggressive NET	Daily oral regime Well tolerated	Early data
Temozolomide/thalidomide [20]	Pancreatic NET	Daily oral regime Good response & survival Minimal toxicity	Early data

Interpretation of these results is difficult as only five patients were treated.

The results of chemotherapy for midgut (jejunum, ileum, appendix, and right and transverse colon) carcinoid tumors are less impressive with only a 15–30% response rate which may only be sustained for 6–8 months [15].

A summary of the cytotoxic chemotherapy available is shown in Table 67.1.

Biotherapy

More recently, biotherapy with interferon-α has been used both as a single agent and in combination with, for example, lanreotide; however, with tumor markers, such as 5-hydroxy-indole acetic acid, reductions may occur in half of the patients and objective responses are seen in only about 15%. Symptomatic benefit is reported in up to 60–70% of patients; however, interferon treatment is frequently associated with considerable side effects and can lead to interruption in therapy. Response durations are also short [1, 16].

Novel therapies

Antiangiogenic agents
Novel agents used in the treatment of other malignancies are being tested in neuroendocrine tumors. Neuroendocrine tumors are very vascular and highly express vascular endothelial growth factor (VEGF) and may well be sensitive to antiangiogenic strategies [17]. Bevacizumab, an intravenous anti-VEGF monoclonal antibody with activity in a number of cancers, has recently been demonstrated to have single agent activity in neuroendocrine tumors [18]. It is felt that bevacizumab may also aid control of hormonal output in patients with octreotide refractory disease. SU11248 is an oral small molecule multitargeted tyrosine kinase inhibitor with anti-VEGF activity and has also shown modest response rates in early clinical trials. It appears to be well tolerated [19]. The antiangiogenic agents have produced better responses in other cancers when used in combination with cytotoxic chemotherapy agents.

A Phase II study of neuroendocrine tumors was recently conducted using temozolomide, an oral alkylating agent similar to dacarbazine but with less reported toxicity, coupled with thalidomide, another oral agent which is thought to have antiangiogenic activity. An overall radiological response rate of 25% was seen and median duration of response was 13.5 months; 2-year survival 61%. Forty-five percent of pancreatic endocrine tumors responded. Toxicity was generally mild [20]. It is likely that further clinical trials will yield results with different cytotoxic/anti-VEGF combinations.

Tyrosine kinase inhibition
The oral small molecule tyrosine kinase inhibitor imatinib mesylate, which is now routinely used in the treatment of chronic myeloid leukemia and gastrointestinal stromal tumors, has shown

inhibition of proliferation and enhanced apoptosis when used to treat neuroendocrine tumor cells *in vitro*, both in c-Kit positive and negative cell lines [21]. This is a well-tolerated treatment which may also show antitumor activity *in vivo*.

Patient selection for chemotherapy

Certain prognostic factors may assist the selection of patients for chemotherapy. Patients with carcinoid tumors that are strongly positive on radioscintigraphy imaging may have a poor response rate, reported as 10% in one paper, whereas patients with a negative scan may have a response rate of greater than 70% [12].

Summary

While standard cytotoxic chemotherapy regimes have been of limited use in the treatment of these tumors, largely due to the significant toxicity outweighing the antitumor activity, novel agents already in the clinic for other cancers are showing potential. They may well be of further benefit when used in combination with systemic chemotherapy or other treatment modalities but the high cost of these agents may limit their widespread use.

References

1. Faiss S, Pape UF, Bohmig M, et al. Prospective, randomized, multicenter trial on the antiproliferative effect of lanreotide, interferon alfa, and their combination for therapy of metastatic neuroendocrine gastroenteropancreatic tumors – the International Lanreotide and Interferon Alfa Study Group. *J. Clin. Oncol.* 2003;21:2689–2696.

2. Bukowski RM, Johnson KG, Peterson RF, et al. A phase II trial of combination chemotherapy in patients with metastatic carcinoid tumors. A Southwest Oncology Group Study. *Cancer* 1987;60:2891–2895.

3. Engstrom PF, Lavin PT, Moertel CG, et al. Streptozocin plus fluorouracil versus doxorubicin therapy for metastatic carcinoid tumor. *J. Clin. Oncol.* 1984;2:1255–1259.

4. Bajetta E, Ferrari L, Procopio G, et al. Efficacy of a chemotherapy combination for the treatment of metastatic neuroendocrine tumours. *Ann. Oncol.* 2002;13:614–621.

5. Moertel CG, Lefkopoulo M, Lipsitz S, et al. Streptozocin-doxorubicin, streptozocin-fluorouracil or chlorozotocin in the treatment of advanced islet-cell carcinoma. *N. Engl. J. Med.* 1992;326:519–523.

6. Kouvaraki MA, Ajani JA, Hoff P, et al. Fluorouracil, doxorubicin, and streptozocin in the treatment of patients with locally advanced and metastatic pancreatic endocrine carcinomas. *J. Clin. Oncol.* 2004; 22:4762–4771.

7. Sun W, Lipsitz S, Catalano P, et al. Phase II/III study of doxorubicin with fluorouracil compared with streptozocin with fluorouracil or dacarbazine in the treatment of advanced carcinoid tumors: Eastern Cooperative Oncology Group Study E1281. *J. Clin. Oncol.* 2005;23: 4897–4904.

8. Bajetta E, Rimassa L, Carnaghi C, et al. 5-Fluorouracil, dacarbazine, and epirubicin in the treatment of patients with neuroendocrine tumors. *Cancer* 1998;83:372–378.

9. Ramanathan RK, Cnaan A, Hahn RG, et al. Phase II trial of dacarbazine (DTIC) in advanced pancreatic islet cell carcinoma. Study of the Eastern Cooperative Oncology Group-E6282. *Ann. Oncol.* 2001;12:1139–1143.

10. Moertel CG. Treatment of the carcinoid tumor and the malignant carcinoid syndrome. *J. Clin. Oncol.* 1983;1:727–740.

11. Mitry E, Baudin E, Ducreux M, et al. Treatment of poorly differentiated neuroendocrine tumours with etoposide and cisplatin. *Br. J. Cancer* 1999;81:1351–1355.

12. Moertel CG, Kvols LK, O'Connell MJ, et al. Treatment of neuroendocrine carcinomas with combined etoposide and cisplatin. Evidence of major therapeutic activity in the anaplastic variants of these neoplasms. *Cancer* 1991;68:227–232.

13. Kulke MH, Wu B, Ryan DP, et al. A phase II trial of irinotecan and cisplatin in patients with metastatic neuroendocrine tumors. *Dig. Dis. Sci.* 2006;51:1033–1038.

14. Mavligit GM, Pollock RE, Evans HL, et al. Durable hepatic tumor regression after arterial chemoembolization-infusion in patients with islet cell carcinoma of the pancreas metastatic to the liver. *Cancer* 1993;72:375–380.

15. Ramage JK, Davies AH, Ardill J, et al. Guidelines for the management of gastroenteropancreatic neuroendocrine (including carcinoid) tumours. *Gut* 2005;54(Suppl 4):iv1–16.

16. Moertel CG, Rubin J, Kvols LK. Therapy of metastatic carcinoid tumor and the malignant carcinoid syndrome with recombinant leukocyte A interferon. *J. Clin. Oncol.* 1989;7:865–868.

17. Terris B, Scoazec JY, Rubbia L, et al. Expression of vascular endothelial growth factor in digestive neuroendocrine tumours. *Histopathology* 1998;32:133–138.

18. Yao J, Ng C, Hoff P, et al. Improved progression free survival (PFS) and rapid, sustained decrease in tumor perfusion among patients with advanced carcinoid treated with bevacizumab. *J. Clin. Oncol.* 2005;23(abstr 4007).

19. Kulke MH, Lenz H, Meropol N, et al. A phase 2 study to evaluate the efficacy and safety of SU11248 in patients (pts) with unresectable neuroendocrine tumors (NETS). *J. Clin. Oncol.* 2005;23(abstr 4008).

20. Kulke MH, Stuart K, Enzinger PC, et al. Phase II study of temozolomide and thalidomide in patients with metastatic neuroendocrine tumors. *J. Clin. Oncol.* 2006;24:401–406.

21. Lankat-Buttgereit B, Horsch D, Barth P, et al. Effects of the tyrosine kinase inhibitor imatinib on neuroendocrine tumor cell growth. *Digestion* 2005;71:131–140.

6 Medical Syndromes and Endocrine Neoplasia

68 Multiple Endocrine Neoplasia Type 1 (MEN 1)

Cornelis J.M. Lips, Koen M.A. Dreijerink, Gerlof D. Valk, and Jo W.M. Höppener

> **Key points**
> - Multiple endocrine neoplasia type 1 is an autosomal dominantly inherited disorder, characterized by the occurrence of tumors of specific endocrine organs, notably the parathyroid glands, the pancreatic islets, the pituitary gland, and the adrenal cortex, as well as neuroendocrine tumors in the thymus, lungs and stomach.
> - Neuroendocrine tumors of the thymus and pancreatic-duodenal gastrinomas are the most harmful multiple endocrine neoplasia type 1 tumor types, since these tumors have malignant potential and curative treatment is difficult to achieve.
> - Multiple endocrine neoplasia type 1 is caused by germline mutations of the *MEN1* tumor suppressor gene. Nucleotide sequence analysis of this gene enables MEN 1 disease gene carriers to be identified presymptomatically.
> - Multiple endocrine neoplasia type 1 patients and their family members, family members of *MEN1* gene mutation carriers and patients who are clinically suspected to be carriers of a *MEN1* gene mutation are eligible for mutation analysis.
> - Multiple endocrine neoplasia type 1-associated tumors can be detected and treated at an early stage through periodic clinical monitoring of *MEN1* gene mutation carriers.

Introduction

Multiple endocrine neoplasia type 1 (MEN 1) is an autosomal dominantly inherited syndrome. MEN 1 is characterized by the occurrence of tumors of the parathyroid glands, the pancreatic islets, the anterior pituitary gland and the adrenal glands, as well as neuroendocrine tumors in the thymus, lungs, and stomach, often at a young age. Non-endocrine manifestations of MEN 1 include angiofibromas, collagenomas, lipomas, leiomyomas, and meningiomas (Table 68.1).

The prevalence of MEN 1 is 2–3 per 100 000, and is equal among males and females. MEN 1 and MEN 2 are two distinct syndromes. In MEN 2, patients frequently develop medullary thyroid carcinoma and adrenal medullary tumors (pheochromocytoma).

MEN 1 is caused by germline mutations of the *MEN1* gene [1]. Since the discovery of the gene in 1997, DNA diagnosis has become available. Carriers of a *MEN1* gene germline mutation can be monitored periodically by targeted clinical examination to identify MEN 1-associated lesions at a presymptomatic stage.

In this review, the recent developments concerning the etiology of MEN 1 as well as the current diagnostic and therapeutic options are presented. Furthermore, guidelines for *MEN1* mutation analysis and periodic clinical monitoring are provided.

Table 68.1 The variable expression of *MEN1*. Percentages of *MEN1* gene germline mutation carriers that develop a MEN 1-associated tumor

Parathyroid adenomas	75–95%
Pancreatic islet cell tumors	55%
Gastrinomas	45%
Insulinomas	10%
Non-functioning (including pancreatic polypeptide-producing tumors)	10%
Other	2%
Pituitary adenomas	47%
Prolactinomas	30%
Non-functioning (i.e., not producing hormone)	10%
ACTH producing	1%
GH producing	3–6%
Adrenal cortical adenomas	20%
NET	18%
Thymus	8%
Bronchial	8%
Stomach	5%
Skin lesions	80%
Angiofibromas	75%
Collagenomas	5%
Lipomas	30%
Leiomyomas	5%
Meningiomas	25%

ACTH, adrenocorticotropic hormone; GH, growth hormone; NET, neuroendocrine tumors.

Clinical Endocrine Oncology, 2nd edition. Edited by Ian D. Hay and John A.H. Wass. © 2008 Blackwell Publishing. ISBN 978-1-4051-4584-8.

Etiology of MEN 1

MEN 1 is caused by inactivating germline mutations of the *MEN1* gene, which is located on chromosome 11q13 [1]. The *MEN1* gene is a tumor suppressor gene. Biallelic inactivation of the *MEN1* gene is required for the development of a tumor cell. Loss of the wild-type allele (loss of heterozygosity) is observed frequently in MEN 1-associated tumors in MEN 1 patients.

Since the discovery of the gene, more than 400 different germline mutations have been identified in MEN 1 families. These mutations are found scattered throughout the gene. Also in sporadic MEN 1-associated tumors, mutations of the *MEN1* gene have been found, which suggests that inactivation of the *MEN1* gene contributes to the development of these tumors.

No clear genotype–phenotype correlation has been established. The expression of the disease is variable, even within families. However, some *MEN1* gene mutations seem to be causing familial isolated hyperparathyroidism or a variant *MEN1* that is characterized by the frequent occurrence of prolactinoma. Thus, additional genetic events may play a role in MEN 1-associated tumorigenesis. The *MEN1* gene encodes the menin protein. Menin is expressed ubiquitously, and performs its tasks predominantly in the nucleus (Plate 68.1a).

Recent observations indicate that normal menin functions in the regulation of gene transcription. This function is linked to modification of histones, cores of proteins wrapped in DNA wound in a double loop. In this capacity, intact menin has a dual function and may serve either as a co-repressor or as a co-activator of gene expression. Co-repressors and co-activators serve as adaptors between nuclear receptors and the general transcription machinery (see Plate 68.1a). Interaction of nuclear receptors with co-activators or co-repressors takes place through LXXLL motifs (where L = leucine and X = any amino acid) present in the co-activator or co-repressor proteins.

Menin interacts with the AP1-family transcription factor JunD, changing it from an oncoprotein into a tumor suppressor protein, putatively by recruitment of histone deacetylase complexes. Recently, the telomerase (*hTERT*) gene was identified as a menin target gene. The ends of chromosomes in a cell, the telomeres, shorten after DNA replication.

Eventually, after several cell divisions, the DNA loses its stability and the cell is subjected to apoptosis. Telomerase is an enzyme that maintains the length of the telomeres. Telomerase is not expressed in normal cells, but it is active in stem cells and tumor cells. Menin is a suppressor of the expression of telomerase. Possibly, inactivation of menin could lead to cell immortalization by telomerase expression, which could allow a cell to develop into a tumor cell (see Plate 68.1b). Besides this corepressor function, intact menin suppresses transforming growth factor-β-mediated signal transduction involved in division of parathyroid hormone- and prolactin-producing cells.

Menin is an integral component of mixed lineage leukemia 1/2 (MLL1/MLL2) histone methyltransferase complexes. In this capacity menin is a co-activator of expression of p18^{INK4C} and p27^{Kip1} cyclin-dependent kinase inhibitors. These proteins usually act as tumor suppressors by causing arrest of the cell cycle, i.e. inhibition of cell division. Furthermore, menin serves as a co-activator of steroid receptor-mediated transcription, as illustrated by recruiting histone H3K4 methyltransferase activity to the estrogen-responsive *TFF1*(*pS2*) gene promoter (see Plate 68.1a) [2, 3].

Menin links histone modification pathways to transcription factor function. Evolutionary conservation indicates that menin plays a role in integrating multiple cellular stimuli at critical transcriptional loci during fundamental developmental processes. Null mutant animals have indicated that menin is essential for viability. Inactivating mutations in both *MEN1* alleles disturb the tight link between chromatin modification and gene expression and are crucial for MEN 1 tumorigenesis (Plate 68.1b).

Further insight into the mechanisms that underlie MEN 1-associated tumorigenesis may provide opportunities for new therapeutic strategies.

Clinical manifestations, diagnosis and treatment

According to the MEN consensus published in 2001, a practical definition of a MEN 1 patient is a patient with at least two of the three main MEN 1-related endocrine tumors (i.e. parathyroid adenomas, enteropancreatic endocrine tumors, and a pituitary adenoma) [4]. Familial MEN 1 is similarly defined as at least one MEN 1 case plus at least one first-degree relative with one of those main MEN 1 tumors. Alternatively, because parathyroid and pituitary adenomas occur relatively frequently in the general population, a MEN 1 patient can be defined more precisely as a patient with three or more of the five major MEN 1-associated lesions (i.e., besides the three tumor types mentioned, adrenal gland tumors, and neuroendocrine tumors in the thymus, lungs, and stomach). A MEN 1-suspected patient is defined as having at least two major MEN 1-associated lesions, multiple lesions within one MEN 1-related organ, and/or a MEN 1-associated lesion at a young age (<35 years) [5]. Such a patient may be considered for DNA analysis (see under *MEN1* mutation analysis below).

Below, for each tumor type the clinical presentation and the diagnostic and therapeutic options are listed. In Fig. 68.1, flow charts are shown for diagnosis and therapy of MEN 1-associated tumors of the pancreatic islets and pituitary adenoma.

Parathyroid adenoma (see also Chapter 21: Parathyroid Adenomas and Hyperplasia)

Parathyroid adenomas are often the first manifestation of MEN 1. About 75–95% of MEN 1 patients develop parathyroid adenomas [6]. Usually, parathyroid adenomas in MEN 1 are multiple and benign. Other forms of familial hyperparathyroidism are found in familial isolated hyperparathyroidism (FIHP), caused by inactivating mutations in the parafibromin gene on chromosome 1 (1q31.2), and in MEN 2A, caused by activating mutations in the

RET proto-oncogene. MEN 1 genotyping appears worthwhile in FIHP families, as the finding of mutation(s) in this gene may predict possible involvement of other organs [7].

The increased production of parathyroid hormone causes hypercalcemia. Symptoms and signs of hypercalcemia include fatigue, depression, constipation, nausea, symptoms caused by nephrolithiasis or nephrocalcinosis, bone pain, myalgia and arthralgia as well as hypertension.

Diagnosis (see also Chapter 14: Thyroid and Parathyroid Imaging)

Laboratory investigation consists of measurement of (ionized) calcium, chloride, phosphate and parathyroid hormone in blood. In addition to this, the 24-h calcium excretion in the urine is measured. Bone densitometry can be used to detect bone mass reduction.

Preoperative localization is useful, because adenomas may be situated in or behind the thyroid lobes. Parathyroid adenomas can be effectively localized by ultrasound (US), supplemented with computerized tomography (CT). To confirm the location, a nuclear scan can be made with ^{99m}Tc- sestamibi that is retained selectively by parathyroid adenomas.

Treatment

If signs of hyperparathyroidism are found it is useful not to postpone surgery for a long time, because continuously elevated calcium levels stimulate secretion and proliferation of pancreatic islet cells and promote bone loss and systemic calcification.

Optimal surgical intervention must balance the risk of recurrent hypercalcemia with the morbidity of permanent hypoparathyroidism. Three-gland (subtotal) parathyroidectomy, transcervical thymectomy, and parathyroid cryopreservation constitute the preferred initial surgical procedure [8]. Another option is total parathyroidectomy with immediate heterotopic autotransplantation of parathyroid tissue into the non-dominant forearm. In selected cases, minimally invasive parathyroidectomy may be preferred. However, one has to realize that after some years a second procedure will be necessary [9]. Surgical treatment should therefore aim to minimize the risk of permanent hypocalcemia and facilitate future surgery. When correctly performed, subtotal parathyroidectomy fulfills these objectives [10].

Tumors of the endocrine duodenum and pancreatic islets (see also Chapter 57: Classification of Neuroendocrine Tumors)

Definition of neuroendocrine tumors

In the past, the classic term "carcinoid" was well established in medical terminology but it is not adequate to cover the entire spectrum of neuroendocrine neoplasms. In 2000, the term neuroendocrine tumors (NET) was suggested by the World Health Organization (WHO) in the new classification of tumors that differ in their morphological and functional features [11].

Divergence in gene expression patterns in the development of the gastroenteropancreatic (GEP) system (divided into NET of jejunum and ileum and pancreaticoduodenal endocrine tumors [PET]) was identified, when they were examined at a molecular level. On the basis of gene expression profiles, neuroendocrine lesions of jejunum and ileum and PET need to be considered as two distinct entities within the group of NET [12].

General

PET develop in about 55% of MEN 1 patients [13, 14]. Multicentric microadenomas are present in 90% of MEN 1 patients [15].

Symptomatology

Hormonal syndromes often occur late and indicate metastases in 50% of patients with this stage of functioning PET [16]. Prospective screening with biochemical markers and endoscopic ultrasound (EUS) is therefore recommended. Prospective endoscopic ultrasonic evaluation reveals that the frequency of non-functioning PET is higher (54.9%) than previously thought (34%) [17].

Diagnosis (see Fig. 68.1a)

Laboratory investigation includes determination of fasting plasma levels of glucose, insulin, C-peptide, glucagon, gastrin, pancreatic polypeptide, and chromogranin A. Pancreatic islet cell tumors can be visualized by US, magnetic resonance imaging (MRI), somatostatin receptor scintigraphy (SRS), CT and F-Dopa positron emission tomography (F-Dopa-PET).

EUS is useful for early detection of PET and will allow early surgery before metastases have developed [14, 16]. EUS is a more sensitive technique for the detection and localization of potentially malignant lesions in patients with MEN 1 than CT or transabdominal US [18].

Treatment

Surgery is required when the tumor is causing a functional syndrome. Local, loco-regional and metastatic disease have to be distinguished. Early diagnosis and surgical excision of MEN 1-related PET improves survival. However, translating these data into a surveillance strategy for the early detection of PET is complex, owing to the potential morbidity of pancreatic resection and the risk of long-term insulin dependence [13].

A conservative approach in treatment of non-functioning tumors of the pancreas (NFTP) is indicated. NFTP are currently the most common tumors of the pancreaticoduodenal region in patients with MEN 1. Prevention of tumor spread by surgery should be balanced with potential operative mortality and morbidity. Routine surgery for NFTP <20 mm is not recommended [19].

Surgical treatment

If an islet cell tumor is larger than 3 cm in diameter and/or is progressively expanding, the tumor and the peripancreatic lymph nodes should be resected and a duodenotomy should be carried out to assess the presence of duodenal tumors. Enucleation of tumors in the head of the pancreas, excision of duodenal gastrinomas together with clearance of lymph node metastases, and distal 80%

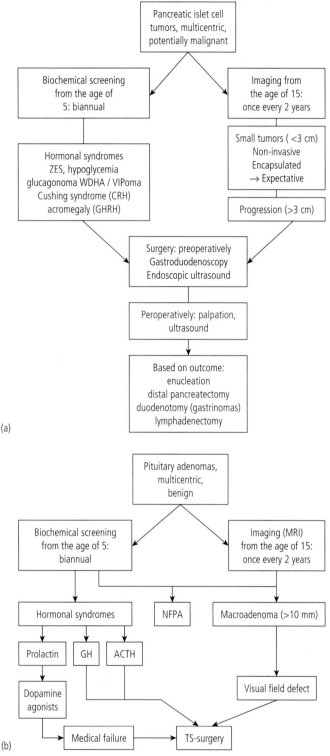

(a)

(b)

Figure 68.1 Recommendations for diagnosis and management of pancreatic islet cell tumors (a), and pituitary adenomas (b) in MEN 1 patients. ACTH, adrenocorticotropic hormone; CT, computerized tomography; GH, growth hormone; NFT, non-functioning tumor; NFPA, non-functioning pituitary adenoma; PRL, prolactin; PTH, parathyroid hormone; SA, somatostatin analogs; TS-surgery, transsphenoidal surgery; VIP, vasoactive intestinal peptide; WDHA, watery diarrhea, hypokalemia, achlorhydria; ZES, Zollinger–Ellison syndrome.

subtotal pancreatectomy may be performed to prevent tumor recurrence [16].

A more aggressive surgical approach is intended to control the functional syndromes and malignant potential for nodal or distant metastasis. This strategy is based on frequent recurrence and some treatment-related morbidity and mortality. Most patients (>50%) eventually demonstrated malignant growth.

Intraoperative ultrasound will give more information about the procedure to follow. If possible, pylorus-preserving pancreatico-duodenectomy (PPPD) is preferred. Early aggressive surgery may prevent development of liver metastases, which are the most life threatening [20].

Medical treatment

Octreotide has antiangiogenic properties. Tyrosine kinase inhibitors may have useful potential in tumors with overexpression of TK receptors (c-kit, EGFR, PDGFR) [21].

Specific syndromes [see also Chapter 60: Gastrinoma (Zollinger–Ellison Syndrome)]

Zollinger–Ellison syndrome (ZES)

Gastrinomas are the most common pancreatic tumors in MEN 1. The elevated levels of ectopic gastrin cause excessive gastric acid production. If untreated, this can lead to the ZES: ulcerations of the digestive tract, diarrhea, and mucosal hypertrophy. Before treatment with proton pump inhibitors became available, the ZES was a frequent cause of death of MEN 1 patients. Gastrinomas are still an important threat to MEN 1 patients, because they are often multicentric and are able to metastasize to the lymph nodes and the liver [6]. The diagnosis is delayed by the widespread use of proton pump inhibitors.

MEN 1 patients frequently develop ZES. About 25% of all ZES patients have MEN 1. Esophageal reflux symptoms are common resulting in strictures and Barrett's esophagus (BE). The frequency of severe peptic esophageal disease, including the premalignant condition BE, was higher in MEN 1 patients with gastrinomas than in patients with sporadic gastrinomas. This higher incidence of severe esophageal disease in MEN 1/ZES was due to delay of diagnosis, more frequent and severe esophageal symptoms, more frequent hiatal hernias, more common pyloric scarring, higher basal acid output, and underdiagnosed hyperparathyroidism [22].

Preoperative selective arterial secretagog injection test (SASI test) with calcium or secretin in the splenic, gastroduodenal or superior mesenteric artery may localize functioning tumors. Preoperative somatostatin receptor scintigraphy and endoscopic US can be useful for the localization of tumors. Intraoperative duodenoscopy (IODS) or intraoperative US (IOUS) may confirm the preoperative findings [23].

The best therapeutic procedure is surgery which, if radical, can be curative. Medical treatment can be the best palliative therapy and should be used, when possible, in association with surgery, in a multimodal therapeutic approach [24].

Eutopic gastrinomas develop from the G-cells in the duodenal and gastric mucosa and generally have a benign course; however, a subgroup of them shows an aggressive behavior and is the cause of death in these patients. If surgery is limited to tumor enucleation or full-thickness duodenal wall resection, the cure rate is low. Pancreatoduodenectomy has a higher chance of cure. For nonfunctioning tumors exceeding 1 cm in diameter prompt treatment is indicated due to their high malignant potential. Gastroscopic surveillance for gastric fundus carcinoids is recommended [25].

Current controversies include the role of pancreaticoduodenectomy (Whipple procedure), surgery and reoperation for metastatic tumor, and the use of minimally invasive surgical techniques to localize and remove gastrinoma.

Other functioning pancreatic islet cell tumors (see also Chapter 59: Insulinomas and Hypoglycemia)

Insulinomas occur in about 10% of all MEN 1 patients. They may present with symptoms of hypoglycemia such as confusion or abnormal behavior due to central nervous system dysfunction at times of exercise or fasting.

Infrequently occurring syndromes are glucagonoma (1.6%), VIPoma (0.98%) and somatostatinoma (0.65%). Glucagonomas can cause skin lesions, whereas tumors producing vasoactive intestinal peptide (VIP), VIPomas, can cause the Verner–Morrison syndrome, also called the watery diarrhea–hypokalemia–achlorhydria (WDHA) syndrome [14]. Surgical excision of insulinomas, glucagonomas, and VIPomas is usually curative. Tumors producing pancreatic polypeptide are common (>80% of PET), but only rarely cause symptoms and therefore do not normally require treatment.

Growth hormone-releasing hormone (GHRH)-producing tumors (see also Chapter 30: Acromegaly)

Acromegaly may be caused by GHRH produced by pancreatic islet cell tumors. GHRH may cause acromegaly indirectly through stimulation of growth hormone (GH) production by the pituitary gland. In more than 50% of MEN 1 patients with acromegaly, a GHRH-producing pancreatic tumor is the cause of the disease.

In MEN 1 patients, acromegaly can also be caused by adenomas in the pituitary gland primarily producing GH and neuroendocrine tumors in the thymus gland producing GHRH.

Pituitary adenomas (see also Chapters 23, 26, 29, 30, 32: on Pituitary adenomas)

Evidence of MEN 1 is found in approximately 2.7% of patients with pituitary adenomas. In addition, somatic mutations in the MEN 1 gene do not play a prominent role in the pathogenesis of sporadic forms of pituitary adenoma (3.7%).

Pituitary tumors in MEN 1 are larger in size and more aggressive than sporadic tumors. MEN 1 must be considered in all children with tumors of the pituitary gland [26].

The most frequently occurring pituitary tumors in MEN 1 are prolactinomas. Prolactinomas occur in approximately 30% of patients with MEN 1 and in this setting, they may be more aggressive than their sporadic counterparts [27].

A MEN 1 variant shows more frequent prolactinoma and less frequent gastrinoma than typical MEN 1 [28]. Non-functioning tumors, growth hormone, or adrenocorticotropic hormone- (ACTH) producing tumors and mixed tumors are seen less frequently.

Symptomatology (Fig. 68.1b)

Elevated levels of prolactin may cause amenorrhea, galactorrhea, and lack of libido in females and hypogonadism in males. Acromegaly, caused by a GH-producing tumor, is observed in 3–6% of MEN 1 patients. Patients present with enlarged hands or feet, coarse facial features or soft tissue growth. Patients with acromegaly have an increased risk of developing cardiovascular disease and malignancy.

Non-functioning pituitary adenomas may grow large without symptoms. Due to compression of the surrounding tissues by the expanding tumor, complaints of visual field defects, headache, or an impairment of other pituitary functions may develop. Gonadotroph tumors occur infrequently but may cause ovarian hyperstimulation [29].

Diagnosis

The diagnosis is confirmed by determining plasma levels of prolactin (prolactinoma), midnight cortisol (Cushing disease), or insulin-like growth factor I (IGF-I) and by an oral glucose tolerance test to demonstrate absence of suppression of growth hormone production (acromegaly). Pituitary adenomas can be detected visually by MR imaging with gadolinium contrast.

Treatment

Dopamine suppresses prolactin secretion. Hence, the primary treatment of prolactinomas consists of dopamine receptor agonists such as bromocriptine, quinagolide or cabergoline. Surgery is required infrequently. For acromegaly, the initial therapy for localized adenomas is transsphenoidal microsurgery because of its rapid reduction of GH levels, low incidence of postoperative hypopituitarism, and low morbidity and high success rate. Patients with persisting GH hypersecretion postoperatively should be treated with sustained-release forms of somatostatin, which represses GH secretion. Radiation therapy should be reserved for patients with inadequate response to surgery and medical therapy.

ACTH-producing adenomas are removed operatively after pretreatment with ketoconazole. If non-functional adenomas have a diameter larger than 10 mm, or if there is visual field loss, or deficiency of other pituitary hormones (gonadotropins), a patient is eligible for transsphenoidal surgery. Radiation therapy is usually required to prevent progression.

Adrenal tumors (see also Chapter 50: Adrenal Incidentalomas)

About 20% of MEN 1 patients develop adrenal tumors. These tumors are often detected early by imaging of the upper abdomen every 2 years. Like sporadic incidentalomas of the adrenals, these tumors usually do not produce hormones and are mostly benign.

Treatment:

When a tumor is larger than 4 cm in diameter, there is an increased risk of malignancy and the tumor should be resected.

NET of thymus, lungs, and stomach (see also Chapter 64: Lung and Thymic Neuroendocrine Tumors, and Chapter 60: Gastrinoma)

In MEN 1, NET arise from cells that are derived from the embryonic foregut. NET in MEN 1 can develop in the thymus (mostly in males), in the lungs (mostly in females), and in the stomach, duodenum or the pancreas (PET).

They do not cause symptoms until at an advanced stage. As these tumors are capable of infiltrating surrounding tissues and metastasizing, and treatment is very difficult, early detection of these tumors is of vital interest (Fig. 68.1) [14].

NET produce a vast spectrum of amines, peptides and prostaglandins. NET in MEN 1 do not release serotonin (5HT), but do produce 5-hydroxytryptophan (5-HTP), the precursor of serotonin. The 5-HTP is partially converted into serotonin in the kidneys. Levels of platelet serotonin and chromogranin A are useful markers. The level of 5-hydroxyindoleacetic acid (5-HIAA) in the 24-h urine of MEN 1 patients with NET is not usually elevated.

Imaging

Tumors can be detected using MRI, SRS or CT scintigraphy, and endoscopy.

Thymus (see also Chapter 64: Lung and Thymic Neuroendocrine Tumors)

Thymic NETs in MEN 1 are associated with a very high lethality. Nearly all thymus carcinoid patients are male smokers. Therefore, prophylactic thymectomy should be considered at neck surgery for primary hyperparathyroidism in male MEN 1 patients, especially for smokers, and, due to the frequent familial clustering of this pathology, in subjects with affected relatives presenting this feature.

In 22 separate MEN 1 families with thymic carcinoids, all but two (91%) have mutations coding for a truncated menin protein. There is clearly a high prevalence of truncating mutations in MEN 1-related thymic carcinoids. Although, when compared with the prevalence of truncating mutations among all reported MEN 1 mutations, it is not significantly higher in MEN 1 families with thymic NETs ($p = 0.39$) [30].

Screening every patient affected with a neuroendocrine thymic neoplasm for MEN 1 syndrome is recommended. Association occurs in approximately 25% [31].

Cushing syndrome due to ACTH-producing thymic carcinoid should also be considered as one phenotype of the MEN 1 spectrum [32].

Lung (see also Chapter 64: Lung and Thymic Neuroendocrine Tumors)

Bronchopulmonary NET are relatively uncommon, occurring in approximately 5% of MEN 1 patients. Hypergastrinemia was significantly more common in patients with pulmonary nodules. No deaths or distant metastases occurred among these patients despite long-term follow-up. They did not appear to predict a poor prognosis in the majority of affected patients [33].

Stomach [see also Chapter 60: Gastrinoma (Zollinger–Ellison Syndrome)]

In MEN 1 patients, gastric NET have their origin in enterochromaffin-like (ECL) cells. Longstanding tumors may become symptomatic, and demonstrate aggressive growth. Patients may have ZES. With increased long-term medical treatment and life expectancy, these tumors will become an important determinant of survival. They require surgical treatment before they metastasize to the liver [34].

MEN1 mutation analysis

MEN1 gene germ line mutations are detected in the vast majority of MEN 1 patients by nucleotide sequence analysis [5]. Besides MEN 1 patients, first-degree family members (parents, brothers, sisters, children) of MEN 1 patients, and family members of *MEN1* gene mutation carriers are eligible for mutation analysis.

With regard to new case-finding, unfortunately, only a small percentage in non-selected patients with apparently sporadic MEN 1-associated tumors turn out to be carriers of a *MEN1* germline mutation (at most 5%). To increase the sensitivity and specificity (cost-effectiveness) for mutation detection and to be able to identify all these MEN 1 patients, without screening the entire group of patients with apparently sporadic tumors, the criteria for MEN 1-suspected patients have been defined. In 60% of MEN 1-suspected patients a germline mutation of the *MEN1* gene has been found [5].

The earliest manifestation of MEN 1 reported is a pituitary adenoma in a 5-year-old boy. Therefore, in principle, mutation analysis should be performed before the age of 5 [35].

Periodic clinical monitoring

MEN 1 patients and their family members have to be monitored periodically. The clinical investigation is aimed at identification of MEN 1-associated lesions and includes, besides the patient's history and physical examination, biochemical screening and imaging. The protocol for periodic clinical monitoring is shown in Table 68.2.

Conclusion

MEN 1 is an inherited disorder with a variable presentation, often already present at a young age. The initial symptoms of MEN 1-associated lesions may be very general. By using stringent criteria, MEN 1 patients can be identified efficiently. Nucleotide sequence

Table 68.2 Criteria for MEN1 mutation analysis and guidelines for periodical clinical monitoring

Criteria for mutation analysis	
MEN1 gene mutation analysis is offered to:	Patients with three of the five major MEN 1-associated lesions: parathyroid adenomas, pancreatic islet cell tumors, pituitary adenomas, adrenal adenomas, NET
	First-degree family members (parents, brothers, sisters, children) of MEN 1 patients with a confirmed *MEN1* gene germline mutation, family members of clinical MEN 1 patients without an identified germline mutation or who declined mutation analysis
	First-degree family members of asymptomatic *MEN1* gene germline mutation carriers
	MEN 1-suspected patients: patients with two of the five major lesions, two MEN 1-associated tumors within one organ and/or a MEN 1-associated lesion at a young age (<35 years)
Periodical clinic monitoring	
MEN 1 patients, *MEN1* gene germline mutation carriers and MEN 1-suspected patients without a confirmed mutation are eligible for periodic clinical monitoring	
Periodical screening includes:	
From the age of 5:	Biannual clinical examination, laboratory investigation including measurement of ionized calcium, chloride, phosphate, parathyroid hormone, glucose, insulin, C-peptide, glucagon, gastrin, pancreatic polypeptide, prolactin, IGF-I, platelet serotonin and chromogranin A
From the age of 15, once every 2 years:	MRI of the upper abdomen
	MRI of the pituitary with gadolinium contrast
	MRI of the mediastinum in males

MRI, magnetic resonance imaging; IGF, insulin-like growth factor.

analysis enables *MEN1* gene mutation carriers to be identified. Gastrinomas and other NET have malignant potential. Periodic clinical monitoring makes presymptomatic detection and treatment of MEN 1-associated tumors possible. This is beneficial for both life expectancy and quality of life of MEN 1 patients.

Acknowledgment

Koen Dreijerink is supported by the Netherlands Organisation for Health Research and Development (ZonMw; AGIKO-stipendium).

References

1. Chandrasekharappa SC, Guru SC, Manickam P, et al. Positional cloning of the gene for multiple endocrine neoplasia type 1. *Science* 1997;276:404–407.
2. Dreijerink KM, Mulder KW, Winkler GS, Höppener JW, Lips CJ, Timmers HT. Menin links estrogen receptor activation to histone H3K4 trimethylation. *Cancer Res.* 2006;66:4929–4935.
3. Dreijerink KMA, Höppener JWM, Timmers HThM, Lips CJM. Mechanisms of disease: multiple endocrine neoplasia type 1-relation to chromatin modifications and transcription regulation. *Nat. Clin. Pract. Endocrinol. Metab.* 2006;2:562–570.
4. Brandi ML, Gagel RF, Angeli A, et al. Consensus. Guidelines for diagnosis and therapy of MEN type 1 and type 2. *J. Clin. Endocrinol. Metab.* 2001;86:5658–5671.
5. Roijers JF, de Wit MJ, van der Luijt RB, Ploos van Amstel HK, Höppener JW, Lips CJ. Criteria for mutation analysis in MEN 1-suspected patients: MEN 1 case-finding. *Eur. J. Clin. Invest.* 2000;30:487–492.
6. Geerdink EA, van der Luijt RB, Lips CJ. Do patients with multiple endocrine neoplasia syndrome type 1 benefit from periodical screening? *Eur. J. Endocrinol.* 2003;149:577–582.
7. Cetani F, Pardi E, Ambrogini E, et al. Genetic analyses in familial isolated hyperparathyroidism: implication for clinical assessment and surgical management. *Clin. Endocrinol.* (Oxf.) 2006;64:146–152.
8. Lambert LA, Shapiro SE, Lee JE, et al. Surgical treatment of hyperparathyroidism in patients with multiple endocrine neoplasia type 1. *Arch. Surg.* 2005;140:374–382.
9. Carling T, Udelsman R. Parathyroid surgery in familial hyperparathyroid disorders. *J. Intern. Med.* 2005;257:27–37.
10. Hubbard JG, Sebag F, Maweja S, Henry JF. Subtotal parathyroidectomy as an adequate treatment for primary hyperparathyroidism in multiple endocrine neoplasia type 1. *Arch. Surg.* 2006;141:235–239.
11. Klöppel G, Anlauf M. Epidemiology, tumour biology and histopathological classification of neuroendocrine tumours of the gastrointestinal tract. *Best Pract. Res. Clin. Gastroenterol.* 2005;19:507–517.
12. Zikusoka MN, Kidd M, Eick G, Latich I, Modlin IM. The molecular genetics of gastroenteropancreatic neuroendocrine tumors. *Cancer* 2005;104:2292–2309.

13. Kouvaraki MA, Shapiro SE, Cote GJ, et al. Management of pancreatic endocrine tumors in multiple endocrine neoplasia type 1. *World J. Surg.* 2006;30:643–653.

14. Levy-Bohbot N, Merle C, Goudet P, et al. Groupe des Tumeurs Endocrines. Prevalence, characteristics and prognosis of MEN 1-associated glucagonomas, VIPomas, and somatostatinomas: study from the GTE (Groupe des Tumeurs Endocrines) registry. *Gastroenterol. Clin. Biol.* 2004;28:1075–1081.

15. Anlauf M, Schlenger R, Perren A, et al. Microadenomatosis of the endocrine pancreas in patients with and without the multiple endocrine neoplasia type 1 syndrome. *Am. J. Surg. Pathol.* 2006;30:560–574.

16. Akerstrom G, Hessman O, Hellman P, Skogseid B. Pancreatic tumours as part of the MEN-1 syndrome. *Best Pract. Res. Clin. Gastroenterol.* 2005;19:819–830.

17. Thomas-Marques L, Murat A, Delemer B, et al. Prospective endzscopic ultrasonographic evaluation of the frequency of nonfunc-tioning pancraeticoduodenal endocrine tumors in patients with multiple endocrine neoplasia type 1. *Am. J. Gastroenterol.* 2006;101:266–273.

18. Hellman P, Hennings J, Akerstrom G, Skogseid B. Endoscopic ultrasonography for evaluation of pancreatic tumours in multiple endocrine neoplasia type 1. *Br. J. Surg.* 2005;92:1508–1512.

19. Triponez F, Goudet P, Dosseh D, et al. Is surgery beneficial for MEN1 patients with small (</=2 cm), nonfunctioning pancreaticoduodenal endocrine tumors? *World J. Surg.* 2006;30:654–662.

20. Bartsch DK, Fendrich V, Langer P, Celik I, Kann PH, Rothmund M. Outcome of duodenopancreatic resections in patients with multiple endocrine neoplasia type 1. *Ann. Surg.* 2005;242:757–764, discussion 764–766.

21. Viola KV, Sosa JA. Current advances in the diagnosis and treatment of pancreatic endocrine tumors. *Curr. Opin. Oncol.* 2005;17:24–27.

22. Hoffmann KM, Gibril F, Entsuah LK, Serrano J, Jensen RT. Patients with multiple endocrine neoplasia type 1 with gastrinomas have an increased risk of severe esophageal disease including stricture and the premalignant condition, Barrett's esophagus. *J. Clin. Endocrinol. Metab.* 2006;91:204–212.

23. Imamura M, KomotoI, Ota S. Changing treatment strategy for gastrinoma in patients with ZES. *World J. Surg.* 2006;30:1–11.

24. Tomassetti P, Campana D, Piscitelli L, et al. Treatment of Zollinger–Ellison syndrome. *World J. Gastroenterol.* 2005;21:5423–5432.

25. Tonelli F, Fratini G, Falchetti A, Nesi G, Brandi ML. Surgery for gastroenteropancreatic tumours in multiple endocrine neoplasia type 1: review and personal experience. *J. Intern. Med.* 2005;257:38–49.

26. Rix M, Hertel NT, Nielsen FC, et al. Cushing's disease in childhood as the first manifestation of multiple endocrine neoplasia syndrome type 1. *Eur. J. Endocr.* 2004;151:709–715.

27. Ciccarelli A, Daly AF, Beckers A. The epidemiology of prolactinomas. *Pituitary* 2005;8:3–6.

28. Hao W, Skarulis MC, Simonds WF, et al. Multiple endocrine neoplasia type 1 variant with frequent prolactinoma and rare gastrinoma. *J. Clin. Endocrinol. Metab.* 2004;89:3776–3784.

29. Benito M, Asa SL, Livolsi VA, West VA, Snyder PJ. Gonadotroph tumor associated with multiple endocrine neoplasia type 1. *J. Clin. Endocrinol. Metab.* 2005;90:570–574.

30. Lim LC, Tan MH, Eng C, Teh BT, Rajasoorya RC. Thymic carcinoid in multiple endocrine neoplasia 1: genotype-phenotype correlation and prevention. *J. Intern. Med.* 2006;259:428–432.

31. Ferolla P, Falchetti A, Filosso P, et al. Thymic neuroendocrine carcinoma (carcinoid) in multiple endocrine neoplasia type 1 syndrome: the Italian series. *J. Clin. Endocrinol. Metab.* 2005;90:2603–2609.

32. Takagi J, Otake K, Morishita M, et al. Multiple endocrine neoplasia type I and Cushing's syndrome due to an aggressive ACTH producing thymic carcinoid. *Intern. Med.* 2006; 45:81–86.

33. Sachithanandan N, Harle RA, Burgess JR. Bronchopulmonary carcinoid in multiple endocrine neoplasia type 1. *Cancer* 2005;103:509–515.

34. Norton JA, Melcher ML, Gibril F, Jensen RT. Gastric carcinoid tumors in multiple endocrine neoplasia-1 patients with Zollinger–Ellison syndrome can be symptomatic, demonstrate aggressive growth, and require surgical treatment. *Surgery* 2004;136:1267–1274.

35. Stratakis CA, Schussheim DH, Freedman SM, et al. Pituitary macroadenoma in a 5-year-old: an early expression of multiple endocrine neoplasia type 1. *J. Clin. Endocrinol. Metab.* 2000;85:4776–4780.

69 Medullary Thyroid Carcinoma and Associated Multiple Endocrine Neoplasia Type 2

Clive S. Grant

Key points
- Medullary thyroid carcinoma most commonly presents as a sporadic malignancy. Approximately 20–25% of MTC patients occur as autosomal dominant hereditary disease:
  Multiple endocrine neoplasia 2A
  Multiple endocrine neoplasia 2B
  Familial medullary thyroid carcinoma.
- Medullary thyroid carcinoma represents one of the prototypically successful examples of translational research:
  The most sensitive and specific tumor marker (calcitonin)
  Hereditary forms can be diagnosed by direct genetic testing
  Genetic testing permits prophylactic surgery to avoid predictable development of cancer
  Genetic–phenotypic linkage in disease prognosis.
- Disease treatment requires consideration of other potential tumors and abnormalities:
  Hyperparathyroidism
  Pheochromocytomas (bilateral)
  Marfanoid habitus
  Ganglioneuromatosis.
- New disease treatments are likely to evolve from genomic profiling of medullary thyriod carcinoma. Gene expression and peptide growth factors that modulate signaling pathways that control cell proliferation, angiogenesis, metastatic spread and apoptosis can be targeted for therapeutic intervention.

Introduction

Despite its rarity, comprising only approximately 5% of thyroid carcinomas, medullary thyroid carcinoma (MTC) has been the focus of intense interest and landmark scientific advances. The impressive sequence of discoveries over the last half century related to MTC is chronicled in Table 69.1. Whereas MTC is seldom cured when it has progressed beyond the confines of the thyroid gland, in striking contrast, disease detection has progressed in MTC to the point where direct genetic screening of a patient's DNA from a blood sample can provide absolute, unambiguous confirmation that the disease will develop, yet it can be prevented by prophylactic thyroidectomy.

MTC, derived from parafollicular or C-cells (neural crest in origin) that produce calcitonin, was first described by Hazard et al. in 1959 [1] and characterized as a solid non-follicular histologic

pattern with amyloid in the stroma. They recognized that despite the undifferentiated histologic pattern, the clinical behavior was intermediate between the low-grade papillary thyroid cancer and the highly malignant anaplastic cancer.

Clinical presentation

Sporadic MTC is non-hereditary, comprises 20–25% of the disease overall, typically is unifocal, and is most commonly encountered in the fifth to sixth decade. Patients most commonly present with a thyroid nodule, or cervical lymphadenopathy which is clinically apparent in up to 50% of patients. Local tumor invasion may become manifest with hoarseness or dysphagia, and distant metastases may be detected in 20% of sporadic MTC patients. Very rarely symptoms of hormonal excess herald the disease such as diarrhea or flushing which are complications of high levels of calcitonin, or Cushing syndrome that can develop from ectopic adrenocorticotropic hormone (ACTH) production when the disease is metastatic.

Hereditary MTC is composed of three forms: multiple endocrine neoplasia (MEN) 2A, MEN 2B, and familial medullary

---

Clinical Endocrine Oncology, 2nd edition. Edited by Ian D. Hay and John A.H. Wass. © 2008 Blackwell Publishing. ISBN 978-1-4051-4584-8.

Table 69.1 History of medullary thyroid cancer

1959	Medullary thyroid cancer first described [1]
1961	Sipple described syndrome of MTC, pheochromocytoma [16]
1962	Calcitonin noted to be secreted by parafollicular cells, called C-cells [17]
1965	Characterization of multiple endocrine neoplasia (MEN 2): MTC, pheochromocytoma, and hyperparathyroidism
1966	MTC originated from parafollicular cells
1968	MTC defined as the reason for excessive calcitonin production
1968	MEN 2B described: MCT, pheochromocytoma, marfanoid habitus, and ganglioneuroma phenotype [18]
1973	C-cell hyperplasia (CCH) defined as the precursor of MTC in familial disease, labeled as "preneoplastic" or "*in situ* cancer"
1977	Calcium and pentagastrin stimulation of calcitonin utilized for diagnostic testing when basal calcitonin normal
1986	Familial medullary thyroid carcinoma (FMTC) without associated endocrinopathies described
1987	MEN 2A locus on chromosome 10 identified by linkage analysis
1993	Germline mutations in the RET proto-oncogene located in the proximal region of the long arm of chromosome 10 are responsible for MEN 2A [19, 20]
1994	Germline mutation in RET responsible for MEN 2B and FMTC
1994	Prophylactic thyroidectomy prevents development of MTC for asymptomatic, gene carriers of hereditary disease, even before elevation of calcitonin
1995	Youngest patients with invasive MEN 2A: 2.7 years; MEN 2B: 7 months
1995	RET mutations associated with sporadic MTC
1996	Gene mutations in MEN 2A and 2B and FMTC convert RET into a dominant transforming gene with oncogenic activity [20]

thyroid carcinoma (FMTC). The germline RET (*re*arranged dur*ing* *t*ransfection) proto-oncogene is responsible for all three forms, and the MTC component has virtually 100% penetrance, but variable expressivity which correlates with the exact codon mutation in the gene. Approximately 20–25% of MTC is hereditary, autosomal dominant, and the pathology is typically multifocal and bilateral in the thyroid gland.

MEN 2A

In MEN 2A carriers, pheochromocytomas develop in 30–50%, and hyperparathyroidism in 10–30%. Adrenomedullary disease is usually bilateral (but pheochromocytomas may present metachronously), multicentric, detected after the onset of MTC, are very rarely malignant or extra-adrenal, and must be screened for and treated before the MTC. Clinical symptoms are variable, but follow the usual pattern of headache, palpitations, marked sweating, and anxiety. Hypertension may not be prominent feature, so screening is crucial.

Hyperparathyroidism in MEN 2A is less serious with fewer complications than sporadic or MEN 1. As such, in contrast to MEN 1 patients, we usually resect only enlarged glands, but have commonly needed to autotransplant normal glands in the course of the total thyroidectomy for MTC.

MEN 2B

Patients with MEN 2B suffer the most aggressive form of MTC and have characteristic phenotypic abnormalities: large lips, mucosal neuromas of lips and tongue, thickened corneal nerves, ganglioneuromas of the gastrointestinal tract, as well as pheochromocytomas. They also have a connective tissue abnormality with excessive growth of the long bones, ribs, and skull that gives them a distinctive marfanoid appearance with long thin extremities and fingers. They often have marked morbidity from their gastrointestinal dysmotility including constipation, diarrhea, abdominal pain, and megacolon. The principal causes of death in MEN 2B patients are MTC and pheochromocytoma, often occurring in their second or third decade of life.

FMTC

Patients with FMTC, by definition, do not have hyperparathyroidism, pheochromocytomas, or any of the phenotypic abnormalities of MEN 2B patients. The MTC is the most indolent of all forms, depending on the specific genetic codon abnormality. Strict guidelines now must be fulfilled to be categorized as FMTC: (1) more than 10 carriers in the kindred, (2) multiple carriers or affected members over the age of 50 years, and (3) an adequate medical history. The specific intent is not to miss a small kindred of MEN 2A patients, presumed to have FMTC but the potentially lethal pheochromocytoma has been overlooked.

Genetics

MEN 2A and 2B and FMTC are caused by germline missense activating mutations in the RET proto-oncogene, located in the proximal region of the long arm of chromosome 10, band q11.2. Mutations in the RET proto-oncogene convert it into a dominant transforming gene with oncogenic activity. It encodes a RET protein receptor tyrosine kinase that includes a cysteine-rich extracellular ligand-binding domain, a transmembrane domain, and an intracellular tyrosine kinase catalytic portion. Approximately 98% of patients with hereditary MTC can now be detected by genetic testing. The sites of mutation are listed in Table 69.2 [2] and gene mutations of MEN 1 and MEN 2 are compared in Table 69.3.

Codon 634 mutations are the most common (at least 50–60%) in MEN 2A, exhibiting a statistically significant association (TGC to CGC) with the presence of pheochromocytoma and hyperparathyroidism. Mutation at codon 918 (ATG to ACG) is responsible for >95% of MEN 2B. Interestingly, somatic mutations of codon 918 have been found in approximately 25% of sporadic MTC [3].

It is clear that not only should patients who have MTC be genetically tested for the presence of hereditary MTC, but relatives who are at risk for inheriting the disease should also undergo DNA testing. This has provided the opportunity to proceed with prophylactic thyroidectomy in gene-positive patients prior to the development even of CCH or the presence of abnormal calcitonin levels. This approach has been successful in preventing the occurrence of MTC in children with RET mutations [4].

Whereas many authors suggest screening for the RET protooncogene by age 5–6 in MEN 2A patients, we have advocated screening during infancy and proceeding to thyroidectomy by age 2. We also

Table 69.2 Specific codon abnormalities in the RET proto-oncogene in MTC

Phenotype	Codon	Phenotype	Codon
Sporadic	768	MEN 2B	883
	918		918*
MEN 2A	609	FMTC	609
	611		611
	618		618
	620		620
	630		630
	634*		634
	666		768
	790		790
	V804L		791
			V804M

*Most common mutations.

Table 69.3 Comparison of the abnormal genes in MEN 1 and MEN 2 syndromes

Category	MEN 1	MEN 2
Gene	*Menin*	*RET*
Location	11q13	Pericentromeric 10
Type of gene	Tumor suppressor	Proto-oncogene
Result of gene mutation	Parathyroid tumor: 95%	Hyperplasia → cancer
Genetic testing?	Sometimes	Standard of care

advise testing for MEN 2B during infancy and proceed surgically within the first year of life. These recommendations are based on the fact that we have cared for children with MEN 2A and 2B with invasive MTC at age 2.7 and 0.7 years respectively.

Diagnosis of MTC

The diagnosis of MTC can be made on the basis of fine needle cytology (FNA), serum calcitonin, or direct genetic testing, depending heavily on the circumstances of the patient. Because the large majority of MTC is sporadic, FNA of a thyroid nodule or metastatic cervical lymph node – the most common presentations of sporadic MTC – is the most common method of diagnosis. The cytologic appearance is characterized by spindle cells, an amorphous amyloid substance that stains with Congo red, and is positive on immunohistochemistry (IHC) staining for calcitonin. The serum calcitonin level is virtually always elevated (greater than 7 ng/L) in patients with clinical MTC. False-positive elevations of calcitonin have led to thyroidectomy, so the preferred methods of testing are cytologic or genetic. The actual levels of calcitonin roughly correlate with the amount of tumor burden, and the doubling time of the calcitonin may be more important for prognosis than the actual value. In some patients, a calcium stimulation test may be indicated for diagnosis (2 mg/kg body weight, intravenously over 1 min). As noted in the previous section, direct genetic testing for abnormal codon changes in the *RET* proto-oncogene is now readily available, accurate, and represents the standard of care in hereditary MTC.

Although some studies have suggested obtaining basal calcitonin levels on all patients with thyroid nodules as a screen to identify patients with MTC at an earlier pathologic stage, we have not embraced this practice because of the significant cost ramifications and the reported problems with false-positive tests.

Carcinoembryonic antigen (CEA) is also a useful tumor marker that is not specific for MTC, but the degree of elevated level correlates with MTC tumor volume and aggressiveness. It is often obtained in combination with serum calcitonin in the follow-up of patients with MTC.

Pathology

MTC develops from C-cells (derived from the neural crest), located predominantly in the junction of the upper and middle thirds of the thyroid lobes. In sporadic MTC, the disease is less commonly multicentric whereas in MEN 2 syndrome, this reaches virtually 100% when gross disease is present. Macroscopically, MTC is solid, white, unencapsulated and gritty. Histologically, the cells have a spindle appearance, and an amyloid-like substance can be identified that stains similar to amyloid, but is actually a prohormone for calcitonin, a polypeptide hormone secreted by the C-cells [5].

C-cell hyperplasia (CCH) comprises multicentric clusters of C cells within the thyroid parenchyma. CCH is the premalignant lesion that precedes the development of hereditary MTC. How-ever, it is not pathognomonic of MTC as 20–30% of the general population has C-cell hyperplasia. When only CCH and not frank MTC is present, calcitonin elevation is detected only with calcium stimulation.

Both lymphatic and hematogenous dissemination as well as aggressive direct local invasion may occur with MTC. The frequency of lymph node metastases correlates with the primary tumor size: tumors ≤1 cm, 20–30%; tumors from 1–4 cm, 50%; and tumors >4 cm, up to 90%. These lymph node metastases occur first in the central compartment (level VI: in the thyroid beds, tracheoesophageal grooves, pretracheal, supraisthmic nodes), then may extend into the lateral jugular nodes (levels II–V) and the upper mediastinal lymph nodes (level VII). The current AJCC staging system reflects the serious prognostic implications of level II–V or VII lymph node metastases (see below). Distant metastases occur most frequently to liver, bone and lung, and are usually diffuse and affect multiple organs. Liver metastases are often small, thin lesions on the liver surface that are easily missed by most imaging techniques, and may require direct visualization with laparoscopy.

Prognostic factors

The overall survival of patients with MTC is 86% at 5 years and 65% at 10 years, but individual patient survival is markedly influenced by several prognostic factors. Whereas some patients,

Staging (TNM – AJCC, 2002)

Tumor (T)

- T1: Tumor ≤2 cm in greatest dimension, limited to the thyroid

- T2: Tumor >2 cm but ≤4 cm in greatest dimension, limited to the thyroid

- T3: Tumor >4 cm in greatest dimension limited to the thyroid or any tumor with minimal extrathyroid extension (e.g., extension to sternothyroid muscle or perithyroid soft tissues)

- T4a: Tumor of any size extending beyond the thyroid capsule to invade subcutaneous soft tissues, larynx, trachea, esophagus, or recurrent laryngeal nerve

- T4b: Tumor invades prevertebral fascia or encases carotid artery or mediastinal vessels

Nodes (N)

- N0: No regional lymph node metastasis

- N1: Regional lymph node metastasis

- N1a: Metastasis to level VI (pretracheal, paratracheal, and prelaryngeal/Delphian lymph nodes)

- N1b: Metastasis to unilateral or bilateral cervical or superior mediastinal lymph nodes

Distant metastases (M)

- M0: No distant metastasis

- M1: Distant metastasis

Staging

- Stage I
  - T1, N0, M0
- Stage II
  - T2, N0, M0
- Stage III
  - T3, N0, M0
  - T1, N1a, M0
  - T2, N1a, M0
  - T3, N1a, M0
- Stage IVA
  - T4a, N0, M0
  - T4a, N1a, M0
  - T1, N1b, M0
  - T2, N1b, M0
  - T3, N1b, M0
  - T4a, N1b, M0
- Stage IVB
  - T4b, any N, M0
- Stage IVC
  - Any T, any N, M1

Used with the permission of the American Joint Committee on Cancer (AJCC), Chicago, Illinois. The original source for this material is the AJCC Cancer Staging Manual, Sixth Edition (2002) published by Springer-Verlag New York, www.springer-ny.com/

even with distant metastases or significant elevation of calcitonin levels, enjoy prolonged survival, others die within a few years of diagnosis. Most authors would sequence the severity of MTC from most favorable to most aggressive as FMTC, MEN 2A, sporadic, and MEN 2B. Other unfavorable risk factors include older age, elevated calcitonin and CEA levels, extrathyroid invasion, regional metastatic nodes or distant metastases, or inability to achieve complete gross resection.

In hereditary MTC the specific mutated codon of *RET* correlates with both the familial variant and the aggressiveness of MTC [6, 7]. On the basis of the reported age of onset of the disease and its aggressiveness, recommendations were generated regarding the optimal age for thyroidectomy.

Level 1 – least high risk

- *RET* codons 609, 768, 790, 791, 804, 891
- Usually grows more slowly, develops at later age
- Can have nodal metastasis, be fatal (except 790, 791)
- Total thyroidectomy by age 5–10

Level 2 – high risk of MTC

- *RET* codons 611, 618, 620, 634
- Total thyroidectomy ± central node dissection by age 5

Level 3 – highest risk, aggressive MTC

- *RET* codons 883, 918, 922
- Thyroidectomy within 1–6 months of life
- Metastasis during first year of life documented

Yip et al. [8] at the MD Anderson Cancer Center have characterized their series of hereditary MTC patients according to the above classification:

Level 1 – 15 patients

- Stages 0–II: 8 (53%)
- Stages III–IV: 3 (20%); unknown stage: IV
- Recurrent disease: 4 (33%)
- Persistent disease: 9 (60%)

Level 2, 53 patients

- Stages 0–II: 22 (42%)
- Stages III–IV: 16 (30%)
- Recurrence: 9 (20%)
- Persistent disease: 37 (70%)

Level 3, 10 patients

- Stages 0–II: 1 (10%)
- Stages III–IV: 5 (50%)
- Recurrence: 4 (44%)
- Persistent disease: 10 (100%)

Treatment

Preoperative management

Once a diagnosis of MTC has been established or genetic confirmation of familial MTC has been confirmed, the next phase is treatment which is predominantly surgical. We have found a preoperative management checklist helpful.

- FNA thyroid nodule, lateral jugular node (± IHC)
- Serum calcitonin, CEA
- 24-hour urine: metanephrines, catecholamines
- Computerized tomography (CT) neck, chest, abdomen if advanced disease
- Obtain blood sample for RET proto-oncogene
- Neck ultrasound (US) to screen for metastatic jugular lymph nodes

Recognizing the high frequency of metastatically involved lateral jugular lymph nodes and the recommendation by others to *routinely* proceed with full modified radical neck dissection, we prefer to screen for metastatically involved jugular lymph nodes utilizing high-resolution ultrasound. Ultrasonography is also utilized as a routine part of follow-up of MTC patients.

Surgical considerations

The primary operative procedure should be appropriate for the type and stage of MTC, which can be subdivided into sporadic and hereditary disease, and for the latter, further subdivided into clinically apparent as opposed to genetically or biochemically detected. Also to be considered with the operative procedure is the management of the parathyroid glands. For palpable MTC, some surgeons have routinely excised and then autotransplanted all four parathyroid glands. We prefer to excise any abnormal parathyroid glands but save those that are normal and can be preserved with their blood supply. Normal parathyroid glands that cannot be saved *in situ* are autotransplanted.

Patient outcome in MTC as in many cancers is influenced by four factors: biology of the disease, stage of the disease, adequacy of operative treatment, and efficacy of other adjuvant treatments. Chemotherapy is largely ineffective in this disease, and radiation treatment is limited to palliation. The biology of the disease is unalterable clinically at present. Disease stage has been dramatically affected by the introduction and now widespread utilization of DNA genetic testing. This has provided a unique opportunity to cure or even prevent cancer in many of these patients. Unfortunately, this benefits only a small minority of MTC patients. Because 70–80% of MTC encountered in most centers is sporadic, the only variable that can be altered is the adequacy of the surgical procedure. Sporadic MTC is often accompanied by metastatic regional lymph nodes. Therefore, considerable recent literature has focused on the indication and extent of lymph node dissections in conjunction with total thyroidectomy.

The extent and indications for lymph node dissection are still the subject of debate. Virtually all surgeons agree that usually the sternocleidomastoid muscle (SCM), jugular vein, and spinal accessory nerve (modified radical neck dissection) should be preserved.

The definition of lymph node compartments can be summarized as follows.
- Central neck: thyroid cartilage superiorly, innominate artery inferiorly, carotid arteries laterally including pretracheal and tracheoesophageal groove nodes.
- Lateral neck: clavicle inferiorly, lateral border of SCM and cervical plexus laterally, digastric muscle superiorly, jugular vein medially.
- Mediastinum: below innominate vein requiring sternal split.

Surgical treatment

RET positive with normal calcitonin level
Total thyroidectomy.

Sporadic or hereditary MTC with elevated calcitonin level
The surgical treatment that is universally accepted includes:
- total thyroidectomy
- central neck node dissection
- modified radical neck dissection (lateral neck) for positive lateral nodes.

Debate centers on whether to undertake lateral neck and mediastinal lymph node dissections based on *probability* of positive nodes rather than definitive evidence. Dralle [9] favors a very aggressive approach, routinely dissecting both lateral compartments if any nodes are positive in the central neck, and adding a sternal split for mediastinal dissection if ≥3 nodes are positive in the central neck or for positive nodes low in the central neck near the sternum. However, interestingly, he recently stated, "Once lymphatic dissemination has occurred, biochemical cure, as defined by a postoperative normalization of serum calcitonin, may be beyond reach despite radical surgery on the neck and mediastinum."

There are a number of considerations that may impact the decision regarding lymph node dissection.
- No treatment other than surgery is as yet proven effective.
- Approximately 50–80% of non-screen detected MTC patients have metastatically involved nodes at diagnosis.
- Serum calcitonin is an extremely sensitive marker of MTC, and even microscopic disease will cause elevated values.
- In a group of patients who had persistently elevated calcitonin levels but with negative results of localization, the 10-year survival exceeded 85% [10].
- Only 3% (1/31) of patients with metastatic lymph nodes had a normal postoperative calcitonin level, yet 50% had 10-year survival at the Memorial Sloan-Kettering Cancer Center.
- No patient with metastatic mediastinal nodes below the innominate vein has been returned to a normal calcitonin level in Dralle's, Moley's or Tissel's experience.
- If extrathyroidal invasion of MTC (pT3) is present, the calcitonin was not returned to normal.
- Most reports suggest that when metastasis are limited to only a few nodes at the original operation, at most 20–33% may have an initial return to normal of their calcitonin level with node dissection.

Lymph node dissection conclusions

• Central neck node dissection should be performed routinely with the exception of early, screen-detected patients.
• Lateral neck dissection will often, but not always, yield positive nodes in patients with positive central neck nodes, palpable primary tumors, or tumors with extrathyroid extension. However, seldom will the calcitonin be returned to normal.
• Long-term survival is common in patients who have elevated calcitonin levels but no detectable disease by imaging studies: US, CT, magnetic resonance imaging (MRI), or positron emission tomography (PET) scan.
• Therefore, our thresholds for dissecting the lateral jugular neck nodes are usually palpable nodes, or suspicious nodes by US or other imaging technique.

Reoperation for MTC

Aggressive reoperation, including extensive neck dissections utilizing microdissection techniques, has been advocated for persistent or recurrent MTC limited to the neck and mediastinum. Following the original description by Tisell [11], Moley [12] has reported the following results in 115 patients.

• 62 (54%) were operative candidates, but 10 had liver metastases (detected by laparoscopy).
• Of 52 resulting patients: 45 underwent curative operation; 7 were palliative.
• 17 (38% of curative intent group; 15% of original patient group) had normal calcitonin level postoperatively.
• 15 (13%) maintained normal calcitonin with short follow-up.

Clark from the University of San Francisco reported on a similar group of 33 patients [13]:

• 2 (6%) achieved a normal calcitonin with reoperation (3 positive nodes in each pt).
• 21 (64%) had <50% decrease in calcitonin level.

The Mayo Clinic approach is:
• aggressive preoperative imaging search for occult persistent/recurrent disease
  • ultrasound of neck
  • PET scan
• CT ± MRI of chest, abdomen.
• *Directed* operative dissection of disease in neck and sometimes in the mediastinum.

External beam radiation; chemotherapy

External beam radiotherapy has been effective in MTC in eradicating small residual disease. However, there is no evidence that it provides survival advantage. It is of value in patients with painful bone metastases. Radioactive iodine has no place in the treatment of patients with MTC. Chemotherapy has been disappointing. A few reports of tumor response have been recorded, but its use, outside of clinical trials, is generally reserved for late, symptomatic disease. Somatostatin analogs have produced inconstant and transient effects when used to palliate hormone-mediated diarrhea. They have not yielded any tumor regression.

Mayo Clinic experience

From 1980 through 2000, 107 patients underwent primary surgical management for resectable medullary thyroid carcinoma (Tables 69.4–69.7). The mean age was 43 years, reflecting the predominance of sporadic disease, whereas the range from 2 to 85 years indicates early age screening for genetically transmitted disease. The gender distribution was nearly equal and the type of disease was only about 50% sporadic, biased by the referral practice. The change in the AJCC staging criteria from the fifth to the sixth edition in 2002 is characterized in Table 69.5. Most notable are the shifts of patients from stage II to stage I, and particularly stage III to stage IV patients, reflecting the stage IV classification of patients with metastatically involved jugular venous nodes. Although about one-third of patients with sporadic disease died from it, and another one-third are living with disease, there is a wide span of survival with a mean of 6 years, ranging from less than a year to 18 years. These are typically extensive operations, as indicated by the intentional sacrifice of the recurrent laryngeal nerve (RLN) in six patients, as well as the need for central and lateral jugular neck dissections. Nevertheless, only a single patient suffered an unintentional RLN paralysis, and <5% had hypoparathyroidism.

Table 69.4 Mayo Clinic series MTC, 1980–2000

Age: mean, range (years)	43; 2–85
Gender: male/female	57/50
Type of disease	
Sporadic	54
MEN 2A	28
MEN 2B	4
FMTC	21
Clinical presentation	
Screening, MEN 2A	24
Screening, FMTC	17
Palpable thyroid and metastatic nodes	5
Palpable metastatic nodes	14
Other	14
Tumor size: mean, range (cm)	1.4; 0.1–7
Surgical complications	
RLN paralysis, unintentional/intentional	1/6
Hypoparathyroidism	1

RLN, recurrent laryngeal nerve.

Table 69.5 TNM staging, Mayo Clinic series, 1980–2000

	Pre 2002 stage (AJCC 5th edn)		Stage, AJCC 6th edn	
	Patients, *n*	%	Patients, *n*	%
I	30	28%	45	42%
II	23	21%	8	7%
III	49	46%	20	19%
IV	5	5%	34	32%
Total	107	100%	107	100%

Table 69.6 Disease status, Mayo Clinic series

Disease status Number of patients	Stages I–IV 107	Sporadic 54	MEN 2A 28	MEN 2B 4	FMTC 21
Dead of disease, *n* (%) F/U mean (range), years	18 (17)	16 (30) 6.5 (0.7–18)	1 (4) 10	1 (25)	0 (0)
Alive, NED, *n* (%)	49 (46)	16 (30)	18 (64)	1 (25)	14 (67)
Alive with disease *n* (%) F/U mean (range), years	34 (32)	18 (33)	8 (29) 12 (6–23)	2 (50)	6 (29) 8 (4–13.5)
Dead, NED	4 (2)	3 (5)	0 (0)	0 (0)	1 (5)
Dead with disease F/U, years	2 (2)	1 (2)	1 (4) 21	0 (0)	0 (0)

F/U, follow-up; NED, no evidence of disease.

Table 69.7 Survival by stage, Mayo Clinic series

Disease status Number of patients	Stage I 45	Stage II 8	Stage III 20	Stage IV 34
Dead of disease *n* (%)	0 (0)	1 (13)	3 (15)	14 (41)
Alive, NED *n* (%)	39 (87)	2 (25)	7 (35)	1 (3)
Alive with disease *n* (%)	3 (7)	4 (50)	8 (40)	19 (56)
Dead, NED *n* (%)	3 (7)	0 (0)	1 (5)	0 (0)
Dead with disease *n* (%)	0 (0)	1 (12)	1 (5)	0 (0)

NED, no evidence of disease.

New treatment possibilities

A large proportion of patients with non-screen detected MTC will have metastatic disease to lymph nodes or distant sites and are quite likely incurable, at least by the criteria of normalizing postoperative calcitonin levels. Current adjuvant treatment is almost always futile. *RET* encodes for the RET receptor tyrosine kinase, which transduces signals for cell growth and differentiation. Protein kinases are involved in transmitting intracellular signals that are involved in multiple processes of cancer cells including growth, survival, motility, invasion and metastasis. Targeting the enzymatic activity of tyrosine kinases by small molecule inhibitors is a promising strategy in human cancer therapy. One of the most successful such agents is imatinib mesylate (Gleevec) for diseases carrying c-Kit point mutations such as gastrointestinal stromal tumors. A compound, ZD6474 (Zactima™), was shown to inhibit thyroid carcinoma cell lines and it also has an inhibitory effect on angiogenesis. In a single-arm Phase II study of 14 patients with metastatic hereditary MTC, two partial responses and nine patients with stable disease were observed [14]. A different tyrosine kinase inhibitor CEP-751 given in combination with irinotecan, a topoisomerase I poison [15], showed a 100% clinical response in xenografts (nude mice) inoculated with human MTC cell line. It is now in Phase II clinical trial for advanced MTC.

References

1. Hazard J, Hawk W, Crile GJ. Medullary (solid) carcinoma of the thyroid; a clinicopathologic entity. *J. Clin. Endocrinol. Metab.* 1959;19:152–161.
2. Gagel R. Molecular abnormalities in thyroid carcinoma. In *Thyroid Cancer and Hyperparathyroidism*. Boston, MA: 2001.
3. Gagel R. Putting the bits and pieces of the RET proto-oncogene puzzle together. *Bone* 1995;17:13S–16S.
4. Wells SJ, Chi D, Toshima K. Predictive DNA testing and prophylactic thyroidectomy in patients at risk for multiple endocrine neoplasia type 2A. *Ann. Surg.* 1994;220:237–247.
5. Wells SJ, Franz C. Medullary carcinoma of the thyroid gland. *World J. Surg.* 2000;24:952–956.
6. Brandi M, Gagel R, Angeli A, et al. Consensus: guidelines for diagnosis and therapy of MEN type 1 and type 2. *J. Clin. Endocrinol. Metab.* 2001;86:5658–5671.
7. Yip L, Cote G, Shapiro S, et al. Multiple Endocrine Neoplasia type 2: evaluation of the genotype-phenotype relationship. *Arch. Surg.* 2003;138:409–416.
8. Yip L, Lee J, Shapiro S, et al. Surgical management of hereditary pheochromocytoma. *J. Am. Coll. Surg.* 2004;198:525–535.
9. Machens A, Gimm O, Hinze R, et al. Genotype–phenotype correlations in hereditary medullary thyroid carcinoma: oncological features and biochemical properties. *J. Clin. Endocrinol. Metab.* 2001;86:1104–1109.
10. van Heerden JA, Grant CS, Gharib H, Hay ID, Ilstrup DM. Long-term course of patients with persistent hypercalcitoninemia after apparent curative primary surgery for medullary thyroid carcinoma. *Ann. Surg.* 1990;212:395–401.
11. Tisell L-E, Hansson G, Hansson S. Reoperation in the treatment of asymptomatic metastasizing medullary thyroid carcinoma. *Surgery* 1986;99:60–66.
12. Moley JF, Dilley WG, DeBenedetti MK. Improved results of cervical reoperation for medullary thyroid carcinoma. *Ann. Surg.* 1997;225:734–743.

13. Kebebew E, Kikuchi S, Duh Q-Y, Clark O. Long-term results of reoperation and localizing studies in patients with persistent or recurrent medullary thyroid cancer. *Arch. Surg.* 2000;135:895–901.

14. Wells S, You Y, Lakhani V, et al. The use of ZACTIMA(TM) (ZD6474) in the treatment of patients with hereditary medullary thyroid carcinoma: AACR-NCI-EORTC; 2005. Report No.: B248.

15. Strock C, Park J-I, Rosen D, et al. Activity of irinotecan and the tyrosine kinase inhibitor CEP-751 in medullary thyroid cancer. *J. Clin. Endocrinol. Metab.* 2006;91:79–84.

16. Sipple J. The association of pheochromocytoma with carcinoma of the thyroid gland. *Am. J. Med.* 1961;31:163–166.

17. Copp D, Cameron E, Cheney B. Evidence for calcitonin – a new hormone from the parathyroid that lowers blood calcium. *Endocrinology* 1962;70:638–649.

18. Schimke R, Hartmann W, Prout T, Rimoin D. Syndrome of bilateral pheochromocytoma, medullary thyroid carcinoma and multiple neuromas: a possible regulatory defect in the differentiation of chromaffin tissue. *N. Engl. J. Med.* 1968;279:1–7.

19. Mulligan L, Kwok J, Healey C, et al. Germline mutations of the RET proto-oncogene in multiple endocrine neoplasia type 2A. *Nature* 1993;363:458–460.

20. Donis-Keller H, Dou S, Chi D, et al. Mutations in the *ret* proto-oncogene are associated with MEN 2A and FMTC. *Hum. Mol. Genet.* 1993;7:851–856.

21. Santoro M, Carlogmagno F, Romano A, et al. Activation of RET as a dominant transforming gene by germline mutations of MEN 2A and MEN 2B. *Science* 1995;267:381–383.

70 von Hippel–Lindau Disease

Shern L. Chew and Eamonn R. Maher

Key points
- von Hippel–Lindau disease is an autosomal dominant familial tumor syndrome.
- The endocrine manifestations are pheochromocytoma and pancreatic cystic disease and islet cell tumors.
- Pheochromocytomas are often bilateral.
- Pancreatic lesions are often asymptomatic.
- Genetic testing and surveillance programs should be offered.

Introduction and background

The most frequent endocrine manifestations associated with von Hippel–Lindau disease (VHL) are pheochromocytomas, pancreatic cystic disease and islet cell tumors. VHL is an autosomal dominant familial tumor syndrome characterized by central nervous system (CNS) and retinal hemangioblastomas, and renal cysts and carcinomas (Table 70.1). von Hippel and others had described the appearance and pathology of the retinal hemangioblastoma by 1911. While studying cerebellar hemangioblastomas, Lindau linked the cerebellar, retinal and visceral components in 1926. The diagnostic criteria of VHL were established by Melmon and Rosen [1]: two or more hemangioblastomas; or one hemangioblastoma and a visceral manifestation; or one hemangioblastoma or visceral lesion and a family history of hemangioblastoma, but a diagnosis of VHL may also be made by molecular genetic analysis in patients who do not satisfy conventional clinical criteria.

Molecular pathogenesis

Linkage of VHL to chromosome 3p25 was reported in 1988 and the VHL tumor suppressor gene was cloned in 1993 (see [2] and references within). The gene behaves similarly to other tumor suppressor genes. Thus, a mutated *VHL* allele is inherited in the germline, and the second allele becomes defective later in the somatic cells. Tumors develop in tissues when both alleles of the gene are inactivated. As predicted by Knudson, sporadic tumors (e.g., clear cell renal cell carcinoma) of the same type as those inherited in VHL sometimes may show abnormalities of the VHL tumor suppressor gene. Germline *VHL* mutations may be detected in the vast majority of patients with VHL disease. Up to 40% of

Table 70.1 Lesions associated with von Hippel–Lindau disease

Major components
  Central nervous system
    Retinal hemangioblastoma
    Cerebellar hemangioblastoma
    Spinal cord hemangioblastoma
    Brain stem hemangioblastoma
  Visceral
    Renal cell carcinoma and cysts
    Pheochromocytoma, paraganglioma
    Pancreatic cysts, serous microcystic adenoma and carcinoma
    Pancreatic islet cell tumors
    Epididymal cystadenoma
Rare lesions
  Central nervous system
    Supratentorial hemangioblastoma
    Endolymphatic sac tumors
  Visceral
    Liver adenoma, hemangioblastoma and cysts
    Lung angioma and cysts
    Splenic angioma

patients have large exonic deletions and most of the remaining mutations are accounted for by small intragenic mutations which result in amino acid substitutions or are predicted to cause truncation of the VHL protein (http://www.umd.be:2020/).

The VHL protein (pVHL) has multiple functions but the best defined is regulation of hypoxia-inducible factors (HIF-1 and HIF-2). HIF-1 and HIF-2 are heterodimeric transcription factors containing α and β subunits that function in conditions of cellular hypoxia. They increase expression of genes involved in angiogenesis and cell proliferation. Under normal oxygen concentrations, the HIF-α subunits are degraded by the proteosome. The degradation is mediated by binding by a pVHL-containing protein complex (Fig. 70.1). The ability of pVHL to bind the HIF-α subunits depends on the hydroxylation status of two key HIF-α proline residues. In

Clinical Endocrine Oncology, 2nd edition. Edited by Ian D. Hay and John A.H. Wass. © 2008 Blackwell Publishing. ISBN 978-1-4051-4584-8.

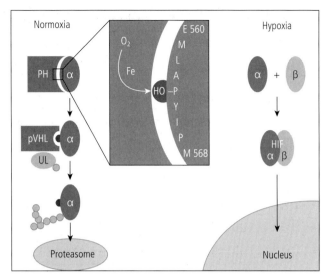

Figure 70.1 A scheme of pVHL and HIF function under conditions of normoxia (left side) and hypoxia (right side). Under normoxia, the hydroxylation to a proline residue on HIF-α allows binding of pVHL (inset box). Under hypoxia, pVHL does not bind and HIF heterodimers are formed. PH, prolyl hydroxylase; UL, ubiquitin ligase. (Redrawn from Zhu and Bunn, Science 2001;292:449, with permission from the AAAS.)

hypoxia, the prolines are not hydroxylated (oxygen is an essential co-factor for the key proline hydroxylating enzymes) and pVHL is unable to bind HIF-α. This leads to stabilization of HIF-1 and HIF-2 with ensuing activation of downstream hypoxia-inducible target genes such as vascular endothelial growth factor [3, 4]. Similarly, mutations that inactivate pVHL cause abnormal HIF stabilization and increased expression of hypoxia response genes – a feature that correlates with the high vascularity of VHL tumors [5]. Most VHL families with pheochromocytoma have missense mutations (particularly protein surface missense mutations), while pheochromocytoma is uncommon with mutations that would be expected to produce a truncated protein or not be associated with protein expression. Although most patients with pheochromocytoma-associated VHL mutations are also at risk of hemangioblastomas and renal cell carcinoma (Type 2B VHL disease), certain mutations (e.g., p.Tyr98His) are associated with a high risk of pheochromocytoma and hemangioblastomas, but a low risk of renal cancer [6]. Furthermore, rare *VHL* mutations can predispose to pheochromocytoma and not hemangioblastomas or renal cell carcinoma (Type 2C mutations). The role of HIF-1 and HIF-2 in the pathogenesis of pheochromocytoma is supported by the finding that pheochromocytomas in patients with germline succinate dehydrogenase (*SDHB* and *SDHD*) mutations demonstrate increased expression of HIF-1, HIF-2 and hypoxia-inducible target genes [7]. However, HIF dysregulation may not be a complete explanation for pheochromocytoma development, as Type 2C (pheochromocytoma only) pVHL mutants retained the ability to regulate HIF-1 appropriately [8, 9]. Other mechanisms include impaired developmental culling of sympathetic neuronal precursor cells in VHL and other familial pheochromocytoma syndromes [10].

Thus, it has been postulated that pheochromocytoma-associated VHL mutations impair (via a HIF-independent mechanism) the normal developmental apoptosis that occurs in response to nerve growth factor withdrawal.

Clinical features

The estimated birth incidence of VHL is 1 in 35 000 [11]. The average age of presentation is about 27 years and practically all patients will have disease manifestations by 65 years of age [12].

Retinal angiomatosis

Over 40% of VHL patients will have retinal hemangioblastomas as the initial manifestation of disease. They are unusual before 10 years of age (<5% occurring at younger ages) but lifetime risk of retinal disease is >70% in most cases. Hemangioblastomas consist predominantly of polygonal stromal cells and capillaries. The lesions are usually situated at the periphery of the retina. The appearance on funduscopy is of a red oval lesion with an associated feeder artery and vein (Fig. 70.2). The lesions may not be seen by funduscopy and, particularly in younger patients, fluorescein angioscopy may be needed. Untreated they tend to grow. The high flow rate of blood through these malformations leads to fluid leakage and exudates. Bleeding may occur, with retinal detachment and scarring as complications. Ultimately, the most serious complication is loss of visual acuity, and the major risk factors for this are large angiomas, presentation at a young age or symptomatic angiomas [13]. Treatment is with laser or cryotherapy, and the treatment of small lesions is more successful than larger tumors.

Cerebellar and other central nervous system hemangioblastomas

About 75% of the hemangioblastomas in VHL occur in the cerebellum; the rest occur in the spinal cord, with rare cases having

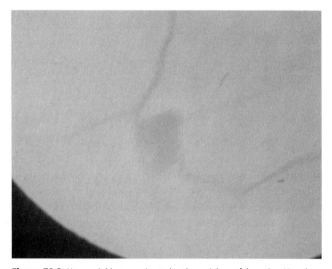

Figure 70.2 Hemangioblastoma situated at the periphery of the retina. Vessels can be seen entering and leaving the lesion.

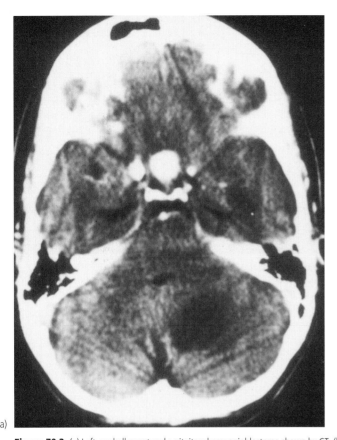

(a)

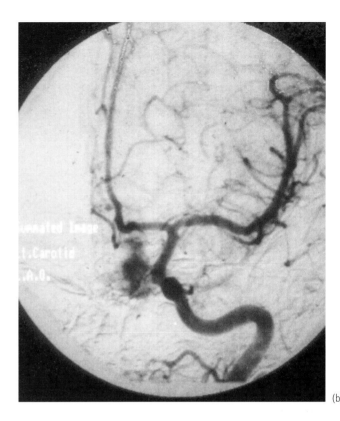

(b)

Figure 70.3 (a) Left cerebellar cyst and a pituitary hemangioblastoma shown by CT. (b) The vascular nature of the pituitary lesion is confirmed by a left carotid angiogram. (Radiographs were kindly provided by Dr C.G.D. Beardwell, Christie Hospital, Manchester, UK.)

supratentorial localizations. Cerebellar hemangioblastomas occur as the first manifestation in about 40% of VHL patients and lifetime risk in most patients is >70%. Cerebellar hemangioblastomas usually presents with symptoms of a mass lesion (morning headaches, vomiting), ataxia and inco-ordination. Magnetic resonance imaging (MRI) may show a solid or cystic lesion (Fig. 70.3). The main treatment is by surgical excision. External beam radiotherapy and Gamma Knife radiosurgery have been used as salvage treatments in patients with recurrent lesions.

Renal cell carcinoma and cysts

Renal cell carcinoma is now the commonest cause of death in VHL patients. The renal carcinomas usually occur at a later age (mean 44 years for symptomatic lesions) than retinal and cerebellar hemangioblastomas. Renal cell carcinomas in VHL tend to be multifocal and occur at an earlier age than in sporadic cases. The probability that a VHL patient will develop a renal cell carcinoma by the age of 60 has been estimated to be 70%. Renal cysts are frequent in VHL patients and renal cell carcinoma can arise within the cyst. Many renal cell carcinomas in VHL patients are diagnosed at a subclinical stage by MRI (or ultrasound) scanning during routine surveillance. Such lesions may be followed until they reach 3 cm diameter and then removed by a nephron-sparing approach [14]. Although there is a low risk of metastatic disease

with such an approach, it minimizes the risks of renal replacement therapy, which arguably carries a poorer prognosis and quality of life.

Pheochromocytoma and other adrenal lesions

Pheochromocytomas occur in approximately 10% of VHL cases, but the prevalence within an affected family can range from 0% to 92%. Bilateral tumors are found in up to 40% of those with pheochromocytomas [15, 16] (Fig. 70.4). Up to 23% of patients presenting with pheochromocytomas had either VHL or multiple endocrine neoplasia when fully investigated [15].

Surveillance programs should detect most pheochromocytomas before patients develop symptoms. Establishing the diagnosis of a pheochromocytoma is complicated by the fact that VHL patients have been reported with a variety of adrenal pathologies including cortical adenomas, hemangioblastomas, and hyperplasia. High-resolution computerized tomography (CT) and ultrasound scanning by a radiologist with an interest in adrenal radiology will detect most lesions. The function and nature of an adrenal lesion are best assessed by a combination of 24-h urinary free catecholamine levels, plasma catecholamines or plasma free normetanephrines (a norepinephrine metabolite), MRI and meta-iodobenzylguanidine (MIBG) isotope scanning. Pheochromocytomas from VHL patients secrete more plasma free

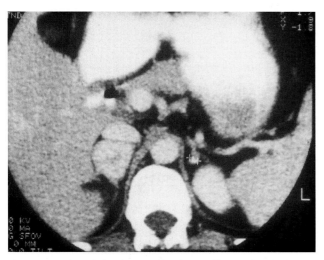

Figure 70.4 Bilateral adrenal tumors shown by CT and both confirmed to be pheochromocytomas by histology. The right-sided lesion is larger (25 mm), while the left adrenal contains a 5 mm nodule.

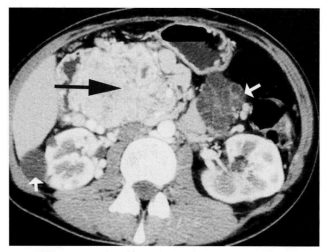

Figure 70.5 A large islet cell tumor (black arrow) arising in the head of the pancreas shown by CT after contrast injection. Note the cystic lesions in the kidney and tail of the pancreas (white arrows).

normetanephrines compared to those from multiple endocrine neoplasia type 2A patients [17]. When the pheochromocytomas are small in size MRI may fail to show the characteristic high T2-weighted signal. Radiolabeled MIBG may be taken up by up to 20% of normal adrenal medullas, again giving uncertainty when lesions are small. If these tests are equivocal or negative, adrenal vein catheterization and catecholamine sampling (by an experienced operator) may help in confirming the presence of a small intra-adrenal pheochromocytoma.

Initial treatment consists of α- and β-adrenoreceptor blockade especially before any invasive test or procedure [18]. Before any procedure we would treat any VHL patient harboring an adrenal lesion with phenoxybenzamine even if catecholamine secretion was apparently normal. This is because we have seen paroxysmal surges of blood pressure and catecholamines occurring only when a patient is stressed by a procedure or operation.

Definitive treatment is by adrenalectomy. Great care must be taken not to miss bilateral disease. Some of these tumors are small and may not be seen or felt macroscopically. Missing these may result in unnecessary repeat adrenalectomies. Conversely, over-aggressive removal of non-pheochromocytoma adrenal masses will result in unnecessary life-long adrenal replacement therapy. Experience is growing with laparoscopic and cortical-sparing adrenalectomy [19–21], but patients will require follow-up for recurrent pheochromocytoma as some adrenal medullary tissue is inevitably left behind. Non-pheochromocytoma and non-functioning adrenal lesions can be observed by scanning and biochemical testing at yearly intervals.

Pancreatic lesions

Pancreatic lesions are common in VHL, but are often asymptomatic and detected on routine scanning. Studies with CT or MRI have shown between 40% and 77% of patients have lesions and they tend to co-exist with renal or adrenal tumors [22–25]. The commonest pancreatic subtypes are serous microcystic adenomas and multiple or single cysts. Solid pancreatic lesions are seen in a substantial minority of patients and most are islet cell tumors (Fig. 70.5). Larger islet cell tumors may be malignant. Hence solid pancreatic lesions >3 cm will usually require surgical excision. Most of the pancreatic islet cell tumors are clinically non-functioning, but secretion of vasoactive intestinal polypeptide, insulin, glucagon and calcitonin has been reported. Pancreatic endocrine dysfunction and secondary diabetes mellitus has been found in a small number of VHL patients with substantial pancreatic microcystic adenomas.

Other visceral manifestations

The other lesions associated with VHL are listed in Table 70.1. In general most cystic lesions can be observed clinically and by yearly MRI or ultrasound scanning.

Diagnostic work-up and disease surveillance

The approaches we recommend are listed in Tables 70.2 and 70.3. Early diagnosis remains fundamental to the well-being of VHL patients. Genetic testing may allow surveillance programs to focus on gene carriers and low-risk relatives to be reassured. Hence molecular genetic diagnosis should be offered to all

Table 70.2 Testing for von Hippel–Lindau disease

Palpate for renal and epididymal lesions
Urinalysis
24 h urine collection for epinephrine, norepinephrine and dopamine
Funduscopy and fluorescein angioscopy
Brain MRI scan
Renal and adrenal MRI/ultrasound/CT

Table 70.3 Surveillance program for von Hippel–Lindau disease

Affected patient
Examination and urinalysis – yearly
24 hour urinary free catecholamines and plasma free normetanephrine – yearly
Direct and indirect funduscopy – yearly
Abdominal MRI scan – yearly
Brain MRI scan – 3 yearly to age 50 then 5 yearly
At-risk relative
Examination and urinalysis – yearly
24 hour urinary free catecholamines and plasma free normetanephrines – yearly
Direct and indirect funduscopy (± fluoroscein angioscopy) – yearly from ages 5 to 60
Abdominal MRI scan – yearly from age 16 to 65
Brain MRI scan – 3 yearly from age 15 to 40 then 5 yearly to age 60

affected patients. Characterization of the familial *VHL* mutation can provide a general guide to the risk of specific tumors such as pheochromocytoma.

References

1. Melmon KL, Rosen SW. Lindau's disease. *Am. J. Med.* 1964;36:595–617.

2. Maher ER. Von Hippel-Lindau disease. *Curr. Mol. Med.* 2004;4:833–842.

3. Ivan M, Kondo K, Yang H, et al. HIFalpha targeted for VHL-mediated destruction by proline hydroxylation: implications for O2 sensing. *Science* 2001;292:464–468.

4. Jaakkola P, Mole DR, Tian YM, et al. Targeting of HIF-alpha to the von Hippel–Lindau ubiquitylation complex by O$_2$-regulated prolyl hydroxylation. *Science* 2001;292:468–472.

5. Maxwell PH, Wiesener MS, Chang GW, et al. The tumour suppressor protein VHL targets hypoxia-inducible factors for oxygen-dependent proteolysis [see comments]. *Nature* 1999;399:271–275.

6. Bender BU, Eng C, Olschewski M, et al. VHL c.505 T>C mutation confers a high age related penetrance but no increased overall mortality. *J. Med. Genet.* 2001;38:508–514.

7. Gimenez-Roqueplo AP, Favier J, Rustin P, et al. Functional consequences of a SDHB gene mutation in an apparently sporadic pheochromocytoma. *J. Clin. Endocrinol. Metab.* 2002;87:4771–4774.

8. Hoffman MA, Ohh M, Yang H, Klco JM, Ivan M, Kaelin WG, Jr. von Hippel–Lindau protein mutants linked to type 2C VHL disease preserve the ability to downregulate HIF. *Hum. Mol. Genet.* 2001;10:1019–1027.

9. Clifford SC, Cockman ME, Smallwood AC, et al. Contrasting effects on HIF-1alpha regulation by disease-causing pVHL mutations correlate with patterns of tumourigenesis in von Hippel–Lindau disease. *Hum. Mol. Genet.* 2001;10:1029–1038.

10. Lee S, Nakamura E, Yang H, et al. Neuronal apoptosis linked to EglN3 prolyl hydroxylase and familial pheochromocytoma genes: developmental culling and cancer. *Cancer Cell* 2005;8:155–167.

11. Maher ER, Iselius L, Yates JR, et al. Von Hippel–Lindau disease: a genetic study. *J. Med. Genet.* 1991;28:443–447.

12. Maher ER, Yates JR, Harries R, et al. Clinical features and natural history of von Hippel–Lindau disease. *Q. J. Med.* 1990;77:1151–1163.

13. Kreusel KM, Bechrakis NE, Krause L, Neumann HP, Foerster MH. Retinal angiomatosis in von Hippel–Lindau disease: a longitudinal ophthalmologic study. *Ophthalmology* 2006;113:1418–1424.

14. Grubb RL, III, Choyke PL, Pinto PA, Linehan WM, Walther MM. Management of von Hippel–Lindau-associated kidney cancer. *Nat. Clin. Pract. Urol.* 2005;2:248–255.

15. Neumann HPH, Berger DP, Sigmund G, et al. Pheochromocytomas, multiple endocrine neoplasia type 2, and von Hippel–Lindau disease. *N. Engl. J. Med.* 1993;329:1531–1538.

16. Chew SL, Dacie JE, Reznek RH, et al. Bilateral phaeochromocytomas in von Hippel–Lindau disease: diagnosis by adrenal vein sampling and catecholamine assay. *Q. J. Med.* 1994;87:49–54.

17. Eisenhofer G, Walther MM, Huynh TT, et al. Pheochromocytomas in von Hippel–Lindau syndrome and multiple endocrine neoplasia type 2 display distinct biochemical and clinical phenotypes. *J. Clin. Endocrinol. Metab.* 2001;86:1999–2008.

18. Chew SL. Recent developments in the therapy of phaeochromocytoma. *Exp. Opin. Investig. Drugs* 2004;13:1579–1583.

19. Baghai M, Thompson GB, Young WF, Jr., Grant CS, Michels VV, van Heerden JA. Pheochromocytomas and paragangliomas in von Hippel–Lindau disease: a role for laparoscopic and cortical-sparing surgery. *Arch. Surg.* 2002;137:682–688.

20. Yip L, Lee JE, Shapiro SE, et al. Surgical management of hereditary pheochromocytoma. *J. Am. Coll. Surg.* 2004;198:525–534.

21. Neumann HP, Reincke M, Bender BU, Elsner R, Janetschek G. Preserved adrenocortical function after laparoscopic bilateral adrenal sparing surgery for hereditary pheochromocytoma. *J. Clin. Endocrinol. Metab.* 1999;84:2608–2610.

22. Delman KA, Shapiro SE, Jonasch EW, et al. Abdominal visceral lesions in von Hippel–Lindau disease: incidence and clinical behavior of pancreatic and adrenal lesions at a single center. *World J. Surg.* 2006;30:665–669.

23. Mukhopadhyay B, Sahdev A, Monson JP, Besser GM, Reznek RH, Chew SL. Pancreatic lesions in von Hippel–Lindau disease. *Clin. Endocrinol. (Oxf.)* 2002;57:603–608.

24. Hough DM, Stephens DH, Johnson CD, Binkovitz LA. Pancreatic lesions in von Hippel–Lindau disease: prevalence, clinical significance, and CT findings. *AJR* 1994;162:1091–1094.

25. Hammel PR, Vilgrain V, Terris B, et al. Pancreatic involvement in von Hippel–Lindau disease. The Groupe Francophone d'Etude de la Maladie de von Hippel–Lindau. *Gastroenterology* 2000;119:1087–1095.

71 Neurofibromatosis Type 1

Vincent M. Riccardi

Key points

- The defining features of neurofibromatosis type 1 are café-au-lait spots, multiple neurofibromas and iris Lisch nodules.
- Neuroficromatosis type 1 also variably involves the brain, bones, vasculature and the adrenal glands.
- Puberty and growth disturbances, sometimes due to chiasmal optic gliomas, are part of neuroficromatosis type 1.
- Neuroficromatosis type 1 molecular (DNA) diagnosis is nearly 98% accurate.

Introduction

The disorder originally known by the eponym Von Recklinghausen disease was first referred to as neurofibromatosis type 1 (NF1) by Riccardi in 1982. This designation was formally adopted by the NIH Consensus Conference on Neurofibromatosis in 1987. NF1 is characterized by patchy hyperpigmentation of the skin, that is, café-au-lait spots, multiple neurofibromas, iris Lisch nodules and the more variable presence of involvement of other tissues, including those of the central nervous system, the skeleton, the vasculature and the endocrine system [1–6]. This chapter will focus on the several ways that NF1 manifests as problems in terms of clinical endocrine oncology.

Overview of NF1

The *NF1* gene locus is on the long arm of chromosome 17; it comprises over 300 kilobases (kb) of genomic DNA, arranged in approximately 50 exons that are transcribed into a mRNA molecule of about 13 kb [7–10]. This transcript has at least two alternative splice sites, allowing for the gene product, neurofibromin, to have at least three different forms. The unmodified protein has 281 eight amino acid residues and a molecular mass of 327 kDa. The neurofibromin has at least one specifically defined function, namely that of a guanosine triphosphate (GTP)-ase-activating protein (GAP). The GAP element presumably accounts for neurofibromas and other tumors by influencing the interaction of guanosine nucleotides with ras oncoproteins. GTP is required for an "active" ras protein; wild-type neurofibromin promotes the cleavage of a phosphate group from GTP to form guanosine diphosphate (GDP), diminishing the growth-promoting activities of ras. The GAP function of neurofibromin has generated much interest in a medicinal approach to treating NF1 tumor growth, specifically, obviating the *NF1* mutation by an opposite effect on the ras control system. A number of knockout mouse models have been developed in attempts to understand more completely the role of the *NF1* gene and neurofibromin in the pathogenesis of NF1 lesions [11].

Confirming the diagnosis of NF1 using molecular (i.e., DNA) markers has had relatively limited use, respecting that by 1 year of age, the diagnosis is almost always readily apparent to the trained professional. However, there are increasing indications for attempting genotype-phenotype correlations. Specifically, deletions of the entire gene may well be associated with a more severe outcome and certain point mutations may be associated with less severe problems. Presently, approximately 95% of all NF1 mutations can be identified at the molecular levels. Prenatal diagnosis and preimplantation diagnosis are considerations for the use of molecular testing and have afforded important opportunities for avoiding the recurrence of the disorder in the offspring of affected patients.

NF1 defining features

Every person with NF1 eventually will have café-au-lait spots, iris Lisch nodules and multiple neurofibromas. The café-au-lait spots are apparent at or shortly after birth. The Lisch nodules generally then become apparent sometime after 5 years of age. The neurofibromas become obvious as a function of age and of the type of neurofibroma. Cutaneous and subcutaneous neurofibromas usually appear at or around the time of puberty. Nodular plexiform neurofibromas tend to become apparent in the late teenage years. Diffuse plexiform neurofibromas are congenital lesions, although they might not be readily obvious until they grow larger or until the appropriate diagnostic studies are done (e.g., radiography). A

Clinical Endocrine Oncology, 2nd edition. Edited by Ian D. Hay and John A.H. Wass. © 2008 Blackwell Publishing. ISBN 978-1-4051-4584-8.

corollary to the congenital nature of diffuse plexiform neurofibromas is that if a person with NF1 does not manifest such a tumor (and it has been realistically looked for it), that person will not develop one subsequently. That is, for such a person there is not a continuing risk for such a development. This fact is a source of solace to many parents.

Although each of these defining features will be present eventually in each typical patient with NF1, there is tremendous variation in the number and severity of the lesions, and severity thus is not predictable from one generation to another, even in a single family. A minimally affected parent can have a child that is severely affected, for example, with very numerous cutaneous neurofibromas.

NF1 general variable features

All the other features of NF1 are variable, not only in terms of their respective levels of severity, but also in terms of their frequencies. It is not possible to itemize all the variable features, although several are chosen here to make some broad general points. For a complete review the reader is referred to the author's monograph [1]. Endocrine features will be discussed later in this chapter.

The frequencies of variable features of NF1 range from somewhere around 0.1% for juvenile chronic myelogenous leukemia through about 0.5% for pheochromocytoma and 15% for optic pathway gliomas to as high as 60% or more for learning disabilities. Many features have a frequency of about 5%, as for example sphenoid wing dysplasia. The sum of these estimated average frequencies makes an important clinical point: it is very unusual for a patient with NF1 to avoid all of the variable features. As a practical matter, it is usual for a patient to have at least two or three such variable features. This is among the reasons why I tend to see NF1 as a relatively serious disorder, not as a disorder that is more often mild than serious.

Optic pathway gliomas
Optic pathway gliomas are symptomatic in no less than 5% of patients with NF1, although the total number of patients with NF1 that have this form of tumor is 15% or more. The symptoms include visual deficits, hypothalamic/pituitary impingement (discussed below) and less specific consequences of an intracranial space-occupying lesion (e.g., hydrocephalus). Several percent of patients with NF1 have non-optic pathway gliomas, most often in the posterior fossa, but occasionally in a cerebral hemisphere. The issue of screening children for optic pathway gliomas prior to the reversible vision loss is controversial presently, although I personally encourage such screening as a realistic alternative to irreversible symptoms of the types described above that occur in at least 5% of these at-risk youngsters.

Neurofibrosarcoma
This malignancy occurs in about 10% of patients with NF1, almost always arising in a diffuse or nodular plexiform neurofibroma.

Based on this observation, the 10% risk may not apply to all patients with NF1. Rather, it would be lower for those without any plexiform neurofibroma and higher for those with such a lesion. This malignancy is very rare in the first decade of life; most of the patients with this feature present with it in the second or third decades.

Skeletal dysplasia
Skeletal dysplasias include pseudarthrosis of the tibia (about 1%) or other tubular bones (less than 0.5%); sphenoid wing dysplasia (5%); vertebral dysplasia and dystrophic scoliosis (5%); and non-specific features including pectus excavatum, angulation deformities at the knees, ankle valgus and pes planus. A key aspect of acknowledging these features is the resultant emphasis on the embryonic and fetal onset of the disorder, as well as its protean nature: NF1 is more than a skin pigmentation and tumor disorder.

Vascular dysplasia
A similar point can be made about the vascular dysplasias. The most frequent portion of the vascular tree to be involved is that feeding the kidneys. Renovascular hypertension afflicts at least 3% of patients with NF1. Another somewhat smaller group of patients with NF1 has involvement of the gastrointestinal or cerebral vascular systems.

Learning disabilities
School performance problems occur in at least 40%, and probably high than 60%, of youngsters with NF1 [12]. Although in some generic sense this is a type of "learning disability," some experts object to applying that phrase in any strict sense to the problems seen in NF1. However, the parents of affected youngsters understand the generic sense and it sums up the situation for them well. The precise basis for this performance abnormality is not known. Efforts to correlate its presence with other variable features of NF1 have been unsuccessful, with particular regard to macrocephaly and to the hyperintense T2-weighted signal seen on cranial magnetic resonance imaging (MRI) scans. Plainly there is no correlation between learning problems and the MRI findings. Early identification is helpful, as remedial intervention is quite salutary.

Seizures
Seizures are emphasized here only because there is no specific anatomic basis to account for this feature, which is present in about 5% of patients with NF1 (i.e., only slightly different from the general population). The types of seizures include all the usual ones, including infantile spasms as seen in tuberous sclerosis.

Short stature and macrocephaly
At least 16% of patients with NF1 have short stature (height 2 or more standard deviations below the mean for age and sex) [1]. Similarly, at least 16% of patients with NF1 have macrocephaly (head circumference 2 or more standard deviations above the mean for age and sex) [1]. In addition, there is probably another

group with relative macrocephaly: less than 2 standard deviations above the mean, but excessively large with respect to the patient's short stature. The short stature is not explained by chiasmal optic gliomas or by unequivocal deficiencies in human growth hormone (hGH), as discussed further below.

NF1 endocrine features

Pregnancy and puberty

Puberty and pregnancy are both associated with changes in the rate of development and size of neurofibromas. In general, the neurofibroma increases precede or accompany puberty rather than necessarily being caused by puberty. Pregnancy also tends to make neurofibromas more obvious on the basis of intercellular turgidity, which dissipates shortly after delivery [1]. It is very possible, if not likely, that the basis for the increase in the number and/or size of cutaneous neurofibromas is the accumulation of subcutaneous fat, both as the prelude to puberty and as part of pregnancy in preparation for lactation. There is no reliable evidence for an adverse effect of birth-control pills in NF1 [1]. The overall severity of NF1 as determined by the number or nature and consequence of neurofibromas is the same for both men and women.

Hypothalamo–pituitary

Optic pathway gliomas involving the optic chiasm not infrequently impinge on the adjacent hypothalamus and/or pituitary gland. It is common in such situations for there to be one of three types of clinical problems: short stature, puberty disturbances and the Russell diencephalic syndrome. However, each of these problems is part of the NF1 picture and may be present without an apparent optic chiasm glioma.

Short stature

Short stature is frequent in NF1, as noted above. It is much more common than tumors involving the optic chiasm or hypothalamus. Moreover, the role of deficient hGH secretion has yet to be defined. No publications have documented that such a deficiency actually accounts for the short stature, although endocrinology specialists in local facilities often interpret hGH (baseline and provocative testing) data to provide a basis for hGH replacement therapy. There have been some claims based on drug company-sponsored studies for a beneficial effect of hGH administration to patients with NF1 and short stature; however, the use of a growth-promoting substance in the setting of the disorder characterized by aberrant growth in multiple tissues is an experiment in nature that warrants thoughtfulness in the extreme.

Puberty disturbances

Premature puberty in NF1 almost always indicates a chiasmal optic pathway glioma, although the hormonal details are usually unclear. Delayed puberty, on the other hand, may have no specific anatomical basis, or there may be a chiasmal glioma or a less

specific brain abnormality, such as ventricle dilation. In general, these cases have not been keenly studied and the "exact" basis for the puberty disturbance is usually not apparent.

Russell diencephalic syndrome

Patients with NF1 and optic chiasm glioma may present with the Russell diencephalic syndrome (hypothalamic syndrome, skin pallor, visual loss). These patients are important for two reasons. First, they document the presence of avoidable symptoms attributable to NF1 chiasmal gliomas. Second, they document how effective radiotherapy can be. Patients have been seen with this syndrome who reverse their downward course within days of initiating radiotherapy. Optic pathway gliomas and their consequences are clearly amenable to treatment.

Pheochromocytoma

Most commonly involving the adrenal medulla, pheochromocytomas probably occur with a frequency of 0.5% among patients with NF1. The involvement of other sites, including the aortic bifurcation (organ of Zuckerkandl), is well known in NF1. The author knows of no patients in their first decade of life who have NF1 and a pheochromocytoma, and the frequency after that age is still about 0.5% (1 in 200), a relatively low likelihood. However, a pheochromocytoma is a key part of NF1 because it represents an avoidable lethal complication. It is essential to consider this diagnosis in all patients with this condition [4].

Neuroendocrine tumors of the gut

Neuroendocrine tumors of the gut probably occur with the frequency of about 1%, although no accurate numbers are known. It may be that the frequency is closer to 2% or 3%. Presentation is usually as an epigastric or pancreatic mass. Serotonin-related symptoms are the exception. The recent interest in the so-called gastrointestinal stromal tumor (GIST) of NF1 is likely to add substantially to this story [13].

Parathyroid glands

Although several groups have published on excessive frequency of parathyroid adenomas among patients with NF1, it is not certain that the frequency represents anything other than an investigator bias [1].

NF2

NF2 is a disorder characterized by intracranial schwannomas, meningiomas and ependymomas, as well as paraspinal schwannomas [14]. Other features include cutaneous schwannomas, subcapsular cataracts and a distinctive pigmentary retinopathy [14]. NF2 is totally distinct from NF1, with the chromosomal location of the NF2 locus being the long arm of chromosome 22. Its gene product, *merlin*, is quite different from the NF1 gene product, neurofibromas. Endocrine oncology problems are not a part of this disorder.

References

1. Riccardi VM. *Neurofibromatosis: Phenotype, Natural History and Pathogenesis*, 2nd edition. Baltimore: Johns Hopkins University Press, 1992.

2. Riccardi VM. Neurofibromatosis: clinical heterogeneity. *Curr. Probl. Cancer* 1982;7:1–34.

3. Al Otibi M, Rutka JT. Neurosurgical implications of neurofibromatosis Type 1 in children. *Neurosurg. Focus* 2006;20:E3.

4. Bausch B, Borozdin W, Neumann HPH. Clinical and genetic characteristics of patients with Neurofibromatosis type 1 and pheochromocytoma. *N. Engl. J. Med.* 2006;354:2729–2731.

5. Lammert F, Friedman JM, Roth HJ, et al. Vitamin D deficiency associated with number of neurofibromas in neurofibromatosis 1. *J. Med. Genet.* 2006;48:810–913.

6. Rawal A, Yin Q, Roebuck M, et al. Atypical and malignant peripheral nerve sheath tumors of the brachial plexus: report of three cases and review of the literature. *Microsurgery* 2006;26:80–86.

7. Jenne DE, Tinschert S, Dorschner MO, Hameister H, Stephens K, Kehrer-Sawatzki H. Complete physical map and gene content of the human NF1 tumor suppressor region in human and mouse. *Genes Chromosomes Cancer* 2003;37:111–120.

8. Gottfried ON, Viskochil DH, Fults DW, Couldwell WT. Molecular, genetic and cellular pathogenesisof neurofibromatosis and surgical implications. *Neurosurgery* 2006;58:1–16.

9. Hanna F, Ho I, Tong JJ, Zhu Y, Nurnberg P, Zhong Y. Effect of neurofibromatosis type 1 mutations on a novel pathway for adenyl cyclase activation requiring neurofibromin and ras. *Hum. Mol. Genet.* 2006;15:1087–1098.

10. Wimmer K, Yao S, Claes K, et al. Spectrum of single- and multiexon NF1 copy number changes in a cohort of 1,100 unselected NF1 patients. *Genes Chromosomes Cancer* 2006;45:256–276.

11. Yang F-C, Ingram DA, Chen S, et al. Neurofibromin-deficient Schwann cells secrete a potent migratory stimulus for Nf1+/− mast cells. *J. Clin. Invest.* 2003;112:1851–1861.

12. Coude FX, Mignot C, Lyonnet S, Munnich A. Academic impairment is the most frequent complication of neurofibromatosis type 1 (NF1) in children. *Behav. Genet.* 2006;11:33–35.

13. Maertens O, Prenen H, Debiec-Rychter M, et al. Molecular pathogenesis of multiple gastrointestinal stromal tumors in NF1. *Hum. Mol. Genet.* 2006;15:1015–1023.

14. Martuza RL, Eldridge R. Neurofibromatosis 2 (bilateral acoustic neurofibromatosis). *N. Engl. J. Med.* 1988;318:684–688.

72 Carney Complex

Constantine A. Stratakis

Key points

- Carney complex is a familial lentiginosis syndrome; these disorders cover a wide phenotypic spectrum ranging from a benign inherited predisposition to develop cutaneous spots not associated with systemic disease to associations with several conditions.
- Carney complex is caused by *PRKAR1A* mutations and perturbations of the cyclic AMP-dependent protein kinase A signaling pathway.
- The main endocrine manifestations of Carney complex are: (1) primary pigmented nodular adrenocortical disease, a bilateral adrenal hyperplasia leading to Cushing syndrome; (2) growth hormone-secreting pituitary adenoma or pituitary somatotropic hyperplasia leading to acromegaly; (3) thyroid and gonadal tumors, including a predisposition to thyroid cancer.
- Other tumors associated with Carney complex include: (1) myxomas of the heart, breast and other sites; (2) psammomatous melanotic schwannomas which can become malignant; (3) a variety of skin and mucosal pigmented and non-pigmented lesions (nevi, macules, epitheliomas, other); (4) a predisposition to a variety of cancers.

Introduction

By 1981, a young man had been in and out the National Institutes of Health (NIH) Clinical Center for a variety of ailments; he had first been diagnosed with a growth hormone-producing tumor but his investigation and treatment were complicated by the baffling concurrent diagnosis of testicular tumors and hypercortisolemia due to adrenal tumors [1]. Before the end of the year, this patient was found dead at his home; ". . . this combination of lesions is best explained by the concept of neurocristopathies" is what the medical examiner in rural Pennsylvania concluded, finishing his report on the autopsy of this 19-year-old, heavily freckled man, who died in 1981 due to malignant, metastatic pigmented melanotic schwannoma. It was clear that he was affected simultaneously by two rare endocrine conditions, acromegaly and Cushing syndrome; several physicians had noted his many "freckles" and other pigmented skin lesions, but his disease was not actually diagnosed until years later. We finally diagnosed him with Carney complex (CNC) in 1995.

The association of myxomas, spotty skin pigmentation (lentigines) and endocrine overactivity (Table 72.1) was first reported by Dr J. Aidan Carney in 1985 and subsequently designated as CNC in 1986 and Carney syndrome by others in 1994 [2, 3]. With the report of this new syndrome it was realized that the majority of patients previously characterized under the separate diagnoses of LAMB (lentigines, atrial myxoma, mucocutaneous myxoma,

Clinical Endocrine Oncology, 2nd edition. Edited by Ian D. Hay and John A.H. Wass. © 2008 Blackwell Publishing. ISBN 978-1-4051-4584-8.

Table 72.1 Clinical manifestations of Carney complex at the time of presentation

Manifestation	Number of patients	Percentage
Spotty skin pigmentation	262	77
Heart myxoma	53	178
Skin myxoma	110	33
PPNAD	88	26
LCCSCT	42	33 (of male patients)
Acromegaly	33	10
PMS	33	10
Thyroid nodules or cancer	11	5
Breast ductal adenoma	6	3 (of female patients)

PPNAD, primary pigmented nodular adrenocortical disease; LCCSCT, large cell calcifying Sertoli cell tumor; PMS, psammomatous melanotic schwannoma.

blue nevi) and NAME (nevi, atrial myxoma, myxoid neurofibroma, ephelides) would now be more appropriately described under CNC [4, 5]. The diagnosis of CNC is made if two of the main manifestations of the syndrome are present (Table 72.2); these need to be confirmed by histology, biochemical testing or imaging; alternatively the diagnosis is made when one of the criteria is present and the patient is a carrier of a known inactivating mutation of the *PRKAR1A* gene [6] (Table 72.2).

Clinical manifestations

The most common features of CNC (Table 72.1) include spotty skin pigmentation (Plate 72.1) (lentigines, freckling, café-au-lait spots, and blue nevi), myxomas of the heart, skin, and breast, and

Table 72.2 Diagnostic criteria for Carney complex

To make a diagnosis of Carney complex, a patient must either: (1) exhibit two of the manifestations of the disease listed below, or (2) exhibit one of these manifestations and meet one of the supplemental criteria (an affected first-degree relative or an inactivating mutation of the *PRKAR1A* gene)

1	Spotty skin pigmentation with a typical distribution (lips, conjunctiva and inner or outer canthi, vaginal and penile mucosa)
2	Myxoma (cutaneous and mucosal)*
3	Cardiac myxoma*
4	Breast myxomatosis* *or* fat-suppressed magnetic resonance imaging findings suggestive of this diagnosis[a]
5	PPNAD* *or* paradoxical positive response of urinary glucocorticosteroids to dexamethasone administration during Liddle's test[b]
6	Acromegaly due to GH-producing adenoma*
7	LCCSCT* *or* characteristic calcification on testicular ultrasonography
8	Thyroid carcinoma* *or* multiple, hypoechoic nodules on thyroid ultrasonography
9	Psammomatous melanotic schwannoma*
10	Blue nevus, epithelioid blue nevus (multiple)*
11	Breast ductal adenoma (multiple)
12	Osteochondromyxoma of bone*

Supplemental criteria	
1	Affected first-degree relative
2	Inactivating mutation of the *PRKAR1A* gene

*With histologic confirmation, [a]see [38], [b]see [10].

Table 72.3 Causes of death among 51 patients with Carney complex

Cause	Number of patients	Percentage
Heart and heart related	29	57
Cardiac myxoma	13	25
Cardiac myxoma emboli	6	12
Heart surgery complications	5	10
Cardiomyopathy	2	4
Probable cardiac arrhythmia	3	6
Psammomatous melanotic schwannoma	7	14
Metastatic PMS	6	12
Intracranial PMS	1	2
Postoperative complications (other than open heart surgery)	6	12
Bilateral adrenalectomy	2	4
Hernia	1	2
Abdominal emergency	2	4
Bilateral oophorectomy	1	2
Carcinoma or other metastatic tumor	7	14
Pancreas	2	4
Other abdominal tumor	3	6
Breast	1	2
Metastatic LCCSCT*	1	2
Other unknown	2	4

*LCCSCT, large cell calcifying Sertoli cell tumor.

primary pigmented nodular adrenal cortical disease (PPNAD) associated with an atypical form of Cushing syndrome (CS) [6, 7]. The breadth of involved organs in CNC is quite unique; CNC is both a multiple endocrine neoplasia (MEN) (along with MEN 1 and 2) and a cardiocutaneous syndrome (such as Noonan syndrome and related conditions) [2, 3, 8]. Of the non-cutaneous lesions found in CNC, cardiac myxomas are the most common [6]. These tumors tend to be of a more aggressive nature when compared to sporadic, non-CNC-associated myxomas; unlike the latter, the former may be in any cardiac chamber and may present multiple times, starting at a very young age (even in infancy) and without any predilection for gender (sporadic myxomas are more common in older women and almost always occur in the left atrium as single one-time tumors). Historically, cardiac myxomas have been reported to be responsible for more than 50% of the disease-specific mortality among CNC patients (Table 72.3).

Endocrine gland involvement includes growth hormone (GH)-secreting pituitary adenomas, thyroid gland disease, adrenocorticotropin (ACTH)-independent CS secondary to PPNAD, and testicular tumors, in particular, large cell calcifying Sertoli cell tumors (LCCSCT) (Fig. 72.1). Overall, PPNAD is the most common endocrine lesion and causes the greatest degree of endocrine-associated morbidity [7]. In male patients, however, the occurrence of LCCSCT may supersede PPNAD in number,

but not in morbidity, as it is typically a benign lesion most often diagnosed during routine testicular ultrasound when microcalcifications are found. Leydig cell tumors and adrenal rests have also been reported. Ovarian cysts are often found by sonographic examination as multiple hypoechoic lesions and although usually clinically insignificant, they may progress, occasionally, to ovarian carcinoma [9, 10].

Thyroid gland disease spans the spectrum from nodular disease to carcinoma, but in contrast to pituitary and adrenal pathology, there does not appear to be an increased risk of hyper- or hypothyroidism [11]. By sonographic examination, more than 60% of children and adults with CNC will be found to have cystic or multinodular disease. On biopsy, follicular adenoma is the most common finding, whereas thyroid cancer, follicular or papillary, may develop in up to 10% of CNC patients with pre-existing thyroid pathology [11]. Of note, recent examination for loss-of-heterozygosity (LOH) at the CNC locus on chromosome 17 (17q22–24) in sporadic thyroid cancer has found increased loss of this region, supporting the hypothesis that thyroid tissue is susceptible to tumorigenesis induced by *PRKAR1A* loss of function [12].

A variety of other tumors and conditions have been associated with CNC (Table 72.4).

Molecular genetics

Genetic linkage analysis has revealed two distinct loci for CNC, one on chromosome 2p16 (*CNC2*) and the other on chromosome

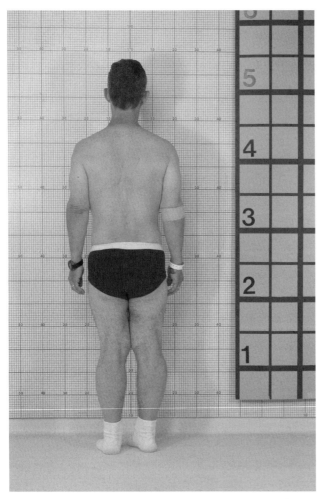

Figure 72.1 Skeletal features of a patient with CNC who ended up with short stature as an adult due to precocious puberty caused by bilateral testicular tumors, followed by Cushing syndrome in childhood; interestingly, now, he has acromegaly evident by the coarseness of his extremities in this picture.

Table 72.4 Findings suggestive of or possibly associated with CNC, but not diagnostic for the disease

Intense freckling (without darkly pigmented spots or typical distribution)

Blue nevus, usual type (if multiple)

Café-au-lait spots or other "birthmarks"

Elevated IGF-1 levels, abnormal oGTT, or paradoxical GH responses to TRH testing *in the absence of clinical acromegaly*

Cardiomyopathy*

Pilonidal sinus†

History of Cushing syndrome, acromegaly, or sudden death in extended family

Multiple skin tags and other skin lesions; lipomas

Colonic polyps (usually in association with acromegaly)

Hyperprolactinemia (usually mild and almost always in association with clinical or subclinical acromegaly)

Single, benign thyroid nodule in a young patient; multiple thyroid nodules in an older patient (detected by ultrasonography)

Family history of carcinoma, in particular of the thyroid, colon, pancreas and the ovary; other multiple benign or malignant tumors‡

*Three cases of hypertrophic cardiomyopathy are known among the 338 patients with CNC reported in reference 8.

†Nine cases of this anatomical anomaly were reported among 338 patients with CNC.

‡Colonic (rectum) (1), ovarian (2), mammary (1), gastric (1), and pancreatic (2) carcinomas, and retroperitoneal malignant fibrous histiocytoma (1) have been reported among 338 patients with CNC.

mutations in the *PRKAR1A* gene result in premature stop codons and predicted mutant protein products are not found in affected cells secondary to nonsense mRNA-mediated decay (NMD) of the mutant sequence [14, 16].

Biochemically, loss of R1α leads to increased cAMP-stimulated total (but not protein kinase A (PKA)-specific) activity that is thought to be secondary to up-regulation of other components of the PKA tetramer, including both type I (*PRKAR1B*) and type II (*PRKAR2A* or *PRKAR2B*) subunits, in a tissue-dependent manner, but how this leads to increased tumorigenesis is currently unknown [15].

Initial data supported the role of *PRKAR1A* as a "classic" tumor suppressor gene with tumors from CNC patients exhibiting germline mutations and subsequent LOH at the *PRKAR1A* locus; however, it now appears that haploinsufficiency of *PRKAR1A* may be sufficient for phenotypic expression of increased PKA activity [16] and the development of certain tumors, such as eyelid myxomas [17]. This concept is exemplified in animal models of CNC: whereas mice homozygous for R1α deletions die early *in utero* [18], transgenic mice with heterogeneous expression of an antisense transgene for exon 2 *of PRKAR1A* exhibit many of the phenotypic characteristics of CNC patients, including thyroid follicular hyperplasia and non-dexamethasone suppressible hypercortisolism [19, 20]. Not all of these lesions exhibited consistent losses of the normal R1α allele.

17q22−24 (*CNC1*) [13, 14]. Inactivating mutations of the gene encoding the protein kinase A type I-α regulatory (R1α) subunit (*PRKAR1A*) were identified in all patients mapping to the chromosome 17 and analysis of families registered in the National Institutes of Health-Mayo Clinic collection has revealed that most CNC patients have mutations at the *CNC1* locus [13]. The gene responsible for CNC at the chromosome 2p16 locus is unknown. At this point, there are no clear phenotypic differences between families mapping to one or the other locus.

The role of R1α in human tumorigenesis has been explored in several different cancer tissues and cell lines. Enhanced expression of R1α has been shown to play a role in colorectal, renal, breast, and ovarian cancer, and malignant osteoblasts, and may be associated with more advanced disease [15]. The notion of reduced R1α activity had not been investigated prior to the discovery of it being the protein that was defective in CNC; CNC represents the first identified human disease associated with a mutation of the PKA heterotetramer [4]. The majority of

Examination of the mechanisms associated with loss of R1α, increased PKA activity, and tumorigenesis is currently underway. PKA is a ubiquitous serine–threonine kinase intimately involved in the regulation of cell growth, including a potential role in chromosome stability [5]. The cross-talk between signal transduction pathways and the tissue-specific effects of altered PKA function are inherently quite complex, reflected by at times conflicting data. For example, alterations of 17q and/or the *PRKAR1A* locus have been found in both sporadic adrenal and thyroid cancers [12] yet allelic loss of 17q in cardiac and skin myxomas from CNC patients, with known germline *PRKAR1A* mutations, have not been found. Interestingly, CNC myxomas appear to have a more aggressive nature when compared to sporadic, non-CNC-associated myxomas, as discussed previously.

The physiologic impact of *PRKAR1A*-inactivating mutations has been most thoroughly studied in PPNAD, a rare form of ACTH-independent CS, which is present in approximately one-third of CNC patients [6]. PPNAD often presents in an indolent fashion and may be difficult to diagnose due to an intermittent or cyclical nature of the associated hypercortisolism. Diagnosis is established using the 6-day Liddle test as patients with PPNAD show a classic paradoxical rise in the 24 h urinary free cortisol and/or 17-hydroxysteroids of more than 50% on the second day of high-dose dexamethasone administration [6, 7]. While this response appears to be pathognomonic for PPNAD it does not appear to be dependent on the presence of *PRKAR1A* mutations as comparative *in vitro* studies between PPNAD cell lines with and without R1α deficiency showed increased cortisol secretion in response to dexamethasone associated with increased expression of the glucocorticoid receptor [7]. The underlying mechanism for this response is not known, however.

Additional studies aimed at elucidating the interrelationship between the *PRKAR1A* status, altered PKA activity, and cellular metabolism, are being aggressively pursued. Microarray analysis of R1α antisense targeted tumor cells has recently been shown to change expression of more than 240 genes, suggesting that altered regulation of a significant number of downstream targets is likely to contribute to the CNC phenotype [5]. Investigation of one of the signaling pathways, the mitogen-activated protein kinase (MAPK) ERK 1/2 pathway, typically inhibited by PKA in many cells, has recently been reported. In this report, the lymphocytes from CNC patients with known *PRKAR1A* mutations showed altered PKA activity and increased ERK 1/2 phosphorylation. Cell metabolism and cell proliferation studies suggested that altered PKA activity is associated with reversal of PKA-mediated inhibition of the MAPK pathway resulting in increased cell proliferation [16].

Laboratory evaluation and genetic testing

The recommended clinical surveillance of patients with CNC differs per age group. For post-pubertal pediatric and adult patients we recommend annual echocardiogram (this study may be needed biannually for adolescent patients with a history of excised myxoma), testicular and thyroid ultrasound, and urinary free cortisol (UFC) and serum insulin-like growth factor-1 (IGF-1) levels. For pre-pubertal pediatric patients, we recommend an annual echocardiogram (biannually for patients with a history of excised myxoma) and testicular ultrasound for boys. If close monitoring of growth rate and pubertal staging indicates other abnormalities, such as possible Cushing syndrome, appropriate testing should be done as needed. For PPNAD leading to Cushing syndrome, in addition to UFC we recommend diurnal cortisol levels (11:30 p.m., 12:00 midnight and 07:30 a.m., 08:00 a.m. sampling) and/or dexamethasone stimulation test (modified Liddle's test, as per Stratakis et al. [10]), and adrenal computerized tomography. For gigantism/acromegaly, in addition to serum IGF-1 levels, pituitary magnetic resonance imaging and a 3-h oral glucose tolerance test (oGTT) may be obtained. For psammomatous melanotic schwannoma, magnetic resonance imaging of the brain, spine, chest, abdomen, retroperitoneum, and/or pelvis may be necessary.

Clinical and biochemical screening for CNC remains the gold standard for the diagnosis of CNC. Molecular testing for *PRKAR1A* mutations is not recommended at present for all patients with CNC, but may be advised for detection of affected patients in families with known mutations of that gene to avoid unnecessary medical surveillance of non-carriers.

References

1. Rosenzweig JL, Lawrence DA, Vogel DL, Costa J, Gorden P. Adrenocorticotropin-independent hypercortisolemia and testicular tumors in a patient with a pituitary tumor and gigantism. *J. Clin. Endocrinol. Metab.* 1982;55:421–427.

2. Bauer AJ, Stratakis CA. The lentiginoses: cutaneous markers of systemic disease and a window to new aspects of tumourigenesis. *J. Med. Genet.* 2005;42:801–810.

3. Rhodes AR. Benign neoplasias and hyperplasias of melanocytes. and dysplastic melanocytic nevi. In Freedberg IM, Eisen AZ, Wolff K, et al. (eds). *Dermatology in General Medicine*, 5th edition. New York: McGraw-Hill, Inc., 1999:1018–1059;1060–1079.

4. Stergiopoulos SG, Stratakis CA. Human tumors associated with Carney complex and germline *PRKAR1A* mutations: a protein kinase A disease ! *FEBS Lett.* 2003;546:59–64.

5. Bossis I, Voutetakis A, Bei T, Sandrini F, Griffin KJ, Stratakis CA. Protein kinase A and its role in human neoplasia: the Carney complex paradigm. *Endocr. Relat. Cancer* 2004;11:265–280.

6. Stratakis CA, Kirschner LS, Carney JA. Clinical and molecular features of the Carney complex: diagnostic criteria and recommendations for patient evaluation. *J. Clin. Endocrinol. Metab.* 2001;86:4041–4046.

7. Bourdeau I, Lacroix A, Schurch W, Caron P, Antakly T, Stratakis CA. Primary pigmented nodular adrenocortical disease: Paradoxical responses of cortisol secretion to dexamethasone occur *in vitro* and are associated with increased expression of the glucocorticoid receptor. *J. Clin. Endocrinol. Metab.* 2003;88:3931–3937.

8. Carney JA, Stratakis CA. Epitheliod blue nevus and psammomatous melanotic schwannoma: the unusual pigmented skin tumors of the Carney complex. *Semin. Diagn. Pathol.* 1998;15:216–224.

9. Stratakis CA, Papageorgiou T, Premkumar A, et al. Ovarian lesions in Carney complex: clinical genetics and possible predisposition to malignancy. *J. Clin. Endocrinol. Metab.* 2000;85:4359–4366.

10. Stratakis CA, Papageorgiou T. Ovarian tumors associated with multiple endocrine neoplasias and related syndromes (Carney complex, Peutz–Jeghers syndrome, von Hippel–Lindau disease, Cowden's disease). *Int. J. Gynecol. Cancer* 2002;12:337–347.

11. Stratakis CA, Courcoutsakis NA, Abati A, et al. Thyroid gland abnormalities in patients with the syndrome of spotty skin pigmentation, myxomas, endocrine overactivity and schwannomas (Carney complex). *J. Clin. Endocrinol. Metab.* 1997;82: 2037–2043.

12. Sandrini F, Matyakhina L, Sarlis NJ, et al. Regulatory subunit type 1-A of protein kinase A (*PRKAR1A*): a tumor suppressor gene for sporadic thyroid cancer. *Genes Chromosomes Cancer* 2002;35:182–192.

13. Stratakis CA, Kirschner LS, Carney JA. Carney complex, a familial multiple neoplasia and lentiginoses syndrome. Analysis of 11 kindreds and linkage to the short arm of chromosome 2. *J. Clin. Invest.* 1996;97:699–705.

14. Kirschner LS, Carney JA, Pack SD, et al. Mutations of the gene encoding the protein kinase A type I-A regulatory subunit in patients with the Carney complex. *Nat. Genet.* 2000;26:89–92.

15. Bossis I, Stratakis CA. *PRKAR1A*: normal and abnormal functions. *Endocrinology* 2004;145:5452–5458.

16. Robinson-White A, Hundley TR, Shiferaw M, Bertherat J, Sandrini F, Stratakis CA. Protein kinase A activity in PRKAR1A-mutant cells and regulation of mitogen-activated protein kinases ERK1/2. *Hum. Mol. Genet.* 2003;12:1475–1484.

17. Tsilou ET, Chan CC, Sandrini F, et al. Eyelid myxoma in Carney complex without PRKAR1A allelic loss. *Am. J. Med. Genet.* 2004;130A: 395–397.

18. Kirschner LS, Kusewitt DF, Matyakhina L, et al. A mouse model for the Carney complex tumor syndrome develops neoplasia in cyclic AMP-responsive tissues. *Cancer Res.* 2005;65:4506–4514.

19. Griffin KJ, Kirschner LS, Matyakhina L, et al. Down-regulation of regulatory subunit type 1A of protein kinase A leads to endocrine and other tumors. *Cancer Res.* 2004;64:8811–8815.

20. Griffin KJ, Kirschner LS, Matyakhina L, et al. A transgenic mouse bearing an antisense construct of regulatory subunit type 1A of protein kinase A develops endocrine and other tumors: comparison to Carney complex and other *PRKAR1A*-induced lesions. *J. Med. Genet.* 2004;41:923–931.

73 McCune–Albright Syndrome

William F. Schwindinger and Michael A. Levine

Key points

- McCune–Albright syndrome is characterized by the clinical triad of polyostotic fibrous dysplasia, café-au-lait pigmented skin lesions, and endocrinopathy.
- While McCune–Albright syndrome is not an inherited disease, it is a genetic disease that arises by somatic mutation soon after fertilization.
- The mutation in *GNAS*, termed *gsp*, results in constitutive activation of $G\alpha_s$, and in turn stimulation of adenylyl cyclase in affected tissues.
- The clinical spectrum of McCune–Albright syndrome is influenced by the timing of the *gsp* mutation, the variable ability of cyclic adenosine monophosphate to induce proliferation in different cells, and the parental origin of the *GNAS* allele that carries the *gsp* mutation.
- The growing understanding of the diverse presentation of McCune–Albright syndrome now compels a more thorough evaluation of patients with fibrous dysplasia or *café-au-lait* pigmented skin lesions to determine whether they have subtle endocrinopathies.

Introduction

McCune–Albright syndrome (MAS) is characterized by the clinical triad of polyostotic fibrous dysplasia, café-au-lait pigmented skin lesions, and endocrinopathy [1, 2]. The endocrinopathies include precocious puberty, hyperthyroidism, growth hormone excess, hyperprolactinemia and hypercortisolism. These endocrine disorders are characterized by autonomous (i.e., trophic hormone independent) proliferation and excessive function of specific hormone-secreting tissues. A variety of less common additional features can occur in patients with MAS, such as hypophosphatemic osteomalacia, cardiomyopathy and hepatitis (Table 73.1). MAS is a sporadic genetic disorder, but it is not inherited. A mutation in the gene (*GNAS*) that encodes the α-subunit of the stimulatory G-protein of adenylyl cyclase, $G\alpha_s$, is present in affected tissues of patients with MAS. The mosaic distribution of cells that contain the *GNAS* mutation is consistent with the hypothesis that MAS results from a somatic mutation that occurs during early embryogenesis. The *GNAS* mutation, termed *gsp*, results in constitutive (i.e., ligand-independent) activation of $G\alpha_s$, and in turn stimulation of adenylyl cyclase, and is the molecular basis for autonomous function and hyperplasia of the affected cells.

Clinical Endocrine Oncology, 2nd edition. Edited by Ian D. Hay and John A.H. Wass. © 2008 Blackwell Publishing. ISBN 978-1-4051-4584-8.

Table 73.1 Clinical manifestations of McCune–Albright syndrome

	Ringel et al. 1996		Lumbroso et al. 2004	
	n = 158	%	*n* = 113	%
Fibrous dysplasia	154	97	52	46
Café-au-lait skin lesions	135	85	60	53
Precocious puberty	82	52	89	79
Growth hormone excess	42	27	5	4
Hyperprolactinemia	23	15	4	4
Hyperthyroidism	30	19	3	3
Hypercortisolism	9	6	7	6
Hyperparathyroidism			1	1
Myxomas	8	5		
Osteosarcoma	3	2		
Rickets/osteomalacia	4	3		
Cardiac abnormalities	17	11		
Hepatic abnormalities	16	10	6	5
Testicular abnormalities	1	1		

Clinical data on 158 cases of MAS identified by a survey of the literature [3], and in a series of 113 patients from a European collaborative study [4]. Because of the clinical variability of MAS, the data provide only a rough estimate of the relative incidences of the more common manifestations.

Clinical features

Café-au-lait pigmented skin lesions

Patients with MAS classically have one or more flat, pigmented skin lesions (café-au-lait macules) with irregular borders (Fig. 73.1).

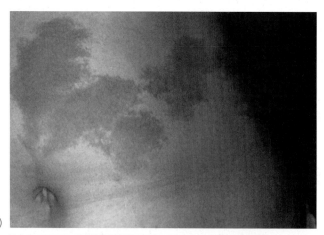

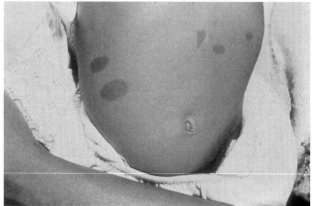

Figure 73.1 Café-au-lait lesion of MAS (a) as compared to that of neurofibromatosis (b). Note the irregular border of the lesion in MAS ("Coast of Maine") as compared to the smooth border in neurofibromatosis ("Coast of California").

Biopsy reveals that the pigment, melanin, is present in both melanocytes and keratinocytes. The irregular border ("Coast of Maine") of these lesions distinguishes them from the pigmented macules of neurofibromatosis, which have a smooth border ("Coast of California"). The distribution of the café-au-lait macules in MAS is also characteristic. Individual lesions on the torso or face rarely extend across the midline. The majority of the skin lesions tends to be on the same side as the most severe skeletal involvement, and may be quite extensive. The macules occur most frequently on the sacrum, buttocks and lumbar region, which may be related to the embryological origin of melanoblasts from the neural crest. Happle [5] noted that the pattern of the cutaneous lesions follows the embryological lines of ectodermal migration described by Blashko, and first suggested that MAS might be a mosaic disorder.

Fibrous dysplasia of bone

Patients with MAS classically develop fibrous dysplasia at one or more skeletal sites, and these expansile lesions can cause skeletal deformities, nerve entrapment, or fracture. Fibrous dysplasia in MAS typically develops before the age of 10 years, in contradistinction to non-syndromic mono-ostotic fibrous dysplasia

lesions, which occurs in the second or third decade [6]. Existing lesions may enlarge and cause progressive deformity, but few new lesions develop over time. In polyostotic fibrous dysplasia, lesions of the proximal femur are likely to progress with pathological fracture and coxa vara deformity (e.g. shepherd's crook deformity). Plain radiographs reveal thinning of the cortex and circumscribed lesions with a characteristic ground glass appearance (Fig. 73.2). The lesions may appear multilocular due to a scalloped pattern of endosteal erosion. Histological sections reveal fibrous tissue with embedded bony trabeculae (Fig. 73.3).

The basis for the unusual cellular changes in fibrous dysplasia is poorly understood. Recent evidence indicates that the fibrotic areas consist of an excess of cells with phenotypic features of pre-osteogenic cells, whereas the lesional bone formed *de novo* within fibrotic areas represents the biosynthetic output of mature but abnormal osteoblasts. It is likely that at least some of the phenotypic changes in affected osteogenic cells result from cyclic adenosine monophosphate (cAMP)-induced increases in expression of interleukin-6 and the *c-fos* protooncogene [8, 9]. Cyclic AMP also plays a major role in regulating growth plate development, with $G\alpha_s$ negatively regulating chondrocyte differentiation [10], but no specific defect in the growth plate has been described in children with MAS. The mosaic distribution of lesions in fibrous dysplasia may also play an important pathogenic role, as close contact between transplanted normal bone cells and osteogenic cells containing the *gsp* mutation is necessary to reproduce the fibrous dysplasia lesion in mice [11].

Radiographs of the femora and pelvis are useful in screening for bone involvement. However, any bone may be involved. Panoramic dental radiographs reveal craniofacial bone involvement in 80% of MAS patients [12]. Although the optic nerves are usually involved and are often encased circumferentially as they pass through the cranial base, optic nerve compression is very unusual [13]. Scintigraphy with ^{99m}Tc methylene diphosphonate is more sensitive than radiography in detecting early lesions, and reveals that spinal involvement is common, with 60% of MAS patients having spinal lesions and 40% showing scoliosis [14]. Scintigraphy is also useful in assessing the total skeletal burden which is correlated with biochemical abnormalities and the clinical severity of the bone disease [15].

Endocrinopathies

Precocious puberty

Precocious puberty is a common initial manifestation of MAS in girls. Cyclical elevation of circulating concentration of estrogen corresponds with the development and involution of ovarian cysts. Early breast development and menstruation may occur as early as 1 year of age. The ovaries are hyperfunctional despite low circulating levels of gonadotropins, and there is a prepubertal response of gonadotropins to gonadotropin-releasing hormone (GnRH). Serum levels of inhibin B are low or normal in girls with MAS-associated precocious puberty, whereas girls with central precocious puberty have inhibin B levels that are elevated in

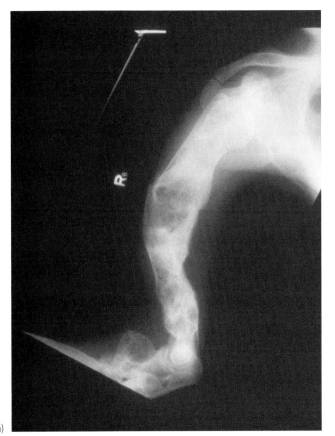

(a)

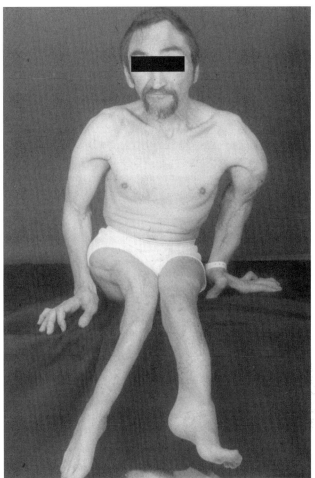

(b)

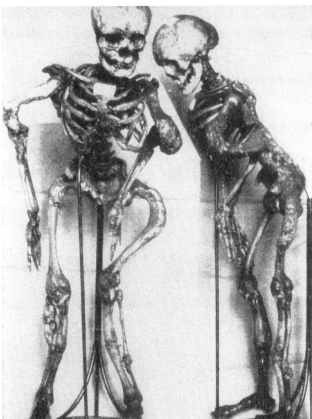

(c)

Figure 73.2 Polyostotic fibrous dysplasia. (a) Plain radiographs reveal expansile lesions that may appear scalloped. (b) Recurrent fractures can lead to progressive deformity. (c) Illustration from von Recklinghausen (1891) cited as an example of osteitis fibrosa generalista, but because of the marked "shepherd's crook" deformities of the femora and the bulge in the occiput; Albright et al. concluded that this is an example of polyostotic fibrous dysplasia [7].

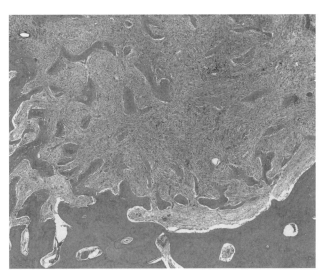

Figure 73.3 Histology of polyostotic fibrous dysplasia. Microscopically, trabeculae of immature non-lamellar (woven) bone are scattered throughout nondescript fibrous tissue having variable cellularity. The margins of the bony fragments are indistinct and have no clear limiting edge of osteoblasts, a feature which distinguishes this lesion from ossifying fibroma. The irregular trabeculae have C- and S-shapes that resemble Chinese script writing. Multinucleated giant cells and cementum-like calcifications may be present.

accor-dance with Tanner maturation stage [16]. Physiological activation of the hypothalamo–pituitary–ovarian axis, with activation of central puberty, occurs as the bone age advances or the child reaches maturity. Although some adult women may experience menstrual irregularities, they are usually fertile. Precocious puberty occurs less frequently in boys with MAS, and testicular biopsy reveals varying degrees of seminiferous tubule development. Testicular enlargement is typically bilateral, but unilateral enlargement without sexual precocity may occur due to restriction of the *gsp* mutation to Sertoli cells [17]. Levels of serum inhibin B are elevated if Sertoli cells are involved. Ultrasound revealed testicular microlithiasis in five of eight boys with MAS [18].

Autonomous thyroid nodules

About 50% of patients with MAS develop excessive thyroid function that ranges from subclinical laboratory abnormalities to hyperthyroidism. MAS patients with hyperthyroidism do not develop orbitopathy or cutaneous features of Graves' disease, and do not have detectable serum levels of thyroid-stimulating immunoglobulins. The hyperthyroidism in MAS is due to autonomous function within regions of the thyroid gland. Clinically evident goiter is present in many MAS patients with hyperthyroidism, and nodules are detected by thyroid ultrasound in essentially all patients. Thyroid function testing reveals suppressed thyroid-stimulating hormone (TSH), a blunted response of TSH to thyrotropin-releasing hormone (TRH), and failure of synthetic liothyronine (T_3) to suppress radioactive iodine uptake. The continuous development of new and autonomous nodules may account for the poor responsiveness of hyperthyroidism to radioactive iodine ablation. Thyroid carcinoma has been described in two MAS patients and may be a rare complication [19].

Growth hormone excess and hyperprolactinemia

About 20% of patients with MAS may develop pituitary-dependent growth hormone (GH) excess. GH excess is associated with attainment of normal adult height despite precocious puberty, and with an increased incidence of hearing and vision defects [20]. GH excess in MAS is indistinguishable biochemically from that which occurs in patients with isolated GH-producing pituitary adenomas. GH secretion is stimulated by growth hormone-releasing hormone (GHRH) and TRH, poorly inhibited by oral glucose, and increased by sleep. However, less than 40% of patients with MAS and GH excess have radiological evidence of a pituitary tumor and over 80% have associated hyperprolactinemia. Pituitary pathology in MAS varies and includes adenoma, nodular hyperplasia or mammosomatotroph hyperplasia.

Hypercortisolism

Patients with MAS occasionally develop hypercortisolism. In most cases hypercortisolism appears to be due to autonomous activity of the adrenal gland. Cortisol levels show no diurnal variation and are not suppressible by dexamethasone. Plasma levels of adrenocorticotropic hormone (ACTH) are undetectable and adrenal biopsy reveals nodular adrenal hyperplasia or adrenal adenoma

[21]. However, an activating mutation of $G\alpha_s$ in an isolated corticotroph-secreting pituitary adenoma has been reported [22].

Hypophosphatemic rickets and osteomalacia

Some patients with MAS develop a generalized metabolic bone disease that is associated with low serum levels of phosphate, low or low-normal serum levels of 1,25-dihydroxyvitamin D, high levels of alkaline phosphatase, and a depressed renal tubular maximum reabsorption of phosphate (TMP)/glomerular filtration rate (GFR). These patients have normal levels of serum calcium, 25-hydroxyvitamin D and parathyroid hormone (PTH). Histology of the bone demonstrates a mineralization defect similar to that which occurs in several other forms of hypophosphatemic bone disease (e.g., hypophosphatemic rickets or oncogenic osteomalacia). Circulating levels of FGF-23, a leading candidate for the phosphate-regulating hormone phosphatonin, are elevated in most patients with MAS [23]. The development of hypophosphatemic rickets in patients with MAS corresponds with the presence of extensive fibrous dysplasia, suggesting that the fibrous dysplasia is the source of the FGF-23 [23]. FGF-23 is believed to be the common mediator of phosphaturia in a growing number of sporadic and inherited hypophosphatemic syndromes. X-linked hypophosphatemic rickets is caused by mutations in a neutral endopeptidase, PHEX, which is thought to be indirectly involved in the degradation of FGF-23. Autosomal dominant hypophosphatemic rickets is caused by mutations that render FGF-23 resistant to proteolytic degradation. Oncogenic osteomalacia is caused by excessive secretion of FGF-23 by tumor cells.

Non-classical features of MAS

Patients with MAS may develop metabolic problems in additional tissues that can lead to hepatobiliary disease (neonatal jaundice, elevated transaminases, hepatomegaly, cholestasis, extramedullary hematopoiesis), cardiac disease (cardiomegaly, tachyarrhythmias, sudden death), gastrointestinal polyps, hyperplasia of the thymus and spleen, acute pancreatitis, failure to thrive, developmental delay, and microcephaly. These disorders may result from expression of the activated $G\alpha_s$ mutation in cells of the affected organ or may develop as a response to an underlying endocrinopathy. Hepatobiliary disease and cardiac disease are particularly common problems in patients with MAS, and are associated with the presence of activating $G\alpha_s$ mutations in the affected tissues. MAS may present as a severe neonatal disease with involvement of multiple endocrine glands and non-endocrine organs that leads to premature death [24].

Pathogenesis

Identification of *GNAS* mutations

Insight into the pathogenesis of MAS came with the identification of mutations in the gene encoding $G\alpha_s$ *(GNAS)* in a subset of GH-secreting pituitary tumors with increased adenylyl cyclase activity. Landis and colleagues [25] established that the molecular

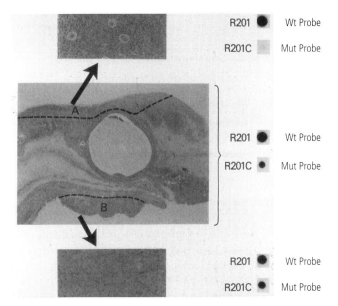

Figure 73.4 Mosaic distribution of activating mutation of Gα$_s$ in the ovary of a patient with MAS. DNA prepared from a histologically normal area of the ovary (above) showed little of the mutant allele (R201C) while DNA prepared from the histologically abnormal area of the ovary (below) revealed almost 50% mutant allele. (Reproduced from Weinstein et al. [26], with permission from the Massachusetts Medical Society.)

basis for this anomaly was a missense mutation that resulted in replacement of either Arg[201] or Gln[227] in the Gα$_s$ protein. This oncogenic form of Gα$_s$, termed *gsp*, lacks GTPase activity and leads to constitutive (i.e., ligand-independent) activation of adenylyl cyclase. Increased intracellular cAMP may account for both autonomous function and proliferation of cells expressing the mutation.

Mutations in Arg[201] of *GNAS* in patients with MAS have been identified in DNA from surgical and autopsy specimens of endocrine tumors [26], a café-au-lait pigmented skin lesion [27], fibrous dysplasia lesions [28], and in peripheral blood cells [29]. These mutations were present in some but not all tissues examined from each patient. Each patient had a single mutation in Gα$_s$, either Arg[201]→Cys or Arg[201]→His. In some cases, the *gsp* mutation was present in abnormal portions of a tissue but not in histologically normal portions of the same tissue (Fig. 73.4). Taken together these observations suggest that somatic mutations in the *GNAS* gene arise as a postzygotic event during early embryogenesis, with mosaic distribution of mutation-bearing cells following a developmental pattern. Other mutations that replace Arg[201] of *GNAS* have been identified only rarely in patients with MAS. Remarkably, to date no mutations in Gln[227] have been reported in patients with MAS.

Genetic modulation – alternative transcripts and imprinting of *GNAS*

GNAS is a highly complex locus that achieves tremendous transcriptional plasticity through the use of alternative exons, generation of antisense transcripts, and reciprocal imprinting [30]. Gα$_s$, the stimulatory G-protein of adenylyl cyclase, is expressed from both the maternal and paternal alleles in most tissues. However, in some cells (e.g. renal proximal tubule cells, thyroid follicular cells, and pituitary somatotrophs) there is preferential expression of the maternal allele [31]. Theoretically, in these tissues, only somatic mutations of the maternal allele will have pathophysiological consequences [32]. This seems to be the case for sporadic GH-secreting pituitary adenomas where activating mutations of Gα$_s$ were found to be on the maternal allele in 21 of 22 cases [33].

One alternative transcript of the GNAS locus worth mentioning is XLα$_s$, which is expressed exclusively from the paternal allele. XLα$_s$ shares carboxyl terminal sequences with Gα$_s$ but has a larger amino terminal end encoded by the alternate first exon. XLα$_s$ is enriched in the golgi of neuroendocrine tissues and functions in G-protein coupled signal transduction. A recent study has shown that *gsp* mutations in XLα$_s$ can affect signal transduction *in vitro* [34] but a role for *gsp* mutations in XLα$_s$ in human disease has yet to be defined.

Pathogenesis – summary

Taken in context, the clinical and endocrinological expression of MAS will be determined by several key variables. (1) Timing of the *gsp* mutation. The number of tissues in which the *gsp* is present, and the proportion and distribution of affected cells in a tissue, will be determined by the precise stage in development in which the mutation occurred. (2) The variable ability of cAMP to induce proliferation in different cells. Mutational activation of Gα$_s$ will have the most significant consequences in those tissues in which cAMP stimulates cellular proliferation and/or hormone secretion. Even in cells in which cAMP is a strong growth stimulator, induction of counter-regulatory responses (such as increased cAMP phosphodiesterase activity [35]) could mitigate or even reverse the effects of the activated Gα$_s$ phenotype. (3) Parental origin of the *GNAS* allele that carries the *gsp* mutation. MAS patients who have a *gsp* mutation of the maternal allele might have a more severe phenotype, particularly with regard to those tissues where imprinting silences expression of the paternal allele of Gα$_s$, e.g. autonomous thyroid nodules or GH-secreting pituitary adenomas.

Patient management

Diagnosis

The diagnosis of MAS is confirmed clinically when a patient is found to have at least two features of the classic triad of polyostotic fibrous dysplasia, café-au-lait pigmented skin lesions, and autonomous endocrinopathy [36]. Recent reports have suggested that the diagnosis should be considered in patients with any one of the three clinical manifestations of the full syndrome. For example, a recent study of children who were evaluated for fibrous dysplasia in orthopedic surgery clinics found that most patients had other clinical or endocrinological features that were consistent with MAS [37]. The identification of specific activating mutations in the

GNAS gene in patients with suspected MAS can provide a laboratory confirmation of the diagnosis, but cannot distinguish between MAS and a more limited disorder in which a *gsp* mutation occurs in only one tissue, such as isolated fibrous dysplasia or an ovarian cyst. Mutations in *GNAS* are more easily identified in affected tissues in which a high proportion of cells carry the *gsp* mutation, such as endocrine tumors and fibrous dysplasia, than in skin or peripheral leukocytes [4]. However, biopsy of affected tissues is only rarely indicated. Newer PCR techniques that utilize PNA (peptide nucleic acid) hybridization probes allow more sensitive detection of mutant alleles [29] or quantification of the mutant: normal alleles ratio [38].

Treatment

Given the variability of the expression and distribution of lesions in patients with MAS, treatment must be individualized for each patient. The history and physical examination should be directed to discovery of clinical features of precocious puberty, hyperthyroidism, hyperprolactinaemia, acromegaly, Cushing syndrome and skeletal deformity. An initial evaluation should include at a minimum: radiographs of affected bones; a ^{99m}Tc bone scan if bone lesions are not clinically evident; a chemistry panel, including liver function tests, calcium, phosphorus, and alkaline phosphatase; and assessment of endocrine function with measurement of serum levels of TSH, insulin-like growth factor-1 (IGF-1) and prolactin.

Bone disease

Polyostotic fibrous dysplasia may be asymptomatic or associated with pathological fractures or progressive deformities that require multiple orthopedic procedures. Craniofacial bone involvement is common in MAS, particularly with encasement of the optic nerves. However, encasement of the optic nerves does not lead to optic neuropathy, and as the condition appears to remain stable over time no specific treatment is indicated [39]. Highly potent nitrogen-containing bisphosphonates, such as intravenous pamidronate and zolendronic acid, remain the primary treatment for fibrous dysplasia, particularly for patients with extensive and/or symptomatic disease or patients who have lesions that threaten to fracture. Bisphosphonates afford considerable pain relief, but histological or radiographic improvement of bone lesions is far more variable, particularly in children and adolescents. There do not appear to be any reliable clinical or biological predictors of a favorable response to bisphosphonate therapy. Surgery may be complicated by heavy bleeding from affected bone. Radiation therapy to fibrous dysplastic lesions has been met with only limited success, and may induce osteosarcoma.

Hypophosphatemic osteomalacia or rickets is usually treated with calcitriol and inorganic phosphate supplements, but bone histology generally shows little improvement.

Endocrinopathies

Treatment of girls with MAS and precocious puberty is challenging. Therapy with GnRH analogs and super-agonists or Provera is not effective unless there has been a progression to central precocious puberty [40]. Past studies of aromatase inhibitors have been disappointing, but newer agents with greater potency (e.g. anastrazole and letrazole) may offer greater hope [41]. More recently a study of the selective estrogen inhibitor (SERM) tamoxifen showed promising results, with significant regression of breast development and reduced rate of advancement of bone age in most patients [42].

Pituitary-independent precocious puberty also occurs in boys with MAS, but it is much less common than in young girls. Approximately 10% of reported MAS patients with precocious puberty are male. Testicular biopsy in these cases reveals variable degrees of seminiferous tube development and Leydig cell hyperplasia. Treatment is similar to that for familial male precocious puberty due to activating mutations of the LH receptor (i.e., testitoxicosis), and consists of the combination of aromatase inhibitors plus spironalactone.

Hyperthyroidism may be treated long term with antithyroid drugs, radioactive iodine ablation, or surgical resection. It is often refractory to treatment and may recur years after successful treatment. Pituitary surgery for GH excess or hyperprolactinemia may be complicated by bleeding from dysplastic bone in the pituitary fossa. GH excess may respond to conventional medical therapy with the long-acting somatostatin analog octreotide and the GH receptor antagonist pegvisomant [43]. Treatment of Cushing syndrome has usually required bilateral adrenalectomy.

Prognosis

Because MAS is expressed in a mosaic distribution, the clinical manifestations extend over a wide spectrum. At one extreme, MAS may occur as a single endocrinopathy or an asymptomatic bone lesion, and the diagnosis of MAS may not be obvious. At the other extreme MAS may present at an early age with jaundice, abnormal liver function tests, persistent tachycardia, hyperthyroidism, Cushing syndrome, and extensive bone deformities, leading to death in childhood. Most patients with MAS live beyond reproductive age. Marked bone deformities may reduce life expectancy because of loss of mobility and attendant risks of thrombosis, infection, or ventilatory problems. Sudden death is an uncommon feature of MAS and may be due to cardiac involvement.

Conclusion

The diagnosis of MAS remains a clinical one, and requires a careful integration of physical findings, biochemical evaluation, and radiological examination. Specific *GNAS* gene mutations are detectable in DNA from affected tissues and in some cases peripheral blood leukocytes, and can confirm a clinical diagnosis of MAS. However, appropriate tissue samples may not be available and the necessary techniques for detection of the mutation are not currently offered by clinical reference laboratories. Recognition of the molecular basis of MAS and careful analysis of the phenotype has led to the appreciation that MAS involves many other tissues, including liver, heart, pancreas and thymus. This has enabled recognition of a severe form of the disease that is fatal in infancy or early childhood. The growing understanding of the diverse presentation of MAS now compels a more thorough evaluation of patients with fibrous dysplasia or café-au-lait pigmented skin lesions to determine whether they have subtle endocrinopathies. Finally, the genetic basis for MAS, mosaicism of a somatic *gsp* mutation, provides new insights into the role of imprinting as a modulator of human phenotype.

References

1. Albright F, Butler AM, Hampton AO, Smith P. Syndrome characterized by osteitis fibrosa disseminata, areas of pigmentation and endocrine dysfunction, with precocious puberty in females. *N. Engl. J. Med.* 1937;216:727–741.

2. McCune DJ, Bruch H. Osteodystrophia fibrosa. *Am. J. Dis. Child.* 1937;54:806–843.

3. Ringel MD, Schwindinger WF, Levine MA. Clinical implications of genetic defects in G proteins. The molecular basis of McCune–Albright syndrome and Albright hereditary osteodystrophy. *Medicine (Baltimore)* 1996;75:171–184.

4. Lumbroso S, Paris F, Sultan C; European Collaborative Study. Activating $G_s\alpha$ mutations: analysis of 113 patients with signs of McCune–Albright syndrome – a European Collaborative Study. *J. Clin. Endocrinol. Metab.* 2004;89:2107–2113.

5. Happle R. The McCune–Albright syndrome: a lethal gene surviving by mosaicism. *Clin. Genet.* 1986;29:321–324.

6. Parekh SG, Donthineni–Rao R, Ricchetti E, Lackman RD. Fibrous dysplasia. *J. Am. Acad. Orthop. Surg.* 2004;12:305–313.

7. Albright FA, Reifenstein EC. *The Parathyroid Glands and Metabolic Bone Disease*. Baltimore: Williams & Wilkins, 1948:282.

8. Candeliere GA, Glorieux FH, Prud'homme J, St-Arnaud R. Increased expression of the c-fos proto-oncogene in bone from patients with fibrous dysplasia. *N. Engl. J. Med.* 1995;332:1546–1551.

9. Motomura T, Kasayama S, Takagi M, et al. Increased interleukin-6 production in mouse osteoblastic MC3T3-E1 cells expressing activating mutant of the stimulatory G protein. *J. Bone Miner. Res.* 1998;13:1084–1091.

10. Sakamoto A, Chen M, Kobayashi T, Kronenberg HM, Weinstein LS. Chondrocyte-specific knockout of the G protein $G_s\alpha$ leads to epiphyseal and growth plate abnormalities and ectopic chondrocyte formation. *J. Bone Miner. Res.* 2005;20:663–671.

11. Bianco P, Kuznetsov SA, Riminucci M, Fisher LW, Spiegel AM, Robey PG. Reproduction of human fibrous dysplasia of bone in immunocompromised mice by transplanted mosaics of normal and Gsalpha-mutated skeletal progenitor cells. *J. Clin. Invest.* 1998;101:1737–1744.

12. Akintoye SO, Otis LL, Atkinson JC, et al. Analyses of variable panoramic radiographic characteristics of maxillo-mandibular fibrous dysplasia in McCune–Albright syndrome. *Oral Dis.* 2004;10:36–43.

13. Lee JS, FitzGibbon E, Butman JA, et al. Normal vision despite narrowing of the optic canal in fibrous dysplasia. *N. Engl. J. Med.* 2002;347:1670–1676.

14. Leet AI, Magur E, Lee JS, Wientroub S, Robey PG, Collins MT. Fibrous dysplasia in the spine: prevalence of lesions and association with scoliosis. *J. Bone Joint Surg. Am.* 2004;86-A:531–537.

15. Collins MT, Kushner H, Reynolds JC, et al. An instrument to measure skeletal burden and predict functional outcome in fibrous dysplasia of bone. *J. Bone Miner. Res.* 2005;20:219–226.

16. Lahlou N, Roger M. Inhibin B in pubertal development and pubertal disorders. *Semin. Reprod. Med.* 2004;22:165–175.

17. Arrigo T, Pirazzoli P, De Sanctis L, et al. McCune–Albright syndrome in a boy may present with a monolateral macroorchidism as an early and isolated clinical manifestation. *Horm. Res.* 2006; 65:114–119.

18. Wasniewska M, De Luca F, Bertelloni S, et al. Testicular microlithiasis: an unreported feature of McCune–Albright syndrome in males. *J. Pediatr.* 2004;145:670–672.

19. Collins MT, Sarlis NJ, Merino MJ, et al. Thyroid carcinoma in the McCune–Albright syndrome: contributory role of activating $G_s\alpha$ mutations. *J. Clin. Endocrinol. Metab.* 2003;88:4413–4417.

20. Akintoye SO, Chebli C, Booher S, et al. Characterization of *gsp*-mediated growth hormone excess in the context of McCune–Albright syndrome. *J. Clin. Endocrinol. Metab.* 2002;87:5104–5112.

21. Fragoso MC, Domenice S, Latronico AC, et al. Cushing's syndrome secondary to adrenocorticotropin-independent macronodular adrenocortical hyperplasia due to activating mutations of *GNAS1* gene. *J. Clin. Endocrinol. Metab.* 2003;88:2147–2151.

22. Riminucci M, Collins MT, Lala R, et al. An R201H activating mutation of the *GNAS1* (Gsα) gene in a corticotroph pituitary adenoma. *Mol. Pathol.* 2002;55:58–60.

23. Riminucci M, Collins MT, Fedarko NS, et al. FGF–23 in fibrous dysplasia of bone and its relationship to renal phosphate wasting. *J. Clin. Invest.* 2003;112:683–692.

24. Shenker A, Weinstein LS, Moran A, et al Severe endocrine and nonendocrine manifestations of the McCune–Albright syndrome associated with activating mutations of stimulatory G protein G_s. *J. Pediatr.* 1993;123:509–518.

25. Landis CA, Masters SB, Spada A, Pace AM, Bourne HR, Vallar L. GTPase inhibiting mutations activate the α chain of G_s and stimulate adenylyl cyclase in human pituitary tumours. *Nature* 1989;340:692–696.

26. Weinstein LS, Shenker A, Gejman PV, Merino MJ, Friedman E, Spiegel AM. Activating mutations of the stimulatory G protein in the McCune–Albright syndrome. *N. Engl. J. Med.* 1991;325:1688–1695.

27. Schwindinger WF, Francomano CA, Levine MA. Identification of a mutation in the gene encoding the alpha subunit of the stimulatory G protein of adenylyl cyclase in McCune–Albright syndrome. *Proc. Natl. Acad. Sci. U S A* 1992;89:5152–5156.

28. Shenker A, Weinstein LS, Sweet DE, Spiegel AM. An activating $G_s\alpha$ mutation is present in fibrous dysplasia of bone in the McCune–Albright syndrome. *J. Clin. Endocrinol. Metab.* 1994;79:750–755.

29. Lietman SA, Ding C, Levine MA. A highly sensitive polymerase chain reaction method detects activating mutations of the GNAS gene in peripheral blood cells in McCune–Albright syndrome or isolated fibrous dysplasia. *J. Bone Joint Surg. Am.* 2005;87:2489–2494.

30. Weinstein LS, Liu J, Sakamoto A, Xie T, Chen M. Minireview: GNAS: normal and abnormal functions. *Endocrinology* 2004;145:5459–5464.

31. Germain-Lee EL, Ding CL, Deng Z, et al. Paternal imprinting of $G\alpha_s$ in the human thyroid as the basis of TSH resistance in pseudohypoparathyroidism type 1a. *Biochem. Biophys. Res. Commun.* 2002;296: 67–72.

32. Mantovani G, Bondioni S, Lania AG, et al. Parental origin of $G_s\alpha$ mutations in the McCune–Albright syndrome and in isolated endocrine tumors. *J. Clin. Endocrinol. Metab.* 2004;89:3007–3009.

33. Hayward BE, Barlier A, Korbonits M, et al. Imprinting of the $G_s\alpha$ gene *GNAS1* in the pathogenesis of acromegaly. *J. Clin. Invest.* 2001;107:R31–36.

34. Linglart A, Mahon MJ, Kerachian MA, et al. Coding GNAS mutations leading to hormone resistance impair *in vitro* agonist- and cholera toxin-induced cAMP formation mediated by human $XL\alpha_s$. *Endocrinology* 2006;147:2253–2262

35. Lania A, Persani L, Ballare E, Mantovani S, Losa M, Spada A. Constitutively active $G_s\alpha$ is associated with an increased phosphodiesterase activity in human growth hormone–secreting adenomas. *J. Clin. Endocrinol. Metab.* 1998;83:1624–1628.

36. Lee PA, Van Dop C, Migeon CJ. McCune–Albright syndrome. Long-term follow-up. *JAMA* 1986; 256:2980–2984.

37. Hannon TS, Noonan K, Steinmetz R, Eugster EA, Levine MA, Pescovitz OH. Is McCune–Albright syndrome overlooked in subjects with fibrous dysplasia of bone? *J. Pediatr.* 2003;142:532–538.

38. Karadag A, Riminucci M, Bianco P, et al. A novel technique based on a PNA hybridization probe and FRET principle for quantification of mutant genotype in fibrous dysplasia/McCune–Albright syndrome. *Nucleic Acids Res.* 2004;32:e63.

39. Cutler CM, Lee JS, Butman JA, et al. Long-term outcome of optic nerve encasement and optic nerve decompression in patients with fibrous dysplasia: risk factors for blindness and safety of observation. *Neurosurgery* 2006;59:1011–1017.

40. Schmidt H, Kiess W. Secondary central precocious puberty in a girl with McCune–Albright syndrome responds to treatment with GnRH analogue. *J. Pediatr. Endocrinol. Metab.* 1998;11:77–81.

41. Roth C, Freiberg C, Zappel H, Albers N. Effective aromatase inhibition by anastrozole in a patient with gonadotropin-independent precocious puberty in McCune–Albright syndrome. *J. Pediatr. Endocrinol. Metab.* 2002;15(Suppl. 3):945–948.

42. Eugster EA, Rubin SD, Reiter EO, Plourde P, Jou HC, Pescovitz OH; McCune–Albright Study Group. Tamoxifen treatment for precocious puberty in McCune–Albright syndrome: a multicenter trial. *J. Pediatr.* 2003;143:9–10.

43. Akintoye SO, Kelly MH, Brillante B, et al. Pegvisomant for the treatment of *gsp*-mediated growth hormone excess in patients with McCune–Albright syndrome. *J. Clin. Endocrinol. Metab.* 2006;91: 2960–2966.

74 Cowden Syndrome

Ingrid Witters and Jean-Pierre Fryns

> **Key points**
> - Cowden syndrome is a multiple hamartoma syndrome affecting derivates of all three germ cell layers with a high risk of benign and malignant tumors of the breast, thyroid and endometrium.
> - Affected individuals usually have macrocephaly, trichilemmomas (benign follicular epithelial neoplasms) and papillomatous papules usually presenting by the late 20s.
> - The lifetime risk for breast cancer is 25–50%, for thyroid cancer (non-medullary) around 10%, and for endometrial cancer 5–10%.
> - Cowden syndrome is caused by a mutation in the tumor suppressor gene *PTEN* (phosphatase and tensin homolog) on chromosome 10q23.
> - At least 80% of Cowden syndrome patients have a phosphatase and tensin homolog mutation.

Disease characteristics

Cowden syndrome is a part of the phosphatase and tensin homolog (PTEN) hamartoma tumor syndrome (PHTS) which also includes Bannayan–Riley–Ruvalcaba syndrome (BRRS, MIM 153480, macrocephaly, hamartomatous intestinal polyposis, lipomas, and pigmented macules of the glans penis), Proteus syndrome (MIM 176920, a highly variable disorder involving congenital malformations, hamartomatous overgrowth of multiple tissues, connective tissue and epidermal nevi and hyperostoses with a mosaic distribution and sporadic occurrence), and Proteus-like syndrome (individuals with significant clinical features of Proteus syndrome who do not meet the diagnostic criteria).

Clinical aspects

Mucocutaneous findings

Most patients with Cowden syndrome present to the physician with mucocutaneous manifestations, occurring in 90–100% of affected individuals. Cutaneous facial lesions are most commonly trichilemmomas (benign follicular epithelial lesions), often multiple and located primarily on and around the eyelids, alae nasi, nasolabial folds, mouth, pinnas, lateral neck, glabella and the dorsa of the hands and forearms.

Oral lesions include benign fibromas, presenting as whitish papules in the gingival, labial and palatal surface of the mouth in more than 80% of patients. The lesions may coalesce and produce a cobblestone appearance. Thickening of the tongue (scrotal tongue) can be present.

Acral keratoses (flesh-colored verrucoid papules) are present in more than 60% of patients on the dorsal hands and feet as well as palmoplantar keratoses (translucent punctuate keratoses) on the palms or soles.

Less frequently noted lesions include subcutaneous lipomas and cutaneous hemangiomas. Squamous cell carcinoma of the skin of the nose and basal cell carcinoma of the face/perianal skin have been reported.

Cranial findings

More than 80% of patients with Cowden syndrome have macrocephaly (Fig. 74.1), and can present with an adenoid face, small jaws and a high arched palate. Lhermitte–Duclos disease, or

Clinical Endocrine Oncology, 2nd edition. Edited by Ian D. Hay and John A.H. Wass. © 2008 Blackwell Publishing. ISBN 978-1-4051-4584-8.

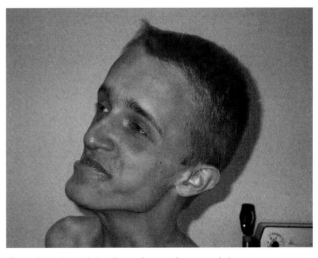

Figure 74.1 Boy with Cowden syndrome with macrocephaly.

dysplastic gangliocytoma of the cerebellum, is considered part of Cowden syndrome. It is characterized by an overgrowth of cerebellar ganglion cells, which replace granular cells and Purkinje cells. The clinical presentation is that of a cerebellar mass with ataxia, intracranial hypertension, and hydrocephalus, often presenting in late childhood or young adulthood.

Meningiomas have been reported, and also astrocytoma and medulloblastoma. Mental retardation and autism/pervasive developmental disorder are present in about 10% of patients.

Thyroid/breast/endometrial cancer

Thyroid lesions, present in approximately 60% of patients, include goiter, benign adenomas and thyroglossal cysts. Thyroid non-medullary cancer develops in about 10% of patients. Breast involvement with fibrocystic dysplasia and fibroadenomas is present in 75% of patients and 25–50% develop a breast carcinoma. As with other hereditary cancer syndromes, the risk of bilateral breast cancer is increased. Breast carcinoma has been reported also in males with Cowden syndrome. Endometrial carcinoma develops in 5–10% of patients with Cowden syndrome.

Other manifestations

Other possible genitourinary manifestations include uterine fibroids and renal cell carcinoma. Further manifestations are gastrointestinal polyps, most common in the colon, with low malignant potential and skeletal manifestations as bone cysts, thoracal kyphoscoliosis [1–4].

Diagnostic criteria

Consensus diagnostic criteria for Cowden syndrome have been developed [2] and updated each year by the National Comprehensive Cancer Network [5] and have been divided in to three categories.

1. *Pathognomonic criteria*

Adult Lhermitte–Duclos disease (LDD), defined as the presence of a cerebellar dysplastic gangliocytoma

Mucocutaneous lesions:

Trichilemmomas (facial)

Acral keratoses

Papillomatous lesions

Mucosal lesions.

2. *Major criteria*

Breast cancer

Thyroid cancer (non-medullary), especially follicular thyroid epithelial cancer

Macrocephaly (occipital frontal circumference ≥ 97th percentile)

Endometrial carcinoma.

3. *Minor criteria*

Other thyroid lesions (e.g., adenoma, multinodular goiter)

Mental retardation (IQ ≤ 75)

Hamartomatous intestinal polyps

Fibrocystic disease of the breast

Lipomas

Fibromas

Genitourinary tumors (especially renal cell carcinoma)

Genitourinary malformation

Uterine fibroids.

An operational diagnosis of Cowden syndrome is made if an individual meets any one of the following criteria:

- Pathognomonic mucocutaneous lesions alone if there are:

  Six or more facial papules, of which three or more must be trichilemmoma, or

  Cutaneous facial papules and oral mucosal papillomatosis, or

  Oral mucosal papillomatosis and acral keratoses, or

  Six or more palmoplantar keratoses

or

- Two or more major criteria

or

- One major and at least three minor criteria

or

- At least four minor criteria.

In a family in which one individual meets the diagnostic criteria for Cowden syndrome listed above, other relatives are considered to have a diagnosis of CS if they meet any one of the following criteria:

- The pathognomonic criteria *or*
- Any one major criterion with or without minor criteria *or*
- Two minor criteria *or*
- History of Bannayan–Riley–Ruvalcaba syndrome.

Prevalence

Because the diagnosis of Cowden syndrome is difficult to establish, the true prevalence is unknown. The prevalence has been estimated at 1 in 200 000 [6, 7], but this is likely an underestimation because of the often subtle external manifestations [8, 9].

Molecular genetics

Approximately 80% of individuals who meet the diagnostic criteria for Cowden syndrome have a detectable *PTEN* gene (phosphatase and tensin homolog) mutation. *PTEN* is a tumor suppressor gene located on 10q23.31.

The *PTEN* gene is responsible in embryonic development for organizing the relationship among different cell types and thegene encodes a dual-specificity phosphatase that plays a broad role in sporadic human malignancy. The wild-type protein is a major lipid phosphatase that downregulates the PI3K/Akt pathway to cause G1 arrest and apoptosis. In addition, the protein phosphatase appears to play an important role in inhibition of cell migration and spreading, as well as downregulating several cell cyclins [1, 10].

Genetically related (allelic) disorders

Bannayan–Riley–Ruvalcaba syndrome is allelic to Cowden syndrome with germline mutations of *PTEN* in approximately 50–60% of individuals with Bannayan–Riley–Ruvalcaba syndrome [11].

Families have been reported with some individuals having Cowden syndrome and others Bannayan–Riley–Ruvalcaba syndrome with germline *PTEN* mutations in >90% of these families [12]. In patients with Bannayan–Riley–Ruvalcaba syndrome and an identified *PTEN* mutation cancer surveillance is therefore mandatory.

In approximately 20% of patients with Proteus syndrome germline *PTEN* mutations have been identified and approximately 50% of patients with a Proteus-like syndrome were also found to have germline *PTEN* mutations [13].

Although Lhermitte–Duclos disease is usually sporadic, PTEN mutations were identified in tissues from Lhermitte–Duclos disease lesions and all these cases had *adult* onset of the disease [14].

In addition, *PTEN* mutations have been identified in patients with macrocephaly and autistic features [15, 16]. Recently, Butler et al. [17] found that approximately 20% of individuals with autism spectrum disorders and macrocephaly have germline *PTEN* mutations.

At least one child with vertebral anomalies, anal atresia, tracheoesophageal fistula and radial and renal anomalies (VATER) association and macrocephaly has been found to have a germline *PTEN* mutation [18] and one child with Bannayan–Riley–Ruvalcaba syndrome-like features and hemimegalencephaly was found to have a germline *PTEN* IVS5+1delG mutation [11].

Management

Because the most important consequences of Cowden syndrome relate to the increased risk of breast, thyroid, and endometrial cancer, increased cancer surveillance is mandatory. Surveillance in general for individuals with *PTEN* mutations (with Cowden syndrome, Bannayan–Riley–Ruvalcaba syndrome, Proteus syndrome, or Proteus-like syndromes) includes annual physical examination from age 18 years, annual urinalysis, and baseline colonoscopy at age 50 years.

Specific surveillance for breast cancer in individuals with Cowden syndrome includes monthly self-examination beginning at age 18 years (for females and males), annual clinical breast examinations beginning at age 25 years, and annual mammography and breast magnetic resonance imaging (MRI) beginning at age 30–35 years [5]. Some patients prefer a bilateral prophylactic mastectomy [19]. The use of tamoxifen for reduction of breast cancer risk is not advised.

Surveillance for thyroid cancer includes annual thyroid ultrasound examination at 18 years and annual thyroid ultrasound examinations.

Surveillance for endometrial cancer includes annual suction biopsies beginning at age 35–40 years for premenopausal women and annual transvaginal ultrasound examination for postmenopausal women with biopsy of suspicious areas. For the mucocutaneous manifestations of Cowden syndrome topical agents (e.g., 5-fluorouracil), curettage, cryosurgery, or laser ablation can be used and excision of lesions is only advised if malignancy is suspected or symptoms are important since excision causes cheloid formation and recurrence risk of lesions is high.

Therapy under investigation: mTOR inhibitors

There are a number of studies under way investigating targeted cancer therapy that inhibits the activity of mTOR (mammalian Target of Rapamycin), a cellular enzyme that plays a key role in cell growth and proliferation.

Indeed, the absence of functional *PTEN* in cancer cells leads to constitutive activation of downstream components of the PI3K pathway including the Akt and mTOR kinases. In model organisms, inactivation of these kinases can reverse the effects of *PTEN* loss. These data raise the possibility that drugs targeting these kinases, or PI3K itself, might have significant therapeutic activity in *PTEN*-null cancers.

Akt kinase inhibitors are still in development; however, as a first test of this hypothesis, Phase I and Phase II trials of inhibitors of mTOR, namely, rapamycin and rapamycin analogs, are under way [20].

Genetic counseling

Inheritance is autosomal dominant with complete penetrance and variable expression. There is an excess of affected females. Only 10–50% of individuals with Cowden syndrome have an affected parent [21]. If neither parent has a *PTEN* mutation and no clinical manifestations, the risk to sibs is low since germline mosaicism has not been reported.

Prenatal diagnosis is possible in families with a known *PTEN* mutation by analysis of DNA extracted from fetal cells obtained by amniocentesis/chorionic villus sampling. Preimplantation genetic diagnosis is at present available in a small number of genetic centers.

References

1. Gorlin RJ, Cohen MMJ, Hennekam RCM. Cowden syndrome. In *Syndromes of the Head and Neck*, 4th edn. Oxford: Oxford University Press, 2001:432–437.

2. Eng C. Will the real Cowden syndrome please stand up: revised diagnostic criteria. *J. Med. Genet.* 2000;37:828–830.

3. Van Calenbergh F, Vantomme N, Flamen P, et al. Lhermitte–Duclos disease: 11C-methionine positron emission tomography data in 4 patients. *Surg. Neurol.* 2006;65:293–296.

4. Brownstein MH, Wolf M, Bikowski JB. Cowden's disease: a cutaneous marker of breast cancer. *Cancer* 1978;41:2393–2398.

5. NCCN. National Comprehensive Cancer Network. Genetic/Familial High-Risk Assessment: Breast and Ovarian. Clinical Practice Guidelines in Oncology – v.1.2006. http://www.nccn.org/professionals/physician_gls/PDF/genetics_screening.pdf

6. Nelen MR, van Staveren WC, Peeters EA, et al. Germline mutations in the PTEN/MMAC1 gene in patients with Cowden disease. *Hum. Mol. Genet.* 1997;6:1383–1387.

7. Nelen MR, Kremer H, Konings IB, et al. Novel PTEN mutations in patients with Cowden disease: absence of clear genotype-phenotype correlations. *Eur. J. Hum. Genet.* 1999;7:267–273.

8. Haibach H, Burns TW, Carlson HE, Burman KD, Deftos LJ. Multiple hamartoma syndrome (Cowden's disease) associated with renal cell carcinoma and primary neuroendocrine carcinoma of the skin (Merkel cell carcinoma). *Am. J. Clin. Pathol.* 1992;97:705–712.

9. Schrager CA, Schneider D, Gruener AC, Tsou HC, Peacocke M. Clinical and pathological features of breast disease in Cowden's syndrome: an underrecognized syndrome with an increased risk of breast cancer. *Hum. Pathol.* 1998;29:47–53.

10. Eng C. PTEN: one gene, many syndromes. *Hum. Mutat.* 2003;22:183–198.

11. Merks JH, de Vries LS, Zhou XP, et al. PTEN hamartoma tumour syndrome: variability of an entity. *J. Med. Genet.* 2003;40:e111.

12. Marsh DJ, Coulon V, Lunetta KL, et al. Mutation spectrum and genotype-phenotype analyses in Cowden disease and Bannayan–Zonana syndrome, two hamartoma syndromes with germline *PTEN* mutation. *Hum. Mol. Genet.* 1998;7:507–515.

13. Zhou X, Hampel H, Thiele H, et al. Association of germline mutation in the PTEN tumour suppressor gene and Proteus and Proteus-like syndromes. *Lancet* 2001;358:210–211.

14. Zhou XP, Marsh DJ, Morrison CD, et al. Germline inactivation of PTEN and dysregulation of the phosphoinositol-3-kinase/Akt pathway cause human Lhermitte–Duclos disease in adults. *Am. J. Hum. Genet.* 2003;73:1191–1198.

15. Dasouki MJ, Ishmael H, Eng C. Macrocephaly, macrosomia and autistic behaviour due to a de novo PTEN germline mutation [abstract 564]. *Am. J. Hum. Genet.* 2001;69S:280.

16. Goffin A, Hoefsloot LH, Bosgoed E, Swillen A, Fryns JP. PTEN mutation in a family with Cowden syndrome and autism. *Am. J. Med. Genet.* 2001;105:521–524.

17. Butler MG, Dasouki MJ, Zhou XP, et al. Subset of individuals with autism spectrum disorders and extreme macrocephaly associated with germline PTEN tumour suppressor gene mutations. *J. Med. Genet.* 2005;42:318–321.

18. Reardon W, Zhou XP, Eng C. A novel germline mutation of the *PTEN* gene in a patient with macrocephaly, ventricular dilatation, and features of VATER association. *J. Med. Genet.* 2001;38:820–823.

19. Hartmann LC, Schaid DJ, Woods JE, et al. Efficacy of bilateral prophylactic mastectomy in women with a family history of breast cancer. *N. Engl. J. Med.* 1999;340:77–84.

20. Sansal I, Sellers WR. The biology and clinical relevance of the PTEN tumor suppressor pathway. *J. Clin. Oncol.* 2004;22:2954–2963.

21. Marsh DJ, Kum JB, Lunetta KL, et al. *PTEN* mutation spectrum and genotype–phenotype correlations in Bannayan–Riley–Ruvalcaba syndrome suggest a single entity with Cowden syndrome. *Hum. Mol. Genet.* 1999;8:1461–1472.

75 Paraneoplastic Syndromes

David William Ray

Key points
- Paraneoplastic syndromes may lead to diagnosis of underlying cancer.
- Paraneoplastic syndromes carry their own burden of morbidity.
- The majority of syndromes have an autoimmune basis.
- Diagnosis depends on exclusion of other cancer-related processes, e.g., metastasis.
- Specific therapy is available for some manifestations, and may improve patient well-being.

Introduction

The term paraneoplastic syndrome refers to symptom complexes and diseases that are associated with the presence of underlying malignancy. It is important to exclude effects caused by toxicity of cancer therapy, co-existent vascular disease, coagulopathies, infection and either toxic or metabolic causes before inferring the presence of a paraneoplastic syndrome. The general principles of the paraneoplastic syndromes are either aberrant protein expression, such as the ectopic adrenocorticotropic hormone (ACTH) syndrome (see Chapter 78), or presentation of protein to the immune system, as in the Lambert–Eaton syndrome, discussed later in this chapter. It has been argued that ectopic hormone production in cancer is rather an accentuated production of low-level gene expression seen in healthy tissue. In this regard it is important that those hormones most frequently found to be expressed in cancer have the widest expression in health, such as ACTH peptides, while those with very restricted expression are only very rarely found to be aberrantly expressed in cancer, for example renin. Therefore, if the cancer cell phenotype results from a pattern of dysdifferentiation of a pleuripotent progenitor cell, the augmented hormone production either results from altered control of its gene or low-level production occurring in a vastly increased number of cells.

In this chapter distant manifestations of cancer caused by either hormonal overproduction or metabolic insult will not be considered – for example, Cushing syndrome (see Chapter 31), hyponatremia (see Chapter 76), hypercalcemia (see Chapter 77) and hypoglycemia (see Chapter 79) – as they are covered elsewhere.

Clinical Endocrine Oncology, 2nd edition. Edited by Ian D. Hay and John A.H. Wass. © 2008 Blackwell Publishing. ISBN 978-1-4051-4584-8.

Paraneoplastic disorders are less common than other distant manifestations of malignancy caused by, for example, metastases in the central nervous system. However, they are important for several reasons. The first reason is that some patients will present with a paraneoplastic syndrome, which will be the first clue of the presence of an underlying malignancy. Second, the paraneoplastic syndrome itself may be the cause of severe morbidity and even premature mortality and therefore merits prompt diagnosis and appropriate treatment in its own right. Third, in patients with a known diagnosis of cancer who are perhaps undergoing treatment the emergence of a paraneoplastic syndrome needs to be recognized, to distinguish it from the presence of disseminated malignancy, which may well carry a widely different prognosis.

Although most types of tumor have been described to be associated with paraneoplastic disorders in the majority of cases there is a clear association between the paraneoplastic syndrome and the tumor type. Neuroblastoma in childhood and small cell lung carcinoma in adults are the most frequently associated with paraneoplastic phenomena. The diversity of paraneoplastic manifestations would suggest a plurality of causative mechanisms. However, although in many cases a precise mechanism has not been identified the majority of neurological and cutaneous paraneoplastic syndromes can be associated with autoimmune phenomena. A common mechanism, therefore, is a host versus tumor immune response which gives rise to circulating antibodies with significant cross-reactivity to self antigens. In one recent study of patients with small cell lung cancer it was found that patients with antibodies to the voltage-gated calcium channel and features of Lambert–Eaton myasthenia syndrome had a significantly better prognosis than antibody-positive patients without the syndrome or patients without antibodies. These data could be interpreted as showing that patients who mounted the most robust antitumor immune response, as manifest by autoimmune disease, had, as a direct result, a better prognosis [1].

Paraneoplastic syndromes are discussed in two sections: neurological manifestations and cutaneous manifestations.

Neurological paraneoplastic syndromes

Paraneoplastic syndromes may affect any part of the central nervous system (CNS) and the peripheral nervous system. It is also important to recognize that although some clinical syndromes, for example the Lambert–Eaton myasthenia syndrome, should always raise suspicion of a paraneoplastic etiology, there is no neurological syndrome that is exclusively seen in the presence of an underlying neoplasm and any of the disorders discussed here may occur in patients without an underlying tumor. The classic neurological paraneoplastic syndromes are listed in Table 75.1.

As discussed above it is thought that the majority of neurological paraneoplastic disorders are autoimmune in nature. Over the last 20 years there has been a steady rise in the number of well-characterized antineuronal antibodies identified in the serum of patients with paraneoplastic disorders. These are summarized in Table 75.2. Using these antibodies as tools, a number of new autoantibody target molecules have been cloned and characterized. Some of the paraneoplastic antibodies have a particular selectivity, for example anti-recoverin antibodies in patients with retinal degeneration. However, the majority of paraneoplastic autoantibodies show a more widespread reactivity with neuronal tissue and are associated with a variety of different neurological syndromes. The most frequently seen antibodies in this context are those directed against Hu and CV2 antigens. Small cell lung cancer is particularly associated with development of such antibodies and many patients with this disorder will have multiple autoantibodies reacting against different target molecules [2]. The target molecules for the common auto antibodies are listed in Table 75.3.

Table 75.1 Classic paraneoplastic neurological syndromes

Encephalomyelitis
Limbic encephalitis
Subacute cerebellar degeneration
Opsoclonus–myoclonus
Subacute sensory neuronopathy
Chronic gastrointestinal pseudo obstruction
Lambert–Eaton myasthenia syndrome
Dermatomyositis

Table 75.2 Paraneoplastic syndromes and associated autoantibodies

Syndrome	Antibody
Lambert–Eaton syndrome	VGCC
Encephalomyelitis	Hu, CV2, ANNA3, amphiphysin
Limbic encephalitis	Tr, ANNA-3, amphiphysin, Hu, CV2, PCA-1, mGluR1, VGKC, Zic4
Opsoclonus–myoclonus	Ri, Yo, Hu, amphiphysin, Ma2
Retinal degeneration	recoverin
Sensorimotor neuronopathy	Hu, CV2, ANNA-3

Table 75.3 Autoantigens implicated in paraneoplastic neurological syndromes

Recoverin	Retinal protein involved in rhodopsin phosphorylation
ANNA-3	170kD protein expressed in hippocampus and cerebellum
Amphiphysin	125kD protein in synaptic vesicles
Hu	RNA binding proteins expressed in neurons
Yo	Purkinje cell protein
Ri	CNS neuron expressed protein
CV2	66kD protein expressed in retina, optic nerve, neurons, and oligodendrocytes
Tr	Purkinje cell expressed protein
VGKC	Voltage-gated potassium channel
Zic4	Cerebellar and hippocampus expressed protein

As with most autoimmune diseases associated with autoreactive antibodies the causative role of the antibodies in the development of the syndrome is relevant. Some neurological paraneoplastic syndromes appear to be directly caused by antibody action. The best characterized example of this is the Lambert–Eaton myasthenia syndrome, which is caused by antibodies reacting with voltage-gated calcium channels at presynaptic neuromuscular junctions. These antibodies may also cause neurological injury in subsets of patients with paraneoplastic cerebellar degeneration. In addition, antirecoverin antibodies almost certainly exert a direct cytotoxic effect to cause carcinoma-associated retinal degeneration. However, it is also likely that some antibodies, for example anti-Hu or anti-Yo, do not directly cause injury, as certainly *in vitro* they do not appear to cause damage to cultured neurons and animals immunized to generate high titer antibodies do not show any clinical or pathological signs of disease. In this case it seems more likely that the development of the autoantibodies is a marker for autoimmune damage caused by T-cells. This is supported by adoptive transfer experiments in which rat T-lymphocytes specific for onconeural proteins cause meningeal inflammation and cell infiltration in recipient animals [3–5].

Patient management

It is important to rationally break down the clinical management of patients with either known or suspected paraneoplastic syndromes. There are four important components which include: first, the appropriate diagnosis of the syndrome; second, diagnosis of the underlying tumor; third, treatment of the underlying tumor; and fourth, consideration of treatment for the autoimmune process causing the paraneoplastic syndrome.

There is a clear difference between investigation of patients with known underlying malignancy and those with a possible paraneoplastic presentation. In patients with a known underlying cancer diagnosis the cell type will influence the level of suspicion. For example, as mentioned above small cell lung cancer is frequently associated with paraneoplastic disorders whereas squamous cell lung carcinoma is not. It is also important to consider if the neurological manifestations are as a result of metastatic disease, therapeutic toxicity, metabolic derangement or CNS infection.

In patients without a previous cancer diagnosis the level of suspicion will be influenced by risk factors for an underlying malignancy including age, smoking history, gender and the neurological syndrome. It is important to recognize that the underlying tumor may remain occult despite repeated search. Therefore, in all patients in whom conventional imaging studies are negative, repeated imaging or fluorodeoxyglucose positron emission tomography should be considered [6].

Classic syndromes

A number of syndromes are often found to be associated with underlying cancer. Identification of such a syndrome should always prompt investigation for an occult tumor. If during such a search a tumor is found that is not usually associated with the syndrome it is recommended that the search be continued to look for a second, more typical, underlying tumor [6]. The classic syndromes are listed in Table 75.1.

Encephalomyelitis
This diagnostic term is used to describe patients with clinical dysfunction at multiple levels of the CNS including dorsal route ganglia or myenteric plexus. In fact, the term is not quite accurate as many patients show involvement of peripheral nerves as well. However, the diagnostic label has become established. Another problem with a diagnostic label of encephalomyelitis is that there is a lack of information on the predominant clinical manifestation seen in an individual patient. Hence, wherever possible, a more precise identification of the main neurological dysfunction should be considered [7, 8].

Limbic encephalitis
This diagnosis is suggested by a progressive neurological syndrome of days to weeks in duration consisting of convulsions, memory disturbance, confusion and multiple psychiatric problems. Definitive diagnosis must also include either neuroradiological evidence of limbic dysfunction such as magnetic resonance imaging (MRI) scanning or neuropathological analysis. In the majority of patients there is cerebrospinal fluid (CSF) evidence of inflammation, which may be used to support the clinical diagnosis. Although high titers of autoantibodies directed to the voltage-gated potassium channel are seen in this syndrome these are not specific enough to be relied on to make a diagnosis [7, 9, 10].

Subacute cerebellar degeneration
This syndrome is characterized by development, in less than 3 months, of a severe cerebellar syndrome with no magnetic resonance evidence of cerebellar atrophy. The severity of the syndrome should be sufficient to significantly interfere with the lifestyle of the patient. Typically isolated or prominent gait ataxia is present in the early stages but truncal and hemispheric

cerebellar dysfunction is required for diagnosis. It is not uncommon for other manifestations outside the cerebellum to be present. In particular, there is a significant association with Lambert–Eaton myasthenia syndrome, particularly in patients with lung cancer [7, 11].

Sensory neuronopathy
This diagnosis is suggested by onset over less than 3 months of severe numbness and pain, often with marked asymmetry, affecting the arms and legs with associated loss of proprioception and electrophysiological evidence that shows involvement of sensory fibers in at least one of the nerves studied. Again, sensory neuronopathy is often not an isolated syndrome and there may be demonstrated involvement of motor nerves, autonomic nervous system or the brain as well [12].

Opsoclonus–myoclonus
Opsoclonus–myoclonus syndrome (OMS) is a rare syndrome that can occur as a paraneoplastic manifestation but also can occur following viral infection. In childhood more than half of cases occur in the presence of underlying neuroblastoma. Characteristic features of OMS are an acute onset of chaotic and rapid eye movements leading to its alternative designation, dancing eyes syndrome. In addition, there is associated myoclonic jerking and often neuro-psychiatric manifestations. The pathogenesis of the condition is not determined but as immunosuppressive therapies may ameliorate the features it seems possible that there is an immune etiology.

Autoantibodies, including antineurofilament, anti-Hu, anti-Ri, and other autoreactive antibodies, have been frequently reported in OMS. Histological examination of the associated tumors often identifies interstitial and perivascular lymphoid infiltrates, with some resemblance to lymphoid follicles. These immunological foci within the tumor may be important for the development of a specific immune response, which generates cross-reacting autoantibodies, and so to the development of the neurological syndrome.

Because of the rarity of the syndrome in the general population and the relatively high rates of association with underlying malignancy, it is particularly important to thoroughly investigate patients presenting with OMS for tumors. There is evidence that repeat evaluation with thin cut computerized tomography (CT) scanning identifies neuroblastoma in a number of cases that have previously escaped detection with conventional imaging procedures. It is also possible that in some of the cases that are apparently idiopathic spontaneous regression of an occult neuroblastoma, tumor may have been the underlying cause.

The diagnostic approach for possible underlying neuroblastoma should include, after exclusion of central nervous system pathology with brain, MRI scan and lumbar puncture, imaging of the adrenal glands with thin cut CT, meta-iodobenzylguanidine (MIBG) and also urinary measurements for catecholamines.

The acute neurological findings of OMS include ataxia, difficulty in walking and irritability. The movement disorder is accompanied by opsoclonus. Opsoclonus is a very distinctive eye movement and is dissimilar to nystagmus. The eye movements tend to be conjugate, non-phasic and multidirectional. The eye movements can often be provoked by changing gaze fixation from far to near and they can occur in bursts. In cases where they are not prominent careful observations with changes in fixation of gaze may be required to unmask them. It is also important to note that OMS may occur as late as a few weeks after the onset of motor systems.

There is little systematic evidence for beneficial effect of specific treatment for OMS. Clearly initial treatment priority should be directed against the underlying tumor, should it be identified. Thereafter there is some evidence of benefit with immunosuppression but such an approach is not without its own risks [13].

Chronic gastrointestinal pseudo-obstruction

Impaired gastrointestinal mobility is a relatively recently recognized paraneoplastic manifestation. It is described to occur with small cell lung cancer and with other tumors including thymoma. In one study 80% of patients with gut dysmotility were found to have autoantibodies present. These antibodies reacted with neurons of the myenteric submucosal plexus in the gut. Antibodies of this type were not found in a control group of patients with non-paraneoplastic pseudo-obstruction [14]. More recently, analysis has identified the specificity of the autoantibodies as being directed against voltage-gated potassium channels. In isolated case reports plasmapheresis had a beneficial effect, suggesting that in fact the circulating antibodies may be playing a causal role in development of the pseudo-obstruction. It has been proposed that the presence of such voltage-gated potassium channel antibodies in a patient presenting with pseudo-obstruction should prompt a search for underlying malignancy [7, 15].

Lambert–Eaton myasthenia syndrome

Lambert–Eaton syndrome is a disorder of the neuromuscular junction. This neurological site lies outside the protection of the blood–brain barrier and therefore is perhaps particularly vulnerable to immunological attack. The other common neuromuscular junction disorder is myasthenia gravis, which is itself frequently found to be associated with underlying thymoma. However, myasthenia will not be considered further here.

The common feature of neuromuscular junction disorders is symptomatic muscle weakness that tends to pick out particular muscles and varies in severity according to muscle usage. It is indeed this characteristic feature, particularly picking out proximal muscle groups, that usually suggests the diagnosis.

Diagnosis of Lambert–Eaton myasthenia syndrome can be confirmed by identification of circulating antibodies directed against the voltage-gated calcium channel and also by electrophysiological analysis [16]. In particular, repetitive nerve stimulation gives a characteristic electrophysiological pattern and single fiber electromyography also demonstrates a characteristic feature in patients with Lambert–Eaton myasthenia syndrome, typically showing abnormal jitter. The magnitude of jitter is frequently found to be far greater than would be predicted by the relatively mild degree of clinical weakness seen.

The underlying malignancy in Lambert–Eaton myasthenia syndrome is most frequently found to be small cell lung cancer. In patients with lung cancer up to 90% will have antibodies detected against the voltage-gated calcium channel on presynaptic nerve terminals. There is, however, no correlation between the titer of antibody and severity of disease and failure to detect such antibodies does not exclude the diagnosis [17]. The action of such antibodies reduces release of acetylcholine from motor terminals, and so impairs neuromuscular transmission. Therapy for paraneoplastic Lambert–Eaton myasthenic syndrome should primarily be directed against the underlying tumor. Specific antitumor therapy will often improve the neurological presentation. However, in patients with severe weakness 3,4-diaminopyridine, or immunosuppressive therapy, with either plasmapheresis or intravenous immunoglobulin treatment, can confer short-term benefits. In addition, glucocorticoid therapy alone or in combination with azathioprine or ciclosporin can have long-term beneficial effects.

Cutaneous paraneoplastic syndromes

In addition to the general definition of paraneoplastic syndromes as symptom complexes that are associated with the presence of malignancy in dermatology this definition has been somewhat modified to include all dermatoses that are associated with internal malignancy. It is proposed that four criteria should be met to fulfill the definition. The skin manifestation should have concurrent onset and show a parallel course to that of the underlying malignancy, the dermatosis should be of a characteristic type associated with malignancy, in epidemiological terms there should be a clear statistical association between the presence of the dermatosis and the malignancy, and there should be a genetic link between the dermatosis and malignancy. The common cutaneous syndromes are listed in Table 75.4.

Acanthosis nigricans

Acanthosis nigricans consists of pigmented velvety plaques typically seen on the sides and the back of the neck and in other skinfold areas. Skin tags frequently arise on pre-existing plaques of acanthosis nigricans. In endocrine terms acanthosis nigricans

Table 75.4 Dermatological paraneoplastic syndromes

Acanthosis nigricans
Acrokeratosis paraneoplastica of Bazex
Dermatomyositis
Erythema gyratum repens
Necrolytic migratory erythema
Paraneoplastic pemphigus
Sweet's syndrome
Pyoderma gangrenosum
Acquired ichthyosis
Hypertrichosis lanuginosa

is most frequently seen in association with obesity and in particular as a sign of insulin resistance. However, extensive and severe acanthosis nigricans is often associated with malignancy. Malignancy-associated acanthosis nigricans may be more widespread and also involve interdigital areas and even mucosal surfaces including the palate [18].

Underlying malignancies associated with acanthosis nigricans are predominantly adenocarcinomas and of these in particular gastrointestinal adenocarcinomas. Other carcinomas that have been reported to be associated include adrenal testicular and thyroid carcinomas and carcinoma of the bile duct, bladder, breast, cervix, endometrium, liver, larynx, lung, ovary, prostate, and kidney.

The underlying mechanism giving rise to acanthosis nigricans in the presence of malignancy is not known. It has been proposed that tumor production of factors that either directly have growth-promoting activity or cause activation of insulin-like growth factors or their receptors in the skin may be causative. In addition, transforming growth factor alpha, which acts on epidermal growth factor receptors in the skin, may be important.

Acrokeratosis paraneoplastica of Bazex

The lesions of this condition are characteristically distributed acrally and exhibit hyperkeratosis, hence the name. The plaques are usually erythematous to violaceous with overlying scaling. These lesions are reminiscent of psoriasis. The distribution of lesions, however, is not found in the typical locations expected of common psoriasis. The most common sites reported in recent studies were ears, nose, fingers, palms, hands, and feet.

The principal differential diagnosis is psoriasis, particularly the acral variants. However, the distinguishing clinical feature which is nearly always present in acrokeratosis paraneoplastica is involvement of the helices of the ear and the tip of the nose. Histologically there are some changes reminiscent of psoriasis but a number of non-psoriatic changes also exist including vacuolar degeneration with melanin-containing macrophages in the dermis and dyskeratotic keratinocytes.

Squamous cell carcinoma is most frequently associated with acrokeratosis paraneoplastica. In addition, associations with tumors in oropharynx, larynx and disseminated squamous cell carcinoma have also been reported.

The mechanism underlying this curious skin eruption is unknown but a similar mechanism to that underlying a number of the neurological manifestations of paraneoplastic syndromes has been proposed, that being mediated by host-generated antibodies against tumor antigens that subsequently cross-react with either keratinocyte or basement membrane antigens. The skin eruption parallels the development and progression of the underlying malignancy and can reappear as tumors recur [18, 19].

Dermatomyositis

The characteristic purplish erythema around the orbits and extensor surfaces can sometimes be difficult to distinguish from cutaneous lupus. Classically, dermatomyositis rashes are described

as being predominantly violaceous erythema while lupus is generally more of a red color. The link between dermatomyositis and malignancy remains controversial despite continuing reports of associations in the literature. In childhood dermatomyositis is generally thought not to be associated with malignancy. The predominant increase in cancer risk seen in patients with either dermatomyositis or isolated polymyositis occurs in men older than 50 years of age. In most reports there is a clearly higher risk in patients with dermatomyositis than in those with isolated polymyositis. In the majority of cases the underlying malignancy is isolated within 2 years of initial presentation with dermatomyositis and for this reason a thorough physical exam and good medical history are essential. The presence of an elevated erythrocyte sedimentation rate (ESR) and cutaneous necrosis are particularly suggestive of underlying malignancy.

The malignancies most commonly associated with dermatomyositis include those of breast, lung, gastric, and genitourinary tumors, particularly ovarian cancer. More recently lymphoma and prostate cancer have been associated [18].

Erythema gyratum repens

This is a rare entity but with a highly distinctive presentation. It consists of concentric bands of erythema on the skin with some associated scaling. The erythematous margin moves very rapidly, at up to 1 cm per day, and the resultant appearance has been described as being reminiscent of a wood grain. There is characteristically a marked eosinophilia but histological analysis is often non-specific. There may be associated hyperkeratosis of palms, ichthyosis and bullous lesions. Interestingly, erythema gyratum repens is usually diagnosed before the underlying malignancy which is most typically of lung, breast or esophageal origin [18].

Necrolytic migratory erythema

This skin disease is almost pathognomonic for the presence of underlying islet cell tumors, typically gluconomas. There may therefore be the typical associated clinical features of glucagonoma including diabetes, weight loss, diarrhea, steatorrhea and psychiatric disturbance.

The clinical appearance of the rash is commonly as an erosive skin lesion with overlying crusting and it is particularly found in skinfold areas such as groin, perineum, and buttocks. In addition to the erosive lesions there may also be scaly papules or plaques. There may be diagnostic confusion with other dermatoses such as pemphigus foliaceus, mucocutaneous candidiasis, psoriasis and severe seborrheic dermatitis [18].

Paraneoplastic pemphigus

Pemphigus has been described in association with a number of different internal malignancies, but association has been complicated by a possible causative role of the immunosuppressive agents typically used to treat the blistering skin disease. However, it is becoming clear that there is a distinct subentity of paraneoplastic pemphigus. It has been proposed that several major criteria should be fulfilled to make this diagnosis and these include a polymorphous mucocutaneous eruption, concurrent internal neoplasm and characteristic serum immunological findings [18].

Painful inflammation of the mouth and lips is the most characteristic skin feature of paraneoplastic pemphigus. In approximately 80% of cases there is associated lymphoma, leukemia or Castleman disease. The antibody response in paraneoplastic pemphigus is dominated by the presence of autoantibodies against desmoglein, but in addition antibodies directed against the plakin family of desmosomal proteins are also described. Development of paraneoplastic pemphigus is usually a catastrophic feature predicting rapid decline and death [20].

Neutrophilic disorders

Sweet syndrome

This disorder is characterized by a neutrophilic leukocytosis and elevated ESR. The cutaneous manifestation is the presence of raised tender plaques on the upper part of the body, particularly in women. Sometimes lesions may be pustular, bullous or ulcerated. The presence of a malignancy is identified in approximately 20% of patients. The most frequently found underlying malignancy is acute myelogenous leukemia but other lympho- and myeloproliferative disorders have also been described [20].

Pyoderma gangrenosum

The skin manifestation of pyoderma is with the onset of a sterile pustule which rapidly develops into a painful ulcer. It may occur following minor trauma and is associated with both inflammatory diseases and myeloproliferative disorders. The histological feature is a dense neutrophilic infiltrate in the dermis without evidence of vasculitis [20].

Acquired ichthyosis

The skin changes of acquired ichthyosis are usually asymptomatic and present after the diagnosis of malignancy. The severity of the skin manifestation tends to parallel that of the underlying cancer. The skin lesions are similar to ichthyosis vulgaris and consist of scaly lesions particularly in the lower portions of the legs. The relevant disease associations are primarily with myelo- and lymphoproliferative disease, although associations with solid tumors have also been described. It is important to note that acquired ichthyosis may occur following an adverse drug reaction and certain infections such as leprosy and acquired immune deficiency syndrome (AIDS) [20].

Hypertrichosis lanuginosa

This is a very rare paraneoplastic disorder but the cutaneous manifestation is striking. There is the appearance of fine, downy hair diffusely over the face, trunk and extremities. It is typically seen in women between the ages of 40 and 70 and in association with carcinomas of the lung, breast, uterus, ovaries, bladder, pancreas, kidney, and the gastrointestinal tract. The skin manifestation is usually of a relatively late onset and is found after dissemination of the underlying malignancy. For this reason patient survival is usually limited [20, 21].

Miscellaneous syndromes

Hypophosphataemic osteomalacia

This disorder of calcium and phosphate metabolism was originally described in childhood where severe symptomatic rickets was accompanied by hypophosphatemia. A child was found to have a chest tumor and the rickets healed spontaneously following its removal.

Most neoplasms found with this syndrome are of mesenchymal origin but it has also been reported in prostatic carcinoma. The characteristic biochemical features are of hypophosphatemia with greatly increased phosphate clearance in the presence of near normal serum calcium concentrations. In addition, in most patients there are low levels of serum 1, 25 dihydroxyvitamin D. Replenishment with 1, 25 dihydroxyvitamin D has a beneficial effect by reducing renal phosphate clearance and raising serum phosphate levels. For this reason it has been proposed that the mechanism is by a tumor product inhibiting renal phosphorylation of vitamin D. However, there is in addition a hypothesis that suggests the elaboration of a phosphaturic factor by the tumors [22].

References

1. Wirtz PW, Lang B, Graus F, et al. P/Q–type calcium channel antibodies, Lambert–Eaton myasthenic syndrome and survival in small cell lung cancer. *J. Neuroimmunol.* 2005;164:161–165.
2. Dropcho EJ. Update on paraneoplastic syndromes. *Curr. Opin. Neurol.* 2005;18:331–336.
3. Dropcho EJ. Neurologic paraneoplastic syndromes. *Curr. Oncol. Rep.* 2004;6:26–31.
4. Pittock SJ, Kryzer TJ, Lennon VA. Paraneoplastic antibodies coexist and predict cancer, not neurological syndrome. *Ann. Neurol.* 2004;56:715–719.
5. Pellkofer H, Schubart AS, Hoftberger R, et al. Modelling paraneoplastic CNS disease: T–cells specific for the onconeuronal antigen PNMA1 mediate autoimmune encephalomyelitis in the rat. *Brain* 2004;127:1822–1830.
6. Candler PM, Hart PE, Barnett M, Weil R, Rees JH. A follow up study of patients with paraneoplastic neurological disease in the United Kingdom. *J. Neurol. Neurosurg. Psychiatry* 2004;75:1411–1415.
7. Graus F, Delattre JY, Antoine JC, et al. Recommended diagnostic criteria for paraneoplastic neurological syndromes. *J. Neurol. Neurosurg. Psychiatry* 2004;75:1135–1140.
8. Graus F, Keime-Guibert F, Rene R, et al. Anti-Hu-associated paraneoplastic encephalomyelitis: analysis of 200 patients. *Brain* 2001;124:1138–1148.
9. Vincent A, Buckley C, Schott JM, et al. Potassium channel antibody-associated encephalopathy: a potentially immunotherapy-responsive form of limbic encephalitis. *Brain* 2004;127:701–712.
10. Pozo-Rosich P, Clover L, Saiz A, Vincent A, Graus F. Voltage-gated potassium channel antibodies in limbic encephalitis. *Ann. Neurol.* 2003;54:530–533.
11. Stich O, Graus F, Rasiah C, Rauer S. Qualitative evidence of anti–Yo–specific intrathecal antibody synthesis in patients with paraneoplastic cerebellar degeneration. *J. Neuroimmunol.* 2003;141:165–169.

12. Chalk CH, Windebank AJ, Kimmel DW, McManis PG. The distinctive clinical features of paraneoplastic sensory neuronopathy. *Can. J. Neurol. Sci.* 1992;19:346–351.

13. Matthay KK, Blaes F, Hero B, et al. Opsoclonus myoclonus syndrome in neuroblastoma a report from a workshop on the dancing eyes syndrome at the advances in neuroblastoma meeting in Genoa, Italy, 2004. *Cancer Lett.* 2005;228:275–282.

14. Lennon VA, Sas DF, Busk MF, et al. Enteric neuronal autoantibodies in pseudoobstruction with small–cell lung carcinoma. *Gastroenterology* 1991;100:137–142.

15. Dalmau J, Gultekin HS, Posner JB. Paraneoplastic neurologic syndromes: pathogenesis and physiopathology. *Brain Pathol.* 1999;9: 275–284.

16. Meriggioli MN, Sanders DB. Advances in the diagnosis of neuromuscular junction disorders. *Am. J. Phys. Med. Rehabil.* 2005;84:627–638.

17. Mareska M, Gutmann L. Lambert–Eaton myasthenic syndrome. *Semin. Neurol.* 2004;24:149–153.

18. Stone SP, Buescher LS. Life-threatening paraneoplastic cutaneous syndromes. *Clin. Dermatol.* 2005;23:301–306.

19. Buxtorf K, Hubscher E, Panizzon R. Bazex syndrome. *Dermatology* 2001;202:350–352.

20. Thomas I, Schwartz RA. Cutaneous paraneoplastic syndromes: uncommon presentations. *Clin. Dermatol.* 2005;23:593–600.

21. Perez-Losada E, Pujol RM, Domingo P, et al. Hypertrichosis lanuginosa acquisita preceding extraskeletal Ewing's sarcoma. *Clin. Exp. Dermatol.* 2001;26:182–183.

22. Fukumoto Y, Tarui S, Tsukiyama K, et al. Tumor-induced vitamin D-resistant hypophosphatemic osteomalacia associated with proximal renal tubular dysfunction and 1,25-dihydroxyvitamin D deficiency. *J. Clin. Endocrinol. Metab* 1979;49:873–878.

76 Syndrome of Inappropriate Antidiuretic Hormone Secretion

Rachel K. Crowley and Chris Thompson

Key points
- Syndrome of inappropriate antidiuretic hormone secretion is the most common cause of euvolemic hyponatremia.
- Syndrome of inappropriate antidiuretic hormone secretion complicates a wide variety of malignancies and treatments for neoplastic disease.
- Strict criteria exist for diagnosis of syndrome of inappropriate antidiuretic hormone secretion, which should be applied when assessing the hyponatremic patient with a diagnosis of malignancy.
- Small cell carcinoma of the lung is the malignancy most frequently associated with syndrome of inappropriate antidiuretic hormone secretion.
- Hyponatremia in malignancy-associated syndrome of inappropriate antidiuretic hormone secretion tends to develop slowly and should be corrected using fluid restriction, demeclocycline or vasopressin antagonists, with careful monitoring of plasma sodium.

Background

The syndrome of inappropriate antidiuresis (SIADH) is the most common cause of euvolemic hyponatremia, and is a well-described complication of malignant disease [1]. The index report of SIADH was the classic description by Bartter and Schwartz in 1956, of two patients with hyponatremia and bronchogenic carcinoma [2]. Bartter and Schwartz identified a state of antidiuresis in both patients, by alternating fluid restriction with fluid loading, and postulated that an excess of circulating "antidiuretic hormone" was responsible for the hyponatremia. Many years later their clinical hypothesis was proven correct, when a radioimmunoassay for arginine vasopressin (AVP) identified high circulating levels of this antidiuretic hormone in patients diagnosed with SIADH [3].

Since Bartter and Schwartz first described SIADH, the syndrome has been reported to occur as a complication of a wide variety of malignancies. In addition, it occurs as a well-recognized complication of the use of chemotherapeutic agents in oncology practice. SIADH is reported to be a complication of other drug treatments, pulmonary diseases and particularly neurosurgical conditions.

In this chapter we will describe the physiology of water balance, the perturbations which occur during SIADH, and an approach to the differential diagnosis and management of hyponatremia in patients with malignant disease.

Clinical Endocrine Oncology, 2nd edition. Edited by Ian D. Hay and John A.H. Wass. © 2008 Blackwell Publishing. ISBN 978-1-4051-4584-8.

Regulation of plasma sodium concentration

Sodium is the most abundant extracellular cation and under physiological conditions its concentration in human plasma remains within a very narrow range. Sodium balance is regulated by a variety of physiological influences, including dietary sodium intake, and the hormonal effect on renal tubular sodium handling of the renin–angiotensin–aldosterone axis and natriuretic peptides. However, plasma sodium concentration is principally dependent upon the regulation of renal water handling by the antidiuretic hormone, AVP.

Increases in plasma osmolality are detected by osmoreceptors located in the anterior hypothalamus, in the organum vasculosum laminae terminalis, the subfornical organ and the median preoptic nucleus, which are collectively known as the circumventricular organs. The osmoreceptors for thirst in the AV3V region are thought to be in close proximity to those for AVP release, because many hypothalamic lesions affect both the release of AVP and the thirst response to increased plasma osmolality [4]. Stimulation of the osmoreceptors causes depolarization of the neural projections to the supraoptic and paraventricular nuclei, where AVP is synthesized. AVP moves from the supraoptic and paraventricular nuclei via axonal transport to the posterior pituitary from where it is released into the circulation.

The site of action of AVP is the V2 receptor (V2R) in the collecting ducts of the kidney. Receptor binding leads to a rise in intracellular cAMP, which causes shuttling of protein water channels called aquaporins (AQP2) to the apical membrane of the collecting ducts, and increased synthesis of AQP2 mRNA. The net effect of V2R activation and AQP2 recruitment is the re-absorption of water from the collecting duct into the circulation, with a consequent reduction in plasma sodium concentration and normalization of plasma osmolality.

Detectable increases in plasma AVP concentration can be measured by sensitive radioimmunoassay once plasma osmolality rises to approximately 285 mOsm/kg (285 mmol/kg). As plasma osmolality increases above this "osmotic threshold," plasma AVP concentration rises in a linear fashion, with subsequent reduction in renal-free water excretion. Conversely, when water intake is excessive, and plasma osmolality falls below the osmotic threshold, AVP secretion is suppressed, with the onset of hypotonic polyuria. Thus, in the setting of hyponatremia, the appropriate physiological response to low plasma osmolality is suppression of AVP secretion, with the development of maximally dilute urine. Therefore, urine osmolality greater than 100 mOsm/kg (100 mmol/kg) when a patient is hyponatremic, is *de facto* evidence of urine concentration that is inappropriate to the clinical setting.

Pathogenesis of SIADH

SIADH is characterized by an excess of extracellular water with subsequent hyponatremia. Urine is inappropriately concentrated due to antidiuretic activity of vasopressin. There is not a wealth of data in the literature but it is known that there are four distinct categories of SIADH, which can be classified according to the pattern of AVP secretion [5] (Fig. 76.1).

Type A

This is the most common pattern of AVP secretion (40%), and is classically associated with small cell lung tumors, which can synthesize and secrete bioactive AVP. Plasma AVP secretion is unregulated, with erratic plasma concentrations which bear no

relationship to ambient plasma osmolality. Plasma AVP secretion is not suppressed as plasma osmolality falls and significant hyponatremia may occur. Data from our own laboratory shows that thirst is not suppressed in this variant of SIADH, and drinking occurs at plasma osmolalities lower than the usual osmotic threshold of 284 mOsm/kg (284 mmol/kg), which means that hyponatremia is not corrected by self-regulated water restriction.

Type B

The second most common pattern of AVP secretion in SIADH is characterized by a lower osmotic threshold for AVP secretion. The threshold is reset to a lower level, and at plasma osmolalities above this threshold, the linear relationship between plasma osmolality and plasma AVP concentration is preserved. However, because AVP secretion is suppressed at plasma osmolalities below the reset threshold, severe hyponatremia is prevented by the development of a hypotonic diuresis. A lowered osmotic threshold for thirst has also been demonstrated in Type B SIADH [6].

Type C

This type is characterized by a rare pattern of AVP secretion. At plasma osmolalities above the usual osmotic threshold of 284 mOsm/kg (284 mmol/kg), the linear relationship between plasma AVP and plasma osmolality is preserved. However, lowered plasma osmolalities do not suppress AVP secretion, so that low plasma concentrations of AVP are always detectable in the plasma,

Type D

This is a very rare variant of SIADH, confined to occasional case reports. Patients develop hyponatremia that satisfies the clinical criteria for the diagnosis of SIADH, but plasma AVP concentrations are undetectable. Type D SIADH may be explained by secretion of an unidentified antidiuretic substance by tumor cells, which is undetectable in assays for vasopressin.

Inappropriate elevation of plasma AVP in SIADH leads to increased expression of AQP2 and AQP2 mRNA in the renal tubule. Sustained stimulation of aquaporins causes re-absorption of water from the renal tubules. The resultant increase in the ratio of total body water to sodium causes hyponatremia. Vasopressin antagonists can reverse the expression of AQP2 proteins and mRNA, demonstrating that such AQP2 activation is dependent on AVP or on a possible AVP analog with action at the V2 receptor [7].

Diagnosis

Hyponatremia is the most common electrolyte imbalance in hospital patients, and can present with a variety of neurological symptoms. In patients with a known diagnosis of malignancy, the differential diagnosis for such symptoms is wide, and hyponatremia may be underrecognized. Hyponatremia may reflect a large number of pathophysiologies other than SIADH and there are strict criteria for diagnosis of the syndrome.

The diagnostic criteria are presented in Table 76.1. The blood volume expansion in SIADH is too minimal to be detected clinically, and so the patient must be clinically euvolemic to diagnose

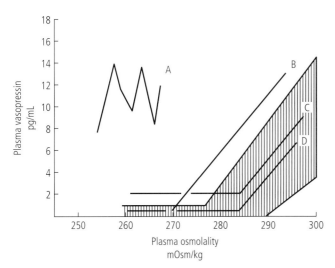

Figure 76.1 Patterns of plasma AVP secretion in SIADH. (Reproduced from Robertson GL et al. Neurogenic disorders of osmoregulation. Am. J. Med. 1982;72:339–353, with permission from Elsevier.)

Table 76.1 Criteria for the clinical diagnosis of SIADH

Essential

Decreased osmolality of the ECF [Posm <275 mOsm/kg (<275 mmol/kg) H₂O]

Inappropriate urinary concentration at some level of hypo-osmolality
[Uosm >100 mOsm/kg (>100 mmol/kg) H₂O, normal renal function]

Clinical euvolemia

Elevated urinary sodium excretion on normal salt and water intake

Absence of other potential causes of euvolemic hypo-osmolality:
hypothyroidism, hypocortisolism and diuretic use

Supplemental

Abnormal water load test [inability to excrete at least 80% of a 20 ml/kg
water load in 4 h and / or failure to dilute Uosm to <100 mOsm/kg
(<100 mmol/kg) H₂O]

Plasma AVP level inappropriately elevated relative to Posm

No significant correction of PNa with volume expansion but improvement
after fluid restriction

Uosm, urinary osmolality; Posm, plasma osmolality; PNa, plasma sodium.
Reproduced from Verbalis JG [8], with permission from Elsevier.

Table 76.2 Causes of SIADH in malignant disease

Malignancy	Lung – small cell, non-small cell, mesothelioma
	GI – esophagus, stomach, pancreas, colon, duodenum
	Hematological – lymphoma, leukemia, myeloma
	Head & neck – tongue, nasopharynx, larynx
	Brain – glioma, medulloblastoma, meningioma, neurofibroma
	Others – breast, prostate, urological, cervix, ovary, melanoma
	Pituitary metastases
Treatment	Cytotoxics – vincristine, vinblastine, cisplatin, cyclophosphamide, melphalan, levamisole
	Adjunctive – morphine, anti-emetics, antidepressants, aminoglutethimide, carbamazepine
	Stem cell transplantation
	Radiotherapy (ACTH deficiency more common)
	Neurosurgery

SIADH. Evaluation of volume status, based on clinical and biochemical criteria, is of paramount importance in establishing the etiology of hyponatremia (Table 76.2), because accurate diagnosis determines appropriate management of the patient [9]. Occasionally, multiple comorbidities may render accurate determination of volume status so difficult that central venous pressure monitoring may be required.

If a patient fits the criteria for euvolemic hyponatremia documented in Table 76.1, it is important to exclude thyroid hormone and glucocorticoid deficiency, as both can mimic SIADH [10, 11]. Thyroxine is necessary for free water clearance and in hypothyroidism mild hyponatremia is not uncommon. Occasionally more severe hyponatremia with neurological sequelae has been reported. Hyponatremia secondary to hypothyroidism responds to thyroxine replacement therapy, and is now also a licensed indication for the use of conivaptan, a vasopressin antagonist, in the USA. Glucocorticoid insufficiency should also be considered as a

cause of hyponatremia. Cortisol is necessary for free water clearance, potentially by both a direct effect on the renal tubules or by inhibition of AVP release from the posterior pituitary. Patients with hyponatremia secondary to hypoadrenalism respond to fluid and hydrocortisone replacement, which can be a life-saving intervention in some cases. Glucocorticoid deficiency as a cause of SIADH in malignant disease is discussed in more detail below.

SIADH in malignant disease

SIADH has been reported in association with a wide variety of malignancies. It has also been reported as a complication of cytotoxic drugs and drugs used as adjunctive therapy, such as morphine, anti-emetics and antidepressants. In addition, SIADH may occur as a complication of surgical intervention, stem cell transplantation and radiotherapy for primary brain tumors.

SIADH has been reported most often in association with lung cancer. It is most common with small cell lung cancer and is reported in various series to occur in 5–38% of cases. Published series have used significant variations in the criteria for diagnosis of SIADH, and many studies omitted details of essential exclusion criteria, such as hypovolemia, thyroid and glucocorticoid deficiency and drugs known to produce SIADH. However, the overall incidence is approximately 15% in reported series. In contrast, the incidence in non-small cell carcinoma of the lung is much lower; there have been fewer large series than for small cell carcinoma, but the incidence in published series varies from 0.4–2% [12].

Other than small cell cancer of the lung, SIADH is probably most common in patients with intracranial malignancy. Data from our own unit show that SIADH is present in 3% of intracranial tumors, but the incidence of hyponatremia rises to 15% after neurosurgical intervention. The majority of cases of hyponatremia are due to SIADH, but the use of hypotonic fluids, drugs such as carbamazepine for seizure control and cerebral salt wasting must be considered. The key differential diagnosis is glucocorticoid deficiency secondary to pituitary damage, particularly if the tumor is parasellar. The co-occurrence of hypotension or hypoglycemia with SIADH in a patient with a parasellar tumor should raise the possibility of acute adrenocorticotropic hormone (ACTH) deficiency.

Tumors of the head and neck have been associated with the development of SIADH. One large series reported an incidence of 3% in 1436 patients with assorted head and neck cancers, though essential diagnostic criteria such as elevated urinary sodium concentration and exclusion of hypovolemia were not described in the methodology [13]. Isolated case reports document SIADH in a very wide spectrum of malignant disease, including hematological malignancy, urological tumors and gastroenterological cancers, but SIADH seems to occur as an idiosyncratic rather than systematic complication of most malignancies.

The pathophysiology of SIADH in malignant disease is varied. The classic paper of George and colleagues in 1972 reported staining for AVP by malignant cells derived from a bronchogenic tumor

[14]. Confirmation that immunohistochemical staining demonstrates synthesis of AVP in cancer cells was subsequently reported in three cases of thymic neuroblastoma [15]. More recently, mRNA for AVP has been demonstrated in tissue obtained from patients with small cell carcinoma of the lung. AVP has been detected in the cerebrospinal fluid of patients with leptomeningeal metastases from small cell carcinoma [16], and in pleural fluid of patients with the same tumor. These data provide strong evidence that SIADH in some malignancies is caused by the synthesis and secretion of AVP from tumor tissue. Hyponatremia and elevated plasma AVP concentrations often return towards normal with regression of small cell lung tumors, though it is unusual for either parameter to completely normalize, even in cases of complete remission. There are conflicting data on the subject of whether SIADH is a negative prognostic indicator in small cell lung cancer.

Not all malignancy-associated SIADH is associated with high or inappropriately high levels of circulating AVP, however. In cases where plasma AVP levels have been checked and found to be low, it is postulated that the state of antidiuresis is secondary to the presence of a different circulating antidiuretic substance, as yet unidentified. High levels of atrial natriuretic peptide (ANP) have been reported in malignancy-associated hyponatremia [17] and mRNA for ANP has been demonstrated in small cell carcinoma cell lines [18]. However, it might be expected that hyponatremia due to excess secretion of natriuretic peptides might occur against a background of volume depletion due to associated diuresis. In addition, the natriuresis and diuresis associated with natriuretic peptides in experimental conditions tend to be self-limiting, which is not the clinical picture of malignancy-associated SIADH. It is also possible that antidiuresis in the absence of circulating AVP is secondary to overactivation of the V2 receptor, or excessive aquaporin recruitment, leading to increased permeability of the renal tubules to water, although a mechanism in malignant disease for the development of such overstimulation is unknown.

Intracranial tumors may produce SIADH by direct physical interference with the osmoregulatory pathways. This is particularly the case in SIADH that complicates neurosurgery. The need to exclude ACTH deficiency in these tumors has already been emphasized. ACTH deficiency occurs in 21% of adults who receive cranial irradiation for treatment of non-pituitary brain tumors [19], and although there were no cases of ACTH deficiency producing SIADH in this series we have observed cases of SIADH due to radiotherapy-induced hypopituitarism (unpublished data).

A wide variety of cytotoxic agents have been documented to cause SIADH, by a variety of mechanisms. Recently, SIADH was reported in 11.4% of 140 pediatric patients who had undergone stem cell transplantation for a variety of diseases, most commonly hematological malignancies. The most important risk factor for development of SIADH was transplantation from an HLA-mismatched donor, and surprisingly, the presence of SIADH was associated with a higher survival rate [20]. The authors were unable to explain this finding.

Management of hyponatremia

The key aspect of management of SIADH associated with malignancy is treatment of the underlying tumor. Hyponatremia associated with small cell tumors of the lung has been shown to regress with surgical or cytotoxic therapy of the underlying malignancy. Treatment of primary or secondary intracranial malignancies with radiotherapy, or dexamethasone to reduce surrounding edema, may occasionally cause resolution of SIADH, though neurosurgical intervention often worsens hyponatremia. Treatment of associated ACTH deficiency with glucocorticoids causes rapid resolution of hyponatremia.

The management of hyponatremia *per se* depends largely on three factors: the severity of symptoms, the degree of hyponatremia and the period of time over which hyponatremia developed. Symptoms of hyponatremia rarely present at plasma sodium concentrations greater than 130 mEq/L (130 mmol/L), whereas seizure risk is substantial at plasma sodium concentrations under 120 mEq/L (120 mmol/L). Cerebral irritation is more likely if hyponatremia is of rapid onset or if there is an intracranial mass lesion or infection. In oncological practice the hyponatremia is usually of gradual onset and hyponatremia is rarely symptomatic unless the tumor is intracranial or the hyponatremia is very severe.

Chronic hyponatremia is arbitrarily defined as developing over a longer time period than 48 h, and is less likely to be symptomatic than acute hyponatremia because the brain adapts by extruding organic solutes into the plasma, preventing the osmotic movement of water from the plasma into the brain. Cerebral edema is thus prevented. In the asymptomatic patient with chronic hyponatremia correction of plasma sodium by fluid restriction to 1 litre or less per day produces a slow, steady increase in plasma sodium concentration in most cases. Long-term fluid restriction is uncomfortable for patients and may be impractical if the patient has a chemotherapy regimen that requires intravenous fluids. Demeclocycline, which promotes clearance of excess free water by inducing a nephrogenic diabetes insipidus, is used in the short to medium term management of patients with SIADH, particularly those with a terminal diagnosis. The use of demeclocycline is limited by its side effect profile, and is likely to be replaced by vasopressin antagonists in the future.

Vasopressin antagonists or "vaptans," are already licensed for use in SIADH in the USA, but have yet to be approved for the European market. They are "aquaretics;" that is, they produce free water clearance without urinary sodium excretion, unlike diuretics. Vaptans are non-peptide antagonists of vasopressin that bind within the V2 receptor, at a site that overlaps slightly with the binding site for AVP. The binding properties of vaptans imply that they could be effective for treatment of Type D as well as the other types of SIADH, because non-competitive antagonists can induce conformational changes in a receptor that may down-regulate its activity. Patients with a re-set osmostat (Type B SIADH) may not have a predictable response to a vasopressin antagonist because vasopressin will start to rise once the threshold osmolality is exceeded, and may have the potential to displace the antagonist from the V2 receptor. An increase in dose may be sufficient to saturate the V2R binding sites in such patients. The main side effect of vaptans identified in the pre-marketing studies is thirst.

Acute hyponatremia, defined as developing in less than 48 h, is unusual in SIADH, but can occur at initiation of cytotoxic therapy. In acute hyponatremia the brain has inadequate time to adapt to changes in plasma sodium, thus rapid correction of plasma sodium is safe. Hypertonic (3%) saline infusion may be required in a case of acute hyponatremia with seizures or depressed level of consciousness. However, hypertonic saline should only be used under the supervision of an experienced physician comfortable with well-published protocols designed to prevent over-rapid correction of plasma sodium.

In summary, SIADH is a fascinating clinical syndrome that is associated with a wide range of malignancy and may complicate treatment. SIADH represents a diagnostic and treatment challenge to the managing physician, as there are strict criteria for diagnosis. Accurate diagnosis and exclusion of differential diagnoses are essential for the institution of appropriate treatment. Treatment of the underlying malignancy is of key importance, but the advent of vasopressin antagonists will expand the therapeutic options for physicians caring for patients with malignancy.

References

1. Crowley RK, Thompson CJ. Syndrome of inappropriate antidiuresis. *Exp. Rev. Endocrinol. Metab.* 2006;1:537–547.
2. Schwartz WB, Bennett W, Curelop S, Bartter FC. A syndrome of renal sodium loss and hyponatremia probably resulting from inappropriate secretion of antidiuretic hormone. *Am. J. Med.* 1957;23:529–542.
3. Zerbe R, Stropes L, Robertson G. Vasopressin function in the syndrome of inappropriate antidiuresis. *Annu. Rev. Med.* 1980;31:315–327.
4. McKinley MJ, Mathai ML, McAllen RM, et al. Vasopressin secretion: osmotic and hormonal regulation by the lamina terminalis. *J. Neuroendocrinol.* 2004;16:340–347.
5. Robertson GL, Aycinena P, Zerbe RL. Neurogenic disorders of osmoregulation. *Am. J. Med.* 1982;72:339–353.
6. Smith D, Moore K, Tormey W, Baylis PH, Thompson CJ. Downward resetting of the osmotic threshold for thirst in patients with SIADH. *Am. J. Physiol. Endocrinol. Metab.* 2004;287:E1019–1023.
7. Smitz S, LeGros JJ, Franchimont P, le Maire M. Identification of vasopressin-like peptides in the plasma of a patient with the syndrome of inappropriate secretion of antidiuretic hormone and an oat cell carcinoma. *Acta Endocrinol.* 1988;119:567–574.
8. Verbalis JG. Disorders of body water homeostasis. *Best Pract. Res. Clin. Endocrinol. Metab.* 2003;17:471–503.
9. Smith D, McKenna K, Thompson CJ. Hyponatraemia. *Clin. Endocrinol.* 2000;52:667–678.
10. Hanna FW, Scanlon MF. Hyponatraemia, hypothyroidism and role of arginine-vasopressin. Lancet 1997;13;350:755–756.
11. Olchovsky D, Ezra D, Vered I, Hadani M, Shimon I. Symptomatic hyponatremia as a presenting sign of hypothalamic–pituitary disease: a syndrome of inappropriate secretion of antidiuretic hormone (SIADH)-like glucocorticosteroid responsive condition. *J. Endocrinol. Invest.* 2005;28:151–156.
12. Sorensen JB, Andersen MK, Hansen HH. Syndrome of inappropriate secretion of antidiuretic hormone (SIADH) in malignant disease *J. Intern. Med.* 1995;238:97–110.
13. Talmi YP, Hoffman HT, McCabe BF. Syndrome of inappropriate secretion of arginine vasopressin in patients with cancer of the head and neck. *Ann. Otol. Rhinol. Laryngol.* 1992;101:946–949.
14. George JM, Capen CC, Philips AS. Biosynthesis of vasopressin in vitro and ultrastructure of a bronchogenic cancer. *J. Clin. Invest.* 1972;51:141–148.
15. Argani P, Erlandson RA, Rosai J. Thymic neuroblastoma in adults: report of three cases with special emphasis on its association with the syndrome of inappropriate secretion of antidiuretic hormone. *Am. J. Clin. Pathol.* 1997;108:537–543.
16. Pederson AG, Hammer M, Hansen M, Sorensen PS. Cerebrospinal fluid vasopressin as a marker of central nervous system metastases from small-cell bronchogenic carcinoma. *J. Clin. Oncol.* 1985;3:48–53.
17. Kamoi K, Ebe T, Hasegawa A, et al. Hyponatraemia in small cell lung cancer. Mechanisms not involving inappropriate ADH secretion. *Cancer* 1987;60:1089–1093.
18. Gross AJ, Steinberg SM, Reilly JG, et al. Atrial natriuretic factor and arginine vasopressin production in tumor cell lines from patients with lung cancer and their relationship to serum sodium. *Cancer Res.* 1993;53:67–74.
19. Agha A, Sherlock M, Brennan S, et al. Hypothalamic–pituitary dysfunction after irradiation of non-pituitary brain tumours in adults. *J. Clin. Endocrinol. Metab.* 2005;90:6355–6360.
20. Kobayashi R, Iguchi A, Nakajima M, et al. Hyponatraemia and syndrome of inappropriate antidiuretic hormone secretion complicating stem cell transplantation. *Bone Marrow Transpl.* 2004;34:975–979.

77 Hypercalcemia of Malignancy

Gregory R. Mundy, Babatunde Oyajobi, Susan Padalecki, and Julie A. Sterling

Key points
- Hypercalcemia is due to malignant disease or primary hyperparathyroidism in 90% of patients.
- Hypercalcemia is always due to a serious underlying condition, and the cause should be searched for diligently.
- The malignancies associated with hypercalcemia are most often lung and breast cancer.
- Occult cancer as a cause of hypercalcemia is rare.
- Hypercalcemia can be reversed in the majority of patients with malignant disease by appropriate use of the powerful bisphosphonates.

Introduction

Hypercalcemia occurs when the normal compensatory mechanisms responsible for the maintenance of the extracellular fluid calcium are overwhelmed. It is usually due to a combination of increased entry of calcium into the extracellular fluid from bone or the gastrointestinal tract, often combined with impaired capacity of the kidney to excrete the calcium load.

Hypercalcemia occurs in most patients with malignancy due to markedly increased bone resorption not balanced by new bone formation, and associated with impaired calcium excretion by the kidney. In some patients, particularly those with myeloma, the latter is due to decreased glomerular filtration, and in most there is also increased renal tubular reabsorption of calcium.

Causes of hypercalcemia [1]

The causes of hypercalcemia and their relative frequency are shown in Tables 77.1 and 77.2. Primary hyperparathyroidism and malignancy comprise approximately 90% of all patients with hypercalcemia. Primary hyperparathyroidism is a common condition and should always be actively excluded in any patient with malignancy and hypercalcemia.

Traditional concepts of calcium homeostasis [2]

The traditional but almost certainly overly simplistic view of calcium homeostasis is that extracellular fluid (ECF) ionized calcium concentration is tightly regulated by the actions of two major hormones (parathyroid hormone (PTH) and 1,25 dihydroxyvitamin

Clinical Endocrine Oncology, 2nd edition. Edited by Ian D. Hay and John A.H. Wass. © 2008 Blackwell Publishing. ISBN 978-1-4051-4584-8.

Table 77.1 Causes of hypercalcemia [1]

Primary hyperparathyroidism
Malignant disease
Hyperthyroidism
Immobilization
Vitamin D intoxication
Vitamin A intoxication
Familial hypocalciuric hypercalcemia (FHH)
Diuretic phase of acute renal failure
Chronic renal failure ± aluminum toxicity
Thiazide diuretics
Sarcoidosis and other granulomatous diseases
Milk-alkali syndrome
Addison's disease
Paget's disease (with immobilization or co-existent primary hyperparathyroidism)
Post partum with lactation

Table 77.2 Relative frequency of causes of hypercalcemia [1]

	No. of patients	Percentage of cases
Primary hyperparathyroidism	111	54
Malignant disease	72	25
Lung	25	35
Breast	18	25
Hematologic (myeloma 5, lymphoma 4)	10	14
Head and neck	4	8
Renal	2	3
Prostate	2	3
Unknown primary	5	7
Others (gastrointestinal 4)	6	8
Other causes – renal failure, sarcoid, thryrotoxicosis, vitamin D intoxication, immobilization)	24	13

D) acting on fluxes of calcium across the gut, kidney and bone. The major storehouse of calcium in the body is the skeleton (which contains approximately 1 kg or 99% of total body calcium). The kidney filters approximately 10 g/day, of which more than 90% is reabsorbed in the proximal convoluted tubules and distal convoluted tubules, (the former influenced by sodium reabsorption, the latter by PTH). In normal adults in zero calcium balance, renal calcium excretion equals net gut absorption. In this view, extracellular fluid calcium is regulated in much the same way as a domestic thermostat ("reactive regulation") by negative feedback loops which control PTH and 1,25 dihydroxyvitamin D production (either directly or indirectly). Calcitonin may also be involved in short-term regulation, although its physiologic role remains unclear 40 years after its discovery. The regulatory controls for this homeostatic system are seemingly overlapping and redundant, but this may be the explanation for control which is so tight.

Frequency of hypercalcemia in patients with malignancy

With the introduction of routine serum calcium measurements by the autoanalyzer in the mid-1970s, hypercalcemia has become recognized as a common electrolyte abnormality in the general population, as well as in hospitalized patients [3]. Estimates of the incidence and prevalence of primary hyperparathyroidism have dramatically risen since that time. In addition, hypercalcemia has also been noted more frequently in patients with malignant disease. Primary hyperparathyroidism and malignant disease are the cause of hypercalcemia in the vast majority of hypercalcemic patients. Other causes of hypercalcemia listed in Table 77.1 are much less common, comprising about 10% of all patients [1].

A relatively small number of specific malignancies are responsible for hypercalcemia in most cancer patients (Table 77.2). Malignant hypercalcemia is frequently caused by squamous cell carcinoma of the lung, whereas anaplastic carcinoma or oat cell carcinoma of the lung is rarely associated with hypercalcemia. Carcinoma of the breast of all types is often responsible for hypercalcemia. Although 20–40% of patients with myeloma developed hypercalcemia during the course of the disease before use of the bisphosphonates became so widespread in this disease, the frequency now is much less. Squamous cell tumors of the head and neck and the upper end of the esophagus are also often associated with hypercalcemia. Many common cancers are almost never associated with hypercalcemia (e.g., carcinoma of the colon and carcinoma of the female genital tract). In contrast, some rare malignancies are frequently associated with hypercalcemia (e.g., cholangiocarcinoma and vasoactive intestinal polypeptide [VIPomas]).

Pathophysiology of hypercalcemia of malignancy

Hypercalcemia of malignancy can be subdivided into three main categories: humoral hypercalcemia of malignancy; hypercalcemia

associated with metastatic bone disease; and myeloma bone disease.

Humoral hypercalcemia of malignancy

The humoral hypercalcemia of malignancy (HHM) syndrome is caused by tumor products that circulate and cause hypercalcemia because of their systemic effects. Although HHM is thought of as being unrelated to local osteolytic bone destruction, many patients with the HHM syndrome also have localized osteolysis. Solid tumors are those most often associated with HHM (e.g., carcinomas of the lung, head and neck, kidney, pancreas, and ovary). Occasionally, patients with malignant lymphomas develop HHM. Most patients with HHM have many of the biochemical features of primary hyperparathyroidism, including hypercalcemia associated with increased urinary excretion of phosphate and cyclic AMP. However, other characteristics of HHM, including decreased calcium absorption from the gut, decreased bone formation, and metabolic alkalosis, are not seen in primary hyperparathyroidism. The variations that occur in these features of HHM are most likely caused by differences in the tumor-derived factors and the variable response of the host immune cells. The most important factor that has been implicated in the pathophysiology of HHM is parathyroid hormone-related protein (PTHrP) [4, 5]. Eight of the first 13 amino acids of PTHrP) are identical to those of PTH. The gene encoding PTHrP is clearly different from the PTH gene and resides on a different chromosome, but probably had a similar evolutionary origin. PTHrP seems to mimic all the biologic effects of PTH and, in addition, has its own unique effects. Like PTH, PTHrP stimulates bone resorption both *in vitro* and *in vivo*, increases renal tubular calcium reabsorption, increases cyclic AMP generation, increases renal phosphate excretion, increases 1,25-dihydroxyvitamin D production, and causes hypercalcemia when given by injection.

Hypercalcemia associated with metastatic bone disease

Hypercalcemia occurs frequently in patients with metastatic bone disease due to solid tumors, and is especially prevalent in those with osteolytic disease. Bone metastases can occur in a number of solid tumor types including breast, prostate, thyroid, lung, colon, and kidney. Bone metastases are especially prevalent in patients with prostate and breast cancer, in which a large portion of the patients develop osteolytic bone metastases at late stages in the disease progression. However, it is important to note that hypercalcemia is common in breast, lung, and renal cancer, but rare in colon, thyroid, or prostate cancer. Most commonly the osteolytic bone metastases are found at highly vascularized areas of the skeleton – the vertebral column, ribs, and long bones. Before the widespread use of bisphosphonates to control osteolytic disease in patients with bone metastases, approximately 30% of all patients with breast cancer developed hypercalcemia at some point in the disease, generally at late stages [6].

Once tumors have established in bone they express factors that stimulate bone resorption. One of the major factors responsible is PTHrP. Immunohistochemistry studies have shown increased expression of PTHrP in bone compared with soft tissue metastases and the primary tumor [7, 8]. Studies in the osteolytic breast cancer cell line, MDA-MB-231, have demonstrated that PTHrP is a major regulator of osteolysis *in vivo* [9]. When cultured human breast cancer cells have been inoculated into nude mice, they increase their expression of PTHrP. Furthermore, when treated with neutralizing antibodies or small molecule inhibitors to PTHrP, tumor-bearing mice have a decrease in osteolysis and tumor burden [9, 10]. PTHrP can stimulate osteoblast expression of receptor activator of nuclear factor (NF)-κB ligand (RANKL) [11]. RANKL then binds to its receptor expressed on the osteoclasts, RANK. This enhances the differentiation of active osteoclasts in the presence of macrophage colony-stimulating factor [11]. In addition, the presence of tumor cells frequently leads to a reduction in the expression of the decoy receptor for RANKL, osteoprotegerin [12]. Alteration of the expression of these proteins by the tumor cells results in an overall increase in RANKL/RANK binding and an increase in osteoclast activation.

While tumor-produced PTHrP has been clearly shown to play a critical role in the activation of RANKL and subsequent osteolysis [11], tumor cells can secrete other factors that stimulate the osteoclasts. One family of cytokines secreted by the tumor cells are the interleukins (IL). IL-1, -6, -8, and -11 are all frequently produced by tumor cells and can lead to osteolysis [13]. Of these, IL-8 expression has been best described in the stimulation of tumor-induced osteolysis.

Tumor–bone interaction: the "vicious cycle"

The presence of many growth factors in the bone matrix provides a fertile environment for tumor cells that have metastasized to bone. Once established in bone, tumors may produce factors such as PTHrP that can stimulate bone resorption. As bone is destroyed by the tumor cells, these growth factors are released from the bone matrix and stimulate tumor cell proliferation and expression of factors that cause further bone destruction. This in turn causes the release of more growth factors and the process continues in a vicious cycle of bone destruction [14, 15].

The major factors, but likely not the only ones, contributing to this cycle of bone destruction are tumor-produced PTHrP and bone-derived transforming growth factor-β (TGF-β). TGF-β released from the bone matrix during osteolysis [16] has been shown to stimulate tumor PTHrP production [17]. This relationship has been clearly shown using MDA-MB-231 cells transfected with a dominant negative TGF-β receptor type II, which leaves the cells non-responsive to TGF-β [17]. In these cells, the production of PTHrP was not enhanced in the bone microenvironment and there was a significant reduction in tumor-induced osteolysis [17]. In addition to TGF-β, there are other growth factors stored in the bone matrix that likely play an important role in this vicious cycle of bone destruction.

Hypercalcemia and myeloma bone disease

Multiple myeloma is the second most common adult hematological malignancy and the most common cancer with the skeleton as its primary site. Myeloma is unique in its propensity to cause osteolysis, with 80% of patients suffering from devastating and progressive bone destruction resulting in severe and unremitting bone pain, pathologic fracture, and spinal cord compression. In addition, until the widespread use of bisphosphonates over the past few years, approximately one-third of patients with myeloma developed hypercalcemia during the course of their disease.

In myeloma patients, the primary cause of the hypercalcemia is widespread bone destruction due primarily to increased osteoclastic bone resorption caused by local cytokines expressed and/or secreted by the myeloma cells (RANKL, OPG, MIP-1α; see below), which in turn leads to efflux of calcium into the extracellular fluid. This, and the irreversible impairment of renal function and the increased renal tubular calcium reabsorption often seen in these patients, overwhelms the capacity to effectively clear excess calcium load from the circulation resulting in elevated serum calcium levels [18]. It remains unclear why myeloma patients present with this increase in renal tubular calcium reabsorption. However, the pathogenesis of hypercalcemia in myeloma is probably more complex than this since not all patients with significant myeloma bone disease develop hypercalcemia, and even then hypercalcemia is often a prominent feature only late in the course of the disease. Nevertheless, hypercalcemia is most common in patients who have the largest tumor burden and is related to the amount of bone-resorbing activity produced by the myeloma cells, as well as glomerular filtration status. Measurements of total body myeloma cell burden together with production of bone resorbing activity by cultured bone marrow myeloma cells *in vitro* do not correlate closely with hypercalcemia, although they do correlate somewhat with extent of osteolytic bone lesions [19]. Thus, there are clearly other factors which are involved in the pathogenesis of hypercalcemia in addition to those that promote osteoclast formation and induce osteoclast activation. There are other differences between hypercalcemia that occurs in myeloma and classic humoral hypercalcemia of malignancy in patients with solid tumors which are sometimes of assistance in the differential diagnosis. Firstly, in patients with hypercalcemia due to myeloma, there is almost always impaired renal function and an increase in serum phosphate that is associated with decreases in glomerular filtration rate. Secondly, markers of bone formation such as serum alkaline phosphatase are usually not increased in patients with myeloma, since bone formation is often not increased and in fact may be suppressed for reasons which are not entirely clear but may involve DKK1 (see below). Thirdly, patients with hypercalcemia due to myeloma usually respond very rapidly to treatment with corticosteroids mainly unlike patients with HHM [20].

Myeloma bone disease

The excessive bone destruction characteristic of myeloma is dependent on osteoclast stimulation [21]. Although it has been known for more than 30 years that osteoclasts are hyperstimulated by cytokines in myeloma, identification of the osteoclast activating factors (OAFs) responsible has proven elusive until the last half-decade. Until recently, the erstwhile approach of identifying such factors by the use of cultured tumor cell lines, followed by protein purification, has not been successful, as it is now apparent that cell–cell interactions involving myeloma cells and other cells in the marrow microenvironment, including stromal cells, cells in the osteoblast lineage, and possibly osteoclasts themselves, are required for the production of OAFs in myeloma. Currently, it seems that the OAFs most likely responsible for bone resorption in myeloma are the cytokine receptor activator of NF-κB ligand (RANKL) and the chemokine macrophage inflammatory protein (MIP)-1α [22, 23]. However, a number of other cytokines, including tumor necrosis factor-α (TNF-α), lymphotoxin (TNF-β) and PTHrP, have been implicated in the disease. There is considerable debate as to whether in myeloma these bone-resorbing cytokines are produced by the tumor cells, accessory cells involved in cell–cell interactions, or both and there is evidence in support of both notions. Myeloma bone disease is also characterized by marked impairment of bone formation, and it appears that a likely mediator of this effect is the soluble antagonist of the wnt pathway, DKK1 [24].

Treatment of hypercalcemia of malignancy

General

Medical therapy for hypercalcemia of malignancy is almost always successful with currently available bone resorption inhibitors. The general principles of therapy for hypercalcemia are: (1) effective treatment of the tumor where possible; (2) use of pharmacologic agents that inhibit bone resorption; (3) treatment of any exacerbating cause that has precipitated hypercalcemia; and (4) treatment of dehydration, which is common in patients with the hypercalcemia of malignancy and may lead to a spiral of disequilibrium hypercalcemia and progressive worsening of the serum calcium. Fluid losses provoke hypercalcemia, which in turn causes nephrogenic diabetes insipidus and consequently further worsens the dehydration.

In patients with malignant disease, hypercalcemia if untreated is usually progressive, and the serum calcium may rise rapidly over a few weeks. This occurs because of progressive increases in bone resorption and overall bone destruction. Because the symptoms of hypercalcemia are unpleasant and can be prevented, all patients with the hypercalcemia of malignancy should be treated actively.

Non-urgent therapy for hypercalcemia

Patients with a serum calcium less than 13 mg/dl at the time of diagnosis usually do not have symptoms related to hypercalcemia or have relatively mild symptoms. A number of agents are satisfactory for this situation. These agents may also be used in patients previously treated for more severe hypercalcemia who have mild residual hypercalcemia. (Conversion of traditional units to SI units: 4 mg/dl = 1 mmol/L.)

Bisphosphonates

Bisphosphonates, analogs of pyrophosphate, bind to mineralized surfaces and inhibit mineral deposition and osteoclastic bone resorption. They have a direct cellular effect to inhibit the bone resorption process, although their precise mechanisms of action are still unclear. Zoledronic acid, pamidronate and clodronate (not available in the US) are the members of this group most widely used. However, it is likely in the next few years that additional members of the bisphosphonate family will be approved. The newer generation bisphosphonates are extremely effective in lowering the serum calcium, usually within 72–96 h. These drugs are effective in more than 95% of patients with the hypercalcemia of malignancy and are the medical agents of first choice. There is some evidence that zoledronic acid may produce greater and longer lasting effects than pamidronate, but these differences are marginal and each of these drugs is very effective in the treatment of hypercalcemia.

Bisphosphonates have been so widely used over the past 30 years, and particularly over the last 10 years, that their side effect profile is now well known. The amino-bisphosphonates may be associated with transient flu-like symptoms that are not serious, and impairment of renal function if the infusion is given too rapidly, particular to a patient with underlying renal disease. The latter is not a problem if lower doses are given according to the labeling information and over appropriate infusion times in the presence of impaired glomerular filtration.

The potential side effect that has received most attention recently has been osteonecrosis of the jaw. Patients with cancer bone disease treated with powerful bisphosphonates, particularly in the presence of underlying dental disease or recent dental extraction, have a propensity to develop avascular exposed bone in the mandible which does not heal within 6 weeks. The condition has been described most frequently with zoledronic acid and pamidronate, but these are also the bisphosphonates most widely used in patients with cancer. It seems all bisphosphonates have been associated with this condition. The frequency is unknown, with reports varying from 0.2% to almost 10% of patients treated with bisphosphonates for cancer bone disease. The cause also remains unknown. Until more information is available, it seems prudent to discontinue bisphosphonates in patients who develop this complication, unless their use is potentially life-saving (for example, in the treatment of hypercalcemia), and to ensure patients do not have active dental disease at the time bisphosphonate therapy is commenced.

Plicamycin

Plicamycin was developed as a cytotoxic drug during the 1960s, and has been used to lower the serum calcium in hypercalcemia of malignancy since that time. It is extremely effective in the treatment of hypercalcemia of malignancy, lowering the serum calcium in greater than 80% of patients. However, it must be given by intravenous infusion over several hours. The infusion should not be repeated until the serum calcium rises again. It is potentially dangerous in patients who have impaired renal function because it has direct nephrotoxic effects and is cleared by the kidney. Other side effects include bone marrow suppression, a non-thrombocytopenic bleeding diathesis, and hepatotoxicity. For these reasons, plicamycin should be reserved for those rare circumstances where other drugs such as the newer bisphosphonates have been unsuccessful, and only in patients with normal renal function.

Calcitonin and glucocorticoids

Glucocorticoids have been used for many years in the treatment of hypercalcemia of malignancy. When used alone they reduce serum calcium in approximately 30% of all patients but rarely to the normal range. They are most likely to be effective in patients with hematologic malignancies such as myeloma or the lymphomas. They are occasionally effective in patients with breast cancer or lung cancer, but it is difficult to predict which patients will respond. Calcitonin is not particularly convenient as it has to be injected. The many chronic side effects of glucocorticoids are not seen in most patients, who in general have no more than 3–6 months of remaining life owing to the progression of the tumor.

Calcitonin alone in many patients produces a transient fall of serum calcium, which is not maintained. This "escape phenomenon" is seen both *in vitro* and *in vivo* [25]. The escape phenomenon can be blocked by concomitant glucocorticoids. The combination of the two drugs is effective in patients who require a rapid fall in serum calcium, particularly in patients with hematologic malignancies. It is an attractive form of treatment in patients with fixed impairment of renal function, in whom most other forms of treatment are either contraindicated or limited. In many patients, it may be necessary to withdraw calcitonin for 48 h every week to avoid escape. There are no significant side effects when calcitonin is used in these doses. We advise reserving this form of medication to patients with hypercalcemia due to myeloma and markedly impaired renal function.

Phosphate

Oral phosphate has been used for many years in the treatment of hypercalcemia. It is only likely to be effective in those patients in whom the serum phosphorus is less than 4 mg/dl. The mechanism of action is complex. Phosphate inhibits osteoclastic bone resorption, decreases calcium absorption from the gut, and promotes soft tissue calcium deposition. Oral phosphate should not be used in patients who have impaired renal function or who have serum phosphorus levels greater than 4 mg/dl. The major side effect of long-term phosphate therapy is troublesome diarrhea, which often limits its usefulness. Intravenous phosphate should only be used after other forms of therapy have failed, and life-saving therapy is required. It frequently provokes extraskeletal calcium deposition, particularly in the presence of impaired renal function.

Gallium nitrate

Gallium nitrate, which was originally used as a cytotoxic agent, inhibits bone resorption *in vitro* and produces prolonged lowering of the serum calcium *in vivo*. It seems to be effective in most forms of hypercalcemia of malignancy with relatively few side effects.

Indometacin and aspirin

Indometacin and aspirin are very effective inhibitors of prostaglandin synthesis and were widely used when prostaglandins were thought to be the major cause of hypercalcemia of malignancy. However, they uncommonly affect serum calcium.

Emergency treatment of hypercalcemia

Emergency treatment for hypercalcemia is necessary in patients with a serum calcium greater than 13 mg/dl. This level of serum calcium is usually associated with severe symptoms, including thirst, nausea, and altered mental status. Such hypercalcemia is potentially life threatening in patients with malignant disease in whom the serum calcium may rapidly rise further, particularly if patients become dehydrated. Other situations that can precipitate severe hypercalcemia include thiazide therapy, treatment with estrogens or antiestrogens in patients with breast cancer, or vomiting with associated dehydration and prerenal azotemia.

Fluids

Patients with severe hypercalcemia are often dehydrated and may require repletion with 6–10 L of normal saline over 24 h. Because severe hypercalcemia is associated with fluid depletion, and calcium and sodium handling by the renal tubules is linked, normal saline should be given to replace fluid losses. Normal saline repletion will lead to a sodium and calcium diuresis, which will help lower the serum calcium. Occasionally, patients will become hypernatremic (excess sodium), and under these circumstances half-normal saline should be substituted for normal saline.

Loop diuretics

Furosemide (frusemide) has been frequently used in the United States for the emergency treatment of hypercalcemia because it promotes a calcium diuresis. However, in the doses used by most clinicians, it is not clear that it produces a significant effect beyond that of saline therapy alone. Moreover, loop diuretics at the required doses may be dangerous and may lead to other electrolyte problems, dehydration, and worsening of hypercalcemia.

Bisphosphonates

The most effective current agents in the emergency treatment of hypercalcemia are the bisphosphonates. Zoledronic acid is effective in approximately 95% of patients and will usually lower the serum calcium to the normal range after 72 h, without serious toxicity. As noted above, the infusion time should not be less than 15 min, it should be avoided in patients with active dental disease or recent tooth extraction, and the dose should be modified in patients with impaired glomerular filtration according to the package insert.

Investigational approaches

The discovery that the RANKL/RANK/OPG pathway is indispensable not only for normal bone resorption but also pathologic bone resorption induced by myeloma and other cancers that metastasize to the skeleton has spurred the clinical development of a number of other types of new anti-resorptive agents. The most advanced of this is a humanized monoclonal antibody to RANKL, denosumab (Amgen). Clinical trials with this agent are on-going in patients with multiple myeloma and bone metastases from breast cancer and recent data suggests that it is efficacious [26].

Acknowledgments

This work was supported by NIH/NCI Program Project Grant PO1 CA40035 (Mundy), an NCI Career Development Award KO1 CA104180 (Oyajobi), and an NIAMS training grant F32 AR05169 (Sterling).

References

1. Mundy GR, Martin TJ. The hypercalcemia of malignancy: pathogenesis and management. *Metabolism* 1982;31:1247–1277.
2. Mundy GR, Guise TA. Hormonal control of calcium homeostasis. *Clin. Chem.* 1999;45:1347–1352.
3. Mundy GR, Cove DH, Fisken R. Primary hyperparathyroidism: changes in the pattern of clinical presentation. *Lancet* 1980;1:1317–1320.
4. Moseley JM, et al. Parathyroid hormone-related protein purified from a human lung cancer cell line. *Proc. Natl Acad. Sci. USA* 1987;84:5048–5052.
5. Yates AJ, et al. Effects of a synthetic peptide of a parathyroid hormone-related protein on calcium homeostasis, renal tubular calcium reabsorption, and bone metabolism in vivo and in vitro in rodents. *J. Clin. Invest.* 1988;81:932–938.
6. Galasko CS, Burn JI. Hypercalcaemia in patients with advanced mammary cancer. *Br. Med. J.* 1971;3:573–577.
7. Powell GJ, et al. Localization of parathyroid hormone-related protein in breast cancer metastases: increased incidence in bone compared with other sites. *Cancer Res.* 1991;51:3059–3061.
8. Southby J, et al. Immunohistochemical localization of parathyroid hormone-related protein in human breast cancer. *Cancer Res.* 1990;50:7710–7716.
9. Guise TA, Yoneda T, Yates AJ, Mundy GR. The combined effect of tumor-produced parathyroid hormone-related protein and transforming growth factor-alpha enhance hypercalcemia in vivo and bone resorption in vitro. *J. Clin. Endocrinol. Metab.* 1993;77:40–45.
10. Gallwitz WE, Guise TA, Mundy GR. Guanosine nucleotides inhibit different syndromes of PTHrP excess caused by human cancers in vivo. *J. Clin. Invest.* 2002;110:1559–1572.
11. Thomas RJ, et al. Breast cancer cells interact with osteoblasts to support osteoclast formation. *Endocrinology* 1999;140:4451–4458.
12. Kong YY, et al. Activated T cells regulate bone loss and joint destruction in adjuvant arthritis through osteoprotegerin ligand. *Nature* 199;402;304–309.
13. Bendre M, Gaddy D, Nicholas RW, Suva LJ. Breast cancer metastasis to bone: it is not all about PTHrP. *Clin. Orthop. Relat. Res.* 2003;S39–45.
14. Mundy GR, Yoneda T. Bisphosphonates as anticancer drugs. *N. Engl. J. Med.* 2002;339:398–400.
15. Mundy GR. Metastasis to bone: causes, consequences and therapeutic opportunities. *Nat. Rev. Cancer* 2202;2:584–593.
16. Pfeilschifter J, Mundy GR. Modulation of type beta transforming growth factor activity in bone cultures by osteotropic hormones. *Proc. Natl Acad. Sci. USA* 1987;84:2024–2028.
17. Yin JJ, et al. TGF-beta signaling blockade inhibits PTHrP secretion by breast cancer cells and bone metastases development. *J. Clin. Invest.* 1999;103:197–206.
18. Tuttle KR, Kunau RT, Loveridge N, Mundy GR. Altered renal calcium handling in hypercalcemia of malignancy. *J. Am. Soc. Nephrol.* 1991;2:191–199.
19. Durie BG, Salmon SE, Mundy GR. Relation of osteoclast activating factor production to extent of bone disease in multiple myeloma. *Br. J. Haematol.* 1981;47:21–30.
20. Mundy GR, Wilkinson R, Heath DA. Comparative study of available medical therapy for hypercalcemia of malignancy. *Am. J. Med.* 1983;74:421–432.
21. Mundy GR, Raisz LG, Cooper RA, Schechter GP, Salmon SE. Evidence for the secretion of an osteoclast stimulating factor in myeloma. *N. Engl. J. Med.* 1974;291:1041–1046.
22. Oyajobi BO, et al. Therapeutic efficacy of a soluble receptor activator of nuclear factor kappaB-IgG Fc fusion protein in suppressing bone resorption and hypercalcemia in a model of humoral hypercalcemia of malignancy. *Cancer Res.* 2001;61:2572–2578.
23. Oyajobi BO, et al. Dual effects of macrophage inflammatory protein-1alpha on osteolysis and tumor burden in the murine 5TGM1 model of myeloma bone disease. *Blood* 2003;102:311–319.
24. Tian E, et al. The role of the Wnt-signaling antagonist DKK1 in the development of osteolytic lesions in multiple myeloma. *N. Engl. J. Med.* 2003;349:2483–2494.
25. Binstock ML, Mundy GR. Effect of calcitonin and glutocorticoids in combination on the hypercalcemia of malignancy. *Ann. Intern. Med.* 1980;93:269–272.
26. Body JJ, et al. A study of the biological receptor activator of nuclear factor-kappaB ligand inhibitor, denosumab, in patients with multiple myeloma or bone metastases from breast cancer. *Clin. Cancer Res.* 2006;12:1221–1228.

78 Syndrome of Ectopic ACTH Secretion

Marie-Laure Raffin-Sanson, Hélène Fierrard, and Xavier Bertagna

Key points

- Ectopic adrenocorticotropic hormone syndrome is a clinically and biologically heterogeneous entity. Rapid onset of a severe Cushing syndrome with weight loss and hypokalemia is a feature of aggressive malignant tumors whereas well-differentiated small carcinoids of the lung display mild and slowly progressive clinical features that mimic Cushing disease.
- At the molecular level also, ectopic adrenocorticotropic hormone syndrome is heterogeneous: pro-opiomelanocortin gene expression and adrenocorticotropic hormone precursor processing are abnormal in malignant tumors whereas a highly differentiated corticotroph phenotype is achieved in adrenocorticotropic hormone-secreting bronchial carcinoids.
- Due to their puzzling clinical and hormonal behavior, these well-differentiated tumors have led to the development of an aggressive investigation procedure, bilateral inferior petrosal sinus sampling, as the best diagnostic approach to recognize the non-pituitary origin of an adrenocorticotropic hormone secretion.
- Thin cut multislice or helical computerized tomography of the thorax and abdomen and magnetic resonance imaging (MRI) of the thorax have the highest detection rate for small occult tumors. The superimposition of ^{111}In-octreotide single photon emission computerized tomography with computerized tomography/magnetic resonance imaging slices may help with localization.
- Treatment of the ectopic adrenocorticotropic hormone syndrome includes different therapeutic options that can be directed towards the non-pituitary tumor and/or the normal adrenals, depending on the nature of the tumor, its localization, and the potential need for rapid control of a life-threatening hypercortisolism.

Introduction

The first case of ectopic adrenocorticotropic hormone (ACTH) syndrome was reported by Brown in 1928 when he described a bearded woman with diabetes who had a small cell carcinoma of the lung (SCCL). Liddle's group [1] subsequently identified cases of patients with Cushing syndrome in whom ACTH was produced by so-called "non-endocrine" tumors. In the initial paper by Meador [2], most patients had lung tumors, the extracts of which contained bioactive ACTH. The concept of "ectopic hormone secretion" was then born. Yet its fine pathophysiological mechanism still remains highly intriguing today, even though much progress has been made, essentially through the recent advances in molecular endocrinology and the unravelling of the details of ACTH biosynthesis.

The ectopic ACTH syndrome: two contrasted clinical presentations

Classically . . .

The first description of the ectopic ACTH syndrome was in patients with obvious and aggressive tumors, mainly SCCLs, most

Table 78.1 Tumors associated with the ectopic ACTH syndrome in a personal series of 43 patients

Small cell lung carcinoma	9	(21%)
Bronchial carcinoid	19	(44%)
Pancreatic tumor	4	(9%)
Pheochromocytoma	3	(7%)
Gastrinoma	2	(4.6%)
Medullary thyroid carcinoma	2	(4.6%)
Ovarian cancer	2	(4.6%)
Neuroblastoma	1	(2.3%)
Thymoma	1	(2.3%)

often leading to fatal outcome [2] (Table 78.1). Here, clinical features of Cushing syndrome have a rapid onset and a severe presentation. Muscle wasting and weight loss can mask fat redistribution. Hyperpigmentation is classic. Severe hypertension is frequent and hypokalemia may be symptomatic. Hormonal investigations most often show that highly elevated ACTH plasma levels and dynamic tests such as the high-dose dexamethasone suppression test, the metyrapone test the vasopressin test, and corticotropin-releasing hormone (CRH) test are typically unresponsive, stressing the autonomous character of ACTH secretion by such tumors [3].

Clinical Endocrine Oncology, 2nd edition. Edited by Ian D. Hay and John A.H. Wass. © 2008 Blackwell Publishing. ISBN 978-1-4051-4584-8.

More recently . . .

Today, there is another set of tumors responsible for what has been denominated the "occult" or the "chronic ectopic ACTH syndrome" [4]. These patients most often bear a small tumor which may escape usual detection means. Further to this diagnostic difficulty, these tumors can behave in a "pituitary-like" manner, leading to the erroneous diagnosis of Cushing disease and eventually to unwarranted and inefficient pituitary surgery. The mild and slowly progressive clinical features resemble that of Cushing disease (Chapter 31) [3, 4] and, what is most intriguing, some of these tumors respond to the classic dynamic tests in a fashion similar to that of a pituitary corticotroph tumor: almost a third suppress cortisol secretion under the high-dose dexamethasone suppression test and some well-documented cases show response to metyrapone and/or CRH stimulation [5, 6].

Carcinoid tumors, especially in the bronchial tree, are the vast majority of these ACTH-secreting non-pituitary tumors responsible for the occult ectopic ACTH syndrome [4] (Table 78.1). These small tumoral lesions display a high degree of neuroendocrine differentiation [7, 8] assessed by the presence of secretory granules, and by their high content in prohormone convertases (PCs) specifically associated with the neuroendocrine cells (i.e., PC1 and PC2), whose function is to process polypeptide precursors to their bioactive peptidic hormones [9, 10].

At the molecular level also, ectopic ACTH syndrome is heterogeneous

How the pro-opiomelanocortin (POMC) precursor and/or its fragments are secreted by non-pituitary tumors

Altered POMC processing is frequent in non-pituitary tumors but not specific. In normal pituitary corticotroph cells POMC is fully processed by the sole PC1: thus, intact ACTH is released [with other fragments resulting from POMC cleavage, such as β- and γ-lipotropin (LPH)]. The precursor itself is not secreted. This is also true in most pituitary corticotroph adenomas. In non-pituitary tumors, the maturation process is often altered, because local PCs are inappropriate to properly process an ectopic precursor like POMC. Hence, an abnormal maturation pattern of POMC is a classic feature of the ectopic ACTH syndrome (Fig. 78.1). Two types of alteration of POMC processing have been shown in these tumors.

• Processing may be incomplete, leading to secretion, sometimes predominant, of the intact precursor (or biosynthetic intermediates to ACTH). Besides chromatographic approaches several groups have developed specific Immuno Radiometric Assays (IRMAs) for POMC or other partially processed precursor fragments, taking advantage of the various antibodies raised against different regions of the POMC molecule to build "sandwich" immunoassays [11, 12].

• Conversely, abnormal fragments such as CLIP (corticotropin-like intermediary lobe peptide) and hβMSH 5–22 may be generated. Recent studies have shown that PC2 was specifically present in

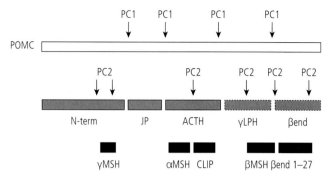

Figure 78.1 ACTH precursor processing in normal corticotroph cells and in aggressive ACTH-secreting tumors. Pro-opiomelanocortin (POMC) is normally processed in corticotroph cells by the propeptide convertase type 1 (PC1) into the peptides indicated in gray: corticotropin (ACTH), lipotropin (LPH), β-endorphin (β-end), joining peptide (JP), N-terminal fragment (N-term). In ACTH-secreting non-pituitary tumors, other peptides may also be produced (indicated in black): unprocessed precursor (POMC) and small fragments resulting from further cleavage of ACTH, N-term and LPH by the action of PC2 or other non-corticotroph enzymes: melanocyte-stimulating hormones (α-, β-, and γMSH), and β-endorphin 1–27.

these tumors which contained CLIP and not in those producing predominantly ACTH [13].

In both cases, these processing abnormalities diminish the tissue's ability to secrete authentic bioactive ACTH and somehow protect the patients from the consequences of the tumor production. They also provide the investigator with subtle molecular clues that an ACTH-dependent Cushing syndrome may originate from a non-pituitary source. Systematic studies of large series of tissues demonstrated that poorly differentiated and aggressive tumors like SCCL preferentially released intact POMC [12], most likely because of a general defect in both PC1 and PC2, whereas carcinoids – which have a high degree of neuroendocrine differentiation – rather overprocess the precursor, releasing ACTH and smaller peptides like CLIP, most probably because of their high content in PCs including PC2 (Fig. 78.2).

Abnormal processing of POMC is not specific to non-pituitary tumors: it is found occasionally in rare pituitary macroadenomas and in some exceptional pituitary cancers. High molecular weight immunoactive ACTH-like materials have been identified in the plasma of such patients. In some cases, a direct POMC IRMA in blood shows that the unprocessed precursor is directly secreted by the pituitary tumor [12]. Thus, defective POMC processing actually indicates an impaired state of neuroendocrine differentiation in aggressive tumors, independent of their pituitary or non-pituitary origin (Fig. 78.2).

How the *POMC* gene is transcribed in non-pituitary tumors

POMC mRNA can be detected in many normal non-pituitary tissues. In most of them, *POMC* gene expression is quantitatively and qualitatively different from that in the pituitary: the tissue concentration of *POMC* mRNA is low and the mRNA is essentially made of short transcripts of about 800 nucleotides (nt) [14].

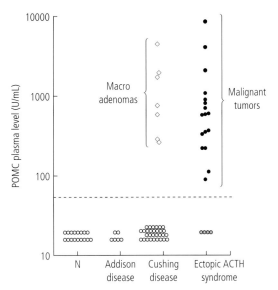

Figure 78.2 POMC plasma level in various causes of Cushing syndrome. POMC plasma levels in: ○ normal controls, patients with Addison disease or corticotroph microadenomas, ◇ corticotroph macroadenomas, ● ACTH-secreting malignant tumors, ACTH-secreting bronchial carcinoids. N, normal subjects. The dotted line indicates the detection limit of the assay.

They are not functional as they cannot be efficiently translated into POMC peptides. Altered *POMC* gene transcription in ACTH-secreting non-pituitary tumors is frequent (see Fig. 78.3); classic Northern blot from ACTH-secreting non-pituitary tumors revealed, besides the normal sized (pituitary like) 1200 nt POMC mRNA, high molecular weight species of about 1450 nt. This material corresponded to a population of three 5′ extended transcripts. By contrast, highly differentiated tumors like bronchial

carcinoids most often contained the pituitary-like 1200 nt POMC nRNA as the highly predominant if not the sole transcript of the *POMC* gene [15].

Different molecular mechanisms may drive *POMC* gene expression in different tumoral entities

The intimate mechanism that triggers *POMC* gene transcription in a non-pituitary tumor remains mysterious. Is it the result of a wide and non-specific molecular turbulence that picks up the POMC gene fortuitously or, alternatively, is it the transposition of a more or less complete corticotroph phenotype out of pituitary limits? The answer to this question may be helped by observations made on the human SCCL cell line DMS79, and by the discovery of markers of the corticotroph phenotype, such as the V3 vasopressin receptor gene.

The *POMC* gene is a target of E2F factors in the POMC-producing human SCCL cell line DMS79

The mechanism of *POMC* gene transcription in aggressive ACTH-producing non-pituitary tumors was addressed using a model of the POMC-producing SCCL cell line: DMS79. Transcription requires the same 417 nt proximal promoter fragment as in the mouse pituitary cell line AtT20 (taken as a model of pituitary corticotroph cells) but the respective contributions of definite regions of this promoter widely vary between the two cell lines [16] indicating that *POMC* gene transcription is achieved in each case through a different set of *trans*-acting factors. A meticulous functional study of the human *POMC* gene promoter allowed identification of a discrete region which was specifically active in

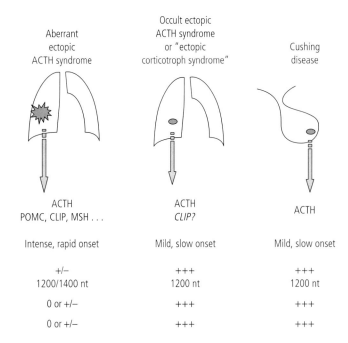

Figure 78.3 Clinical and molecular features of ACTH-secreting tumors. CLIP, corticotropin-like intermediary lobe peptide; POMC, pro-opiomelanocortin; MSH, melanocyte-stimulating hormone; ACTH, corticotropin; V3 R, vasopressin receptor type 3; nt, nucleotides.

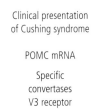

DMS79 and not in AtT20 corticotroph cells. Sequence analysis and functional studies revealed that this element was a target for E2F transcription factors that specifically bound this sequence and enhanced POMC gene transcription [17]. E2F factors are known as regulators of the activity of several cell cycle-regulating genes. Their activity in quiescent cells is normally blocked through their binding of the retinoblastoma proto-oncogene *pRb*. The inhibitory effect of *pRb* can be released when *pRb* is phosphorylated, absent or mutated. The latest situation is the rule in SCCLs including DMS79. The fortuitous activation of the human *POMC* promoter by a mechanism involving protein associated with malignant transformation and proliferation would explain why *POMC* gene expression is so frequent in aggressive tumors. As *POMC* gene expression is not constant in SCCLs and other tumors associated with *pRb* alterations, other mechanisms must modulate the activity of the *POMC* promoter in those cells. A role for epigenetic modifications has been proposed. Methylation of specific sites within the *POMC* promoter (E2F- and PTX1-binding sites, for example) in normal *POMC* non-expressing tissues has been shown to suppress *POMC* transcription activity. These sites are unmethylated in tumors as well as in the DMS79 cell line [18]. The physiological relevance of these observations must, however, be confirmed.

A highly differentiated corticotroph phenotype is achieved in ACTH-secreting bronchial carcinoids

A pituitary-specific receptor called V3 (or V1b) is responsible for ACTH secretion in response to vasopressin. Tissue distribution studies indicated that V3 is highly specific for the anterior pituitary corticotroph cells and thus constitutes, like POMC, a marker of the corticotroph phenotype in a given tumor. Expression of V3 receptor and *POMC* genes was examined simultaneously in various types of ACTH-secreting tumors using a comparative reverse transcriptase–polymerase chain reaction approach. Bronchial carcinoid responsible for the ectopic ACTH syndrome had both POMC and V3 receptor signals as high as those in pituitary corticotroph adenomas. In contrast, no POMC signal and only very faint V3 receptor signal were detected in non-secreting bronchial carcinoids [19]. Other types of aggressive non-pituitary tumors responsible for ectopic ACTH syndrome presented much lower levels of both *POMC*-mRNA, and V3 receptor gene expression was almost undetectable [19].

Thus, bronchial carcinoids constitute a particular subset of tumors where both V3 receptor and *POMC* genes may be expressed in a pattern qualitatively and quantitatively indistinguishable from that in pituitary corticotroph adenomas. They process the precursor to release large amounts of bioactive ACTH in a pituitary manner. The apparent co-ordinated expression of two different genes that characterize the pituitary corticotroph cells suggested the expression of a "master gene" driving corticotroph differentiation. The expression of the newly discovered corticotroph transcription factor *Tpit* [20] was examined in ACTH-secreting non-pituitary tumors. *Tpit* encodes a T box transcription factor restricted to the corticotroph lineage [21] and necessary for terminal differentiation of pituitary POMC-expressing cells [23]. In fact *Tpit* gene is expressed in ACTH-secreting as well as in non-secreting carcinoids, suggesting that some aspects of the pituitary corticotroph phenotype may belong to general carcinoid differentiation. More generally, ACTH-positive carcinoids do not share a characteristic expression pattern of the corticotroph-associated transcription factor genes. Thus, the transcriptional mechanisms of the ACTH-precursor gene differ from those in normal pituitary corticotrophs [21].

Two different entities for the syndrome of ectopic ACTH secretion? (Fig. 78.3)

Thus the ectopic ACTH syndrome appears to be made of two different entities. The first is due to indolent and highly differentiated tumors, that have high content of biochemical neuroendocrine markers, produce large amounts of normal (pituitary-like) POMC mRNA and express high levels of the "corticotroph-specific" V3 receptor. An example of this is bronchial carcinoids (this might be best called "ectopic corticotroph syndrome"). In contrast, when ectopic ACTH syndrome is due to highly malignant, poorly differentiated tumors producing low levels of altered molecular forms of *POMC* mRNA and POMC peptides, with much lower V3 receptor, it might be best called "aberrant ACTH secretion syndrome" (Fig. 78.3).

Clinical implications

Bilateral inferior petrosal sinus sampling

Due to the puzzling clinical and hormonal behavior of the "ectopic corticotroph syndrome," these tumors have led to the development of an aggressive investigation procedure, bilateral inferior petrosal sinus sampling (IPS), as the best diagnostic approach to recognize the non-pituitary origin of an ACTH secretion [4]. In fact, when response to dynamic testing is discordant, and/or when pituitary magnetic resonance imaging (MRI) is normal in an ACTH-dependent Cushing syndrome, sampling of the gradient of corticotropin from the pituitary gland to the periphery is the most reliable means of discriminating between Cushing disease and ectopic ACTH syndrome. Corticotropin concentration is measured simultaneously in left and right IPS as well as in a peripheral vein (P) before and after intravenous injection of ovine or human CRH. An IPS/P ratio <2 before CRH and <3 after CRH indicates an extrapituitary ACTH secretion. This procedure is efficient and safe if performed by experienced hands. Remission of an intermittent ACTH secretion must be ruled out before the test is performed. In these conditions, sensitivity and specificity are excellent [22, 23].

Altered POMC processing could help to diagnose an ectopic source of ACTH production

POMC is the substrate of two enzymes (PC1 and PC2), which are markers of a more or less achieved neuroendocrine phenotype and POMC and/or its fragments are secreted. Thus analysis of POMC and its fragments in a simple peripheral plasma collection allows exploration of the degree of neuroendocrine differentiation of the responsible tumor. Clearly, detectable plasma POMC levels are encountered more often in ectopic ACTH syndromes than in Cushing disease. In this last case, high plasma POMC levels are associated with aggressive macroadenomas, easily detected by usual imaging means. Thus, if POMC plasma levels are high and pituitary MRI is normal, ectopic ACTH syndrome is likely [11, 12]. Unfortunately, POMC immunoassays are not routinely available.

Because some tumors overprocess POMC, CLIP may be a predominant secretory product. There is currently no commercial CLIP assay, either radioimmunoassay or IRMA. The presence of circulating CLIP may be suspected when ACTH IRMAs with different specificities for CLIP give dissociated results in the same plasma sample, or when the LPH/ACTH ratio increases. This may be confirmed by more sophisticated approaches (high pressure liquid chromatography). The availability of a specific CLIP assay would be of great interest to pick up these "occult" tumors that have a tendency to overprocess POMC (Fig. 78.3).

Imaging techniques

Once the non-pituitary origin of the secretion has been established, localization of the small ACTH-secreting tumor is another challenge. Some ACTH-secreting tumors are easy to detect: large invasive carcinoma of the lung or pancreas, pheochromocytoma, medullary thyroid carcinoma. However, about 30% of the patients harbor small neuroendocrine tumors that escape standard imagery (Table 78.1). Thin cut multislice computerized tomography (CT) of the thorax and abdomen and if possible helical CT, MRI of the thorax, or both procedures have the highest detection rate for ectopic ACTH syndrome [24, 25], allowing correct localization in about 75% of the patients. New developments in thoracic MRI may improve diagnostic performance in the detection of small bronchial carcinoids: these tumors are of high signal intensity on T2-weighted and STIR images ("short tau inversion recovery," a T2 weighted sequence with fat suppression), allowing the distinction between a small mass and the pulmonary vasculature.

When the cause of corticotropin production remains occult, it may be tempting to take advantage of the neuroendocrine phenotype of these lesions to disclose small tumors which have escaped the CT scan. Somatostatin (SS) agonists specifically bind with high affinity to receptor subtypes 2 and 5 which are found in most of these neuroendocrine tumors. The most commonly used SS analog, octreotide, may be conjugated with DTPA (diethylene-triamine-penta-acetic acid) or DOTA (tetra-azacyclododecane tetra-acetic acid) as a way of coupling the SS receptor ligand with various radioisotopes, mainly [111]In. Most centers use ^{111}In-DTPA-D Phe1-octreotide (or ^{111}In-pentetreotide). Several studies reported successful localization of small carcinoid tumors by somatostatin scintigraphy [29]. However, although standard somatostatin scintigraphy may confirm the functionality for a lesion seen on classic imaging, it has only rarely been shown to disclose occult tumors

non-visible on CT scan [25, 26]. Using higher than standard doses of radionucleotide may in some cases improve sensitivity. Finally, the superimposition of ^{111}In-octreotide SPECT (single photon emission CT) with CT/MRI slices (anatomical–functional image fusion) has shown improved localization and characterization of some neuroendocrine tumors [27] (Fig. 78.4). Positron emission tomography (PET) with ^{18}F-labelled de-oxyglucose (FDG) is of little benefit since ACTH-secreting occult tumors are slow growing and have a low metabolic activity. The use of C-5-hydroxytryptophan has been proposed in the localization of small neuroendocrine tumors. However, further experience is needed to evaluate its potential value.

Even if several imaging procedures are successively used to investigate these tumors, corticotropin production remains occult in 5–15% of patients who will need symptomatic treatment of hypercortisolism and continued follow-up.

Overview: diagnosis of ectopic ACTH syndrome (Fig. 78.5)

Once a diagnosis of corticotropin-dependent Cushing syndrome is established, the next step is to determine the pituitary (90%) or non-pituitary (10%) origin of ACTH secretion. Sometimes, clinical and biological presentation indicates an obvious ACTH-secreting malignant tumor. No dynamic testing is indicated. Priority is given to the rapid control of hypercortisolism and malignant disease. Treatment will usually associate surgery and/or cytotoxic chemotherapy with adrenolytic drugs.

However, carcinoid tumors can be clinically indistinguishable from Cushing disease and are frequently difficult to identify with imaging, whereas pituitary MRI is normal in 40% of patients with Cushing disease. Dynamic tests (high-dose dexamethasone suppression test, CRH test) and pituitary MRI should be evaluated together. If corticotropin secretion is responsive to both CRH and dexamethasone and pituitary MRI shows a lesion of 6 mm or more, ectopic ACTH syndrome can be ruled out. If not, IPS is indicated. A basal central/peripheral ACTH ratio of more than 2/1 or a ratio of more than 3/1 after CRH injection indicates Cushing disease. The absence of corticotropin gradient is consistent with an ectopic source of ACTH secretion. Axial imaging must be performed, completed by SS. Usefulness of other imaging techniques must be evaluated. When the ACTH secretion remains occult, direct actions at the adrenal level are mandatory to control hypercortisolism. Continued follow-up often allows localization of the tumor, sometimes after several years.

Treatment

Treatment of the ectopic ACTH syndrome includes different options that can be directed towards the non-pituitary tumor, the normal adrenals or the glucocorticoid receptor, sometimes in a combined manner.

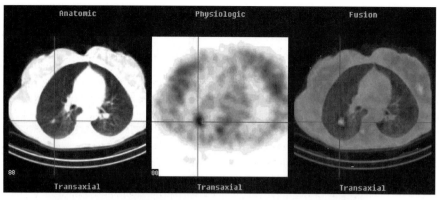

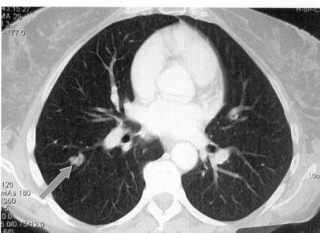

Figure 78.4 Characterization of a bronchial carcinoid by superimposition of ^{111}In-octreotide SPECT with CT/MRI slices (anatomical–functional image fusion).

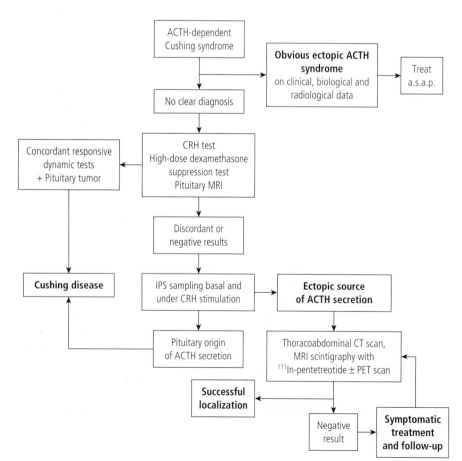

Figure 78.5 Overview: diagnosis of ectopic ACTH syndrome. IPS, inferior petrosal sinus sampling; ACTH, corticotropin; CRH, corticotropin-releasing hormone; PET, positron emission tomography.

Treatment options for the non-pituitary tumor

Surgery of the non-pituitary tumor

Removing the source of ectopic ACTH secretion is the ideal treatment. When feasible it can lead to complete recovery of a normal pituitary–adrenal axis. Two conditions are mandatory to reach this goal:

• that the source of non-pituitary ACTH be precisely localized
• that the non-pituitary tumor be entirely removed with no risk of recurrence or distant metastases.

These two conditions can be met in some favorable situations like a typical bronchial carcinoid that has been readily identified with no metastatic nodes or a rare ACTH-secreting pheochromocytoma that can be easily removed leaving one normal adrenal gland. In an exceptional case, surgical removal of an ACTH-secreting bronchial carcinoid was helped by radioguidance using ^{111}In-penetreotide detection during the operation [28]. Removal of the ACTH source will immediately create a state of adrenal insufficiency since the normal pituitary corticotroph function will be suppressed. The patient will require immediate glucocorticoid coverage at surgery, and substitutive therapy will need to be monitored afterwards.

In many cases, however, things are more difficult, either because an indolent tumor cannot be localized as in "occult ectopic ACTH syndrome," or because the tumor behaves in an aggressive manner as in SCCL.

Cytotoxic chemotherapy

Successful cytotoxic therapy of an ACTH-secreting non-pituitary tumor will eventually control ACTH oversecretion in the same time when the tumor shrinks. Under such treatment it is mandatory to assess corticotroph function, and anticipate glucocorticoid coverage. It might not be always easy to clinically distinguish between side effects of the cytotoxic drugs (gastrointestinal symptoms, fatigue, malaise), and the occurrence of adrenal insufficiency. There is no specific chemotherapeutic regimen directed against an ACTH-secreting non-pituitary tumor; the choice of the treatment will be made according to the type of tumor.

Somatostatin analogs

Because many ACTH-secreting non-pituitary tumors are endocrine tumors with a well-differentiated endocrine phenotype, many of them will share some common characteristics. Among them is the possibility to express genes coding for the receptor(s) to somatostatin. This feature can be utilized to locate such tumors, using scintigraphic approaches with labeled somatostatin analogs. In some of these tumors, the somatostatin receptors are expressed and also functionally coupled to pathways that regulate the biosynthesis/secretory mechanisms. One of these pathways is the cAMP pathway that normally regulates *POMC* gene expression in the normal corticotroph cell. It was thus hypothesized that suppression of the cAMP pathway, by activating functional somatostatin receptor(s) in "non-pituitary" tumors, might suppress ACTH oversecretion. ACTH suppression was indeed induced by octreotide administration in a patient with ectopic ACTH secretion due to a pancreatic endocrine tumor. Since this first observation [29], several other reports have confirmed the efficacy of this pharmacologic approach in various types of endocrine tumor; yet it is not constant, and not predicted by somatostatin imaging. Combined treatment with the dopamine agonist cabergoline has been proposed as a synergistic approach, although the exact role of dopamine agonists in the treatment of the ectopic ACTH syndrome is not fully established and appears occasional [30].

Unfortunately, this approach, almost invariably, only has a clear action on ACTH biosynthesis/secretion, and no definitive action on the tumor growth. Yet, because it can act very quickly, and has few, if any, untoward effects, it is very helpful, and can be administered in a combined fashion, for example with drugs directed at the adrenals, in order to obtain a rapid control in cases with severe, life-threatening hypercortisolism.

Treatment options for the normal adrenals

Whenever treatments directed at the source of ectopic ACTH secretion fail or are not feasible, or when control of hypercortisolism is urgently needed, direct action at the adrenal level may be unavoidable.

Anticortisolic drugs

There are two different types of pharmacologic agents that can act directly at the adrenals to suppress corticosteroid secretion.

• Some are direct enzyme inhibitors: they block the biosynthesis of cortisol. Their action is immediate. Yet, because the ACTH drive from the non-pituitary tumor is not modified, their action is often only transient. Ketoconazole, aminoglutethimide, metyrapone and etomidate are examples of such drugs, and have all been used in this setting, with variable success, mostly in rather short series. Etomidate intravenously has been reported to allow rapid control of severe hypercortisolism in exceptional cases, under close monitoring because of its anesthetic effect [31].
• By contrast, Op'DDD (Mitotane, Lysodren) is an adrenolytic drug which provokes the destruction of the adrenal cortex. For that reason it can obtain a very efficient control of the hypercortisolism, with no "escape." Yet, it has two drawbacks: its delayed action, as anticipated by its mode of action, which may require weeks or months; and a number of side effects that require close monitoring by experienced endocrinologists and the help of plasma Op'DDD measurements.

In some cases, combined treatment with Op'DDD and an enzyme inhibitor allows a quick control, and secondary adrenal destruction.

Adrenal surgery

Total bilateral adrenalectomy allows immediate control of hypercortisolism, with 100% success rate! This strategy is generally discussed when other options have failed. It has to be considered in relation to different factors:

• the severity of the hypercortisolism, which may be a threat to the surgical risk

• the availability of a highly experienced team of surgeon and anesthesiologist, ready to perform a "rescue" operation in an extremely fragile patient
• the nature of the non-pituitary tumor, which may determine the ultimate prognosis for the patient.

It may be a very difficult decision to take when the other options have failed, and to go on to adrenal surgery in a patient whose condition is deteriorating!

Cortisol antagonists: RU486

RU486 (Mifepristone) antagonizes cortisol action at the receptor level. In that setting it has been used in an occasional patient with the ectopic ACTH secretion syndrome, with an apparent success [32]. This approach has several difficulties.

• Because ACTH secretion is not modified, cortisol secretion will remain unchanged and its effects at the mineralocorticoid receptor will not be antagonized by RU486, and therefore hypertension and hypokalemia might not be controlled.
• Monitoring the treatment is extremely difficult. How to titrate the amount of RU486? How to diagnose adrenal crisis in a patient who may also have symptoms in relation to the tumor burden when plasma cortisol measurement is of no help? How to counteract the likelihood of adrenal crisis, with what amount of glucocorticoids?

For all these reasons, and although an occasional patient seems to have benefited from it, RU486 is not recommended as a routine approach in such patients. It is possible that further studies will better delineate the practical modalities of the pharmacologic approach.

References

1. Liddle GW, Nicholson WE, Island DP, Orth DN, Abe L, Lowder SC. Clinical and laboratory studies of ectopic humoral syndromes. *Rec. Prog. Horm. Res.* 1969;25:283–314.
2. Meador CK, Liddle GW, Island DP, et al. Cause of Cushing syndrome in patients with tumors arising from "nonendocrine" tissue. *J. Clin. Endocrinol. Metab.* 1962;22:6893–6703.
3. Wajchenberg BL, Mendonca BB, Liberman B, et al. Ectopic adrenocorticotropic hormone syndrome. *Endocr. Rev.* 1994;15:752–787.
4. Newell-Price J, Bertagna X, Grossman AB, Nieman LK. Cushing syndrome. *Lancet* 2006;367:1605–1617.
5. Nieman LK, Chrousos GP, Oldfield EH, Avgerinos PC, Cutler GB, Loriaux DL. The ovine corticotropin-releasing hormone stimulation test and the dexamethasone suppression test in the differential diagnosis of Cushing syndrome. *Ann. Intern. Med.* 1986;105:862–867.
6. de Keyzer Y, Clauser E, Bertagna X. The pituitary V3 vasopressin receptor and the ectopic ACTH syndrome. *Curr. Opin. Endocrinol. Diab.* 1996;3:125–131.
7. Vieau D, Linard CG, Mbikay M, et al. Expression of the neuroendocrine cell marker 7B2 in human ACTH secreting tumors. *Clin. Endocrinol.* 1992;36:597–603.
8. Vieau D, Rojas-Miranda A, Verley JM, Lenne F, Bertagna X. The secretory granule peptides 7B2 and CCB are sensitive biochemical markers of neuro-endocrine bronchial tumors in man. *Clin. Endocrinol.* 1991;35:319–325.
9. Scopsi L, Gullo M, Rilke F, Martin S, Steiner DF. Proprotein convertases (PC1/PC3 and PC2) in normal and neoplastic human tissues: their use as markers of neuroendocrine differenciation. *J. Clin. Endocrinol. Metab.* 1995;80:294–301.
10. Vieau D, Seidah NG, Chrétien M, Bertagna X. Expression of the prohormone convertase PC2 correlates with the presence of CLIP in human ACTH secreting tumors. *J. Clin. Endocrinol. Metab.* 1994;79:1503–1509.
11. Crosby SR, Stewart MF, Ratcliffe JG, White A. Direct measurement of the precursors of adrenocorticotropin in human plasma by two-site immunoradiometric assay. *J. Clin. Endocrinol. Metab.* 1988;67:1272–1277.
12. Raffin-Sanson M-L, Massias JF, Dumont C, et al. High plasma proopiomelanocortin in aggressive ACTH-secreting tumors. *J. Clin. Endocrinol. Metab.* 1996;81:4272–4277.
13. Vieau D, Massias JF, Girard F, Luton J-P, Bertagna X. Corticotropin-like intermediary lobe peptide as a marker of alternate proopiomelanocortin processing in ACTH-producing non-pituitary tumours. *Clin. Endocrinol.* 1989;31:691–700.
14. Lacaze-Masmonteil T, de Keyzer Y, Luton J-P, Kahn A, Bertagna X. Characterization of proopiomelanocortin transcripts in human non-pituitary tissues. *Proc. Natl Acad. Sci. U S A* 1987; 84:7261–7265.
15. de Keyzer Y, Bertagna X, Luton J-P, A Kahn A. Variable modes of proopiomelanocortin gene transcription in human tumors. *Mol. Endocrinol.* 1989;3:215–223.
16. Picon A, Leblond-Francillard M, Raffin-Sanson M-L, Lenne F, Bertagna X, de Keyzer Y. Functional analysis of the human proopiomelanocortin promoter in the small cell lung carcinoma cell line DMS 79. *J. Mol. Endocrinol.* 1995;15:187–194.
17. Picon A, Bertagna X, de Keyzer Y. Analysis of proopiomelanocortin gene transcription mechanisms in bronchial tumor cells. *Mol. Cell. Endocrinol.* 1999;147:93–102.
18. Newell-Price J. Proopiomelanocortin gene expression and DNA methylation: implications for Cushing syndrome and beyond. *J. Endocrinol.* 2003;177:365–372.
19. de Keyzer Y, Lenne F, Auzan C, et al. The pituitary V3 vasopressin receptor and the corticotroph phenotype in ectopic ACTH syndrome. *J. Clin. Invest.* 1996;97:1311–1318.
20. Lamolet B, Pulichino AM, Lamonerie T, et al. A pituitary cell-restricted T box factor, Tpit, activates POMC transcription in cooperation with Pitx homeoproteins. *Cell* 2001;104:849–859.
21. Messager M, Carriere C, Bertagna X, de Keyzer Y. RT-PCR analysis of corticotroph-associated genes expression in carcinoid tumours in the ectopic-ACTH syndrome. *Eur. J. Endocrinol.* 2006;154:159–166.
22. Lindsay JR, Nieman LK. Differential diagnosis and imaging in Cushing syndrome. *Endocrinol. Metab. Clin. North Am.* 2005;34:403–421.
23. Swearinggen B, Katznelson I, Miller K, et al. Diagnostic errors after inferior petrosal sinus sampling. *J. Clin. Endocrinol. Metab.* 2004;89:3752–3763.
24. Ilias I, Torpy DJ, Pacak K, Mullen N, Wesley RA, Nieman LK. Cushing syndrome due to ectopic corticotropin secretion: twenty years' experience at the National Institutes of Health. *J. Clin. Endocrinol. Metab.* 2005;90:4955–4962.
25. Isidori AM, Kaltsas GA, Grossman AB. Ectopic ACTH syndrome. *Front. Horm. Res.* 2006;35:143–156.
26. Granberg D, Sundin A, Janson ET, Oberg K, Skogseid B, Westlin JE. Octreoscan in patients with bronchial carcinoid tumours. *Clin. Endocrinol.* 2003;59:793–799.

27. Pfannenberg AC, Eschmann SM, Horger M, et al. Benefit of anatomical-functional image fusion in the diagnostic work-up of neuroendocrine neoplasms. *Eur. J. Nucl. Med. Mol. Imaging* 2003;30:835–843.

28. Grossrubatscher E, Vignati F, Dalino P, et al. Use of radioguided surgery with [111In]-pentetreotide in the management of an ACTH-secreting bronchial carcinoid causing ectopic Cushing syndrome. *J. Endocrinol. Invest.* 2005;28:72–78.

29. Phlipponneau M, Nocaudie M, Epelbaum J, et al. Somatostatin analogs for the localization and preoperative treatment of an adrenocorticotropin-secreting bronchial carcinoid tumor. *J. Clin. Endocrinol. Metab.* 1994;78:20–24.

30. Pivonello R, Ferone D, Lamberts SW, Colao A. Cabergoline plus lanreotide for ectopic Cushing syndrome. *N. Engl. J. Med.* 2005;352: 2457–2458.

31. Krakoff J, Koch CA, Calis KA, Alexander RH, Nieman LK. Use of a parenteral propylene glycol-containing etomidate preparation for the long-term management of ectopic Cushing syndrome. *J. Clin. Endocrinol. Metab.* 2001;86:4104–4108.

32. Nieman LK, Chrousos GP, Kellner C, et al. Successful treatment of Cushing syndrome with the glucocorticoid antagonist RU 486. *J. Clin. Endocrinol. Metab.* 1985;61:536–540.

Insulin-like Growth Factors and Tumor Hypoglycemia

Robert C. Baxter

Key points
- Non-islet cell tumor hypoglycemia results from the overproduction of precursor forms of insulin-like growth factor-II ("big" IGF-II) by the tumor.
- Serum IGF-I levels are suppressed in this condition, and an abnormally low ratio of immunoreactive IGF-I:IGF-II is a useful diagnostic marker.
- Growth hormone-dependent proteins which transport IGF in the circulation – IGF binding protein-3 and the acid-labile subunit – are also markedly suppressed, resulting in abnormal IGF transport complexes and increased IGF bioavailability.
- Serum IGF binding protein-2 and -6 levels are also typically elevated in non-islet cell tumor hypoglycemia, though their role in the pathology of this condition is poorly understood.
- While surgery may be the treatment of choice, treatment with either human growth hormone or corticosteroids can reverse the hypoglycemia by restoring IGF transport complexes, although only corticosteroids suppress tumor IGF-II production.

Introduction

Metabolic disturbances occur commonly in cancer patients. Hypoglycemia related specifically to cancer is regarded as rare [1], and may have diverse etiology: high tumor metabolic activity causing increased glucose utilization, liver failure causing decreased gluconeogenesis, insulin hypersecretion from an insulinoma, or the secretion of another hypoglycemic agent from a non-pancreatic tumor. The term non-islet cell tumor hypoglycemia, or NICTH, is commonly used to describe the latter condition [2].

It is over three decades since Megyesi and colleagues reported that hypoglycemia in association with non-pancreatic tumors was sometimes accompanied by elevated plasma levels of an incompletely characterized growth factor, named for its biological activity as NSILAs (non-suppressible insulin-like activity, soluble) [3]. This insulin-like bioactivity, unable to be suppressed by insulin antibodies, was eventually attributed to two distinct polypeptides with a structural relationship to insulin: insulin-like growth factor-I (IGF-I) and IGF-II.

IGFs and their binding proteins

IGF-I and IGF-II are relatively abundant growth factors that occur ubiquitously in the body. In healthy adults, IGF-II circulates at about three times higher concentration than IGF-I. The liver is recognized as the source of most of the circulating IGF-I, but no single tissue has been shown to be the predominant source of IGF-II. Acting through a common tyrosine kinase receptor, the type 1 IGF receptor (or IGF-I receptor), the IGFs stimulate cell proliferation, metabolism, differentiation and survival. They are also relatively weak agonists at the insulin receptor, through which they can xert insulin-like metabolic effects when they are present at high concentration [4]. Since the total serum IGF concentration [about 750 µg/L or (100 nmol/L)] is up to 1000 times greater than that of insulin, the potential to exert such insulin-like actions is considerable.

Protection from the hypoglycemic effects of the IGFs is afforded by the IGF binding proteins (IGFBPs), to which IGF-I and IGF-II bind with high affinity [5]. Of the six members of the IGFBP family, the most abundant is IGFBP-3, a growth hormone (GH)-dependent protein which circulates at a sufficiently high concentration 3–4 mg/L (75–100 nmol/L) to bind almost all of the circulating IGFs [6]. It is not coincidental that IGFBP-3 is equimolar with the total IGF concentration; the proteins form high-affinity complexes which then bind to a third protein, termed the acid-labile subunit or ALS (also growth hormone (GH) dependent), to form heterotrimeric complexes which act as stable circulating reservoirs of almost all of the circulating IGFs. Free IGFs (i.e., uncomplexed to any binding protein) may comprise only about 1% of the total, and are cleared from the circulation with a half-life of a few minutes, whereas IGFBPs alone or complexed to IGFs have half-lives of 15–30 min. In contrast, ternary complexes containing IGF, IGFBP-3 and ALS are restricted in their ability to cross the capillary endothelial barrier and are thus very stable in the circulation,

Clinical Endocrine Oncology, 2nd edition. Edited by Ian D. Hay and John A.H. Wass. © 2008 Blackwell Publishing. ISBN 978-1-4051-4584-8.

with half-lives estimated as 16 h or greater. Among the other five IGFBPs, only IGFBP-5 resembles IGFBP-3 in its ability to form ternary complexes with IGFs and ALS. IGFBP-5 circulates at only about one-tenth the concentration of IGFBP-3 [6].

What is the hypoglycemic agent in NICTH?

A considerable body of evidence supports the concept that incompletely processed forms of the IGF-II precursor polypeptide (pro-IGF-II) make a major contribution to the cause of hypoglycemia in this condition. Many reports describe increased levels of IGF-II gene expression in tumors associated with hypoglycemia, compared to control non-tumor tissue [7–9]. The high level of IGF-II mRNA frequently results in high IGF-II secretion from the tumor, much of it in atypical high molecular weight forms. Mature IGF-II is a single-chain polypeptide of approximately 7.5 kDa, which can be thought of as having four structural domains termed the B, C, A, and D domains, of which the B and A domains correspond in structure to the B and A chains of insulin. Unprocessed precursor or pro-IGF-II includes an 89-residue extension, called the E-domain, on the carboxyterminus of the 67-residue IGF-II. Intact pro-IGF-II thus contains 156 amino acids and has an expected molecular weight of 17.6 kDa. The presence of O-linked glycosylation, which has been detected on pro-IGF-II, would further increase this size.

Circulating IGFs in NICTH – utility in diagnostic testing

Immunoreactive IGF-II forms in the serum of patients with NICTH have been described over a wide size range, typically 11–18 kDa [10] or 15–25 kDa [11], suggesting the presence of proteolytically cleaved precursor forms. These variant IGF-II forms are collectively described by some authors as "big IGF-II." Apart from the aberrant molecular size of serum IGF-II in patients with NICTH, the serum immunoreactive IGF-II levels in these patients may be elevated [9, 12]. However, this is by no means a universal finding, and it is not uncommon for circulating IGF-II values determined by immunological methods to fall within the expected range for healthy subjects [12, 13], or even below the normal range [14–16]. The most likely explanation for these discrepant findings is that immunoassays for IGF-II may recognize the high molecular weight forms poorly. Thus, whereas big IGF-II levels are very commonly elevated, mature 7.5 kDa IGF-II may be normal or suppressed, and total immunoreactive IGF-II may not appear high.

Although serum IGF-II measurement alone is not a sensitive diagnostic method to detect patients with NICTH, the typical suppression of serum IGF-I levels in these patients has led to the proposal that the ratio of IGF-I to IGF-II may be a useful diagnostic tool. Teale and Marks [17] studied eight patients with hypoinsulinemic hypoglycemia associated with non-islet cell tumors. The IGF-I:IGF-II ratio was uniformly below 0.2 in these subjects, compared to a mean ratio in healthy subjects of 1.10 (note that these

are not molar or true concentration ratios since arbitrary standards were used in both assays). Many other studies show very low IGF-I levels in NICTH patients [18, 19], and a low IGF-I:IGF-II ratio [20], and it appears that the IGF-I:IGF-II ratio may be a simple diagnostic marker for this condition, once appropriate reference ranges have been established in each laboratory. Since serum IGF-I levels are largely dependent on the hepatic action of GH, one explanation for the low IGF-I level is the characteristic low serum GH level seen in NICTH. This results from suppression of pituitary GH secretion by the high circulating IGF-II isoforms, since IGF-II, like IGF-I, suppresses GH release from anterior pituitary cells [21].

Big IGFs and free IGFs

Several laboratories have produced antibodies directed against various regions of the E-domain, with the aim of developing an analytical method specific for pro-IGF-II forms [22, 23]. A radioimmunoassay directed against the first 21 amino acids of the E-domain detected very high levels of immunoreactivity in several subjects with non-pancreatic hypoglycemia, but also in subjects on renal dialysis, suggesting that this assay may be useful to detect NICTH in patients without renal failure [22]. Since this assay could not distinguish between free E-domain peptide and big IGF-II, van Doorn et al. developed a two-site enzyme-linked immunosorbent assay which only detected E-domain residues as part of pro-IGF-II. In this more specific assay, big IGF-II in plasma from NICTH patients (22.6 nmol/L) was about six-fold higher than that found in normal subjects (3.8 nmol/L), whereas values were low in renal failure [23]. This method, though not yet widely available, appears to have utility as a simple diagnostic test for NICTH. Immunoblot analysis after sodium dodecyl sulfate-polyacrylamide gel electrophoresis has also been adapted as a direct approach for detecting abnormally elevated big IGF-II forms in serum [24]. In this study the authors compared the size distribution of immunoreactive IGF-II by immunoblot to that determined by gel permeation chromatography, followed by immunoassay of each fraction. This technique showed about two-thirds of IGF-II in "big" forms in NICTH sera, compared to 20–25% in the sera of healthy subjects.

As noted above, free IGFs (i.e., not complexed to IGFBPs) are rather transient species in the circulation, with half-lives estimated at just a few minutes. Although low in concentration relative to protein-bound forms, they could exert a considerable hypoglycemic potential as they are not restricted to the vascular compartment. To investigate whether free IGFs might contribute to the hypoglycemia of NICTH, Frystyk et al. applied well-characterized free IGF assays to patient sera [25]. Surprisingly, free IGF-I levels were four-fold elevated in NICTH despite greatly decreased total IGF-I levels, and free IGF-II levels were 20-fold higher than in healthy subjects. This suggests that free IGF-II measurement might be another valuable diagnostic tool in this condition, though currently difficult to measure reliably.

IGFBP-3 in NICTH

In addition to the marked disturbances of IGF-I and IGF-II described above, circulating IGFBPs in NICTH patients show characteristic changes in both concentration and molecular distribution. The most distinctive change is the redistribution of IGFBP-3 from its characteristic 150 kDa ternary complexes with ALS, to binary complexes of approximately 50 kDa, lacking ALS [26]. This aberrant size distribution, readily visualized by size-fractionating serum proteins chromatographically, reflects a failure to form ternary complexes in addition to a decrease in total IGFBP-3 levels, which decline in NICTH up to 60% compared to values in healthy subjects [25, 26] in some but not all studies [27]. Surgical removal of the tumor in three cases resulted in a clear redistribution of IGFBP-3 back to more normal, 150 kDa complexes [26]. Since ALS is required for ternary complex formation, a low serum ALS value might contribute to the poor ternary complex formation, and indeed ALS can be very low in such subjects, with a mean value reported to be decreased by about 60% compared to normal values [18, 26], increasing to within the normal range after surgical tumor removal.

Although serum ALS levels are undoubtedly low in NICTH, ALS normally circulates at about threefold molar excess over the IGFBP-3 concentration, so that a reduction in ALS concentration would not necessarily mean that there was insufficient for ternary complex formation. To test this, exogenous ALS has been added to NICTH patient sera, and the size distribution of IGFBP-3 compared to that before the addition of ALS [28]. This treatment increased the proportion of IGFBP-3 that complexed with ALS, indicating that ALS might indeed be limiting in these sera. However, a substantial proportion of IGFBP-3 still failed to bind to ALS, raising the possibility of alternative explanations why IGFBP-3 forms ternary complexes poorly in this condition. In a comparison of the ability of tumor- and serum-derived big IGF-II preparations to form complexes with IGFBPs, all six IGFBPs were shown to bind big IGF-II similarly to normal IGF-II. However, big IGF-II extracted from an IGF-II-secreting tumor, although binding normally to IGFBP-3, was only able to form a complex with ALS very poorly [29], and a similar result has been reported with serum-derived big IGF-II [19], suggesting that impaired ternary complex formation caused by big IGF-II might contribute to the abnormal size distribution of IGFBP-3. Regardless of the biochemical explanation for the poor complex formation, IGFs that are predominantly bound in binary complexes would be expected to leave the circulation much more readily than those sequestered in 150 kDa ternary complexes, and might thus contribute to the characteristic hypoglycemia.

Other IGFBPs

Radioimmunoassay for IGFBP-2 in the serum of 11 subjects with NICTH showed extremely high levels [30]. Other studies have reported IGFBP-2 values over 2.5 mg/L, 10-fold above the normal mean value [19, 25]. It is unclear whether this IGFBP-2 is predominantly or even partially tumor derived, since mRNA analyses of tumors causing hypoglycemia have failed to demonstrate any IGFBP-2 gene expression [9, 18]. Based on data from fasting and hypopituitary subjects, it has been speculated that IGFBP-2 levels may rise, in non-tumor subjects, in response to conditions where

there is insufficient binding capacity in IGFBP-3 complexes to carry all of the available IGFs [31]. NICTH represents such a condition, since IGFBP-3 and ALS levels are low, ternary complexes form poorly, IGF-II isoforms are hypersecreted by the tumor, and free IGF levels are elevated. Thus the marked elevation in IGFBP-2, which may certainly contribute to the diagnostic profile for NICTH, probably reflects the metabolic abnormality associated with this condition rather than a tumor-secreted biomarker.

In contrast to IGFBP-2, elevated serum levels of IGFBP-6 may reflect tumor hypersecretion of this protein. IGFBP-6 is unique among the six IGFBPs in having a greatly increased binding affinity for IGF-II compared to IGF-I. The author's laboratory first reported IGFBP-6 levels some four-fold above the normal mean value [19, 28], falling in response to tumor removal. High serum IGFBP-6 levels have been confirmed by others [32], and mRNA analysis of a hypoglycemia-causing hemangiopericytoma revealed high tumor IGFBP-6 gene expression [32]. While the authors of the latter study proposed that the co-production of IGF-II and IGFBP-6 could be important in the pathophysiology of NICTH, the exact mechanism by which this might occur is as yet unknown.

Treatment options for NICTH

NICTH is most commonly seen in patients with large mesenchymal tumors such as fibromas and fibrosarcomas, but may also occur in patients with epithelial carcinomas (Table 79.1). Clinical and laboratory features of a series of 78 patients have recently been summarized [33]. Numerous case reports describe complete alleviation of symptoms following surgical resection of the tumor, and resection or debulking may be the treatment of choice when possible [34, 35]. In other cases, or while waiting for surgery, pharmacological treatment can be very effective (Table 79.1). Among the less frequently reported treatments are glucagon [36] and octreotide which, although often used successfully to alleviate hypoglycemia due to insulinoma, does not appear effective in hypoglycemia of non-islet cell origin [37]. Because proteins of the GH-IGF-IGFBP network are down-regulated in NICTH, treatment with human growth hormone (hGH) has been proposed. Teale et al. reported that hGH alleviated the hypoglycemia in three patients and restored serum IGFBP-3 to normal levels [38]. Others have similarly described the effectiveness of hGH treatment [19, 39, 40], including the long-term treatment of a child with congenital neuroblastoma [39]. In other studies glucocorticoids, used alone or in combination with hGH [19, 27, 40], have been found to effectively alleviate the hypoglycemia (Table 79.1).

Analyses in the author's laboratory of a patient treated with graded doses of prednisolone over 20 days followed by graded doses of hGH over 80 days revealed that both agents relieved the hypoglycemia, restored some insulin secretion, and increased serum IGF-I, IGFBP-3 and ALS levels (Fig. 79.1). Serum IGF-II, which was elevated pre-treatment, was suppressed by prednisolone but not hGH despite alleviation of the hypoglycemia. IGFBP-2 showed a reciprocal pattern to that of serum glucose and

Table 79.1 Examples of non-pancreatic tumor types causing hypoglycemia, and treatment options

Tumor type	Treatment	Reference
Leiomyosarcoma	Surgery	7
Hemangiopericytoma Fibrosarcoma Malignant mesenchymal tumor	Surgery	8
Renal cell carcinoma	Surgery	9
Mesothelioma Hepatic tumor Renal carcinoma Epithelioid leiomyosarcoma Breast tumor Hepatic fibrosarcoma Prostatic carcinoma Retroperitoneal tumor Hepatocellular carcinoma Gastric carcinoma	Surgery	10
Hemangiopericytoma	Surgery	18
Mesenchymal tumor of the thorax Hemangiopericytoma	Surgery	25
Hepatocellular carcinoma Colon carcinoma Meningeal sarcoma Hemangiopericytoma	Glucagon	36
Gastric adenocarcinoma	Octreotide (ineffective), prednisolone	37, 38
Neuroblastoma	Growth hormone	39
Retroperitoneal fibrous tumor	Growth hormone	41
Metastatic lung carcinoma Fibroma Spindle cell tumor Prostate carcinoma	Prednisolone	35
Pleural fibrous tumor	Prednisolone, growth hormone	19
Fibroma with liver metastasis	Prednisone, growth hormone	40

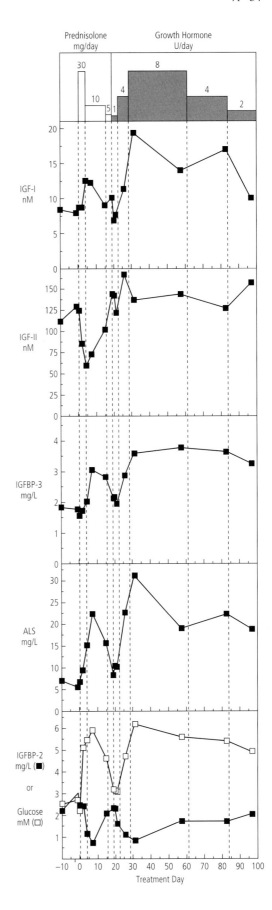

Figure 79.1 Changes in the serum levels of IGF-I, IGF-II, IGFBP-3, ALS, IGFBP-2 and glucose in response to graded doses of prednisolone followed by graded doses of human growth hormone in an 87-year-old woman with hypoglycemia due to a fibrous tumor of the pleura. (Modified from Baxter RC et al. [19], with permission from the Endocrine Society.)

IGFBP-complex proteins, whereas IGFBP-6 levels were elevated but unaffected by treatment [19]. Both treatments also partially restored the size distribution of IGFBP-3 from binary complexes to high molecular weight ternary complexes (i.e., those also containing ALS). This case study graphically illustrates that normoglycemia can be restored by normalizing the IGF-IGFBP complexes, even in the face of continuing IGF-II hyperproduction. The very marked increase in serum ALS seen on high-dose hGH treatment (8 U/day) may be interpreted as decreasing IGF bioavailability, notably that of IGF-II, to an extent where hypoglycemia could be controlled by the body's normal counterregulatory mechanisms. Whether changes in hepatic glucose output accompanied these treatments was not determined in this study.

Conclusion

The hypersecretion of precursor forms of IGF-II by a variety of tumors is accompanied by a complex network of endocrine changes, which may result primarily from the suppression of insulin and GH secretion. Decreased levels of the GH-dependent proteins IGFBP-3 and ALS lead to less ability to form IGF transport complexes, which normally regulate tissue IGF bioavailability. That normoglycemia can be re-established either by GH or corticosteroid treatment, both of which restore IGF transport complexes even though only the latter affects tumor IGF-II production, points to the importance of IGF transport proteins in glycemic regulation, but at the same time indicates that there is still much to be discovered about the underlying metabolic complexities of NICTH.

References

1. Spinazze S, Schrijvers D. Metabolic emergencies. *Crit. Rev. Oncol. Hematol.* 2006;58:79–89.
2. Daughaday WH, Kapadia M. Significance of abnormal serum binding of insulin-like growth factor II in the development of hypoglycemia in patients with non-islet-cell tumors. *Proc. Natl Acad. Sci. USA* 1989; 86:6778–6782.
3. Megyesi K, Kahn CR, Roth J, et al. Hypoglycemia in association with extrapancreatic tumors: demonstration of elevated plasma NSILAs by a new radioreceptor assay. *J. Clin. Endocrinol. Metab.* 1974;38:931–934.
4. Russo VC, Gluckman PD, Feldman EL, et al. The insulin-like growth factor system and its pleiotropic functions in brain. *Endocr. Rev.* 2005;26:916–943.
5. Baxter RC. Insulin-like growth factor (IGF) binding proteins: Interactions with IGFs and intrinsic bioactivities. *Am. J. Physiol.* 2000;278: E967–E976.
6. Rajaram S, Baylink DJ, Mohan S. Insulin-like growth factor binding proteins in serum and other biological fluids: Regulation and functions. *Endocr. Rev.* 1997;18:801–831.
7. Daughaday WH, Emanuele MA, Brooks MH, et al. Synthesis and secretion of insulin-like growth factor II by a leiomyosarcoma with associated hypoglycemia. *N. Engl. J. Med.* 1988;319:1434–1440.

8. Lowe WL Jr, Roberts CT Jr, LeRoith D, et al. Insulin-like growth factor-II in nonislet cell tumors associated with hypoglycemia: increased levels of messenger ribonucleic acid. *J. Clin. Endocrinol. Metab.* 1989;69:1153–1159.
9. Holt RI, Teale JD, Jones JS, et al. Gene expression and serum levels of insulin-like growth factors (IGFs) and IGF-binding proteins in a case of non-islet cell tumour hypoglycaemia. *Growth Horm. IGF Res.* 1998;8:447–454.
10. Hizuka N, Fukuda I, Takano K, et al. Serum high molecular weight form of insulin-like growth factor II from patients with non-islet cell tumor hypoglycemia is O-glycosylated. *J. Clin. Endocrinol. Metab.* 1998;83:2875–2877.
11. Zapf J, Futo E, Peter M, et al. Can "big" insulin-like growth factor II in serum of tumor patients account for the development of extrapancreatic tumor hypoglycemia? *J. Clin. Invest.* 1992;90:2574–2584.
12. Hizuka N, Fukuda I, Takano K, et al. Serum insulin-like growth factor II in 44 patients with non-islet cell tumor hypoglycemia. *Endocr. J.* 1998;45(Suppl):S61–65.
13. Zapf J, Walter H, Froesch ER. Radioimmunological determination of insulin-like growth factors I and II in normal subjects and in patients with growth disorders and extrapancreatic tumor hypoglycemia. *J. Clin. Invest.* 1981;68:1321–1330.
14. Merimee TJ. Insulin-like growth factors in patients with nonislet cell tumors and hypoglycemia. *Metabolism* 1986;35:360–363.
15. Shapiro ET, Bell GI, Polonsky KS, et al. Tumor hypoglycemia: relationship to high molecular weight insulin-like growth factor-II. *J. Clin. Invest.* 1990;85:1672–1679.
16. Baig M, Hintz RL, Baker BK, et al. Hypoglycemia attributable to insulin-like growth factor-II prohormone-producing metastatic leiomyosarcoma. *Endocr. Pract.* 1999;5:37–42.
17. Teale JD, Marks V. Inappropriately elevated plasma insulin-like growth factor II in relation to suppressed insulin-like growth factor I in the diagnosis of non-islet cell tumour hypoglycaemia. *Clin. Endocrinol.* (Oxf.) 1990;33:87–98.
18. Hoekman K, van Doorn J, Gloudemans T, et al. Hypoglycaemia associated with the production of insulin-like growth factor II and insulin-like growth factor binding protein 6 by a haemangiopericytoma. *Clin. Endocrinol.* (Oxf.) 1999;51:247–253.
19. Baxter RC, Holman SR, Corbould A, et al. Regulation of the insulin-like growth factors and their binding proteins by glucocorticoid and growth hormone in nonislet tumor hypoglycemia. *J. Clin. Endocrinol. Metab.* 1995;80:2700–2708.
20. Fukuda I, Hizuka N, Takano K, et al. Characterization of insulin-like growth factor II (IGF-II) and IGF binding proteins in patients with non-islet-cell tumor hypoglycemia. *Endocr. J.* 1993;40:111–119.
21. Ceda GP, Davis RG, Rosenfeld RG, et al. The growth hormone (GH)-releasing hormone (GHRH)-GH–somatomedin axis: evidence for rapid inhibition of GHRH-elicited GH release by insulin-like growth factors I and II. *Endocrinology* 1987;120:1658–1662.
22. Daughaday WH, Trivedi B. Measurement of derivatives of proinsulin-like growth factor-II in serum by a radioimmunoassay directed against the E-domain in normal subjects and patients with nonislet cell tumor hypoglycemia. *J. Clin. Endocrinol. Metab.* 1992;75:110–115.
23. van Doorn J, Hoogerbrugge CM, Koster JG, et al. Antibodies directed against the E region of pro–insulin-like growth factor-II used to evaluate non-islet cell tumor-induced hypoglycemia. *Clin. Chem.* 2002;48:1739–1750.
24. Miraki-Moud F, Grossman AB, Besser M, et al. A rapid method for analyzing serum pro–insulin-like growth factor-II in patients

with non-islet cell tumor hypoglycemia. *J. Clin. Endocrinol. Metab.* 2005;90:3819–3823.

25. Frystyk J, Skjaerbaek C, Zapf J, et al. Increased levels of circulating free insulin-like growth factors in patients with non-islet cell tumour hypoglycaemia. *Diabetologia* 1998;41:589–594.

26. Baxter RC, Daughaday WH. Impaired formation of the ternary insulin-like growth factor-binding protein complex in patients with hypoglycemia due to nonislet cell tumors. *J. Clin. Endocrinol. Metab.* 1991;73:696–702.

27. Teale JD, Marks V. Glucocorticoid therapy suppresses abnormal secretion of big IGF-II by non-islet cell tumours inducing hypoglycaemia (NICTH). *Clin. Endocrinol. (Oxf.)* 1998;49:491–498.

28. Baxter RC. The role of insulin-like growth factors and their binding proteins in tumor hypoglycemia. *Horm. Res.* 1996;46:195–201.

29. Bond JJ, Meka S, Baxter RC Binding characteristics of pro–insulin-like growth factor-II from cancer patients: Binary and ternary complex formation with IGF binding protein-1 to -6. *J. Endocrinology.* 2000;165:253–260.

30. Blum WF, Horn N, Kratzsch J, et al. Clinical studies of IGFBP-2 by radioimmunoassay. *Growth Reg.* 1993;3:100–104.

31. Baxter RC. Physiological roles of IGF binding proteins. In Spencer EM (ed.). *Modern Concepts of Insulin-like Growth Factors.* New York: Elsevier, 1991:371–380.

32. Van Doorn J, Ringeling AM, Shmueli SS, et al. Circulating levels of human insulin-like growth factor binding protein-6 (IGFBP-6) in health and disease as determined by radioimmunoassay. *Clin. Endocrinol. (Oxf.)* 1999;50:601–609.

33. Fukuda I, Hizuka N, Ishikawa Y, et al. Clinical features of insulin-like growth factor-II producing non-islet–cell tumor hypoglycemia. *Growth Horm. IGF Res.* 2006;16:211–216.

34. Rose MG, Tallini G, Pollak J, et al. Malignant hypoglycemia associated with a large mesenchymal tumor: case report and review of the literature. *Cancer J. Sci. Am.* 1999;5:48–51.

35. Teale JD, Wark G The effectiveness of different treatment options for non-islet cell tumour hypoglycaemia. *Clin. Endocrinol. (Oxf.)* 2004;60:457–460.

36. Hoff AO, Vassilopoulou-Sellin R. The role of glucagon administration in the diagnosis and treatment of patients with tumor hypoglycemia. *Cancer* 1998;82:1585–1592.

37. Morbois-Trabut L, Maillot F, De Widerspach-Thor A, et al. "Big IGF-II"-induced hypoglycemia secondary to gastric adenocarcinoma. *Diabetes Metab.* 2004;30:276–279.

38. Teale JD, Blum WF, Marks V Alleviation of non-islet cell tumour hypoglycaemia by growth hormone therapy is associated with changes in IGF binding protein-3. *Ann. Clin. Biochem.* 1992;29(Pt 3):314–323.

39. Katz LE, Liu F, Baker B, et al. The effect of growth hormone treatment on the insulin-like growth factor axis in a child with nonislet cell tumor hypoglycemia. *J. Clin. Endocrinol. Metab.* 1996;81:1141–1146.

40. Bourcigaux N, Arnault-Ouary G, Christol R, et al. Treatment of hypoglycemia using combined glucocorticoid and recombinant human growth hormone in a patient with a metastatic non-islet cell tumor hypoglycemia. *Clin. Ther.* 2005;27:246–251.

41. Silveira LF, Bouloux PM, MacColl GS, et al. Growth hormone therapy for non-islet cell tumor hypoglycemia. *Am. J. Med.* 2002;113:255–257.

80 Metastatic and Other Extraneous Neoplasms in Endocrine Organs

Ian D. Buley

> **Key points**
> - Metastases are common in the endocrine organs of patients who have died with disseminated malignancy.
> - In life, symptoms and signs of endocrine disease due to metastasis are uncommon.
> - The first presentation of malignancy with a metastasis in an endocrine organ is generally rare but this depends on the site and subtype of tumor.
> - The distinction of a metastasis from a primary tumor of an endocrine organ can be a challenging imaging, histopathological or cytopathological problem.
> - Treatment of a metastasis can palliate symptoms and signs of endocrine malfunction and longer survival can be gained.

Introduction

The endocrine organs can be involved by neoplasms originating in other sites by direct extension or by embolism of metastatic tumor in the blood or lymphatic system. Detection of metastases in endocrine organs at autopsy, in patients who have died of disseminated malignancy, is common. In life, symptoms and signs of endocrine malfunction as a consequence of a metastasis are uncommon. Resection or radiotherapy of pituitary metastases can be carried out for palliation of symptoms and longer survival can be gained by resection of isolated endocrine metastases in some malignancies. The first presentation of malignancy with a metastasis in an endocrine organ is rare but can provide a challenging imaging and tissue diagnostic problem particularly as a fine needle aspiration cytology specimen [1, 2].

The broad subtypes of tumor which may metastasize include carcinomas, sarcomas and melanoma. Leukemias and lymphomas can also involve endocrine organs.

Seminal work on metastatic disease was described by Willis [3]. Endocrine organs are relatively vascular as a consequence of their mode of secretion but the distribution of metastases is not simply a reflection of relative blood flow. The likelihood of the establishment of a secondary deposit of tumor at any particular site depends on the genetic and biochemical characteristics of the tumor and the host site enabling the multifactorial processes of tumor invasion, embolization and the establishment of a distant colony to take place. This "seed and soil" hypothesis explains why the thyroid, which is one of the most richly arterialized tissues in the body, is

infrequently a site of metastasis. It also explains why certain tumors have a propensity to spread to particular sites, for example bronchial tumors forming secondary deposits in the adrenals, and similarly may explain why those metastases are often bilateral. Gastric carcinomas have a tendency to bilateral ovarian metastases or Krukenberg tumors and yet these tumors less commonly yield metastases in the liver. The "seed and soil" hypothesis may also explain why metastatic tumors in the thyroid can occupy adenomas and thyroid carcinomas and metastases in the adrenal cortex show a predilection for cortical adenomas and pheochromocytomas.

The adrenal glands

Of all the endocrine organs the adrenal, predominantly the medulla but also the cortex, is the most frequently affected by metastatic tumor (Table 80.1). In unselected series of death due to malignancy the adrenal is involved in up to 30% of cases [4]. Direct spread from neighboring tumors occurs infrequently but it can occur in carcinoma of the kidney, stomach, pancreas, and from metastases in retroperitoneal lymph nodes. Spread via lymphatics has been recorded from carcinoma of the stomach and retrograde spread via the adrenal vein can occur from tumor in the inferior vena cava or renal vein. This form of retrograde spread has been described from a left-sided testicular teratoma. Most metastases are embolic, arriving in arterial blood. They can present simulating a primary adrenal neoplasm though they are frequently bilateral. If the metastases are sufficiently extensive and destroy more than 80–90% of the adrenal glands they can cause Addison disease [5].

The most common sites of the primary tumor are carcinomas of the breast, bronchus (particularly small cell carcinoma), kidney,

Clinical Endocrine Oncology, 2nd edition. Edited by Ian D. Hay and John A.H. Wass. © 2008 Blackwell Publishing. ISBN 978-1-4051-4584-8.

Table 80.1 The most common extraneous tumors of the adrenal gland

Primary site	Tumor type
Lung	Small cell carcinoma
	Large cell undifferentiated
	carcinoma
	Squamous carcinoma
	Adenocarcinoma
	Carcinoid
Breast	Ductal carcinoma
	Lobular carcinoma
Kidney	Renal cell carcinoma
Stomach	Adenocarcinoma
Pancreas	Adenocarcinoma
Colon	Adenocarcinoma
Ovary	Adenocarcinoma
Skin	Melanoma
Liver	Hepatocellular carcinoma
Biliary tract	Adenocarcinoma
Lymph node	Non-Hodgkin and Hodgkin
	lymphoma

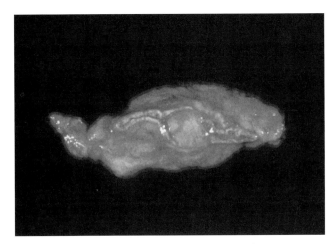

Figure 80.1 The adrenal medulla contains a small metastasis from a primary bronchial small cell carcinoma.

stomach, pancreas, ovary, colon and skin malignant melanomas (Fig. 80.1). Small cell carcinoma and bronchial carcinoid tumors can be endocrinologically active, secreting adrenocorticotropic hormone (ACTH) and causing hyperplasia of the adjacent adrenocortical cells. Histologically or cytologically the origin of the tumor can be deduced from its appearance and its immunophenotype. Renal adenocarcinoma metastases can be bilateral or unilateral and either ipsilateral or contralateral. Grossly and microscopically they can mimic adrenocortical carcinoma. Both are clear cell tumors and can have a similar morphology. The presence of abundant cytoplasmic glycogen favors a renal primary. Electron microscopic evidence of steroid production with mitochondrial tubular cristae and abundant smooth endoplasmic reticulum favors an adrenocortical tumor. The most discriminative immunostains include positive staining for cytokeratins,

epithelial membrane antigen, the RCC antigen and CD10 favoring renal adenocarcinoma. Positivity for inhibin, Melan-A clone A103 and synaptophysin favor the diagnosis of an adrenocortical tumor [6–8]. Large cell lung carcinomas and hepatocellular carcinoma can also mimic the microscopic appearances of adrenocortical carcinoma.

Involvement of the adrenals by non-Hodgkin or Hodgkin lymphoma is usually in the context of disseminated disease and is seen at autopsy in up to 25% of patients. Massive bilateral involvement can lead to Addison disease in life and treatment of the lymphoma can lead to some recovery of adrenal function [9]. Extranodal lymphoma presenting as solitary disease in the adrenal gland is rare. The adrenals are rarely involved by metastatic sarcomas though this can be seen in metastatic leiomyosarcoma and angiosarcoma.

The thyroid gland

At autopsy the frequency of involvement of the thyroid in deaths due to malignancy is of the order of 5–10% in series where the thyroid is carefully examined [3, 10, 11] (Table 80.2). The thyroid may be involved by direct invasion from primary carcinomas of the pharynx, larynx, trachea or esophagus and by extension from metastatic carcinomas in cervical lymph nodes (Fig. 80.2). Blood-borne metastases originate most frequently from renal, breast, bronchial, gastrointestinal, head and neck carcinoma and from malignant melanoma. These metastases cause clinically detectable thyroid enlargement or functional disturbance in less than 25% of cases. Secondary deposits can be solitary or multiple and show an interstitial pattern of infiltration. Presentation with a secondary in the thyroid and an occult primary is rare but occurs particularly

Table 80.2 The most common extraneous tumors of the thyroid gland

Primary site	Tumor type
Pharynx	Squamous carcinoma
Larynx	Squamous carcinoma
Trachea	Squamous carcinoma
Esophagus	Squamous carcinoma
Kidney	Renal cell carcinoma
Breast	Ductal carcinoma
	Lobular carcinoma
Lung	Small cell carcinoma
	Large cell undifferentiated
	carcinoma
	Squamous carcinoma
	Adenocarcinoma
	Carcinoid
Stomach	Adenocarcinoma
Pancreas	Adenocarcinoma
Colon	Adenocarcinoma
Skin	Melanoma
Lymph node	Non-Hodgkin and Hodgkin
	lymphoma

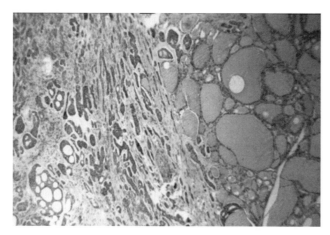

Figure 80.2 The thyroid is directly infiltrated by an adjacent adenoid cystic carcinoma of the trachea. (Courtesy of Dr NG Ryley, Torbay Hospital, UK.)

with renal cell carcinoma, carcinoma of the colon and in malignant melanoma. In one series of nearly 25 000 fine needle aspirates of the thyroid only 25 cases of metastatic malignancy were found. In 11 of these cases there was a known previous history and in the absence of such a history only five cases were correctly identified as metastatic malignancy rather than a thyroid primary [2].

Clear cell carcinoma of the thyroid is rare and whenever it is diagnosed the possibility of metastatic renal carcinoma should be considered and favored if there is a history of a previous renal tumor (Fig. 80.3). There are subtle morphological differences between the tumors and immunostaining with an appropriate panel of antibodies can help to resolve this differential diagnosis. Thyroglobulin staining can be misleading as this soluble antigen can diffuse into a renal metastasis from adjacent thyroid tissue and give false-positive staining. More discriminative staining is provided by positivity for TTF-1 and CD117 in primary thyroid carcinomas and CD10 positivity in renal adenocarcinoma [8, 12]. Primary squamous carcinoma of the thyroid is also rare,

particularly if it appears well differentiated, and the possibility of metastasis or direct invasion from the adjacent aerodigestive tract should be considered. Metastatic lung or gastrointestinal carcinoid tumor in the thyroid mimics primary medullary carcinoma of the thyroid. Poorly differentiated metastatic carcinoma or amelanotic melanoma can mimic primary anaplastic carcinoma. The presence of mucin in poorly differentiated adenocarcinomas favors a secondary tumor and immunostaining again contributes to resolving the differential diagnosis in difficult cases.

Lymphoma in the thyroid is usually primary and typically is a low-grade marginal zone B-cell non-Hodgkin lymphoma also termed a low-grade B cell lymphoma of MALT (mucosa-associated lymphoid tissue) type. Diffuse large B-cell non-Hodgkin lymphoma also occurs and is thought to arise from pre-existing low grade lymphoma. These primary lymphomas often arise on the background of autoimmune thyroiditis. Systemic non-Hodgkin lymphoma presenting with thyroid involvement is less common and Hodgkin disease involving primarily the thyroid is very rare though involvement together with cervical lymph nodes occurs. Plasmacytoma and Langerhans cell histiocytosis can also affect the thyroid either as a solitary deposit or in conjunction with widespread disease. Metastatic sarcoma in the thyroid is exceptionally rare [13].

The pituitary gland

The pituitary can be affected by direct extension of adjacent tumors including nasopharyngeal carcinoma, tumors of bone at the base of the skull and a range of vascular and neural neoplasms (see Part 3, Pituitary and Hypothalamic Lesions). Blood-borne metastases are most frequently from metastatic carcinoma of the breast, lung, kidney, prostate or gastrointestinal tract. The prevalence at autopsy in disseminated malignancy is of the order of 5% (Table 80.3). Metastases occur more frequently in the neurohypophysis than the adenohypophysis though this disparity

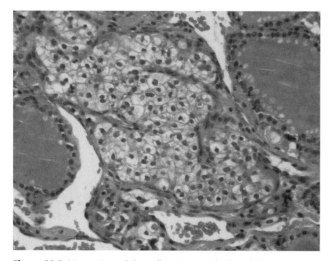

Figure 80.3 Metastatic renal clear cell carcinoma in the thyroid. This tumor may present many years after removal of the primary and resection of isolated metastatic deposits can result in prolonged disease-free survival.

Table 80.3 The most common extraneous tumors of the pituitary gland

Primary site	Tumor type
Adjacent to sella turcica	Nasopharyngeal carcinoma
	Neural, bony and vascular tumors
Breast	Ductal carcinoma
	Lobular carcinoma
Lung	Small cell carcinoma
Kidney	Renal cell carcinoma
Gastrointestinal tract	Adenocarcinoma
Prostate	Adenocarcinoma
Skin	Melanoma
Lymph node	Non-Hodgkin and Hodgkin lymphoma
Bone marrow	Leukemia
	Langerhans cell histiocytosis

is less evident in breast malignancy [14–16]. Most pituitary metastases are found in the context of widespread known malignancy, are microscopic in nature and are asymptomatic. Diabetes insipidus and hyperprolactinemia due to pituitary stalk compression can occur and symptomatic pituitary metastasis can be the first presentation of malignancy. Since the metastases are usually centered on the posterior pituitary they differ in their presentation from pituitary adenomas by the prominence of diabetes insipidus and space-occupying lesion effects including headache and visual disturbance rather than hypopituitarism. The histological appearances of metastatic renal adenocarcinoma can mimic a pituitary adenoma resulting in misdiagnosis. Metastasis into a pre-existing pituitary adenoma can occur, leading to a rapid increase in tumor size and worsening symptoms.

Hematological malignancies including leukemias, particularly acute lymphoblastic and acute myeloid leukemia, can affect the pituitary. The pituitary can be involved by Langerhans cell histiocytosis, with diabetes insipidus a component of Hand–Schüller–Christian syndrome. Non-Hodgkin lymphoma invading the pituitary is rare and Hodgkin disease even rarer. Plasmacytomas in the adjacent sphenoid bone can mimic pituitary adenoma.

The pineal gland

The pineal region is an unusual site for metastasis. A solitary mass in the pineal is more likely to be a primary pineal parenchymal tumor but in those with a previous history of malignancy or in the older age group, a secondary deposit of tumor should be considered. If a primary germ cell tumor of the pineal is diagnosed the rather remote possibility of a metastasis from a gonadal or mediastinal primary should be considered. The most common primary site for a secondary in the pineal is carcinoma of the lung, particularly small cell carcinoma. Metastatic carcinoma of the breast and a range of individual case reports of primary tumors from various sites are also recorded as causing presentation with a pineal mass [17].

The parathyroid glands

The parathyroids can be involved by tumors extending from adjacent tissues, particularly thyroid and laryngeal carcinomas. Blood-borne metastases can be found at autopsy in at least one parathyroid in 6–12% of cases of disseminated malignancy [18]. Hypoparathyroidism as a result of destruction of the parathyroid glands by metastatic malignancy is rare. The most common primary sites documented are carcinomas of the breast and lung, melanoma metastasis and leukemic infiltration.

The testis

The testis can be involved by extraneous neoplasms by direct extension of tumors in the epididymis or spermatic cord or by

Table 80.4 The most common extraneous tumors of the testis

Primary site	Tumor type
Lymph node	Non-Hodgkin lymphoma, particularly diffuse large B-cell type
Bone marrow	Leukemia, particularly acute lymphoblastic, acute myeloid and chronic lymphocytic types
Prostate	Adenocarcinoma
Stomach	Adenocarcinoma
Pancreas	Adenocarcinoma
Colon	Adenocarcinoma
Lung	Small cell carcinoma
Kidney	Renal cell carcinoma
Skin	Melanoma

metastasis. Retrograde extension, or embolism, along the spermatic veins can occur resulting in spread of tumors from the left kidney, either primary renal tumors or metastases. Spread to the testis can also be by retrograde lymphatic extension from the para-aortic lymph nodes. Other postulated routes include retrograde spread along the vas deferens from prostate cancer and spread of tumor from the peritoneal cavity via a patent tunica vaginalis. The usual mode of spread is by arterial embolism (Table 80.4).

Metastatic tumors of the testis most frequently arise from carcinomas of the prostate, lung, colon, stomach, kidney and pancreas and secondary melanoma of the skin. It is rare for a secondary testicular tumor to be the first presentation of a cancer. Secondary adenocarcinoma can mimic primary Sertoli cell tumors, carcinomas of the rete testis and Leydig cell tumors though appropriate immunostaining should enable correct diagnosis. In children acute lymphoblastic leukemia affects the testis histologically in more than 20% of cases. Secondary neuroblastoma can also metastasize to this site providing a differential diagnosis with other small round blue cell tumors. Acute myeloid leukemia can affect the testis giving a microscopic differential diagnosis with large cell non-Hodgkin lymphoma. Malignant lymphoma is the most common testicular tumor in the elderly and overall comprises approximately 5% of testis malignancies. Presentation may be with a testicular mass but this represents metastatic disease as there is usually co-existing lymph node involvement. Bilaterality occurs in approximately 20% of cases. Nearly all cases are non-Hodgkin lymphoma mainly of diffuse large B-cell type. Plasmacytoma of the testis can occur as a manifestation of multiple myeloma or as an isolated lesion [19].

The ovary

The ovary is a common site of involvement by extraneous neoplasms [20] (Table 80.5). It can be involved by direct spread in

Table 80.5 The most common extraneous tumors of the ovary

Primary site	Tumor type
Stomach	Adenocarcinoma
Colon	Adenocarcinoma
Breast	Lobular carcinoma
	Ductal carcinoma
Uterus	Endometrial adenocarcinoma
	Endometrial stromal sarcoma
	Leiomyosarcoma
Lymph node	Non-Hodgkin lymphoma
Bone marrow	Leukemia, particularly endemic
	Burkitt lymphoma
Skin	Melanoma

pelvic intestinal or gynecological malignancy. Metastatic spread can be transcelomic via the peritoneal cavity or fallopian tubes, hematogenous or by retrograde lymphatic involvement. The age distribution of ovarian secondary malignancies is lower than the peak age distribution of the corresponding primary tumors. One explanation may be that the functionally active ovary is more prone to metastasis than the postmenopausal atrophic ovary. Ovarian metastasis occurs in 30% of women dying of cancer and approximately 7% of adnexal masses detected clinically are metastases and may be the first presentation of malignancy. Occasionally metastases in the ovary can produce estrogenic or androgenic effects by stimulating the adjacent ovarian stromal tissue. Ovarian metastases, in comparison with primary ovarian neoplasms, are characteristically bilateral (70% of cases), multinodular, associated with extra-ovarian spread, have unusual histological features, show lymphatic and vascular invasion and have a desmoplastic reaction.

Metastases occur most frequently from gastric, sigmoid colon, rectal and breast carcinomas. Of breast carcinomas the lobular subtype is the most frequent. Spread from mucinous tumors of the appendix, pancreas and biliary tract also occurs. Secondary tumors from all of these sites can mimic primary ovarian tumors. Lymphoma, leukemia, melanoma and metastatic sarcomas can also colonize the ovary.

Metastases can be cystic or solid. A solid pattern is characteristically seen in the Krukenberg tumor which is a diffusely infiltrative bilateral mucinous or signet ring carcinoma. This originates most frequently from carcinoma of the stomach though primaries in the colon and occasionally breast can be responsible. The malignant cells are associated with a stromal spindle cell proliferation. Krukenberg tumors of gastrointestinal origin are frequently the first presentation of malignancy and in only 35% of cases the diagnosis of the primary precedes detection of the ovarian disease.

The histological distinction between primary adenocarcinoma of the ovary and secondary adenocarcinoma of the colon can be aided by immunostaining for carcinoembryonic antigen, CA125, cytokeratin 7 and cytokeratin 20 as each tumor has a characteristic immunophenotype. Endometrial adenocarcinoma can metastasize

to the ovaries. Since the microscopic appearance and known immunophenotype of tumors from these sites can be identical it can be difficult to discern which tumor is primary or whether both are independent primaries. There are other areas of diagnostic difficulty; metastatic carcinoid tumors can be confused with primary ovarian carcinoid though other teratomatous elements are usually present in that instance. They can also be confused with sex-cord stromal tumors including granulosa cell tumors. Metastatic goblet cell carcinoid has a similar appearance to Krukenberg secondary adenocarcinoma. Krukenberg tumors with few signet-ring cells can mimic ovarian fibromas. Renal cell carcinoma rarely metastasizes to the ovary but mimics primary ovarian clear cell carcinoma. Metastatic thyroid carcinoma can be confused with struma ovarii in ovarian teratoma. Primary transitional cell carcinoma of the ovary can appear identical to metastatic urothelial carcinoma.

Melanoma of the ovary can be secondary or arise as a component of an ovarian teratoma. Melanoma can resemble a range of ovarian tumors including granulosa cell tumors, steroid cell tumors and small cell carcinoma. Immunostaining can be helpful in elucidating this differential diagnosis. Metastatic sarcoma can affect the ovary particularly those of gynecological origin including endometrial stromal sarcoma and leiomyosarcoma. B-cell non-Hodgkin lymphoma and leukemias can affect the ovary though rarely, with one exception, are the first manifestation of disease. The exception is Burkitt's lymphoma in endemic areas where this tumor constitutes half of cases of malignant ovarian tumors in childhood. Lymphomas and granulocytic sarcoma can mimic primary dysgerminoma, carcinoid and small cell carcinoma though selection of appropriate immunostains makes this distinction straightforward.

References

1. Buley ID. Other endocrine organs, Section 10 Endocrine System. In Gray W, McKee GT (eds). *Diagnostic Cytopathology*, 2nd edition. London: Churchill Livingstone, 2003:608.
2. Buley ID. The thyroid gland, Section 10 Endocrine System. In Gray W, McKee GT (eds). *Diagnostic Cytopathology*, 2nd edition. London: Churchill Livingstone, 2003:597–598.
3. Willis RA. *The Spread of Tumours in the Human Body*, 3rd edition. London: Butterworths, 1973.
4. Lack EE. Tumors metastatic to adrenal glands. In *Tumors of the Adrenal Gland and Extra Adrenal Paraganglia*. AFIP Fascicle 19. Washington DC, 1997.
5. Lam KY, Lo CY. Metastatic tumours of the adrenal glands; a 30 year experience in a teaching hospital. *Clin. Endocrinol. (Oxf.)* 2002;56; 95–101.
6. Rosai J. Adrenal gland and other paraganglia. In *Rosai and Ackerman's Surgical Pathology*, Vol 1, 9th edition. London: Mosby, 2004:1123.
7. McGregor DK, Khurana KK, Cao C, et al. Diagnosing primary and metastatic renal cell carcinoma: the use of the monoclonal antibody "renal cell carcinoma marker". *Am. J. Surg. Pathol.* 2001;25:1485–1492.
8. Chu P, Arber DA. Paraffin-section detection of CD10 in 505 nonhematopoietic neoplasms. Frequent expression in renal cell

carcinoma and endometrial stromal sarcoma. *Am. J. Clin. Pathol.* 2000;3:374–382.

9. Carey RW, Harris N, Kliman B. Addison's disease secondary to lymphomatous infiltration of the adrenal glands. Recovery of adrenocortical function after chemotherapy. *Cancer* 1987;59:1087–1090.

10. Wood K, Vini L, Harmer C. Metastases to the thyroid gland: the Royal Marsden experience. *Eur. J. Surg. Oncol.* 2004;30:583–588.

11. Nakhjavani MK, Gharib H, Goellner JR, van Heerden JA. Metastasis to the thyroid gland. A report of 43 cases. *Cancer* 1997;79: 574–578.

12. Kaufmann O, Dietel M. Thyroid transcription factor-1 is the superior immunohistochemical marker for pulmonary adenocarcinomas and large cell carcinomas compared to surfactant proteins A and B. *Histopathology* 2000;36:8–16.

13. Rosai J. Thyroid gland. In *Rosai and Ackerman's Surgical Pathology*, Vol 1, 9th edition. London: Mosby, 2004:564–567.

14. Fassett DR, Couldwell WT. Metastases to the pituitary gland. *Neurosurg. Focus* 2004;16:E8.

15. Teears RJ, Silverman EM. Clinicopathologic review of 88 cases of carcinoma metastatic to the pituitary gland. *Cancer* 1975;36:216–220.

16. Branch CL Jr, Laws ER Jr. Metastatic tumors of the sella turcica masquerading as primary pituitary tumors. *J. Clin. Endocrinol. Metab.* 1987;65:469–474.

17. Vaquero J, Martinez R, Magallon R, Ramiro J. Intracranial metastases to the pineal region. Report of three cases. *J. Neurosurg. Sci.* 1991;35: 55–57.

18. Horwitz CA, Myers WP, Foote FW Jr. Secondary malignant tumors of the parathyroid glands. Report of two cases with associated hypoparathyroidism. *Am. J. Med.* 1972;52:797–808.

19. Dutt N, Bates AW, Baithun SI. Secondary neoplasms of the male genital tract with different patterns of involvement in adults and children. *Histopathology* 2000;37:323–331.

20. Prat J, Morice P. Secondary tumours of the ovary. In Tavassoli FA, Devilee P (eds). *WHO Classification of Tumours. Pathology and Genetics of Tumours of the Breast and Female Genital Organs.* Lyon: IARC Press, 2003:193–196.

81 Endocrine Late Effects of Cancer Therapy

Robert D. Murray

Key points

- Five-year survival for childhood cancer now exceeds 70%, and in the UK around one in 715 young adults will be a survivor of childhood cancer by the year 2010. Despite survival of more than 5 years these patients remain at risk of significant premature mortality (SMR 10.8) and morbidity.
- It is estimated that 40–50% of childhood cancer survivors develop an endocrine late effect as a consequence of their treatment regimen.
- Endocrine late effects result from both chemotherapy and radiotherapy.
- Cranial and spinal irradiation have an adverse effect on growth and may lead to skeletal disproportion; cranial irradiation is associated with a variable degree of hypopituitarism, but may also result in precocious puberty; neck irradiation frequently causes thyroid dysfunction, in addition to benign and malignant thyroid nodules, although hyperparathyroidism is an uncommon sequela; gonadal irradiation and various chemotherapeutic agents may result in subfertility and sex steroid deficiency.
- Late endocrine effects of multi-modality cancer therapy occur up to 10–15 years after the putative insult warranting long-term surveillance of individuals at risk.

Introduction

Over the past 40 years cure rates for childhood malignancies have improved at a remarkable pace. Overall 5-year survival has improved from less than 30% in 1960 to more than 70% in 1990. Since the mid-1980s, however, the increase in 5-year survival rates has been only modest. When the overall data are stratified it is clear that long-term survival is dependent on a multitude of dependents including age, gender, genetic factors, and tumor characteristics (tumor type, location, size, metastasis). With increasing cure rates came recognition of the long-term detrimental effects of radiotherapy and chemotherapy on multiple organ systems, commonly known as "late effects". To improve further upon current successes, given that 5-year survival has altered little over the last decade, will undoubtedly necessitate the use of even more complex treatment regimens resulting in a higher prevalence of late effects in these individuals.

The impact of late effects of childhood cancer treatment on health services in the future is likely to be significant. It is estimated that one in 640 adults aged 20–39 years in the USA is currently a survivor of childhood cancer, and in the UK one in 715 young adults will be a survivor of childhood cancer by the year 2010. Epidemiological data from the Childhood Cancer Survivors Study (CCSS) in the USA reported survivors of more than 5 years

to have a 10.8-fold excess in overall mortality [1]. The majority of deaths (67%) relate to recurrence of the original tumor. After exclusion of deaths relating to recurrence or progression of the original tumor, mortality rates remained significantly increased. Standardized mortality rates for second malignancies (SMR 19.4), cardiac disease (SMR 8.2), pulmonary disease (SMR 9.2), and other causes (SMR 3.3) were significantly elevated.

Endocrine late effects are particularly prevalent in childhood cancer survivors with 43% of the CCSS cohort reporting one or more endocrinopathies [2]. Endocrine late effects include disturbances of growth and puberty, hypothalamo–pituitary dysfunction, hypogonadism, subfertility, thyroid dysfunction, benign and malignant thyroid nodules, and reduced bone mass (Tables 81.1–81.3).

Growth

The impact of childhood cancer and treatment thereof has long been recognized to impair height velocity and final height (Table 81.1). A number of studies have attempted to isolate causative factors. Radiation-induced growth hormone deficiency (GHD) and spinal irradiation are two major adverse factors that contribute to the short stature achieved by patients who receive cranial or craniospinal irradiation for treatment of intracranial or hematological malignancies. A subanalysis of the CCSS survivors with brain tumors revealed 40% of patients to have a final height below the 10th percentile [3].

Spinal irradiation in most cases is undertaken concomitantly with cranial irradiation as craniospinal irradiation. To disentangle

Clinical Endocrine Oncology, 2nd edition. Edited by Ian D. Hay and John A.H. Wass. © 2008 Blackwell Publishing. ISBN 978-1-4051-4584-8.

the independent effect of spinal irradiation on growth has depended on comparison of individuals who received cranial with those who received craniospinal irradiation. Spinal irradiation has a negative impact on growth above that of cranial irradiation alone, and relates to reduced spinal growth. Leg length standard deviation score (SDS) in patients who received cranial and craniospinal irradiation is equivalent, whereas spinal growth is impaired only in the latter patients. The greater impairment of spinal growth results in disproportion, reflected by an increase in leg length to sitting height ratio. The impact of spinal irradiation correlates with age. In general, the younger the individual is at the time of irradiation the greater is the impairment of spinal growth and the greater the degree of disproportion. This observation simply reflects the fact that the younger an insult to growth occurs then the greater the loss in growth potential. Disproportion may be further amplified by the use of growth hormone (GH) replacement therapy in patients found to be GHD as although GH replacement will impact favorably on growth of the long bones, the spine remains relatively resistant to the growth-promoting effects of GH. In children who received spinal irradiation growth should be monitored by leg length velocity.

Growth velocity is frequently impaired at the time of diagnosis and during treatment of childhood malignancy, reflecting the acute illness, poor nutritional status, radiation-induced hypothyroidism, and ongoing cancer therapy. Catch-up growth is frequently observed, without growth, promoting intervention, once active treatment has been completed and remission achieved. Although the effect of cytotoxic chemotherapy on growth remains contentious, there is a suggestion that subsequent growth is attenuated. Additionally, chemotherapy may potentiate the growth impairment resulting from craniospinal irradiation. Although the pathophysiological mechanism by which chemotherapy influences growth is unclear a reduction in growth factors including insulin-like growth factor (IGF-I), increased sensitivity of bone to irradiation damage, and a direct action on the growth plate have been postulated. High-dose cranial irradiation leads to gonadotropin deficiency; however, at lower doses it results in early onset of puberty. The age of onset of puberty in children correlates to age at cranial irradiation. Early age at onset of puberty leads to completion of puberty at an early age thereby restricting the time for growth and growth-promoting therapy in these individuals.

Table 81.1 Overview of the primary effects of multi-modality cancer therapy on growth and hypothalamo–pituitary function in cancer survivors

Physiological system	Insult	Pathology	
Growth	Cranial XRT	Impaired GH secretion Precocious puberty	All insults culminate in reduced height velocity and final height. There are no robust data supporting a direct action of chemotherapy on growth.
	Spinal XRT	Impaired spinal growth Disproportion	The ultimate impact on height is dependent on age at XRT, dosage and schedule.
	Chemotherapy	?Potentiation of XRT effects ?Direct effect on growth plate	Puberty occurs earlier, spinal growth is more attenuated, and GH deficiency is more prevalent if XRT occurs at a younger age, in fewer fractions, and at higher dosage.
Growth hormone & IGF-I axis	Cranial XRT	GH deficiency (GHD) (a) Childhood – reduced growth velocity (b) Transition – impaired somatic development (c) Adult – impaired quality of life, adverse body composition and vascular risk profile	Cranial XRT doses as low as 18 Gy given during childhood result in GHD in around a third of individuals by 5 yrs post treatment, whereas doses of 30–40 Gy result in GHD in 60–100% of patients by 5 yrs [4]. Prevalence of GHD is dependent on age at irradiation, fractionation schedule and dose.
Hypothalamo–pituitary axis	Cranial XRT	LH/FSH deficiency ACTH deficiency TSH deficiency Hyperprolactinemia	Additional anterior pituitary hormone deficits are generally observed with XRT doses >30 Gy and are dependent on dose, fractionation schedule, and time since XRT [4]. In most cases the progression of hormone loss follows the pattern GH ⇒ LH/FSH ⇒ ACTH ⇒ TSH. Other than GHD, additional deficits are unusual within the first 2 years following XRT except with exposure to very high doses. Transient hyperprolactinemia is frequently observed following XRT, resolving over the following few years.
Hypothalamo–pituitary axis	Cranial XRT	Early/precocious puberty	Early puberty is a consequence of disinhibition of cortical influences on the GnRH pulse generator. The earlier the age at XRT (25–50 Gy), the earlier puberty occurs [8]. Early puberty effectively foreshortens the time available for growth-promoting interventions when growth is impaired.

ACTH, adrenocorticotropin hormone; FSH, follicle-stimulating hormone; GH, growth hormone; LH, luteinizing hormone; TSH, thyroid secreting hormone; XRT, radiotherapy.

Table 81.2 Overview of the effects of multi-modality cancer therapy on the reproductive system of cancer survivors

Physiological system	Insult	Pathology	
Male reproductive system	Local XRT, spinal XRT, TBI	Oligo – azoospermia Subfertility/sterility Leydig cell insufficiency	Primary insult to germ cells of testis – azoospermia occurring within 2 months from XRT doses as low as 2 Gy. Recovery occurs a mean of 30 months and >5 years following 2–3 or 4–6 Gy respectively [10]. Impaired spermatogenesis leads to small testis which should not be used to stage puberty. Leydig cell function rarely compromised with doses <20 Gy. Puberty progresses normally and secondary sexual characteristics are maintained, despite subfertility.
Ovarian function	Local XRT, spinal XRT, TBI	Transient amenorrhea Premature ovarian failure Subfertility/sterility Estrogen deficiency	Insult reflects damage to a fixed pool of oocytes. Impact of XRT on ovarian function is age and dose dependent [14]. XRT doses >6 Gy result in a premature menopause in women over 40 years of age; however, in young women a dose of 20 Gy leads to premature ovarian failure in only ~50%. Recovery is infrequent, usually transient, and occurs almost exclusively in younger women. Concurrent estrogen deficiency results in failure of puberty to progress.
Uterine function	Pelvic XRT	Immature uterus Failure to carry a child	Irradiation (>20–30 Gy) of the uterus during childhood results in impaired growth, reduced uterine blood flow, and failure of the endometrium to respond to estrogen and progesterone. The impact is greatest the younger the patient at XRT. With egg donation, the impaired uterine function reduces the likelihood of carrying a child through pregnancy.
Male reproductive system	Chemotherapy	Oligo – azoospermia Subfertility/sterility Leydig cell insufficiency	Gonadal toxic agents include the alkylating agents, procarbazine, cisplatin, vinblastine and cytosine. Damage dependent on cumulative dosage. Multiagent chemotherapy is generally more gonadotoxic than single agents. Primary insult is to the germ cells with high-dose therapy additionally resulting in compensated hypogonadism [18]. Recovery frequently occurs, the speed of which is dependent on the regimen administered.
Ovarian function	Chemotherapy	Transient amenorrhea Premature ovarian failure Subfertility/sterility Estrogen deficiency	Insult reflects damage to a fixed pool of oocytes. Ovarian toxicity occurs with similar agents to testis. Impact of chemotherapy on ovarian function is dependent on age and the cumulative dose [20]. Recovery of ovarian function is frequently observed, but these individuals may undergo a premature menopause.

TBI, traumatic brain injury; XRT, radiotherapy.

Table 81.3 Overview of the effects of multi-modality cancer therapy on the thyroid and parathyroid glands of cancer survivors

Physiological system	Insult	Pathology	
Thyroid nodules	Neck XRT or TBI	Malignant nodules	Significant increased risk following neck XRT (RR ~15) [22]. Incidence increases from 5–10 years post XRT. Possible "cell kill" effect at doses above 30 Gy [23]. Risk significantly greater in children compared with adults, and females compared with males [23].
		Benign nodules	Increased prevalence of all benign thyroid disease [22]. Palpable nodules in 20–30% patients who received neck XRT. Prevalence dependent on time since XRT, female gender, and XRT dose.
Thyroid dysfunction	Neck XRT or TBI	Hypothyroidism	Frank or compensated hypothyroidism occurs in 20–30% of patients who receive TBI, and 30–50% of those who received neck irradiation (30–50 Gy) [22]. Hypothyroidism generally occurs within 5 years of XRT. Thyroxine therapy should be instituted early because of the hypothesis that an elevated TSH may drive early thyroid cancers.
		Hyperthyroidism	Graves disease is reported to occur at increased frequency (RR ~8) [22].
Parathyroid	Neck XRT	Late-onset hyperparathyroidism	Latency of 25–47 years. Dose dependency observed [24].

TBI, traumatic brain injury; XRT, radiotherapy.

Hypopituitarism

Radiation-induced hypopituitarism of varying degrees is a well-recognized sequela of external beam irradiation when the hypothalamo–pituitary axis falls within the field of treatment (Table 81.1). Hypopituitarism has been reported in patients irradiated for pituitary and parasellar tumors, intracranial malignancies, soft tissue sarcomas of the facial bones, and nasopharyngeal carcinomas, as well as patients who received cranial irradiation as part of their regimen for treatment of hematological malignancies, or total body irradiation (TBI) as preconditioning for bone marrow transplantation (BMT).

Growth hormone secretion is almost exclusively the first of the anterior pituitary hormones to be affected. Prospective data following irradiation of pituitary tumors and nasopharyngeal tumors suggest that deficiency of the gonadotropins occurs next, followed by corticotropin, with thyrotropin being relatively resistant to irradiation damage. This sequence is evident in around 60% of patients; however, variations occur, the most notable being corticotropin deficiency occurring before loss of the gonadotropins. Transiently elevated prolactin levels are frequently observed after hypothalamo–pituitary irradiation, and tend to return to baseline values over the following few years.

The radiobiological impact of a radiation schedule on hypothalamo–pituitary function is dependent on the total dose, fractionation, and duration over which the radiation is administered. Whilst isolated GHD is frequently observed in children with radiation doses used in preconditioning for BMT (9.0–15.5 Gy) and prophylactic cranial irradiation in the treatment of acute lymphocytic leukemia (ALL; 18–24 Gy), higher doses used in the treatment of pituitary and brain tumors (30–50 Gy) may result in additional pituitary hormone deficits, whereas doses in excess of 60 Gy frequently cause panhypopituitarism. The proportion of patients 5 years post-irradiation of the hypothalamo–pituitary axis when administered a fractionated dosage of ~40 Gy would be expected to be in the region of 60–100%, 30–60%, 20–40%, and 5–25% for GH, gonadotropin, corticotropin, and thyrotropin deficiency respectively (Fig. 81.1). In addition to the incidence of anterior pituitary hormone deficits, radiation dose also determines the speed of onset and severity of hormone deficits [4]. Posterior pituitary dysfunction following irradiation is not described.

As previously mentioned it is an oversimplification to consider only the total dose of irradiation. Fractionation is an important factor to be considered, as a dose divided into a greater number of fractions of smaller size and administered over a longer time period is less likely to result in hypopituitarism. Age at irradiation is an important factor and is best exemplified by the dichotomy between children and adults. Children who receive TBI (9.0–15.5 Gy) as preconditioning for BMT frequently develop GHD, whereas adults treated with a similar regimen show normal GH status up to 4 years later. The prevalence and severity of hormone deficits following irradiation to a previously normal hypothalamo–pituitary axis are a function of time since irradiation and the rate of occurrence is dependent primarily on the dosage received.

Although reported, deficits within the first 12–24 months are infrequent due to significant redundancy in pituitary hormone secretion. The mean peak GH response to the insulin tolerance test (ITT) in healthy young adults is in excess of 30 µg/L, whereas an adult is only considered severely GHD once their peak GH response is <3 µg/L. The progressive nature of hormone deficits following hypothalamo–pituitary radiation is attributable to the cumulative damage resulting from irradiation and pituitary atrophy secondary to hypothalamic damage (Fig. 81.1). This phenomenon necessitates prolonged follow-up with yearly assessment of pituitary function in patients who have received cranial radiation.

The deleterious effect of radiation to the hypothalamo–pituitary axis is thought to be primarily to the hypothalamus with doses of less than 50 Gy. Higher doses are thought to additionally damage the pituitary directly. Support for the hypothesis that the hypothalamus is more vulnerable to radiation than the pituitary is derived from several sources. Following radiation normal GH responses to GH-releasing hormone (GHRH) may be seen in the setting of impaired GH responses to the ITT, and subnormal gonadal function may be observed in the presence of a normal gonadotropin response to gonadotropin-releasing hormone (GnRH). Prolactin levels are frequently transiently elevated, suggesting a reduction in hypothalamic dopaminergic tone. Insertion of ^{90}Y implants (500–1500 Gy) in to pituitary adenomas results in a lower prevalence of anterior pituitary hormone deficits compared with conventional external beam irradiation (37.5–42.5 Gy); the likely explanation for this observation is that the field for conventional irradiation includes the hypothalamus, which is relatively spared with ^{90}Y. The pathophysiological mechanism responsible for radiation-induced hypothalamic damage is unclear and may reflect either vascular or direct neuronal damage. Hypothalamic blood flow declines with time following irradiation; however, there was no change in hypothalamic/occipital blood flow ratio between 6 months and 5 years following irradiation. This was in contrast to the progressive endocrine dysfunction.

Growth hormone deficiency (GHD)

In contrast to higher irradiation doses where the majority of children develop severe GHD within 5 years of irradiation, lower irradiation doses (9.0–24 Gy) leave the majority of patients with "normal" stimulated GH responses. Studies of spontaneous GH release in these latter children, however, frequently show subnormal levels with failure of the expected increase in GH secretion at puberty. The phenomenon of impaired spontaneous GH secretion and normal stimulated GH levels is termed neurosecretory dysfunction, the clinical relevance of which is currently unknown, but has been associated with an attenuated pubertal growth spurt.

GH replacement is commonly used to optimize final height in children diagnosed with radiation-induced GHD. Most studies have shown improvements in height velocity but the most robust data come from studies analyzing final height, or the change in height SDS from initiation of therapy until completion

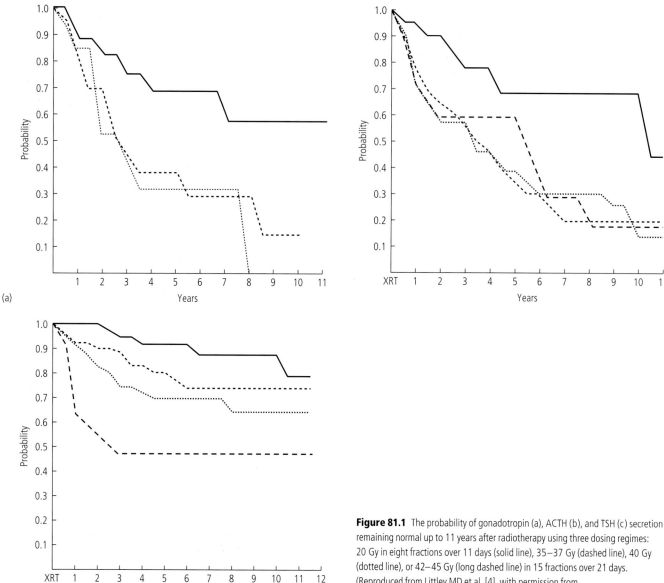

Figure 81.1 The probability of gonadotropin (a), ACTH (b), and TSH (c) secretion remaining normal up to 11 years after radiotherapy using three dosing regimes: 20 Gy in eight fractions over 11 days (solid line), 35–37 Gy (dashed line), 40 Gy (dotted line), or 42–45 Gy (long dashed line) in 15 fractions over 21 days. (Reproduced from Littley MD et al. [4], with permission from Blackwell Publishing.)

of growth, in patients treated with GH compared with those who did not receive GH therapy. Early studies showed disappointingly small differences in the height loss prevented by the use of GH replacement, and much less than observed in children treated for idiopathic GHD. A number of factors contributed to these suboptimal results including spinal irradiation, early puberty, a prolonged interval between irradiation and initiation of GH therapy, and inadequate GH schedules. The predominant factor likely relates to the interval between hypothalamo–pituitary irradiation and initiation of GH therapy. Since the risk of recurrence of childhood brain tumors is relatively low more than 2 years out from treatment and there is no evidence that GH therapy increases the risk of recurrence of brain tumors, it is reasonable to consider GH replacement at this time. The approach of clinicians is vari-

able with some offering GH replacement only to children who demonstrate a reduced peak GH response to stimulation in association with a reduced height velocity, whereas others offer GH replacement on the basis of the biochemistry alone on the premise of preventing height loss which, once established, may not be fully remediable. Where growth velocity and GH stimulation tests are normal at 2 years post treatment growth should be monitored and the GH stimulation tests repeated annually.

Following completion of growth, GH plays an important role in optimizing somatic development, a time frequently referred to as transition. GHD during this time results in reduced muscle and bone mass, along with increased fat mass which is predominantly truncal in distribution. A significant relationship is observed between the degree by which a child fails to achieve final height and the adverse body composition, implying a critical role for growth as a surrogate for normalization of body composition. GH replacement from completion of growth through to the mid-20s ensures somatic development continues and genetically predetermined muscle and bone mass are reached. It is unclear whether GH replacement, if reinstituted later in adult life, will fully reverse the adverse body composition changes resulting from a prolonged period of GHD. To date there are no data specific to transitional use of GH in adults with radiation-induced GHD; however, it is intuitive to surmise that the beneficial effects of GH replacement in these individuals would be similar to GHD hypopituitary adults of other etiologies. Before committing an individual who received childhood GH replacement for radiation-induced GHD to transitional GH replacement it is essential to reassess the GH axis. This necessity is derived from the fact that all degrees of GHD are treated during childhood and only those with severe GHD qualify for treatment as an adult. Furthermore, the reproducibility of GH stimulation tests is poor and recent data reassessing GH status in childhood brain tumor survivors showed that only 61% retested severe GHD at final height [5]. GH doses used to treat GHD adults during transition should be aimed at normalizing the IGF-I level in contrast to the weight-based regimens used during childhood.

Adult GHD is characterized by impaired quality of life, reduced lean body mass, increased fat mass, insulin resistance, an adverse lipid profile, elevated procoagulant factors and osteopenia, culminating in a three-fold increase in fracture rates and a two- to three-fold increase in mortality. GHD survivors of childhood cancer are phenotypically indistinguishable from GHD hypopituitary adults. In the former group the relative contribution of GHD is difficult to disentangle from the direct effects of the primary pathology, irradiation, chemotherapy, high-dose glucocorticoids, insufficient exercise and excess caloric intake. Physiological GH replacement in adult GHD survivors of childhood cancer significantly improves quality of life, with the greatest benefit occurring in the domain of vitality. Beneficial effects on body composition, serum lipids, and bone density were minor [6]. No beneficial effect of 18 months' GH replacement was observed on the spinal bone density of patients who previously received spinal irradiation. It could be deduced, therefore, that the adverse sequelae observed in GHD survivors of childhood cancer, with the exception of quality of life, are not primarily the consequence of radiation-induced GHD. Following the NICE review of adult GH replacement in the UK, severely impaired quality of life was deemed the only cost-effective indication for the use GH replacement in severely GHD adults irrespective of the underlying etiology [7]. A trial of therapy is therefore appropriate in GHD adult survivors of cancer where quality of life is impaired.

Disturbances of gonadotropin secretion

Following cranial irradiation gonadotropin secretion is the most frequently affected anterior pituitary hormone after GH. The incidence of gonadotropin deficiency is dose and time dependent. Gonadotropin deficiency following irradiation is present in a

continuum from subtle abnormalities resulting in low normal sex hormone levels to severe deficiency with clearly subnormal sex hormone levels. In the first year following irradiation of the hypothalamo–pituitary axis when treating men with nasopharyngeal carcinoma a rise in basal and stimulated follicle-stimulating hormone (FSH) with no change in either luteinizing hormone (LH) or testosterone levels has been reported. After the first year a progressive decline in both the FSH and LH occurs. The underlying mechanism has been suggested to represent an initial decline in pulse frequency of hypothalamic GnRH, followed by a progressive reduction in GnRH pulse amplitude.

In addition to gonadotropin deficiency cranial irradiation doses of less than 50 Gy can result in precocious or early puberty in children (Table 81.1). Both genders are affected with irradiation doses employed in the treatment of brain tumors (25–50 Gy), whereas lower doses used for prophylaxis in treatment of ALL result in a predominance of girls developing precocious puberty. There is a linear association between age at irradiation and the age at onset of puberty in patients who received cranial irradiation for brain tumors distant to the hypothalamo–pituitary axis. The onset of puberty occurs at a mean of 8.51 years in girls and 9.21 years in boys plus 0.29 years for every year of age at irradiation [8]. The mechanism responsible for early puberty is thought to result from disinhibition of cortical influences on the hypothalamus allowing GnRH pulse frequency and amplitude to increase prematurely. It has been postulated that the cortical restraint on the onset of puberty is more easily disrupted in girls than boys by any insult, including irradiation. The impact of early puberty in a child with radiation-induced GHD is to foreshorten the time available for GH therapy and thereby restrict the therapeutic efficacy of this intervention. It is for this reason that children with early puberty are treated with a combination of GnRH analogs and GH replacement. Studies examining the effect of GnRH analogs on final height in GHD patients treated with cranial irradiation have generally reported improvements in auxological outcome. The majority of studies compare a group treated with GnRH analogs with a group who did not receive this intervention. The decision to initiate GnRH analogs is frequently based on the child having a poorer final height prediction. Direct comparison of GnRH-treated and untreated individuals therefore almost certainly underestimates the beneficial impact of GnRH analogs on final height.

Adrenocorticotropic hormone (ACTH) deficiency

ACTH is more resilient to irradiation-induced damage than either the GH and gonadotropin axes. A clear dose dependency in damage to this axis is observed. There are few reports of ACTH deficiency following TBI (9.0–15.0 Gy) used as preconditioning before BMT. Children who received cranial irradiation (18–24 Gy) as part of their treatment for ALL infrequently develop ACTH deficiency. In survivors of childhood brain tumors ACTH deficiency tends to occur late, necessitating continued awareness and screening beyond 10 years after treatment of the primary disease (Fig. 81.1).

Thyroid-stimulating hormone (TSH) deficiency

TSH is the least vulnerable of the anterior pituitary axes to radiation-induced damage (Fig. 81.1). Diagnosis of central hypothyroidism is notoriously difficult as the TSH can lie within, below, or slightly above the normal range, with free thyroxine levels in the lower reaches of the normative range or only slightly below. The slightly elevated TSH levels seen in central hypothyroidism are thought to be the consequence of an alteration in the predominant form of TSH secreted, resulting in an alteration in the ratio of bioactive/immunoreactive TSH. There is no convincing evidence to support the routine use of the TRH test to improve the diagnostic sensitivity and specificity of central hypothyroidism.

Gonadal damage

As a result of the multi-modality treatment regimens employed in the treatment of cancer, damage to the gonadal axis can occur directly at the level of the gonad and centrally at the hypothalamus and pituitary as previously discussed. Damage to the gonads and central structures is not mutually exclusive and it is not uncommon for an individual to have involvement at both levels. Damage to the gonads can occur from irradiation exposure and cytotoxic chemotherapy (Table 81.2). Irradiation of the gonads occurs as a consequence of irradiation for gonadal tumors and testicular relapses of hematological malignancies, as a result of pelvic irradiation, TBI, and scatter from spinal irradiation. Damage from cytotoxic chemotherapy is most frequently described following alkylating agents including cyclophosphamide, chlorambucil, and mustine; however, nitrosoureas, procarbazine, vinblastine, cytosine arabinoside, and cisplatin have also been incriminated. In a large retrospective study of female childhood cancer survivors 6.3% developed ovarian failure within 5 years of diagnosis. Independent risk factors for ovarian failure were increasing age, exposure to ovarian irradiation, and treatment with procarbazine or cyclophosphamide. Of the patients with ovarian failure 54% had received ovarian irradiation in excess of 10 Gy [9].

Radiation and the testis (Table 81.2)

The testis is one of the most radiosensitive tissues in the body. A dichotomy between damage to the germinal epithelium and the Leydig cells is observed, very low doses of irradiation causing significant impairment of spermatogenesis whereas sex hormone production is impaired only with high radiation doses. As a consequence puberty progresses normally in children and secondary sexual characteristics are maintained in the adult. Testicular volumes are small, reflecting damage to the germinal epithelium, and should not be relied upon for staging puberty. In contrast to most other tissues dose fractionation increases gonadal toxicity. The effect of single fraction radiotherapy on spermatogenesis is well documented. In general, the most immature cells, spermatogonia, are the most radiosensitive with doses as low as 0.1 Gy causing a significant reduction in sperm count and morphological changes in the spermatozoa. Higher doses of 2–3 Gy are required to kill spermatocytes leading to a reduction in spermatid number. Doses of 4–6 Gy significantly reduce the number of spermatozoa implying direct damage to the spermatids (Fig. 81.2) [10]. A fall in the number of spermatozoa is seen 60–70 days following damage to immature cells from irradiation doses of up to 3 Gy. At higher doses the reduction in sperm count occurs earlier, reflecting damage to the spermatids. As a guide, doses of less than 0.8 Gy tend to result in oligospermia and doses above 0.8 Gy in azoospermia. At the doses discussed recovery of spermatogenesis occurs from proliferation of surviving stem cells. Complete recovery of the germinal epithelia and achievement of pre-morbid sperm counts occurs 9–18 months, 30 months, and 5 years or more following radiation doses of <1 Gy, 2–3 Gy, and >4 Gy respectively (Fig. 81.2) [10].

The majority of testicular radiation exposure occurs as a consequence of fractionated irradiation. In 10 patients who received a testicular dose of 1.2–3.0 Gy over 14–26 fractions during irradiation for Hodgkin disease no recovery of spermatogenesis was observed in those who received 1.4–2.6 Gy after 17–43 months, but a return to fertility occurred in the two patients who received 1.2 Gy [11]. These data suggest a threshold for permanent testicular damage of 1.2–1.4 Gy. In eight patients who received 0.28–0.9 Gy

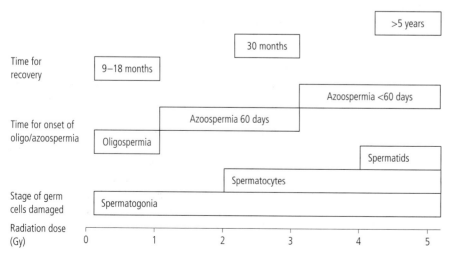

Figure 81.2 Impairment of spermatogenesis following single dose irradiation. The effect of radiation dose on stage of germ cell damage and time for onset and recovery from germ cell damage (adapted from data of Rowley et al. *Radiat. Res.* 1974;59;665–678, by Howell et al. *Int. J. Androl.* 2002;25:269–276 with permission from Allen Press Inc.).

for a diagnosis of testicular seminoma a return of spermatogenesis was reported in all, and four of five assessed at 12 months had normal sperm counts [12]. Fractionated radiotherapy doses of <0.2 Gy have no significant effect on spermatogenesis, doses of 0.2–0.7 Gy cause a dose-dependent increase in FSH and transient reduction in spermatogenesis that recovers within 12–24 months, and doses of 2.0–3.0 Gy frequently result in azoospermia with recovery of spermatogenesis often delayed for 10 years or more.

At the irradiation doses discussed Leydig cell function is relatively spared, the vast majority of patients having normal testosterone levels albeit at the cost of an elevated LH level in some. With time the elevated LH level gradually returns to normal. Higher irradiation doses (20–30 Gy) used for carcinoma *in situ* in the contralateral testis following unilateral orchidectomy during adulthood result in significant Leydig cell dysfunction characterized by a fall in testosterone and a compensatory increase in LH levels. The fall in testosterone, however, is not so great as to require replacement therapy in the majority of adults. In contrast there is a suggestion that individuals who have undergone a similar treatment regimen for testicular cancer during childhood may be more vulnerable to radiation-induced Leydig cell damage and frequently require testosterone replacement as an adult. It is noteworthy that an irradiation dose of 20–30 Gy will completely ablate the germinal epithelium.

Following TBI during childhood (9.0–15.5 Gy) FSH is elevated in the majority (68–90%) of pubertal and peripubertal boys and LH is elevated in 40–50%, whereas testosterone levels are infrequently low (0–16%). There are no robust data documenting sperm counts in adult life to determine the proportion that would be spontaneously fertile or fertile with assisted fertility techniques.

Radiation and the female reproductive tract

The effect of irradiation and chemotherapy on the ovary can best be explained by loss of oocytes from a fixed population, which once destroyed cannot be replaced (Table 81.2). The natural history of the healthy ovary is for oocyte number to fall exponentially with aging. Ovaries of older females are therefore much more sensitive to radiation-induced damage, and a dose of 6 Gy is liable to result in a permanent menopause in women aged 40 years or more. In contrast, in young women it is estimated that 20 Gy over a 6-week period will result in permanent sterility in around 50%. Consistent with this, 97% of 2068 women who received an estimated ovarian dose of 3.6–7.2 Gy in two to four fractions failed to menstruate again [13]. In childhood, the LD_{50} of the oocyte has been estimated to be 4 Gy [14], and may present as failure to enter or complete puberty, or later in life with a premature menopause. Ovarian recovery following childhood irradiation has been reported, but is often temporary with the onset of secondary amenorrhea usually ensuing within the following few years.

The ovaries are irradiated in management of pelvic tumors, lymphoma, during the spinal component of craniospinal irradiation, and during TBI preconditioning prior to BMT. Treatment of Hodgkin disease involves local irradiation of involved lymph nodes, including those along the iliac vessels. The ovaries lie adjacent to the iliac vessels and will receive a dose of ~35 Gy inevitably resulting in premature ovarian failure. Oophoropexy before irradiation, combined with shielding, can reduce the dose of irradiation received by the ovaries to less than 6 Gy over 12–45 days thereby reducing the incidence of amenorrhea by around 50%. The exact reduction in risk of amenorrhea as a consequence of oophoropexy is controversial and needs to be assessed in the context of disease extent, patient age and surgical expertise.

Pelvic irradiation during childhood that involves the uterus within the irradiation field leads to changes that result in failure to carry a child. In those patients who do conceive the risk of miscarriage and low birth weight infants is greatly increased [15]. An irradiation dose of 20–30 Gy during childhood leads to a reduction in adult uterine length and failure of the endometrium to respond to physiological estrogen and progesterone therapy (Table 81.2). Uterine blood flow is reduced in the post-irradiation uterine arteries on Doppler ultrasound. An adequate blood flow is essential to uterine function, particularly endometrial proliferation, implantation and successful continuation of pregnancy. It is unlikely that an adult who has received a significant irradiation dose to the uterus during childhood would be able to carry a child to term. Uterine irradiation not only impacts on patients who retain normal ovarian function, but also on those who request *in vitro* fertilization with donor oocytes for concomitant ovarian failure.

Chemotherapy and the testis (Table 81.2)

The adverse impact of chemotherapeutic agents on the testis is directed primarily at the germinal epithelium. The extent of damage and potential for recovery of spermatogenesis is dependent on the chemotherapeutic agents used and the cumulative dosage. It has also been suggested that the adult testis is more susceptible to damage than that of the prepubertal testis. In general combination chemotherapy is more toxic than single agents and the induced azoospermia is less likely to recover. Of 116 men treated with cyclophosphamide alone 45% showed evidence of testicular dysfunction. The incidence of gonadal dysfunction correlated with the cumulative dose of cyclophosphamide. Over 80% of post-pubertal males who received a total dose of >300 mg/kg showed evidence of testicular dysfunction [16]. The use of MVPP (mustine, vinblastine, procarbazine, prednisolone) in treatment of Hodgkin disease renders almost all males azoospermic after the first cycle, and less than 5% will have a normal sperm count 5 years after receiving six or more cycles [17]. Despite rendering the majority of patients azoospermic following use of CVB (cisplatin, vinblastine, bleomycin) in the treatment of metastatic testicular cancer the outlook for fertility is much better than for MVPP, with 50% of men having a normal sperm count 3 years following this schedule.

Although subnormal testosterone levels <200 ng/dL (<7 nmol/L) are infrequent following chemotherapy there is irrefutable evidence for a more subtle impact on Leydig cell function. The most frequent abnormalities of Leydig cell function are an elevated basal and GnRH-stimulated LH level in the setting of a normal or low normal testosterone level. Physiologically LH pulse amplitude is increased whilst pulse frequency remains unaltered. The compensatory increase in LH means testosterone replacement is rarely necessary. In 135 men treated with high-dose chemotherapy for Hodgkin disease 31% were found to have an elevated LH in association with a testosterone level in the lower half of the normal range or frankly subnormal, and a further 7% showed an isolated raised LH level [18]. These biochemical abnormalities support the hypothesis that a significant proportion of men treated with cytotoxic chemotherapy have mild testosterone deficiency. Studies of testosterone replacement in these individuals with elevated LH and testosterone levels within the lower reaches of the normative range have failed to showed significant benefits to date [19].

Chemotherapy and the ovary (Table 81.2)

Ovarian damage presents clinically with amenorrhea with or without symptoms of estrogen deficiency, or failure to progress through puberty. Hormonally, the gonadotropins may be grossly elevated with an unrecordable estradiol level, or show moderate elevation of the gonadotropins in association with a mid-follicular estradiol level. The majority of accumulated data relates to toxicity from cyclophosphamide. Similar to irradiation-induced ovarian damage the susceptibility of the ovary to chemotherapeutic damage, speed of onset of amenorrhea, and the potential for recovery are dependent on age and cumulative dosage. In women with breast cancer treated with multi-agent chemotherapy including cyclophosphamide, the average dose of cyclophosphamide to induce amenorrhea in women in their 20s, 30s and 40s was 20.4, 9.3, and 5.2 g respectively [20]. Intuitively prepubertal and pubertal girls would be assumed to be at lower risk of ovarian damage; however, clinical and morphological studies reveal that although infrequent, they are not totally resistant to cytotoxic ovarian damage. Following treatment of Hodgkin disease with MVPP (mustine, vincristine, procarbazine, prednisolone) or MOPP (mustargen, oncovin, procarbazine, prednisolone) 15–62% of survivors develop amenorrhea. In many the onset is abrupt, whilst in others there is progression to oligomenorrhea with later development of a premature menopause.

Sex steroid replacement and fertility

Strategies aimed at prevention of gonadal damage have led to the use of chemotherapeutic regimens, such as AVBD (adriamycin, vinblastine, bleomycin, dacarbazine) for the treatment of Hodgkin disease, that have equivalent cure rates but significantly less impact on gonadal function. Suppression of the gonadal axis with GnRH analogs prior to cancer therapy has shown gonadal protection in animal models; however, there is no convincing evidence for benefit in either sex in the human. Males at risk of azoospermia due to their impending treatment schedule can have sperm frozen for future use. Sperm storage is most effective where the sperm concentration, motility and morphology are not affected by the primary disease process. A significant proportion of men with Hodgkin disease and testicular tumors are oligospermic at presentation.

Recovery of ovarian function in amenorrheic women and the possibility of a premature menopause in women retaining a normal cycle is difficult to predict accurately following an insult to the gonads received during the treatment of cancer. The use of transvaginal ultrasound to accurately quantitate ovarian volume, and measurement of inhibin B and anti-Müllerian hormone have been proposed as guides of future reproductive potential following cancer therapy. Preservation of fertility in women who are to undergo intense treatment likely to result in infertility is a significant growth area. Both oocytes and embryos can be frozen with successful implantation occurring in around 10% and 20–25% of cycles respectively. Despite advances with the former, this technique is still regarded as experimental and has significantly lower success rate than embryo storage. Embryo storage requires the patient to be in a stable relationship and undergo controlled stimulation of the ovary for several weeks, along with regular ultrasonograph monitoring and aspiration of follicles. These techniques are time-consuming when there is a pressing need to start treatment, are invasive, do not permit natural conception, and are not applicable to prepubertal females. Recently, interest has been directed towards cryopreservation of ovarian strips that are later grafted back in to the patient at the original site (orthotopic) or elsewhere (heterotopic) [21]. Several large centers are now storing ovarian strips; however, there are limited data following regrafting of the tissue and only time will tell if this technique will improve the fertility prospects of women who are to undergo multi-modality cancer therapy.

In women under the age of 50 who have developed gonadal failure sex steroid replacement is recommended to alleviate symptoms and prevent loss of bone mass. The impact of sex steroid replacement on cardiovascular events remains controversial in patients below the age of 50 in light of recent data showing an increase in vascular events in post-menopausal women treated with hormone replacement therapy.

Thyroid damage

Thyroid nodules

Large-scale epidemiological studies have unequivocally confirmed a causal relationship between external beam irradiation of the neck and the development of thyroid cancer (Table 81.3). The thyroid is most commonly irradiated in treatment of lymphomas, head and neck tumors, and during spinal irradiation in the treatment of some brain tumors and hematological malignancies. Some of the most robust data are derived from individuals who received mantel irradiation in the treatment of Hodgkin disease. The increased incidence of thyroid carcinogenesis appears 5–10 years after irradiation and remains elevated for at least several decades. The actuarial risk of thyroid carcinoma in survivors of Hodgkin disease has been calculated as 1.7%, equivalent to a relative risk of 15.6 [22]. Histologically, the majority of radiation-induced thyroid carcinomas are well-differentiated papillary carcinomas (~80%), with follicular carcinomas accounting for almost all remaining neoplasms. The risk of developing thyroid carcinoma following neck irradiation is greater in children compared with adults, and young children are more vulnerable than older children. The odds ratio for development of thyroid carcinoma following 10–20 Gy irradiation to the thyroid in children diagnosed <10 years at their first cancer compared with those diagnosed >10 years at their first cancer has been estimated to be 16.3 and 2.9 respectively [23]. The risk of developing thyroid cancer has been assumed to be linearly associated with dose. More recent data confirm this to be true for radiation doses up to 20–29 Gy; however, at doses greater than 30 Gy a fall in the dose response is observed consistent with a cell-killing effect of radiation at high doses (Fig. 81.3) [23]. Women are at greater risk of developing thyroid cancer than men at all doses of radiation. No definite association of chemotherapy with an increased risk of thyroid cancer has been shown, and neither does chemotherapy modify the carcinogenic effect of radiotherapy. Most thyroid cancers are in the main eminently curable, but in an individual previously treated for cancer, the diagnosis can be a substantial psychological and physical burden. Long-term surveillance with yearly examination of the neck and thyroid in survivors of cancer who received irradiation to the neck is essential. Controversy remains as to the best method to accomplish this as ultrasound will detect neoplasms earlier than palpation, including many small benign lesions of no clinical significance.

In addition to thyroid carcinomas, thyroid irradiation is also associated with an increased incidence of benign thyroid nodules including focal hyperplasia, adenomas, colloid nodules, lymphocytic thyroiditis and fibrosis (Table 81.3). Studies suggest palpable thyroid abnormalities to be present in 20–30% of the irradiated population compared with 1–5% in the general population. Time since irradiation, female gender, and dose of irradiation to the thyroid are independently associated with a greater risk of developing benign thyroid nodules. Recurrence rates are high following surgical removal of radiation-induced benign thyroid nodules, similar to the non-irradiated gland. Following surgery, thyroxine therapy aimed at TSH suppression reduces the rate of recurrence of benign radiation-induced nodules.

Thyroid dysfunction

In addition to thyroid nodules patients who receive irradiation to the thyroid have a greatly increased risk of thyroid dysfunction (Table 81.3). Compensated or frank hypothyroidism is reported to occur in 20–30% following preconditioning with TBI (9.0–15.0 Gy) prior to BMT. Patients treated for lymphoma or head and neck cancers receive a dose of 30–50 Gy to the thyroid over several weeks. The cumulative probability of developing hypothyroidism in these individuals is 30–50%. The majority of cases develop within the first 5 years with the incidence declining thereafter. Younger age at irradiation, female gender, time since irradiation and radiation dose all increase the prevalence of hypothyroidism. There is no conclusive evidence that any cytotoxic chemotherapy alters thyroid function. Treatment of compensated and frank hypothyroidism with thyroxine is warranted when the thyroid has been irradiated as TSH is known to promote thyroid tumor growth.

The prevalence of Graves disease and Graves ophthalmopathy is increased in patients who receive a radiation dose >30 Gy to the thyroid. The relative risk of Graves disease is around eight-fold higher than the normal population.

Hyperparathyroidism

Neck irradiation has been associated with an increased risk of hyperparathyroidism (Table 81.3). The absolute increase in incidence is difficult to quantitate as a consequence of the long latency period between irradiation and the development of hyperparathyroidism (25–47 years). Schneider et al. determined the prevalence of hyperparathyroidism in 2555 individuals who underwent neck irradiation for benign conditions before age 16 years. The relative risk of hyperparathyroidism increased by 0.11 per cGy; however, the data were based upon only 36 confirmed cases of hyperparathyroidism [24]. The presence of a dose relationship between irradiation and development of hyperparathyroidism supports the previous observational data of a causal association.

Conclusion

Endocrine late effects in survivors of cancer can lead to abnormalities of all endocrine axes. Both chemotherapy and radiotherapy play a role in the etiology of the adverse sequelae observed. All individuals involved in the care of cancer survivors need to be vigilant to the development of late effects which can occur even decades after completing cytotoxic therapy.

References

1. Mertens AC, Yasui Y, Neglia JP, et al. Late mortality experience in five-year survivors of childhood and adolescent cancer: the Childhood Cancer Survivor Study. *J. Clin. Oncol.* 2001;19:3163–3172.
2. Gurney JG, Kadan-Lottick NS, Packer RJ, et al. Endocrine and cardiovascular late effects among adult survivors of childhood brain tumors: Childhood Cancer Survivor Study. *Cancer* 2003;97:663–673.

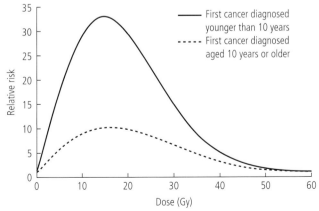

Figure 81.3 Thyroid cancer risk by radiation dose according to age at diagnosis of first cancer (Reproduced from Sigurdson AJ et al. [23], with permission from Elsevier.)

3. Gurney JG, Ness KK, Stovall M, et al. Final height and body mass index among adult survivors of childhood brain cancer: childhood cancer survivor study. *J. Clin. Endocrinol. Metab.* 2003;88:4731–4739.

4. Littley MD, Shalet SM, Beardwell CG, Robinson EL, Sutton ML. Radiation-induced hypopituitarism is dose-dependent. *Clin. Endocrinol. (Oxf.)* 1989;31:363–373.

5. Gleeson HK, Gattamaneni HR, Smethurst L, Brennan BM, Shalet SM. Reassessment of growth hormone status is required at final height in children treated with growth hormone replacement after radiation therapy. *J. Clin. Endocrinol. Metab.* 2004;89:662–666.

6. Murray RD, Darzy KH, Gleeson HK, Shalet SM. GH-deficient survivors of childhood cancer: GH replacement during adult life. *J. Clin. Endocrinol. Metab.* 2002;87:129–135.

7. NICE. Technology appraisal #64. Human growth hormone (Somatotropin) in adults with growth hormone deficiency. London: Department of Health, 2003.

8. Ogilvy-Stuart AL, Clayton PE, Shalet SM. Cranial irradiation and early puberty. *J. Clin. Endocrinol. Metab.* 1994;78:1282–1286.

9. Chemaitilly W, Mertens AC, Mitby P, et al. Acute ovarian failure in the childhood cancer survivor study. *J. Clin. Endocrinol. Metab.* 2006;91:1723–1728.

10. Rowley MJ, Leach DR, Warner GA, Heller CG. Effect of graded doses of ionizing radiation on the human testis. *Radiat. Res.* 1974;59:665–678.

11. Speiser B, Rubin P, Casarett G. Aspermia following lower truncal irradiation in Hodgkin's disease. *Cancer* 1973;32:692–698.

12. Centola GM, Keller JW, Henzler M, Rubin P. Effect of low-dose testicular irradiation on sperm count and fertility in patients with testicular seminoma. *J. Androl.* 1994;15:608–613.

13. Doll R, Smith PG. The long-term effects of x irradiation in patients treated for metropathia haemorrhagica. *Br. J. Radiol.* 1968;41:362–368.

14. Wallace WH, Shalet SM, Hendry JH, Morris-Jones PH, Gattamaneni HR. Ovarian failure following abdominal irradiation in childhood: the radiosensitivity of the human oocyte. *Br. J. Radiol.* 1989;62:995–998.

15. Li FP, Gimbrere K, Gelber RD, et al. Outcome of pregnancy in survivors of Wilms' tumor. *JAMA* 1987;257:216–219.

16. Rivkees SA, Crawford JD. The relationship of gonadal activity and chemotherapy-induced gonadal damage. *JAMA* 1988;259:2123–2125.

17. Whitehead E, Shalet SM, Blackledge G, Todd I, Crowther D, Beardwell CG. The effects of Hodgkin's disease and combination chemotherapy on gonadal function in the adult male. *Cancer* 1982;49:418–422.

18. Howell SJ, Radford JA, Ryder WD, Shalet SM. Testicular function after cytotoxic chemotherapy: evidence of Leydig cell insufficiency. *J. Clin. Oncol.* 1999;17:1493–1498.

19. Howell SJ, Radford JA, Adams JE, Smets EM, Warburton R, Shalet SM. Randomized placebo-controlled trial of testosterone replacement in men with mild Leydig cell insufficiency following cytotoxic chemotherapy. *Clin. Endocrinol. (Oxf.)* 2001;55:315–324.

20. Koyama H, Wada T, Nishizawa Y, Iwanaga T, Aoki Y. Cyclophosphamide-induced ovarian failure and its therapeutic significance in patients with breast cancer. *Cancer* 1977;39:1403–1409.

21. Radford JA, Lieberman BA, Brison DR, et al. Orthotopic reimplantation of cryopreserved ovarian cortical strips after high-dose chemotherapy for Hodgkin's lymphoma. *Lancet* 2001;357:1172–1175.

22. Hancock SL, Cox RS, McDougall IR. Thyroid diseases after treatment of Hodgkin's disease. *N. Engl. J. Med.* 1991;325:599–605.

23. Sigurdson AJ, Ronckers CM, Mertens AC, et al. Primary thyroid cancer after a first tumour in childhood (the Childhood Cancer Survivor Study): a nested case–control study. *Lancet* 2005;365:2014–2023.

24. Schneider AB, Gierlowski TC, Shore-Freedman E, Stovall M, Ron E, Lubin J. Dose–response relationships for radiation-induced hyperparathyroidism. *J. Clin. Endocrinol. Metab.* 1995;80:254–257.

7 Endocrine-responsive Tumors and Female Reproductive Hormone Therapy

82 Endocrine-responsive Tumors: Prostate Cancer

Sarah Ngan, Ana Arance, and Jonathan Waxman

Key points

- The androgen receptor is pivotal in the pathogenesis of prostate cancer and hormone resistance.
- Molecular mechanisms of hormone resistance include mutations in the androgen receptor, co-regulator imbalance, and androgen receptor activation by other signaling pathways.
- Androgen deprivation therapy is the cornerstone in the management of advanced prostate cancer.
- In androgen-independent prostate cancer secondary hormonal therapy along with chemotherapy may be considered.
- New targeted therapies may provide hope for patients with hormone-refractory prostate cancer.

Introduction

Prostate cancer is the most frequently diagnosed malignancy among men in the Western world, affecting 25 000 men in the United Kingdom annually. Androgens regulate the growth, development and differentiation of the normal prostate. Their effects are mediated by the androgen receptor (AR), a member of a superfamily of ligand-activated nuclear transcription factors. In the 1940s Higgins and Hodges demonstrated that prostate cancer is androgen dependent and tumor regression could be induced with androgen ablation by castration. Since then, chemical castration utilizing gonadotropin-releasing hormone receptor (GnRH) agonists and anti-androgens have become the accepted treatment for non-organ confined disease. The majority of patients (85%) have an initial response to hormonal therapy. However, after 18–24 months many patients become refractory to hormonal treatment due to selection of resistant cells and tumor adaptation. Palliative chemotherapy at this point achieves responses in 50–70% of patients, but most will die from their disease within 1–2 years. Since the majority of these androgen-independent prostate cancers (AIPC) continue to express the AR there has been much interest in the AR pathway and more recently other molecular pathways, which modulate AR function in an androgen-deprived environment. This chapter describes the current status of research into the role of the AR in prostate cancer, the molecular biology of resistance to hormonal treatment and prostate cancer treatment options, including the potential role of novel treatments.

Clinical Endocrine Oncology, 2nd edition. Edited by Ian D. Hay and John A.H. Wass. © 2008 Blackwell Publishing. ISBN 978-1-4051-4584-8.

Androgen synthesis and the androgen receptor

Testosterone is the main circulating androgen in men and is primarily produced by the Leydig cells in the testes. Its release is influenced by the pituitary hormones, luteinizing hormone (LH) and follicle-stimulating hormone (FSH). Testosterone is transported in the circulation by steroid hormone-binding globulin (SHBG) and is converted intracellularly by the enzyme 5α-reductase to the more powerful androgen dihydrotestosterone (DHT) in target organs. A small amount of testosterone is additionally produced by the adrenal glands (Fig. 82.1).

The AR is a member of the nuclear receptor superfamily of ligand-activated transcription factors. The AR is a member of the class I receptor group, which also includes other steroid receptors such as the estrogen receptor α (ERα), the progesterone receptor (PR), the glucocorticoid receptor (GR), and the mineralocorticoid receptor (MR). The AR acts as a transcription factor to regulate the expression of genes required for normal male sexual development and maintenance of accessory sexual organ function [1].

The unliganded AR is localized to the cytoplasm, where it is sequestered by binding to heat-shock proteins (hsp): hsp 90, hsp 70 and hsp 56 [2]. Androgen binding causes a conformational change that releases the hsps, allows AR translocation to the nucleus, receptor phosphorylation and dimerization [2]. The AR then binds to specific androgen response elements, in the promoter and enhancer regions of target genes. This is the first step in the sequential assembly and dissociation of a series of protein complexes on the DNA, which include co-activators, co-repressors, RNA polymerase II and associated factors, ultimately leading to the stimulation of transcription of androgen-regulated genes (Fig. 82.2).

Prostate cancer and hormone resistance

Several mechanisms have been proposed to be responsible for the emergence of hormonal resistance in prostate cancer. These can broadly be divided into those which bypass the AR, and those that involve the AR signaling pathway (Fig. 82.3).

AR mutations

One of the first AR mutations identified was in the LNCaP prostate cancer cell line, which was derived from a lymph node deposit from a patient with hormone-refractory prostate cancer (HRPC). Sequencing of the AR cDNA from this cell line revealed a single point mutation in the ligand-binding domain of the receptor,

resulting in the substitution of threonine at amino acid position 877 to alanine. The resultant receptor is promiscuous in its ligand binding, with an affinity for estrogenic and progestogenic steroids, adrenal androgens, as well as the non-steroidal anti-androgens hydroxyflutamide and nilutamide. AR mutations are rare in patients with primary prostate cancer but are found in up to 30% of metastases that are resistant to hormone therapy, suggesting that they play a role in tumor progression [3]. The majority of reported mutations are in the ligand-binding domain and as in the LNCaP cell line produce a receptor which is more sensitive to androgen and activated by other steroid hormones and/or anti-androgens which are used to treat the disease. Further evidence of abnormal AR function has been provided by reports of clinical improvement in patients with HRPC following

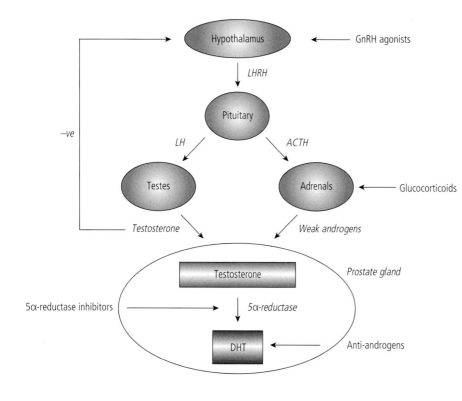

Figure 82.1 The hypothalamo–pituitary–gonadal axis and hormonal treatment targets. ACTH, adrenocorticotropic hormone; −ve, negative feedback. For explanation of other abbreviations see text.

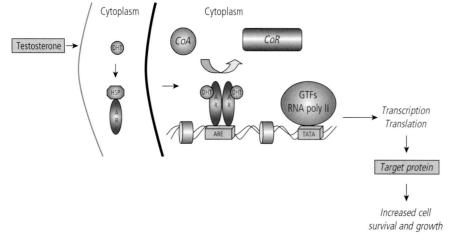

Figure 82.2 Model of the AR transcription complex. CoA, co-activator; CoR, co-repressor; ARE, androgen response element; GTFs, general transcription factors. For explanation of other abbreviations see text.

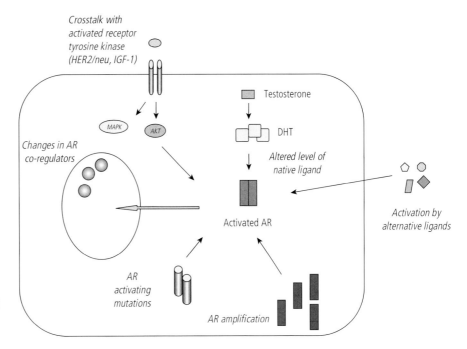

Figure 82.3 Mechanisms of resistance to hormonal treatment in prostate cancer, which involve the AR. For abbreviations see text.

withdrawal of anti-androgen treatment [4]. It has been postulated that this may be due to receptor mutation leading to activation or stabilization of the receptor by the anti-androgen itself as an adaptation to long-term androgen ablation.

AR expression

Amplification of the androgen receptor gene, leading to over-expression of the receptor, is another postulated mechanism for the development of AIPC, by increasing the sensitivity of prostate cancer cells to low circulating levels of androgen. A number of studies have reported no AR gene amplification in pretreatment tissue specimens from whom AR gene amplifications developed. This suggests that gene amplification may be an adaptive response [5]. This is consistent with the finding that patients with AR amplification at the time of recurrence on androgen deprivation therapy (ADT) have a higher chance of responding to second-line hormonal treatment than those without amplification. In addition these patients with receptor amplification have a better prognosis than those with receptor mutations [5].

Increased bioavailability of circulating androgen

Long-term androgen ablation therapy may select tumor cells, which have acquired mechanisms to accumulate intracellular concentrations of androgen, for example sequestration of androgens by SHBG or by altered regulation of enzymes involved in steroid hormone synthesis and metabolism. A recent study using comparative gene expression microarray analysis of castration-resistant and naïve tumor samples detected an increased expression of enzymes in the steroid precursor pathway in the castration-resistant samples [6]. Further evidence supporting the role of steroid-synthesizing enzymes in prostate cancer, includes the high incidence of polymorphisms in the 5α-reductase gene in

men of African descent, which can result in higher levels of 5α-reductase activity and a higher incidence of tumors with a poor prognosis.

AR co-regulators

A large number of steroid receptor co-regulator molecules have been recently identified, which are recruited to the promoters of steroid receptor target genes after ligand binding and via protein–protein interactions augment or reduce steroid receptor transcriptional activity. Although more *in vivo* confirmatory studies are awaited, there is now strong *in vitro* evidence implicating the role of AR co-factors in the development of androgen-resistance. These AR co-factors exert their effects via three main mechanisms: by increasing AR transcriptional activity in the presence of low levels of ligand; by altering the ligand specificity of AR allowing anti-androgens and other steroid hormones to act as agonist; and by facilitating AR nuclear translocation in the absence of androgen.

Co-activators that lead to enhanced AR activity include the p160 family of co-activators, p300 and c-jun [7]. The p160 co-factor family is made up of SRC-1, 2 and 3, which are commonly over-expressed in hormone-refractory prostate cancer. SRC-1 has been found in LNCaP cells to enhance ligand-dependent activation of AR by binding to its N-terminal domain (NTD). In the absence of androgen, if SRC-1 is phosphorylated by mitogen-activated protein kinase (MAPK), interaction of SRC-1 with the AR results in the same magnitude of AR activation that is obtained with DHT. Expression of the AR co-activator p300 is associated with a high Gleason score and prostate cancer progression. It is also associated with prostate cancer cell proliferation and is believed to be involved with cell cycle. c-jun binds to the AR NTD domain and by promoting the N-C domain interaction, promotes

AR homodimerization and so allows AR to act as a transcription factor in the absence of ligand.

A number of co-activators have been found to alter the ligand specificity of the AR. The androgen-associated proteins ARA 54 and ARA 70 can selectively augment the activity of the AR to alternative ligands such as hydroxyflutamide and estradiol, sensitize the receptor to lower concentrations of androgen and allow ligand-independent activation of the receptor by receptor tyrosine kinases such as HER2 [6]. A change in the balance of co-activators to co-repressors can alter AR transactivation activity in the presence of low concentrations of ligand. In addition, since co-repressors are thought to mediate in part the antagonist actions of bicalutamide and flutamide, an imbalance between co-regulator proteins may explain the paradoxical agonist effects of anti-androgens on prostate cancer growth in some cases of HRPC.

AR activation by other signaling pathways

In prostate cancer cell lines there is increasing evidence of AR activation in the absence of ligand, by several factors and signaling pathways acting in an independent or combined manner. Peptide growth factors such as epidermal growth factor (EGF), insulin-like growth factor (IGF-1) and keratinocyte growth factor (KGF) all activate the AR. These growth factors act as ligands for membrane receptor tyrosine kinases (TK) and act through several tyrosine pathways to promote AR activation and growth in an androgen-deprived environment. The stimulatory effect of IGF-1 on AR activation is blocked completely by the AR antagonist bicalutamide, indicating that this activation is AR dependent. HER2, a member of the EGF receptor family of membrane-bound TK receptors, has also been implicated in prostate cancer progression, since it is over-expressed more frequently in HRPC as opposed to hormone-naïve tumors. It is thought to act by promoting AR phosphorylation, stability, translocation to the nucleus and DNA binding via MAPK and Akt activity [6]. This therefore provides a rationale for targeting HER2 in clinical practice.

Crosstalk between the AR and the phosphatidylinositol 3-kinase (PI3K)/Akt pathway is another example of ligand-independent AR activation. The PI3K/Akt pathway links cell growth and survival signals received by cell surface TK receptors to internal cell control mechanisms. Activation of these membrane-bound TK re-ceptors leads to the recruitment of PI3K to the cell membrane, which in turn stimulates the generation of phosphatidylinositol-3-phosphate (PIP3). PIP3 then activates Akt and through phosphorylation activates AR activity. In addition, it also modulates a number of other downstream pathways involved in the cell survival and proliferation, such as FOXO1A, BAD, GSK3 and TSC2/mTOR pathways [7]. The PI3K/Akt pathway inhibitor phosphatase and tensin homolog (PTEN) on the other hand represses AR activity and cell proliferation. Loss of PTEN is therefore thought to be important in prostate cancer development. PTEN mutations have been identified in up to a third of HRPCs and the loss of PTEN expression has been found to correlate with a high Gleason score and advanced stage [7].

AR-independent pathways

In certain tumors the AR pathway may be bypassed altogether, especially since foci of AR-negative cells are often detected in prostate cancer specimens, in particular those samples from patients with HRPC. Possible mechanisms for bypassing the AR pathway include mutations, in oncogenes or tumor suppressor genes and blocking apoptosis by enhancing anti-apoptotic genes or depleting pro-apoptotic genes.

Protein concentration of the anti-apoptotic gene *bcl-2* has been correlated to the development of androgen resistance and treatment with *bcl-2* anti-sense in a prostate cancer animal model has been found to delay the emergence of androgen resistance [8]. Other anti-apoptotic proteins may also be important such as survivin and the caspase group of proteins.

The *p53* gene encodes a phosphoprotein which is crucial in regulating cell proliferation and apoptosis. In prostate cancer, *p53* mutations are rarely seen in benign prostatic hypertrophy and the incidence in localized untreated specimens is approximately 20% [9]. In metastatic or HRPC, however, the incidence reaches 50–75%. This suggests that mutations of the *p53* gene are a late development in prostate cancer progression.

In addition to the involvement of the MAPK and PI3K pathways in ligand-independent activation of the AR, there is increasing evidence of the involvement of these pathways in the development of hormone escape independent of the AR. For example, components of the MAPK pathway may influence cell cycle regulation and cell proliferation via AP-1, c-myc and nuclear factor-κB transcription factors. Similarly PI3K/Akt has been shown in prostate cancer cell lines to inhibit apoptosis by suppressing the pro-apoptotic functions of BAD [7].

Prostate cancer – hormonal therapy

The basis for endocrine treatment of prostate cancer is to deprive the cancer cells of androgens. Regression of an androgen-dependent tumor can be induced by any procedure that reduces intracellular concentration of dihydrotestosterone by 80% or more. This can be done by elimination of testicular testosterone production by orchidectomy or medically, using GnRH agonists. Alternatively the androgen receptors of the prostate cancer can be blocked with androgen antagonists. It is important to achieve serum testosterone concentrations as low as possible for ADT to minimize stimulation of prostate cancer cells.

GnRH agonists and antagonists

Medical castration with GnRH agonists in prostate cancer patients was first introduced in 1982, and is now the treatment of choice for men needing testicular androgen deprivation for the treatment of prostate cancer. This is especially the case since medical castration with GnRH agonists is equivalent in efficacy to orchidectomy.

Endogenous GnRH is a small hypothalamic hormone, composed of 10 amino acids, that controls the secretion of LH and FSH by the gonadotropic cells in the anterior pituitary gland.

Table 82.1 Hormonal therapy for prostate cancer

Orchidectomy
GnRH agonists: leuprolide, goserelin
GnRH antagonists: abarelix
Anti-androgens: flutamide, bicalutamide

Continuous stimulation of the pituitary with high concentrations of GnRH agonists appears to induce downregulation of GnRH receptors. This results in receptor desensitization and inhibition of LH release, which in turn inhibits the production of testosterone by the testes within 3 weeks. In normal prostate tissue and prostatic tumors, GnRH-like peptides and GnRH receptors have been identified indicating that GnRH agonists also have a direct effect at the level of the tumor.

Leuprolide and goserelin are two commonly used GnRH agonists and are administered in the form of 1-, 3-, and 6-month depot injections. It is well recognized that GnRH agonists cause an initial stimulation of LH release, with a corresponding increase in serum testosterone lasting 10 to 20 days. This may stimulate prostate cancer growth with a worsening of related symptoms, which is known as the "flare" phenomenon. In order to prevent this, administration of an anti-androgen is recommended before and during the first few weeks of GnRH agonist therapy to block the effects of this testosterone surge on peripheral androgen receptors.

GnRH receptor antagonists have recently been developed for androgen deprivation. These compounds, such as abarelix, have the advantage that they act as competitive inhibitors of the GnRH receptor without any agonist activity and so produce a rapid decline in serum LH, FSH and testosterone without the initial flare phenomenon. Recent clinical studies have demonstrated that abarelix monotherapy achieves medical castration and a reduction of serum prostate-specific antigen (PSA) levels to the same extent achieved by GnRH agonists. However, they have a 3.7% incidence of anaphylaxis and long-term follow-up studies are necessary to determine whether GnRH antagonists can be routinely used for advanced prostate cancer.

Maximum androgen blockade

The adrenal glands secrete inactive androgen precursors that are converted into active androgens in peripheral tissues as well as in the prostate. Thus, men who undergo ADT still have relatively high levels of adrenal androgens, which could have a stimulatory effect on the tumor. The basis of maximum androgen blockade (MAB) is to neutralize both testicular and adrenal sources of androgens. MAB consists of GnRH agonist combined with a non-steroidal anti-androgen such as flutamide or bicalutamide. Anti-androgen compounds competitively inhibit binding of testosterone or its metabolite, dihydrotestosterone, to the AR in the target cell, which ultimately prevents the activation of AR pathways in those cells.

A debate exists on the use of MAB as first-line therapy in patients with non-organ confined disease; randomized controlled trials have shown a survival advantage of around 7 months with combination treatment [10, 11] and a meta-analysis which looked at 5-year survival rates found a small but significant benefit for combined androgen blockade [12]. As the median survival of these patients is only 3 years it would have been more helpful if overall survival had been used as a primary end point in these studies. Therefore, MAB appears the most effective treatment for patients with advanced prostate cancer.

Side effects of androgen deprivation therapy

The most common adverse events of medical or surgical castration include loss of libido, erectile dysfunction, and hot flushes. Other adverse events, such as fatigue, anemia, and loss of cognitive function, can also have a profound negative impact on quality of life. In addition, ADT has been associated with an increased risk of cardiovascular disease and osteoporosis. Accordingly, the risk of osteoporotic fractures is increased in men undergoing ADT. Both prevalence of osteoporosis and relative risk of hip fracture increase according to the length of androgen suppression. Bisphosphonates have been shown to prevent bone loss and increase bone mineral density in men treated with ADT but they have a limited effect in the relief of pain secondary to bone metastases and in preventing bone metastasis in prostate cancer. The beneficial effect of bisphosphonates on preventing bone loss has been demonstrated using an annual 4 mg infusion of zoledronic acid in postmenopausal women [13] but this approach has yet to be verified in prostate cancer patients.

Intermittent androgen deprivation

The proliferation of androgen-independent cancer cells limits the long-term efficacy of ADT. Data indicate that androgen-independent progression may begin early after the start of hormonal treatment, coinciding with the cessation of androgen-induced differentiation of stem cells. It is possible that if ADT were stopped prior to the development of androgen-independent cells, any subsequent tumor growth would be due to the proliferation of androgen-dependent stem cells, which would be susceptible once again to androgen withdrawal.

Serial determinations of serum PSA levels make intermittent androgen deprivation possible since it provides an easy method for early detection of tumor growth during periods of no treatment. There are several potential advantages to this approach. Libido and potency could be recovered during off-treatment periods, and also other long-term side effects like osteoporosis, muscle atrophy and depression may be avoided. In addition, intermittent ADT might improve outcome by delaying the development of hormonal resistance, although this is merely speculative. A number of Phase II single institution studies have been undertaken to establish the feasibility of this approach and many have demonstrated beneficial effects in terms of quality of life and morbidity reduction. Given the heterogeneity of patients and the differences in second-line treatments used in these studies, there is to date little meaningful survival data regarding this approach. Three multicenter randomized Phase III studies are currently ongoing in order

Table 82.2 Secondary hormonal manipulations for prostate cancer

Anti-androgen withdrawal
Adrenal androgen synthesis inhibition: hydrocortisone, prednisolone,
  dexamethasone

Table 82.3 Systemic therapy for hormone-refractory prostate cancer

Chemotherapy: mitroxantrone, docetaxel
Novel agents under investigation
Chemotherapy: ixabepilone, satraplatin
Targeted molecular agents: cetuximab, trastuzamab, gefitimib, imatinib, RAD-001

confirm the efficacy and survival impact of intermittent androgen deprivation.

Secondary hormonal manipulations

Patients who fail initial ADT despite castrate testosterone levels and demonstrate evidence of disease progression, such as increasing PSA levels, progressive disease on imaging studies and progression of symptoms, may be treated with secondary hormonal therapy.

Anti-androgen withdrawal

The anti-androgen withdrawal response was first recognized in 1993 when Kelly and Scher observed a PSA decline in men receiving MAB when flutamide was discontinued at the time of disease progression [4]. Although the mechanism of anti-androgen withdrawal is unclear, androgen receptor mutations, such as the point mutation at codon 877 in LNCaP cells, and AR co-regulatory factor involvement may be responsible. These data indicate a trial of anti-androgen withdrawal before evaluating other therapeutic agents. Around one-third of patients will respond to this approach, with a decrease in PSA lasting 4–6 months.

Adrenal androgen synthesis inhibition

Drugs that inhibit adrenal steroidogenesis can induce clinical responses in some patients. Inhibitors of adrenal steroidogenesis include aminoglutethimide, ketoconazole, and corticosteroids. Corticosteroids inhibit secretion of adrenocorticotropic hormone through a negative feedback loop, thereby decreasing androgen production in the adrenal glands. Hydrocortisone, prednisone and dexamethasone have all produced clinical responses. Aminoglutethimide plus hydrocortisone provided a partial response rate of 9% but with accompanying fatigue, nausea, skin rash, orthostatic hypotension, and ataxia. The effects of aminoglutethimide have subsequently been found to be transient due to its catabolism secondary to liver enzyme induction; the steroid component is therefore primarily responsible for the efficacy of this approach. Studies using ketoconazole in combination with replacement hydrocortisone have reported response rates ranging from 15% to 63%. Toxicities include nausea, diarrhea, fatigue, and skin changes that require stopping the drug.

Role of continued androgen suppression

Most data support the maintenance of castrate testosterone levels in the androgen-independent patient up to the time that death appears imminent. A retrospective analysis of 341 patients has been reported, with 287 continuing ADT while 54 did not. Patients

who continued ADT achieved a 2-month extension of median survival. In contrast, the Southwest Oncology Group (SWOG) report of 205 patients, of whom 172 continued ADT while 33 did not, revealed no differences in survival between the groups. Although inconclusive, these data suggest a benefit for continued androgen suppression.

Systemic chemotherapy for hormone-refractory prostate cancer

Median survival for patients with HRPC ranges from 7 to 16 months. Until recently, the role of chemotherapy was limited to palliation; however, results of recent clinical trials have renewed the enthusiasm for developing effective chemotherapy treatments for this disease.

Mitoxantrone

Mitoxantrone is an anthracycline that has been extensively evaluated in HRPC. Several randomized studies have shown that mitoxantrone plus corticosteroids confers a palliative benefit including reduced pain, improved quality of life, and decreased need for analgesia but without any survival improvement.

A Phase III study randomized hormone-refractory patients with pain to receive mitoxantrone plus prednisone (MP) or prednisone alone [14]. Palliative response was observed in 29% of patients who received MP, and in 12% who received prednisone alone ($p = 0.01$). The duration of palliation was longer in patients who received MP (46 vs. 18 weeks, $p < 0.0001$) with no difference in overall survival. Similarly, the Cancer and Leukemia Group B randomized patients with HRPC to receive mitoxantrone plus hydrocortisone or hydrocortisone alone [15]. Again, the combination yielded no improvement in median survival.

Docetaxel

Docetaxel-based chemotherapy has been evaluated in two randomized Phase III trials that demonstrated an improvement in survival for the docetaxel arms.

The TAX 327 study compared two schedules of docetaxel with mitoxantrone in a large randomized trial with 1006 patients [16]. HRPC patients were randomized to docetaxel 3-weekly, docetaxel weekly, or mitoxantrone. A survival benefit was shown for docetaxel every 3 weeks relative to mitoxantrone (18.9 vs. 16.5 months, $p = 0.009$), but not for the weekly docetaxel group (17.4 months, $p = 0.36$). More patients in the 3-weekly docetaxel arm experienced a reduction in pain compared with mitoxantrone (35% vs. 22%, $p = 0.01$). Patients in each docetaxel arm (22% for 3-weekly and

23% for weekly) had a significant improvement in quality of life compared with mitoxantrone (13%). Hematological toxicity occurred more commonly in patients treated with the 3-weekly docetaxel.

The SWOG-9916 trial also demonstrated a superior median survival for docetaxel and estramustine compared with mitoxantrone and prednisone (17.5 vs. 15.6 months, $p = 0.02$). Greater gastrointestinal, cardiovascular and hematological toxicity was observed in the docetaxel-estramustine arm [17].

Both trials reported significant improvements in overall survival, time to disease progression, pain control, and PSA response with docetaxel-based chemotherapy. Given the toxicities of estramustine, it is reasonable to conclude that treatment with docetaxel plus prednisone is the preferred regimen for the first-line treatment of HRPC.

Novel prostate cancer treatments

As we understand more about the molecular biology of prostate cancer, the development of targeted therapies with improved efficacy and minimal toxicity has become more of a reality. There is also considerable interest in combining these biological agents with cytotoxic chemotherapy.

Chemotherapy agents

A novel group of microtubule inhibitors know as the epothilones have shown activity at a cellular level in taxane-resistant tumors. A Phase II study comparing ixabepilone, an epothilone-B analog, with or without estramustine in patients with chemotherapy-naïve HRPC, demonstrated PSA responses of 48% in the ixabepilone arm and 69% in the combination arm. As a result of this study a Phase III study is under way comparing ixabepilone with mitoxantrone. A novel platinum compound, satraplatin, has also been evaluated in patients with HRPC [18]. A Phase III study comparing satraplatin and prednisolone with prednisolone alone demonstrated better progression-free survival (5.2 vs. 2.5 months) and PSA response (33.3% vs. 8.7%) in the combination arm.

Targeted molecular agents that affect the AR signaling pathway

Along with anti-androgen treatment, a number of strategies targeting the AR itself are being developed such as double stranded RNA interference, microinjection of anti-AR antibodies, and anti-sense oligonucleotides. Agents targeting the hsp 90 chaperone protein, such as ansamycin antibiotics, are also under evaluation [6]. By targeting hsp 90, these antibiotics induce the degradation of the AR and affect other hsp client proteins such as HER2 and Akt which are expressed more frequently in hormone-resistant as opposed to hormone-naïve tumors.

Targeted molecular agents that affect other pathways

A number of inhibitors of the HER kinase signaling axis have been evaluated as single agents in patients with HRPC, such as cetux-imab, a monoclonal antibody directed against EGF receptor, and trastuzumab, a monoclonal antibody directed against HER2. Other small molecule inhibitors of receptor TK such as gefitinib and imatinib have also been evaluated [6]. Unfortunately as single agents they have shown limited activity (although it should be noted that the patients in these studies were not selected on the basis of their receptor status) and they may still have a role in combination with docetaxel or other chemotherapy agents. In addition to this, preclinical models have indicated that PTEN-deficient tumors do not require HER-kinase signaling for growth or survival. Up to 80% of prostate cancers have reduced levels of PTEN; an alternative strategy, therefore, is to sensitize the tumor cells to EGFR inhibitors by inhibition of PI3K and so make the cell dependent on the normal default pathway. The combination of gefitinib and the PI3K inhibitor RAD-001 is currently under evaluation. Studies comparing docetaxel in combination with molecular targets such as imatinib (InterSPORE prostate cancer trial) and bevacizumab (CALGB 11570) are also underway.

Other drugs which may show promise in combination with taxane chemotherapy include: atrasentan (an endothelin receptor antagonist), G3139 (a *bcl-2* anti-sense inhibitor) and vaccine immunotherapy.

Conclusion

ADT is the most widely used systemic treatment for prostate cancer. Once patients develop hormone-resistant disease treatment options are limited. Docetaxel-based chemotherapy is now the new standard of care for these patients. Advances in the treatment of prostate cancer will depend on a better understanding of molecular pathways leading to androgen-independent cellular proliferation. In the future the combination of targeted therapies with chemotherapy agents may improve the outlook for these patients.

References

1. Gelmann EP. Molecular biology of the androgen receptor. *J. Clin. Oncol.* 2002;20:3001–3015.
2. Taplin ME, Balk SP. Androgen receptor: a key molecule in the progression of prostate cancer to hormone independence. *J. Cell. Biochem.* 2004;91:483–490.
3. Tilley WD, Buchanan G, Hickey TE, et al. Mutations in the androgen receptor gene are associated with progression of human prostate cancer to androgen independence. *Clin. Cancer Res.* 1996;2:277–285.
4. Kelly WK, Scher HI. Prostate specific antigen decline after anti-androgen withdrawal: the flutamide withdrawal syndrome. *J. Urol.* 1993;149:607–609.
5. Koivisto P, Kononen J, Palmberg C, et al. Androgen receptor gene amplification: a possible molecular mechanism for androgen deprivation therapy failure in prostate cancer. *Cancer Res.* 1997;57:314–319.
6. Scher HI, Sawyers CL. Biology of progressive, castration-resistant prostate cancer: directed therapies targeting the androgen-receptor signaling axis. *J. Clin. Oncol.* 2005;23:8253–8261.

7. Edwards J, Bartlett JM. The androgen receptor and signal-transduction pathways in hormone-refractory prostate cancer. Part 2: Androgen-receptor cofactors and bypass pathways. *BJU Int.* 2005;95:1327–1335.

8. Foley R, Hollywood D, Lawler M. Molecular pathology of prostate cancer: the key to identifying new biomarkers of disease. *Endocr. Relat. Cancer* 2004;11:477–488.

9. Rau KM, Kang HY, Cha TL, et al. The mechanisms and managements of hormone-therapy resistance in breast and prostate cancers. *Endocr. Relat. Cancer* 2005;12:511–532.

10. Crawford ED, Eisenberger MA, McLeod DG, et al. A controlled trial of leuprolide with and without flutamide in prostatic carcinoma. *N. Engl. J. Med.* 1989;321:419–424.

11. Eisenberger MA, Blumenstein BA, Crawford ED, et al. Bilateral orchiectomy with or without flutamide for metastatic prostate cancer. *N. Engl. J. Med.* 1998;339:1036–1042.

12. Prostate Cancer Trialists' Collaborative Group. Maximum androgen blockade in advanced prostate cancer: an overview of the randomised trials. *Lancet* 2000;355:1491–1498.

13. Reid IR, Brown JP, Burckhardt P, et al. Intravenous zoledronic acid in postmenopausal women with low bone mineral density. *N. Engl. J. Med.* 2002;346:653–661.

14. Tannock IF, Osoba D, Stockler MR, et al. Chemotherapy with mitoxantrone plus prednisone or prednisone alone for symptomatic hormone-resistant prostate cancer: a Canadian randomized trial with palliative end points. *J. Clin. Oncol.* 1996;14:1756–1764.

15. Kantoff PW, Halabi S, Conaway M, et al. Hydrocortisone with or without mitoxantrone in men with hormone-refractory prostate cancer: results of the cancer and leukemia group B 9182 study. *J. Clin. Oncol.* 1999;17:2506–2513.

16. Tannock IF, de Wit R, Berry WR, et al. Docetaxel plus prednisone or mitoxantrone plus prednisone for advanced prostate cancer. *N. Engl. J. Med.* 2004;351:1502–1512.

17. Petrylak DP, Tangen CM, Hussain MH, et al. Docetaxel and estramustine compared with mitoxantrone and prednisone for advanced refractory prostate cancer. *N. Engl. J. Med.* 2004;351:1513–1520.

18. Sonpavde G, Hutson TE, Berry WR. Hormone refractory prostate cancer: Management and advances. *Cancer Treat. Rev.* 2006;32:90–100.

83 Endocrine Therapy in Breast Cancer Management

Andrew M. Wardley

Key points

- Estrogen is pivotal in the pathogenesis of breast cancer.
- Targeting the estrogen is pivotal to the management of estrogen receptor-positive breast cancer and has resulted in significant improvement in disease-free survival and overall survival for patients with this type of breast cancer.
- Aromatase inhibitors represent an important advance in the treatment of post-menopausal women with steroid hormone receptor-positive breast cancer.
- Better understanding of molecular changes in breast cancer is required to improve endocrine treatment in the future.

Introduction

Routine application of adjuvant systemic therapy has been one of the major factors contributing to improvements in breast cancer outcomes in recent decades, significantly prolonging disease-free and overall survival in women with early-stage breast cancer (EBC); for instance in the UK, deaths from breast cancer have declined by 20–30% since the early 1980s, despite an increasing incidence of more than 25% to more than 43 500 [1]. Endocrine therapy targets the estrogen receptor. As understanding of the biology of breast cancer (BC) improves through molecular classification [2] better understanding and choice of treatments will become possible [3].

Historically there was a tendency for premenopausal women to receive chemotherapy and post-menopausal women to receive tamoxifen. The importance of endocrine therapy in steroid hormone receptor-positive breast cancer (SHR+BC) is emphasized by an analysis of 3700 pre-menopausal women treated with CMF (cyclophosphamide, methotrexate, 5-fluorouracil) chemotherapy in trials conducted by the International Breast Cancer Study Group (IBCSG). Paradoxically, in very young women (<35 years) the prognosis after CMF was worse for those that had estrogen receptor positive (ER+) BC than those in whom the BC was estrogen receptor negative (ER−) [4]. In older premenopausal women disease-free survival (DFS) was similar for ER+ and ER−. This further emphasizes the peril of omitting adequate endocrine therapy in patients with SHR+BC.

Ovarian ablation/ovarian function suppression improves DFS and overall survival (OS) in premenopausal women with SHR+ BC. Chemotherapy-induced amenorrhea by adjuvant cytotoxic chemotherapy is associated with a better outcome in SHR+BC [5]. Several trials have shown that hormone therapy with gonadotropin-releasing hormone (GnRH) analogs ± tamoxifen has similar efficacy to CMF chemotherapy alone [6–8]. These provocative trials indicate some issues with trials that recruit slowly: the control arm omits tamoxifen at the time of design but this is no longer the case in current practice; the chemotherapy regimen has been superseded.

The addition of tamoxifen to CAF (cyclophosphamide, doxorubicin, 5-fluorouracil) chemotherapy and goserelin (CAF-ZT) resulted in significant improvement in DFS compared to CAF alone of CAF with goserelin (CAF-T) in a randomized trial of CAF alone, CAF-Z, and CAF-ZT in premenopausal women with node-positive, receptor-positive BC [9]. This trial and the IBCSG VIII trial in node-negative pre-menopausal women suggest an advantage for goserelin in addition to chemotherapy in women less than 40 years of age at diagnosis with SHR+BC [10]. These patients are less likely to have chemotherapy-induced menopause.

Endocrine therapy

For nearly 30 years tamoxifen was the gold standard for hormone therapy in SHR+BC. The routine use of adjuvant tamoxifen was largely a result of the Early Breast Cancer Trialists' Collaborative Group (EBCTCG) and support for the use of tamoxifen was established a decade earlier than for chemotherapy [11]. The most recent EBCTCG analysis shows that 5 years of tamoxifen reduces

Clinical Endocrine Oncology, 2nd edition. Edited by Ian D. Hay and John A.H. Wass. © 2008 Blackwell Publishing. ISBN 978-1-4051-4584-8.

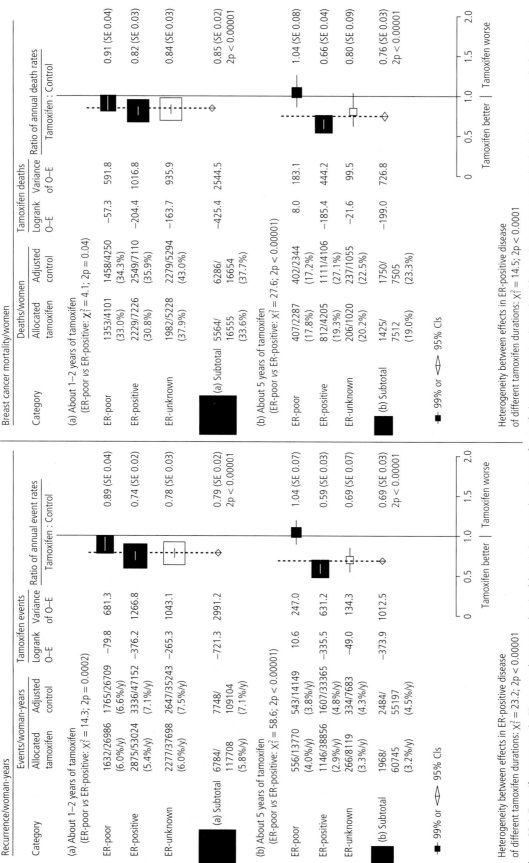

Figure 83.1 Tamoxifen versus not, by ER status and treatment duration (about 1–2 years or about 5 years of tamoxifen): event rate ratios. (Reproduced from Early Breast Cancer Trialists' Collaborative Group [12], with permission from Elsevier.)

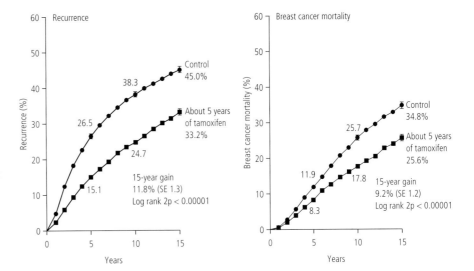

Figure 83.2 About 5 years of tamoxifen versus not in ER-positive (or ER-unknown) disease: 15-year probabilities of recurrence and of BC mortality. (10 386 women: 20% ER-unknown, 30% node-positive. Error bars are ±1SE.) (Reproduced from Early Breast Cancer Trialists' Collaborative Group [12], with permission from Elsevier.)

the risk of BC recurrence by 41% (recurrence rate ratio 0.59 [SE 0.03]) and the risk of death from BC by one-third (death rate ratio 0.66 [0.04]: see Fig. 83.1). Despite these benefits a substantial number of women relapse with and die from BC, and tamoxifen treatment is associated with rare but serious toxicities, including endometrial cancer and thromboembolism [12].

The majority of the difference in recurrence occurs in the first 5 years and this leads to an increasing benefit in survival in the decade after the 5 years of tamoxifen treatment, indicating a common truism of adjuvant treatment that reducing (potentially eradicating) undetectable BC prolongs survival (see Fig. 83.2).

Tamoxifen, because of its mode of action, has partial agonist activity, accounting for some of its known side effects, including stimulation of endometrium causing vaginal bleeding and endometrial cancer. Tamoxifen also increases the risk of venous thromboembolic events.

Tamoxifen increases the risk of endometrial carcinoma by about 2.5 times. The annual rate of endometrial carcinoma was 2.3 per 1000 in the tamoxifen arm compared to 0.91 per 1000 in the placebo control arm of the P-1 prevention trial, leading to a 5-year cumulative incidence of 5.4 per 1000 women and 13.0 per 1000 women. The ER-agonist activity of tamoxifen has potentially beneficial effects, particularly in the skeleton where it reduces bone resorption and reduces the rate of osteoporotic fractures by about 19% (4.29 vs. 5.28 per 1000 women annual rate: hazard ratio [HR] 0.81; 95% confidence interval [CI] 0.63–1.05), with a particularly pronounced effect on the important and potentially fatal hip fracture rate, reducing this by 45% (HR 0.55; 95% CI 0.25–1.15) [13]. Because tamoxifen delays or prevents BC recurrence, tamoxifen-treated patients have a greater chance of death before recurrence (61 000 woman-years vs. 55 000 woman-years) [12]. Correcting for this reveals a non-significant excess of only about seven non-BC deaths, which can be accounted for by the small excesses of deaths from thromboembolic disease and from uterine cancer, both non-significant.

Aromatase inhibitors result in better efficacy lower side-effects than tamoxifen

In postmenopausal women aromatase inhibitors (AIs) represent an improvement on 5 years adjuvant tamoxifen and have changed the standard of care. Aromatase inhibitors block the conversion of androgens to estrogens in postmenopausal women and reduce estrogen levels in tissue and plasma [14, 15]. Third-generation AIs include the non-steroidal inhibitors letrozole and anastrozole, and the steroidal inactivator exemestane. With daily oral administration, anastrozole and exemestane inhibit aromatase activity *in vivo* by 97–98%, and letrozole inhibits aromatase by more than 99% [16–19].

Several very large randomized controlled trials comparing AIs to tamoxifen for 5 years have been published, the two most relevant strategies for newly diagnosed patients being immediate treatment with an AI or switching to an AI after 2–3 years of tamoxifen.

Two trials involving 13 226 (5216 and 8010) patients with SHR+BC indicate that the immediate use of an AI improves DFS by 17–19% for patients with SHR+BC. The Arimidex, Tamoxifen, Alone or in Combination (ATAC) trial (Table 83.1), a double-blind randomized trial, compared 5 years of the AI anastrozole alone with tamoxifen alone, or the combination, as adjuvant therapy in 9366 postmenopausal women with localized BC. The combination treatment arm was closed because of low efficacy [20]. At a median follow-up of 68 months anastrozole improved DFS by 17% (HR 0.83; 95% CI 0.73–0.94; p = 0.005) and time-to-recurrence (TTR) by 26% (HR 0.74; 95% CI 0.64–0.87; p = 0.0002) in patients with SHR+BC [21]. This represents a 67% risk reduction for TTR compared to no hormone therapy (26% over tamoxifen + 41% risk reduction previously shown for 5 years of tamoxifen versus placebo) [12, 21].

Results of the comparison of immediate letrozole vs. immediate tamoxifen as adjuvant treatment for SHR+BC from the Breast International Group (BIG) Trial 1-98 with a median follow-up of

Table 83.1 Pre-specified toxicity of anastrozole compared to tamoxifen from ATAC trial

	Number of patients (%)		Odds ratio, anastrozole vs. tamoxifen (95% CI)	p
	Anastrozole (*n* = 3092)	Tamoxifen (*n* = 3094)		
Hot flushes	1104 (35.7%)	1264 (40.9%)	0.80 (0.73−0.89)	<0.0001
Nausea and vomiting	393 (12.7%)	384 (12.4%)	1.03 (0.88−1.19)	0.7
Fatigue/tiredness	575 (18.6%)	544 (17.6%)	1.07 (0.94−1.22)	0.3
Mood disturbances	597 (19.3%)	554 (17.9%)	1.10 (0.97−1.25)	0.2
Arthralgia	1100 (35.6%)	911 (29.4%)	1.32 (1.19−1.47)	<0.0001*
Vaginal bleeding	167 (5.4%)	317 (10.2%)	0.50 (0.41−0.61)	<0.0001
Vaginal discharge	109 (3.5%)	408 (13.2%)	0.24 (0.19−0.30)	<0.0001
Endometrial cancer†	5 (0.2%)	17 (0.8%)	0.29 (0.11−0.80)	0.02
Fractures‡	340 (11.0%)	237 (7.7%)	1.49 (1.25−1.77)	<0.0001*
Hip	37 (1.2%)	31 (1.0%)	1.20 (0.74−1.93)	0.5
Spine	45 (1.5%)	27 (0.9%)	1.68 (1.04−2.71)	0.03*
Wrist/Colles	72 (2.3%)	63 (2.0%)	1.15 (0.81−1.61)	0.4
All other sites$	220 (7.1%)	142 (4.6%)	1.59 (1.28−1.98)	<0.0001*
Ischemic cardiovascular disease	127 (4.1%)	104 (3.4%)	1.23 (0.95−1.60)	0.1
Ischemic cerebrovascular events	62 (2.0%)	88 (2.8%)	0.70 (0.50−0.97)	0.03
Venous thromboembolic events	87 (2.8%)	140 (4.5%)	0.61 (0.47−0.80)	0.0004
Deep venous thromboembolic events	48 (1.6%)	74 (2.4%)	0.64 (0.45−0.93)	0.02
Cataracts	182 (5.9%)	213 (6.9%)	0.85 (0.69−1.04)	0.1

*In favor of tamoxifen. †*n* = 2229 for anastrozole, 2236 for tamoxifen, excluding patients with hysterectomy at baseline, recorded at any time. ‡Patients with one or more fractures occurring at any time before recurrence (includes patients no longer receiving treatment). $Patients may have had one or more fractures at different sites. (Reproduced from ATAC Trialist's Group [21], with permission from Elsevier.)

25.8 months showed that patients randomized to letrozole were 19% less likely to suffer invasive cancer recurrence or death than patients receiving tamoxifen (HR 0.81; 95% CI 0.70 to 0.93; *p* = 0.003) [22, 23]. The trial was initiated as a direct comparison of letrozole vs. tamoxifen in March 1998, and amended to a four-arm randomization (5 years tamoxifen (A), 5 years letrozole (B), 2 years tamoxifen followed by 3 years letrozole (C) or 2 years letrozole followed by 3 years tamoxifen (D), each with reciprocal placebo) in September 1999. There was overlap of the two- and four-arm enrolment in different centers with a total of 1835 patients entering the former up to March 2000 and 6193 patients the latter up to May 2003. Events and follow-up occurring more than 30 days after switching treatments are excluded from this analysis. The first presentation was based on analysis after 779 DFS events released by the IDMC to the steering committee. The 3-year and 5-year DFS differences were 1.5% (L 90.5% vs. T 89.0%) and 2.6% (L 84.0% vs. T 81.4%), respectively (see Table 83.2 and Fig. 83.3). These results are very similar to original and mature results of the ATAC trial for anastrozole vs. tamoxifen.

In ATAC absolute differences in recurrence rates increased over time, and beyond 5 years of scheduled treatment, suggesting a carry-over effect for anastrozole similar to that observed for tamoxifen, at least in the short term [12, 21].

The BIG 1–98 trial shows a significant improvement in reducing the number of patients suffering a distant recurrence and therefore destined to die from metastatic breast cancer. This is

Table 83.2 Incidence of efficacy end-point events

Event	Letrozole (*n* = 4003)	Tamoxifen (*n* = 4007)
	Number (percent)	
Primary end-point		
Disease-free survival event*	351 (8.8)	428 (10.7)
Local recurrence	21 (0.5)	37 (0.9)
Contralateral breast cancer	16 (0.4)	27 (0.7)
Regional recurrence	13 (0.3)	12 (0.3)
Distant recurrence	177 (4.4)	232 (5.8)
Soft tissue	11 (0.3)	19 (0.5)
Bone	80 (2.0)	99 (2.5)
Viscera	86 (2.1)	114 (2.8)
Second, non-breast cancer	69 (1.7)	82 (2.0)
Death without prior cancer event	55 (1.4)	38 (0.9)
Secondary end-points		
Death from any cause	166 (4.1)	192 (4.8)
Systemic disease-free survival events (excluding local and contralateral breast events)	323 (8.1)	383 (9.6)

*A disease-free survival event was defined as the first of any of the following events: any breast cancer recurrence; a new, invasive cancer in the contralateral breast; a second, non-breast cancer; or death without a prior cancer event. (Reproduced from The Breast International Group 1–98 Collaborative Group [22], with permission from the Massachusetts Medical Society.)

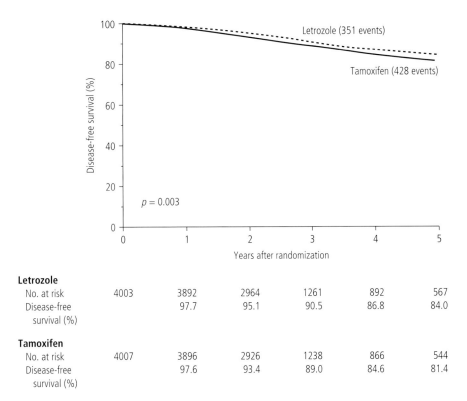

Figure 83.3 Comparison of letrozole and tamoxifen: differences in disease-free survival. Reproduced from The Breast International Group 1-98 Collaborative Group [22], with permission from the Massachusetts Medical Society.

Letrozole						
No. at risk	4003	3892	2964	1261	892	567
Disease-free survival (%)		97.7	95.1	90.5	86.8	84.0
Tamoxifen						
No. at risk	4007	3896	2926	1238	866	544
Disease-free survival (%)		97.6	93.4	89.0	84.6	81.4

supported by a borderline significant improvement in the ATAC trial. In ATAC time-to-distant-recurrence for anastrozole in the subset of SHR+BC patients was improved by 16% (HR 0.84; 95% CI 0.70–1.00; $p = 0.06$), and in BIG1-98 distant DFS (DDFS) events occurred 24% less frequently (HR 0.76, L4.4% vs. T 5.8%; $p = 0.005$) [21, 22].

Both anastrozole and letrozole significantly reduced the cumulative incidence of BC relapse compared with tamoxifen, with the difference becoming evident after 1 year from randomization, and an absolute difference of 1.6% and 2.5% at 3 and 5 years for anastrozole and 1.9% at 3 years and 3.4% at 5 years for letrozole, respectively [21, 22].

The incidence of contralateral BC was substantially reduced by anastrozole compared with tamoxifen (all patients 35 vs. 59, 42% reduction, 95% CI 12–62; $p = 0.01$; hormone receptor-positive patients 53%, 95% CI 25–71; $p = 0.001$) [21]. Early follow-up of BIG1-98 shows a trend to reduction of contralateral invasive BC 0.4% vs. 0.7% of similar magnitude (43% less) [22]. Since tamoxifen shows a 50% reduction in the occurrence of these tumors compared with placebo [12], the findings from the ATAC and BIG1-98 studies suggest that AIs might prevent 70–80% of SHR+BC in women at high risk of BC.

To date there is no difference in OS between upfront AIs and tamoxifen. There was no difference in OS for patients treated with anastrozole or tamoxifen (HR 0.97; 95% CI 0.85–1.12; $p = 0.7$) [21]. In BIG1-98, at 25.8 months' follow-up there were more deaths in the tamoxifen-treated patients than the letrozole-treated patients (L 166 [4.1%] vs. T 192 [4.8%], HR 0.86; $p = 0.176$). Most deaths were due to BC (L 111 [2.8%] vs. T 154 [3.8%], HR 0.86;

$p = 0.176$), but there was a non-significant increase in the cumulative incidence of deaths without prior BC event in the letrozole group (L 55 [1.4%] vs. T 38 [0.9%]; $p = 0.077$) [22]. The significant reductions in recurrence and distant recurrence associated with AIs suggest that a reduction in deaths from BC will eventually be seen.

Other adjuvant trials of AIs of EBC in post-menopausal women have compared switching on to an AI after 2–3 years of tamoxifen to continuation of tamoxifen. Most of the benefit of tamoxifen appeared to be obtained in the first 2 years [24, 25]. Several reasons suggest a benefit of sequential endocrine therapy involving switching from tamoxifen to an AI after 2–3 years. Many patients with BC have a relapse and die within 5 years after the initial diagnosis. Both EBC and MBC patients develop tamoxifen resistance as early as 12–18 months after the initiation. Serious side effects of tamoxifen increase with longer exposure. Since tamoxifen reduces bone resorption in postmenopausal women a combination of tamoxifen and AI may have less impact on long-term skeletal health [26].

Two large datasets have shown approximately 24–40% reduction in risk in patients randomized to an AI after 2–3 years of tamoxifen. In the Intergroup Exemestane Study (IES) postmenopausal women with EBC who were free of disease after 2–3 years were randomized to exemestane (25 mg) or tamoxifen (20 mg) daily to complete a total of 5 years of adjuvant endocrine treatment [27].

The second large dataset is from a prospectively planned analysis of two trials – ABCSG trial 8 and the ARNO 95 trial by the German Adjuvant Breast Cancer Group (GABG). None of the patients in this dataset had received adjuvant chemotherapy [28].

Switching to exemestane improved DFS by 42% (odds ratio (OR) 0.68; 95% CI, 0.56 to 0.82; $p = 0.00005$ by the log-rank test), corresponding to an absolute improvement of 4.7% (95% CI 2.6–6.8) (exemestane 91.5%; 95% CI 90.0–92.7) and tamoxifen 86.8% (95% CI 85.1–88.3) [27]. Recently updated results with 55.7 months median follow-up and 808 DFS events show 25% improvement in DFS (95% CI 0.65–0.87) with an absolute difference at 5 years of 3.5% in the patients with SHR + BC [29]. Similar results were obtained in the combined Austro-German analysis (HR 0.60; 95% CI 0.44–0.81; $p = 0.0009$), corresponding to an absolute event-free survival benefit at 3 years of 3.1% (anastrozole group 95.8% [standard deviation (SD) 0.65]; tamoxifen group 92.7% [SD 0.81]) [28].

Distant metastases were reduced by 34% with exemestane (HR 0.66; 95% CI 0.52 to 0.83; $p = 0.0004$) and by 46% with anastrozole in chemotherapy-naive patients (HR 0.54; 95% CI 0.37–0.80; $p = 0.0016$) [27–29]. Contralateral BC was approximately halved with an AI [27–29].

The most recent data from IES, with median follow-up of 55.7 months, 808 DFS events and 483 deaths, show that the improvement in DFS translated into a borderline significant OS benefit, with a 17% reduction in risk of death (95% CI 0.69–1.0; $p = 0.05$) in the patients with SHR+/unknown BC [29].

What is the role for extending adjuvant hormone therapy?

SHR+BC has a very protracted risk period [30].

The improvement in DFS with 5 years' tamoxifen continues for about a year after cessation – the so-called "carry-over effect" of tamoxifen. Numerically more recurrences and most of the deaths occur in the years 5–15. There is clearly a rationale for treatment after 5 years, particularly in SHR+BC.

The MA.17 trial, a randomized, double-blind, placebo-controlled trial of letrozole (2.5 mg orally daily) after 4.5–6 years of tamoxifen, has shown a significant improvement for patients randomized to letrozole.

The trial results greatly exceeded the prespecified notification boundaries. Letrozole improved 4-year DFS by 42% (OR 0.58; 95% CI 0.45–0.76) from 89.9% in placebo arm to 94.4% in letrozole-treated patients at a median follow-up of 2.5 years [31]. Overall 4-year survival was 95.4% for letrozole and 95.0% for placebo. Pre-planned subgroup analysis showed a significant 39% (HR 0.61; 95% CI 0.38–0.98; $p = 0.04$) improvement in OS in patients who had node-positive BC at the outset (45% of the study population) [31].

Supporting evidence for extended adjuvant AI comes from the small ABCSG 6a trial, which randomized 856 post-menopausal women who had completed adjuvant tamoxifen and/or aminoglutethimide to receive 3 years anastrozole ($n = 387$) or no therapy ($n = 469$). With 60 months follow-up the risk of recurrence was reduced by 36% (HR 0.64; 95% CI 0.41–0.99; $p = 0.047$) for pati-

ents receiving anastrozole (30/387) compared to those receiving nothing (56/486) [32]. Further support for extended adjuvant aromatase inhibitor therapy is provided by the NSABP-B33 trial that randomized postmenopausal patients with clinical stage T1-3 N0-1 M0 breast cancer, who were disease free after 5 years of tamoxifen, to receive exemestane or placebo for 5 years [33]. The results of NCIC MA.17 in October 2003, showing benefit from extended adjuvant letrozole after 5 years of tamoxifen, necessitated closure of accrual, treatment unblinding, and offering exemestane to placebo patients in NSABP-B33. At the time of unblinding, 560 out of 783 patients on exemestane continued exemestane and 344 of the 779 patients allocated to placebo switched to exemestane. Despite the crossover, with median follow-up of 30 months there was a borderline statistically significant improvement in DFS in favor of the exemestane arm (91% vs. 89%, RR = 0.68; $p = 0.07$) and a statistically significant improvement in RFS (96% vs. 94% RR = 0.50; $p = 0.03$) but no difference in OS [33].

Has the optimal duration of hormone treatment been determined?

The optimal duration of hormone therapy is unknown. Tamoxifen was recommended for 5 years based on data showing 5 years to be superior to 2 years. There is, however, no trial to address whether 3–4 years might be adequate/optimal and trials addressing the question of up to 10 years tamoxifen compared to 5 years are ongoing.

There are no data to support continuing tamoxifen as the problem of tamoxifen resistance is more likely to explain failure than discontinuation [34].

Analysis of duration of letrozole therapy in MA.17 suggests that, at least out to about 48 months, longer duration of letrozole treatment is associated with greater benefit in the extended adjuvant therapy setting. After discontinuation of tamoxifen the hazard ratio for recurrence progressively increases for patients randomized to placebo. On the contrary, for patients receiving letrozole the HR is lower at 6 months than the placebo group and reduces over the ensuing 48 months. There is therefore increasing separation of the hazard ratios for DFS and DDFS which progressively decreased over time, favoring letrozole, with the trend being significant ($p < 0.0001$ and $p = 0.0013$, respectively). For the 2360 patients with node-positive status, the HRs for DFS, DDFS and OS all decreased over time with tests for trend all showing significance ($p = 0.0004$, 0.0005 and 0.038, respectively) [35].

The difficult question of how long after adjuvant tamoxifen extended adjuvant letrozole should be considered remains unanswered. When MA.17 was unblinded in October 2003 after the first interim analysis, 1601 of the 2247 women originally assigned to placebo crossed over to letrozole. These women had 69% reduction in BC recurrence and 72% reduction of distant metastases [36]. Overall survival was improved by 47% ($p = 0.05$). This suggests that commencing an AI some time after completion of adjuvant tamoxifen can improve outcomes.

What are the side effects of AIs?

The ATAC trial has the longest follow-up and provides the best data with respect to the effects of long-term treatment with AIs. AIs cause less endometrial cancer, thromboembolic events, ischemic cerebrovascular events, vaginal bleeding, hot flashes, and vaginal discharge than tamoxifen. Vaginal bleeding was halved with AI compared with tamoxifen. The rate increases with time; 3.3% letrozole vs. 6.6% tamoxifen at 25.8 months, 4.5% anastrozole vs. 8.2% tamoxifen at 33.3 months and 5.4% anastrozole vs. 10.2% tamoxifen (OR 0.5; 95% CI 0.41–0.61) at 68 months. Vaginal bleeding on an AI is most likely due to endometrial atrophy [37]. The rate of endometrial carcinoma increases with increasing time on tamoxifen from 0.5% (25.8–33 months) to 0.8% at 68 months. The rate on an AI is 20–40% of that for tamoxifen and does not apparently increase over time (0.2% at 25.8 months, 0.1% at 33 months, 0.2% at 68 months).

In all trials AIs were associated with significantly fewer venous thromboembolic events with these being 40–60% less for immediate AI than tamoxifen and 42–77% less in the switching trials.

The problem for AI is increased bone mineral loss and the attendant increased risk of osteoporosis and fractures. In the ATAC trial there were fracture rates per 1000 woman-years of 22.6 for anastrozole and 15.6 for tamoxifen (HR 1.44; 95% CI 1.21–1.68; $p < 0.0001$) [20, 21]. The bone fracture rates were almost identical for the AIs and tamoxifen in the BIG1-98 trial [22].

Another consideration when prescribing AIs is hypercholesterolemia and cardiac health. This was first demonstrated in BIG1-98, the only study to include regular cholesterol monitoring [22]. Hypercholesterolemia was observed in more patients on letrozole, but was rarely higher than grade 2. More grade 3–5 cardiovascular events were seen in patients on letrozole than tamoxifen. The IES study showed a non-significant increase in myocardial infarction on exemestane 0.9% (0.7% on treatment) compared to tamoxifen 0.4% (0.3% on treatment) ($p = 0.02$ and 0.13 on treatment) [29]). As AIs do not appear to directly affect lipid levels, the difference in serum cholesterol between letrozole- and tamoxifen-treated patients may be due to absence of the beneficial effect of tamoxifen on lipid profile [31, 37, 39]. Further investigation is needed to clarify the role of all AIs and tamoxifen on lipids, coagulation and endothelial cells.

Bone and cardiovascular health need to be considered when prescribing adjuvant endocrine therapy. Patients should routinely have their cholesterol monitored and treated appropriately, as well as bone density checks. One of the spin-offs of these important trials may be a more holistic approach to patient care.

Is there an optimal strategy for introduction of AIs?

There remains uncertainty whether immediate use of an AI for 5 years or a sequential approach combining tamoxifen and AI (AIs) represents the optimal strategy. The results of the sequencing arms of BIG1-98, as well as the TEAM trial, will hopefully answer this issue in due course.

The individual patient's BC risk as well as competing health issues should clearly be considered when prescribing adjuvant endocrine therapy. Patients with greater risk from BC derive more benefit from more active treatments. To this end there was apparently greater benefit for letrozole in patients who had node-positive BC [22].

The optimum timing and duration of therapy for AIs remain uncertain. The role of tamoxifen for 5 years in post-menopausal women is being replaced by incorporation of AIs into the endocrine therapy plan. Immediate or sequential use of AIs is the most difficult decision many face. Identifying a group at highest risk of early relapse may be important in this respect. In view of the long-term risk from SHR+BC there may be an advantage to prolonging treatment plan for many patients whereas for those at risk of early recurrence and with tamoxifen-resistant BC-early introduction of an AI would be beneficial.

The American Society of Clinical Oncology recommends that based on results from multiple large randomized trials, adjuvant therapy for postmenopausal women with hormone receptor-positive BC should include an AI in order to lower the risk of tumor recurrence [39]. It does not make any recommendations with respect to optimal timing or duration of AIs therapy. It suggests that AIs are appropriate as initial treatment for women with contraindications to tamoxifen, and that for all other postmenopausal women, treatment options include 5 years of AIs treatment or sequential therapy consisting of tamoxifen (for either 2–3 years or 5 years) followed by AIs for 2–3 or 5 years. Patients intolerant of AIs should receive tamoxifen. There are no data on the use of tamoxifen after an AI in the adjuvant setting. Women with hormone receptor-negative tumors should not receive adjuvant endocrine therapy. The ASCO agrees that the role of other biomarkers such as progesterone receptor and HER2 status in selecting optimal endocrine therapy remains controversial. Aromatase inhibitors are contraindicated in premenopausal women; there are limited data concerning their role in women with treatment-related amenorrhea. The side effect profiles of tamoxifen and AIs differ. The late consequences of AI therapy, including osteoporosis, are not well characterized. The conclusion of this panel was that optimal adjuvant hormonal therapy for a postmenopausal woman with receptor-positive BC includes an AI as initial therapy or after treatment with tamoxifen. Women with BC and their physicians must weigh the risks and benefits of all therapeutic options.

Recently in the UK the National Institute of Clinical Excellence (NICE) has assessed the effectiveness and cost-effectiveness of AIs [40]. It recommends AIs (anastrozole, exemestane and letrozole) within their licenced indications as options for the adjuvant treatment of early estrogen receptor-positive invasive BC in postmenopausal women. The choice of treatment strategy (that is, primary adjuvant treatment with an AI, switching from tamoxifen to an AI or use of an AI after completion of 5 years of tamoxifen treatment) should be made after discussion between the responsible clinician and the patient about the risks and benefits of the options available. Consideration of the strategy to be adopted should include whether the patient has received tamoxifen as part of their treatment so far, the side effect profiles of the individual drugs and, in particular, the assessed risk of recurrence.

References

1. Toms JE. *CancerStats Monograph*. London: Cancer Research UK, 2004. (http://info.cancerresearchuk.org/cancerstats/types/breast/incidence/)

2. Perou CM, Sorlie T, Eisen MB, et al. Molecular portraits of human breast tumours. *Nature* 2000;406:747–752.

3. Rouzier R, Perou CM, Symmans WF, et al. Breast cancer molecular subtypes respond differently to preoperative chemotherapy. *Clin Cancer Res* 2005;11:5678–5685.

4. Aebi S, Gelber S, Castiglione-Gertsch M, et al. Is chemotherapy alone adequate for young women with oestrogen-receptor-positive breast cancer? *Lancet* 2000;355:1869–1874.

5. Poikonen P, Saarto T, Elomaa I, Joensuu HCB. Prognostic effect of amenorrhoea and elevated serum gonadotropin levels induced by adjuvant chemotherapy in premenopausal node-positive breast cancer patients. *Eur. J. Cancer* 2000;36:43–48.

6. Jakesz R, Hausmaninger H, Kubista E, et al. Randomized adjuvant trial of tamoxifen and goserelin versus cyclophosphamide, methotrexate, and fluorouracil: evidence for the superiority of treatment with endocrine blockade in premenopausal patients with hormone-responsive breast cancer – Austrian Breast and Colorectal Cancer Study Group Trial 5. *J. Clin. Oncol.* 2002;20:4621–4627.

7. Kaufmann M, Jonat W, Blamey R, et al. Survival analyses from the ZEBRA study: goserelin (Zoladex(TM)) versus CMF in premenopausal women with node-positive breast cancer. *Eur. J. Cancer* 2003;39:1711–1717.

8. Baum M, Hackshaw A, Houghton J, et al. Adjuvant goserelin in premenopausal patients with early breast cancer: results from the ZIPP study. *Eur. J. Cancer* 2006;42:895–904.

9. Davidson NE, O'Neill AM, Vukov AM, et al. Chemoendocrine therapy for premenopausal women with axillary lymph node-positive, steroid hormone receptor-positive breast cancer: results From INT 0101 (E5188). *J. Clin. Oncol.* 2005;23:5973–5982.

10. International Breast Cancer Study Group. Adjuvant chemotherapy followed by goserelin versus either modality alone for premenopausal lymph node-negative breast cancer: a randomized trial. *J. Natl Cancer Inst.* 2003:1833–1846.

11. Early Breast Cancer Trialists' Collaborative Group. Effects of adjuvant tamoxifen and of cytotoxic therapy on mortality in early breast cancer. An overview of 61 randomized trials among 28 896 women. Early Breast Cancer Trialists' Collaborative Group. *N. Engl. J. Med.* 1988;319:1681–1692.

12. Early Breast Cancer Trialists' Collaborative Group. Effects of chemotherapy and hormonal therapy for early breast cancer on recurrence and 15-year survival: an overview of the randomised trials. *Lancet* 2005;365:1687–1717.

13. Fisher B, Costantino JP, Wickerham DL, et al. Tamoxifen for the prevention of breast cancer: current status of the National Surgical Adjuvant Breast and Bowel Project P-1 Study. *J. Natl Cancer Inst.* 2005;97:1652–1662.

14. Osborne C. Tamoxifen in the treatment of breast cancer. *N. Engl. J. Med.* 1998;339:1609–1618.

15. Smith IE, Dowsett M. Aromatase inhibitors in breast cancer. *N. Engl. J. Med.* 2003;348:2413–2442.

16. Dowsett M, Jones A, Johnston SR, et al. *In vivo* measurement of aromatase inhibition by letrozole (*CGS 20267*) in postmenopausal patients with breast cancer. *Clin. Cancer Res.* 1995;1:1511–1515.

17. Geisler J, King N, Dowsett M, et al. Influence of anastrozole (Arimidex), a selective nonsteroidal aromatase inhibitor, on *in vivo* aromatisation and plasma oestrogen levels in postmenopausal women with breast cancer. *Br. J. Cancer* 1996;74:1286–1291.

18. Geisler J, King N, Anker G, et al. *In vivo* inhibition of aromatization by exemestane, a novel irreversible aromatase inhibitor, in postmenopausal breast cancer patients. *Clin. Cancer Res.* 1998;4:2089–2093.

19. Lonning PE. Aromatase inhibitors in breast cancer. *Endocr. Relat. Cancer* 2004;11:179–189.

20. ATAC Trialists' Group. Anastrozole alone or in combination with tamoxifen versus tamoxifen alone for adjuvant treatment of postmenopausal women with early breast cancer: first results of the ATAC randomised trial. *Lancet* 2002;359:2131–2139.

21. ATAC Trialists' Group. Results of the ATAC (Arimidex, Tamoxifen, Alone or in Combination) trial after completion of 5 years' adjuvant treatment for breast cancer. *Lancet* 2005;365:60–62.

22. Breast International Group 1-98 Collaborative Group. A comparison of letrozole and tamoxifen in postmenopausal women with early breast cancer. *N. Engl. J. Med.* 2005;353:2747–2757.

23. Thurlimann BJ, Keshaviah A, Mouridsen H, et al. BIG 1-98: randomized double-blind phase III study to evaluate letrozole (L) vs. tamoxifen (T) as adjuvant endocrine therapy for postmenopausal women with receptor-positive breast cancer. *ASCO 2005. J. Clin. Oncol.* 2005;23(16S):511 (Abstract).

24. Current Trials Working Party of the Cancer Research Campaign Breast Cancer Trials Group. Preliminary results from the cancer research campaign trial evaluating tamoxifen duration in women aged fifty years or older with breast cancer. *J. Natl Cancer Inst.* 1996;88:1834–1839. Erratum, *J. Natl Cancer Inst.* 1997;89:590.

25. Swedish Breast Cancer Cooperative Group. Randomized trial of two versus five years of adjuvant tamoxifen for postmenopausal early stage breast cancer. *J. Natl Cancer Inst.* 1996;88:1543–1549.

26. Love RR, Barden HS, Mazess RB, Epstein S, Chappell RJ. Effect of tamoxifen on lumbar spine bone mineral density in postmenopausal women after 5 years. *Arch. Intern. Med.* 1994;154:2585–2588.

27. Coombes RC, Hall E, Gibson LJ, et al. A randomized trial of exemestane after two to three years of tamoxifen therapy in postmenopausal women with primary breast cancer. *N. Engl. J. Med.* 2004;350:1081–1092.

28. Jakesz R, Jonat W, Gnant M, et al. for ABCSG and the GABG. Switching of postmenopausal women with endocrine-responsive early breast cancer to anastrozole after 2 years' adjuvant tamoxifen: combined results of ABCSG trial 8 and ARNO 95 trial. *Lancet* 2005;366:455–462.

29. Coombes RC, Kilburn LS, Snowdon CF, et al. Survival and safety of exemestane versus tamoxifen after 2–3 years' tamoxifen treatment (Intergroup Exemestane Study): a randomised controlled trial. *Lancet* 2007;369:559–570.

30. Saphner T, Tormey DC, Gray R. Annual hazard rates of recurrence for breast cancer after primary therapy. *J. Clin. Oncol.* 1996;14:2738–2746.

31. Goss PE, Ingle JN, Martino S, et al. Randomized trial of letrozole following tamoxifen as extended adjuvant therapy in receptor-positive breast cancer: updated findings from NCIC CTG MA.17. *J. Natl Cancer Inst.* 2005;97:1262–1271.

32. Jakesz RSH, Greil R, Gnant M, et al., on behalf of the ABCSG. Extended adjuvant treatment with anastrozole: results from the Austrian Breast and Colorectal Cancer Study Group Trial 6a (ABCSG–6a). ASCO 2005. *J. Clin. Oncol.* 2005;23:527.

33. Mamounas E, Jeong J-H, Wickerham L, et al. NSABP Benefit from exemestane (EXE) as extended adjuvant therapy after 5 years of tamoxifen (TAM): intent-to-treat analysis of NSABP B-33 SABCS General Session 3, Friday, December 15, 2006, Abstract 49.

34. Clarke R, Leonessa F, Welch J, Skaar T. Cellular and molecular pharmacology of antiestrogen action and resistance. *Pharmacol. Rev.* 2001;53:25–71.

35. Ingle J, Tu D, Pater J, et al. Duration of letrozole treatment and outcomes in the placebo–controlled NCIC CTG MA.17 extended adjuvant therapy trial. *Breast Cancer Res. Treat.* 2006;99:295–300 (Epub 2006 Mar 16).

36. Goss PE, Ingle J, Palmer M, Shepherd L, Tu D. Updated analysis of NCIC CTG MA.17 (letrozole vs. placebo to letrozole vs placebo) post unblinding. *Breast Cancer Res. Treat.* 2005;94:S10.

37. Gerber B, Krause A, Reimer T, et al. Anastrozole versus tamoxifen treatment in postmenopausal women with endocrine-responsive breast cancer and tamoxifen-induced endometrial pathology. *Clin. Cancer Res.* 2006;12:1245–1250.

38. Kumar N, Lyman G. Serum cholesterol reduction with tamoxifen. Breast Cancer Res. Treat. 1990;17:3–7.

39. Chlebowski RT, Col N, Winer EP, et al. American Society of Clinical Oncology Technology Assessment of Pharmacologic Inter-ventions for Breast Cancer Risk Reduction Including Tamoxifen, Raloxifene, and Aromatase Inhibition. *J. Clin. Oncol.* 2002; 20:3328–3343.

40. http://guidance.nice.org.uk/TA112/guidance/pdf/English

84 Female Reproductive Hormone Therapy: Risks and Benefits

Toral Gathani, Jane Green, and Valerie Beral

> **Key points**
> - Use of hormone treatments for contraception and relief of menopausal symptoms is widespread.
> - Users of hormone therapy are at an increased risk of developing breast cancer.
> - The oral contraceptive pill is a safe and effective method of contraception.
> - The evidence available should be used to allow women to make informed choices about their own treatments.

Introduction

The reproductive life of women is marked by menarche at puberty and the menopause in middle age. The use of exogenous hormones in the form of oral contraception in reproductive life and hormone replacement therapy in post-reproductive life is widespread. This chapter provides a brief overview of the evidence about the major risks and benefits associated with the use of these drugs as researched through epidemiological studies.

Hormone replacement therapy

Hormone replacement therapy (HRT) has been available for use for several decades to alleviate the symptoms associated with the menopause that arise as a result of ovarian failure. Initial HRT preparations contained only estrogen as the active ingredient. Evidence in the late 1970s suggested that use of unopposed estrogen in postmenopausal women with an intact uterus led to an increased risk of endometrial hyperplasia and carcinoma. As a result, newer preparations of HRT were developed which contained synthetic progesterone to confer protection to the postmenopausal uterine lining against estrogen. An individual woman's gynecological history has a strong bearing on which type of HRT she will use. Broadly, estrogen-alone is used by women without a uterus following hysterectomy and the combined estrogen–progesterone preparations are used by those with an intact uterus.

Following the introduction of the combined preparations the popularity of HRT rose once again, having fallen in the late

Clinical Endocrine Oncology, 2nd edition. Edited by Ian D. Hay and John A.H. Wass. © 2008 Blackwell Publishing. ISBN 978-1-4051-4584-8.

1970s. The 1980s saw the publication of observational data suggesting that HRT conferred protection to postmenopausal women against adverse cardiovascular outcomes [1]. On the background of this evidence the popularity of HRT grew not only as a treatment for the symptoms of the menopause but also as a secondary preventative measure against future disease such as cardiovascular disease and osteoporosis in postmenopausal women [2].

During the early to mid-1990s doubts had begun to surface in the epidemiological community about the validity of those studies that suggested that HRT conferred apparent protection to postmenopausal women against adverse cardiovascular outcomes. It was suggested that the apparent protective effect seen was due to selection bias and a "healthy user effect," in that hormone replacement therapy was more likely to be prescribed to healthier women [3]. By the mid-1990s one-third of women aged 50–64 in the UK were estimated to be using HRT. Furthermore, estimates suggested that somewhere between 20–30% of women aged 45–64 in developed countries were using HRT and since at that the time the population of women in those age groups was about 100 million women, it was estimated that in the 1990s 20 million women were using HRT [4].

Several large research studies set up in the early 1990s have recently reported results and there has been a substantial rise in the availability of information about the effects of HRT on the risk of major illnesses developing in postmenopausal women. The largest trial and the most influential is the Women's Health Initiative study, a United States-based multicenter randomized controlled trial, which was set up specifically to investigate whether the use of HRT reduced the incidence of coronary heart disease in otherwise healthy women [5]. The Million Women Study is a UK-based multicenter cohort study which was set up to investigate the relationship of HRT use and breast cancer risk [6]. These studies and others have provided valuable information about the effect of HRT use on various aspects of women's health and are discussed in more detail below.

The results of these studies were widely publicized and for the most part, accepted. Indeed, in light of these findings the prescribing guidance for the use of HRT in postmenopausal women was reviewed and subsequently amended by the Food and Drug Administration in the US [7], the Committee for the Safety of Medicines in the UK [8] and the European Union. Since 2002 prescription rates for HRT have fallen substantially, but it is estimated that still about 1 million UK women continue to use HRT [9].

Hormone therapy and treatment of the symptoms of the menopause

The main indication for the use of HRT has been for the relief of menopausal symptoms. The symptoms of the menopause including vasomotor symptoms occur as a result of lack of endogenous estrogen. Hot flushes are the most characteristic manifestation of the menopause. The effect of HRT on vasomotor symptoms has been evaluated by a Cochrane review [10] and the review concludes that the use of oral HRT is highly effective compared to placebo in controlling the vasomotor symptoms of the menopause. The menopause is also associated with loss of libido and other sexual dysfunction. It is obviously very difficult to accurately evaluate the effect of a treatment on these symptoms as studies are reliant on questionnaires as opposed to any objective measurements. Standard HRT preparations have not been demonstrated to improve libido per se; however, in symptomatic women HRT does improve well-being and therefore improves libido indirectly.

Hormone therapy and risk of cancer

There is consistent evidence both from observational studies and from randomized controlled trials that users of HRT are at an increased risk of developing breast cancer and that the risk is greater for users of estrogen–progesterone combined HRT than for users of estrogen-only HRT [11, 12]. Overall the evidence suggests that the risk is increased whilst the women are taking HRT and that the effect wears off quickly once use has ceased. In current users, increasing duration of use increases the risk of developing breast cancer. Furthermore women who have previously been diagnosed with breast cancer are at increased risk of developing the disease again if they use HRT [13].

HRT is also known to decrease the sensitivity and specificity of mammography, thereby increasing the rate of interval cancers detected within a breast cancer screening program [14]. It is unclear as to what the effect of HRT is on the pathology of the cancers that arise on the background of HRT use. Some observational studies, but not all have suggested that breast cancers that arise on the background of HRT were more likely to have characteristics associated with a favorable prognostic outcome. However, the tumors diagnosed in the treatment group of the combined estrogen–progesterone arm of the Women's Health Initiative Trial were on average significantly larger and more likely to have spread beyond the breast than the cancers diagnosed in non-users of HRT [11].

The association of use of HRT and the subsequent development of endometrial hyperplasia and carcinoma was probably the first serious risk identified with HRT use. Combined preparations containing both estrogens and progesterones were referred to as "cyclical" or "sequential" HRT and involve monthly bleeding for most women. The acceptability of HRT increased with the introduction of the "continuous combined" regimens for postmenopausal women as this allowed most women to be free of bleeding. The epidemiological evidence is consistent and shows that whilst estrogens increase the risk of endometrial cancer substantially, progestogens counteract the adverse effect of estrogens on the endometrium [15].

The effect of HRT on the incidence of ovarian cancer in postmenopausal women is less clear. Evidence from observational studies suggests a possible slight increase in the incidence of ovarian cancer associated with use of HRT, and evidence from the Women's Health Initiative trial reported an increased risk of ovarian cancer in the HRT user group but the numbers were small and the result not statistically significant. More information is required before this association can be clarified [16].

With regard to colorectal carcinoma, evidence from both observational studies and randomized trials suggests that use of HRT reduces the incidence of disease. The effect of HRT on other cancers which are generally rarer than the ones already discussed has been little studied.

It is important to bear in mind that the absolute effect of HRT use on cancer risk overall, and the relative effects of estrogen-only and combined preparations, depend not only on the relative risks associated with HRT use for each cancer but also on cancer prevalence. For example, in postmenopausal women breast cancer is far more common than endometrial cancer and so the effects of HRT on BC risk predominate when both cancers are considered together, the risk of both cancers combined being higher for estrogen–progestogen than for estrogen-only HRT despite the protective effect of progestogens on endometrial cancer [15].

Hormone therapy and osteoporosis

Ovarian failure at the menopause results in decreasing levels of circulating estrogens which in turn is associated with accelerated bone loss. Osteoporosis is a known risk factor for fractures. HRT replaces estrogen in postmenopausal women and results in a decreased rate of bone loss. The evidence from both randomized trials and from observational studies shows that current (but not past) use of HRT in postmenopausal women is associated with a substantially decreased incidence of fracture, including hip fracture [17, 18]. The data from observational studies show that most of the commonly used HRT preparations both estrogen-only and combined confer a similar degree of protection against fracture.

Hormone therapy and cardiovascular disease

As previously mentioned, observational data in the 1980s suggested that postmenopausal women who used HRT were at a lower risk of developing cardiovascular disease compared to those women who did not.

Evidence from the recent randomized controlled trials, however, suggests that there is no significant difference in the incidence of coronary heart disease between women taking placebo and those using either estrogen-only HRT or combined estrogen progesterone HRT preparations. With regard to stroke, current users of both of estrogen-alone HRT and estrogen–progesterone combined HRT were at a significantly increased risk of developing a stroke compared to those women who were allocated placebo. The risk of pulmonary embolism is significantly elevated in women who use HRT, with no significant difference observed between the results for estrogen alone preparations and combined estrogen–progesterone HRT [19]. The discrepancy between the results of the trials and those from observational studies is likely to be due to prescribing bias within the observational studies. This is particularly relevant for conditions such as coronary heart disease (CHD), for which risk factors such as hypertension and diabetes are well identified and commonly measured. In contrast, the results from observational studies and randomized trials agree well for conditions such as cancer where prescribing is less likely to be biased by prior disease.

Balance of risk and benefit

To appreciate the impact of use of HRT on disease incidence, it is important to keep in perspective the absolute frequency of these conditions among women in their 50s and 60s. Among women aged 50–59 years, breast cancer is by far the most common and major potentially life-threatening condition with around 12 per 1000 women who are not using HRT expected to develop the condition over a 5-year period. Among the same 1000 women over a 5-year period, around five would be expected to experience incident coronary heart disease and the incidence of stroke, colorectal cancer, pulmonary embolism and hip fracture is each estimated at around 1–3 per 1000. Among women aged 60–69 years not using HRT the incidence of breast cancer and CHD is similar at around 15 and 16.5 per 1000, respectively. The incidence of stroke is around 10–11 per 1000, the incidences of colorectal cancer and hip fracture are each about 7–8 per 1000, and 4 per 1000 would be expected to have a pulmonary embolism (PE).

Robust assessment of the effect of HRT on the risk of major disease is possible for combined HRT preparations using randomized controlled trial data. Among 1000 postmenopausal women aged 50–59 years who have never used HRT an estimated 26.5 women would develop one of the six conditions of interest over a 5-year period (breast cancer, fracture, CHD, PE, colorectal cancer, stroke). If these same women used combined HRT for 5 years, the number diagnosed with these conditions would increase to an estimated 31.9 per 1000 women, resulting from an excess of breast cancer, stroke, CHD and PE of around 7.1 per 1000 women and a deficit of colorectal cancer and hip fracture of around 1.7 per 1000. For 1000 women aged 60–69 years who have never used HRT, an estimated 61.5 women would develop one of the six conditions of interest over a 5-year period. If these women used combined HRT for 5 years, the number diagnosed would increase to 71.5 per 1000 women, resulting from an extra 15.5 cases of breast cancer, CHD, stroke and PE and 5.5 fewer cases of colorectal cancer and hip fracture [20]. Table 84.1 summarizes the risks and benefits of HRT.

Table 84.1 Risks and benefits of hormone replacement therapy

Benefits
Relief of acute symptoms of menopause
Reduced risk of osteoporosis
Reduced risk of colorectal cancer

Risks
Increased risk of breast cancer
Increased risk of endometrial cancer
Increased risk of ovarian cancer
Increased risk of stroke
Increased risk of pulmonary embolism

Summary

There is a role for HRT for the treatment of the acute symptoms of the menopause. The evidence suggests that the use of HRT to prevent secondary disease is not justifiable as the risks outweigh benefit. Current guidelines advise the prescribing of HRT for relief of the acute symptoms of the menopause and in all patients one should prescribe the lowest dose possible and for the shortest period of time and use should be reviewed annually.

Oral contraceptive pill

The combined oral contraceptive pill has been in widespread use since the 1960s. Several generations of the pill have been formulated with each new generation of the pill containing a lower dose of the active ingredients, estrogen and progesterone. In the following discussion combined oral contraceptive pills are referred to as oral contraceptives throughout.

Oral contraceptive pill and risk of cancer

The Collaborative Group on Hormonal Factors in Breast Cancer was formed in 1992 with the aim of bringing together, reanalyzing and publishing the worldwide epidemiological evidence on breast cancer risk in relation to hormonal factors, including hormonal contraceptives. The main findings of the study were that firstly there is a small increase in the risk of having breast cancer diagnosed in women currently using oral contraceptives or who had stopped use in the preceding 10 years and secondly there is no evidence to suggest that an increased risk of breast cancer exists in women who stopped using oral contraceptives more than 10 years previously [21].

It has been hypothesized that the development of ovarian cancer is related to the number of ovulations of a woman's lifetime. The risk of disease increases with increasing number of ovulation cycles. Therefore pregnancy and oral contraceptive use would be associated with a lower risk of developing ovarian cancer. A review and meta-analysis of 20 epidemiological studies published in 1992 confirmed a reduction in the risk of ovarian cancer associated with oral contraceptive use and furthermore that risk decreases with increasing duration of use [21]. The risk reduction of ovarian cancer observed with increasing duration of use has also been confirmed in more recent studies with longer follow-up and the studies also observe a persistent effect of past use [22].

The risk of endometrial cancer is increased by increased exposure to unopposed estrogen. The use of combined oral contraceptives provides protection to the uterine lining, as is the case with combined HRT preparations. Use of combined oral contraceptives has been shown to reduce the risk of developing endometrial carcinoma [23] and there is a persistent effect of past use.

The relationship between oral contraceptive use and cervical cancer is complex. Oral contraceptive use and risk of developing cervical cancer is difficult to study because there is a positive association between oral contraceptive use and the frequency of Pap screening, and furthermore there is also a positive association with oral contraceptive use and the significant sexual risk factors for developing cervical cancer, i.e. exposure to human papilloma virus. A recent systematic review of published evidence, taking these factors into account, found an independent association between use of oral contraceptives and increased risk of cervical cancer; and combined oral contraceptives have been classed as carcinogenic to the cervix by the World Health Organization (WHO) [24, 25].

Oral contraceptives and cardiovascular disease

Since the introduction of the oral contraceptives in the late 1960s, the use of high-dose oral contraceptives was associated with increased rates of acute myocardial infarction, fatal and non-fatal thrombotic and hemorrhagic stroke, venous thromboembolism and elevated systolic blood pressure.

The effect of oral contraceptives on the development of deep vein thrombosis has been evaluated through a WHO-commissioned collaborative study, the results of which were published in 1995. The study suggested that current users of the oral contraceptive pill had a higher odds ratio of developing deep vein thrombosis compared to non-users and furthermore, the risk was highest for women who used combination oral contraceptives containing desogestrel or gestodene [26]. The increased risk of deep vein thrombosis translates to 1–2 additional cases of deep vein thrombosis per 10 000 users per year.

Acute myocardial infarction is rare among young women (<35 years) and is not significantly increased in current users of combined oral contraceptives who do not smoke and who do not have any other cardiac disease risk factors. However, women who are older (>35 years) and who smoke have a substantially increased risk of disease [27].

The findings for stroke are similar to that for the risk of acute myocardial infarction, in that in young users of the oral contraceptive pill, the incidence of stroke is small and is not significantly increased compared with non-users, but for older women who smoke and who have not been assessed for hypertension prior to commencing oral contraceptive use, the risk of stroke is significantly elevated with OC use [26]. Other studies have suggested that the risk of stroke is estrogen dose dependent with higher risks seen in users of higher dose oral contraceptives.

Table 84.2 Risks and benefits of oral contraceptives

Benefits
Effective and reliable contraception
Relief of dysmenorrhea and menorrhagia
Reduced risk of ovarian cancer
Reduced risk of endometrial cancer

Risks
Increased risk of deep vein thrombosis
Increased risk of myocardial infarction and stroke in older (>35 years) women
Increased risk of breast cancer but not persistent

Older generation oral contraceptives containing higher doses of estrogen were associated with an increased risk of hypertension. The modern low-dose oral contraceptives appear to raise blood pressure but not significantly. However, as risk of myocardial infarction is increased in women with higher blood pressure, regular monitoring of blood pressure is advocated in all users of oral contraceptives.

The evidence further suggests that the risk of these adverse cardiovascular effects does not persist after use of combined oral contraceptives is discontinued.

Gynecological benefits of oral contraceptive use

There are several benefits associated with the use of combined oral contraceptives. The most obvious benefit of oral contraceptive use is the prevention of pregnancy. Used correctly, the failure rate is less than 1%. Additional gynecological benefits include control of menorrhagia and hence reduction of the incidence of iron-deficiency anemia. Regular oral contraceptive use is also known to ameliorate dysmenorrhea.

Summary

Use of oral contraceptive pills is associated with adverse side effects including an increased risk of deep vein thrombosis, stroke and, among older women who smoke, myocardial infarction (Table 84.2). Long-term benefits include a reduced risk of developing ovarian cancer. However, the most important benefit is the avoidance of pregnancy using a method that is acceptable and effective. For the majority of women the benefit of avoiding pregnancy with its attendant health risks outweighs the risks of oral contraceptive use.

References

1. Bush TL, Barrett-Connor E. Noncontraceptive estrogen use and cardiovascular disease. *Epidemiol. Rev.* 1985;7:89–104.
2. Grady D, Rubin SM, Petitti DB, et al. Hormone therapy to prevent disease and prolong life in postmenopausal women. *Ann. Intern. Med.* 1992;117:1016–1037.
3. Matthews KA, Kuller LH, Wing RR, Meilahn EN, Plantinga P. Prior to use of estrogen replacement therapy, are users healthier than nonusers? *JAMA* 1996;143:971–978.

4. Beral V, Banks E, Reeves G, Appleby P. Use of HRT and the subsequent risk of cancer. *J. Epidemiol. Biostat.* 1999;4:191–215.

5. Women's Health Initiative Study Group. Design of the Women's Health Initiative clinical trial and observational study. *Control Clinical Trials* 1998;19:61–109.

6. Million Women Study Collaborative Group. The Million Women Study: design and characteristics of the study population. *Breast Cancer Res.* 1999;1:73–80.

7. Food and Drug Administration. Questions and answers for estrogen and estrogen with progestin therapies for postmenopausal women. http://www.fda.gov/cder/drug/infopage/estrogens_progestins/Q&A. htm.

8. Medicines and Healthcare Products Regulatory Agency. Use of hormone replacement therapy in the prevention of osteoporosis: important new information, 2003. Access via: http://medicines. mhra.gov.uk

9. Hersh A, Stefanick M, Stafford R. National use of postmenopausal hormone therapy – annual trends and response to recent evidence. *JAMA* 2004;291:47–53.

10. MacLennon A, Lester S, Moore V. Oral oestrogen replacement therapy versus placebo for hot flushes. Cochrane Databse Systematic Review 1: CD002978, 2001.

11. Chlebowski RT, Hendrix SL, Langer RD. Influence of estrogen plus progestin on breast cancer and mammography in healthy postmenopausal women. The Women's Health Initiative Randomized Trial. *JAMA* 2003;289:3243–3253.

12. Million Women Study Collaborators. Breast cancer and hormone replacement therapy in the Million Women Study. *Lancet* 2003;362: 419–427.

13. Holmberg L, Anderson H. HABITS (hormone replacement therapy after breast cancer – is it safe), a randomised comparison: trial stopped. *Lancet* 2004;363:453–455.

14. Banks E, Reeves G, Beral V, et al. Hormone replacement therapy and false positive recall in the Million Women Study: patterns of use, hormonal constituents and consistency of effect. *Breast Cancer Res.* 2005;8:R8–17.

15. Million Women Study Collaborators. Endometrial cancer and hormone-replacement therapy in the Million Women Study. *Lancet* 2005;365:1543–1551.

16. Anderson GL, Judd HL, Kaunitz AM, et al. Effects of estrogen plus progestin on gynecologic cancers and associated diagnostic procedures: the Women's Health Initiative randomised trial. *JAMA* 2004;291:42.

17. Writing Group for the Women's Health Initiative Investigators. Risks and benefits of estrogen plus progestin in healthy postmen-opausal women. *JAMA* 2002;288:321–333.

18. Banks E, Beral V, Reeves G, Balkwill A, Barnes I. Fracture incidence in relation to the pattern of use of hormone therapy in postmenopausal women. *JAMA* 2004;291:2212–2220.

19. Beral V, Reeves G, Banks E. Current evidence about the effect of hormone replacement therapy on the incidence of major conditions in postmenopausal women. *Br. J. Obstet. Gynaecol.* 2005;112:692–695.

20. Banks E, Reeves G, Evans S. Disease incidence associated with long-term use of HRT. In Critchley H, Gebbie A, Beral V (eds). *Menopause and Hormone Replacement.* London: RCOG Press, 2004:241–254.

21. Collaborative Group on Hormonal Factors in Breast Cancer. Breast cancer and hormonal contraceptives: collaborative reanalysis of individual data on 53239 women with breast cancer and 100239 women without breast cancer from 54 epidemiological studies. *Lancet* 1996; 347:1713–1727.

22. Hankinson SE, Colditz G, Hunter DJ, et al. A quantitative assessment of oral contraceptive use and risk of ovarian cancer. *Obstet. Gynecol.* 1992;80:708–714.

23. Ness RB, Grisso JA, Klapper JJ, et al. Risk of ovarian cancer in relation to estrogen and progestin dose adn use characteristics of oral contraceptives. *Am. J. Epidemiol.* 2000;152:233–241.

24. Henderson BE, Casagrande MC, Pike MC, et al. The epidemiology of endometrial cancer in young women. *Br. J. Cancer* 1983;47:749–756.

25. Cogliano V, Grosse Y, Baan R, et al. Carcinogenicity of combined oestrogen–progestogen contraceptives and menopausal treatment. *Lancet Oncol.* 2005;6(8):552–553.

26. World Health Organization Collaborative Study of Cardiovascular Disease and Steroid Hormone Contraception. Venous thromboembolic disease and combined oral contraceptives: results of international multicentre case–control study. *Lancet* 1995;346:1575–1582.

27. World Health Organization Collaborative Study of Cardiovascular Disease and Steroid Hormone Contraception. Acute myocardial infarction and combined oral contraceptives: results of an international multicentre case–control study. *Lancet* 1997;1997:1202–1209.

Appendix

Reference ranges for results of endocrinological laboratory investigations.

A1
Reference ranges for thyroid function – hormones (collection method: routine serum)

Test	Traditional units	Conversion factor	SI units
TSH	0.4–5.0 mU/L	1	0.4–5.0 mU/L
Total T_4	5–12 mcg/dL	12.9	58–174 nmol/L
Free T_4	0.8–1.8 ng/dL	12.9	10–22 pmol/L
Total T_3	70–220 ng/dL	0.015	1.07–3.18 nmol/L
Free T_3	3.5–6.5 pg/mL	1.54	5–10 pmol/L
Thyroglobulin	<1.2 ng/mL		N/A

A2
Reference ranges for prolactin and gonadotropins (collection method: routine serum)

Test	Traditional units	Conversion factor	SI units
Prolactin	<18 ng/mL	20	<360 mU/L
Women			
FSH			
Follicular	2.5–10 mU/mL	1	2.5–10 µ/L
Mid-cycle	25–70 mU/mL		25–70 µ/L
Luteal	0.3–2.1 mU/mL		0.3–2.1 µ/L
Postmenopausal	>30 mU/mL		>30 µ/L
Prepubertal	<5 mU/mL		<5 µ/L
LH			
Follicular	2.5–10 mU/mL	1	2.5–10 µ/L
Mid-cycle	25–70 mU/mL		25–70 µ/L
Luteal	<1–13 mU/mL		<1–13 µ/L
Postmenopausal	>30 mU/mL		>30 µ/L
Prepubertal	<5 mU/mL		<5 µ/L
Men			
FSH	1–7 mU/mL		1–7 µ/L
LH	1–10 mU/mL		1–10 µ/L

A3
Reference ranges for adrenal and gonadal steroids (collection method: routine serum)

Test	Traditional units	Conversion factor	SI units
0900 cortisol	7–25 ng/dL	27.6	200–700 nmol/L
Supine aldosterone (30 min)	5–14.5 ng/dL	27.7	135–400 pmol/L
Standing aldosterone	12–30 ng/dL	27.7	330–830 pmol/L
DHEAS			
Women	1100–4400 ng/mL	0.0027	3–12 nmol/L
Men	750–3700 ng/mL	0.0027	2–10 nmol/L
Prepubertal	<185 µg/mL		<0.5 µmol/L
Androstenedione	0.9–2.3 Ug/L	3.49	3–8 nmol/L
Prepubertal	<0.3 mcg/L		<1 nmol/L
17-hydroxyprogesterone			
Follicular	0.33 Ug/L	3.3	1–10 nmol/L
Luteal	3–6 Ug/L	3.3	10–20 nmol/L
Neonatal	<24 Ug/L	3.3	<80 nmol/L
Estradiol (women)			
Follicular	55–110 pg/mL	3.6	200–400 pmol/L
Mid-cycle	110–330 pg/mL	3.6	400–1200 pmol/L
Luteal	110–275 pg/mL	3.6	400–1000 pmol/L
Prepubescent	<6 pg/mL	3.6	<20 pmol/L
Postmenopausal	<30 pg/mL	3.6	<100 pmol/L
Estradiol (men)	<50 pg/mL	3.6	<180 pmol/L
Progesterone			
Follicular	<3 ng/mL	3.2	<10 nmol/L
Luteal	>10 ng/mL	3.2	>30 nmol/L
Men	<2 ng/mL		<6 µmol/L
Testosterone			
Men	2.5–10 ng/mL	3.46	9–35 nmol/L (median 18 nmol/L)
Women	0.14–0.87 ng/mL	3.46	0.5–3 nmol/L (median 1.5 nmol/L)
Prepubertal	<0.2 ng/mL		<0.8 nmol/L
Dihydrotestosterone			
Men	0.29–0.76 ng/mL	3.44	1–2.6 nmol/L
Women	0.087–0.27 ng/mL	3.44	0.3–93 nmol/L

A4
Reference ranges for growth hormone and insulin-like growth factor (IGF-1) (collection method: routine serum)

Test	Traditional units (ng/mL)	Conversion factor	SI units (nmol/L)
Basal, fasting	<0.5	2	<1 mU/L
GH during ITT-induced hypoglycaemia	>20		>40 mU/L
IGF-1 (years)			
0–3	7–100		0.9–13.3
4–6	14–175		1.9–23.3
7–9	42–210		6.6–28.0
10–12	50–280		6.7–37.3
13–18	70–420		9.3–56.0
19–29	125–329		16.6–43.8
30–39	120–330		16.0–44.0
40–49	126–369		16.8–49.2
50–59	108–263		14.4–35.0
60–70	108–229		14.4–30.0

A5
Reference ranges for plasma ACTH and catecholamines (collection method: lithium heparin tube cold spun immediately and freeze)

Test	Traditional units	Conversion factor	SI units
0900 ACTH	<80 pg/mL	0.22	<18 pmol/L
Adrenaline	0.01–0.25 ng/mL	5.46	0.03–1.31 nmol/L
Noradrenaline	0.08–0.75 ng/mL	5.99	0.47–4.14 nmol/L

NB: Catecholamine samples: patient lying; collect through venous cannula placed 30 min prior to sampling.

A6
Reference ranges for calcium, parathyroid hormone, vitamin D, and calcitonin

Collection method:
(a) Total calcium, routine serum (correct for serum albumin by adding 0.02 mmol/L for every g/L that albumin falls below 47 g/L.
(b) Parathyroid hormone: serum, cold spun and flash frozen.
(c) Calcitonin: plasma, lithium heparin; cold spun and flash frozen.
(d) Vitamin D: measured as 25 hydroxyvitamin D in serum; cold spun and flash frozen.

Test	Traditional units	Conversion factor	SI units
Total calcium	8.9–10.5 mg/dL	0.25	2.23–2.63 mmol/L
Parathyroid hormone	9–54 ng/L	0.1	0.9–5.4 pmol/L
Vitamin D metabolites	4.40 mg/L		
Calcitonin	<80 pg/L	1	<80 ng/L

A7
Reference ranges for plasma pancreatic and gut hormone profile (collection method; fast overnight, trasylol [200 µL of 500 000 KIU], plasma [lithium heparin], cold spun, flash frozen)

Test	Traditional units	Conversion factor	SI units
Insulin			
Fasting	<16 µU/mL	7.18	<114 µmol/L
During hypoglycaemia (blood glucose <2.2 mmol/L)	<3 µU/mL	7.18	21 µmol/L
Gastrin	<120 pg/mL	0.45	<55 pmol/L
Vasoactive intestinal polypeptide (VIP)	<72 pg/mL	0.42	< 30 pmol/L
Pancreatic polypeptide (PP)	<1260 pg/mL	0.24	<300 pmol/L
Glucagon	<175 pg/mL	0.28	< 50 pmol/L

NB: Vacuum will be lost from vacutainers if opened to add trasylol.

A8
Reference ranges for 24-h urinary catecholamines and 5-hydroxyindoleacetic acid (5-HIAA) [collection method: 24-h urine collection with acid in container (30 ml 6N HCl)]

Test	Traditional units	Conversion factor	SI units
Adrenaline	<10 µg/24 h	5.91	8–144 nmol/24 h (95% confidence limits)
Noradrenaline	<97 µg/24 h	5.46	<570 nmol/24 h (95% confidence limits)
Dopamine	<588 µg/24 h	5.27	<3100 nmol/24 h (95% confidence limits)
Metanephrines	<12 mg/24 h	5.46	<63 µmol/24 h
5-HIAA	<9 mg/24 h	5.24	<75 µmol/24 h

A9
Reference range for 24-h urinary cortisol and calcium (collection method: 24-h urine collection. Normal container [no acid])

Test	Traditional units	Conversion factor	SI units
Cortisol	20–100 µg/24 h	2.76	55–250 nmol/24 h
Calcium	<300 mg/24 h	0.025	<7.5 mmol/24 h

A10

Reference ranges for blood glucose HbA$_{1c}$ and lipids (glucose and HbA$_{1c}$ in plasma [using fluoride], lipids in serum)

Test	Traditional units	Conversion factor	SI units
Fasting glucose (plasma)	60–108 mg/100 mL	0.056	3.3–5.9 mmol/L
HbA$_{1c}$	DCC target	<7%	
Cholesterol	200 mg/100 mL	0.026	<5.2 mmol/L (desirable)
HDL cholesterol	>34.8 mg/100 mL	0.02586	>0.9 mmol/L (desirable)
Triglyceride (fasting)	<250 mg/100 mL	0.0113	<2.83 mmol/L (normal)

LDL cholesterol calculated as
total cholesterol − (HDL chol + triglyceride / 2.2)

<3.4 mmol/L (desirable)

NB: Friedwald's calculation is only valid if Tg rich lipoproteins + VLDL are at average concentration and of predictable composition; not valid if total Tg is beyond 5 mmol/L; fasting serum is of course required.

Common tumor markers

Total B-HCG	0–4 mU/mL
Carcinoid embryonic antigen	0–9 µg/mL
Alpha fetoprotein	0–10 kU/L
Prostate-specific antigen	0–4 ng/mL

Index

Note: page numbers in *italics* represent figures, those in **bold** represent tables.

17-AAG, thyroid tumors **152**
abarelix, prostate cancer 604–5, **605**
aberrant ACTH secretion syndrome *569*, 570
absolute enhancement washout 349
acanthosis nigricans 552–3
ACE inhibitors
    catecholamine assay interference **354**
    MIBG uptake **356**
acetaminophen, catecholamine assay interference **354**
acidophil stem cell adenoma 218
acral keratoses 545
acrokeratosis paraneoplastica of Bazex 553
acromegaly 246–52, 275
    Carney complex *534*
    clinical presentation 246–8, *247, 248*
    confirmation of 248–9, *248, 249*
    definition of cure 249–50
    epidemiology 246
    etiology 249
    medical therapy 250–1
    MEN 1 511
    pituitary function tests 249
    pituitary radiotherapy 251, *251*
    radiological assessment 249, *249*
    radiotherapy 231–2
    somatostatin analog therapy 62–3
    surgery 228
    transsphenoidal surgery 250
    treatment 250, *250*
    treatment aims 249–50
    visual field testing 249
ACTH **6, 92,** 194, 353
    adenomas producing 218–19
    big *see* pro-opiomelanocortin
    drugs lowering 258, *259*
    ectopic secretion *see* ectopic ACTH syndrome
    pituitary carcinoma 274
    reference range **624**
    see also Cushing syndrome
ACTH deficiency, radiation-induced 593
ACTH-dependent Cushing syndrome 342, *342, 343*
ACTH-independent macronodular adrenal
    hyperplasia 342
actinomycin

gestational trophoblastic tumor 433
ovarian germ cell tumor 409
sex cord–stromal tumors 407
activin 7
adamantinomatous craniopharyngioma *209, 283*
Addison disease
    and hypercalcemia **561**
    POMC in *569*
ADH *see* vasopressin
adipocytokines 39
adiponectin 39
adipostatin 16
adrenal androgen synthesis inhibition 606
adrenal cortex 7
    primary pigmented nodular adrenocortical disease
    28
adrenal cyst 350
adrenal glands 13–14, *14*
    18-FDG positron emission tomography 340
    computerized tomography 339, 393
    Conn syndrome *see* Conn syndrome
    Cushing syndrome *see* Cushing syndrome
    magnetic resonance imaging 340
    metastatic tumors 582–3, *583*, **583**
    radiological anatomy 341
    scintigraphy 340
    venous sampling 71–2, *72*, 340
    virilization 344, *344*
adrenal hyperplasia
    ACTH-independent macronodular 342
    bilateral 343, 371, *371*
    congenital 344, *344*
adrenal lesion–spleen ratio 340
adrenal medulla 7
adrenal suppression 393
adrenal tumors
    cortical 392
        adenoma 341, 346–9, *347–9*, **507**
        carcinoma *see* adrenocortical carcinoma
        primary pigmented nodular adrenocortical
            disease 341–2, *342*
        incidentalomas 346–50, 384–9
            causes and prevalence 384–6, *385*, **385**
            clinical aspects 386

computerized tomography 346–9, *347–9*
histological diagnosis *385*
hormonal assessment 386–7
imaging studies 387–8, *387*
magnetic resonance imaging 349, *350*
pathogenesis 386
percutaneous adrenal biopsy 349
surgery 82–3
treatment and follow-up 388–9, *388*
medullary 344–6
    ganglioneuroblastoma 345–6
    hypoadrenalism 346, *346*
    neuroblastoma **28**, 345–6, *346*
    paraganglioma 344–5
    pheochromocytoma 14, 22, **28**, 344–5, *345*,
        352–9
MEN 1 511–12
myelolipoma 350
surgery 82–4, *82*
    metastatic tumors 83–4
    pheochromocytoma 83
    primary hyperaldosteronism 83
virilizing 344
adrenal venous sampling 71–2, *72*
adrenaline *see* epinephrine
adrenocortical carcinoma **28**, 341, *341*
    NIS gene therapy 55
    surgery 83
adrenocorticotropic hormone *see* ACTH
AGES score 132
agouti-related protein 8
aldosterone 7
    reference range **623**
    regulation of secretion 370
aldosteronoma 72, 343, 370–1, *371*
alendronate, hyperparathyroidism 176
alpha fetoprotein 311, **312**
    reference range **625**
alpha-subunit **93**
alpha1-adrenoceptor blockers
    catecholamine assay interference **354**
    MIBG uptake **356**
alpha2-adrenoceptor agonists, catecholamine assay
    interference **354**

amenorrhea 237, 318, 319, **331**
American Society of Clinical Oncology 88
  evidence rankings for tumor markers **90**
amiloride, Conn syndrome 376
amitriptyline **103**
amphetamines, catecholamine assay interference 354
amphiphysin 550
amyloid β precursor protein 182
analgesics **103**
anaplastic ependymoma 298
anaplastic thyroid carcinoma 80, 155–61
  cause of death 156
  diagnosis and histology 156–7
  epidemiology 155–6, *156*
    Arthur G. James Cancer Hospital experience 155–6, *156*
    Ohio State University Experience 155–6, *156*
    worldwide experience 155
  etiology 156
  pathogenesis 127–8, *128*
  presentation 156
  staging and prognostic features 157
  surgery 80
  therapy 157–60, *159*
  tumor characteristics 155–6, *156*
  ultrasound 118
anastrozole
  breast cancer **612**
  precocious puberty 542
androblastoma *see* Sertoli–Leydig cell tumor
androgens 7
  adrenal synthesis inhibition 606
  and breast cancer 35
  intermittent deprivation 605–6
  maximum androgen blockade 605
  and prostate cancer 36–7
  synthesis 601
androgen biosynthesis defect **421**
androgen excess **421**
androgen insensitivity syndrome 424
androgen receptor 601
  activation 604
  co-regulation 603–4
  expression 603
  mutations 602–3, *602*
androgen receptor-independent pathways 604
androgen-secreting tumors 390–5
  adrenocortical tumors 392
  clinical presentation 392
  epidemiology and pathology 390
  granulosa cell tumors 391
  management 394
  ovarian tumors 390
    with functioning stroma 392
  prognosis 394
  sclerosing stromal cell tumors 391
  screening and diagnosis 392–4
    adrenal suppression 393
    endocrine evaluation 393
    imaging 393
    ovarian suppression and stimulation 393
    venous sampling 393–4
  Sertoli–Leydig cell tumors 391
  sex cord tumors with annular tubules 391–2
  sex cord-stromal tumors 390–1, **390**

steroid cell tumors 391
  thecoma 391
androstenedione 7
  breast cancer **34**
  reference range **623**
aneuploidy 362
aneurysm 211
angiofibroma, *MEN1* expression 507
angiogenesis 51, 189–90
angular cheilitis, in glucagonoma 475
ANNA3 550
anorexia–cachexia syndrome 104
anti-androgen withdrawal 606
antiangiogenic agents 503
  gene therapy 51–2
  peripheral neuroblastic tumors 368
antibodies
  encephalomyelitis 550
  heterophile 88, *88*
  insulin 458
  Lambert–Eaton syndrome 550
  limbic encephalitis 550
  monoclonal *see* monoclonal antibodies
  opsoclonus–myoclonus 550
  retinal degeneration 550
  sensorimotor neuronopathy 550
  thyroglobulin **91**, 98–100, *99*
anticortisolic drugs 573
antidiuretic hormone *see* vasopressin
antipsychotics
  catecholamine assay interference 354
  MIBG uptake 356
antithyroid peroxidase 112
appendiceal tumors
  carcinoid 444, 498–501
    clinical features and management 500
    etiopathogenesis 498
    macroscopic appearances 499
    microscopic appearances 499–500, *499, 500*
    relative frequency 499
  neuroendocrine 442
appendix 498
aquaporins 556, 557
arachnoid cyst 289–90, *290*
arcuate nucleus 8
arginine vasopressin 556
arginine-GHRH test 197
aromatase inhibitors 611–14
  introduction of 615–16
  side effects 615
arrhenoblastoma *see* Sertoli–Leydig cell tumor
arteriography 459
aryl hydrocarbon receptor interacting protein gene 192
Aschheim Zondek test 412
aspirin
  catecholamine assay interference 354
  hypercalcemia 565
assay interferences 88, *88*
  catecholamines 354
astrocytoma 210
ataxia 327
ATRX 423
attenuation values 339
autoantibodies 88, *88*
autoantigens, paraneoplastic syndromes 550

AXD6244, thyroid tumors **152**
axitinib, thyroid tumors **152**
azathioprine, sarcoidosis 333

B-Raf 125
Bannayan–Riley–Ruvalcaba syndrome 545, 547
basal corticoid test 195
Beckwith–Wiedemann syndrome 381
beta-adrenoceptor blockers, catecholamine assay interference 354
bevacizumab **503**
  carcinoid syndrome 495–6, **495**
  complications 106, **106**
  peripheral neuroblastic tumors 368
bicalutamide, prostate cancer 604–5, **605**
bilateral adrenal hyperplasia 343, 371, *371*
biliary tumors
  carcinoid 444
  metastatic adenocarcinoma 583
biological agents *see* biotherapy
biopsy
  adrenal 349
  image-guided 70
biotherapy 503
  complications 106, **106**
  see also individual drugs
BIPSS 257–8
Birbeck granules 327
bisphosphonates
  hypercalcemia 564, 565
  hyperparathyroidism 176
  McCune–Albright syndrome 542
  side effects 564
  see also individual drugs
bleomycin
  craniopharyngioma 285
  ovarian germ cell tumor 409
  sex cord-stromal tumors 407
  testicular germ cell tumors 416
blood glucose, reference range **625**
blue nevus 534
bone marrow tumors, metastases 584, 585, 586
bone morphogenetic protein 10
bone scintigraphy 447–8
bortezomib, thyroid tumors **152**
brachytherapy, craniopharyngioma 284–5
BRAF, thyroid cancer 125, *126*, 128
brain stem hemangioblastoma, von Hippel–Lindau disease 523
BRCA1 29
BRCA2 29
breast cancer
  androgens 35
  androstenedione 34
  Cowden syndrome 546
  DHEA-sulfate 34
  estrogens 32–3, *33*, **33**
  hypercalcemia **561**
  metastases 583, 584, 586
  NIS gene therapy 55
  progestins 33–5, *35*
  prolactin 37
  sex steroid associations **34**
  treatment 579
    aromatase inhibitors 611–14, **612**, *613*, 615–16

extension of adjuvant hormone therapy 614
optimal duration of hormone therapy 614
tamoxifen 609–11, *610*, *611*
unopposed estrogen hypothesis 33, **33**
Brenner tumor 390, 401
bridging vascular sign 401
British Thyroid Association 136
bromocriptine
catecholamine assay interference **354**
prolactinoma 241
thyrotropinoma 272
bronchial carcinoids 482–5
clinical presentation 483
diagnosis 483–4
differential diagnoses 484
ectopic ACTH syndrome **567**
epidemiology 482
etiology 482
genetic alterations 483
histopathology 483
immunohistochemistry 483
pathology 482–3
prognosis 484–5
survival **489**
treatment 484, **484**
tumorlets 482
buprenorphine 103

C-cell hyperplasia 517
c-Kit ligand 425
C-peptide 37–8
cabergoline
prolactinoma 241–2
thyrotropinoma 272
café-au-lait spots
Carney complex **534**
Coast of California border 538
Coast of Maine border 538
McCune–Albright syndrome 537–8, **537**, *538*
neurofibromatosis type 1 528
caffeine, catecholamine assay interference **354**
calcimimetics 184
calcitonin 6, 14, **91**, 96–8, *97*, 353
and calcium regulation 562
hypercalcemia 565
reference range **624**
calcitonin escape 11
calcitonin gene-related peptide 353
calcitriol, rickets 542
calcium
reference range **624**
selective arterial injection 458
calcium channel blockers
catecholamine assay interference **354**
MIBG uptake 356
pheochromocytoma 357
Call–Exner bodies 405
cancer predisposition syndrome 42
capecitabine, thyroid tumors **152**
Cappabianca, P. 223
carbamazepine 103
carboplatin
bronchial carcinoids 484, **484**
testicular germ cell tumors 417, **417**
carcinoembryonic antigen 86, **93**, 100, 517

carcinoid crisis 490
carcinoid heart disease 490
carcinoid syndrome 437–8, 488–97
appendiceal 444, 498–501
clinical features and management 500
etiopathogenesis 498
macroscopic appearances 499
microscopic appearances 499–500, *499*, *500*
relative frequency 499
biliary 444
bronchial 482–5
clinical presentation 483
diagnosis 483–4
differential diagnoses 484
epidemiology 482
etiology 482
genetic alterations 483
histopathology 483
immunohistochemistry 483
pathology 482–3
prognosis 484–5
treatment 484, **484**
tumorlets 482
clinical presentation 489–90, *489*
colonic 445, 498–501
clinical features and management 500
etiopathogenesis 498
macroscopic appearances 499
microscopic appearances 499–500, *499*, *500*
relative frequency 499
diagnosis 490–2, *491*
biochemical 490–1
imaging studies 491–2
duodenal 444
epidemiology 488–9, **489**
gastric 444, *444*
hepatic metastases 492
metastatic 445, 447–8, *447*
bone scintigraphy 447–8, *447*
MIBG scintigraphy 447, *447*
PET-CT 448
somatostatin receptor scintigraphy 445, *446*
prognosis 488–9, **489**
rectal 445, 498–501
clinical features and management 500–1
etiopathogenesis 498
macroscopic appearances 499
microscopic appearances 499–500, *499*, *500*
relative frequency 499
small bowel 444–5
survival **489**
thymic 485–6
clinical presentation 485–6
diagnosis 486
epidemiology 485
etiology 485
genetic alterations 485
histopathology 485
immunohistochemistry 485
prognosis 486
treatment 486
treatment 492–6
ablative therapy 493
chemoembolization 493
chemotherapy 495

combination therapy 494–5
hepatic artery embolization 493
interferons 494
novel therapies 495–6, **495**
somatostatin analogs 493–4, **494**
surgery 492–3
tumor markers *94*, *95*, 501
see also neuroendocrine tumors
carcinoid tumors *see* carcinoid syndrome
cardiomyopathy **534**
cardiovascular disease
and hormone therapy 619–20
and oral contraceptive pill 621
Carney complex **26**, 144, 263, 274, 380, **381**, 532–6
causes of death **533**
clinical manifestations 532–3, **532**
diagnostic criteria **533**
genetic testing **46**, 535
laboratory evaluation 535
molecular genetics 533–5, *534*, **534**
caspase 8, epigenetic silencing 362
catechol-*o*-methyltransferase 353
catecholamines 5, **91**, 95–6
plasma 354
urinary 354
drugs affecting 354
cavernous sinus hemangioma 318–24, *318*, *319*
differential diagnosis 321, *322*
endocrine implications 319
neuroimaging findings 319–21, *320*, *321*
patient demographic characteristics 319
treatment 321, 323
microsurgery 321, 323
stereotactic radiosurgery and fractionated
radiotherapy 323
CCKB receptor radiotherapy 61
cecal neuroendocrine tumors 440, 442
celecoxib, thyroid tumors **152**
cerebellar hemangioblastoma, von Hippel–Lindau
disease **523**, 524–5, *525*
cerebrospinal fluid examination, sarcoidosis 332
cetuximab, complications 106, **106**
Charing Cross Scoring System 433, **433**
chemoembolization 502–3
carcinoid syndrome 493
transarterial 74–5, *75*
see also hepatic arterial embolization
chemotherapy 502–4
antiangiogenic agents 503
biotherapy 503
carcinoid syndrome 495
bronchial 484, **484**
combination 502
cytotoxic 502–3, **503**
complications 104, **105**
germ cell tumors 409–10
germinoma 314
non-germinomatous germ cell tumors 315
parathyroid carcinoma 183
patient selection 504
peripheral neuroblastic tumors 367
sex cord-stromal tumors 407
thyroid lymphoma 163
tyrosine kinase inhibition 503–4
see also individual drugs

Chernobyl accident 167, 168–9
chiasmatic cistern
  inflammation of 212
  lesions of 211, *212*
children, genetic testing 45
Children's Cancer and Leukaemia Group 313
chlorambucil, sarcoidosis 333
chloroquine, sarcoidosis 334
cholecystokinin 7, 440
cholecystokinin receptors 59
cholelithiasis 480
cholesterol 5
  reference range **625**
chondrosarcoma 304, *304*
chordoma 302–4, *303*
  etiology 302–3
  pathology 303
  presentation 303
  prognosis 304
  radiology 303, *303*
  treatment 303
choriocarcinoma 408, 431
  tumor markers **312**
chromaffin cells 353
chromogranins 5, 13, 275, 489
chromogranin A 90, **91**
  carcinoid syndrome 490
    bronchial 483–4
  gastrinoma 464
  neuroendocrine tumors 438
  pheochromocytoma 355
Chvostek's sign 373
ciclosporin A, sarcoidosis 333
cisplatin 316, **503**
  adrenocortical carcinoma 382
  bronchial carcinoids 484, **484**
  ovarian germ cell tumor 409
  sex cord-stromal tumors 407
  testicular germ cell tumors **416**
CITED1 147
cladribine, sarcoidosis 333
Claude Bernard Horner syndrome *363*
cloacal exstrophy 421
clodronate
  hypercalcemia 564
  hyperparathyroidism 176
cocaine, MIBG uptake **356**
codeine phosphate **103**
coefficient of variation 88
cold intolerance 331
collagenoma, *MEN1* expression **507**
colon 498
colonic tumors
  adenocarcinoma 390
  carcinoid 445, 498–501
    clinical features and management 500
    etiopathogenesis 498
    macroscopic appearances 499
    microscopic appearances 499–500,
      499, 500
    relative frequency 499
    survival **489**
  carcinoma 579
  metastases 583, 585, **586**
  neuroendocrine 440, 442

complete androgen insensitivity syndrome 424, 425,
  427
complications
  of cancer 102–4, **103**
    anorexia–cachexia syndrome 104
    infection 103–4
    pain 102–3, **103**
    psychological morbidity 104
  of therapy 104–6, **105, 106**
    biological agents 106, **106**
    cytotoxic therapy 104, **105**
    radiation therapy 104–6
computerized tomography
  adrenal glands 339, 393
  adrenal tumors
    adenoma 346–9, *347–9*
    adrenocortical carcinoma *387*
    pheochromocytoma 357
  carcinoid syndrome 491
    gastric *444*
    ileal *446*
  Conn syndrome 374
  craniopharyngioma 283
  Cushing syndrome *258*, 379
  granulosa cell tumor *398*
  insulinoma 459
  islet cell tumors *449, 450*
  pituitary gland 202–3, *203*
  Sertoli–Leydig cell tumors 397
  thecoma *400*
  thyroid 112–13
  VIPoma **471**
Conn syndrome 14, 21, 343–4, *343*, 370–7
  adrenal vein sampling 375–6
  aldosterone-producing adenoma 370–1, *371*
  assessment *375*
  bilateral adrenal hyperplasia 371, *371*
  clinical features 372–3
  diagnosis 373
    confirmation of 374
  differential diagnosis 373
  glucocorticoid-remediable aldosteronism 371–2,
    372
  radiological investigations 374–5
  screening 373–4, **373**
  subtypes and localization 374
  treatment 376
corpus luteum 7
corrective gene therapy 49, 50–1
  thyroid cancer 50–1
corticosteroids, sarcoidosis 333
corticotropin-like intermediary lobe peptide 568
corticotropin-releasing hormone 5, **6**
corticotropin-releasing hormone test 257
cortisol 7
  late night salivary 256
  midnight plasma 256
  reference range **623, 624**
  urinary free 255
cortisol antagonists 574
cortisol-binding globulin 195, 255
Cowden syndrome **26**, 144, 545–8
  cranial findings 545–6, *545*
  diagnostic criteria 546
  disease characteristics 545

genetic counselling 547
genetic testing **46**
genetically related disorders 547
  management 547
  molecular genetics 546–7
  mucocutaneous findings 545
  phenotypic characteristics *42*
  prevalence 546
  thyroid/breast/endometrial cancer 546
cranial nerve
  compression 263
  schwannoma 321
craniopharyngioma 10, 210, **238**, 282–7
  adamantinomatous *209*, 283
  clinical, hormonal and imaging features 283–4,
    284
  differential diagnosis 279
  epidemiology 282
  imaging 208–9, *209*
  intracystic therapy 69
  morbidity and mortality 285–6
  papillary *283*
  pathogenesis 282–3, *283*
  pathology 282–3, *283*
  treatment 284–5
    brachytherapy 284–5
    stereotactic radiosurgery 285
    stereotactic radiotherapy 285
    surgical removal 284
  treatment algorithm 286–7, *286*
craniotomy 227–8
Crooke's hyalinization 218–19, 275
cryoablation 75
cryptorchidism 423, 427
CT *see* computerized tomography
Cushing, Harvey 378
Cushing syndrome 14, 21, 208, 218, 253–61, 341–3
  ACTH-dependent 257, 342–3, *342*
    ectopic ACTH source 342, *343*
    pituitary-dependent 342
  ACTH-independent 341–2, 378
    adrenal adenoma 341
    adrenal carcinoma 341, *341*
    macronodular adrenal hyperplasia 342
    primary pigmented nodular adrenocortical
      disease 341–2, *341*
  adrenal 378–83
    etiology **378**
    pathophysiology and molecular biology 380–1,
      381
    treatment 381–2
  biochemical assessment 255
  biochemical diagnosis 255, *255*
  Carney complex **534**
  causes 253–4, *254*
  clinical features 254–5, **254**
  differential diagnosis 379–80, *380*
  dynamic non-invasive tests 257–8
  epidemiology 253
  etiology 256–7, *256*
  imaging 258, *258*
  invasive testing 257–8
  late night salivary cortisol 256
  low-dose dexamethasone suppression test 255–6
  management 258–9

midnight plasma corticol 256
pathogenesis 254
pituitary surgery 228
POMC in 569
presentation 378–9
prognosis 253
radiotherapy 232
steroid cell tumors 401
surgery 259–60, 259
    adrenal 260
    fractionated external pituitary radiotherapy 260
    stereotactic radiosurgery 260, 260
    transsphenoidal 259–60
thymic carcinoids 485
urinary free cortisol 255
cutaneous paraneoplastic syndromes 552–4, 552
    acanthosis nigricans 552–3
    acrokeratosis paraneoplastica of Bazex 553
    dermatomyositis 553
    erythema gyratum repens 553
    necrolytic migratory erythema 553
    paraneoplastic pemphigus 553–4
CV2 550
Cyberknife 67
cyclins 187, 189
cyclophosphamide
    bronchial carcinoids 484, 484
    gestational trophoblastic tumor 433
    ovarian germ cell tumor 409
    sarcoidosis 333
    sex cord-stromal tumors 407
cysts
    adrenal 350
    arachnoid 289–90, 290
    dermoid 283, 290–1, 291
    epidermoid 283, 291
    Rathke's cleft see Rathke's cleft cysts
    thyroid 289
cytokeratin-19 147
cytokines 3, 5
cytokine storm 325
cytoreductive gene therapy 49, 51–2
cytotoxic drugs 502–3, 503
    complications 104, 105
    ectopic ACTH syndrome 573
    and SIADH 558, 559
    see also chemotherapy; and individual drugs

dacarbazine 502, 503
    carcinoid syndrome 495
    glucagonoma 477
dancing eyes/dancing feet syndrome 364
Dax1 190, 423
decitabine, thyroid tumors 152
dehydroepiandrosterone see DHEA
denosumab 565
Denys–Drash syndrome 423, 424
depsipeptide, thyroid tumors 152
dermatomyositis 553
dermoid cyst 283, 290–1, 291
    differential diagnosis 283
desmopressin testing 257
dexamethasone 103
dexamethasone suppression tests 372
    high-dose 257

low-dose 255–6
DHEA 13, 33
    adrenal incidentaloma 387
    breast cancer 34
DHEA-sulfate 7, 33
    breast cancer 34
    reference range 623
Dhh 423
diabetes insipidus 327, 328, 331, 332
    risk factors 329
diabetes mellitus, glucagonoma 475, 477
diamorphine 103
diarrhea
    carcinoid syndrome 490
    differential diagnosis 470
diclofenac 103
diffuse reticuloendotheliosis see Langerhans cell
    histiocytosis
DiGeorge syndrome 13
dihydrocodeine 103
dihydrotestosterone 15
    reference range 623
dihydroxyphenylalanine 5
Dmrt1 423
docetaxel
    bronchial carcinoids 484, 484
    prostate cancer 606–7
dopamine 5, 6, 8
    reference range 624
dopamine agonists
    acromegaly 250
    effect on fetus 244
    PRL cell adenoma 216–17
    withdrawal 242–3
    see also individual drugs
dopamine β-hydroxylase 5
dopamine receptors 189
Dott, Norman 222, 223
doxazosin, pheochromocytoma 357, 389
doxorubicin
    adrenocortical carcinoma 382
    carcinoid syndrome 495
        bronchial 484, 484
    glucagonoma 477
DSD see sexual development, disorders of
duodenal tumors
    carcinoid 444
    neuroendocrine 440
    somatostatinoma 480–1
dysarthria 327
dysgerminoma 238, 408
dysphagia 327

E-cadherin 182
ectopic ACTH syndrome 567–75
    classic presentation 567
    clinical implications 570–1
        altered POMC processing in diagnosis 570–1
        bilateral inferior petrosal sinus sampling 570
    diagnosis 571, 572
    imaging techniques 571, 572
    occult/chronic presentation 568
    POMC gene
        expression 569–70
        transcription 568–9, 569

POMC secretion 568, 568
    treatment 571, 573–4
        cytotoxic chemotherapy 573
        normal adrenals 573–4
        somatostatin analogs 573
        surgery 573
    tumors associated with 567
ectopic corticotroph syndrome 570
embolization
    transarterial 74–5, 75
    see also chemoembolization; hepatic arterial
        embolization
Embospheres 484
embryonal carcinoma 408
    tumor markers 312
empty sella syndrome 238
encephalomyelitis 551
    antibodies 550
endocrine evaluation 393
endocrine pancreas see pancreas; pancreatic
endocrine system 3–17
endocrine tumors
    adrenal cortical see adrenal tumors
    epidemiology 18–23
    genetic susceptibility 24–9, 25–8, 29–31, 30
    incidence 18, 22
    neuroendocrine see neuroendocrine tumors
    ovarian cancer see ovarian tumors
    parathyroid see parathyroid tumors
    pheochromocytoma see pheochromocytoma
    pituitary adenoma see pituitary adenoma
    testicular cancer 19–20, 19
    thyroid cancer see thyroid tumors
endocrinopathy 300
endodermal sinus tumor 408
Endogenous Hormones and Breast Cancer
    Collaborative Group 33
endometrial cancer
    Cowden syndrome 546
    role of sex steroids 35–6, 36
enterochromaffin cells 7, 16, 90
enterochromaffin-like cells 440
enteroglucagon 7
eosinophilic granuloma see Langerhans cell
    histiocytosis
ependymoma 10, 210, 298–301
    anaplastic 298
    diagnosis 299
    molecular and cellular genetics 299
    myxopapillary 298
    pathology 298–9
    prognosis 300
    treatment 299–300
ephedrine, catecholamine assay interference 354
epidemiology 18–23
epidermal growth factor 39–40, 187, 189, 604
epidermal growth factor receptor 187, 189, 276
epidermoid cyst 291
    differential diagnosis 283
epinephrine 7
    reference range 624
    see also catecholamines
epithelial membrane antigen 298
eplerenone, Conn syndrome 376
erbB-2 189

erlotinib, complications 106, **106**
erythema gyratum repens 553
escape phenomenon 373
esophageal tumors, metastases **583**
estradiol
    breast cancer **34**
    reference range **623**
estrogen augmented by progesterone hypothesis 33
estrogens 7
    and breast cancer 32–3, *33*, **33**
estrone, breast cancer **34**
estrone sulfate, breast cancer **34**
ethanol, percutaneous injection 75
etidronate, hyperparathyroidism 176
etoposide **503**
    adrenocortical carcinoma 382
    bronchial carcinoids 484, **484**
    gestational trophoblastic tumor 433
    ovarian germ cell tumor 410
    sex cord-stromal tumors 407
    testicular germ cell tumors 416
everolimus, carcinoid syndrome 495–6, **495**
exemestane, breast cancer 614
external beam radiotherapy 64–5

factitial hypoglycemia 456
familial hyperparathyroidism syndromes 177–8
    hyperparathyroidism–jaw tumor syndrome 177–8
    multiple endocrine neoplasia syndromes 177
familial hypocalciuric hypercalcemia 176–7, **561**
familial isolated primary hyperparathyroidism 178
familial paraganglioma syndrome **353**
family2 182
famotidine, gastrinoma 465
feeding strategies 106
female reproductive hormone therapy 618–22
    hormone replacement 618–20, **620**
    oral contraceptive pill 620–1, **621**
fetal zone 7, 13
fibroblast growth factor 9, 15
    pituitary adenoma 190
    thyroid cancer 128
fibroma, oral 545
fibronectin-1 147
fibrosarcoma
    hepatic **579**
    treatment **579**
fibrothecoma 400–1, *400, 401*
    endocrine aspects 405–6
    stained-glass appearance 401
fibrous dysplasia of bone 537, **538**, *539*
fine needle aspiration biopsy
    parathyroid carcinoma 181
    thyroid tumors 113–14, **113**, 118–19
flare phenomenon 605
fludrocortisone suppression test 374
fluid-attenuated inversion recovery (FLAIR) MRI,
    sarcoidosis 332, *334*
5-fluorouracil 502, **503**
    adrenocortical carcinoma 382
    bronchial carcinoid 484, **484**
    glucagonoma 477
    pituitary carcinoma 276
    sex cord-stromal tumors 407
flutamide, prostate cancer 604–5, **605**

FNAB *see* fine needle aspiration biopsy
focal radiation therapy 233
folate receptor 187, 192
follicle-stimulating hormone 5, 6, 194
    adenomas producing 219
    reference range **623**
follicular thyroid carcinoma 78–9, 143–54
    advanced disease 151–2, *152*
    diagnosis **146**, 147–8, *148*
    epidemiology 143
        chronic iodine deficiency 143–4
        genetic syndromes 144
    etiology 143–4
    long-term follow-up 151
    non-syndromic forms 144–7, *145*, **146–7**
    pathogenesis 126–7
    pathology 144–5, *145*, **145**
    staging and prognosis 148–9
    TNM staging **146–7**
    treatment 149–51
        surgery 149–50
        TSH suppressive therapy 150
    tumor biomarkers 99
        systemic iodine-131 therapy 150–1
    ultrasound 117–18, *118*
follistatin 7, 15
fractionated external pituitary radiotherapy 260
Frasier syndrome 423, *424*
FSH *see* follicle-stimulating hormone
furosemide, hypercalcemia 565
fusion proteins, peripheral neuroblastic tumors 368

G cells 440
gabapentin **103**
GADD45- **187**, 191
Gal-3 **187**
galactorrhea 331
galectin-3 147, 182, 191
gallium nitrate, hypercalcemia 565
Gamma Knife radiosurgery 66
    cavernous sinus hemangioma 323
    chordoma 303
    Cushing syndrome 260, *260*
    hamartoma 295
    pituitary 233
ganciclovir 51
gangliocytic paraganglioma 440
gangliocytoma 296–7, **296**
    clinical and laboratory findings 296–7
    pathogenesis 296
    therapy 297
ganglioneuroblastoma 345–6, 361
ganglioneuroma 14, 361
gastric tumors
    adenocarcinoma **579**
    carcinoid 444, *444*
        survival **489**
    metastases 583, 585, 586
    neuroendocrine 440
    treatment **579**
gastrin 6, 92, 353, 462, *463*
    reference range **624**
gastrin-releasing peptide 59, 462
gastrinoma 439, **439**, 440, 462–8
    conditions associated with **463**

    diagnosis 463–4, **464**
    duodenal 466
    ectopic ACTH syndrome **567**
    MEN 1 466–7, 510–11, 512
    MEN1 expression **507**
    provocative tests 464, *464*
    somatostatin receptor scintigraphy **451**
    staging 467, **467**
    surgery 84
    treatment
        medical 465
        palliative 466
        surgical 465–6
    tumor localization 464–5, *465*
gastrointestinal neuroendocrine tumors 440, 442
    appendix 442
    cecum 440, 442
    colon 440, 442
    duodenum 440
    jejunum 440
    gastric 440
    imaging 443–4
        algorithms 451–3, **451**, *452, 453*
        carcinoid syndrome 444–5, *444*
        islet cell tumors 448–51, **448**, *449, 450*
        metastatic carcinoid syndrome 445, 447–8, *447*
    rectum 440, 442
gastrointestinal peptide 7
gastrointestinal pseudo-obstruction 552
gastrointestinal stroma tumor 530
gastrointestinal tract **6**
    endocrine tissue 16
gefitinib, carcinoid syndrome 495–6, **495**
gelastic seizures 294
gene therapy 49–50, *50*
    adrenocortical carcinoma 55
    antiangiogenic 51–2
    corrective 49, 50–1
    cytoreductive 49, 51–2
    immunomodulatory 49, 52
    NIS 52–5, *53, 54*
    peripheral neuroblastic tumors 368
    pituitary adenoma 192–3
    thyroid cancer 50–1
    virus-mediated oncolysis 49, 52
genetic counselling 42–3
    Cowden syndrome 547
genetic registers 47
genetic susceptibility
    endocrine neoplasia 29–31, *30*
    endocrine tumors 24–9, **25–8**
genetic testing 44–5, **45**, 46
    Carney complex 46, 535
    children 45
    Cowden syndrome **46**
    and insurance 45
    sporadic testing 46–7
germ cell tumors 307, 310–17, *311*, 390
    classification **407**
    clinical presentation 312–13
        pineal tumors 312
        suprasellar tumors 312–13
    follow-up 315–16
    germinomas 314
    histology 310–12, *312*, **312**

incidence 310
investigations 313
metastatic 585
non-germinomatous 315
ovarian 407
　chemotherapy 409–10
　radiotherapy 410
　surgery 409
teratomas *see* teratoma
testicular 412–20
　clinical behavior and response to treatment 416
　clinical management 415–16
　early-stage 417–18, **417**, **418**
　epidemiology 412–14, **413**
　future trials 418
　good-risk patients 417, **417**
　immune response and prognosis 415
　intrauterine exposure to "xeno-estrogens" 415
　metastatic disease 416, **416**
　pathology 414–15, **414**
　poor-risk patients 416–17
treatment 313
germinoma 10, 314
　differential diagnosis 283
　tumor markers **312**
gestational choriocarcinoma 430
gestational trophoblastic tumors 430–4
　Charing Cross Scoring System 433, **433**
　epigenetics 431–2, **432**
　genetics 431
　human chorionic gonadotrophin 432
　investigations and treatment 432–3, **433**
　long-term outlook 433
GH *see* growth hormone
ghrelin 8, 16
GHRH *see* growth hormone-releasing hormone
glial cell line-derived neurotropic factor 127
glial fibrillary acid protein 296, 298
glicentin 498
glioma 10, 210
　differential diagnosis 279, 283
　hypothalamic 306
　optic nerve 211, 306, 529
glomus tumors 306–7
　etiology 306–7
　pathology 307
　presentation 307
　prognosis 307
　radiology 307
　treatment 307
glossitis, in glucagonoma 475
glucagon 6, **92**, 438, **579**
　excess, metabolic effects 474
　reference range **624**
glucagon stimulation test **195**, 196, **197**
glucagon-like peptide 16, 59, 474
glucagonoma 439, **439**, 474–8
　clinical features 474–5
　diabetes mellitus 475, 477
　histopathology 476
　hypoaminoacidemia 475–6, 477
　imaging 476, *476*
　laboratory features 475–6
　and MEN 1 475
　MEN 1 475

necrolytic migratory erythema 474, 475
pathogenesis 476–7
prognosis 478
somatostatin receptor scintigraphy **451**
treatment
　hepatic embolization for metastatic disease 477
　medical 477
　surgical 477
glucocorticoids, hypercalcemia caused by 565
glucocorticoid-remediable aldosteronism 371–2
GNAS mutation 537
　alternative transcripts and imprinting 541
　identification of 540–1, *541*
　see also McCune–Albright syndrome
GnRH *see* gonadotropin-releasing hormone
goiter 11
　Cowden syndrome 546
　multinodular **28**
Golgi apparatus 5
gonadal atrophogens 413–14, **413**
gonadal dysgenesis **421**, 424
gonadal endocrine tissue 14–16
gonadal stroma tumor of android type *see*
　　Sertoli–Leydig cell tumor
gonadal tumors 424
　classification 424
　clinical disorders 424
　disorders of sex determination 424, **425**
　origin of 424–6, **425**
gonadoblastoma 409
gonadotroph adenomas 219
gonadotropin deficiency, radiation-induced 593
gonadotropin-releasing hormone 6, 8
　sex cord-stromal tumors 407
gonadotropin-releasing hormone
　agonists/antagonists, in prostate cancer 604–5
gonadotropinoma
　non-functioning 262–7
　　clinical presentation 263–4
　　diagnosis 264–5, *264*
　　epidemiology 262
　　management 265–6, *265*
　　pathology and pathogenesis 262–3
gonocytes 425
goserelin, prostate cancer 604–5, **605**
gossypol, adrenocortical carcinoma 382
granulosa cells 7
granulosa cell tumor 391, 397–400, *398–400*, **398**
　adult 398, 404–5
　androgen-secreting 391, 398
　computerized tomography *398*
　endocrine aspects 404–5
　juvenile 398, 405
　magnetic resonance imaging *399*
　ultrasound *398*, *399*
Graves disease 269
　and radiotherapy 597
Greig cerebropolysyndactyly syndrome 293
GRIM19, thyroid cancer 126
growth, cancer treatment effects 588–90, **589**, **590**
growth hormone 5, **6**, 10, **92**, 194, **579**
　adenomas producing 215–16
　deficiency, radiation-induced 588, 591–3, *592*
　excess 537, 540
　mixed GH/PRL adenoma 218

reference range **624**
growth hormone-insulin-like growth factor-1 axis
　196–7, **197**
　normal physiology 196
　provocative tests 196–7, **197**
growth hormone-releasing hormone 6, 8, **92**
　tumors producing *see* acromegaly
growth hormone-releasing hormone receptor **187**, 189
Gsp **187**, 189
GTPase activating protein 528
gynandroblastoma 402

hamartoma *211*, 293–6, *294*
　clinical manifestations 294–5
　　central precocious puberty 295
　　seizures 294–5
　diagnosis 295
　differential diagnosis 279, 283
　therapy 295–6
　　precocious puberty 295–6
　　seizures 295
Hand–Schüller–Christian disease *see* Langerhans
　　cell histiocytosis
Hardy, Jules 223
Hashimoto thyroiditis 80, 125, 162
HbA1c, reference range **625**
HBME1 147
HDL cholesterol, reference range **625**
head and neck tumors
　hypercalcemia **561**
　and SIADH 558
headache **331**
Helicobacter pylori 462
hemangioblastoma 210
hemangiopericytoma 305–6
　etiology 305–6
　pathology 306
　prognosis 306
　radiology 306
　treatment 306, **579**
hepatic arterial embolization
　bronchial carcinoids 484
　carcinoid syndrome 493
　glucagonoma 477
hepatic fibrosarcoma, treatment **579**
hepatocellular carcinoma
　metastases **583**
　treatment **579**
hereditary pheochromocytoma-paraganglioma
　　syndrome **26**, **27**, 30
heterophile antibodies 88, **88**
5-HIAA 90–1, **91**, 94–5, *94*, *95*, 501
　reference range **624**
High Mobility Group A2 gene 192
Hirsch, Oskar 223
histiocytosis X *see* Langerhans cell histiocytosis
histon-1 182
HMGA2 **187**
holoprosencephaly 293
Homer–Wright pseudorosette 361
homovanillic acid **91**, 95–6
hook effect 151, 239
hormones 4–8
　ACTH *see* ACTH
　catecholamines 5

cellular mechanisms of secretion *4*
corticotropin-releasing hormone 5, **6**
FSH *see* follicle-stimulating hormone
GnRH **6**, 8, 407
growth hormone *see* growth hormone
LH *see* luteinizing hormone
parathyroid hormone *see* parathyroid hormone
peptide/protein/glycoprotein group 4–5
steroids 5
thyroid-releasing 6
thyrotropin 6, 10, 112, 219
thyrotropin-releasing hormone 8, *271*
thyroxine 6, 112, **623**
treatment of, sex cord-stromal tumors 407
vasopressin 6, 557
see also individual hormones
hormone replacement therapy 618–20, **620**
cancer risk 619
and cardiovascular disease 619–20
menopause 619
and osteoporosis 619
risk–benefit balance 620, **620**
hormone-secreting cells 6–7
Horsley, Victor 222
Hounsfield units 339, 349
HRPT2 gene 180, 182
5-HT *see* serotonin
Hu **550**
human chorionic gonadotrophin **92**, 312
gestational trophoblastic tumors 432
reference range **625**
human telomere reverse transcriptase 299
humoral hypercalcemia of malignancy 562
hungry bones syndrome 175
Huntington disease 25
Hürthle cell carcinoma 79, 126, 147, 149
hydatidiform mole 430, **430**
hydralazine, catecholamine assay interference 354
hydrocephalus 283, *311*
treatment 313
hydroxychloroquine, sarcoidosis 334
5-hydroxyindole acetic acid *see* 5-HIAA
17-hydroxyprogesterone, reference range **623**
hyperaldosteronism
surgery 83
see also Conn syndrome
hyperandrogenism 392
ovarian causes 396
hypercalcemia 470, 509
calcium homeostasis 561–2
causes 561, **561**
emergency treatment 565–6
of malignancy 561–6
frequency of 562
humoral 562
metastatic bone disease 562–3
myeloma bone disease 563–4
pathophysiology 562–4
tumor–bone interaction 563
management 183–4
treatment 564–6
hypercortisolemia 255, *255*
ACTH-independent 380
McCune–Albright syndrome 537, 540
see also Cushing syndrome

hyperestrogenism, ovarian causes 396
hypergastrinemia 464
see also gastrinoma
hyperglycemia 470
hyperparathyroidism 172–6
clinical manifestations 173–4
familial isolated primary 178
and hypercalcemia 561
imaging *175*
laboratory findings 174
medical management 176
pathogenesis 172–3
pathology
parathyroid adenoma 173
parathyroid hyperplasia 173
radiation-induced 597
surgery 80–1, 174–5
hyperparathyroidism–jaw tumor syndrome 27, 177–8, 180
genetic testing **46**
hyperprolactinemia 237–8
Carney complex **534**
differential diagnosis **238**
drug-induced **238**
McCune–Albright syndrome 537, 540
see also prolactinoma
hyperreflexia 327
hypertensive crisis 358, *358*
hyperthyroidism
Graves disease 269
and hypercalcemia 561
McCune–Albright syndrome 537, 540
treatment 542
hypertrichosis lanuginosa 554
hypoadrenalism 346
hypoaminoacidemia 475–6, 477
hypochlorhydria 470
hypoglycemia
factitial 456
insulin autoimmune 456
non-islet cell 576–81
hypoglycemic disorders
causes
insulin autoantibody hypoglycemia 456
insulinoma 456
pancreatogenous hypoglycemia syndrome 456
classification 456
diagnostic tests 456–8
72-h fast 456–8, *457*
insulin antibodies 458
mixed meal test 458
selective arterial calcium injection 458
hypogonadotropic hypogonadism **331**
hypokalemia 257, 470
hypomagnesemia 470
hyponatremia 470, 557–8
malignancy-associated 558–9, **558**
management of 559–60
see also SIADH
hypopituitarism 263–4
radiation-induced 591–4, *592*
hypospadias **421**
hypothalamic glioma 306
hypothalamic hamartoma 210
hypothalamo-pituitary neurosarcoidosis 332

hypothalamo-pituitary-adrenal axis 194–6
basal corticoid test 195
glucagon stimulation test **195**, 196
insulin tolerance test 195–6, **195**
short Synacthen test **195**, 196
hypothalamo-pituitary-gonadal axis 197–8, *602*
hypothalamo-pituitary-thyroid axis 197
thyrotropinoma *268*
hypothalamus 6, 8–10, *8*, *9*
imaging 200–14
hypothyroidism, radiation-induced 597
hypovitaminosis B 476
hypoxia-inducible factors 523–4

ichthyosis, acquired 554
IGF 15, *38*, 48, 576–81
big 577
free 577
non-islet cell tumor hypoglycemia 577–8
reference range **624**
IGF binding proteins 576–7
IGF-1 7, 197
ileal neuroendocrine tumors 440, 442
image-guided biopsy 70
imantinib mesylate
carcinoid syndrome 495–6, **495**
peripheral neuroblastic tumors 368
immobilization, hypercalcemia caused by **561**
immunomodulatory agents, sarcoidosis 333–4
immunomodulatory gene therapy 49, 52
immunosuppressants, sarcoidosis 333
imperforate anus 293
impotence 331
incidentaloma 18, 82–3
adrenal 346–50, 384–9
causes and prevalence 384–6, *385*, **385**
clinical aspects 386
computerized tomography 346–9, *347–9*
histological diagnosis *385*
hormonal assessment 386–7
imaging studies 387–8, *387*
magnetic resonance imaging 349, *350*
pathogenesis 386
percutaneous adrenal biopsy 349
surgery 82–3
treatment and follow-up 388–9, *388*
pituitary 278–81
alternative diagnoses 279–80
definition 278, *278*
evaluation 280
incidence 278–9, *279*
management 280–1
presentation 280
indometacin, hypercalcemia 565
infection 103–4
inferior petrosal sinus sampling 71
infliximab, sarcoidosis 334
inhibin 7
insulin 6, 37–8, **92**, 438
reference range **624**
insulin antibodies 458
insulin autoimmune hypoglycemia 456
insulin tolerance test 195–6, **195**, 197
insulin–IGF axis 37–8
insulin-like growth factor *see* IGF

insulinoma *439*, **439**, 455–61
  arteriography 459
  computerized tomography 459
  hypoglycemic disorders
    causes 456
    classification 456
    diagnosis 456–8, *457*
  malignant 459–60, *460*
  MEN 1 459, *459*, 511
  MEN1 expression **507**
  somatostatin receptor scintigraphy **451**
  surgery 84
  ultrasound
    endoscopic 459
    intraoperative 459
    transabdominal 458
  Whipple's triad 455–6
insurance 45
interferons
  carcinoid syndrome 494
  complications 106, **106**
interferon-α 503
  bronchial carcinoids 484, **484**
interferon-γ 462
interleukin-1β 462
interleukin-2 52
interleukin-12 52
internal jugular venous sampling 258
International Neuroblastoma Pathology
    Classification 361
International Neuroblastoma Staging System **366**
interventional radiology 70–7
  image-guided biopsy 70
  metastatic neuroendocrine tumors 74–6
    cryoablation 75
    percutaneous ethanol injection 75
    radiofrequency ablation 75–6, *76*
    transarterial embolization/chemoembolization
      74–5, *75*
  selective internal radiation therapy 76
  venous sampling
    adrenal 71–2, *72*
    hepatic with intra-arterial stimulation 73
    inferior petrosal sinus 71
    islet cell tumors 72–3, *73*
    parathyroid 70–1, *71*
    transhepatic portal vein 73
intracranial tumors, and SIADH 558
iodine deficiency 143–4
iodine-123, thyroid tumors 119–20
iodine-124, thyroid tumors 120
iodine-131
  thyroid tumors 119
    follicular thyroid cancer 150–1
iodothyronines 5, 11
irinotecan **503**
irofulven, thyroid tumors 152
islet cell tumors
  imaging 448–51
    computerized tomography *449*, 450
    functional 451
    magnetic resonance imaging 450–1, *450*
    metastatic tumors 451
    ultrasound 449–50
  MEN1 expression **507**

subtypes **448**
  venous sampling 72–3, *73*
islets of Langerhans 16, 438
Ivalon 484
ixabepilone, prostate cancer 607

jejunal neuroendocrine tumors 440
Jho, H. 223
jugulotympanic tumors 307

kallikrein 489
Kallman syndrome 9
Karnofsky Performance Scale 285
keratin, wet 282, *283*
keratinocyte growth factor 604
ketoconazole, Cushing syndrome 258
Ki67 276, 438
Klinefelter syndrome 421, **421**
Krukenberg tumor 390, 586

labetalol
  catecholamine assay interference **354**
  MIBG uptake **356**
LAMB 532
Lambert–Eaton myasthenia syndrome 550, 552
  antibodies **550**
Langerhans cell histiocytosis 325–30
  diagnosis 327, *328*
  differential diagnosis 283
  disease involvement 325–7, *326*
  disease sequelae 328–30, **329**
  endocrine and central nervous system disease 327
  endocrine deficiencies in **329**
  epidemiology 325
  etiology 325
  multisystem disease 326–7
  polyostotic *326*
  prognosis 328
  staging 327, *327*
  symptoms 325–7, *326*
  treatment
    hypothalamo-pituitary axis 328
    local 327–8
    systemic 328
lanreotide 62–3
  acromegaly 250
  radiolabeled 68
  thyrotropinoma 272
laryngeal tumors, metastases 583
late night salivary cortisol 256
Laws, E.R. 223
LDL cholesterol, reference range **625**
learning disabilities 529
leiomyoma, *MEN1* expression **507**
leiomyosarcoma
  epithelioid 579
  treatment **579**
lentigenes 534
leptin 39
letrozole
  breast cancer *613*
  precocious puberty 542
Letterer–Siwe disease *see* Langerhans cell histiocytosis
leuprolide, prostate cancer 604–5, **605**
Leydig cells 7, 14, 313, 422

Leydig cell hypoplasia **421**
LH *see* luteinizing hormone
Lhermitte–Duclos disease 545–6, 547
Li–Fraumeni syndrome 381
libido, loss of **331**
limbic encephalitis 551
  antibodies **550**
linear accelerators 65, *65*
lingual thyroid 11
lipoma 210
  MEN1 expression **507**
Lisch nodules 528
liver transplantation, carcinoid syndrome 492–3
lomustine, pituitary carcinoma 276
loop diuretics, in hypercalcemia 565
low-density lipoprotein 5
lung tumors
  bronchial carcinoids 482–5
    clinical presentation 483
    diagnosis 483–4
    differential diagnoses 484
    ectopic ACTH syndrome 567
    epidemiology 482
    etiology 482
    genetic alterations 483
    histopathology 483
    immunohistochemistry 483
    pathology 482–3
    prognosis 484–5
    survival **489**
    treatment 484, **484**
    tumorlets 482
  ectopic ACTH syndrome 567
  hypercalcemia **561**
  metastases 579, 583, 584, 585
  SIADH in 558
luteinizing hormone 5, 6, 194
  adenomas producing 219
  reference range **623**
lymphocytic hypophysitis 238
  differential diagnosis 279
lymphoma 211
  hypercalcemia **561**
  metastases 583, 584, 585, 586
  thyroid 80, 162–5
    chemotherapy 163
    clinical presentation and staging 162–3, *162*,
      162, 163
    etiology and pathogenesis 162
    radiation dose 164
    radiotherapy 163
    surgery 80, 163
    survival *164*
    treatment 163–4, **164**
    treatment outcome 163–4

Ma2 **550**
McCune–Albright syndrome 263, 381, 537–44
  clinical features 537–40, **537**
    autonomous thyroid nodules 540
    café-au-lait spots 537–8, *538*
    fibrous dysplasia of bone 538, *539*
    growth hormone excess 540
    hypercortisolism 540
    hyperprolactinemia 540

hypophosphatemic rickets and osteomalacia 540
  non-classical 540
  precocious puberty 538–9
  diagnosis 541–2
  pathogenesis 540–1
    genetic modulation of *GNAS* 541
    GNAS mutations 540–1, *541*
  prognosis 542
  treatment 542
    bone disease 542
    endocrinopathies 542
macrocephaly
  Cowden syndrome 545, *545*
  neurofibromatosis type 1 529–30
macroprolactinemia 239
Maffuci syndrome 398
magnetic resonance imaging
  acromegaly 249
  adrenal glands 340
  adrenal tumors
    adenoma 349
    cortical carcinoma 388
  carcinoid syndrome 491
  contrast media 201–2
  Cushing syndrome 258, 379
  granulosa cell tumor *399*
  islet cell tumors 450–1, *450*
  pheochromocytoma 357, *357*
  pituitary carcinoma 275
  pituitary gland 200–2, *201*, *202*
  sarcoidosis 332, *332*, *334*
  Sertoli–Leydig cell tumors 397
  thecoma *401*
  thyroid gland 112–13
  thyrotropinoma 270
major histocompatibility complex 52
malaise 331
mammalian Target of Rapamycin (mTOR) inhibitors 547
Marie, Pierre 246
maximum androgen blockade 605
  side effects 605
medullary thyroid carcinoma 79–80, 515–22
  clinical presentation 515–16, **516**
  diagnosis 517
  ectopic ACTH syndrome **567**
  genetics 516–17, **517**
  history **516**
  pathogenesis 127
  pathology 517
  prognostic factors 517–18
  staging 518
  surgery 79–80
  treatment 519–21, **520**, **521**
    chemotherapy 520
    lymph node dissection 520
    preoperative management 519
    reoperation 520
    surgery 519
    surgical considerations 519
  tumor markers 97
  ultrasound 117, *118*
MEG3 191–2
MEG3a **187**
α-melanocyte-stimulating hormone 8

melanoma, metastastatic **583**, **584**, **585**, **586**
MEN 1 *see* multiple endocrine neoplasia, type 1
MEN1
  expression **507**
  mutation analysis 512, **513**
menin 508
menin gene 269, 392
meningeal sarcoma **579**
meningioma 211, **238**, 304–5, *305*
  Cowden syndrome 546
  differential diagnosis 279, 283
  etiology 304–5
  MEN1 expression **507**
  pathology 305
  presentation 305
  prognosis 305
  radiology 305, *305*
  treatment 305
menopause 619
6-mercaptopurine, Langerhans cell histiocytosis 328
merlin 530
mesothelioma, treatment **579**
MET, thyroid cancer 126
metabolic acidosis **470**
metaiodobenzylguanidine *see* MIBG
metanephrines **91**, 95–6, 353
  plasma free 354–5
  reference range **624**
  urinary 354–5
metastatic bone disease, and hypercalcemia 562–3
metastatic tumors
  adrenal glands 83–4, 582–3, *583*, **583**
  neuroendocrine
    interventional radiology 74–6
      cryoablation 75
      percutaneous ethanol injection 75
      radiofrequency ablation 75–6, *76*
      transarterial embolization/
        chemoembolization 74–5, *75*
  ovary 585–6, **586**
  parathyroid glands 585
  pineal gland 585
  pituitary gland 584–5, *584*
  testis 585, *585*
  thyroid gland 583–4, *583*, *584*
methotrexate
  gestational trophoblastic tumor 433
  sarcoidosis 333
metyrapone
  adrenocortical carcinoma 382
  Cushing syndrome 258
mGluR1 **550**
MIBG 59–60, 61–2
  carcinoid syndrome 447
  drugs interfering with uptake **356**
  pheochromocytoma 356–7
  radiolabeled 68
midnight plasma cortisol 256
milk–alkali syndrome **561**
mitotane, Cushing syndrome 258
mitoxantrone, prostate cancer 606
mixed adenoma 218
mixed meal test 458
moles 430, **430**
monoamine oxidase 353

monoclonal antibodies
  complications 106, **106**
  peripheral neuroblastic tumors 368
  radiolabeled 68–9
morphine sulfate **103**
mosaicism 47
motesanib, thyroid tumors **152**
motilin 7, 440
MRI *see* magnetic resonance imaging
mucinous cysadenocarcinoma 390
Müllerian-inhibiting factor 14
multiple endocrine neoplasia 177
  genetic testing 46
  pheochromocytoma risk 353
multiple endocrine neoplasia type 1 25, 263, **381**,
    507–14
  acromegaly 511
  adrenal tumors 511–12
  clinical monitoring 512
  etiology 508
  gastrinoma 466–7, 510–11, 512
  glucagonoma 475
  insulinoma 459, *459*, 511
  lung tumors 512
  MEN1 expression **507**
  MEN1 mutation analysis 512, **513**
  neuroendocrine tumors 509–10, *510*
  parathyroid adenoma 508–9
  thymic tumors 512
    carcinoid 485
multiple endocrine neoplasia type 2A 25
  genetics 516–17, **517**
  medullary thyroid carcinoma 516
multiple endocrine neoplasia type 2B 25
  genetics 516–17, **517**
  medullary thyroid carcinoma 516
MYCN gene amplification 362
mycophenolate mofetil, sarcoidosis 333
myelolipoma, adrenal 350
myeloma
  bone disease 563–4
  hypercalcemia **561**, 563
myxoma, McCune–Albright syndrome **537**
myxopapillary ependymoma 298

NAME 532
National Thyroid Cancer Treatment Cooperative
    Study Group 135
necrolytic migratory erythema 474, 475, 553
Nelson syndrome 218, 260, 275
nephrocalcinosis 180
nephrolithiasis 180
nestin 298
neuroblastoma 28, 345–6, *346*, 361
  ectopic ACTH syndrome **567**
  and paraneoplastic disorders 549
  treatment **579**
neuroendocrine tumors 21, 437–42
  carcinoid *see* carcinoid syndrome
  chemotherapy 502–4
  classification 436–7, **441**
  epidemiology 436
  gastrointestinal 440, 442
    appendix 442
    duodenum and upper jejunum 440

gastric 440
   ileum, cecum, colon and rectum 440, 442
   imaging 443–54
  MEN 1 509–10, *510*
  metastatic *see* metastatic tumors
  NIS gene therapy 55
  pancreas 438–40, *439*, **439**
  pathology and biology 438
  somatostatin analog therapy 63
  see also individual tumors
neurofibromatosis type 1 27, 528–31
  defining features 528–9
  endocrine features
    hypothalamo-pituitary 530
    neuroendocrine tumors of gut 530
    parathyroid glands 530
    pheochromocytoma 530
    pregnancy and puberty 530
  general variable features
    learning disabilities 529
    neurofibrosarcoma 529
    optic pathway gliomas 529
    seizures 529
    short stature and macrocephaly 529–30
    skeletal dysplasia 529
    vascular dysplasia 529
  genetic testing **46**
  pheochromocytoma risk **353**
neurofibromatosis type 2 530
neurofibromin 528
neurofibrosarcoma 529
neurokinins 489
neuron-specific enolase **93**, 438
neuropeptide Y 8, 353
neurosteroids 3
neurotensin **93**
nicardipine, pheochromocytoma 357
NIS gene therapy 52–5, *53*, *54*
  adrenocortical cancer 55
  breast cancer 55
  neuroendocrine tumors 55
  ovarian cancer 55
  prostate cancer 55
  thyroid cancer 53–5, *54*
non-functioning pituitary adenoma 262–7
  clinical presentation 263–4
    hypopituitarism 263–4
    visual field disturbance 263
  diagnosis 264–5, *264*
  epidemiology 262
  management 265–6, *265*
  pathology and pathogenesis 262–3
non-germinomatous germ cell tumors 315
non-islet cell tumor hypoglycemia 576–81
  cause of 577
  circulating IGFs in 577–8
  treatment 578–80, *579*, **579**
noradrenaline *see* norepinephrine
norepinephrine 7
  reference range **624**
  see also catecholamines
normetanephrine 353
Notch signaling 16
notochord 302
null cell adenoma 219

obesity **331**
  and breast cancer 33
  and cancer risk 38, *38*
OCT3/4 426
Octreoscan *see* scintigraphy
octreotide 62–3, **579**
  acromegaly 250
  carcinoid syndrome 493–4, **494**
    bronchial 484, **484**
  gastrinoma 465
  glucagonoma 477
  radiolabeled 68
  thyrotropinoma 272
  VIPoma 472
Ollier disease 398
oncocytoma 219
oncogenes, pituitary adenoma **187**
ONYX-015 virus 52
Op'DDD 573
opioids, MIBG uptake 356
opsoclonus–myoclonus 551–2
  antibodies **550**
optic chiasm, tumors of 210
optic nerve glioma 211, 306, 529
oral contraceptive pill 620–1, **621**
  cancer risk 620–1
  and cardiovascular disease 621
  risks and benefits 621, **621**
orexin 8
organ of Zuckerkandle 13
organic anion transporters 5
osmoreceptors 556
osteoclast activating factors 563–4
osteomalacia, hypophosphatemic 554
  McCune–Albright syndrome **537**, 540
osteoporosis, and hormone therapy 619
osteosarcoma, McCune–Albright syndrome **537**
ovarian cancer 19
  ectopic ACTH syndrome **567**
  NIS gene therapy 55
ovarian suppression/stimulation 393
ovarian tumors 390
  androgen-secreting 390
    with functioning stroma 392
  choriocarcinoma 408
  differential diagnosis 402
  dysgerminoma 408
  embryonal carcinoma 408
  endocrine aspects 404–11
  endodermal sinus tumor 408
  fibrothecoma 400–1, *400*, *401*
    endocrine aspects 405–6
    stained-glass appearance 401
  functional 392, 396–403, **396**
  functioning stroma 402
  germ cell tumors 407, **407**
    chemotherapy 409–10
    radiotherapy 410
    surgery 409
  gonadoblastoma 409
  granulosa cell tumor 391, 397–400, *398–400*, **398**
    adult 398, 404–5
    androgen-secreting 391, 398
    computerized tomography *398*
    endocrine aspects 404–5

    juvenile 398, 405
    magnetic resonance imaging *399*
    ultrasound *398*, *399*
  gynandroblastoma 402
  metastases **583**
  polyembryoma 408
  in pregnancy 402
  sclerosing stromal tumor 401–2
    androgen-secreting 391
    endocrine aspects 406
  Sertoli–Leydig cell tumor 397
    androgen-secreting 391
    endocrine aspects 406
  sex cord tumor with annular tubules 402
    androgen-secreting 391–2
    endocrine aspects 406–7
  sex cord-stromal tumors 396–7
    androgen-secreting 390–1, **390**
    chemotherapy 407
    endocrine aspects 404, **404**
    hormonal therapy 407
    prognostic factors 407
    radiotherapy 407
    surgery 407
  staging **399**
  steroid cell tumors 401
  teratoma 409
  thecoma 391, 400–1, *400*, *401*
    androgen-secreting 391
    computerized tomography *400*
    endocrine aspects 405–6
    luteinized 400
    magnetic resonance imaging *401*
ovary 7
  cancer therapy effects **590**
  chemotherapy effects 596
  imaging 393
  metastatic tumors 585–6, **586**
  radiation effects 595
ovotesticular DSD **421**, 427
oxytetracycline, catecholamine assay interference 354
oxytocin 6, 7, 8

1p deletion 362
P16INK4a **187**, 188
P27KIP1 **187**, 188
p53 50, 189, 604
paclitaxel, bronchial carcinoids 484, **484**
Paget disease, and hypercalcemia 561
pain 102–3, **103**
  acute 102
  chronic 102
pain relief **103**
Pallister–Hall syndrome 293, 294
pamidronate **103**
  hypercalcemia 564
  McCune–Albright syndrome 542
pancreas, endocrine 16, **28**
  carcinoid **28**
  tumor **28**
pancreatic islets 6
pancreatic polypeptide 6, **93**, 438
  reference range **624**
pancreatic tumors

ectopic ACTH syndrome **567**
  metastases **583**, **585**
  neuroendocrine 438–9
  somatostatinoma 480, *480*, **480**
  surgery 84
pancreatogenous hypoglycemia syndrome 456
panhypopituitarism **331**
papillary craniopharyngioma *283*
papillary thyroid carcinoma 78–9, 130–42
  long-term surveillance 137–8
  metastasis 138–9
  molecularly targeted treatments 139–40
  mortality 131, *131*
  outcome prediction 131–2, *132*
  pathogenesis 124–6, *125*, **126**
  presenting features 130–1
  primary surgery 133–4, *133*
  radioiodine remnant ablation 134–6, *134–6*, **134**
  recurrence 131, *131*, 138–9
  risk-group stratification 131–2, *132*
  thyroxine suppressive therapy 134
  ultrasound 117, *117*, *118*
parafibromin 182
parafollicular C-cells 11–12
paraganglioma 344–5
  genetic testing **46**
  parasympathetic **28**
  sympathetic **28**
paraneoplastic pemphigus 553–4
paraneoplastic syndromes 549–55
  classic 551–2
    chronic gastrointestinal pseudo-obstructin 552
    encephalomyelitis 551
    Lambert–Eaton myasthenia syndrome 552
    limbic encephalitis 551
    opsoclonus–myoclonus 551–2
    sensory neuropathy 551
    subacute cerebellar degeneration 551
  cutaneous 552–4, **552**
    acanthosis nigricans 552–3
    acrokeratosis paraneoplastica of Bazex 553
    dermatomyositis 553
    erythema gyratum repens 553
    necrolytic migratory erythema 553
    paraneoplastic pemphigus 553–4
  hypophosphatemic osteomalacia 554
  neurological 550, **550**
  neutrophilic disorders
    acquired ichthyosis 554
    hypertrichosis lanuginosa 554
    pyoderma gangrenosum 554
    Sweet syndrome 554
  patient management 550–1
parasellar pituitary tumors 210–11
parathyroid glands 6, 12–13
  cancer therapy effects **590**
  familial hyperparathyroidism syndromes 177–8
  familial hypocalciuric hypercalcemia 176–7
  hyperparathyroidism 172–6
  hyperplasia 173
  imaging 121–2, *122*
  metastatic tumors 585
  venous sampling 70–1, *71*
parathyroid hormone 5, **6**, 353
  reference range **624**

thymic carcinoids 485
parathyroid hormone-related protein 13, **92**
  thymic carcinoids 485
parathyroid tumors 21
  adenoma 28, 172–9, **172**
    MEN 1 508–9
    neurofibromatosis type 1 530
    pathology 173
  atypical parathyroid adenoma 181
  carcinoma 28, 180–4
    chemotherapy 183
    clinical presentation 180–1
    diagnosis 181
    etiology 180
    histopathology 181–2, *181*, *182*
    management of hypercalcemia 183–4
    molecular oncogenesis 182–3
    radiotherapy 183
    surgery 81–2, 183
  surgery 80–2, *81*
    parathyroid carcinoma 81–2, 183
    parathyromatosis 81
    primary hyperparathyroidism 80–1
    recurrent/persistent disease 81
    secondary hyperparathyroidism 81
parathyromatosis, surgery 81
paraventricular nucleus 8
Parinaud syndrome 10, 312
partial androgen insensitivity syndrome 424
pasireotide, carcinoid syndrome 494
Paul, F.T. 222
pazopanib, thyroid tumors **152**
PCA-1 **550**
pedigree drawing 43, *43*
pegvisomant 251
pemphigus, paraneoplastic 553–4
pentoxifylline, sarcoidosis 334
peptic ulcer disease, and gastrinoma **463**
peptide receptor imaging 58–60
peptide receptor radiation therapy 60–1, **61**
peptide receptor therapy 62–3
peptide YY 498
percutaneous ethanol injection 75
pergolide, prolactinoma 242
peripheral neuroblastic tumors 360–9
  clinical presentation 362–6, *362*, *363–5*
  diagnosis 365–6, *365*, *366*, 366
  epidemiology 360–1, *361*
  etiology 360
  genetics 361–2
    1p deletion 362
    17q gain 362
    aneuploidy 362
    epigenetic silencing of caspase 8 362
    MYCN gene amplification 362
  pathology 361
  staging 366–7, **366**, *367*
  treatment 367–9
    anti-angiogenesis 368
    chemotherapy 367
    gene therapy 368
    liposomal tumor and vascular targeting 368–9
    radiotherapy 367
    retinoids 368
    risk-guided therapy 367–8, **368**

  surgery 367
  tumor antigen-specific monoclonal antibodies 368
perisellar tumors 302–9
  chondrosarcoma 304, *304*
  chordoma 302–4, *303*
  differential diagnosis **302**
  glomus tumors 306–7
  hemangiopericytoma 305–6
  meningioma *see* meningioma
  optic nerve and hypothalamic gliomas 211, 306
  surgery 307–8, *308*
peroxisome proliferator-actived receptor *see* PPAR
persistent Müllerian duct syndrome **421**
PET *see* positron emission tomography
Peutz–Jeghers syndrome 391, 402, 406
pharyngeal tumors, metastases **583**
phenoxybenzamine, pheochromocytoma 357
phenylethanolamine-*N*-methyl transferase 13
pheochromocytoma 14, 22, 28, 344–5, *345*, 352–9
  diagnosis 354–7, *355*
    plasma catecholamines 354
    plasma chromogranin A 355
    plasma free and urinary metanephrines 354–5
    radiological localization 356–7, *356*, **356**, *357*
    urinary catecholamines 354
    venous sampling 355–6
  ectopic ACTH syndrome **567**
  genetic testing **46**
  hypertensive crisis 358, **358**
  magnetic resonance imaging 345, *345*
  malignant 358
  molecular genetics 352–3, *353*
  neurofibromatosis type 1 530
  pathology 353
  in pregnancy 352
  presentation 353–4
  risk factors **353**
  screening for **354**
  surgery 83
  treatment 357–8
    intraoperative management 357
    postoperative management 357–8
    preoperative management 357
  von Hippel–Lindau disease 525–6, *526*
phosphate, in treatment of hypercalcemia 565
phosphatidylinositol 3-kinase/Akt pathway 604
PIC3CA, thyroid cancer **126**
pilonidal sinus **534**
pineal gland 10
  tumors *see* germ cell tumors
pineoblastoma 10
Pit-1 190
  thyrotropinoma 269
Pit-1-independent thyrotrophs 10
pituicytes 10
pituicytoma 10
pituitary adenoma 22, 28, 187–93, **187**
  ACTH-producing 218–19
  angiogenesis 189–90
  aryl hydrocarbon receptor interacting protein gene 192
  cell cycle regulation 188–9
  differential diagnosis 283
  folate receptor 192

FSH/LH-producing 219
GADD45- 191
galectin-3 191
gene therapy 192–3
GH/PRL-producing 218
growth hormone-producing 215–16
High Mobility Group A2 gene 192
imaging 203–5, *204, 205*
MEG3 191–2
MEN1 expression **507**
non-functioning *see* non-functioning pituitary
    adenoma
null cell 219
oncocytoma 219
pathology 215–21
pituitary transcription factors 190
pituitary tumor transforming gene 190–1
predisposition **27**
PRL cell 216–18, *217*
signaling pathways 189
transgenic mouse models **188**
TSH-producing 219
pituitary adenylate cyclase-activating peptide 59
pituitary apoplexy 263–4
surgery 229
pituitary carcinoma 220, 274–7
clinical presentation 275
definition 274
diagnostic investigations 275
epidemiology 274–5
hormonal profile **274**
incidence 274–5
pathogenesis 275–6
pathology 275–6
predictors of development 275–6
prognosis 276
risk factors 274–5
treatment 276
pituitary function tests 249
pituitary gland 9
adenohypophysis **6**
functional assessment 194–9
growth hormone-insulin-like growth factor-1 axis
    196–7, **197**
hypothalamo-pituitary-adrenal axis 194–6
hypothalamo-pituitary-gonadal axis 197–8
hypothalamo-pituitary-thyroid axis 197
imaging 200–14
    CT 202–3, *203*
    inflammatory disease 212
    MRI 200–2, *201, 202*
    nuclear isotope 211–12, *212*
    pituitary microadenoma 203–5, *204, 205*
    postoperative/follow-up scanning 205–6, *206*
    suprasellar and parasellar tumors 210–11
metastatic tumors 584–5, **584**
post-radiotherapy endocrine surveillance 199
prolactin 197–8
surgery
    perioperative steroid management 198–9, *198*
    postoperative pituitary assessment 199
pituitary glycoprotein hormone α-subunit *271*
pituitary incidentaloma 278–81
alternative diagnoses 279–80
definition 278, *278*

evaluation 280
incidence 278–9, *279*
management 280–1
presentation 280
pituitary microadenoma 206–8, *207, 208*
pituitary radiotherapy 231–6
acromegaly 231–2, 251, *251*
complications 233–5
    late hypopituitarism 234
    radiation oncogenesis 234–5
    visual impairment 233–4
conventional 232–3
Cushing syndrome 232
focal 233
Gamma Knife therapy 233
non-functioning tumors 232
prolactinoma 231
pituitary resistance to thyroid hormones **270**
pituitary surgery 222–30
advances in 229
choice of approach 225–7, **225–7**
    endonasal 226
    endoscopic 226–7, *227*
    extended transsphenoidal 227
    transsphenoidal 226
complications 227, **227**
contraindications 224
craniotomy 227–8
history 222–3
indications 223–4
    biopsy of sellar/suprasellar lesion 224
    normalization of pituitary hypersecretion 224
    pituitary apoplexy 223–4
    progressive mass effect of tumor 224
preoperative investigations 224–5, *225*, **225**
    anatomical diagnosis 224–5, *225*, **225**
    endocrine diagnosis 224
    minimizing risks of treatment 225
results 228–9
    acromegaly 228
    Cushing syndrome 228
    non-functioning adenomas 228
    pituitary apoplexy 229
    prolactinoma 228–9
pituitary transcription factors 190
pituitary tumor transforming gene **187**, 190–1
placental-like alkaline phosphatase 426
placental-site trophoblastic tumor 431
platelet-derived growth factor 15
plicamycin, hypercalcemia 564–5
plurihormonal adenoma 238
Pneumocystis jiroveci 379
polycystic ovary syndrome 36, *36*
polydactyly 293
polydipsia 181, **331**
polyembryoma 408
polyostotic Langerhans cell histiocytosis *326*
polyuria 181
POMC *see* pro-opiomelanocortin
POMC gene
    expression 569–70
    transcription 568–9, *569*
positron emission tomography 60
    adrenal glands 340
    carcinoid syndrome 492

Cushing syndrome 380
pheochromocytoma 357
positron emission tomography-computed
    tomography, carcinoid syndrome 448
post-partum hypercalcemia 561
PPAR 50
    Cushing syndrome 259
    thyroid cancer **126**
PPoma 439
prazosin, pheochromocytoma 357, 389
precocious puberty 295, 344, *344*
    hamartoma 295
    McCune–Albright syndrome **537**, 538, 540
    neurofibromatosis type 1 530
    therapy 295–6
prednisolone **579**
prednisone **579**
pregnancy
    functional ovarian tumors 402
    neurofibromatosis type 1 530
    pheochromocytoma 352
    post-partum hypercalcemia **561**
    prolactinoma 243–4, **243**
pregranulosa cells 15
preimplantation genetic diagnosis 45–6
prenatal diagnosis 45–6
preprogastrin 462
PRKAR1A 534, 535
PRL *see* prolactin
pro-opiomelanocortin 10
    secretion by non-pituitary tumors 568, *568*
procalcitonin 91, 96–8, *97*
prodrugs 51
progastrin 462
progesterone 7
    breast cancer **34**
    reference range **623**
    sex cord-stromal tumors 407
progesterone-binding protein **7**
progestins, and breast cancer 33–5, *35*
prohormones 4
prohormone convertase 5
prolactin 6, 10, 194, 197–8
    and breast cancer 37
    mixed GH/PRL adenoma 218
    pituitary carcinoma 274
    reference range **623**
prolactin cell adenoma 216–19, *217*
    dopamine agonist treatment 216–17
prolactinoma 237–45
    clinical manifestations 237–8
    differential diagnosis 238–9, **238**
    epidemiology 237
    evaluation 239
    MEN1 expression **507**
    pathogenesis 237
    in pregnancy 243–4, **243**
    surgery 228–9
    treatment 239–40
        medical therapy 241–3
        radiotherapy 240–1
        surgery 240
prostate cancer 55, 601–8
    androgen receptors in
        activation 604

androgen receptor-independent pathways 604
    co-regulators 603–4
    expression 603
    mutations 602–3, *602*
androgens in 36–7
    increased bioavailability of 603
chemotherapy 606–7
    docetaxel 606–7
    mitoxantrone 606
    novel agents 607
hormonal therapy 604–6, **605**
    GnRH agonists/antagonists 604–5
    intermittent androgen deprivation 605–6
    maximum androgen blockade 605
hormone resistance 602–4, *602*, *603*
hypercalcemia **561**
metastases **585**
secondary hormonal manipulations 606, **606**
treatment **579**
prostate-specific antigen, reference range **625**
proteomic multiplexing 100
Proteus syndrome 545
Proteus-like syndrome 545
proton beam therapy 66–7
proton pump inhibitors, gastrinoma 465
pseudoglucagonoma syndrome 474
psycho-affective change 331
psychological morbidity 104
PTEN
    Cowden syndrome 546, 547
    thyroid cancer **126**
pyoderma gangrenosum 554

17q gain 362
quality of life 107
quality-adjusted life-years 280
quinagolide, prolactinoma 242

R1α 534
radiation medicine 64–9
    external beam radiotherapy 64–5
    Gamma Knife radiosurgery 66
    intracystic therapy for craniopharyngioma 69
    linear accelerators 65, *65*
    metaiodobenzylguanidine 68
    proton beams 66–7
    radio-iodine 67–8
    radioisotope therapy 67
    radiolabeling
        monoclonal antibodies 68–9
        somatostatin analogs 68
    tomotherapy 65–6, *66*
radiation oncogenesis 234–5
radiation-induced thyroid tumors 166–71
    Chernobyl accident 168–9
    diagnostic evaluation 169–70, **170**
    environmental exposure 167–8
    features of 169, **169**
    high-dose radiation 168
    low-dose radiation 167–8
    risk factors 166–7, **167**
    treatment 170–1
radiofrequency ablation 75–6, *76*
    carcinoid syndrome 493
radioimmunoscintigraphy 68

radioimmunotherapy 68
radioiodine 67–8
    anaplastic thyroid carcinoma 159
    remnant ablation in papillary thyroid carcinoma 134–6, *134–6*, **134**
    see also various iodine isotopes
radioisotope therapy 67
radiotherapy
    bronchial carcinoids 484
    cavernous sinus hemangioma 323
    chordoma 303
    complications 104–5
    craniopharyngioma 285
    endocrine late effects 588–98
        gonadal damage 594–6, *594*
        growth 588–90, **589**, **590**
        hypopituitarism 591–4, *592*
        thyroid damage 596–7, *597*
    ependymoma 299
    fractionated external pituitary 260
    germ cell tumors 410
    germinoma 314
    lymphoma, thyroid 163
    non-functioning 265–6
    non-germinomatous germ cell tumors 315
    parathyroid carcinoma 183
    peripheral neuroblastic tumors 367
    pituitary adenoma 231–6
        acromegaly 231–2
        complications 233–5
        conventional 232–3
        Cushing syndrome 232
        focal 233
        Gamma Knife therapy 233
        non-functioning tumors 232
        prolactinemia 240–1
    prolactinoma 231
    sex cord-stromal tumors 407
    thyrotropinoma 271–2, **271**
raloxifene, hyperparathyroidism 176
ranitidine, gastrinoma 465
RANKL 563, 564
Ras
    thyroid cancer 125, **126**
    thyrotropinoma 269
Ras proteins 125
RASSF1A, thyroid cancer 126
Rathke's cleft cysts **238**, 288–9, *289*
    differential diagnosis 279, 283
    imaging 210, *210*
Rathke's pouch 9, 10
recoverin **550**
rectal tumors
    carcinoid 445, 498–501
        clinical features and management 500–1
        etiopathogenesis 498
        macroscopic appearances 499
        microscopic appearances 499–500, *499*, *500*
        relative frequency 499
        survival **489**
    neuroendocrine 440, 442
rectum 498
regions of interest 340
relative enhancement washout 349
relaxin 7

renal carcinoma
    hypercalcemia **561**
    treatment **579**
renal cell carcinoma 30, 525
    Cowden syndrome 546
    metastases **583**, **584**, **585**
    treatment **579**
renal failure, and hypercalcemia **561**
renin–angiotensin–aldosterone axis 556
reproductive system, cancer therapy effects 590, 594–6, *594*
reserpine, MIBG uptake 356
RET proto-oncogene 50–1
    thyroid cancer 125, **126**, 127, 169
retinal angiomatosis 524, *524*
retinal degeneration, antibodies 550
retinal hemangioblastoma, von Hippel–Lindau disease **523**
retinoblastoma 41
    proto-oncogene 570
    susceptibility gene **187**, **188**
retinoids, peripheral neuroblastic tumors 368
retroperitoneal tumor **579**
Ri 550
rickets, McCune–Albright syndrome 537, 540
Rieger syndrome 10
risedronate, hyperparathyroidism 176
risk advice 43–4
rosiglitazone, Cushing syndrome 259
RU486 574
Russell diencephalic syndrome 530

S100 protein 298
saline load test 374
salmon calcitonin, hyperparathyroidism 176
sarcoidosis 331–5
    diagnosis and investigations 332–3, *332*, **332**, **333**
    differential diagnosis 279, 283
    endocrine manifestations 331–2, **331**
    and hypercalcemia **561**
    prognosis 335
    treatment 333–4
        corticosteroids 333
        immunomodulatory agents 333–4
        immunosuppressive agents 333
satraplatin, prostate cancer 607
Schiller–Duval bodies 408
Schoffler, Herman 223
schwannoma 211
Schwartz–Bartter syndrome 10
scintigraphy
    adrenal glands 340
    adrenocortical cancer 388
    bone 447–8
    bronchial carcinoids 483
    carcinoid syndrome
        MIBG 447, *447*
        somatostatin receptor 445, *447*
    Conn syndrome 374–5
    Cushing syndrome 379
    hyperparathyroidism *175*
    parathyroid glands 121–2, *122*
    pituitary carcinoma 275
    somatostatin receptor
        carcinoid syndrome 445, *447*, 491–2

gastrinoma 464
glucagonoma 451
somatostatinoma 451
VIPoma **471**
thyroid tumors 112, 119–20, **119**
iodine-123 119–20
iodine-124 120
iodine-131 119
Tc-99m pertechnetate 119
sclerosing stromal tumor 391, 401–2
androgen-secreting 391
endocrine aspects 406
screening
Conn syndrome 373–4, **373**
pheochromocytoma **354**
scrotal tongue 545
secretin 440
selective arterial injection 465
secretin stimulation test *464*
secretion **7**
seizures 294–5, 529
therapy 295
selective internal radiation therapy 484
seminoma 311
sensorimotor neuronopathy, antibodies **550**
sensory neuronopathy 551
serotonin 7, 90–1, **91**, 94–5, *94, 95*, 353
synthesis *489*
see also carcinoid syndrome
serotoninoma 439
Sertoli cells 14, 422
Sertoli–Leydig cell tumor 391, 397
androgen-secreting 391
endocrine aspects 406
sestamibi, parathyroid glands 121–2, *122*
sex chromosome DSD **421**
sex cord tumor with annular tubules 391–2, 402
androgen-secreting 391–2
endocrine aspects 406–7
sex cord-stromal tumors 390–1, **390**, 396–7
androgen-secreting 390–1, **390**
chemotherapy 407
endocrine aspects 404, **404**
hormonal therapy 407
prognostic factors 407
radiotherapy 407
surgery 407
sex determination 421–2
sex hormone-binding globulin *see* SHBG
sex steroids
and breast cancer **34**
and endometrial cancer 35–6, *36*
replacement, effects on fertility 596
sexual development, disorders of 421–9
classification **421**
gonadal tumors 424
classification 424
clinical disorders 424
origin of 424–6, **425**
management 426–7
normal sex determination 421–4, *422*
tumor markers 426, **426**
SHBG
breast cancer **34**
thyrotropinoma *271*

shepherd's crook deformity 538, *539*
short stature 529–30
short Synacthen test **195**, 196
short tau inversion recovery 571
SIADH 556–60
diagnosis 557–8, **558**
in malignant disease 558–9, **558**
management 559–60
pathogenesis 557–8, *557*, **558**
regulation of plasma sodium 556–7
type A 557
type B 557
type C 557
type D 557
signal intensity index 340
silent adenoma 219
silent "corticotroph" adenoma 220
skeletal dysplasia 529
skin cancer, metastatic **583, 584, 585, 586**
skin tags **534**
small bowel carcinoids 444–5
survival **489**
sodium iodide symporter *see* NIS
sodium, regulation of plasma concentration 556–7
somatomammotropinoma **238**
somatostatin 6, 7, 8, 16, **92**, 438
actions of 479, **480**
somatostatin analogs 62–3
acromegaly 62–3, 250
carcinoid syndrome 493–4, **494**
bronchial 484, **484**
complications 106, **106**
ectopic ACTH syndrome 573
gastrinoma 465
glucagonoma 477
neuroendocrine tumors 63
radiolabeled 67–8, 495
thyrotropinoma 270
VIPoma 472
somatostatin cell tumors 440
somatostatin receptors 189
distribution **59**
radiotherapy 61, **61**
somatostatin receptor scintigraphy
carcinoid syndrome 445, *447*, 491–2
gastrinoma 464
glucagonoma 451
somatostatinoma 451
VIPoma 471
somatostatin receptor targeting 58–9, **58, 59**
somatostatinoma 439, 479–81
duodenal 480–1
pancreatic 480, **480**, *481*
somatostatin receptor scintigraphy 451
survival rates 481
sonic hedgehog 302
sorafenib
carcinoid syndrome 495–6, **495**
thyroid tumors 152
SOX9 423
sphenoid air sinus 9
sphenoid ostium 227
sphenoid sinus, mucocele 289, *290*
spinal cord hemangioblastoma, von Hippel–Lindau
disease **523**

spindle cell tumor **579**
spironolactone, Conn syndrome 376
Spongostan 484
Sry 423
stage specific duality 40
stained-glass appearance 401, 402
standard deviation 88, **88**
stellate reticulum 282
steroid acute regulatory protein 5
steroid cell tumors 391, 401
androgen-secreting 391
steroid hormone-binding globulin 601
steroidogenic factor 1 423
streptozocin 502, **503**
carcinoid syndrome 495
bronchial 484, **484**
glucagonoma 477
stromal carcinoids 390
stromal luteoma 401
struma ovarii 409
SU11248 **503**
subacute cerebellar degeneration 551
subependyomoma 298
substance P 7, 14
suicide gene therapy 49, 51
NIS 52–5, *53, 54*
sunitinib
carcinoid syndrome 495–6, **495**
thyroid tumors **152**
support groups 47
suprasellar aneurysm, differential diagnosis 283
suprasellar pituitary tumors 210–11, 312–13
surafinib, complications 106, **106**
suramin, adrenocortical carcinoma 382
surgery 78–85
adrenal tumors 82–4, *82*
adrenocortical carcinoma 83
incidentaloma 82–3
metastatic tumors 83–4
pheochromocytoma 83
primary hyperaldosteronism 83
androgen-secreting tumors 394
carcinoid syndrome 492–3
bronchial 484
Conn syndrome 376
craniopharyngioma 284
ectopic ACTH syndrome 573
gastrinoma 465–6
germ cell tumors 409
glucagonoma 477
non-germinomatous germ cell tumors 315
pancreatic neuroendocrine tumors 84
gastrinoma 84
insulinoma 84
parathyroid tumors 80–2, *81*
parathyroid carcinoma 81–2, 183
parathyromatosis 81
primary hyperparathyroidism 80–1
recurrent/persistent disease 81
secondary hyperparathyroidism 81
peripheral neuroblastic tumors 367
perisellar tumors 307–8, *308*
pituitary adenoma 222–30
advances in 229
choice of approach 225–7, **225–7**

complications 227, **227**
contraindications 224
craniotomy 227–8
history 222–3
indications 223–4
non-functioning 265
preoperative investigations 224–5, *225*, **225**
results 228–9
prolactinoma 240
sex cord-stromal tumors 407
thymic carcinoids 486
thyroid tumors 78–80, *79*
anaplastic 80
differentiated 78–9
lymphoma 80, 163
medullary carcinoma 79–80, 519
thyrotropinoma 271–2, **271**
Surveillance Epidemiology and End Results (SEER)
Program 488, 489
Sweet syndrome 554
Swyer syndrome 421
sympathomimetics, MIBG uptake 356
synaptophysin 275, 438
syncytiotrophoblasts 312
syndrome of inappropriate antidiuretic hormone
secretion *see* SIADH

T3 *see* triiodothyronine
tachykinins 489
tamoxifen
breast cancer 609–11, *610*, *611*, *613*
carry-over effect 615
precocious puberty 542
sex cord-stromal tumors 407
taxanes, sex cord-stromal tumors 407
Tc-99m pertechnetate, thyroid 119
telomerase 508
temozolomide **503**
bronchial carcinoids 484, **484**
pituitary carcinoma 276
temsirolimus, carcinoid syndrome 495–6, **495**
teratoma 314–15, 409, 424
tumor markers 312
terazosin, pheochromocytoma 357
testicular cancer 19–20, *19*
testicular DSD 421
testicular dysgenesis syndrome 20
testicular germ cell tumors 412–20
clinical behavior and response to treatment 416
clinical management 415–16
early-stage 417–18, **417**, **418**
epidemiology 412–14, **413**
atrophy-induced gonadotropin drive 413,
413
exogenous atrophogens acting post-puberty
413–14, **413**
geographical 412, **413**
future trials 418
good-risk patients 417, **417**
immune response and prognosis 415
intrauterine exposure to "xeno-estrogens" 415
metastatic disease 416, **416**
oncofetal markers 415–16
pathology 414–15, **414**

poor-risk patients 416–17
risk factors **414**
semen analysis **413**
testis 7
chemotherapy effects 595–6
metastatic tumors 585, **585**
radiation effects 594–5
testosterone 7
breast cancer 34
reference range 623
tetracycline, catecholamine assay interference 354
thalidomide **503**
carcinoid syndrome 495–6, **495**
sarcoidosis 334
theca interna cells 7
thecoma 391, 400–1, *400*, *401*
androgen-secreting 391
computerized tomography *400*
endocrine aspects 405–6
luteinized 400
magnetic resonance imaging *401*
thiazide diuretics, and hypercalcemia **561**
thoracic mesenchymal tumor 579
thymic carcinoids 485–6
clinical presentation 485–6
diagnosis 486
epidemiology 485
etiology 485
genetic alterations 485
histopathology 485
immunohistochemistry 485
prognosis 486
treatment 486
thymic tumors
ectopic ACTH syndrome 567
MEN 1 **507**, 512
thymopoietin 13
thymosin 13
thymus 12–13
thyroglobulin 11, **91**, 98–100, *99*
antibodies **91**, 98–100, *99*
mRNA 98–100, *99*
reference range 623
thyroglossal cyst 546
thyroid cyst *117*
thyroid gland 6, 11–12, *12*
C-cell hyperplasia 28
cancer therapy effects 590
goiter 11, 28
medullary carcinoma 28
metastatic tumors 583–4, **583**, *584*
papillary carcinoma 28
radiation-induced damage 596–7, *597*
"thyroid map" *116*
thyroid nodules, radiation-induced 596–7
thyroid transcription factors 11
thyroid tumors 20–1, *20*, 111–15
anaplastic thyroid carcinoma 155–61
cause of death 156
diagnosis and histology 156–7
epidemiology 155–6, *156*
etiology 156
pathogenesis 127–8, *128*
presentation 156

staging and prognostic features 157
surgery 80
therapy 157–60, *159*
tumor characteristics 155–6, *156*
ultrasound 118
assessment 111–14, 118–19
clinical evaluation 111–12, **112**
differentiated, surgery 78–9
FNAB 113–14, **113**, 118–19
follicular thyroid adenoma
pathogenesis 126–7
ultrasound 117–18, *118*
follicular thyroid carcinoma 78–9, 143–54
advanced disease 151–2, **152**
diagnosis 147–8, *148*
epidemiology 143
etiology 143–4
long-term follow-up 151
non-syndromic forms 144–7, *145*, 146–7
pathogenesis 126–7
staging and prognosis 148–9
treatment 149–51
tumor biomarkers 99
ultrasound 117–18, *118*
follow-up of thyroid enlargement 114
gene therapy 50–1
NIS 53–5, *54*
laboratory investigations 112
lymphoma 162–5
clinical presentation and staging 162–3, *162*,
162, **163**
etiology and pathogenesis 162
surgery 80
survival *164*
treatment 163–4, *164*, **164**
treatment outcome 163–4
medullary carcinoma 79–80, 515–22
clinical presentation 515–16, **516**
diagnosis 517
ectopic ACTH syndrome 567
genetics 516–17, **517**
history **516**
pathogenesis 127
pathology 517
prognostic factors 517–18
staging 518
surgery 79–80
treatment 519–21, **520**, **521**
tumor markers 97
ultrasound 117, *118*
microcarcinomas 114
micronodules 114
papillary thyroid carcinoma 78–9, 130–42
long-term surveillance 137–8
metastasis 138–9
molecularly targeted treatments 139–40
mortality 131, *131*
outcome prediction 131–2, *132*
pathogenesis 124–6, *125*, **126**
presenting features 130–1
primary surgery 133–4, *133*
radioiodine remnant ablation 134–6, *134–6*,
134
recurrence 131, *131*, 138–9

risk-group stratification 131–2, *132*
thyroxine suppressive therapy 134
ultrasound 117, *117*, *118*
pathogenesis 124–9
postoperative surveillance 120–1, *121*
prediction of malignancy 114–15
prognosis 163–4
radiation-induced 166–71
Chernobyl accident 168–9
diagnostic evaluation 169–70, **170**
environmental exposure 167–8
features of 169, **169**
high-dose radiation 168
low-dose radiation 167–8
risk factors 166–7, *167*
treatment 170–1
scintigraphy 112, 119–20, **119**
iodine-123 119–20
iodine-124 120
iodine-131 119
Tc-99m pertechnetate 119
surgery 78–80, *79*
ultrasound 112, 116–18, *116–18*
thyroid-releasing hormone 6
thyroid-stimulating hormone *see* thyrotropin
thyrotropin 6, 10, 112
adenomas producing 219
deficiency, radiation-induced 594
reference rage 623
suppressive therapy 150, 159
thyrotropin-releasing hormone 8, *271*
thyrotropinoma 268–73, *268*
diagnostic procedures 269–70, **270**
differential diagnosis 270–1, *271*
molecular studies 269
pathogenesis 269
treatment 271–2
medical 272, **272**
surgery and irradiation 271–2, **271**
thyroxine 6, 112
reference range 623
suppressive therapy 134
tomotherapy 65–6, *66*
topotecan, peripheral neuroblastic tumors 367
toxic goiter 269
TP53, thyroid cancer **126**, 127
Tpit 570
Tr **550**
tracheal tumors, metastases **583**
transcription factors activator protein-2 426
transforming growth factor beta 40
transhepatic portal venous sampling 73
with intra-arterial stimulation 73
transsphenoidal surgery 226
acromegaly 250
complications 227, **227**
Cushing syndrome 259–60
extended 227
trichilemmoma 545
tricyclic antidepressants
catecholamine assay interference 354
MIBG uptake 356
triglyceride, reference range **625**
triiodothyronine 6, 112

reference range **623**
toxicosis 112
Trousseau's sign 373
tryptophan metabolism *489*
TSPY 424, 426
tuberculosis 307
differential diagnosis 279, 283
tumor markers 86–101
analytical considerations 87–8, *87*, **88**, 89
carcinoid syndrome 94, 95
characteristics of 86–7
clinical validation 88–9, **90**
definition and applications 86
endocrine 89–100
5-HIAA 90–1, **91**, 94–5, *94*, *95*
5-HT 90–1, **91**, 94–5, *94*, *95*
calcitonin 6, 14, **91**, 96–8, **97**
catecholamines 5, **91**, 95–6
chromogranin A 90, **91**
features of 89–90, **91–3**
homovanillic acid **91**, 95–6
metanephrines **91**, 95–6
procalcitonin **91**, 96–8, **97**
thyroglobulin 11, **91**, 98–100, *99*
thyroglobulin antibodies **91**, 98–100, *99*
thyroglobulin mRNA 98–100, *99*
vanillylmandelic acid **91**, 95–6
evidence-based use 88–9, **90**
gonadal tumors 426, **426**
reference range **625**
tumor necrosis factor-α 52, 462
myeloma 564
tumor suppressor genes 41
pituitary adenoma **187**
tumor targeting 58–63
CCKB receptor radiotherapy 61
future directions 63
MIBG therapy 61–2
peptide receptor imaging 58–60
peptide receptor radiation therapy 60–1, **61**
peptide receptor therapy 62–3
positron emission tomography 60
Turner syndrome 319, 421, **421**, 427
tyrosine kinase inhibition 503–4

ultrasound
gastrinoma 465
granulosa cell tumor *398*, *399*
insulinoma
endoscopic 459
intraoperative 459
transabdominal 458
islet cell tumors 449–50
parathyroid glands 122
thyroid tumors 112, 116–18, *116–18*
anaplastic carcinoma 118
follicular adenoma/carcinoma 117–18, *118*
medullary carcinoma 117, *118*
papillary thyroid carcinoma 117, *117*, *118*
VIPoma **471**
United Kingdom Children's Cancer Study Group 313
unopposed estrogen hypothesis 33, **33**
urapidil, pheochromocytoma 357

urinary catecholamines 354
drugs affecting 354
urinary free cortisol 255
uterine tumors, metastatic **586**
uterus, cancer therapy effects **590**

V2 receptor 556
V3 receptor 570
vaginal atresia **421**
vandetanib, thyroid tumors 152
vanillylmandelic acid **91**, 95–6, 353
vascular dysplasia 529
vascular endothelial growth factor 39, 51
pituitary adenoma 190
thyroid cancer 128
vasoactive intestinal peptide 6, 7, 14, **92**, 353, 462, 470
reference range **624**
see also VIPoma
vasopressin **6**, 557
vasopressin antagonists (vaptans) 559
vatalanib, carcinoid syndrome 495–6, **495**
venous sampling
adrenal 71–2, *72*, 340, 393–4
Conn syndrome 375–6
hepatic with intra-arterial stimulation 73
inferior petrosal sinus 71
islet cell tumors 72–3, *73*
ovarian 393–4
parathyroid 70–1, *71*
pheochromocytoma 355–6
transhepatic portal vein 73
Verner–Morrison syndrome 469
VGCC **550**
VGKC **550**
VHL protein 523, *524*
Vibrio cholerae 469
vimentin 298
vinblastine
Langerhans cell histiocytosis 328
ovarian germ cell tumor 409
sex cord-stromal tumors 407
testicular germ cell tumors 416
vincristine
adrenocortical carcinoma 382
bronchial carcinoids 484, **484**
gestational trophoblastic tumor 433
ovarian germ cell tumor 409
sex cord-stromal tumors 407
VIPoma 439, **439**, 469–73
biochemical abnormalities **470**
clinical features **469**
diagnosis 470–1, **471**
pathophysiology 470, **470**
somatostatin receptor scintigraphy 451
treatment 472
tumor localization 471–2, **471**
and WDHHA syndrome 469–70, **469**, **470**
virilization 344, *344*
virus-mediated oncolysis 49, 52
visual defects **331**
visual field disturbance in non-functional pituitary adenoma 263
visual field testing 249

vitamin A intoxication **561**

vitamin D **38–9**
  intoxication **561**
  reference range **624**

von Hippel–Lindau disease **25**, **26**, 43, 443, 480, 523–7
  clinical features 524–6
    cerebellar hemangioblastoma 524–5, *525*
    pancreatic lesions 526
    pheochromocytoma 353, 525–6, *526*
    renal cell carcinoma/cysts 525
    retinal angiomatosis 524, *524*
  diagnostic work-up 526–7, **526**
  genetic testing **46**
  lesions associated with **523**
  molecular pathogenesis 523–4, **523**, *524*
  surveillance 526–7, **527**

vorinostat, thyroid tumors **152**

watery diarrhea, hypochlorhydria, hypokalemia and severe hyperchloremic metabolic acidosis (WDHHA) 469–70, **469**, **470**
weight gain **331**
weight loss **331**
Weiss, M. 223
Whipple's triad 455–6
Wilms tumor 14
Wnt4 423
World Health Organization, evidence rankings for tumor markers **90**

X-linked lissencephaly 423
X-rays 65
xeno-estrogens 415

46,XX DSD **421**
46,XY DSD **421**

Yo **550**
yolk sac tumor 424
  tumor markers 312

Zic4 **550**
zinc deficiency, and glucagonoma 476
zoledronic acid **103**
  hypercalcemia 564
  McCune–Albright syndrome 542
Zollinger–Ellison syndrome *see* gastrinoma
zona fasciculata 7, 13
zona glomerulosa 7
zone reticularis 7